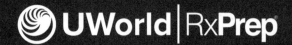 **THE REVIEW PROGRAMS TRUSTED** BY TOP STUDENTS, SCHOOLS AND EMPLOYERS

The UWorld RxPrep® Difference

NAPLEX®, MPJE® & CPJE Reviews

Not sure how to learn it all? The comprehensive UWorld RxPrep online course can help you prepare for the NAPLEX the smart way. It includes access to our online QBank and video lectures that match each chapter in this course book. You can watch lectures at your own pace, create tests, track your progress and assess your readiness prior to exam day.

READ

The UWorld RxPrep course book
The course book is the student-preferred resource for the NAPLEX. It includes all topics tested, with must-know key drugs and study tips as well as the simplest and most complete calculations and biostatistics reviews.

WATCH

The online video lectures
Pair the course book with video lectures that emphasize the required drug information. Focus on topics that need a review, or jump to a video segment for a quick refresher of a tough concept.

PRACTICE

The question bank (QBank)
Over 3,400 questions are available in the QBank, including a cumulative practice exam. Apply what you've learned and assess your performance using case-rich, exam-style questions that simulate the NAPLEX. You have the flexibility to create your own tests and integrate content across multiple topics.

UPDATED

Current, complete and ready for exam preparation
The course book is updated annually and QBank edits are made in real-time when guidelines or drug information changes. Updated videos are released on a rolling basis to those with an active subscription.

PURCHASE THE VIDEO LECTURES AND QBANK ONLINE AT PHARMACY.UWORLD.COM

CONTACT UWORLD RxPrep FOR LIVE OR STREAMING REVIEWS AND GROUP RATES

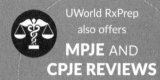
UWorld RxPrep also offers **MPJE** AND **CPJE REVIEWS** Course manual, QBank, video lectures and state-specific flashcards

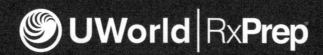

2025 NAPLEX® COURSE BOOK

Editors

Meera Aggarwal, PharmD, BCPS

Chelsea Bombatch, PharmD, BCPS

Katherine Brontoli, PharmD, BCPS, BCOP

Peter Colley, PharmD, BCIDP, AAHIVE

Adrienne DeBerry, PharmD, CPh, BCACP, CSP

Stephanie Garrett, PharmD, BCPS

Melissa Sandler, PharmD, BCCCP

Yasar Tasnif, PharmD, BCPS, FAST

Angie Veverka, PharmD, BCPS

Contributors

Ayesha Araya
PharmD, BCPS

Caitlin Davis
PharmD, BCPS

Stephanie Weightman
PharmD, BCPS,
BCPPS, BCEMP

Book design and
production
Joni Hutton

CHAPTER TABLE OF CONTENTS
INCLUDING REQUIRED FORMULAS

CHAPTER TABLE OF CONTENTS
INCLUDING REQUIRED FORMULAS

CONTENT LEGEND

⚏ = Required Formula

KEY DRUG GUY AND STUDY TIP GAL
PAGE NUMBERS

CONTENT LEGEND

Study Tip Gal   Key Drug Guy

KEY DRUG GUY AND STUDY TIP GAL
PAGE NUMBERS CONT.

CONTENT LEGEND

🔔 Study
Tip Gal

🔑 Key Drug
Guy

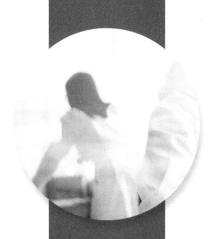
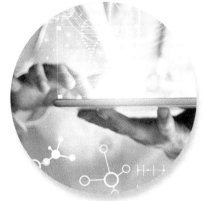
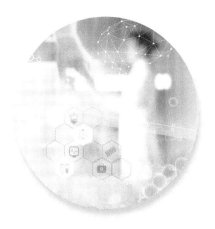

PREPARING FOR THE NAPLEX®

CONTENTS

CHAPTER CONTENT

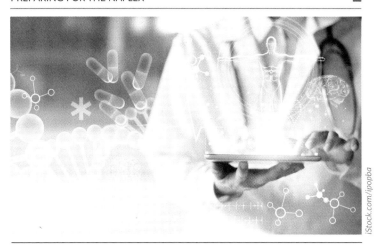

iStock.com/ipopba

CHAPTER 1
PREPARING FOR THE NAPLEX®
WITH UWORLD RxPREP

UWORLD RxPREP STUDY MATERIALS

There is no such thing as luck when taking licensure exams; there is only drug knowledge and the skill required to apply the knowledge to case-based questions. All topics must be mastered, and all calculations must be completed with adequate speed and accuracy. Thorough preparation is necessary to pass the NAPLEX®; apply the tips provided in this chapter to have the greatest chance of passing.

The UWorld RxPrep online course includes a question bank (or QBank for short) and video lectures that are used in conjunction with this course book. These materials are available online at pharmacy.uworld.com. The online course includes everything you need to be successful on the NAPLEX.

COURSE BOOK UPDATES AND ERRATA

The course book is updated annually to be current for the pharmacist licensure exam. It is best to study from the most current edition available for your period of testing.

New drug information and guidelines are continuously published, and pharmacists must remain current in their drug knowledge. The UWorld RxPrep pharmacists review new drug approvals and new guidelines on an ongoing basis; most new information will be added into the next edition of the course book, but some time-sensitive information that is relevant for testing in between book publications will be summarized online.

Refer to the "Resources" section at pharmacy.uworld.com to find relevant updates for the NAPLEX. Any course book corrections are posted in the same location.

HOW TO USE THE UWORLD RxPREP COURSE BOOK

The UWorld RxPrep course book includes several tools to simplify the information. Drugs are bolded if they are top sellers or have major safety issues. These are important drugs for the NAPLEX and should be known well (including the brand name, if bolded). If information is underlined, it is essential to know for the exam.

Study Tip Gals and Key Drug Guys are used to highlight important information. Study Tip Gals contain an explanation, simplification or summary of points, and Key Drug Guys are there to help you learn drugs with similar traits. Do not skip these; they contain highly testable information! These are marked with a light bulb (for a Study Tip Gal) or a key (for a Key Drug Guy) on the table of contents for the chapter. You can also find them using the table of contents for the course book.

Example Drug Table

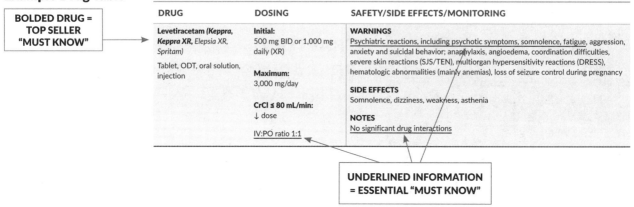

Study Tip Gal Box

STUDY TIP GAL

- The gal with the light bulb points out a study tip. This information is MUST KNOW for testing.

- The study tips include an approach to complex concepts, a way to organize the information or a way to remember the information.

Select Guidelines/References
This box highlights the main guidelines/references for the topic. The main source of information about the medications in this course book is the FDA-approved package labeling (package inserts).

Key Drug Guy Box

OTHER DRUGS

The drugs in the back box have the same concern, but are less well known.

KEY DRUGS

The guy with the key points out key drugs.

Drugs in this front box are MUST KNOW for testing (e.g., drugs that cause hypoglycemia).

FOUNDATION CHAPTERS

There are foundation chapters at the beginning and end of the course book (in the sections titled Pharmacy Foundations Part 1 and Part 2). Information in these chapters will apply to other topics. Complete these early; learning this material will help you throughout your studies. Then, revisit them at the end of your studies to make sure the information was retained. Foundation material may be required to answer questions in any QBank.

PRACTICE CASES, QUESTIONS AND CASE SCENARIOS

You will need to obtain information from a case to answer questions on the NAPLEX. For example, how many grams of protein per day are being provided by the patient's parenteral nutrition order? Or, which drug is the best option to treat the patient's infection? Practice cases and sample questions that are designed to be similar to cases you might see on the exam can be found in several chapters. They allow you to test your knowledge. Look for case scenarios in grey shaded boxes. These are a complement to the QBank, which is the best place to apply what you have learned to case-based scenarios.

GETTING STARTED WITH A STUDY SCHEDULE

Begin by creating a study schedule. To help you get started, the UWorld RxPrep pharmacists have organized the course book topics based on the time it usually takes to complete them (see table below). Three sample study planners can be found online at pharmacy.uworld.com on the NAPLEX Study Guide page, found under the "About Exams" dropdown.

HELPFUL POINTERS FOR CREATING YOUR STUDY SCHEDULE

- Fill in the schedule by allocating adequate time for each of the topics. Use the time estimates below, with your best guess if you will need more or less time to complete a topic.
- Include math early in your study schedule and allow time to practice frequently. Repetition is required for mastery.
- Alternate between math, foundation and clinical topics to stay engaged, or integrate topics using the QBank.
- Always leave weekly catch-up time. It is normal to fall behind; catch-up time will keep you on track. If you fall behind on your study schedule and are unable to catch up, it may be best to postpone your exam. Do not skip chapters or QBanks as any topic can appear on the exam.

- Leave the two weeks before your estimated test date open. The last two weeks are used to take the UWorld RxPrep Practice Exam, remediate any missed areas, and review the math and other topics that may have been forgotten.

Alternate your study time between math and clinical topics, or integrate multiple topics using the QBank.

Estimated Topic Completion Time		
1-2 hours per Topic	**2-4 hours per Topic**	**> 4 hours per Topic**
Allergic Rhinitis, Cough & Cold	Acute & Critical Care Medicine	Anticoagulation
Alzheimer's Disease	Acute Coronary Syndromes	Biostatistics
Anemia	ADHD	Calculations II
Answering Case-Based Exam Questions	Arrhythmias	Calculations III
Anxiety Disorders	Asthma	Calculations IV
Basic Science Concepts	Calculations I	Common Skin Conditions
Benign Prostatic Hyperplasia (BPH)	Calculations V	Diabetes
Bipolar Disorder	Chronic Heart Failure	Dyslipidemia
Common Conditions of the Eyes & Ears	Compounding with Hazardous Drugs	HIV
Constipation & Diarrhea	Contraception & Infertility	Infectious Diseases I
COPD	Depression	Infectious Diseases II
Cystic Fibrosis	Dietary Supplements, Natural & Complementary Medicine	Oncology
Drug Allergies & Adverse Drug Reactions	Drug Interactions	Osteoporosis, Menopause & Testosterone Use
Drug Formulations & Patient Counseling	GERD & PUD	Pain
Drug References	Hepatitis & Liver Disease	Seizures/Epilepsy
Drug Use in Pregnancy & Lactation	Hypertension	Systemic Steroids & Autoimmune Conditions
Gout	Immunizations	
Infectious Diseases IV	Infectious Diseases III	
Intravenous Medication Principles	Inflammatory Bowel Disease	
Migraine	Lab Values & Drug Monitoring	
Motion Sickness	Medication Safety & Quality Improvement	
Parkinson Disease	Nonsterile Compounding	
Pediatric Conditions	Pharmacokinetics	
Pharmacogenomics	Renal Disease	
Pulmonary Arterial Hypertension	Schizophrenia/Psychosis	
Sexual Dysfunction	Sterile Compounding	
Sickle Cell Disease	Transplant	
Sleep Disorders		
Stable Angina		
Stroke		
Thyroid Disorders		
Tobacco Cessation		
Toxicology & Antidotes		
Travelers		
Urinary Incontinence		
Weight Loss		

TIPS FOR STUDYING

STUDYING CLINICAL CHAPTERS

- If you know a topic well, review the course book chapter quickly with a focus on bolded drugs, underlined information, Study Tip Gals and Key Drug Guys. Then proceed to the QBank to test your knowledge.

- If you are not confident with a topic, you will need to review it before proceeding to the QBank. Read the chapter, or watch the video lecture while following along with the chapter. Highlight the information you will need to review and review it before attempting the questions in the QBank.

- After completing the QBank questions on a topic, review any questions you answered incorrectly. Use the available QBank tools to make flashcards or notes for content you want to revisit later.

STUDYING CALCULATIONS

Math is an important part of the exam, and calculations are best mastered through repetition. Start by completing the Calculations chapters in the course book, then move on to the QBank. There are five Calculations chapters. Calculations I, II, III and IV can be completed in any order. The last Calculations chapter (Calculations V) contains exam-style math practice; review this chapter after the other four have been completed.

Other essential calculations are found in these chapters:

- Biostatistics
- Pharmacokinetics
- Select clinical chapters (e.g., corrected phenytoin in Seizures/Epilepsy, insulin math in Diabetes).

Use the Required Formulas Sheet (found in the quick guides and the end of the course book) while you are learning. Repeat each of the calculations questions in the QBank until you can do all of the problems with decent speed and accuracy. You can complete the questions in the QBank by chapter or integrate them across chapters.

As your scores improve, shift to completing the QBanks without using the Required Formulas Sheet. Turn off "Tutor" mode so you can assess your timing. The goal is to complete each question in ~1 minute and 36 seconds to mimic timing on the NAPLEX.

Test Your Knowledge

The formulas on the Required Formulas Sheet must be memorized. To assess what you know, take the Required Formulas Practice Test and check off items on the Required Formulas Checklist as you go (see next page) if you have memorized the formula.

INTEGRATING CONTENT

At any point in your studies, you can create integrated tests in the QBank by mixing questions from multiple chapters (including calculations). Using this feature can increase engagement and retention, and it makes your studies more challenging, as you will not know what chapter a question is coming from on an individual test. This also better simulates what to expect on the NAPLEX. In addition, the QBank has helpful tools to assess your performance and quickly identify your most challenging areas; see pharmacy.uworld.com for details.

ASSESSING READINESS FOR THE NAPLEX

You will know you are ready for the NAPLEX when the following conditions are met:

- Each calculation on the Required Formulas Checklist is marked off, indicating the formula is memorized, and the math can be completed flawlessly and efficiently.

- All topics in the course book have been reviewed. Any topic can appear on the NAPLEX; skipping topics and taking a chance on the NAPLEX is not advised.

- All questions in the QBank show as "used" (indicating they have been completed), and questions answered incorrectly have been reviewed.

THE UWORLD RxPREP PRACTICE EXAM

Once you have completed your studies and feel prepared to take the NAPLEX, take the UWorld RxPrep Practice Exam (found under "Assessments"). The questions on this exam have been selected to align with the NAPLEX Competency Statements (discussed in the next section).

- The Practice Exam has 150 questions. To have the same time per question as the NAPLEX, it should be taken as a timed, 4-hour exam.

- Use a calculator only. Do not use your course book, notes or the Required Formula Sheet.

Evaluate your performance on the Practice Exam to determine your readiness to take the NAPLEX. If you did not score well, you may need to postpone your exam to allow for additional time to study. If you feel ready to take the NAPLEX, use your remaining time to review missed information from the Practice Exam and items that are easily forgotten, such as math (including clinical math, biostatistics and pharmacokinetics) and compounding. If you did not score well in a few areas, review those topics more thoroughly using the course book, video lectures and QBank.

REQUIRED FORMULAS CHECKLIST

Calculations
- ❏ Liquid (Volume) Conversions p. 105
- ❏ Solid (Weight) Conversions p. 105
- ❏ mEq to mmol Conversion p. 105
- ❏ Height Conversions p. 105
- ❏ Percentage Strength p. 117
- ❏ Ratio Strength p. 121
- ❏ Parts Per Million (PPM) p. 123
- ❏ Specific Gravity (SG) p. 124
- ❏ Dilution & Concentration (Q1C1, Changing Strength or Quantity) p. 125
- ❏ Alligation p. 126
- ❏ Osmolarity p. 129
- ❏ Isotonicity (E Value) p. 132
- ❏ Moles and Millimoles p. 133
- ❏ Milliequivalents p. 135
- ❏ Determining Fluid Needs p. 139
- ❏ Total Energy Expenditure p. 140
- ❏ Parenteral Nutrition Calories p. 141
- ❏ Enteral Nutrition Calories p. 141
- ❏ Grams of Nitrogen From Protein p. 142
- ❏ Corrected Calcium for Albumin < 3.5 p. 149
- ❏ Body Mass Index (BMI) p. 158
- ❏ Ideal Body Weight (IBW) p. 159
- ❏ Adjusted Body Weight (AdjBW$_{0.4}$) p. 159
- ❏ Which Weight to Use for Drug Dosing (mg/kg) p. 160
- ❏ Flow Rates/Drop Factor p. 161 & p. 164
- ❏ Dehydration p. 166
- ❏ Cockcroft-Gault Equation p. 167
- ❏ Arterial Blood Gas (ABG) p. 169
- ❏ Anion Gap p. 170
- ❏ pH Calculations p. 171
- ❏ Percent Ionization p. 174
- ❏ Absolute Neutrophil Count (ANC) p. 176

Answering Case-Based Exam Questions
- ❏ Temperature Conversions p. 97

Biostatistics
- ❏ Mean, Median and Mode p. 192
- ❏ Risk, Relative Risk (RR) p. 197
- ❏ Relative Risk Reduction (RRR) p. 198
- ❏ Absolute Risk Reduction (ARR) p. 198
- ❏ Number Needed to Treat (NNT) p. 199
- ❏ Number Needed to Harm (NNH) p. 200
- ❏ Odds Ratio (OR) p. 200
- ❏ Hazard Ratio (HR) p. 201
- ❏ Incremental Cost-Effectiveness Ratio p. 211

Nonsterile Compounding
- ❏ Minimum Weighable Quantity (MWQ) p. 216

Dyslipidemia
- ❏ Friedewald Equation p. 395

Common Skin Conditions
- ❏ Time to Burn (TTB) p. 532

Tobacco Cessation
- ❏ Pack-Year Smoking History p. 569

Diabetes
- ❏ Initiating Basal-Bolus Insulin in Type 1 Diabetes p. 589
- ❏ Insulin-to-Carbohydrate Ratio: Rule of 500 for Rapid-Acting Insulin p. 591
- ❏ Insulin-to-Carbohydrate Ratio: Rule of 450 for Regular Insulin p. 591
- ❏ Correction Factor: 1,800 Rule for Rapid-Acting Insulin p. 591
- ❏ Correction Factor: 1,500 Rule for Regular Insulin p. 591
- ❏ Correction Dose p. 591

Acute & Critical Care Medicine
- ❏ Mean Arterial Pressure (MAP) p. 685

Oncology
- ❏ Body Surface Area (Mosteller) p. 763

Seizures/Epilepsy
- ❏ Phenytoin Correction for Albumin < 3.5 p. 853

Pharmacokinetics
- ❏ Bioavailability (F) p. 919
- ❏ Volume of Distribution (Vd) p. 920
- ❏ Clearance p. 922 & p. 924
- ❏ Elimination Rate Constant (ke) p. 924
- ❏ Predicting Drug Concentrations p. 924
- ❏ Half-Life ($t_{1/2}$) p. 925
- ❏ Loading Dose (LD) p. 927

Drug-Dose Conversions
- ❏ KCl Solution (Oral) to Tablets p. 136
- ❏ Calcium Salts p. 175
- ❏ Aminophylline ↔ Theophylline p. 175
- ❏ Statins p. 398
- ❏ Metoprolol p. 417
- ❏ Loop Diuretics p. 443
- ❏ Insulin p. 592
- ❏ Levothyroxine p. 601
- ❏ Steroids p. 608
- ❏ Opioids (methodology) p. 732
- ❏ Lithium p. 813

NOTE: The required formulas can be found in the quick guides section at the end of this chapter, plus in an easy "tear out" page at the end of the course book.

NAPLEX COMPETENCY STATEMENTS

The NAPLEX Competency Statements are available on the National Association of Boards of Pharmacy (NABP) website at https://nabp.pharmacy. The Competency Statements provide a blueprint (outline) of tested items, split into six "areas" or sections.

AREA	TITLE
1	Obtain, interpret, or assess data, medical, or patient information
2	Identify drug characteristics
3	Develop or manage treatment plans
4	Perform calculations
5	Compound, dispense, or administer drugs or manage delivery systems
6	Develop or manage practice or medication-use systems to ensure safety and quality

The key points for each competency area are summarized below, but you are encouraged to read the complete Competency Statements on the NABP website.

AREA #1 (~18% OF THE EXAM)

- Questions are largely asked in a case-based format. It will be important to quickly identify pertinent information from a case (e.g., abnormal labs, past medical history, medication use history, diagnostic tests) or an abstract (e.g., results from a study). It is critical to master the Lab Values & Drug Monitoring chapter; lab reference ranges will be provided.

AREA #2 (~14% OF THE EXAM)

- This section includes pharmacology, mechanism of action, therapeutic class, boxed warnings, safety in pregnancy or lactation and prescription vs. OTC status.

- Brand/generics are tested, along with common dosage forms.

AREA #3 (~35% OF THE EXAM)

- This area focuses on defining therapeutic goals, outcomes and clinical endpoints. You should be able to identify medications without an indication, untreated conditions, and duplications of therapy. Drug dosing, dosing adjustments and duration of therapy may be tested.

- Strong knowledge of drug contraindications, precautions, adverse effects and drug interactions is essential.

- The ability to apply guidelines to patient care (e.g., evidence-based practice) is covered in Area #3.

AREA #4 (~14% OF THE EXAM)

- Calculations involving patient parameters (e.g., BSA, body weight) and laboratory measures (e.g., CrCl, corrected phenytoin, ANC) are essential to making drug therapy decisions.

- The ability to calculate quantities of drugs to be dispensed or ingredients to be compounded is tested in this section.

- Nutritional calculations, rates of administration (e.g., flow rates), dose conversions and drug concentrations are covered.

- Biostatistics and pharmacokinetic calculations are included in Area #4.

AREA #5 (~11% OF THE EXAM)

- Techniques, procedures and equipment used for sterile and nonsterile compounding, including hazardous drugs, are a requirement.

- Properties of drug products that affect compatibility/stability, onset/duration or pharmacokinetics are covered.

- Familiarity with proper storage, packaging, handling and medication disposal is expected.

- Instructions and techniques for medication administration are tested in this section.

AREA #6 (~7% OF THE EXAM)

- Medication safety concepts, including the role of pharmacy informatics in the medication-use system, are included in Area #6.

- Disease prevention, screening programs and stewardship are covered. Knowledge of vaccinations will be important.

THE FORMAT OF THE NAPLEX

The NAPLEX is a 6-hour exam with 225 questions. Of these, 200 questions are used to determine the exam result (pass or fail). The other 25 questions are pretest questions that are being evaluated for inclusion on future exams. Pretest questions are interspersed throughout the exam; it is not possible to identify them.

- The majority of the questions (including calculations) are asked in a case-based format (such as patient profiles with an accompanying question). There are also stand-alone questions without a case.

- All questions must be answered in the order they are presented. You cannot skip questions or go back to a question at a later time.

The computer screen will display a prompt for two optional 10-minute breaks; these do not count towards the 6-hour time limit. Any other non-scheduled breaks that you request will be subtracted from the total test time.

QUESTION TYPES

The NABP website includes samples of three question types that may be encountered on the NAPLEX:

- Multiple-Choice: select the one correct answer.
- Multiple-Response: select all of the correct responses and no incorrect response for credit.
- Constructed-Response: enter the answer using the computer keyboard (usually for math problems).

There are two additional question types in the UWorld RxPrep QBank (as these were historically tested on NAPLEX and are good for learning the material):

- Ordered-Response: put the items in a specified order.
- Hot Spot: identify the correct area on a diagram or picture.

CALCULATORS

- Personal calculators are not permitted during the exam. The Pearson VUE testing center dashboard uses an on-screen calculator that is similar to the Texas Instruments TI-30XS Multiview and other comparable hand-held, non-graphing calculators. The on-screen calculator can be opened in a pop-up window during the exam at any time.

- A candidate requesting a handheld calculator will be given a basic, non-scientific calculator. Some of the calculations may require advanced functions that require the use of the on-screen calculator (e.g., order of operands, exponents and multi-step problems). Refer to the Calculations chapters for detailed information.

- Pearson VUE offers a demo test on their website, available at: home.pearsonvue.com/nabp.

ARRIVAL DETAILS, TUTORIAL

On the day of the exam, arrive at least 30 minutes prior to your appointment for check-in procedures (ID verification, digital signature and photograph). Review the Candidate Application Bulletin on the NABP website for details on acceptable forms of ID, prohibited items and exam misconduct.

- If you arrive more than 30 minutes after your scheduled appointment and are refused admission to sit for the exam, you will be required to forfeit your appointment.

- Take the online exam tutorial before starting the exam. The tutorial will explain how to navigate the cases, enter answers, etc. The tutorial is important and does not take away from your test time.

PHARMACY LAW EXAMS

MPJE®

Many people study for the MPJE after the NAPLEX has been completed. There is little overlap between the NAPLEX and MPJE.

Depending on a person's prior knowledge and work experience, MPJE preparation will take about 2 – 5 weeks. The UWorld RxPrep MPJE course and state-specific flashcard decks will provide the content needed to do well.

CPJE

Unlike the MPJE, the law exam in California (the CPJE), contains clinical content that overlaps with the NAPLEX. The UWorld RxPrep course book includes the topics that overlap with the CPJE (Medication Safety, Infectious Diseases, Immunizations, HIV, others). The clinical topics not covered on the NAPLEX that are tested on the CPJE are included in the separate CPJE course (e.g., therapeutic interchange). California law is covered completely in the CPJE course.

Best wishes for your exam preparation,

The UWorld RxPrep Pharmacy Team

REQUIRED FORMULAS

Calculations

Liquid (Volume) Conversions p. 105
1 tsp (t) = 5 mL, 1 tbsp (T) = 15 mL
1 fl oz = 30 mL
1 cup = 8 oz, 240 mL
1 pint = 16 oz, 480 mL
1 quart = 2 pints, 960 mL
1 gallon = 4 quarts, 3,840 mL

Solid (Weight) Conversions p. 105
1 kg = 2.2 pounds (lbs)
1 oz = 28.4 grams (g)
1 lb = 454 g, 16 oz
1 grain = 65 mg
mEq to mmol is 1:1 for monovalent ions, 1:0.5 for divalent ions

Height Conversions p. 105
1 inch (in) = 2.54 centimeters (cm)
1 meter (m) = 100 cm

Percentage Strength p. 117

$$\% \text{ w/v} = \frac{X \text{ g}}{100 \text{ mL}} \qquad \% \text{ v/v} = \frac{X \text{ mL}}{100 \text{ mL}} \qquad \% \text{ w/w} = \frac{X \text{ g}}{100 \text{ g}}$$

Ratio Strength p. 121
Percentage strength = 100 / Ratio strength
Ratio strength = 100 / Percentage strength

Parts Per Million (PPM) p. 123
PPM → Percentage strength   Move the decimal left 4 places
Percentage strength → PPM   Move the decimal right 4 places

Specific Gravity (SG) p. 124

$$SG = \frac{\text{weight of substance (g)}}{\text{weight of equal volume of water (g)}} \quad \text{or} \quad SG = \frac{g}{mL}$$

Dilution & Concentration (Changing Strength or Quantity) p. 125
Q1 x C1 = Q2 x C2   Q1 = old quantity   Q2 = new quantity
C1 = old concentration   C2 = new concentration

Alligation p. 126

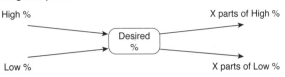

High %   X parts of High %

                          Desired
                            %

Low %   X parts of Low %

Use proportions to calculate amount of high % and/or low % required

Osmolarity p. 129

$$\text{mOsmol/L} = \frac{\text{Wt of substance (g/L)}}{\text{MW (g/mole)}} \times (\text{\# of particles}) \times 1{,}000$$

Isotonicity (E Value) p. 132

$$E = \frac{(58.5)(i)}{(\text{MW of drug})(1.8)}$$

Moles and Millimoles p. 133

$$\text{mols} = \frac{g}{MW} \quad \text{or} \quad \text{mmols} = \frac{mg}{MW}$$

Milliequivalents p. 135

$$\text{mEq} = \frac{mg \times valence}{MW} \quad \text{or} \quad \text{mEq} = \text{mmols} \times valence$$

Enteral Nutrition Calories p. 141
Carbs, Protein = 4 kcal/gram   Fat = 9 kcal/gram

Parenteral Nutrition Calories p. 141
Dextrose monohydrate = 3.4 kcal/gram   ILE 10% = 1.1 kcal/mL
Amino acid solutions = 4 kcal/gram   ILE 20% = 2 kcal/mL
                                        ILE 30% = 3 kcal/mL

Determining Fluid Needs p. 139
When weight > 20 kg: 1,500 mL + (20 mL)(weight in kg − 20)
Can estimate using 30-40 mL/kg/day

Total Energy Expenditure p. 140
TEE = BEE x activity factor x stress factor

Grams of Nitrogen From Protein p. 142

$$\text{Nitrogen (g)} = \frac{\text{protein intake (g)}}{6.25}$$

Corrected Calcium for Albumin < 3.5 (not needed with ionized Ca) p. 149
$Ca_{corrected}$ (mg/dL) = $calcium_{reported(serum)}$ + [(4.0 − albumin) x (0.8)]

Body Mass Index (BMI) p. 158

$$\text{BMI (kg/m}^2) = \frac{\text{weight (kg)}}{[\text{height (m)}]^2} \quad \text{or} \quad \frac{\text{weight (lbs)}}{[\text{height (inches)}]^2} \times 703$$

Ideal Body Weight (IBW) p. 159
IBW (males) = 50 kg + (2.3 kg)(number of inches over 5 feet)
IBW (females) = 45.5 kg + (2.3 kg)(number of inches over 5 feet)

Adjusted Body Weight (AdjBW$_{0.4}$) p. 159
AdjBW$_{0.4}$ = IBW + 0.4(TBW − IBW)

Which Weight to Use for Drug Dosing (mg/kg) p. 160
All drugs (if underweight)   Total Body Weight (TBW)
Most drugs (if normal weight or obese)   TBW
Exceptions
Acyclovir, Aminophylline, Levothyroxine, IBW
Theophylline (normal weight, obese)
Aminoglycosides (obese)   AdjBW$_{0.4}$

Flow Rates/Drop Factor (drops/min) p. 161 & p. 164

$$\frac{\text{\# drops}}{mL} \times \frac{mL}{hr} \times \frac{hr}{60 \text{ min}} = \frac{\text{\# drops}}{min}$$

Dehydration p. 166
BUN:SCr > 20:1

Cockcroft-Gault Equation p. 167

$$\frac{CrCl}{(\text{mL/min})} = \frac{140 - (\text{age of patient})}{72 \times SCr} \times \text{weight (kg)} (\times 0.85 \text{ if female})$$

Arterial Blood Gas (ABG) p. 169
ABG: pH/pCO$_2$/pO$_2$/HCO$_3$/O$_2$ Sat
1. pH < 7.35 → acidosis, pH > 7.45 → alkalosis
2. Respiratory: pCO$_2$ < 35 → alkalosis, pCO$_2$ > 45 → acidosis
   Metabolic: HCO$_3$ > 26 → alkalosis, HCO$_3$ < 22 → acidosis
3. Which abnormal value (pCO$_2$ or HCO$_3$) matches the pH from Step #1?
   Ex: ↓ pH + ↑ pCO$_2$ → <u>respiratory</u> acidosis
   Ex: ↓ pH + ↓ HCO$_3$ → <u>metabolic</u> acidosis

Anion Gap p. 170
Anion gap (AG) = Na − Cl − HCO$_3$

pH Calculations p. 171
Weak acid   Weak base

$$pH = pK_a + \log\left[\frac{salt}{acid}\right] \qquad pH = pK_a + \log\left[\frac{base}{salt}\right]$$

Percent Ionization p. 174
Weak acid   Weak base

$$\% \text{ ionization} = \frac{100}{1+10^{(pKa-pH)}} \qquad \% \text{ ionization} = \frac{100}{1+10^{(pH-pKa)}}$$

Absolute Neutrophil Count (ANC) p. 176
ANC (cells/mm^3) = WBC x [(% segs + % bands)/100]

Answering Case-Based Exam Questions
Temperature Conversions (Fahrenheit ↔ Celsius) p. 97
°C = (°F − 32)/1.8   °F = (°C x 1.8) + 32

Common Skin Conditions
Time to Burn (TTB) p. 532
TTB (with sunscreen in min) = SPF x TTB (without sunscreen)

Biostatistics

Mean, Median and Mode p. 192

Mean - average value

Median - value in the middle of an ordered list

Mode - value that occurs most frequently

Risk, Relative Risk (RR) p. 197, Relative Risk Reduction (RRR), Absolute Risk Reduction (ARR) p. 198

$$\text{Risk} = \frac{\text{Number of subjects in group with an unfavorable event}}{\text{Total number of subjects in group}}$$

$$\text{RR} = \frac{\text{Risk in treatment group}}{\text{Risk in control group}}$$

$$\text{RRR} = \frac{(\% \text{ risk in control group} - \% \text{ risk in treatment group})}{\% \text{ risk in the control group}}$$

$$\text{ARR} = (\% \text{ risk in control group}) - (\% \text{ risk in treatment group})$$

Number Needed to Treat or Harm (NNT, NNH) p. 199-200

$$\text{NNT or NNH} = \frac{1}{\text{ARR*}}$$

*expressed as decimal

Odds Ratio (OR) p. 200

Exposure	Outcome Present	Outcome Absent
Present	A	B
Absent	C	D

$$\text{OR} = \frac{AD}{BC}$$

Hazard Ratio (HR) p. 201

$$\text{HR} = \frac{\text{Hazard rate in the treatment group}}{\text{Hazard rate in the control group}}$$

Incremental Cost-Effectiveness Ratio p. 211

$$\text{Incremental cost ratio} = \frac{(C_2 - C_1)}{(E_2 - E_1)} \quad C = \text{costs, } E = \text{effects}$$

Tobacco Cessation

Pack-Year Smoking History p. 569

$$\text{Pack-year smoking history} = \text{Cigarette packs / day} \times \text{years smoked}$$

Diabetes

Initiating Basal-Bolus Insulin in Type 1 Diabetes p. 589

1. Calculate total daily dose (TDD) of 0.5 units/kg/day using TBW.
2. Divide into 1/2 basal & 1/2 rapid-acting.
3. Split rapid-acting among meals.

Insulin-to-Carbohydrate Ratio: Rule of 450 for Regular Insulin p. 591

$$\frac{450}{\text{total daily dose of insulin (TDD)}} = \text{grams of carbohydrate covered by 1 unit of regular insulin}$$

Insulin-to-Carbohydrate Ratio: Rule of 500 for Rapid-Acting Insulin p. 591

$$\frac{500}{\text{total daily dose of insulin (TDD)}} = \text{grams of carbohydrate covered by 1 unit of rapid-acting insulin}$$

Correction Factor: 1,500 Rule for Regular Insulin p. 591

$$\frac{1,500}{\text{total daily dose of insulin (TDD)}} = \text{correction factor for 1 unit of regular insulin}$$

Correction Factor: 1,800 Rule for Rapid-Acting Insulin p. 591

$$\frac{1,800}{\text{total daily dose of insulin (TDD)}} = \text{correction factor for 1 unit of rapid-acting insulin}$$

Correction Dose p. 591

$$\frac{(\text{blood glucose now}) - (\text{target blood glucose})}{\text{correction factor}} = \text{correction dose}$$

Dyslipidemia

Friedewald Equation p. 395

$$\text{LDL} = \text{TC} - \text{HDL} - \frac{\text{TG*}}{5}$$

*do not use if TG > 400

Nonsterile Compounding

Minimum Weighable Quantity (MWQ) p. 216

$$\text{MWQ} = \frac{\text{Sensitivity requirement}}{\text{Acceptable error rate (usually 0.05)}}$$

Oncology

Body Surface Area (Mosteller) p. 763

(review use of Du Bois and Du Bois)

$$\text{BSA (m}^2) = \sqrt{\frac{\text{Ht (cm)} \times \text{Wt (kg)}}{3,600}}$$

Pharmacokinetics

Bioavailability (F) p. 919

$$F (\%) = 100 \times \frac{\text{AUC}_{\text{extravascular}}}{\text{AUC}_{\text{intravenous}}} \times \frac{\text{Dose}_{\text{intravenous}}}{\text{Dose}_{\text{extravascular}}}$$

Volume of Distribution (Vd) p. 920

$$\text{Vd} = \frac{\text{Amount of drug in body}}{\text{Concentration of drug in plasma}}$$

Clearance p. 922 & p. 924

$$\text{Cl} = \frac{F \times \text{dose}}{\text{AUC}} \quad \text{or} \quad \text{Cl} = ke \times \text{Vd}$$

Elimination Rate Constant (ke) p. 924

$$ke = \frac{\text{Cl}}{\text{Vd}}$$

Predicting Drug Concentrations p. 924

$$C_2 = C_1 \times e^{-kt} \qquad ke = \frac{\ln(C_1/C_2)}{t}$$

Half-Life (t½) p. 925

$$t_{\frac{1}{2}} = \frac{0.693}{ke}$$

Loading Dose (LD) p. 927

$$\text{LD} = \frac{\text{Desired concentration} \times \text{Vd}}{F}$$

Acute & Critical Care Medicine

Mean Arterial Pressure (MAP) p. 685

$$\text{MAP} = [(2 \times \text{diastolic pressure}) + \text{systolic pressure}] / 3$$

Seizures/Epilepsy

Phenytoin (Total) Correction for Albumin < 3.5 p. 853

$$\text{Phenytoin}_{\text{corrected}} \text{ (mcg/mL)} = \frac{\text{Total phenytoin measured}}{(0.2 \times \text{albumin}) + 0.1}$$

DRUG-DOSE CONVERSIONS

KCl Solution (Oral) to Tablets p. 136 (see problem #61)
KCl 10% = 20 mEq/15 mL

Calcium Salts p. 175
Calcium carbonate = 40% elemental calcium
Calcium citrate = 21% elemental calcium

Aminophylline ↔ Theophylline p. 175
Aminophylline to **T**heophylline: **M**ultiply by 0.8 (remember: **ATM**)
Theophylline to Aminophylline: Divide by 0.8

Statins p. 398

Pitavastatin	2 mg	Lovastatin	40 mg
Rosuvastatin	5 mg	Pravastatin	40 mg
Atorvastatin	10 mg	Fluvastatin	80 mg
Simvastatin	20 mg		

Metoprolol p. 417
IV:PO = 1:2.5

Loop Diuretics p. 443

Ethacrynic acid	50 mg	Bumetanide	1 mg
Furosemide	40 mg	Furosemide	IV:PO = 1:2
Torsemide	20 mg	Other Loops	IV:PO = 1:1

Insulin p. 592
Usually, 1:1 conversion
Exceptions:
NPH dosed BID → glargine dosed daily, use 80% of NPH dose
Toujeo → other forms of glargine or detemir, use 80% of *Toujeo* dose

Levothyroxine p. 601
IV:PO = 0.75:1

Steroids p. 608

Cortisone	25 mg	Methylprednisolone	4 mg
Hydrocortisone	20 mg	Triamcinolone	4 mg
Prednisone	5 mg	Dexamethasone	0.75 mg
Prednisolone	5 mg	Betamethasone	0.6 mg

Opioids (methodology) p. 732

Lithium p. 813
5 mL lithium citrate syrup = 300 mg lithium carbonate = 8 mEq Li⁺ ion

TOP PRESCRIPTION DRUGS

Top-selling/must-know prescription drugs are included in this list and bolded throughout the course book. Refer to the clinical chapters for essential underlined information about them. These are oral formulations unless otherwise noted. Top prescription drugs that are injectable only and top OTC medications are listed separately. Note that some prescription medications are also available OTC (see Top OTC Drugs list).

DRUG	BRAND NAME
Abacavir	
Abacavir/Lamivudine	*Epzicom*
Acetaminophen	*Tylenol* (oral), generics (suppository, injection)
Acetaminophen/ Codeine	
Acyclovir	*Zovirax* (topical), generics (oral, injection)
Adapalene	*Differin* (topical)
Albuterol	*ProAir HFA, ProAir RespiClick, Proventil HFA, Ventolin HFA* (inhalation)
Albuterol/Ipratropium	*Combivent Respimat* (inhalation)
Alendronate	*Fosamax*
Allopurinol	*Zyloprim* (oral), *Aloprim* (injection)
Alprazolam	*Xanax*
Alvimopan	*Entereg*
Amiodarone	*Pacerone* (oral), *Nexterone* (injection)
Amitriptyline	
Amlodipine	*Norvasc*
Amlodipine/Benazepril	*Lotrel*
Amoxicillin	
Amoxicillin/ Clarithromycin/ Lansoprazole	*Prevpac*
Amoxicillin/Clavulanate	*Augmentin*
Amphetamine/ Dextroamphetamine	*Adderall*
Ampicillin	Generics (oral, injection)
Anastrozole	*Arimidex*
Apixaban	*Eliquis*

DRUG	BRAND NAME
Aprepitant	*Emend*
Aripiprazole	*Abilify*
Atazanavir	*Reyataz*
Atenolol	*Tenormin*
Atenolol/Chlorthalidone	*Tenoretic*
Atomoxetine	*Strattera*
Atorvastatin	*Lipitor*
Azelastine	*Astepro* (nasal), generics (ophthalmic)
Azithromycin	*Zithromax* (oral, injection), *Z-Pak* (oral)
Bacitracin/Neomycin/ Polymyxin B/ Hydrocortisone	*Cortisporin* (topical)
Baclofen	*Lioresal* (intrathecal), generics (oral)
Beclomethasone	*QVAR RediHaler* (inhalation)
Benazepril	*Lotensin*
Benzonatate	*Tessalon Perles*
Benztropine	*Cogentin*
Betamethasone dipropionate	Generics (topical)
Betamethasone/ Clotrimazole	*Lotrisone* (topical)
Bictegravir/ Emtricitabine/Tenofovir alafenamide	*Biktarvy*
Bimatoprost	*Lumigan, Latisse* (ophthalmic)
Bismuth/ Metronidazole/ Tetracycline	*Pylera*
Bisoprolol/ Hydrochlorothiazide	*Ziac*
Brompheniramine/ Pseudoephedrine/ Dextromethorphan	*Bromfed DM*

DRUG	BRAND NAME
Budesonide	*Pulmicort, Pulmicort Flexhaler* (inhalation), *Entocort EC, Uceris* (oral)
Budesonide/Formoterol	*Symbicort, Breyna* (inhalation)
Bumetanide	*Bumex* (oral), generics (injection)
Buprenorphine	*Belbuca* (buccal film), *Butrans* (patch)
Buprenorphine/ Naloxone	*Suboxone* (SL film), *Zubsolv* (SL tablet)
Bupropion	*Wellbutrin SR, Wellbutrin XL*
Buspirone	
Butoconazole	*Gynazole-1* (topical)
Calcitonin	*Miacalcin* (injection), generics (nasal)
Canagliflozin	*Invokana*
Canagliflozin/ Metformin	*Invokamet*
Cannabidiol	*Epidiolex*
Capecitabine	*Xeloda*
Carbamazepine	*Tegretol*
Carbidopa/Levodopa	*Sinemet*
Cariprazine	*Vraylar*
Carisoprodol	*Soma*
Carvedilol	*Coreg, Coreg CR*
Cefdinir	
Cefuroxime	Generics (oral, injection)
Celecoxib	*Celebrex*
Cephalexin	
Chlorpheniramine/ Hydrocodone	*TussiCaps*

Top Prescription Drugs Continued

DRUG	BRAND NAME
Chlorthalidone	
Cholecalciferol, vitamin D3	
Cinacalcet	*Sensipar*
Ciprofloxacin	*Cipro* (oral), generics (injection)
Ciprofloxacin/ Dexamethasone	*Ciprodex* (otic)
Citalopram	*Celexa*
Clarithromycin	
Clindamycin	*Cleocin* (injection, oral), *Cleocin-T, Clindagel* (topical)
Clobetasol	*Clobex, Temovate, Olux* (topical)
Clonazepam	*Klonopin*
Clonidine	*Kapvay* (oral), *Catapres-TTS* (patch)
Clopidogrel	*Plavix*
Clozapine	*Clozaril*
Cobicistat	*Tybost*
Codeine	
Codeine/Promethazine	
Colchicine	*Colcrys*
Colesevelam	*Welchol*
Cyanocobalamin, vitamin B12	Generics (injection, nasal)
Cyclobenzaprine	*Amrix, Fexmid*
Cyclophosphamide	Generics (oral, injection)
Cyclosporine	*Neoral, Gengraf* (modified; oral) *Sandimmune* (non-modified; oral, injection), *Restasis* (ophthalmic)
Dabigatran	*Pradaxa*
Dapagliflozin	*Farxiga*
Darunavir	*Prezista*
Darunavir/Cobicistat/ Emtricitabine/Tenofovir alafenamide	*Symtuza*

DRUG	BRAND NAME
Desvenlafaxine	*Pristiq*
Dexamethasone	Generics (oral, injection)
Dexlansoprazole	*Dexilant*
Dextromethorphan/ Promethazine	
Diazepam	*Valium* (oral), *Diastat AcuDial* (rectal gel), generics (injection)
Diclofenac	*Voltaren* (topical), generics (oral, patch)
Dicyclomine	*Bentyl*
Digoxin	*Digitek* (oral), *Lanoxin* (oral, injection)
Dihydroergotamine	*D.H.E. 45* (injection), *Migranal* (nasal)
Diltiazem	*Tiazac, Cardizem* (oral), generics (injection)
Diphenhydramine	*Benadryl* (oral, topical, injection)
Diphenoxylate/Atropine	*Lomotil*
Dipyridamole/Aspirin	*Aggrenox*
Dolutegravir	*Tivicay*
Dolutegravir/Abacavir/ Lamivudine	*Triumeq*
Dolutegravir/ Lamivudine	*Dovato*
Donepezil	*Aricept* (oral), *Adlarity* (patch)
Donepezil/Memantine	*Namzaric*
Dornase alfa	*Pulmozyme* (inhalation)
Doxazosin	*Cardura*
Doxepin	
Doxycycline	*Vibramycin* (oral), generics (injection)
Dronabinol	*Marinol*
Duloxetine	*Cymbalta*
Efavirenz	

DRUG	BRAND NAME
Elvitegravir/Cobicistat/ Emtricitabine/Tenofovir alafenamide	*Genvoya*
Elvitegravir/Cobicistat/ Emtricitabine/Tenofovir disoproxil fumarate	*Stribild*
Empagliflozin	*Jardiance*
Emtricitabine	
Emtricitabine/Tenofovir alafenamide	*Descovy*
Emtricitabine/Tenofovir disoproxil fumarate	*Truvada*
Enalapril	*Vasotec*
Entecavir	*Baraclude*
Ergocalciferol, vitamin D2	*Calciferol*
Erythromycin	*E.E.S., Ery-Tab* (oral), *Erythrocin* (oral, injection)
Escitalopram	*Lexapro*
Esomeprazole	*Nexium, Nexium 24HR* (oral), *Nexium IV* (injection)
Estradiol	*Estrace* (vaginal cream), *Estring* (vaginal ring), *Vagifem* (vaginal tablet), *Vivelle-Dot, Climara* (patch)
Estrogens, conjugated (equine)	*Premarin* (vaginal cream, oral, injection)
Estrogens, conjugated (equine)/ Medroxyprogesterone	
Eszopiclone	*Lunesta*
Ethinyl estradiol/ Drospirenone	*Yasmin, Yaz*
Ethinyl estradiol/ Etonogestrel	*NuvaRing* (vaginal ring)
Ethinyl estradiol/ Levonorgestrel	*Seasonique*
Ethinyl estradiol/ Norethindrone	*Junel, Loestrin, Lo Loestrin, Microgestin*
Ethinyl estradiol/ Norgestimate	*Tri-Sprintec, Sprintec 28*
Ethosuximide	*Zarontin*
Ezetimibe	*Zetia*

Top Prescription Drugs Continued

DRUG	BRAND NAME
Famotidine	*Pepcid* (oral, injection), *Zantac 360*
Fenofibrate	*Tricor, Trilipix*
Fentanyl	*Sublimaze* (injection), generics (patch)
Fidaxomicin	*Dificid*
Finasteride	*Proscar, Propecia*
Fluconazole	*Diflucan* (oral, injection)
Fluocinonide	*Vanos* (topical)
Fluoxetine	*Prozac*
Fluticasone	*Flovent Diskus, Flovent HFA, Arnuity Ellipta* (inhalation)
Fluticasone/Salmeterol	*Advair Diskus, Advair HFA* (inhalation)
Fluticasone/Vilanterol	*Breo Ellipta* (inhalation)
Formoterol	Inhalation
Furosemide	*Lasix* (oral), generics (injection)
Gabapentin	*Neurontin*
Gemfibrozil	*Lopid*
Glecaprevir/Pibrentasvir	*Mavyret*
Glimepiride	*Amaryl*
Glipizide	
Glyburide	
Glyburide, micronized	*Glynase*
Glycopyrrolate/Formoterol/Budesonide	*Breztri Aerosphere* (inhalation)
Granisetron	*Sancuso* (patch), generics (injection, oral)
Guanfacine ER	*Intuniv*
Haloperidol	Generics (oral, injection)
Hydralazine	Generics (oral, injection)
Hydralazine/Isosorbide dinitrate	*BiDil*

DRUG	BRAND NAME
Hydrochlorothiazide	
Hydrocodone/Acetaminophen	
Hydrocortisone	*Solu-Cortef* (injection), generics (oral)
Hydromorphone	*Dilaudid* (oral, injection)
Hydroxychloroquine	*Plaquenil*
Hydroxyurea	
Hydroxyzine	*Vistaril*
Ibandronate	Generics (oral, injection)
Ibuprofen	*Advil, Motrin IB* (oral)
Icosapent ethyl	*Vascepa*
Imatinib	*Gleevec*
Indomethacin	*Indocin* (oral, injection, suppository)
Influenza vaccine, live attenuated (LAIV4)	*FluMist Quadrivalent* (nasal)
Ipratropium bromide	*Atrovent HFA* (inhalation)
Irbesartan	*Avapro*
Isocarboxazid	*Marplan*
Isoniazid (INH)	
Isosorbide mononitrate	
Isotretinoin	*Absorica, Amnesteem*
Ketoconazole	Generics (oral, topical)
Ketorolac	Generics (oral, injection, nasal), *Acular* (ophthalmic)
Labetalol	Generics (oral, injection)
Lacosamide	*Vimpat* (oral, injection)
Lactulose	
Lamivudine	
Lamotrigine	*Lamictal, Lamictal ODT, Lamictal Starter Kit*

DRUG	BRAND NAME
Lansoprazole	*Prevacid, Prevacid 24HR, Prevacid SoluTab*
Latanoprost	*Xalatan, Xelpros* (ophthalmic)
Levetiracetam	*Keppra* (oral, injection)
Levofloxacin	Generics (oral, injection)
Levothyroxine	*Levoxyl, Synthroid, Unithroid* (oral), generics (injection)
Lidocaine	*Lidoderm* (patch), generics (oral solution, topical)
Linaclotide	*Linzess*
Linagliptin	*Tradjenta*
Linezolid	*Zyvox* (oral, injection)
Liothyronine	*Cytomel*
Lisdexamfetamine	*Vyvanse*
Lisinopril	*Zestril*
Lisinopril/Hydrochlorothiazide	*Zestoretic*
Lithium	*Lithobid*
Lorazepam	*Ativan* (oral, injection)
Losartan	*Cozaar*
Losartan/Hydrochlorothiazide	*Hyzaar*
Lovastatin	*Altoprev*
Lubiprostone	*Amitiza*
Lurasidone	*Latuda*
Medroxyprogesterone	*Provera* (oral), *Depo-Provera* (injection)
Meloxicam	*Mobic*
Memantine	*Namenda*
Meperidine	*Demerol* (oral, injection)
Mesalamine	*Asacol HD, Pentasa* (oral), *Canasa* (suppository), *Rowasa* (enema)

Top Prescription Drugs Continued

DRUG	BRAND NAME
Metformin	Fortamet, Glumetza
Metformin/Pioglitazone	Actoplus Met
Metformin/Sitagliptin	Janumet
Methadone	
Methimazole	
Methocarbamol	Robaxin
Methotrexate	Trexall (oral), Otrexup, Rasuvo (injection)
Methylnaltrexone	Relistor (oral, injection)
Methylphenidate	Concerta, Ritalin, Ritalin LA (oral), Daytrana (patch)
Methylprednisolone	Medrol (oral), Solu-Medrol (injection)
Metoclopramide	Reglan (oral), generics (injection)
Metoprolol succinate ER	Toprol XL
Metoprolol tartrate IR	Lopressor (oral), generics (injection)
Metronidazole	Flagyl (oral, injection)
Minocycline	Solodyn (oral), Minocin (oral, injection)
Mirtazapine	Remeron, Remeron SolTab
Mometasone	Generics (topical)
Mometasone/Formoterol	Dulera (inhalation)
Montelukast	Singulair
Morphine	MS Contin (oral), Duramorph, Infumorph (injection)
Moxifloxacin	Vigamox (ophthalmic), generics (oral, injection)
Mupirocin	Generics (topical)
Mycophenolate mofetil	CellCept (oral, injection)
Mycophenolic acid	Myfortic

DRUG	BRAND NAME
N-acetylcysteine	Acetadote (injection), generics (oral)
Nabilone	Cesamet
Nadolol	Corgard
Naloxegol	Movantik
Naloxone	Narcan, RiVive (nasal), generics (injection)
Naproxen	Aleve
Naproxen/Esomeprazole	Vimovo
Nebivolol	Bystolic
Neomycin/Polymyxin B/Dexamethasone	Maxitrol (ophthalmic)
Niacin	
Nifedipine ER	Procardia XL
Nitrofurantoin	Macrobid, Macrodantin
Nitroglycerin	Nitro-BID (ointment), Nitrostat (SL tablet), Nitrolingual, NitroMist (SL spray), generics (injection)
Norethindrone	Errin, Camila, Nora-BE
Nortriptyline	Pamelor
Nystatin	
Ofloxacin	Ocuflox (ophthalmic)
Olanzapine	Zyprexa
Olmesartan	Benicar
Olmesartan/Hydrochlorothiazide	Benicar HCT
Olopatadine	Pataday (ophthalmic)
Omega-3 fatty acids	Lovaza
Omeprazole	Prilosec, Prilosec OTC
Ondansetron	Zofran (oral), generics (injection)
Orlistat	Xenical, Alli

DRUG	BRAND NAME
Oseltamivir	Tamiflu
Oxcarbazepine	Trileptal
Oxybutynin	Ditropan XL (oral), Oxytrol, Oxytrol for Women (patch)
Oxycodone	Oxycontin (ER; oral), Roxicodone (IR; oral)
Oxycodone/Acetaminophen	Percocet, Endocet
Paliperidone	Invega
Pancrelipase	Creon, Viokace, Zenpep
Pantoprazole	Protonix (oral, injection)
Paroxetine	Paxil
Penicillin VK	
Phenazopyridine	Pyridium
Phenelzine	Nardil
Phenobarbital	Generics (oral, injection)
Phentermine	Adipex-P
Phenytoin	Dilantin, Dilantin Infatabs (oral), generics (oral, injection)
Pioglitazone	Actos
Polyethylene glycol 3350	MiraLax
Polyethylene glycol-electrolyte solution	Colyte, GoLytely
Polymyxin/Trimethoprim	Polytrim (ophthalmic)
Posaconazole	Noxafil (oral, injection)
Potassium chloride	Klor-Con, K-Tab, Micro-K (oral), generics (oral, injection)
Pramipexole	Mirapex, Mirapex ER
Prasugrel	Effient
Pravastatin	
Prednisolone	Millipred, Orapred ODT (oral), Pred Forte, Pred Mild (ophthalmic)

Top Prescription Drugs Continued

DRUG	BRAND NAME
Prednisone	
Pregabalin	*Lyrica*
Progesterone, micronized	*Prometrium*
Prochlorperazine	Generics (oral, injection)
Promethazine	Generics (oral, injection, suppository)
Propranolol	*Inderal LA, Inderal XL* (oral), generics (injection)
Propylthiouracil (PTU)	
Quetiapine	*Seroquel*
Quinapril	*Accupril*
Raloxifene	*Evista*
Raltegravir	*Isentress, Isentress HD*
Ramipril	*Altace*
Rifampin	
Rifaximin	*Xifaxan*
Rilpivirine	
Rilpivirine/Emtricitabine/Tenofovir alafenamide	*Odefsey*
Rilpivirine/Emtricitabine/Tenofovir disoproxil fumarate	*Complera*
Risperidone	*Risperdal*
Ritonavir	*Norvir*
Rivaroxaban	*Xarelto*
Rivastigmine	*Exelon* (patch), generics (oral)
Ropinirole	
Rosuvastatin	*Crestor*
Rotavirus 1 vaccine	*Rotarix*
Rotavirus 5 vaccine	*RotaTeq*
Sacubitril/Valsartan	*Entresto*
Salmeterol	*Serevent Diskus* (inhalation)
Scopolamine	*Transderm Scop* (patch)

DRUG	BRAND NAME
Selenium sulfide	*Selsun* (topical)
Sertraline	*Zoloft*
Sevelamer carbonate	*Renvela*
Sevelamer hydrochloride	*Renagel*
Sildenafil	*Viagra* (oral), *Revatio* (oral, injection)
Simvastatin	*Zocor*
Sitagliptin	*Januvia*
Sodium phosphates	*OsmoPrep* (oral), generics (injection)
Sodium polystyrene sulfonate	*SPS* (oral, enema)
Sodium/Potassium/Magnesium sulfate	*Suprep Bowel Prep Kit*
Sofosbuvir/Velpatasvir	*Epclusa*
Solifenacin	*Vesicare*
Spironolactone	*Aldactone*
Sucralfate	*Carafate*
Sulfamethoxazole/Trimethoprim	*Bactrim DS, Bactrim* (oral), generics (injection)
Sumatriptan	*Imitrex* (oral, injection, nasal), *Imitrex STATdose* (injection), *Onzetra Xsail* (nasal)
Sumatriptan/Naproxen	*Treximet*
Tacrolimus	*Envarsus XR* (oral), *Prograf* (oral, injection)
Tadalafil	*Cialis, Adcirca*
Tamoxifen	
Tamsulosin	*Flomax*
Temazepam	*Restoril*
Tenofovir alafenamide	*Vemlidy*
Tenofovir disoproxil fumarate	*Viread*
Terazosin	

DRUG	BRAND NAME
Terbinafine	Generics (oral)
Terconazole	Generics (topical, vaginal)
Testosterone	*AndroGel, AndroGel Pump* (topical)
Theophylline	
Thyroid, desiccated	*Armour Thyroid*
Ticagrelor	*Brilinta*
Timolol	*Timoptic, Istalol, Timoptic-XE* (ophthalmic)
Timolol/Dorzolamide	*Cosopt, Cosopt PF* (ophthalmic)
Tiotropium	*Spiriva HandiHaler, Spiriva Respimat* (inhalation)
Tizanidine	*Zanaflex*
Tobramycin	Generics (inhalation, injection)
Tolterodine	*Detrol*
Tolvaptan	*Samsca*
Topiramate	*Topamax*
Torsemide	
Tramadol	
Tranexamic acid	Generics (oral, injection)
Tranylcypromine	*Parnate*
Travoprost	*Travatan Z* (ophthalmic)
Trazodone	
Tretinoin	*Atralin, Altreno, Renova, Retin-A, Retin-A Micro* (topical)
Triamcinolone	*Kenalog* (topical, injection)
Triamterene/Hydrochlorothiazide	*Maxzide*
Ulipristal	*Ella*
Umeclidinium/Vilanterol/Fluticasone	*Trelegy Ellipta* (inhalation)
Valacyclovir	*Valtrex*

Top Prescription Drugs Continued

DRUG	BRAND NAME
Valganciclovir	*Valcyte*
Valproic acid/ Divalproex	*Depakote, Depakote ER, Depakote Sprinkle,* (oral), generics (injection)
Valsartan	*Diovan*
Valsartan/Amlodipine	*Exforge*
Valsartan/ Hydrochlorothiazide	*Diovan HCT*
Vancomycin	*Vancocin* (oral, injection)
Varenicline	
Venlafaxine	*Effexor XR*
Verapamil	*Calan SR*
Vitamin K, phytonadione	*Mephyton* (oral), generics (injection)
Voriconazole	*Vfend* (oral), *Vfend IV* (injection)
Warfarin	*Jantoven*
Zidovudine	Generics (oral, injection)
Ziprasidone	*Geodon* (oral, injection)
Zolpidem	*Ambien* (oral), *Edluar* (SL tablet)

TOP PRESCRIPTION DRUGS: INJECTABLE ONLY

Top-selling/must-know prescription drugs that are injectable only are included in this list and are bolded throughout the course book. Refer to the clinical chapters for essential underlined information about them.

DRUG	BRAND NAME	DRUG	BRAND NAME	DRUG	BRAND NAME
Adalimumab	Humira	Cefotetan		Eptifibatide	
Albumin	Albutein, AlbuRx	Cefoxitin		Ertapenem	Invanz
Alirocumab	Praluent	Ceftaroline	Teflaro	Esmolol	Brevibloc
Alteplase	Activase	Ceftazidime		Etanercept	Enbrel
Amikacin		Ceftriaxone		Evolocumab	Repatha
Amphotericin B, conventional		Certolizumab pegol	Cimzia	Factor VIIa recombinant	NovoSeven RT
Amphotericin B, liposomal	Ambisome	Cetuximab		Ferumoxytol	Feraheme
Ampicillin/Sulbactam	Unasyn	Cisatracurium	Nimbex	Filgrastim	Neupogen
Andexanet alfa	Andexxa	Cisplatin		Flumazenil	
Antithymocyte globulin (equine)	Atgam	Crotalidae polyvalent immune Fab	CroFab	Fluorouracil, 5-FU	
Antithymocyte globulin (rabbit)	Thymoglobulin	Dextrose 5% in water (D5W)		Fosaprepitant	Emend
Argatroban		Daptomycin	Cubicin	Fosphenytoin	Cerebyx
Aztreonam	Azactam	Darbepoetin alfa	Aranesp	Four factor prothrombin complex concentrate	Kcentra
Belimumab	Benlysta	Denosumab	Prolia, Xgeva	Fulvestrant	
Bempedoic acid		Dexmedetomidine	Precedex	Ganciclovir	
Bevacizumab	Avastin	Digoxin immune Fab	DigiFab	Gentamicin	
Nirsevimab	Beyfortus	Diphtheria and tetanus toxoids, acellular pertussis (Tdap) vaccine	Adacel, Boostrix	Glatiramer acetate	Copaxone
Bivalirudin	Angiomax	Dopamine		Golimumab	Simponi
Bleomycin		Doxorubicin		Goserelin	Zoladex
Busulfan		DTaP-HepB-IPV vaccine	Pediarix	Hepatitis A vaccine	Havrix, Vaqta
Cabotegravir	Apretude	Dulaglutide	Trulicity	Hepatitis B vaccine	Engerix-B, Heplisav-B, Recombivax HB
Cabotegravir/Rilpivirine	Cabenuva	Enalaprilat	Vasotec IV	Human papillomavirus (HPV) vaccine (9-valent)	Gardasil 9
Carmustine		Enoxaparin	Lovenox	Idarucizumab	Praxbind
Caspofungin	Cancidas	Epinephrine	Adrenalin, EpiPen	Ifosfamide	
Cefazolin		Epoetin alfa	Epogen, Procrit		
Cefepime		Epoprostenol	Flolan		
Cefotaxime					

Top Prescription Drugs: Injectable Only Continued

DRUG	BRAND NAME
Immunoglobulin	*Gammagard, Octagam, Privigen, Gamunex-C*
Inactivated influenza quadrivalent vaccine (IIV4)	*Afluria Quadrivalent, Fluad Quadrivalent, Fluarix Quadrivalent, FluLaval Quadrivalent, Flucelvax Quadrivalent, Fluzone Quadrivalent, Fluzone High-Dose Quadrivalent*
Inclisiran	
Infliximab	*Remicade*
Insulin aspart	*Novolog*
Insulin detemir	*Levemir*
Insulin glargine	*Lantus, Toujeo*
Insulin lispro	*Humalog*
Insulin NPH	*Humulin N, Novolin N*
Insulin regular	*Humulin R, Novolin R*
Insulin, premixed (70% NPH/30% regular)	*Humulin 70/30, Novolin 70/30*
Irinotecan	
Iron sucrose	*Venofer*
Lactated Ringer's	
Leuprolide	*Lupron Depot*
Liraglutide	*Victoza, Saxenda*
Measles-Mumps-Rubella vaccine (MMR)	*M-M-R II*
Measles-Mumps-Rubella-Varicella vaccine (MMRV)	*ProQuad*
Meningococcal conjugate vaccine, quadrivalent (MenACWY)	*MenQuadfi, Menveo*
Meningococcal serogroup B vaccine (MenB)	*Bexsero, Trumenba*

DRUG	BRAND NAME
Meningococcal conjugate vaccine, pentavalent (MenABCWY)	*Penbraya*
Meropenem	
Micafungin	*Mycamine*
Midazolam	
Mitoxantrone	
Natalizumab	*Tysabri*
Nicardipine	*Cardene IV*
Nitroprusside	*Nipride*
Norepinephrine	*Levophed*
Normal saline (NS), ½NS, ¼NS	
Octreotide	*Sandostatin*
Omalizumab	*Xolair*
Paclitaxel	
Palivizumab	*Synagis*
Palonosetron	
Pamidronate	
Pegfilgrastim	*Neulasta*
Penicillin G benzathine	*Bicillin L-A*
Piperacillin/Tazobactam	*Zosyn*
Plasma-Lyte A	
Pneumococcal conjugate vaccine, 15-valent (PCV15)	*Vaxneuvance*
Pneumococcal conjugate vaccine, 20-valent (PCV20)	*Prevnar 20*
Pneumococcal polysaccharide vaccine, 23-valent (PPSV23)	*Pneumovax 23*
Propofol	*Diprivan*
Protamine sulfate	
Rabies vaccine	*RabAvert*

DRUG	BRAND NAME
Rasburicase	*Elitek*
Rituximab	*Rituxan*
Respiratory syncytial virus (RSV) vaccine	*Abrysvo*
Semaglutide	*Ozempic, Wegovy*
Succinylcholine	
Tenecteplase	*TNKase*
Testosterone cypionate	
Tigecycline	*Tygacil*
Tirzepatide	*Zepbound*
Trastuzumab	*Herceptin*
Unfractionated heparin	
Varicella virus (chickenpox) vaccine	*Varivax*
Vasopressin	
Vedolizumab	*Entyvio*
Vincristine	
Zoledronic acid	*Reclast, Zometa*
Zoster virus (shingles) vaccine	*Shingrix*

TOP OTC DRUGS

For drugs that are available in both OTC and Rx (prescription) versions, the Rx doses are generally higher than the OTC doses. The brand names can be different [e.g., orlistat OTC (*Alli*) is 60 mg/dose, orlistat Rx (*Xenical*) is 120 mg/dose] and are provided as a study aid (generic may be the top-seller).

DRUG

ALLERGIC RHINITIS, COUGH AND COLD

Antihistamines, Non-Sedating

Cetirizine (*Zyrtec Allergy, Zyrtec Childrens Allergy*)

Fexofenadine (*Allegra Allergy, Allegra Allergy Childrens*)

Levocetirizine (*Xyzal Allergy 24HR, Xyzal Allergy 24HR Childrens*)

Loratadine (*Claritin, Claritin Childrens*)

Antihistamines, Sedating

Chlorpheniramine

Diphenhydramine (*Benadryl*), OTC and Rx

Doxylamine

Cough Suppressant

Dextromethorphan (*Delsym, Robitussin*)

Mucolytic-Expectorant

Guaifenesin (*Mucinex, Robafen*)

Cough Suppressant/Mucolytic-Expectorant

Dextromethorphan/Guaifenesin (*Robafen DM, Robitussin DM*)

Decongestants

Oxymetazoline (*Afrin*) – nasal

Phenylephrine (*Sudafed PE*) – systemic

Pseudoephedrine (*Sudafed, Nexafed, Zephrex-D*) – systemic, behind the counter

Decongestants/Antihistamines, Non-Sedating

Cetirizine/Pseudoephedrine (*Zyrtec-D*)

Fexofenadine/Pseudoephedrine (*Allegra-D*)

Loratadine/Pseudoephedrine ER (*Claritin-D*)

Nasal Steroid Inhalers

Budesonide (*Rhinocort Allergy*)

Fluticasone (*Flonase Allergy Relief, Flonase Sensimist, Children's Flonase*)

Triamcinolone (*Nasacort Allergy 24HR, Nasacort Allergy 24HR Children*)

Nasal Mast Cell Stabilizer

Cromolyn (*NasalCrom*)

DRUG

COMMON SKIN CONDITIONS

Acne

Adapalene (*Differin*), OTC and Rx

Azelaic acid

Benzoyl peroxide

Salicylic acid

Alopecia

Minoxidil (*Rogaine*) – topical

Cold Sores, for Herpes Simplex

Docosanol (*Abreva*)

Dandruff Shampoos

Coal tar (*T/Gel*)

Ketoconazole 1% (*Nizoral A-D*)

Pyrithione zinc (*Head & Shoulders*)

Selenium sulfide (*Selsun*)

Diaper Rash

Petrolatum/Zinc Oxide (*Desitin*)

Topical Antifungals, for *Tinea* Infections

Butenafine (*Lotrimin Ultra*) – cream

Clotrimazole (*Lotrimin AF*) – cream

Miconazole (*Lotrimin AF*) – powder and spray

Terbinafine (*Lamisil AT*) – cream

Tolnaftate (*Tinactin*) – cream, powder and spray

Undecylenic acid

Vaginal Antifungals, for *Candida* Infections

Clotrimazole

Miconazole (*Monistat*)

Hemorrhoids

Phenylephrine (*Preparation H*)

Lice

Permethrin 1% (*Nix*)

Piperonyl butoxide/Pyrethrin (*RID*)

DRUG

Minor Wounds

Polymyxin/Bacitracin/Neomycin (*Neosporin*) – topical antibiotic

Pinworm

Pyrantel pamoate

Inflammation and Rash

Hydrocortisone cream 0.5% and 1% (*Cortizone-10*) – topical, OTC and Rx

CONSTIPATION AND DIARRHEA

Antidiarrheals

Bismuth subsalicylate (*Pepto-Bismol*)

Loperamide (*Imodium A-D*)

Constipation

Bisacodyl (*Dulcolax*) – oral, enema, suppository

Calcium polycarbophil (*FiberCon*)

Docusate sodium (*Colace*) – oral, enema

Glycerin – suppository

Magnesium hydroxide (*Milk of Magnesia*)

Methylcellulose (*Citrucel*)

Polyethylene glycol 3350 (*MiraLax*), OTC and Rx

Psyllium (*Metamucil*)

Sodium phosphates (*Fleet Enema*) – enema

Senna (*Ex-Lax, Senokot*)

Senna/Docusate (*Senokot S, Senna S*)

Wheat dextrin (*Benefiber*)

CONTRACEPTION

Condoms

Diaphragm

Nonoxynol-9 spermicide

Emergency Contraception

Levonorgestrel (*Plan B One-Step*), OTC and Rx

Top OTC Drugs Continued

DRUG

DIABETES: INSULIN, OTC and Rx

NPH Insulin

Humulin N, Novolin N

Premixed Insulins

Humulin 70/30, Novolin 70/30

Regular Insulin

Humulin R, Novolin R

DIETARY SUPPLEMENTS, NATURAL & COMPLEMENTARY MEDICINE

Calcium carbonate *(Tums)*

Calcium carbonate/Cholecalciferol *(Caltrate)*

Calcium citrate *(Cal-Citrate)*

Calcium citrate/Cholecalciferol *(Citracal)*

Coenzyme Q10

Ferrous sulfate

Omega-3 fatty acids (fish oils)

Magnesium citrate

Magnesium oxide

Probiotics

Lactobacillus (Culturelle)

Bifidobacterium longum (Align)

Saccharomyces boulardii (Florastor)

Vitamins

Niacin controlled release *(Slo-Niacin)*

Multivitamin *(One-A-Day,* others)

Prenatal multivitamin, OTC and Rx

Vitamin B complex

Vitamin B12, cyanocobalamin, OTC and Rx

Vitamin B9, folic acid, folate, OTC and Rx

Vitamin C, ascorbic acid

Vitamin D2, ergocalciferol, OTC and Rx

Vitamin D3, cholecalciferol, OTC and Rx

GASTROESOPHAGEAL REFLUX DISEASE & PEPTIC ULCER DISEASE

Proton Pump Inhibitors, OTC and Rx

Esomeprazole 20 mg *(Nexium 24HR)*

Omeprazole 20 mg *(Prilosec OTC)*

Lansoprazole 15 mg *(Prevacid 24HR)*, Lansoprazole 15 mg ODT

DRUG

H2-Receptor Antagonists, OTC and Rx

Famotidine 10-20 mg *(Pepcid AC, Zantac 360)*

Antacids & Antigas

Aluminum/Magnesium/Simethicone *(Mylanta Maximum Strength)*

Calcium carbonate *(Tums)*

Calcium carbonate/Magnesium *(Mylanta Supreme)*

Calcium carbonate/Simethicone *(Maalox Advanced Maximum Strength)*

Anhydrous citric acid/Aspirin/Sodium bicarbonate *(Alka-Seltzer)*

Simethicone *(Gas-X)*

Alpha-galactosidase enzyme *(Beano)*

Lactase enzyme *(Lactaid)*

MOTION SICKNESS

Dimenhydrinate *(Dramamine)*

Meclizine *(Dramamine Less Drowsy)*

OPHTHALMICS AND OTICS

Artificial tears *(Systane, Refresh)* – dry eye

Carbamide peroxide *(Debrox)* – ear wax removal

Ketotifen *(Alaway, Zaditor)* – red eyes/allergies

Naphazoline *(Clear Eyes Redness Relief)* – red eye

Naphazoline/Pheniramine *(Naphcon-A, Visine-A)* – red eyes/allergies

Olopatadine *(Pataday)* – red eyes/allergies, OTC and Rx

Tetrahydrozoline *(Visine)* – red eye

PAIN

Acetaminophen 325/500/650 mg *(Tylenol, FeverAll* rectal suppository)

Acetaminophen/Caffeine *(Excedrin Tension Headache)*

Acetaminophen/Aspirin/Caffeine *(Excedrin Extra Strength, Excedrin Migraine)*

Acetaminophen/Caffeine/Pyrilamine *(Midol Complete)*

Aspirin *(Ecotrin, Bufferin, Ascriptin)*

Capsaicin 0.025% and 0.075% cream *(Zostrix, Zostrix HP)*

Diclofenac gel *(Voltaren)*, OTC and Rx

Ibuprofen 200 mg *(Motrin IB, Advil)*, OTC and Rx

DRUG

Lidocaine patches, OTC and Rx

Magnesium salicylate *(Doan's Extra Strength)*

Methyl salicylate and menthol topical *(BenGay, Salonpas, IcyHot)*

Naproxen sodium 220 mg *(Aleve)*, OTC and Rx

Trolamine salicylate *(Aspercreme)*

Opioid Reversal

Naloxone *(Narcan, RiVive)*

SLEEP DISORDERS

Diphenhydramine *(Benadryl)*, OTC and Rx

Doxylamine *(Unisom SleepTabs)*

Melatonin

TOBACCO CESSATION

Nicotine gum *(Nicorette)*

Nicotine lozenge *(Nicorette Mini)*

Nicotine transdermal patch *(Nicoderm CQ)*

URINARY INCONTINENCE

Oxybutynin *(Oxytrol for Women)*, OTC and Rx

WEIGHT LOSS

Orlistat *(Alli)*, OTC and Rx

DIAGNOSTIC TESTS

DISORDER/CONDITION	DIAGNOSTIC TESTS (REFER TO SPECIFIC CHAPTER FOR MORE INFORMATION)
AUTOIMMUNE CONDITIONS	
Autoimmune, Various	↑ erythrocyte sedimentation rate **(ESR)**, ↑ C-reactive protein **(CRP)**, positive rheumatoid factor **(RF)** antibodies, positive anti-nuclear antibody **(ANA)**
Rheumatoid Arthritis (RA)	Above autoimmune tests plus positive anti-citrullinated peptide antibody (ACPA)
Systemic Lupus Erythematosus (SLE)	Above autoimmune tests plus positive anti-dsDNA antibodies
Multiple Sclerosis	Magnetic resonance imaging **(MRI)**
ANTICOAGULATION AND BLOOD DISORDERS	
Anemia	All: **↓ Hgb/Hct/RBCs**
	Microcytic (or iron deficiency): ↓ MCV (cell size is smaller, MCV < 80 fL)
	Macrocytic (or B12 or folate deficiency): ↑ MCV (cell size is larger, MCV > 100 fL), Schilling test
Venous Thromboembolism (VTE)	**D-dimer** test (marker of fibrinolysis)
	Deep vein thrombosis (DVT): **ultrasound (US),** venography, MRI
	Pulmonary embolism (PE): pulmonary computed tomographic angiography (CTA)
Stroke Prevention	**CHA$_2$DS$_2$-VASc** scoring system (score directs need for anticoagulation in patients with atrial fibrillation)
Heparin-Induced Thrombocytopenia (HIT)	Unexplained **↓ platelets (> 50% drop from baseline)** 5-14 days after starting heparin, positive antibodies based on a heparin-platelet factor 4 (PF4) enzyme-linked immunosorbent assay (ELISA) test and/or serotonin release assay (SRA)
CARDIOVASCULAR CONDITIONS	
Acute Coronary Syndromes (ACS)	Electrocardiogram **(ECG or EKG),** cardiac enzymes [creatine kinase muscle/brain (CK-MB), **troponin** I and T]
Arrhythmias	**ECG** (or EKG), **Holter monitor** (a portable ECG device), heart rate (HR)
Cerebrovascular Accident (CVA, or Stroke)	Computed tomography **(CT), MRI**
Chronic Heart Failure	Echocardiogram **(echo),** ↑ B-type natriuretic peptide (BNP), ↑ N-terminal proBNP (NT-proBNP)
Stable Angina	**Cardiac stress test,** angiography
Dyslipidemia	**↑ TC, Non-HDL, LDL, TGs,** coronary artery calcium (CAC, a non-invasive CT scan of the heart that measures calcium-containing plaque)
Hypertension	↑ systolic blood pressure (SBP)/diastolic blood pressure (DBP)
Hypertensive Emergency or Urgency	Emergency: **↑ BP (≥ 180/120 mmHg) with acute target organ damage**
	Urgency: **↑ BP (≥ 180/120 mmHg) without acute target organ damage**
10-Year Risk for Atherosclerotic Cardiovascular Disease (ASCVD)	10-year **ASCVD risk tool** [use if no history of ASCVD (ACS/IHD, stroke, PAD)]
ENDOCRINE CONDITIONS	
Diabetes, Prediabetes	Fasting plasma glucose **(FPG),** oral glucose tolerance test **(OGTT),** hemoglobin A1C **(A1C)**
Hyperthyroidism	↓ thyroid stimulating hormone **(TSH),** ↑ free T4 **(FT4)**
Hypothyroidism	**↑ TSH, ↓ FT4**
FEMALE HEALTH	
Ovulation	Luteinizing hormone **(LH),** peak value provides optimal timing for intercourse to become pregnant
Pregnancy	Positive human chorionic gonadotropin **(hCG)** in urine (outpatient test kit) or in blood
Bacterial Vaginitis	Clear, white or gray vaginal discharge, with a **fishy odor** and **pH > 4.5,** little or no pain
Candida Vaginitis	**White, thicker** vaginal discharge, **pruritus**
Trichomoniasis	**Yellow, green frothy,** foul-smelling vaginal discharge, **pH > 4.5,** soreness and pain with intercourse

Diagnostic Tests Continued

DISORDER/CONDITION	DIAGNOSTIC TESTS (REFER TO SPECIFIC CHAPTER FOR MORE INFORMATION)
GASTROINTESTINAL DISORDERS	
Peptic Ulcer Disease (PUD)	Upper gastrointestinal endoscopy (mouth to small intestine) **Duodenal ulcer:** pain 2-3 hrs after eating **(without food in stomach), pain relief** with food/antacids **Gastric ulcer:** pain right after eating **(with food in stomach), little/no pain relief** with food/antacids
GERD	**Esophageal pH monitoring,** endoscopy
H. pylori	**Urea breath test (UBT),** fecal antigen test
Inflammatory Bowel Disease (Ulcerative Colitis, Crohn's Disease)	Endoscopy (for Crohn's disease, which affects more of the GI tract) Sigmoidoscopy (for ulcerative colitis, which affects the colon and rectum) For both: colonoscopy, biopsy, CT, MRI
PULMONARY DISORDERS	
Bronchospastic Diseases	**Spirometry,** measures three main variables: **FEV1:** how much air can be forcefully exhaled in one second **FVC:** the maximum amount of air that can be forcefully exhaled **FEV1/FVC:** the percentage of total air capacity ("vital capacity") that can be forcefully exhaled in one second
Asthma	**FVC, FEV1** and peak expiratory flow rate (PEFR) Allergic asthma: **skin test** (to detect an allergen)
Chronic Obstructive Pulmonary Disease (COPD)	**Post-bronchodilator FEV1/FVC < 0.7** Eosinophils ≥ 300 cells/µL indicates inflammation and better response to inhaled corticosteroids
ACID/BASE DISORDERS	
Metabolic Acidosis	**Arterial blood gas,** measures **pH, pCO2, HCO3** ↓ pH, ↓ HCO3; compensation: respiratory alkalosis
Respiratory Acidosis	↓ pH, ↑ pCO2; compensation: metabolic alkalosis
Metabolic Alkalosis	↑ pH, ↑ HCO3; compensation: respiratory acidosis
Respiratory Alkalosis	↑ pH, ↓ pCO2; compensation: metabolic acidosis
Anion Gap Metabolic Acidosis	Anion gap > 12 mEq/L
INFECTIONS	
General Infection	**Fever** (temperature ≥ 100.4°F or 38°C), ↑ **WBC** count, left shift (↑ bands, or immature neutrophils)
C. difficile	**Positive *C. difficile* stool toxin** [enzyme immunoassay plus glutamate dehydrogenase (GDH) test] or **PCR**
HIV	**HIV antigen/antibody immunoassay, HIV-1/HIV-2 antibody** differentiation immunoassay, **HIV RNA viral load,** nucleic acid test
Infective Endocarditis	Echo (to check for vegetation), blood culture (to identify causative organism)
Lyme Disease	Round, red bullseye rash, **ELISA** test
Meningitis	**Lumbar puncture (LP),** plus symptoms of severe headache, stiff neck and altered mental status
Onychomycosis (Fungal Infection of Toenail or Fingernail)	**20% KOH** (potassium hydroxide) **smear**
Lice (*Pediculosis*)	**Pruritus,** visible lice on the scalp and **nits (eggs)** on hair shafts
Pinworm (*Vermicularis*)	**Tape test** (on skin adjacent to anus to check presence of eggs), **helminths** (worms) in blood, feces or urine
Pneumonia	**Chest X-ray** showing infiltrates, consolidations or opacities
Syphilis	Positive nontreponemal assay [rapid plasma reagin **(RPR)** or Venereal Diseases Research Laboratory **(VDRL)** blood test] and treponemal assay
***Toxoplasma gondii* Encephalitis**	Toxoplasma IgM and IgG test
Tuberculosis (TB)	Latent TB: positive tuberculin skin test **(TST)** [also known as a purified protein derivative **(PPD)],** or interferon-gamma release assay **(IGRA)** blood test Active TB: positive sputum **acid-fast bacilli (AFB) stain** and culture, chest X-ray with cavitation
Urinary Tract Infection (UTI)	**Urinalysis** (positive leukocyte esterase or WBC > 10 cells/mm³, nitrites, bacteria), urine culture

Diagnostic Tests Continued

DISORDER/CONDITION	DIAGNOSTIC TESTS (REFER TO SPECIFIC CHAPTER FOR MORE INFORMATION)
CANCER Initial screenings; all followed by biopsy (tissue sample sent to pathology)	
Breast	**Mammogram, ultrasound, MRI**
Cervical	**Pap smear, HPV test**
Colon	**Colonoscopy, sigmoidoscopy**, double-contrast barium enema, CT colonography, stool DNA, fecal occult blood test (FOBT), fecal immunochemical test
Lung	**CT chest**
Skin	Skin biopsy
Prostate	**Digital rectal exam (DRE), prostate-specific antigen (PSA)**
General	Carcinoembryonic antigen (CEA) test (a marker to identify cancer), positron emission tomography (PET)
ADDITIONAL COMMON CONDITIONS	
Allergic Reactions	**Skin prick** (scratch) test (immediate), immunoglobulin E **(IgE) antibodies** (blood)
Bleeding	↓ Hgb/Hct, visible blood or bruising, coffee ground emesis or dark/tarry stools (upper GI bleeding), red blood in stool (lower GI bleeding or hemorrhoid)
Cholestasis (Bile Duct Blockage)	↑ alkaline phosphatase (Alk Phos), ↑ total bilirubin (Tbili), ↑ gamma-glutamyltransferase (GGT)
Cognitive Impairment **(e.g., Alzheimer's)**	Mini-mental state exam **(MMSE),** score < 24 indicates impairment
Cystic Fibrosis	**Sweat test**
Glaucoma	↑ intraocular pressure **(IOP),** visual field test (to identify optic nerve damage)
Gout	↑ uric acid **(UA)** level
Liver Disease	Liver function tests **(LFTs): ↑ AST/ALT, ↑ Alk Phos, ↑ Tbili,** ↑ lactate dehydrogenase (LDH) **Cirrhosis** (chronic liver disease): **↑ PT/INR, ↓ Albumin** Alcoholic liver disease: ↑ AST > ↑ ALT, ↑ GGT **Hepatic encephalopathy: ↑ ammonia** level (blood)
Movement Disorders **(e.g. Parkinson Disease)**	**Abnormal involuntary movement scale (AIMS),** rating scale used to measure involuntary movements, or tardive dyskinesias, as monitoring for patient improvement
Myopathy	↑ creatine kinase or **creatine phosphokinase (CPK)**
Neuropathy, Peripheral	Assess sensation with **10-g monofilament,** pinprick, temperature and/or vibration tests
Osteoarthritis	X-ray, MRI
Osteoporosis	Bone mineral density **(BMD)** using dual energy X-ray absorptiometry **(DEXA** or DXA), **T-score ≤ -2.5** **Osteopenia: T-score -1 to -2.4**
Pain	**Pain scales,** non-verbal signs (e.g., moaning, grimacing, agitation)
Pancreatitis	**↑ amylase/lipase**
Psychiatric Disease **(e.g., Depression, Schizophrenia)**	**DSM-5** diagnostic criteria Depression-specific: **Ham-D or HDRS assessment scale**
Renal Disease	**↑ BUN/SCr,** creatinine clearance **(CrCl),** glomerular filtration rate **(eGFR), urine albumin** **Dehydration: BUN/SCr ratio > 20:1,** plus symptoms (e.g., ↓ urine output, dry mucus membranes, tachycardia)
Seizures/Epilepsy	Electroencephalogram **(EEG)**
Weight: Underweight, Normal Weight, Overweight, Obesity	BMI (plus **waist circumference** for risks associated with overweight/obesity), ideal body weight **(IBW),** total body weight **(TBW)**

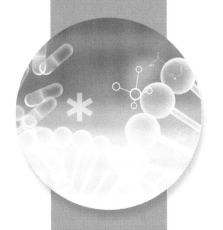
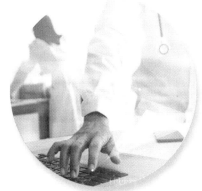
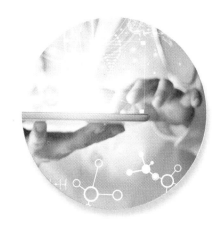

PHARMACY FOUNDATIONS PART 1

CONTENTS

CHAPTER CONTENT

Acetylsalicylic Acid

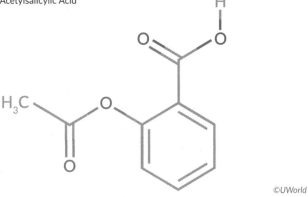

©UWorld

CHAPTER 2
BASIC SCIENCE CONCEPTS

BACKGROUND

An understanding of basic science concepts is essential to a pharmacist's role as the drug information expert. This chapter describes common terminology and foundational concepts that should be known for the NAPLEX. They may be tested directly, or application of knowledge may be required when answering case-based drug therapy questions.

Important drug mechanisms are reviewed in more detail in the specific disease state chapters.

DEFINITIONS

Substrate (or Ligand)
A substance that creates a signal or produces an effect by binding to a receptor, enzyme or transporter.

Endogenous
A substance that is produced by the body (such as a naturally-produced substrate).

Exogenous
A substance that is produced outside of the body (such as a drug or other chemical).

Agonist
A substance that combines with a receptor to initiate a reaction.
Can be endogenous or exogenous (i.e., mimicking an endogenous substrate).

Antagonist
A substance that reduces or blocks a reaction. Can be endogenous or exogenous.

Induction
When a substance increases the activity of an enzyme.

Inhibition
When a substance decreases or blocks the activity of an enzyme.

CONTENT LEGEND

= Study
  Tip Gal

OVERVIEW OF THE NERVOUS SYSTEM

The central nervous system (CNS) includes the brain and the spinal cord. The CNS controls the functions of the rest of the body by sending signals to the peripheral nervous system (PNS). The PNS has two main systems (somatic and autonomic). The somatic nervous system (voluntary) controls muscle movement while the autonomic nervous system (involuntary) controls other bodily functions, such as digestion, cardiac output and blood pressure (BP).

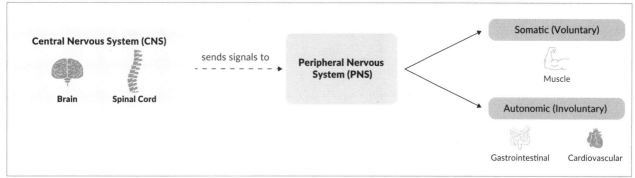

©UWorld

iStock.com/Alex_Doubovitsky, ambassador806, Mack15, sabelskaya

NEUROTRANSMITTERS

Signal transmission in the CNS and PNS is accomplished by neurotransmitters (NTs), which are the body's chemical messengers (i.e., substrates/ligands). NTs are released from presynaptic neurons into the synaptic cleft, then they travel to postsynaptic neurons or other parts of the body to exert their effect (see image).

Common NTs discussed in this chapter include acetylcholine (ACh), epinephrine (Epi), norepinephrine (NE), dopamine (DA) and serotonin (5-HT).

ACh is the primary NT involved in the somatic nervous system. It is released in response to neuron signals and binds to nicotinic receptors (Nn) in skeletal muscles to affect muscle movement. Neurotransmitters involved in the autonomic nervous system are discussed below.

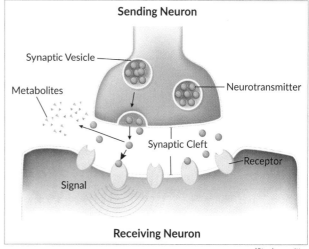

iStock.com/ttsz

AUTONOMIC NERVOUS SYSTEM

There are two main divisions of the autonomic nervous system, parasympathetic and sympathetic (see the diagram on the following page). The parasympathetic nervous system (PSNS) is known as the "rest and digest" system. The PSNS works by releasing ACh, which binds to muscarinic receptors located throughout the body, including the GI tract, the bladder and the eyes. This results in a physiologic response known as SLUDD (salivation, lacrimation, urination, defecation and digestion).

The sympathetic nervous system (SNS) is known as the "fight or flight" system. The SNS works by releasing Epi and NE, which act on adrenergic receptors (alpha-1, beta-1 and beta-2) in the cardiovascular and respiratory systems. Activation of the SNS results in increased BP, HR and bronchodilation. Stimulation of beta-2 receptors in the GI tract increases glucose production to provide muscles with oxygen and energy. When the SNS is activated, functions like digestion and urination are minimized to focus on the more important bodily functions for "fight or flight."

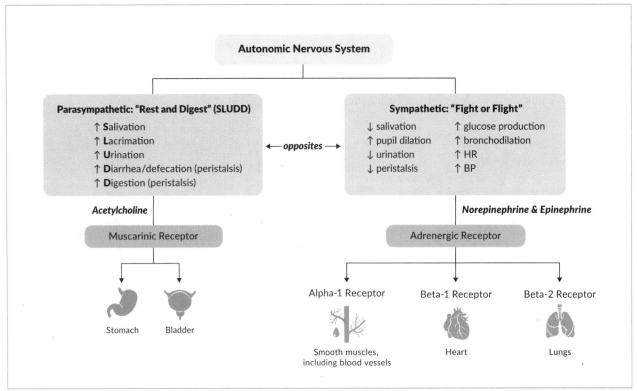

RECEPTORS AND SUBSTRATES

Chemical substances (e.g., neurotransmitters) released by cells in the body act as substrates (or ligands) by interacting with other cells to communicate and send signals. The substrate binds to receptors on the receiving cell to cause a signal or change. Substrates can be endogenous or exogenous. Once bound, the receptor-substrate complex causes some change that results in a biological effect (e.g., secretion of a hormone, contraction of a muscle, activation of an enzyme).

Substrates that bind to receptors can be agonists or antagonists. An agonist is a substance that binds to and activates a receptor, producing some type of response. An antagonist (sometimes called a blocker or inhibitor) binds to a receptor but does not produce a subsequent reaction; the antagonist blocks the agonist from binding and inhibits the subsequent reaction.

The interaction of an antagonist with a receptor can be competitive or non-competitive. Competitive inhibition

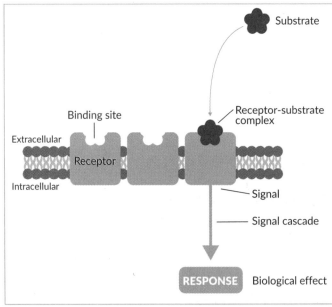

occurs when an antagonist binds to the same active site of a receptor as the endogenous substrate, preventing it from binding and causing a reaction. With non-competitive inhibition, the antagonist binds to the receptor at a site other than the active site (called the allosteric site), which changes the shape of the active site and prevents the endogenous substrate from binding.

DRUG-RECEPTOR INTERACTIONS

Drugs are exogenous substances that can act as agonists or antagonists. An example of a drug agonist and antagonist includes:

- Albuterol, a beta-2 agonist that behaves similarly to epinephrine. It binds to beta-2 receptors in the lungs, which activates several steps [e.g., increased cyclic adenosine monophosphate (cAMP) production and decreased intracellular calcium] and results in bronchial smooth muscle relaxation.

- Beta-1 blockers, which prevent adrenergic neurotransmitters (e.g., epinephrine) from binding to beta-1 receptors in the heart. Epinephrine normally increases heart rate and contractility when it binds to beta-1 receptors. By blocking the receptor, beta-1 blockers decrease heart rate and contractility.

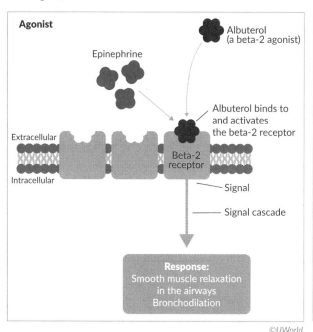

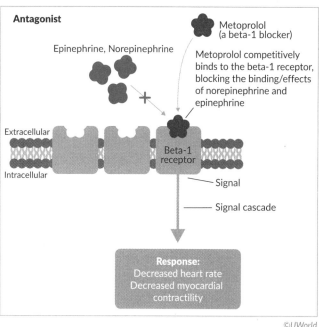

COMMON DRUG RECEPTOR TARGETS

The Study Tip Gal on the following page lists receptors that are common drug targets along with their endogenous substrates. Example drugs that have an agonist or antagonist effect at the receptor, along with the resulting biological effect, are included. How drugs work at these receptors is closely related to the conditions they treat. For example, muscarinic and alpha-1 receptors are targets for medications used to reduce bladder contractions (e.g., oxybutynin) and to relax the bladder (e.g., doxazosin) (see the Urinary Incontinence and Benign Prostatic Hyperplasia chapters). Terbutaline is a beta-2 agonist used in acute, severe asthma exacerbations.

Some medications affect multiple receptors. Isoproterenol is a mixed beta-1 and beta-2 agonist; it is used for bradycardia and causes bronchodilation. Carvedilol inhibits alpha-1, beta-1 and beta-2 receptors. It is used to decrease BP (by causing peripheral vasodilation and a decrease in HR), but it can cause bronchoconstriction. Some vasopressors (e.g., epinephrine, norepinephrine) stimulate multiple receptors, such as alpha-1 and beta-1, leading to increased vasoconstriction, HR and BP.

Other medications work in the CNS to affect the amount of neurotransmitter released and available to act on PNS receptors. Clonidine is a centrally-acting alpha-2 adrenergic agonist. When it binds to (i.e., stimulates) presynaptic alpha-2 receptors located in the brain, there is a decrease in overall sympathetic output (i.e., neurotransmitter release). Decreased release and availability of NE and Epi to bind to adrenergic receptors results in vasodilation (decreased BP) and a decrease in HR. Refer to the Overview of the Nervous System section for more on this process.

COMMON RECEPTORS, SUBSTRATES AND DRUG EXAMPLES

RECEPTOR	ENDOGENOUS SUBSTRATE	AGONIST ACTION	DRUG AGONISTS	ANTAGONIST ACTION	DRUG ANTAGONISTS
Muscarinic	Acetylcholine	↑ SLUDD*	Pilocarpine, bethanechol	↓ SLUDD*	Atropine, oxybutynin
Nicotinic	Acetylcholine	↑ HR, BP	Nicotine	Neuromuscular blockade	Neuromuscular blockers (e.g., rocuronium)
Alpha-1 (mainly peripheral)	Epinephrine, norepinephrine	Smooth muscle vasoconstriction, ↑ BP	Phenylephrine, dopamine (dose-dependent)	Smooth muscle vasodilation, ↓ BP	Alpha-1 blockers (e.g., doxazosin, carvedilol, phentolamine)
Alpha-2 (mainly brain; central)	Epinephrine, norepinephrine	↓ release of epinephrine and norepinephrine, ↓ BP, HR	Clonidine, brimonidine (ophthalmic, for glaucoma)	↑ BP, HR	Ergot alkaloids, yohimbine
Beta-1 (mainly heart)	Epinephrine, norepinephrine	↑ myocardial contractility, CO, HR	Dobutamine, isoproterenol, dopamine (dose-dependent)	↓ CO, HR	Beta-1 selective blockers (e.g., metoprolol) and non-selective beta-blockers (e.g., propranolol, carvedilol)
Beta-2 (mainly lungs)	Epinephrine	Bronchodilation	Albuterol, terbutaline, isoproterenol	Bronchoconstriction	Non-selective beta-blockers (e.g., propranolol, carvedilol)
Dopamine	Dopamine	Many, including renal, cardiac and CNS effects	Levodopa, pramipexole	Many, including renal, cardiac and CNS effects	First-generation antipsychotics (e.g., haloperidol), metoclopramide
Serotonin	Serotonin	Many, including platelet, GI and psychiatric effects	Triptans (e.g., sumatriptan)	Many, including platelet, GI and psychiatric effects	Ondansetron, second-generation antipsychotics (e.g., quetiapine)

*SLUDD = salivation, lacrimation, urination, diarrhea/defecation and digestion (see Autonomic Nervous System section).

ENZYMES

Enzymes are compounds that speed up (catalyze) a reaction (e.g., creating a new compound or breaking down a compound into smaller parts). The interaction of a substrate with an enzyme can be agonistic or antagonistic, competitive or non-competitive (similar to receptors).

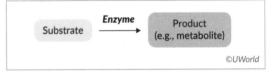

An example enzyme is monoamine oxidase (MAO), which is responsible for breaking down catecholamines (e.g., dopamine, norepinephrine, epinephrine and serotonin) as shown in the pathway below. The Study Tip Gal on the following page describes common enzyme systems and drug targets that alter enzyme effects.

Catecholamine Metabolism: Endogenous Pathways

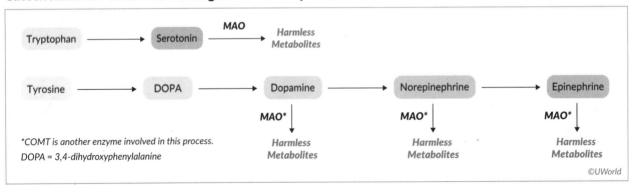

*COMT is another enzyme involved in this process.
DOPA = 3,4-dihydroxyphenylalanine

©UWorld

COMMON ENZYME TARGETS FOR MEDICATIONS

ENZYME	ENDOGENOUS EFFECTS	DRUG EXAMPLES	DRUG ACTION
Acetylcholinesterase	Breaks down acetylcholine	Acetylcholinesterase inhibitors: donepezil, rivastigmine, galantamine	Block acetylcholinesterase, resulting in ↑ ACh levels; used to treat Alzheimer's disease.
Angiotensin-converting enzyme (ACE)	Converts angiotensin I to angiotensin II (a potent vasoconstrictor)	ACE inhibitors (e.g., lisinopril, ramipril)	Inhibit production of angiotensin II, resulting in ↓ vasoconstriction and ↓ aldosterone secretion; used to treat hypertension, heart failure and kidney disease.
Catechol-O-methyltransferase (COMT)	Breaks down levodopa	COMT inhibitor: entacapone	Blocks COMT enzyme to prevent peripheral breakdown of levodopa, resulting in ↑ duration of action of levodopa; used to treat Parkinson disease.
Cyclooxygenase (COX)	Converts arachidonic acid to prostaglandins (cause inflammation) and thromboxane A2 (causes platelet aggregation)	NSAIDs (e.g., aspirin, ibuprofen)	Block COX enzymes to ↓ prostaglandins and thromboxane A2; used to treat pain/inflammation and ↓ platelet activation/aggregation (aspirin).
Monoamine oxidase (MAO)	Breaks down catecholamines (e.g., DA, NE, Epi, 5-HT)	MAO inhibitors: phenelzine, isocarboxazid, tranylcypromine, selegiline, rasagiline	Block MAO which ↑ catecholamine levels; used to treat depression. If catecholamines ↑ too much (due to additive effects with other drugs or foods), toxic effects can occur, such as hypertensive crisis or serotonin syndrome (see MAO Inhibitors, Hypertensive Crisis and Serotonin Syndrome section below).
Phosphodiesterase (PDE)	Breaks down cyclic guanosine monophosphate (cGMP), a smooth muscle relaxant	PDE-5 inhibitors (e.g., sildenafil, tadalafil)	Competitively bind to the same active site as cGMP on the PDE-5 enzyme, preventing the breakdown of cGMP and prolonging smooth muscle relaxation (e.g., in the arteries of the penis); used to treat erectile dysfunction.
Vitamin K epoxide reductase	Converts vitamin K to the active form required for production of select clotting factors	Warfarin	Blocks vitamin K epoxide reductase enzyme which ↓ production of clotting factors II, VII, IX and X; used to treat or prevent blood clots.
Xanthine oxidase	Breaks down hypoxanthine into xanthine and xanthine into uric acid	Xanthine oxidase inhibitor: allopurinol	Blocks xanthine oxidase enzyme which decreases uric acid production; used to prevent gout attacks.

MAO INHIBITORS, HYPERTENSIVE CRISIS AND SEROTONIN SYNDROME

When multiple drugs work similarly at the same receptor or enzyme, additive effects can occur, which can be detrimental. For example, when MAO is blocked by an MAO inhibitor, there is a buildup of catecholamines. This is beneficial for treating depression, but if too many catecholamines accumulate (e.g., due to multiple drugs being used together that increase catecholamines), hypertensive crisis or serotonin syndrome can develop. The diagrams on the following page list the key drugs and foods that contribute to either hypertensive crisis or serotonin syndrome, along with the symptoms indicative of each condition. These types of additive drug interactions are discussed further in the Drug Interactions and Depression chapters.

Catecholamine Metabolism: Additive Effects with MAO Inhibitors

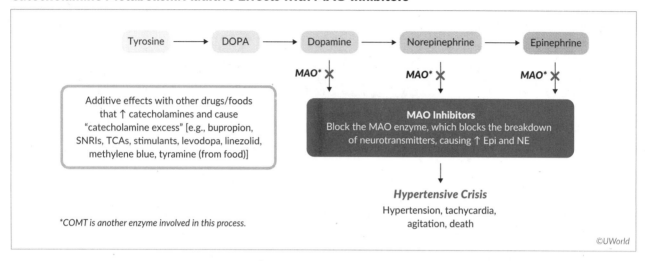

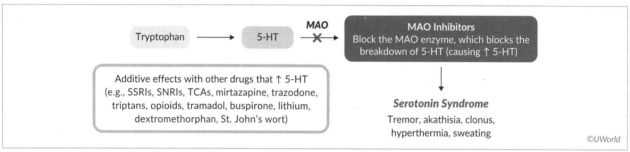

CHEMICAL STRUCTURES

The expected <u>effect</u> of a drug can be <u>predicted</u> from its mechanism of action and chemical structure. The relationship between the structure of a compound and its activity is referred to as the <u>structure-activity relationship</u>.

The common functional groups and <u>drug structures that should be recognized</u> for the exam are shown in the tables starting on the following page. Knowledge of these functional groups allows a pharmacist to predict certain effects or adverse effects of drugs. For example, identification of the <u>sulfonamide</u> functional group on the <u>celecoxib</u> compound (enclosed in the dotted lines of the structure below) explains why celecoxib is contraindicated in patients with a history of hypersensitivity (e.g., allergic reaction) to sulfonamides.

Differences in functional groups within a drug class can be important. If a patient has a hypersensitivity reaction to one type of drug in the class (e.g., an ester-type anesthetic such as procaine), other drugs in the class with the same functional group (e.g., benzocaine) should be avoided due to the potential for cross-reactivity. Selection of an anesthetic with a different functional group (e.g., an amide-type anesthetic such as lidocaine) would be reasonable. Amide-type anesthetics can be recognized by the "i" in their name (e.g., <u>li</u>docaine, bup<u>i</u>vacaine, rop<u>i</u>vacaine).

Celecoxib (Celebrex)

Procaine

Lidocaine

©UWorld

COMMON FUNCTIONAL GROUPS

Neutral Functional Groups

HYDROXYL OR ALCOHOL (PRIMARY)	KETONE	ALDEHYDE	AMIDE

NITRATE	NITRO	AROMATIC (BENZENE) RING	UREA

CARBONATE	CARBAMATE	ETHER	THIOETHER

Acidic Functional Groups

CARBOXYL	PHENOL	IMIDE	SULFONAMIDE

Basic Functional Groups

AMINE (PRIMARY)	AMINE (TERTIARY)	IMINE	AMIDINE

ESSENTIAL DRUG STRUCTURES

Beta-Lactam Antibiotics

AMOXICILLIN

Beta-lactam, penicillin antibiotic

Contains a beta-lactam ring fused to a 5-sided ring

Hypersensitivity: cross-reactive to other drugs with a beta-lactam ring
(see ceftriaxone and ertapenem)

CEFTRIAXONE

Beta-lactam, cephalosporin antibiotic

Contains a beta-lactam ring fused to a 6-sided ring

Hypersensitivity: cross-reactive to other drugs with a beta-lactam ring
(see amoxicillin and ertapenem)

ERTAPENEM

Beta-lactam, carbapenem antibiotic

Contains a beta-lactam ring fused to a 5-sided ring

Hypersensitivity: cross-reactive to other drugs with a beta-lactam ring
(see amoxicillin and ceftriaxone)

Other Antibiotics

AZTREONAM

Monobactam antibiotic

Contains a lactam ring not fused to another ring (note "mono" in
monobactam means one)

Hypersensitivity: not cross-reactive with beta-lactam antibiotics

GENTAMICIN

Aminoglycoside antibiotic

Contains an amine (amino) group* and a sugar (glycoside) group**

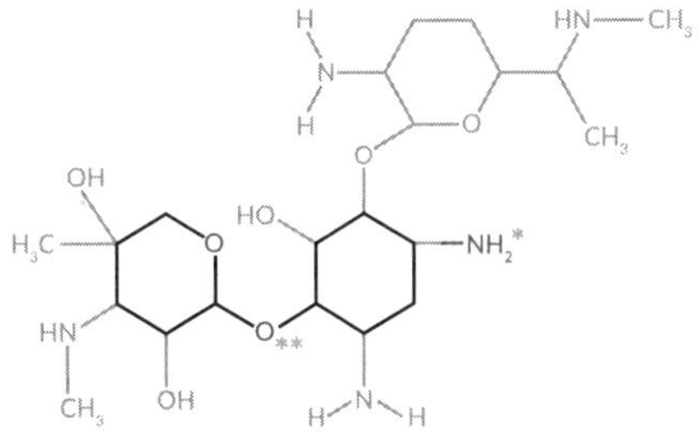

SULFAMETHOXAZOLE

Sulfonamide antibiotic

Contains a sulfonamide group

Hypersensitivity: cross-reactive to other drugs containing a sulfonamide group (e.g., celecoxib)

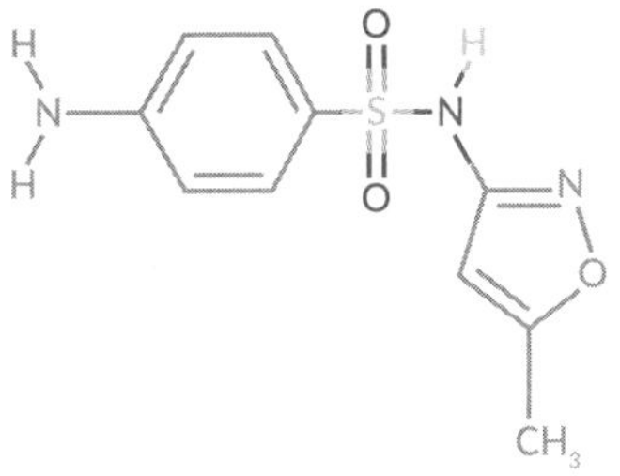

Non-Steroidal Anti-Inflammatory Drugs (NSAIDs)

ASPIRIN

Salicylate non-steroidal anti-inflammatory analgesic

Contains an acidic, carboxyl group

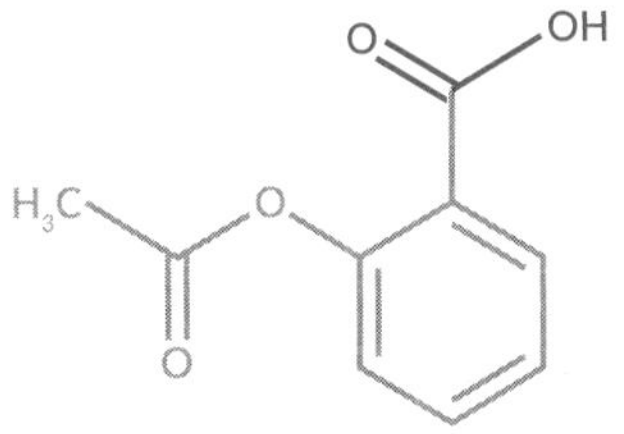

IBUPROFEN

Non-steroidal anti-inflammatory analgesic

Contains a carboxyl group

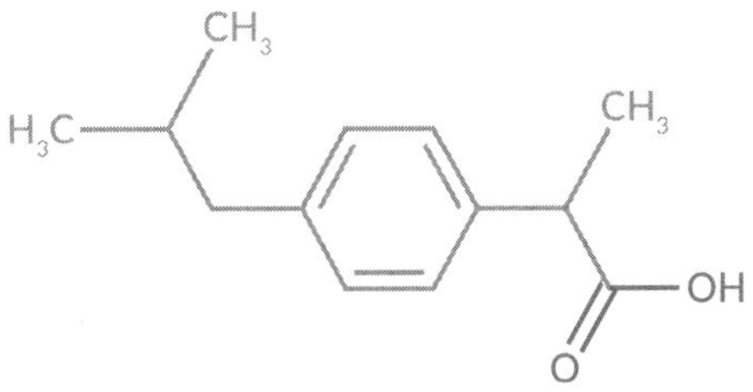

Other Well-Known Structures

AMPHETAMINE

Stimulant

Contains a primary amine functional group (note "amine" in the name)

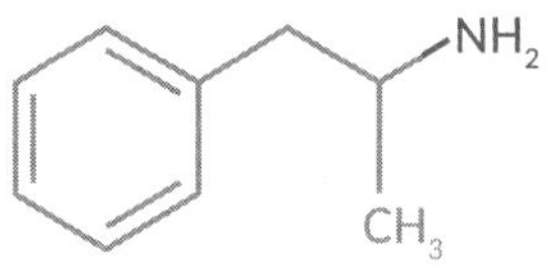

LEVOTHYROXINE

Thyroid hormone (T4)

Contains four iodine molecules in the structure (note the "4" in T4); converted to T3 (triiodothyronine) in the body (note "tri" meaning 3 and "iod" for iodine)

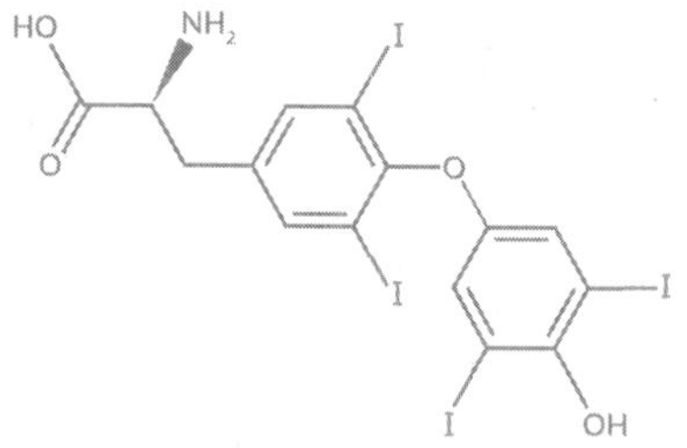

AMIODARONE

Class III antiarrhythmic

Contains two iodine molecules in the structure (note "iod" in the name)

Explains the hyper- and hypothyroid effects and contraindication in patients with an iodine allergy

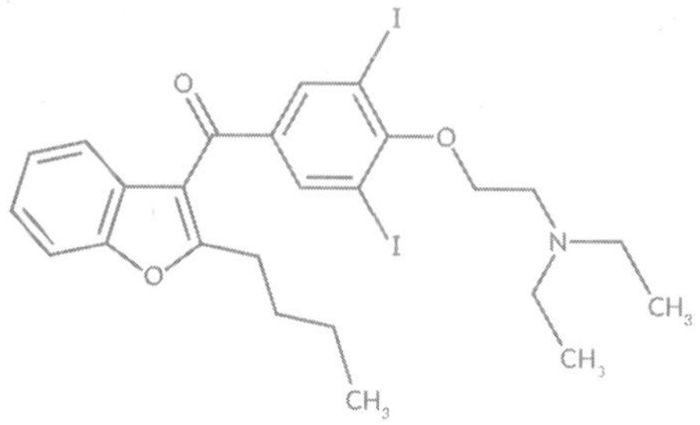

FENOFIBRATE

Fibrate, for high cholesterol

Contains ketone groups

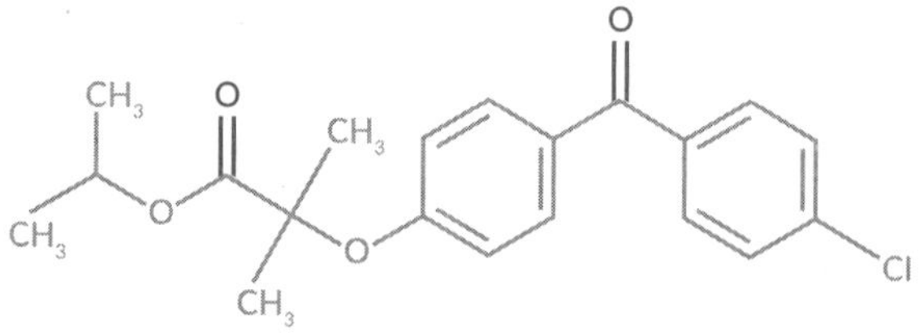

AMITRIPTYLINE

Tricyclic antidepressant

Contains three rings in the structure (note the "tri" in the name)

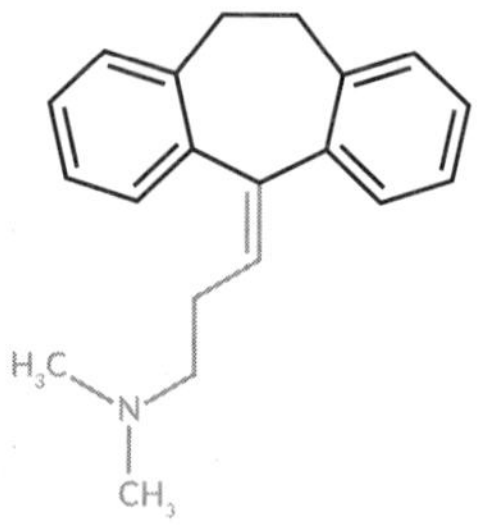

CHLORPROMAZINE

Phenothiazine antipsychotic

Contains a thioether group

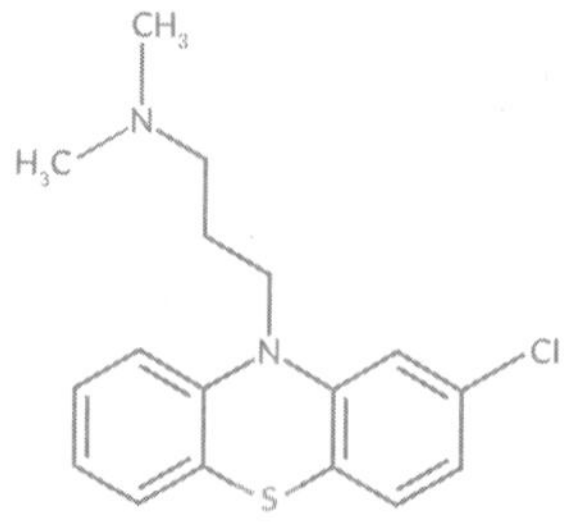

DRUG STABILITY AND DEGRADATION

STABILITY

Stability is the extent to which a product retains, within specified limits, and throughout its period of storage and use (i.e., the shelf-life), the same properties and characteristics it possessed at the time it was made. Drug stability can be compromised during manufacturing (or preparation, for compounded products) and storage, and can be recognized by changes in texture, color, smell or the development of precipitates.

DEGRADATION

The differences between drugs with similar chemical structures lies in the functional groups (see Chemical Structures section) that are attached to the compound's core structure and the bonds that hold the compound together. Reactions involving functional groups are common causes of drug degradation and can make the drug ineffective, unpalatable and/or toxic.

Reactions that Cause Drug Degradation

The three types of chemical reactions that cause most drug products to become unstable and degrade include:

- Oxidation-Reduction
- Hydrolysis
- Photolysis

The following sections describe each of these reactions and methods (e.g., light and moisture protection) that reduce their likelihood. Drug degradation in the body (i.e., metabolism) is reviewed in the Drug Interactions and Pharmacokinetics chapters.

OXIDATION

A compound is oxidized when it loses electrons and is reduced when it gains electrons. Oxidation and reduction reactions occur together; when one compound is oxidized, another must be reduced at the same time. This is called the re-dox reaction. With some drugs, oxidation is visible with a color change, such as epinephrine becoming amber-colored (yellow/orangish). Other compounds turn pink/reddish when oxidized.

The molecular structures most likely to oxidize are those with a hydroxyl (–OH) group directly bonded to an aromatic ring, such as catecholamines (e.g., epinephrine), phenols (e.g., phenylephrine) and aldehydes (e.g., various structures used as flavorings).

Example: Oxidation of Epinephrine
The presence of the hydroxyl groups on the ring make oxidation more likely.

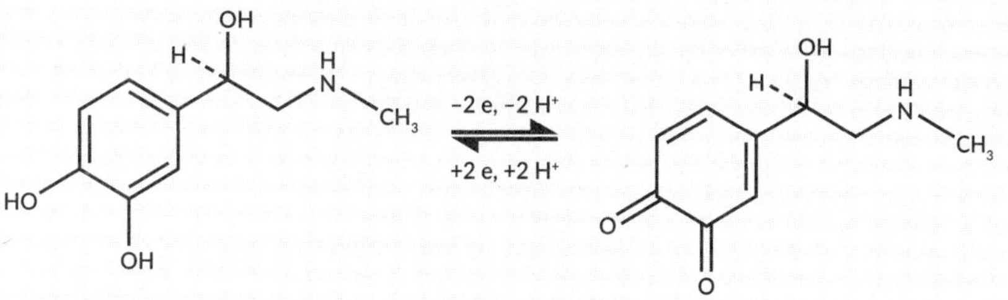

Epinephrine

Preventing Oxidation

Oxidation is catalyzed by heat, light and metal ions. Oxidation produces free radicals, which are highly reactive and can cause an oxidation chain reaction that damages the drug. Autoxidation is when oxidation reactions occur routinely during drug preparation and storage. Methods to prevent oxidation are described in the table below.

Light protection	With amber glass, UV light-blocking containers (e.g., plastic) and light-protective sleeves (bags) for IV bags, IV lines and syringes.
Temperature control	Store drugs according to their instructions (e.g., room temperature, refrigerater, freezer). Temperature ranges for each environment should comply with USP recommendations.
Antioxidants (also called free radical scavengers)	Inhibit free radicals. Common antioxidants include ascorbic acid (vitamin C), tocopherols (vitamin E), ascorbyl palmitate, Na ascorbate, Na bisulfate, Na sulfoxylate and Na thiosulfate.
Chelating agents	Chelate metal ions that have an unshared electron in the outer shell (these are free radicals). The chelating agent ties up the catalyst, preventing the reaction. Common chelators have the letters **ED**: EDetate disodium (EDTA), EDetate calcium disodium and EDetic Acid.
pH control	Maintain pH with a buffer (e.g., acetic acid/sodium acetate).

HYDROLYSIS

Hydrolysis occurs when water causes the cleavage of a bond in a molecule. The most common functional groups susceptible to hydrolysis are esters, amides and lactams; the carbonyl component of these structures is most likely to be subjected to hydrolysis.

Ester Carbonyl group bonded to an OR group	
Amide Carbonyl group bonded to a nitrogen	
Lactam, a cyclic amide This is a beta-lactam ring (present in penicillins, carbapenems, cephalosporins and monobactam)	

Example: Hydrolysis of Acetylsalicylic Acid (Aspirin)
The ester group is hydrolyzed to form acetic acid and salicylic acid. In this case, hydrolysis is beneficial. The analgesic is salicylic acid, which is formed by hydrolysis of the prodrug acetylsalicylic acid.

Aspirin - acetylsalicylic acid   Salicylic acid   Acetic acid

Preventing Hydrolysis

Methods to reduce hydrolysis are described in the table below. Some are similar to those used to reduce oxidation. An important preventative method is to protect the drug from moisture (water). For this reason, patients should be counseled to avoid storing medications in the bathroom and to close drug containers tightly.

Adsorbents (desiccants)	Adsorb any moisture that enters the container.
Lyophilized powders	Drugs stored as a lyophilized (freeze-dried) powder that are only reconstituted into a solution shortly before use have a lower risk of hydrolysis.
Hygroscopic salt	Hygroscopic means water-absorbing. In some cases, a salt form of the drug can be chosen that is less hygroscopic (i.e., will absorb less water and be less likely to degrade from hydrolysis).
Light protection, chelating agents, temperature control, pH control	See Preventing Oxidation table on prior page.

PHOTOLYSIS

Many drugs are sensitive to UV light exposure, which causes photolysis (breakage) of covalent bonds and drug degradation. Photolysis can be prevented with light protection. Compounds that are sensitive to light include ascorbic acid, folic acid, nitroprusside and phytonadione injection. Intravenous drugs that require light protection are discussed in the Intravenous Medication Principles chapter.

CONTENT LEGEND

= Study Tip Gal

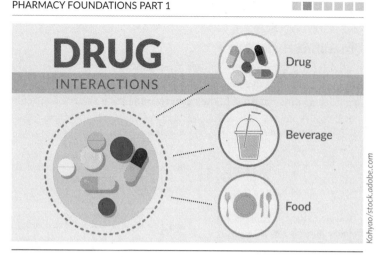

DRUG
INTERACTIONS

Drug

Beverage

Food

Kohyao/stock.adobe.com

CHAPTER 3
DRUG INTERACTIONS

TYPES OF DRUG INTERACTIONS

PHARMACODYNAMIC DRUG INTERACTIONS

Pharmacodynamics refers to the effect or change that a drug has on the body or some other type of organism (see Study Tip Gal below). A pharmacodynamic (PD) drug interaction occurs when two or more drugs are given together, and their end effects impact each other.

PHARMACODYNAMICS: PHARMACO + DYNAMICS

"Pharmaco" refers to a drug. "Dynamic" refers to an activity, such as a type of process or change.

Pharmacodynamics = the effect that a drug has on the body. The effect can be therapeutic (e.g., morphine provides pain relief when it binds to the mu receptor) or toxic (excessive morphine can be fatal).

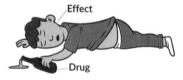

Effect

Drug

PD drug interactions can occur when two or more drugs are given together. The effects can be additive (such as more sedation), antagonistic (one drug blocks the effect of another drug) or synergistic, with an amplified (more than additive) effect.

iStock.com/sirichata

Additive Effects: Agonists Binding to the Same Receptor

Multiple drugs that are agonists at the same receptor can cause additive effects.

Example: opioids are mu-receptor agonists, providing analgesia, but with a risk of fatal toxicity when overdosed. If two opioids (e.g., morphine and oxycodone) are taken together, the effects would be additive, with increased side effects (e.g., excessive sedation, respiratory depression and death).

Additive Effects: Agonists Binding to Different Receptors

Drugs that have similar end effects through different mechanisms/receptors can cause additive effects.

Example: benzodiazepines are sedating and can suppress respiration. The effects are similar to opioids but caused by a different mechanism. Benzodiazepines bind to and enhance the effect of the endogenous inhibitory neurotransmitter gamma-aminobutyric acid (GABA), causing anxiolytic, hypnotic, anticonvulsant and muscle relaxant effects (including relaxing the diaphragm, which is how respiration becomes suppressed). When taken concurrently with opioids, the additive effects increase the risk of a fatal overdose. Drugs in both classes have a boxed warning about this risk (see Study Tip Gal below).

RISK WITH CONCURRENT USE OF BENZODIAZEPINES AND OPIOIDS

Due to the heightened fatality risk when opioids and benzodiazepines are taken together, the FDA added a boxed warning to all drugs in both classes.

WARNING: RISKS FROM CONCOMITANT USE WITH OPIOIDS
Concomitant use of benzodiazepines and opioids may result in profound sedation, respiratory depression, coma and death.

- Limit concomitant prescribing of these drugs to patients for whom alternative treatment options are inadequate.
- Restrict dosages and durations to the minimum required.
- Monitor patients for signs and symptoms of respiratory depression and sedation.

Another example: warfarin causes anticoagulation through inhibition of vitamin K-dependent clotting factors. Aspirin blocks the effects of platelets. Although they work through different mechanisms, both can cause increased bleeding, and when used together, the risk is greater.

Antagonists Block the Action of Agonists

An antagonist blocks the agonist from binding to its receptor. The agonist is unable to initiate a change that would have resulted in some effect (e.g., analgesia from an opioid, or respiratory depression when the opioid dose is excessive).

Example: naloxone is a mu-receptor antagonist; it saturates mu-receptors and blocks the opioid from binding. Naloxone is used to reverse respiratory depression, but will also reverse the analgesic effect.

Synergistic Effects

Synergy occurs when two drugs taken in combination have a greater effect than that obtained by simply adding the two individual effects together.

Example: oxycodone provides analgesia as a mu-receptor agonist. Acetaminophen provides analgesia by a different mechanism, which is not fully understood (some of the analgesic effect is thought to occur via inhibition of prostaglandin synthesis in the central nervous system). The mechanisms that produce analgesia with opioids and acetaminophen do not overlap. Acetaminophen taken with oxycodone produces more analgesia than the effect that would be expected from adding together the analgesic effects provided by each drug.

PHARMACOKINETIC DRUG INTERACTIONS

Pharmacokinetics (PK) refers to the effect or change that the body has on a drug (see Study Tip Gal below).

PHARMACOKINETICS: PHARMACO + KINETICS

"Pharmaco" refers to a drug. "Kinetics" refers to motion.

Pharmacokinetics = the effect the body has on the drug as it goes through the absorption, distribution, metabolism and excretion (ADME) processes.

- **A**bsorption (typically occurring in the small intestine with oral drugs)
- **D**istribution (through the blood and dispersed throughout the tissues)
- **M**etabolism (including enzymatic reactions)
- **E**xcretion [removal of the drug or end products (metabolites) from the body]

PK drug interactions occur when one drug alters the absorption, distribution, metabolism or excretion of another drug. PK drug interactions can be beneficial or harmful.

Reduced Absorption

Chelation occurs when a drug binds to polyvalent cations (e.g., Mg^{++}, Ca^{++}, Fe^{++}) in another compound (e.g., antacids or iron supplements). The chelated complex cannot dissolve in the gut fluid and will pass out in the stool.

Example: quinolone antibiotics can bind to calcium-containing drugs, dairy products or calcium-fortified foods. When taken together, the antibiotic will not dissolve, will not be absorbed, and the infection may not be adequately treated.

Drugs with polyvalent cations or other binding properties (e.g., antacids, multivitamins, sucralfate, bile acid resins, aluminum, calcium, iron, magnesium, zinc, phosphate binders) should be separated from quinolones, tetracyclines, levothyroxine and oral bisphosphonates.

Some drugs require an acidic gut for adequate absorption. If gastrointestinal pH is increased, absorption will be decreased.

Example: acid-suppressing drugs (e.g., H2RAs, proton pump inhibitors) decrease the absorption of some antifungals (e.g., itraconazole) if taken together. This can result in untreated or resistant infections.

The Gastroesophageal Reflux Disease (GERD) & Peptic Ulcer Disease (PUD) chapter contains a more comprehensive list of the most common drugs that have binding interactions or require an acidic gut for absorption.

Induction or Inhibition of Metabolism

The majority of PK drug interactions occur during metabolism (e.g., Phase I or Phase II reactions) in the liver. Drug-drug interactions can be harmful or beneficial.

Example of a beneficial interaction: ritonavir and darunavir are used together. Ritonavir inhibits the metabolism of darunavir, which "boosts" darunavir levels and increases its efficacy in treating HIV.

Examples of harmful interactions: clarithromycin inhibits warfarin metabolism (which increases the INR and risk of bleeding), and rifampin induces warfarin metabolism (which decreases the INR and increases the risk for blood clots). Both reactions are potentially harmful, but treatment with these drug combinations may be necessary. The dose of warfarin can be decreased (with clarithromycin) or increased (with rifampin) to keep the INR in the desired range.

Decreased or Increased Excretion

Renal excretion is the primary route of drug excretion. Drug interactions can block or enhance renal excretion.

Example of decreased renal excretion: probenecid blocks the renal excretion of penicillin. Giving probenecid with penicillin can be beneficial when high penicillin levels are needed to cross the blood-brain barrier (BBB) and provide effective treatment of neurosyphilis.

Example of increased renal excretion: salicylate (e.g., aspirin) overdose results in toxicity (tinnitus, metabolic acidosis). Intravenous sodium bicarbonate alkalinizes the urine, which causes the salicylate to become ionized. Ionized compounds are more hydrophilic (water-loving) and will stay in the urine. Less will be reabsorbed through the renal tubules (i.e., across a lipid membrane) back into the blood. Compounds that stay in the urine will be renally excreted.

ENZYME SYSTEMS, DRUG METABOLISM AND DRUG INTERACTIONS

CYTOCHROME P450 ENZYMES

The purpose of cytochrome P450 (CYP450) enzymes is to catalyze Phase I reactions that either produce essential compounds (e.g., cholesterol and cortisol) or uncover or insert a polar (i.e., water-loving) group on a compound to facilitate renal excretion. CYP450 enzymes are primarily expressed in the liver.

How CYP450 Enzymes Metabolize Drugs

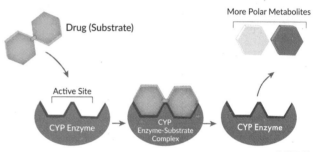

©UWorld
iStock.com/ttsz

More than 50 CYP enzymes have been identified, with six of them metabolizing most drugs. CYP3A4 metabolizes ~34% of all CYP450 drug substrates. The function of CYP450 enzymes can be affected by genetics (see Pharmacogenomics chapter) and other drugs that act as enzyme inhibitors or inducers.

A table of common CYP450 enzyme substrates, inducers and inhibitors is provided at the end of the chapter.

PRODRUGS: INACTIVE DRUGS CONVERTED BY CYP ENZYMES TO ACTIVE DRUGS

Prodrugs are taken by the patient in an inactive form and are converted by CYP450 enzymes into the active form.

How CYP450 Enzymes Metabolize Prodrugs

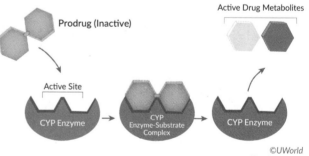

©UWorld
iStock.com/ttsz

Prodrugs are used by drug manufacturers to:

- Increase bioavailability. An example of this is valacyclovir, which is metabolized to the active drug acyclovir. Valacyclovir has higher bioavailability than acyclovir and is dosed less frequently.
- Prevent drug abuse. An example of this is lisdexamfetamine *(Vyvanse)*, which is formulated with an amino acid (lysine) attached to the amphetamine. This renders the amphetamine inactive, until the lysine is detached by enzymatic cleavage, which prevents the crushing and snorting of the drug.

The Study Tip Gal below lists some common prodrugs and their active metabolites along with some example safety concerns that can arise when a prodrug is used in patients with altered drug metabolism (e.g., due to genetics or a drug interaction).

COMMON PRODRUGS AND EXAMPLE SAFETY CONSIDERATIONS

PRODRUG AND ACTIVE METABOLITE	EXAMPLE SAFETY CONSIDERATIONS
Capecitabine → Fluorouracil	Codeine, by itself, and in combination products such as *Tylenol #3*:
Clopidogrel → Active metabolite	■ Risk of toxicity with ultra-rapid metabolizers (UMs)* of CYP2D6 due to a more rapid conversion to morphine.
Codeine → Morphine	
Colistimethate → Colistin	❑ Do not use codeine in UMs of 2D6.
Cortisone → Cortisol	■ Risk of poor analgesia with poor metabolizers (PMs)* of CYP2D6.
Famciclovir → Penciclovir	❑ Use an alternative analgesic in patients identified as PMs of 2D6.
Fosphenytoin → Phenytoin	
Isavuconazonium sulfate → Isavuconazole	Clopidogrel *(Plavix)*:
Levodopa → Dopamine	■ Risk with CYP2C19 inhibitors, which can block conversion to the active form.
Lisdexamfetamine → Dextroamphetamine	❑ Do not use with CYP2C19 inhibitors, including omeprazole and esomeprazole (can decrease antiplatelet effects).
Prednisone → Prednisolone	
Primidone → Phenobarbital	■ Risk with PMs of CYP2C19 (low conversion to the active form, with reduced antiplatelet activity).
Tramadol → Active metabolite	❑ Use an alternative P2Y12 inhibitor in patients identified as PMs of 2C19.
Valacyclovir → Acyclovir	
Valganciclovir → Ganciclovir	

*See Pharmacogenomics chapter.

NON-CYP450 ENZYMES

CYP450 enzymes are involved in Phase I reactions. Other enzymes, including those active in Phase II reactions, can also alter drug levels. For example, bictegravir, an antiretroviral drug for HIV, is a substrate of CYP3A4 and the Phase II enzyme uridine diphosphate glucuronosyltransferase (UGT) 1A1. Inducers or inhibitors of CYP3A4 or UGT1A1 will change the metabolism of bictegravir.

Another type of Phase II enzyme, N-acetyltransferase (NAT), is well known due to its identification early in the history of pharmacogenomic studies. NATs are highly polymorphic; differences in the degree of isoniazid toxicity were found to be due to differences in the rate of acetylation by NAT.

CYP ENZYME INHIBITORS INCREASE THE CONCENTRATION OF SUBSTRATE DRUGS

Drugs that are CYP enzyme <u>inhibitors</u> decrease enzyme function and the ability to metabolize compounds. Drugs that are <u>substrates</u> for the same enzyme as a CYP inhibitor will have a <u>decreased rate of drug metabolism</u> and an <u>increased serum drug level</u>. In some cases, <u>less drug</u> will be <u>lost to first-pass</u> metabolism. <u>Enzyme inhibition is fast</u>; effects are seen within a few days and will end quickly when the inhibitor is discontinued.

With <u>prodrugs</u>, inhibitors and inducers have an <u>opposite</u> effect on drug levels. With an <u>inhibitor</u>, there are less functional enzymes to convert the prodrug and the <u>concentration</u> of the <u>active drug decreases</u> (see clopidogrel example in the Common Prodrugs Study Tip Gal on the previous page).

The FDA labels enzyme inhibitors as strong, moderate or weak, based on the effect on metabolism of substrate drugs. The <u>Study Tip Gal</u> below describes CYP inhibitors that are commonly involved in <u>drug interactions</u>. For most, the interaction occurs because the drug listed is a <u>moderate or strong CYP3A4 inhibitor</u>. For others (e.g., amiodarone), interactions occur due to the drug's ability to <u>inhibit multiple CYP enzymes</u> (e.g., 3A4, 2C9, 2D6).

COMMON CYP INHIBITORS INVOLVED IN DRUG INTERACTIONS

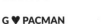

G ♥ PACMAN

Grapefruit

♥

Protease inhibitors (PIs), especially ritonavir, but many PIs are potent inhibitors

Azole antifungals (fluconazole, itraconazole, ketoconazole, posaconazole, voriconazole and isavuconazonium)

Cyclosporine, cobicistat

Macrolides (clarithromycin and erythromycin, **not** azithromycin)

Amiodarone (and dronedarone)

Non-DHP CCBs (diltiazem and verapamil)

Effect on Substrates
- Decreased metabolism
- Increased serum levels and clinical effects
- **IN**hibitors = **IN**creased effects/levels/ADRs/toxicities

Effect on Prodrugs
- Decreased conversion to the active drug (↓ serum levels and clinical effects)

Recognizing the Problem
- Perform therapeutic drug monitoring
- Monitor for therapeutic effect, ADRs, toxicity

Possible Actions: decrease dose of substrate (unless a prodrug), use alternate drug to avoid combination

---

CASE SCENARIO: TOXICITY WITH AN INHIBITOR

A 76-year-old male presents to the pharmacy with a voriconazole prescription to treat aspergillosis.

His medication profile includes betaxolol 1 drop OU BID, simvastatin 40 mg PO QHS and hydrochlorothiazide 25 mg PO QAM.

Recognizing the Problem
Voriconazole is a strong CYP3A4 inhibitor and simvastatin is a major CYP3A4 substrate. Voriconazole will increase the simvastatin level, increasing the risk of muscle toxicity and rhabdomyolysis.

Pharmacist Actions
The combination of voriconazole and simvastatin is contraindicated.

Ensure that the drugs are not used concurrently. Recommend an alternative statin, such as rosuvastatin.

CYP ENZYME INDUCERS DECREASE THE CONCENTRATION OF SUBSTRATE DRUGS

Drugs that are CYP enzyme <u>inducers</u> increase enzyme production or activity. Drugs that are <u>substrates</u> for the same enzyme as a CYP inducer will have an <u>increased rate of drug metabolism</u> and a <u>decreased serum drug level</u>. In some cases, <u>more drug</u> will be <u>lost to first-pass</u> metabolism. Inducers can cause therapeutic failure.

With an <u>inducer</u>, there are more enzymes to catalyze the conversion of a prodrug and the <u>concentration</u> of the <u>active drug</u> <u>increases</u>.

Similar to inhibitors, the FDA labels enzyme inducers as strong, moderate or weak, based on the effect on metabolism of substrate drugs. The <u>Study Tip Gal</u> below describes CYP inducers that are commonly involved in <u>drug interactions</u>. For most, the interaction occurs because the drug listed is a <u>moderate or strong CYP3A4 inducer</u> and/or it <u>induces multiple CYP enzymes</u> (e.g., rifampin).

COMMON CYP INDUCERS INVOLVED IN DRUG INTERACTIONS

PS PORCS

Phenytoin

Smoking

Phenobarbital

Oxcarbazepine

Rifampin (and rifabutin, rifapentine)

Carbamazepine (also an auto-inducer)

St. John's wort

Effect on Substrates
- Increased metabolism
- Decreased serum levels and clinical effects
- In**D**ucers = **D**ecreased effects/levels

Effect on Prodrugs
- Increased conversion to the active drug (↑ serum levels and clinical effects)

Recognizing the Problem
- Perform therapeutic drug monitoring
- Monitor for therapeutic effect

Possible Actions: increase dose of substrate (unless a prodrug), use alternate drug to avoid combination

CASE SCENARIO: SUBTHERAPEUTIC LEVEL WITH AN INDUCER

A 34-year-old female with a mechanical mitral valve has been taking warfarin chronically to prevent thrombosis.

Warfarin dose: 5 mg PO daily

INR range for the past 6 months: 2.6-3.1 (INR goal 2.5-3.5)

She was admitted for infective endocarditis and started on gentamicin, ceftriaxone, rifampin and vancomycin.

Recognizing the Problem
Rifampin is an inducer of P-gp, CYP2C9, 3A4, 1A2 and 2C19.

Warfarin is metabolized by CYP2C9 (major), 1A2, 2C19 and 3A4.

Pharmacist Actions
Monitor INR more frequently; increase warfarin dose as needed.

"Lag" Time for Enzyme Induction

<u>Induction</u> most often requires additional enzyme production, which <u>takes time</u>. The full effect on drug levels may not be seen for up to four weeks. When <u>the inducer is stopped</u>, it could take <u>2 – 4 weeks</u> for the induction effects to <u>disappear completely</u>; the excess enzymes will degrade based on their half-lives.

GUT EXCRETION BY DRUG TRANSPORTERS

P-GLYCOPROTEIN EFFLUX PUMPS

Permeability glycoprotein (P-gp) efflux pumps (or transporters) are located in many tissue membranes where they protect against foreign substances by moving them out of critical areas. The term efflux means to flow out, and P-gp pumps in the cell membranes of the GI tract transport drugs and their metabolites out of the body by pumping them into the gut, where they can be excreted in the stool.

When a drug blocks (or inhibits) P-gp, a drug that is a P-gp substrate will have increased absorption (less drug is pumped into the gut) and the substrate drug level will increase. There are other transporters in other parts of the body that are not described here, including efflux pumps that cause resistance by pumping chemotherapeutics out of cancer cells, and the organic ion transporter OATP1B1/3, which pumps drugs and other compounds from the blood into the liver.

There is overlap among the enzymes and transporters that protect the body from perceived toxins, including drugs. Many drugs which are substrates, inhibitors or inducers of P-gp have the same effect on CYP450 enzymes. The table below lists common P-gp substrates, inducers and inhibitors. A chart of common CYP450 substrates, inducers and inhibitors can be found at the end of the chapter.

P-gp Common Substrates, Inducers and Inhibitors

SUBSTRATES	INDUCERS	INHIBITORS
Anticoagulants (apixaban, edoxaban, dabigatran, rivaroxaban) **Cardiovascular drugs** (digoxin, diltiazem, carvedilol, ranolazine, verapamil) **HCV drugs** (sofosbuvir) **Immunosuppressants** (cyclosporine, sirolimus, tacrolimus) **Others** (atazanavir, colchicine, dolutegravir, posaconazole, raltegravir, saxagliptin)	Carbamazepine, dexamethasone, phenobarbital, phenytoin, rifampin, St. John's wort, tipranavir	**Anti-infectives** (clarithromycin, itraconazole, posaconazole) **Cardiovascular drugs** (amiodarone, carvedilol, conivaptan, diltiazem, dronedarone, quinidine, verapamil) **HCV drugs** (ledipasvir) **HIV drugs** (cobicistat, ritonavir) **Others** (cyclosporine, flibanserin, ticagrelor)

ENTEROHEPATIC RECYCLING

After a drug has been metabolized in the liver, it can be transported through the bile back to the gut. From the gut, the drug can be reabsorbed (primarily in the small intestine, where most drugs are absorbed), enter into the portal vein and travel back to the liver. The recycling of an already-metabolized drug is called enterohepatic recycling, which increases the duration of action of many drugs, including some antibiotics, some NSAIDs, mycophenolate and the cholesterol-lowering drug ezetimibe.

COMMON DRUG INTERACTIONS

Drug interactions are an important part of pharmacy practice. This chapter covers common drug interactions that involve major drug classes (e.g., CNS depressants) or drugs with specific properties (e.g., QT-prolonging drugs). Other important drug interactions involving specific drugs (e.g., warfarin, lithium, theophylline and more) are discussed in depth in their respective chapters (e.g., Anticoagulation, Bipolar Disorder, Asthma).

The major categories of drug interactions discussed in the tables that follow include:

- Common Cardiovascular Drug Interactions
- Inhibitors Increase Substrate Drugs
- Inducers Decrease Substrate Drugs
- Drugs with Additive Risks

COMMON CARDIOVASCULAR DRUG INTERACTIONS

INTERACTION	RISK	ACTIONS BY PHARMACIST/NOTES
AMIODARONE **+ Warfarin** Can be used together for atrial fibrillation treatment: amiodarone (for rhythm control), warfarin (to reduce clot risk). Dronedarone has similar drug interaction issues.	Amiodarone inhibits multiple enzymes, including CYP2C9, which metabolizes the more potent warfarin isomer. ↓ warfarin metabolism causes ↑ INR and bleeding risk.	**If using amiodarone 1st and adding warfarin** ■ Start warfarin at a lower dose of ≤ 5 mg. **If using warfarin 1st and adding amiodarone** ■ ↓ warfarin dose 30-50%, depending on the INR. **Taking both** ■ Monitor INR; adjust as needed.
AMIODARONE **+ Digoxin** Can be given together for atrial fibrillation treatment: amiodarone (for rhythm control), digoxin [for rate control (↓ HR), or for symptom improvement in a patient with HF].	Amiodarone inhibits P-gp; digoxin is a P-gp substrate. ↓ digoxin excretion, ↑ ADRs/toxicity. Amiodarone and digoxin both ↓ HR, ↑ risk of bradycardia, arrhythmia, fatality.	**If using amiodarone 1st and adding digoxin** ■ Start oral digoxin at a low dose, such as 0.125 mg daily. **If using digoxin 1st and adding amiodarone** ■ ↓ oral digoxin dose 50% (e.g., change 0.25 mg daily to 0.125 mg daily, or change 0.125 mg daily to 0.125 mg every other day). **Taking both amiodarone and digoxin** ■ Instruct patient to monitor for symptoms of digoxin toxicity: nausea, vomiting, vision changes; if present, contact prescriber.
DIGOXIN **+ Loop diuretic** Can be given together for heart failure treatment: digoxin (for symptom improvement), loop diuretics (to alleviate symptoms due to fluid overload).	Loop diuretics ↓ K, Mg, Ca and Na. Low K, Mg or Ca will worsen arrhythmias. Digoxin toxicity risk is increased with ↓ K and Mg levels and ↑ Ca levels. Caution: HF and renal impairment often occur together. Digoxin is cleared by P-gp and excreted by the kidneys; renal impairment (which can be exacerbated by loop diuretics) ↑ digoxin levels and toxicity risk.	■ Monitor HR; normal is 60-100 BPM (can be lower, based on patient's history and physical state). Check for other drugs that ↓ HR: beta-blockers, clonidine, diltiazem, verapamil, dexmedetomidine (Precedex). ■ If digoxin is being used for rate control, inform prescribers to consider beta-blockers or non-DHP CCBs instead. **Taking digoxin and a loop diuretic** ■ Monitor electrolytes and correct if abnormal. ■ Renal impairment: ↓ digoxin dose or frequency, or discontinue.
DRUGS THAT DECREASE HEART RATE Diltiazem/verapamil or beta-blockers for rate control; clonidine and beta-blockers to lower blood pressure.	Additive effects when drugs that ↓ HR are used together, including amiodarone, digoxin, beta-blockers, clonidine, diltiazem, verapamil and dexmedetomidine (Precedex).	Monitor HR; normal is 60-100 BPM (can be lower, based on patient's history and physical state).
STATINS **+ Strong CYP3A4 inhibitors** Inhibitors: protease inhibitors (including ritonavir), cobicistat, clarithromycin, erythromycin, azole antifungals, cyclosporine, grapefruit/grapefruit juice	↑ levels of CYP3A4 substrates: lovastatin, simvastatin, atorvastatin. ↑ myopathy risk; if severe (with high CPK), can cause rhabdomyolysis with acute renal failure (ARF).	Simvastatin and lovastatin are contraindicated with strong CYP3A4 inhibitors. Recommend a statin not metabolized by CYP450 enzymes (e.g., pitavastatin, pravastatin, rosuvastatin).
WARFARIN **+ CYP2C9 inhibitors and inducers** Inhibitors: azole antifungals, sulfamethoxazole/trimethoprim, amiodarone, metronidazole Inducers: rifampin, St. John's wort	CYP2C9 inhibitors: ↑ levels of warfarin (↑ INR and bleeding risk). CYP2C9 inducers: ↓ levels of warfarin (↓ INR and ↑ clotting risk).	Monitor INR; therapeutic range is 2-3 for most conditions (2.5-3.5 for some high-risk indications, such as mechanical mitral valve). Some drugs (e.g., amiodarone) require prophylactic warfarin dose adjustment when started (see above).

INHIBITORS INCREASE SUBSTRATE DRUGS

INTERACTION	RISK	ACTIONS BY PHARMACIST/NOTES
CYP3A4 INHIBITORS **+ CYP3A4 substrates (many)** Includes the opioids fentanyl, hydrocodone, oxycodone, methadone.	↓ CYP3A4 substrate (i.e., drug) metabolism will cause ↑ drug levels and ↑ ADRs/toxicity.	Do not use a CYP3A4 inhibitor with an opioid metabolized by CYP3A4; the combination will cause increased ADRs, including sedation, and can be fatal. Grapefruit/grapefruit juice: do not take with CYP3A4 substrates. Drugs that specifically include instructions not to take with grapefruit include amiodarone, simvastatin, lovastatin, nifedipine and tacrolimus; many other drugs have similar risk.
VALPROATE **+ Lamotrigine** Valproate is an inhibitor of lamotrigine metabolism.	Valproate ↓ lamotrigine metabolism and ↑ lamotrigine levels causing ↑ risk of serious skin reactions, including SJS/TEN (can be fatal).	Initiate lamotrigine using the starter kit that begins with lower lamotrigine doses. Titrate carefully every 2 weeks. Counsel patients to get emergency help if rash develops.
MONOAMINE OXIDASE (MAO) INHIBITORS Isocarboxazid, phenelzine, tranylcypromine, rasagiline, selegiline, linezolid, methylene blue + **Drugs/foods that ↑ epinephrine (Epi), norepinephrine (NE), dopamine (DA)** SNRIs, TCAs, bupropion, levodopa, stimulants, including amphetamines used for ADHD (e.g., methylphenidate, lisdexamfetamine, dextroamphetamine), tyramine (from foods) + **Drugs that ↑ serotonin (5-HT)** Antidepressants: SSRIs, SNRIs, TCAs, mirtazapine, trazodone Opioids and analgesics: fentanyl, methadone, tramadol Others: buspirone, dextromethorphan (when high doses taken as drug of abuse), lithium, St. John's wort	The MAO enzyme metabolizes Epi, NE, DA, tyramine and 5-HT. Blocking MAO with an MAO-inhibitor will ↑ Epi, NE, DA and 5-HT. High Epi, NE and DA can cause hypertensive crisis. High 5-HT can cause serotonin syndrome; see Serotonergic Toxicity in the Drugs with Additive Risks section.	Do not use together. Use a 2-week washout period when switching between drugs with MAO inhibition or serotonergic properties (except with fluoxetine, wait 5 weeks). Tyramine-rich foods have been aged, pickled, fermented or smoked, including aged cheeses, air-dried meats, sauerkraut, some wines and beers.
CYP2D6 INHIBITORS Amiodarone, fluoxetine, paroxetine, fluvoxamine **+ CYP2D6 substrates** Many, including codeine, meperidine, tramadol, tamoxifen	↓ drug substrate metabolism, ↑ ADRs/toxicity (or decreased clinical efficacy if a prodrug).	Avoid using together if possible.
CYP3A4, P-GP INHIBITORS + **Calcineurin inhibitors (CNIs)** Tacrolimus, cyclosporine or **mTOR kinase inhibitors** Sirolimus, everolimus	↓ drug substrate metabolism, ↑ ADRs/toxicity, including ↑ blood pressure, nephrotoxicity, metabolic syndrome and other adverse effects (see Transplant chapter).	Avoid using together or ↓ dose of CNI or mTOR kinase inhibitor cautiously and based on drug levels. Monitor transplant drug levels.

INDUCERS DECREASE SUBSTRATE DRUGS

INTERACTION	RISK	ACTIONS BY PHARMACIST/NOTES
ANTISEIZURE MEDICATION (ASM) CYP INDUCERS Phenytoin, phenobarbital, primidone, carbamazepine, oxcarbazepine **+** **Other drugs metabolized by CYP enzymes** Oral contraceptives, other ASMs, carbamazepine (auto-inducer, induces its own metabolism), others	↑ substrate (drug) metabolism will cause ↓ drug levels. ↓ drug effects; with ASMs, loss of seizure control.	Monitor drug levels; induction takes up to 4 weeks for the full effect. Consider increasing the dose of the substrate drug. If substrate is lamotrigine, use the starter kit that begins with higher lamotrigine doses.
RIFAMPIN **+ CYP and P-gp substrates**	↑ substrate (drug) metabolism will cause ↓ drug levels.	Monitor drug levels or other appropriate monitoring parameters, such as an INR with warfarin. Increase the dose of the substrate drug as necessary.
CYP3A4 INDUCERS **+** **Opioids that are CYP3A4 substrates** Fentanyl, hydrocodone, oxycodone, methadone	↑ metabolism results in ↓ opioid concentration; analgesia (pain relief) will decrease.	Assess the patient's use of breakthrough pain medication to determine if an increased maintenance dose is necessary. Use caution; opioids cause respiratory depression when overdosed, and induction has a lag time.
CYP3A4, P-GP INDUCERS **+** **Calcineurin inhibitors (CNIs)** Tacrolimus, cyclosporine **or** **mTOR kinase inhibitors** Sirolimus, everolimus	↑ drug metabolism results in ↓ transplant drug level and ↑ risk of transplant (organ) rejection.	Avoid using together or ↑ dose of CNI or mTOR kinase inhibitor carefully. Monitor transplant drug levels for efficacy.
SMOKING Primarily induces CYP1A2; includes smoking tobacco and marijuana **+** **Some antipsychotics, antidepressants, hypnotics, anxiolytics, caffeine, theophylline, warfarin (R-isomer)**	**Current smoker** CYP1A2 substrates (i.e., drugs) will have ↓ levels. **Smokers who quit** When the inducer (cigarettes) is stopped, drug concentrations of CYP1A2 substrates will ↑, causing toxicity.	When a current smoker starts a drug that is a CYP1A2 substrate, a higher dose can be required. Counsel/advocate for smoking cessation. When a smoker quits, monitor the INR if taking warfarin; the R-isomer of warfarin (less potent isomer) is metabolized by CYP1A2, but the therapeutic range is narrow and could be affected. Nicotine replacement products (NRT, such as the patch and gum) do not induce CYP enzymes.

DRUGS WITH ADDITIVE RISK

ADDITIVE SIDE EFFECT	RISK	ACTIONS BY PHARMACIST/NOTES
SEROTONERGIC TOXICITY		
Antidepressants SSRIs, SNRIs, TCAs, mirtazapine, trazodone **MAO inhibitors** Antidepressants: isocarboxazid, phenelzine, tranylcypromine Selective MAO-B inhibitors: selegiline, rasagiline Others: linezolid, methylene blue **Opioids** Fentanyl, meperidine, methadone, tramadol, tapentadol (though there is risk when any opioid is used in combination with serotonergic drugs) **Triptans** Occasional (PRN) triptan use may be safe; more frequent use can increase risk **Natural products** St. John's wort, L-tryptophan **Others** Buspirone, lithium, dextromethorphan (when taken in excess as a drug of abuse)	Serotonin syndrome risk increases when <u>two or more drugs</u> that affect serotonin are used <u>together</u>. Higher doses ↑ risk. Symptoms range from mild to severe and fatal: ■ Autonomic dysfunction (diaphoresis, nausea, vomiting, hyperthermia) ■ Altered mental status (akathisia, anxiety, <u>agitation</u>, delirium) ■ Neuromuscular excitation (hyperreflexia, tremor, <u>rigidity</u>, tonic-clonic <u>seizures</u>)	<u>Avoid using serotonergic drugs together</u>; if used, doses should be within recommended ranges. Check for inhibitors of serotonergic drugs. Counsel patients to report symptoms, even if mild. If severe symptoms, counsel to go to the emergency department. Recommend eliminating an initial serotonergic drug prior to starting a new serotonergic drug by using a <u>washout period</u>: use <u>2 weeks</u> between the drugs, or use <u>5 weeks</u> for drugs with a longer duration of action, such as <u>fluoxetine</u>.
BLEEDING		
Anticoagulants Warfarin, dabigatran, apixaban, edoxaban, rivaroxaban, heparin, enoxaparin, dalteparin, fondaparinux, argatroban, bivalirudin **Antiplatelets** Salicylates (including aspirin), dipyridamole, clopidogrel, prasugrel, ticagrelor **NSAIDs** Ibuprofen, naproxen, diclofenac, indomethacin, others **SSRIs, SNRIs** Citalopram, escitalopram, fluoxetine, paroxetine, sertraline, duloxetine, venlafaxine, others **Natural products** 5G's: garlic, ginger, ginkgo biloba, ginseng, glucosamine Vitamin E, willow bark, fish oils (high doses)	↑ <u>bleeding risk</u>; can occur with or without changing an anticoagulation monitoring parameter, such as the INR (with warfarin).	<u>Avoid using in combination</u>, with a few exceptions: ■ Aspirin (for cardioprotection) and occasional NSAID use for pain, fever or inflammation. ■ SSRI/SNRI use and occasional NSAID use for pain, fever or inflammation. ■ Dual antiplatelet therapy may be recommended for select patients (e.g., to prevent cardiac stent thrombosis). ■ Bridging/overlap treatment, such as enoxaparin + warfarin, until INR therapeutic ≥ 24 hrs.
HYPERKALEMIA		
Renin-angiotensin-aldosterone system (RAAS) drugs ACE inhibitors, ARBs, aliskiren, sacubitril/valsartan, spironolactone, eplerenone (highest risk with ARBs) **Potassium-sparing diuretics** Amiloride, triamterene **Others** Salt substitutes (KCl), calcineurin inhibitors (tacrolimus and cyclosporine), SMX/TMP, canagliflozin, drospirenone-containing oral contraceptives	Hyperkalemia; symptoms include weakness, heart palpitations, arrhythmia. Higher risk with renal impairment.	Do not use ACE inhibitors with ARBs. <u>Do not use sacubitril/valsartan with ACE inhibitors or ARBs</u>. If risk of hyperkalemia, suggest alternatives to canagliflozin (for diabetes), SMX/TMP (for infection) or drospirenone-containing oral contraceptives. Counsel patient to <u>avoid salt substitutes</u> that contain KCl. Monitor potassium.

ADDITIVE SIDE EFFECT	RISK	ACTIONS BY PHARMACIST/NOTES
QT PROLONGATION		
Antiarrhythmics Class 1a, 1c and III (see Arrhythmias chapter) **Anti-infectives** Antimalarials (e.g., hydroxychloroquine) Azole antifungals, except isavuconazonium Lefamulin Macrolides Quinolones **Antidepressants** SSRIs: highest risk with citalopram, escitalopram TCAs Others: mirtazapine, trazodone, venlafaxine **Antipsychotics** First-generation (e.g., haloperidol, thioridazine) Second-generation: highest risk with ziprasidone **Antiemetics** 5-HT3 receptor antagonists (e.g., ondansetron) Others: droperidol, metoclopramide, promethazine **Oncology medications** Androgen deprivation therapy (e.g., leuprolide) Tyrosine kinase inhibitors (e.g., nilotinib) Arsenic trioxide **Others** Cilostazol, donepezil, fingolimod, hydroxyzine, loperamide, ranolazine, solifenacin, methadone	QT prolongation ↑ the risk of torsades de pointes (TdP), an often fatal arrhythmia. The risk increases with: ■ Higher doses. ■ Higher drug levels due to concurrent enzyme inhibitors. ■ Higher drug levels due to reduced drug clearance, such as with renal or liver disease. ■ Multiple QT-prolonging drugs used together. ■ Elderly (> 60 years) and patients with CVD, including arrhythmias, HF, MI.	With all QT-prolonging drugs, avoid/reduce risk of TdP: ■ Limit use of QT-prolonging drugs or select drugs with lower QT risk, especially with arrhythmias, CVD or CVD risk (exception: amiodarone is the drug of choice to treat an arrhythmia in patients with HF). ■ Carefully dose QT-prolonging drugs; use lower doses/caution in elderly patients. ❑ Do not exceed citalopram 40 mg daily or 20 mg daily in elderly (> 60 years), liver disease or with enzyme inhibitors that decrease clearance. ❑ Do not exceed escitalopram 20 mg daily or 10 mg daily in elderly. ❑ Among SSRIs, sertraline is considered safest in patients with CVD. ■ Avoid concurrent QT-prolonging drugs, if possible. ■ Avoid use of inhibitors that block a QT-prolonging drug's metabolism. ■ Do not use droperidol for inpatient N/V (droperidol is injection only and has restricted use due to QT prolongation risk).
CNS DEPRESSION		
Many Drugs/Drug Classes Opioids Skeletal muscle relaxants Antiseizure medication Benzodiazepines Barbiturates Hypnotics Antidepressants: mirtazapine, trazodone Antihypertensives: propranolol, clonidine Cannabis-related drugs: dronabinol, nabilone Sedating antihistamines Cough syrups with an antihistamine or opioid Some NSAIDs **Highest risk for fatality when used in combination:** Opioids + Benzodiazepines or other CNS depressants	CNS depressant-effects: somnolence, dizziness, confusion/cognitive impairment, altered consciousness/delirium, gait instability/imbalance/risk of falls/accidents, including motor vehicle accidents. Benzodiazepines are drugs of abuse, and are often prescribed inappropriately (for anxiety or insomnia), adding unnecessary risk of CNS depression. Benzodiazepines are appropriate for status epilepticus, alcohol withdrawal, as an antidote for stimulant overdose, prior to medical procedures, in acute high-anxiety situations and for anticipatory emesis with chemotherapy. Opioids: due to the risks of abuse, dependence and addiction, reserve for severe pain that is not responsive to other measures.	Provide patient counseling: ■ Do not use alcohol. ■ Do not operate a car or other vehicles/machines. ■ Can increase risk of falls, confusion. Monitor for sedation, slow and shallow breathing, and shortness of breath. Avoid combining CNS depressants when possible. Suggest alternatives for anxiety (e.g., SSRI, SNRI), insomnia (lifestyle treatments preferred) or pain (e.g., acetaminophen, NSAIDs, antidepressants). **For opioids specifically:** ■ Do not use in combination with benzodiazepines; use of other CNS depressants, including alcohol, have a high risk of fatality with opioids. ■ Extended-release formulations have additional risk: several become shorter-acting when taken with alcohol, which increases the risk of fatality. ■ Recommend naloxone for at-risk patients, including use of high doses, rapid dose increases or reduced clearance (e.g., renal impairment with morphine). ■ Avoid codeine if pharmacogenomic profile is unknown (highest risk with CYP2D6 UMs). ■ See other CYP3A4 and 2D6 interaction information discussed previously.

ADDITIVE SIDE EFFECT	RISK	ACTIONS BY PHARMACIST/NOTES
OTOTOXICITY		
Aminoglycosides Gentamicin, tobramycin, amikacin, others **Cisplatin** **Loop diuretics (especially rapid IV administration)** Furosemide, bumetanide, ethacrynic acid **Salicylates** Aspirin, salsalate, magnesium salicylate, others **Vancomycin**	Hearing loss, tinnitus, vertigo.	▪ Consider an audiology consult at start of treatment for baseline hearing assessment; continue to monitor. ▪ Avoid using multiple ototoxic drugs at the same time, when possible.
NEPHROTOXICITY		
Anti-infectives Aminoglycosides, amphotericin B, polymyxins, vancomycin **Cisplatin** **Calcineurin inhibitors** Cyclosporine, tacrolimus **Loop diuretics** Furosemide, torsemide, bumetanide, ethacrynic acid **NSAIDs** **Radiographic-contrast dye**	Worsening renal function/ acute renal failure (ARF), can be evidenced by ↓ in urine output and ↑ SCr/BUN.	▪ Cisplatin: use amifostine (Ethyol) to protect kidneys. ▪ Maintain adequate hydration (dehydration can worsen kidney function). ▪ Monitor drug levels (e.g., aminoglycosides, vancomycin, tacrolimus), as appropriate. ▪ Discontinue offending drugs if acute renal failure occurs. ▪ Monitor urine output, SCr/BUN.
ANTICHOLINERGIC TOXICITY		
Antidepressants/antipsychotics Paroxetine, TCAs, first-generation antipsychotics **Sedating antihistamines** Diphenhydramine, brompheniramine, chlorpheniramine, doxylamine, hydroxyzine, cyproheptadine, meclizine **Centrally-acting anticholinergics** Benztropine, trihexyphenidyl **Muscle relaxants** Baclofen, carisoprodol, cyclobenzaprine **Antimuscarinics (for urinary incontinence)** Oxybutynin, darifenacin, tolterodine **Others** Atropine, belladonna, dicyclomine	Anticholinergic symptoms: CNS depression, including sedation, and peripheral anticholinergic side effects of dry mouth, dry eyes, blurry vision, constipation, urinary retention. Highest risk in elderly.	▪ Recommend alternatives to sedating antihistamines, such as loratadine, fexofenadine, cetirizine, or suggest saline nasal spray/drops that clear allergens out of the nasal passages. ▪ If using diphenhydramine or other sedating antihistamines for sleep, suggest lifestyle changes (sleep hygiene). ▪ Recommend treatments for dry mouth, dry eyes (see Sjogren's Syndrome in the Systemic Steroids & Autoimmune Conditions chapter); recommend laxatives for constipation (see Constipation & Diarrhea chapter).
HYPOTENSION/ORTHOSTASIS		
PDE-5 inhibitors Sildenafil, tadalafil, avanafil, vardenafil + **CYP3A4 inhibitors** or **Nitrates** or **Alpha-1 blockers** Non-selective (e.g., doxazosin, terazosin) or selective (e.g., tamsulosin)	With CYP3A4 inhibitors: ↓ PDE-5 inhibitor metabolism causes ↑ side effects, including headache, dizziness, flushing (causing ↑ risk of falls/injury). PDE-5 inhibitors, nitrates and alpha-1 blockers all cause vasodilation. Additive effects can lead to hypotension/orthostasis, dizziness and falls. With nitrates, severe hypotension can cause chest pain and CV events, which can be fatal.	**If taking a CYP3A4 inhibitor** ▪ Start with half the usual starting dose of the PDE-5 inhibitor (see Sexual Dysfunction chapter). **PDE-5 inhibitors and nitrates** ▪ Do not use together (contraindicated); check for use of sublingual nitroglycerin PRN for chest pain; can consider use of nitroglycerin in emergent situations (UA/NSTEMI/STEMI) with close monitoring. **PDE-5 inhibitors and alpha-1 blockers** ▪ Start with a low dose when adding a drug from either class (e.g., if taking an alpha-1 blocker, start at half the usual PDE-5 inhibitor starting dose). Do not start a PDE-5 inhibitor unless stable (e.g., no symptoms of hypotension) on an alpha-1 blocker.

CYP450 ENZYMES: COMMON SUBSTRATES, INDUCERS AND INHIBITORS

CYP	SUBSTRATES	INDUCERS	INHIBITORS
3A4	**Analgesics** (buprenorphine, diclofenac, fentanyl, hydrocodone, meloxicam, methadone, oxycodone, tramadol) **Anticoagulants** (apixaban, rivaroxaban, R-warfarin) **Cardiovascular drugs** (amiodarone, amlodipine, bosentan, diltiazem, eplerenone, ivabradine, nifedipine, quinidine, ranolazine, tolvaptan, verapamil) **Immunosuppressants** (cyclosporine, tacrolimus, sirolimus) **Statins** (atorvastatin, lovastatin, simvastatin) **Key HIV drugs** (atazanavir, efavirenz and other NNRTIs, ritonavir, tipranavir) **PDE-5 inhibitors** (avanafil, sildenafil, tadalafil, vardenafil) **Others** (alfuzosin, aprepitant, aripiprazole, benzodiazepines, brexpiprazole, buspirone, carbamazepine, citalopram, clarithromycin, colchicine, dapsone, dutasteride, erythromycin, escitalopram, ethinyl estradiol, felbamate, haloperidol, ketoconazole, levonorgestrel, mirtazapine, modafinil, ondansetron, progesterone, quetiapine, tamoxifen, trazodone, venlafaxine, zolpidem)	Carbamazepine, efavirenz, etravirine, oxcarbazepine, phenobarbital, phenytoin, primidone, rifabutin, rifampin, rifapentine, smoking, St. John's wort	**Anti-infectives** (clarithromycin, erythromycin, azole antifungals, isoniazid) **Cardiovascular drugs** (amiodarone, diltiazem, dronedarone, quinidine, ranolazine, verapamil) **Key HIV drugs** (cobicistat, efavirenz, ritonavir and other protease inhibitors) **Others** (aprepitant, cimetidine, cyclosporine, fluvoxamine, grapefruit juice, haloperidol, nefazodone, sertraline)
1A2	Alosetron, amiodarone, aprepitant, clozapine, cyclobenzaprine, duloxetine, ethinyl estradiol, fluvoxamine, methadone, mirtazapine, olanzapine, ondansetron, pimozide, propranolol, rasagiline, ropinirole, theophylline, tizanidine, R-warfarin, zolpidem	Carbamazepine, phenobarbital, phenytoin, primidone, rifampin, ritonavir, smoking, St. John's wort	Atazanavir, cimetidine, ciprofloxacin, fluvoxamine, zileuton
2C8	Amiodarone, pioglitazone, repaglinide	Phenytoin, rifampin	Amiodarone, atazanavir, clopidogrel, gemfibrozil, ketoconazole, trimethoprim/sulfamethoxazole, ritonavir
2C9	Alosetron, carvedilol, celecoxib, diazepam, diclofenac, fluvastatin, glyburide, glipizide, glimepiride, meloxicam, nateglinide, phenytoin, ramelteon, S-warfarin, tamoxifen, zolpidem	Aprepitant, carbamazepine, phenobarbital, phenytoin, primidone, rifampin, rifapentine, ritonavir, smoking, St. John's wort	Amiodarone, atazanavir, capecitabine, cimetidine, efavirenz, etravirine, gemfibrozil, fluconazole, fluvoxamine, fluorouracil, isoniazid, ketoconazole, metronidazole, oritavancin, tamoxifen, trimethoprim/sulfamethoxazole, valproic acid, voriconazole, zafirlukast
2C19	Amiodarone, clopidogrel, phenytoin, thioridazine, voriconazole	Carbamazepine, phenobarbital, phenytoin, rifampin	Cimetidine, esomeprazole, efavirenz, etravirine, fluoxetine, fluvoxamine, isoniazid, ketoconazole, modafinil, omeprazole, topiramate, voriconazole
2D6	**Analgesics** (codeine, hydrocodone, meperidine, methadone, oxycodone, tramadol) **Antipsychotics/Antidepressants** (aripiprazole, brexpiprazole, doxepin, fluoxetine, haloperidol, mirtazapine, risperidone, thioridazine, trazodone, tricyclic antidepressants, venlafaxine) **Others** (amiodarone, atomoxetine, carvedilol, dextromethorphan, flecainide, methamphetamine, metoprolol, propafenone, propranolol, tamoxifen)		Amiodarone, bupropion, cimetidine, cobicistat, darifenacin, dronedarone, duloxetine, fluoxetine, mirabegron, paroxetine, propafenone, quinidine, ritonavir, sertraline

iStock.com/Michael Burrell

CHAPTER 4
LAB VALUES &
DRUG MONITORING

BACKGROUND

Laboratory values assist healthcare providers in diagnosing and monitoring diseases and drug therapies. Blood or other samples can be sent to a hospital or an outside laboratory for analysis. Alternatively, point-of-care (POC) testing provides rapid results at the site of patient care. There are many POC tests, including tests for cardiac enzymes, A1C, INR, and various infections. Home testing kits, many of which are available OTC, provide convenience and privacy and are available to test for pregnancy, ovulation, HIV infection, herpes, fecal occult blood or the presence of illicit substances or opioids.

Therapeutic drug monitoring (TDM) involves obtaining a drug level or other relevant labs to monitor efficacy and safety. TDM is reviewed in detail at the end of this chapter.

Pharmacists in many states can order and interpret lab tests for a variety of purposes, including screening for and diagnosing disease, monitoring drug levels and other related lab values, checking for medication adherence or screening for drugs of abuse.

DEFINITIONS

COMPLETE BLOOD COUNT

The complete blood count (CBC) is a commonly ordered lab panel that analyzes white blood cells (WBCs), red blood cells (RBCs) and platelets (PLTs). The CBC includes hemoglobin (oxygen-carrying protein in RBCs) and hematocrit (the level of RBCs in the fluid component of the blood, or plasma). When a CBC with differential is ordered, the types of WBCs are analyzed.

CONTENT LEGEND

 = Key Drug Guy

BASIC METABOLIC PANEL/COMPREHENSIVE METABOLIC PANEL

The basic metabolic panel (BMP) includes seven to eight tests that analyze electrolytes, glucose, renal function and acid/base (with HCO3, or bicarbonate) status. Some labs calculate and report an anion gap along with the BMP (see Calculations IV chapter).

A comprehensive metabolic panel (CMP) includes the tests in a BMP plus albumin, alanine aminotransferase (ALT), aspartate aminotransferase (AST), total bilirubin and total protein. The additional tests are used primarily to assess liver function. The BMP and CMP are groups of labs that are ordered together for convenience.

The stick diagrams below are used in practice when writing a paper chart note to denote the primary components of the CBC or BMP. Pharmacists should know which values are contained in the stick diagrams below.

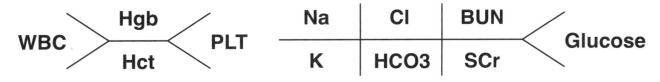

BLOOD CELL LINES

Stem cells in the bone marrow produce red blood cells, white blood cells and platelets (see figure). White blood cells can be called leukocytes, and red blood cells can be called erythrocytes. An immature red blood cell is called a reticulocyte (discussed in the Anemia section of the Common Laboratory Reference Ranges table).

Changes in Blood Cell Lines

Increase in Individual Cell Lines	
↑ WBC	Leukocytosis
↑ RBC	Polycythemia
↑ Platelets	Thrombocytosis
Decrease in Individual Cell Lines	
↓ WBC	Leukopenia
↓ RBC (or ↓ Hgb)	Anemia
↓ Platelets	Thrombocytopenia
Decrease in Multiple Cell Lines	
Myelosuppression	↓ WBCs, RBCs and platelets
Agranulocytosis	
Drug causes: clozapine, propylthiouracil, methimazole, procainamide, carbamazepine, isoniazid, sulfamethoxazole/ trimethoprim	↓ granulocytes (WBCs that have secretory granules in the cytoplasm); includes ↓ neutrophils, basophils and eosinophils

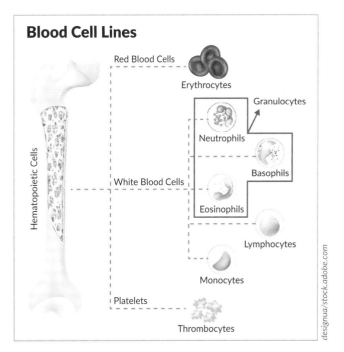

Blood Cell Lines

LAB RESULTS

Lab results are usually reported as a numerical value (e.g., sodium = 139 mEq/L). Some are reported as "positive" or "negative" or indicate a specific finding, such as "gram-positive cocci." Reference ranges can vary slightly from one facility to another (due to slight variances in products and techniques) and between pediatric and adult populations. A patient's lab results may be within the reference ranges (normal) or outside of the reference ranges (can indicate a condition that needs to be addressed). A value that is termed critical can be life-threatening unless corrective action is taken quickly. The Joint Commission requires that all accredited facilities create and follow a protocol to identify and report critical values to the responsible healthcare provider, who has an established time frame to manage the result. This applies to critical lab values and diagnostic procedure results.

COMMON LABORATORY REFERENCE RANGES – ADULT

Reference ranges for labs are generally provided on the NAPLEX, but may not be provided on the California Practice Standards and Jurisprudence Exam (CPJE). Familiarity with lab tests and their interpretation will greatly reduce the time required to evaluate cases on the exam. "Must know" labs for pharmacists are bolded in the following table, though others may be included in patient cases. The reference range for a healthy adult is provided unless otherwise noted. Drugs specifically indicated to treat a lab abnormality (e.g., urate-lowering therapies) are included in the respective chapters (e.g., the Gout chapter). Studying this table will be much easier after mastering all of the associated disease state chapters in this book.

ITEM	COMMON REFERENCE RANGE	NOTES
BMP and Electrolytes		
Calcium (Ca), total Ca, ionized	8.5–10.5 mg/dL 4.5–5.1 mg/dL	Calculate corrected calcium if albumin is low (see Calculations III chapter for formula). Correction is not needed for ionized calcium. ↑ due to calcium supplementation, vitamin D, thiazide diuretics. ↓ due to long-term heparin, loop diuretics, bisphosphonates, cinacalcet, systemic steroids, calcitonin, foscarnet, topiramate. Supplement calcium in pregnancy, osteoporosis/osteopenia and with certain drugs (see Dietary Supplements, Natural & Complementary Medicine chapter).
Chloride (Cl)	95–106 mEq/L	Used with other labs to assess acid-base status and fluid balance.
Magnesium (Mg)	1.3–2.1 mEq/L	↑ due to magnesium-containing antacids and laxatives (higher risk with renal impairment). ↓ due to PPIs, diuretics, amphotericin B, foscarnet, echinocandins, diarrhea, chronic alcohol intake.
Phosphate (PO4)	2.3–4.7 mg/dL	↑ in chronic kidney disease. ↓ due to phosphate binders, foscarnet, oral calcium intake.
Potassium (K)	3.5–5 mEq/L	↑ due to ACE inhibitors, ARBs, aldosterone receptor antagonists (ARAs), aliskiren, canagliflozin, cyclosporine, tacrolimus, potassium supplements, sulfamethoxazole/trimethoprim, drospirenone-containing oral contraceptives, chronic heparin use, mycophenolate, NSAIDs, pentamidine. ↓ due to beta-2 agonists, diuretics, insulin, sodium polystyrene sulfonate, steroids, conivaptan, mycophenolate (both ↑ and ↓ reported).
Sodium (Na)	135–145 mEq/L	↑ due to hypertonic saline, tolvaptan, conivaptan. ↓ due to carbamazepine, oxcarbazepine, SSRIs, diuretics, desmopressin. Sodium level may require correction when hyperglycemia is present (see Diabetes chapter).
Bicarbonate **(HCO3 or "bicarb")**	Venous: 24–30 mEq/L Arterial: 22–26 mEq/L (varies by method)	Used to assess acid-base status. ↑ due to loop diuretics, systemic steroids. ↓ due to topiramate, zonisamide, salicylate overdose.
Blood Urea Nitrogen **(BUN)**	7–20 mg/dL	↑ in renal impairment and dehydration. Used with SCr (e.g., BUN:SCr ratio) to assess fluid status and renal function.
Serum Creatinine **(SCr)**	0.6–1.3 mg/dL	↑ due to many drugs that impair renal function (e.g., aminoglycosides, amphotericin B, cisplatin, colistimethate, cyclosporine, loop diuretics, polymyxin, NSAIDs, radiocontrast dye, tacrolimus, vancomycin). False ↑ due to sulfamethoxazole/trimethoprim, H2RAs, cobicistat. ↓ with low muscle mass, amputation, hemodilution.
Glucose	70-110 mg/dL	See Diabetes section of this table for details on glucose thresholds used in the diagnosis and management of diabetes.
Anion Gap (AG)	5–12 mEq/L	A calculated value, but often reported on the BMP (see Calculations IV chapter). An ↑ anion gap suggests metabolic acidosis.

ITEM	COMMON REFERENCE RANGE	NOTES
WBC Count and Differential		
White Blood Cells (WBCs)	4,000–11,000 cells/mm³	Used to diagnose and monitor infection/inflammation. Can ↑ as an acute phase reactant, indicating a systemic reaction to inflammation or stress (e.g., surgery). ↑ due to systemic steroids, colony stimulating factors, epinephrine. ↓ due to clozapine, chemotherapy that targets the bone marrow, carbamazepine, cephalosporins, immunosuppressants (e.g., DMARDs, biologics), procainamide, vancomycin.
Neutrophils	45–73%	Neutrophils and bands are used with clinical signs and symptoms to assess the likelihood of acute infection. They are also used (with WBCs) in the absolute neutrophil count (ANC) calculation (see Calculations IV chapter) to assess for neutropenia (see Oncology chapter).
Bands	3–5%	Neutrophils are also called polymorphonuclear cells (PMNs or polys) or segmented neutrophils (segs). Bands are immature neutrophils released from the bone marrow to fight infection (called a "left shift" when elevated).
Eosinophils	0–5%	↑ in drug allergy, asthma, inflammation, parasitic infection.
Basophils	0–1%	↑ in inflammation, hypersensitivity reactions, leukemia.
Lymphocytes	20–40%	↑ in viral infections, lymphoma. ↓ in bone marrow suppression, HIV or due to systemic steroids.
Monocytes	2–8%	↑ in chronic infections, inflammation, stress.
Anemia		
Red Blood Cells (RBCs)	Males: 4.5–5.5 x 10⁶ cells/μL Females: 4.1–4.9 x 10⁶ cells/μL	RBCs have an average life span of 120 days. ↑ due to erythropoiesis-stimulating agents (ESAs), smoking and polycythemia (a condition that causes high RBCs). ↓ due to chemotherapy that targets the bone marrow, low production, blood loss, deficiency anemias (e.g., B12, folate), hemolytic anemia, sickle cell anemia.
Hemoglobin (Hgb, Hb)	Males: 13.5–18 g/dL Females: 12–16 g/dL	Hgb is the iron-containing protein that carries oxygen in RBCs. The Hct mirrors the Hgb result (providing the same clinical information). ↑ due to ESAs (see Anemia chapter).
Hematocrit (Hct)	Males: 38–50% Females: 36–46%	↓ in anemias and bleeding (drug-induced causes include anticoagulants, antiplatelets, fibrinolytics).
Mean Corpuscular Volume (MCV)	80–100 fL	Reflects the size and average volume of RBCs. ↑ (macrocytic anemia) due to B12 or folate deficiency. ↓ (microcytic anemia) due to iron deficiency.
Mean Corpuscular Hemoglobin (MCH)	26–34 pg/cell	Additional tests used in an anemia workup. Together MCV, MCHC and RDW are called "RBC indices."
Mean Corpuscular Hgb Concentration (MCHC)	31–37 g/dL	
RBC Distribution Width (RDW)	11.5–14.5%	RDW measures the variability in RBC size.
Iron	65–150 mcg/dL	↑ due to iron supplementation. ↓ due to blood loss or poor nutrition.
Total Iron Binding Capacity (TIBC)	250–400 mcg/dL	Monitored as part of the workup and treatment for iron deficiency anemia or anemia of chronic disease (e.g., CKD). See Anemia chapter for details.
Transferrin	> 200 mg/dL	
Transferrin Saturation (TSAT)	Males: 15–50% Females: 12–45%	
Ferritin	11–300 ng/mL	
Erythropoietin	2–25 mIU/mL	

ITEM	COMMON REFERENCE RANGE	NOTES
Folic Acid (folate)	5–25 mcg/L	B12 and folate are ordered for further workup of <u>macrocytic anemia</u>. ↓ due to <u>phenytoin/fosphenytoin, phenobarbital, primidone</u>, <u>methotrexate</u>, sulfamethoxazole/trimethoprim, sulfasalazine. Supplement folate in women of <u>childbearing age</u> and alcohol use disorder (see Dietary Supplements, Natural & Complementary Medicine chapter).
Vitamin B12	> 200 pg/mL	↓ due to <u>PPIs, metformin</u>, colchicine, chloramphenicol.
Methylmalonic acid (MMA)	Varies	Used for further workup of macrocytic anemia when B12 deficiency is suspected.
Reticulocyte Count	0.5–2.5%	Measures the amount of reticulocytes (immature red blood cells) being made by the bone marrow ↑ with blood loss and hemolysis. ↓ <u>in untreated anemia</u>, due to iron, folate or B12 deficiency, and with <u>bone marrow suppression</u>.
Coombs Test, Direct Also known as: Direct Antiglobulin Test (DAT)	Negative	Used in the diagnosis of immune-mediated <u>hemolytic anemia</u> (see Anemia chapter). Drugs that can cause immune-mediated hemolytic anemia include <u>penicillins and cephalosporins</u> (prolonged use/high concentrations), <u>isoniazid, levodopa, methyldopa, quinidine, quinine, rifampin and sulfonamides</u>. If a drug-induced cause is suspected and the Coombs test is positive, <u>discontinue</u> the offending drug.
Glucose-6-Phosphate Dehydrogenase **(G6PD)**	5–14 units/gram	Used to determine if <u>hemolytic anemia</u> is due to G6PD deficiency (see Anemia chapter). RBC destruction with G6PD deficiency is triggered by stress, foods (<u>fava beans</u>) or these drugs: <u>dapsone, methylene blue, nitrofurantoin, pegloticase, primaquine, rasburicase, quinidine, quinine, and sulfonamides</u>.

Anticoagulation
These tests evaluate different aspects of clotting and are used to monitor specific drugs.

ITEM	COMMON REFERENCE RANGE	NOTES
Anti-Factor Xa Activity **(Anti-Xa)**	Therapeutic doses of <u>LMWH</u> (obtain a <u>peak</u> anti-Xa level <u>4 hours</u> after a SC LMWH dose): 1.0-2.0 IU/mL Unfractionated <u>heparin</u> (obtain <u>6 hours</u> after IV infusion starts and every 6 hours until therapeutic): 0.3-0.7 IU/mL	Used to <u>monitor low molecular weight heparins</u> (LMWHs) and <u>unfractionated heparin</u> (UFH). Monitoring for LMWH is <u>recommended in pregnancy</u> and may be used in obesity, low body weight, pediatrics, elderly, renal insufficiency (see Anticoagulation chapter).
Prothrombin Time / International Normalized Ratio **(PT / INR)**	PT: 10–13 seconds (varies) INR: < 1.2 (if not on warfarin)	Used to <u>monitor warfarin</u>. INR ↑ (without taking warfarin) is typically due to <u>liver disease</u>. <u>False</u> ↑ can occur with <u>daptomycin, oritavancin, telavancin</u>. Drug interactions can cause an ↑ or ↓ INR (see Anticoagulation chapter).
Activated Partial Thromboplastin Time **(aPTT or PTT)**	22–38 seconds (varies, this is called the "control") <u>UFH</u>: obtain <u>6 hours</u> after IV infusion starts and every 6 hours until therapeutic Goal (on UFH): 1.5–2.5x control	Used to <u>monitor UFH</u> and parenteral direct thrombin inhibitors (e.g., argatroban). <u>False</u> ↑ can occur with <u>oritavancin, telavancin</u>.
Activated Clotting Time (ACT)	70–180 seconds (varies)	Used to monitor anticoagulation in the cardiac catheterization lab during percutaneous coronary intervention (PCI) and surgery.
Platelets **(PLTs)**	150,000–450,000 cells/mm³	Platelets have an average life span of <u>7-10 days</u>. Platelets are required for clot formation. Spontaneous bleeding can occur when platelets are < 20,000 cells/mm³. ↓ due to <u>heparin, LMWHs, fondaparinux</u>, glycoprotein IIb/IIIa receptor antagonists, <u>linezolid, valproic acid</u>, chemotherapy that targets the bone marrow.
Heparin-Induced Platelet Antibodies: ELISA test 1st, then an SRA (serotonin release assay)	Negative	<u>Heparin-induced thrombocytopenia (HIT)</u> is suspected when <u>platelets drop > 50%</u> from baseline as a result of treatment with UFH or LMWH. Antibody testing is used to confirm a diagnosis of HIT. If the ELISA test is positive, a positive <u>SRA is confirmatory</u>.

ITEM	COMMON REFERENCE RANGE	NOTES
Liver and Gastroenterology		
Albumin	3.5–5 g/dL	↓ due to cirrhosis and malnutrition. Serum levels of highly protein-bound drugs (e.g., warfarin, calcium, phenytoin) are impacted by low albumin. Phenytoin and calcium serum concentrations require correction for low albumin (see Seizures/Epilepsy, Pharmacokinetics and Calculations III chapters). A "free" phenytoin level or ionized calcium does not require adjustment.
Alkaline Phosphatase (Alk Phos or ALP)	33–131 IU/L	Used with other labs to assess liver, biliary tract (cholestatic) and bone disease.
Aspartate Aminotransferase (AST)	10–40 units/L	AST and ALT are enzymes released from injured hepatocytes (liver cells). Numerous medications and herbals can ↑ AST and ALT (see Hepatitis & Liver Disease chapter).
Alanine Aminotransferase (ALT)	10–40 units/L	
Gamma-Glutamyl Transpeptidase (GGT)	9–58 units/L	Used with other labs to assess liver, biliary tract (cholestasis) and pancreas.
Bilirubin, total (Tbili)	0.1–1.2 mg/dL	Used along with other liver tests to determine causes of liver damage and detect bile duct blockage.
Ammonia	19–60 mcg/dL	Though not diagnostic, often measured in suspected hepatic encephalopathy (HE). ↑ due to valproic acid, topiramate. ↓ due to lactulose.
Hepatic (liver) panel AST, ALT, Tbili, Albumin and Alk Phos	See above	A group of liver function tests (LFTs) ordered together to assess acute and chronic liver inflammation/disease and baseline and routine monitoring of hepatotoxic drugs. The panel can include other tests to evaluate liver function (e.g., PT/INR, total protein).
Pancreatic Enzymes		
Amylase	60–180 units/L	↑ in pancreatitis, which can be caused by didanosine, stavudine, GLP-1 agonists, DPP-4 inhibitors, valproic acid, hypertriglyceridemia.
Lipase	5–160 units/L	
Cardiovascular		
Creatine Kinase or **Creatine Phosphokinase (CK** or **CPK)**	Males: 55–170 IU/L Females: 30–135 IU/L	Used to assess muscle inflammation (myositis), or more serious muscle damage, and to diagnose cardiac conditions. ↑ due to daptomycin, statins, fibrates (especially if given with a statin), emtricitabine, tenofovir, tipranavir, raltegravir, dolutegravir.
CK-MB Isoenzymes, total	≤ 6.0 ng/mL	As a group, these are called "cardiac enzymes." CK-MB, TnT and TnI are used in the diagnosis of MI. Troponins can be elevated with a few other conditions (e.g., sepsis, PE, CKD).
Troponin T (TnT)	0–0.1 ng/mL (assay dependent)	
Troponin I (TnI)	0–0.5 ng/mL (assay dependent)	BNP and NT-proBNP are both markers of cardiac stress. They are not heart failure (HF) nor heart disease-specific, but higher values indicate a higher likelihood of HF when consistent with HF symptoms. Renal failure is the second most common cause of ↑ BNP and NT-proBNP.
B-Type Natriuretic Peptide (BNP)	< 100 pg/mL or ng/L	
N-Terminal-ProBNP (NT-proBNP)	Males: < 61 pg/mL Females: 12–151 pg/mL	Myoglobin and CK-MB are not interchangeable; they are two separate markers. Myoglobin is a sensitive marker for muscle injury but has relatively low specificity for acute MI and therefore is not routinely used for diagnosis (see Acute Coronary Syndromes chapter).
Respiratory		
Eosinophil Count	< 100 cells/mcL	Used, along with a history of COPD exacerbations, to determine if inhaled corticosteroids (ICS) will be beneficial in COPD treatment [See Chronic Obstructive Pulmonary Disease (COPD) chapter].

ITEM	COMMON REFERENCE RANGE	NOTES
Lipids and Cardiovascular Risk		
Total Cholesterol (TC)	< 200 mg/dL	For complete discussion, see Dyslipidemia chapter. Fasting begins 9-12 hours prior to lipid blood draw.
Low Density Lipoprotein (LDL)	≤ 100 mg/dL, desirable	Non-HDL = TC – HDL. Guidelines do not support specific TC, HDL or TG goals; they recommend a statin intensity level for LDL-C reduction based on patient risk. Additional treatments may be added in high-risk patients (e.g., ASCVD) if LDL-C remains elevated (e.g., ≥ 70 mg/dL) on the maximum statin dose tolerated.
High Density Lipoprotein (HDL)	< 40 mg/dL, low (male) ≥ 60 mg/dL, desirable	
Non-HDL	< 130 mg/dL, desirable	
Triglycerides (TG)	< 150 mg/dL	
Lipid panel **TC, HDL, LDL, TG**	See above	A group of labs ordered together to assess the major cholesterol types and determine cardiovascular risk. A fasting lipid panel is preferred.
Lipoprotein-a, Lp(a) Apoliprotein-B, Apo B	< 10 mg/dL < 130 mg/dL	↑ Lp(a) and ↑ ApoB are associated with ↑ coagulation and ↑ risk of CVD.
C-reactive Protein (CRP)	0–0.5 mg/dL	↑ CRP indicates inflammation, which could be due to many conditions (infection, trauma, malignancy). Higher levels indicate ↑ risk. High-sensitivity CRP (hs-CRP) is more sensitive for CVD.
Coronary Artery Calcium score	< 300 Agatston units or < 75th percentile for age, sex and ethnicity; higher score indicates a higher risk	The coronary artery calcium score measures calcium build-up in the coronary arteries.
Ankle Brachial Index (ABI)	1–1.4	The ankle brachial index measures the ratio of the BP in the lower legs to the BP in the arms. It is used to assess severity of peripheral artery disease (PAD). An ABI < 1 indicates some degree of PAD.
Diabetes		
Fasting Plasma Glucose (FPG)	≥ 126 mg/dL is positive for diabetes 100–125 mg/dL is positive for prediabetes	Fasting begins ≥ 8 hours prior to the blood draw. See Diabetes chapter for complete discussion and medications that can cause hyper- and hypoglycemia.
Hemoglobin A1C (A1C)	≤ 7% (ADA), ≤ 6.5% (AACE)	Average blood glucose over the past 3 months; based on attachment of glucose to hemoglobin; ↑ glucose = ↑ BG attached to Hgb = ↑ A1C.
Estimated Average Glucose (eAG)	≤ 154 mg/dL (ADA)	Used to correlate a finger stick glucose with an A1C; an eAG of 126 mg/dL corresponds to an A1C of 6%.
Preprandial Blood Glucose	80–130 mg/dL (ADA) < 110 mg/dL (AACE)	Blood glucose measurement taken before a meal.
Postprandial Blood Glucose	≤ 180 mg/dL (ADA) < 140 mg/dL (AACE)	Blood glucose measurement taken after a meal (1-2 hours after the start of eating).
C-Peptide (fasting)	0.78–1.89 ng/mL	Insulin breakdown product used to evaluate beta-cell function (distinguishes type 1 from type 2 diabetes). ↓ or absent in type 1 diabetes.
Urine Albumin to Creatinine Ratio or Albumin to Creatinine Ratio (UACR or ACR) or	Males: < 17 mg/gram Females: < 25 mg/gram	See Diabetes and Renal Disease chapters.
Urinary Albumin Excretion (UAE)	< 30 mg/24 hours	

ITEM	COMMON REFERENCE RANGE	NOTES
Thyroid Function		
Thyroid Stimulating Hormone **(TSH)**	0.3–3 mIU/L	TSH is used with FT4 to diagnose hypothyroidism and hyperthyroidism, and is used alone (sometimes with FT4) to monitor patients being treated. ↑ TSH = hypothyroidism, ↓ TSH = hyperthyroidism. ↑ or ↓ due to amiodarone, interferons. ↑ (hypothyroidism) due to tyrosine kinase inhibitors, lithium, carbamazepine.
Total Thyroxine (T4)	4.5–10.9 mcg/dL	T4 and FT4 are two of several tests used for a detailed assessment of thyroid function (see Thyroid Disorders chapter).
Free Thyroxine (FT4)	0.9–2.3 ng/dL	
Uric Acid/Gout		
Uric Acid	Males: 3.5–7.2 mg/dL Females: 2–6.5 mg/dL	Used in the diagnosis and treatment of gout. ↑ due to diuretics, niacin, low doses of aspirin, pyrazinamide, cyclosporine, select pancreatic enzyme products, select chemotherapy (due to tumor lysis syndrome).
Inflammation/Autoimmune Disease		
C-Reactive Protein **(CRP)**	Normal: 0–0.5 mg/dL High risk: > 3 mg/dL	Nonspecific tests used in autoimmune disorders, inflammation, infections. If ANA is positive, an anti-dsDNA test will help establish a diagnosis of systemic lupus erythematosus, which can be drug-induced (see below).
Rheumatoid Factor **(RF)**	Negative, or ≤ upper limit of normal (ULN) for the lab (usually < 20 IU/mL)	Drug-induced lupus erythematosus (DILE) can be caused by many drugs. More likely with anti-TNF agents, hydralazine, isoniazid, methimazole, methyldopa, minocycline, procainamide, propylthiouracil, quinidine, terbinafine. The causative drug must be discontinued (see Systemic Steroids & Autoimmune Conditions chapter).
Erythrocyte Sedimentation Rate **(ESR)**	Males: ≤ 20 mm/hr Females: ≤ 30 mm/hr	
Antinuclear Antibodies **(ANA)**	Negative (titers may be provided)	
Antihistone Antibodies (Detected by ELISA)	Negative	
HIV		
CD4 T Lymphocyte Count	Immunocompromised state: < 200 cells/mm^3	Used to diagnose HIV and monitor treatment (see HIV chapter). CD4 count is an indicator of immune function and helps establish the need for opportunistic infection prophylaxis.
HIV RNA Concentration **(Viral Load)**	Undetectable Measured in copies/mL	
HIV Antibody (Ab)	Negative (non-reactive)	Detects infection with the virus; may not become positive until several weeks after exposure.
HIV DNA PCR	Negative	Useful for early detection.
HIV p24 Antigen	Undetectable	
Acid-Base (Arterial Sample)		
pH	7.35–7.45	Together these values make up an arterial blood gas (ABG). This blood must be drawn from an artery (not a vein, as with other labs). Often written in chart notes with a stick diagram: pH/pCO2/pO2/HCO3/O2 Sat (see Calculations IV chapter for ABG interpretation). Bicarbonate on the ABG is a calculated value, and the reference range may differ from venous samples (reported with a BMP).
pCO2	35–45 mmHg	
pO2	80–100 mmHg	
HCO3	22–26 mEq/L	
O2 Sat	> 95%	

ITEM	COMMON REFERENCE RANGE	NOTES
Hormonal		
Testosterone total, free	Males: 300–950 ng/dL	↑ with testosterone supplementation.
Prostate-Specific Antigen (PSA)	< 4 ng/mL	Can ↑ with testosterone supplementation. Used in detecting prostate cancer and BPH.
Human Chorionic Gonadotropin (hCG)	Varies by test	A positive result from a blood or urine test indicates pregnancy.
Luteinizing Hormone (LH)	Varies during cycle	Rises mid-cycle, causing egg release from the ovaries (ovulation). Tested in urine with ovulation predictor kits for women attempting pregnancy.
Parathyroid Hormone (PTH)	Varies	Used in evaluation of parathyroid disorders, hypercalcemia and chronic kidney disease (CKD) (see Renal Disease chapter).
Other		
Cosyntropin Stimulation Test	Baseline and timed increase are measured	Used to test for adrenal suppression; medications that affect baseline cortisol or suppress adrenal response will impact test and may need to be held prior (e.g., steroids).
Lactic Acid (lactate)	0.5–2.2 mEq/L	Lactic acidosis indicates anaerobic metabolism, which occurs in long-distance running and in certain medical conditions (e.g., sepsis). ↑ due to NRTIs (see HIV chapter), metformin (low risk/mostly with renal disease and heart failure), alcohol use, cyanide.
Procalcitonin	≤ 0.15 ng/mL	↑ due to systemic bacterial infections or severe localized infections.
Prolactin	1–25 ng/mL	Secretion is regulated by dopamine; can ↑ with haloperidol, risperidone, paliperidone, methyldopa. Can ↓ with bromocriptine.
Purified Protein Derivative (PPD) or Tuberculin Skin Test (TST)	No induration (raised area); induration is measured to assess exposure to *Mycobacterium tuberculosis*	Tuberculin skin test (TST) administered by intradermal injection to assess for latent TB. Response is measured by diameter (mm) of induration at 48-72 hours (see ID II: Bacterial Infections chapter).
Interferon-Gamma Release Assay (IGRA)	Negative (for exposure to *Mycobacterium tuberculosis*)	Preferred test (instead of TST/PPD) for most patients (does not require follow-up or cause false-positive result if history of BCG vaccination).
Rapid Plasma Reagin (RPR) or Venereal Diseases Reseach Laboratory (VDRL)	Negative	Non-treponemal antibody tests used to screen for syphilis. If the RPR or VDRL is positive, confirmatory testing with a treponemal assay is performed. Titers may be reported and are used to monitor response to therapy.
Serum Osmolality	275–290 mOsm/kg H2O	Used with Na, BUN/SCr, and clinical volume status to evaluate hypo/hypernatremia. ↑ due to mannitol, toxicities (e.g., ethylene glycol, methanol, propylene glycol).
Thiopurine Methyltransferase (TPMT)	≥ 15 units/mL	Those with a genetic deficiency of TPMT are at ↑ risk for myelosuppression (bone marrow suppression) and may require lower doses of azathioprine and mercaptopurine.
Vitamin D, serum 25(OH)	> 30 ng/mL	↓ levels increase risk of osteoporosis, osteomalacia (rickets), CVD, diabetes, hypertension, infectious diseases and other conditions. Supplement vitamin D with various conditions and drugs (see Dietary Supplements, Natural & Complementary Medicine chapter).

ASSESSING PATIENT CASES QUICKLY

Cases can be evaluated more quickly by recognizing lab patterns and signs and symptoms that provide a clue to the patient's diagnosis. Watch for drug-induced signs/symptoms and lab changes. Look for lab contraindications to drugs (e.g., +hCG, hyperkalemia). Additional information can be found in the disease state chapters (e.g., lab patterns due to an infectious disease can be found in the Infectious Diseases chapters).

THERAPEUTIC DRUG MONITORING

Drug levels or other monitoring parameters (such as anti-Xa levels for LMWHs) are used to reach dosing goals and avoid toxicity. Therapeutic drug monitoring (TDM) is increasingly common due to the need to target highly resistant infectious organisms and dose medications properly in overweight and obese patients. The peak level is the highest concentration of a drug in the blood; it requires time for the drug to distribute to body tissues. The trough level is the lowest concentration of a drug in the blood and is drawn right before the next dose or some short period of time before the next dose (30 minutes is common). This allows time to assess the level before another dose is given, so the next dose can be withheld if the level is high. The time that drug levels are drawn is critical for accurate interpretation. For example, a tobramycin level of 6 mcg/mL would be interpreted differently if the level was a trough versus a peak. Obtaining drug levels at steady state is often (but not always) preferred. See the Pharmacokinetics chapter for further discussion.

Narrow therapeutic index (NTI) drugs have a narrow separation between the subtherapeutic (low), therapeutic (desired) and supratherapeutic (high) drug levels. Supratherapeutic drug levels can be toxic.

TDM is commonly performed by pharmacists. The following Key Drugs Guy lists drugs that are routinely monitored. Making treatment recommendations to address high and low drug levels is essential for the NAPLEX.

THERAPEUTIC DRUG LEVELS

DRUG	USUAL THERAPEUTIC RANGE
Carbamazepine	4–12 mcg/mL
Digoxin	0.8–2 ng/mL (AF)
	0.5–0.9 ng/mL (HF)
Gentamicin (traditional dosing)	Peak: 5–10 mcg/mL
	Trough: < 2 mcg/mL
Lithium	0.6–1.2 mEq/L (up to 1.5 mEq/L for acute symptoms), drawn as a trough
Phenytoin/Fosphenytoin	10–20 mcg/mL; if albumin is low, calculate a corrected level; see Seizures/Epilepsy chapter
Free Phenytoin	1–2 mcg/mL
Procainamide	4–10 mcg/mL
NAPA (procainamide active metabolite)	15–25 mcg/mL
Combined	10–30 mcg/mL
Theophylline	5–15 mcg/mL
Tobramycin (traditional dosing)	Peak: 5–10 mcg/mL
	Trough: < 2 mcg/mL
Valproic acid	50–100 mcg/mL (up to 150 mcg/mL in some patients); see Seizures/Epilepsy chapter
Vancomycin	Serious infections (e.g., pneumonia, endocarditis, osteomyelitis, meningitis, bacteremia): AUC/MIC ratio of 400–600 recommended (associated with improved outcomes and less toxicity) or trough: 15–20 mcg/mL
	Other infections: trough: 10–15 mcg/mL
Warfarin	Goal INR is 2–3 for most indications, use higher range (2.5–3.5) for high-risk conditions, such as mechanical mitral valves

Select Guidelines/References
Testing.com. www.testing.com (accessed 2023 Nov 17).
Lee M. Basic Skills in Interpreting Laboratory Data. 7th ed. Betheseda, MD: ASHP; 2022.
Schmidt J, Wieczorkiewicz J. Interpreting Laboratory Data: A Point-of-Care Guide. Betheseda, MD: ASHP; 2011.

CHAPTER CONTENT

> ❝
> Pharmacists respond to drug
> questions around the clock.
> Knowing where to locate drug
> information is essential in all
> practice settings.

CONTENT LEGEND

🌣 = Study
     Tip Gal

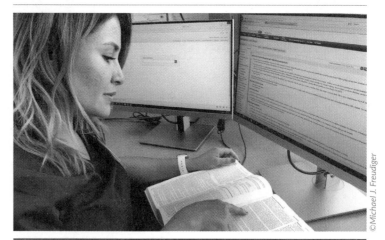

©Michael J. Freudiger

CHAPTER 5
DRUG REFERENCES

BACKGROUND

Providing drug information to patients and other healthcare professionals is a critical function of pharmacists, the drug therapy experts. Pharmacists need to select appropriate resources and provide accurate responses that reflect the most current drug information.

This chapter covers the essential content contained in a package insert (PI) and other general drug information resources used in pharmacy practice. It also includes the most common resources for locating specialty healthcare content (e.g., drug shortages, travel vaccines) and consumer information, as well as databases to retrieve clinical studies.

CASE SCENARIO

MJ presents with a prescription for *Keppra* 500 mg tablets by mouth BID for her 5-year-old, 40 lb daughter. She asks the pharmacist a few questions:

- Is the medication dosed properly for her daughter's age and weight?
- Is it possible to crush the tablets or switch to a liquid?
- Is it safe to take melatonin for sleep with *Keppra*?

RESOURCES

- Drug dosing for a child may (or may not) be in the drug's PI, which includes only FDA-approved indications. It may be included in the off-label section of a general drug information resource, such as *Lexicomp*. A pediatric resource such as *The Harriet Lane Handbook* includes pediatric dosing that might otherwise be unavailable. The clinical guidelines for the condition might have recommended dosing for children, especially for common pediatric conditions, such as epilepsy and various infectious diseases.

- Administration recommendations (e.g., if the tablets can be crushed) and the product formulations available (e.g., a solution) will be reflected in the PI and general drug information resources. If a formulation is not available, it can possibly be prepared by a compounding pharmacist, following the preparation recommendations in USP 795 and the master formula (recipe) (i.e., for oral *Keppra* liquid).

- A drug-natural product interaction tool (found in most general drug information resources), or a specific natural medicine resource, can be used to evaluate the safety of taking melatonin and *Keppra*.

PACKAGE INSERTS

The PI is the <u>FDA-approved drug information</u> that is part of the drug's official labeling. The example PI below shows the common categories included (which are also found in drug monographs from general drug information resources, discussed later in the chapter). The table at the bottom of the page describes methods for locating a PI.

The FDA approves drugs and their labeling. The PI is part of the labeling. PIs contain only the information approved by the FDA. They do not include, for example, off-label uses or drug costs.

COMMON CONTENT CATEGORIES IN A DRUG PACKAGE INSERT

PRESCRIBING INFORMATION
EVISTA (raloxifene hydrochloride) Tablet for Oral Use

BOXED WARNING
Increased Risk of Venous Thromboembolism and Death from Stroke.

------------------------Recent Major Changes------------------------
None.

------------------------Indications and Usage------------------------
EVISTA is an estrogen agonist/antagonist indicated for:
- Treatment and prevention of osteoporosis in postmenopausal women.
- Reduction in risk of invasive breast cancer in postmenopausal women.

------------------------Dosage and Administration------------------------
60 mg tablet orally once daily.
Calcium and vitamin D should be added if insufficient.

------------------------Dosage Forms and Strengths------------------------
Tablets (not scored) 60 mg.

------------------------Contraindications------------------------
- Active or past venous thromboembolism.
- Pregnancy.

------------------------Warnings and Precautions------------------------
- Venous thromboembolism.
- Death due to stroke in patients with cardiovascular disease.
- Do not use to prevent cardiovascular disease.
- Hypertriglyceridemia.

------------------------Adverse Reactions------------------------
Adverse reactions (> 2% and more common than with placebo) include: hot flashes, leg cramps, peripheral edema, arthralgia...

------------------------Drug Interactions------------------------
- Cholestyramine: use with EVISTA is not recommended. Reduces raloxifene absorption.
- Warfarin: monitor prothrombin time.

------------------------Use in Specific Populations------------------------
Renal impairment: EVISTA should be used with caution in patients with moderate or severe renal impairment.

------------------------Drug Abuse and Dependence------------------------
Not applicable.

------------------------Overdosage/Toxicology------------------------
In an 8-week study of 63 postmenopausal women, a dose of raloxifene 600 mg/day was safely tolerated.
In clinical trials, no raloxifene overdose has been reported.

------------------------Pharmacology/Mechanism of Action------------------------
Raloxifene is an estrogen agonist/antagonist, commonly referred to as a selective estrogen receptor modulator (SERM). The biological actions of raloxifene are largely mediated through binding to estrogen receptors.

------------------------Additional Categories------------------------
Description (active and inactive ingredients)

Pharmacokinetics and Pharmacodynamics

Clinical Studies

How Supplied/Storage and Handling

Patient Counseling Information

Revised; not the actual Evista Package Insert.

PACKAGE INSERT LOCATIONS	FORMATS	WEBSITE
DailyMed (NLM)	Online	dailymed.nlm.nih.gov
Drugs@FDA	Online and Mobile App	accessdata.fda.gov/scripts/cder/daf
The Drug Manufacturer's Website	Online	The manufacturer's website (e.g., pfizer.com) or the drug-specific website (common with newer drugs; the website URL will be the drug's brand name, such as eliquis.com)
Attached to the physical product (e.g., the bottle or box)	Printed	N/A

THE PI INCLUDES THE DRUG'S SAFETY INFORMATION

All drugs, OTC and prescription, have some degree of risk. When a decision is made to prescribe a drug (and the patient agrees to take the drug), the benefit must outweigh the risk. Important drug safety information in the PI is split into the categories below. Dispensing of the drug may require separate patient handouts alerting to the drug's toxicity (Medication Guides) and/or a strategy to manage the risk (REMS). These are discussed in the Drug Allergies & Adverse Drug Reactions chapter.

When drug safety information changes (e.g., new warnings, withdrawal from the market), the FDA publishes a safety communication or alert on their website, and an updated PI will reflect the drug's safety-related labeling changes.

- Boxed Warnings: the strictest warnings. The black box around the warning (see example on previous page) alerts prescribers to the risk of death or permanent disability (e.g., increased risk of venous thromboembolism and death from stroke with raloxifene).

- Contraindications: when a patient has a contraindication to a drug, the drug cannot be used in that patient. The risk will outweigh any possible benefit (e.g., a history of venous thromboembolism is a contraindication to the use of raloxifene). If there are no known contraindications for a drug, the section will state "None."

- Warnings and Precautions: includes serious reactions that can result in death, hospitalization, medical intervention, disability or teratogenicity (e.g., raloxifene has a warning for venous thromboembolism). Warnings and precautions may or may not change a prescribing decision.

- Adverse Reactions: refers to undesirable, uncomfortable or dangerous effects from a drug (e.g., arthralgia from raloxifene). The risk-benefit assessment is patient-specific (e.g., arthralgia from raloxifene will be a concern for a patient with chronic joint pain versus a patient with no joint pain).

GENERAL DRUG INFORMATION RESOURCES

General drug information resources rely on the PI for much of their drug monograph content. The table on the following page describes the general drug information resources commonly used by pharmacists. These resources are managed by different companies, and the additional information they contain beyond standard package labeling content varies (see the Unique Features table).

Most general drug information resources require a paid subscription, but a few (e.g., *Drugs.com, RxList*) can be accessed by anyone at no cost to the user. Many resources are available online (as websites, electronic books or comprehensive, searchable databases). Some can be used as a mobile application to help direct real-time patient care decisions.

> General drug information resources contain monographs on each drug. The monographs include the FDA-approved information from the drug's PI, plus additional items, depending on the resource.

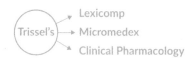

Commonly used drug monograph databases collate information from the PI and other sources and include *Clinical Pharmacology, Facts and Comparisons, Lexicomp* and *Micromedex*. Each contains information that pharmacists find useful, including *Trissel's* IV drug compatibility and stability data, drug class comparisons, natural products, drug identification (tablet/capsule) and international drug names. Most databases provide drug pricing, with either the drug's average wholesale price (AWP), which is usually reported by the manufacturer, or the average price charged at pharmacies, which tends to be lower (~17% less than the AWP).

The *American Hospital Formulary Service (AHFS) Clinical Drug Information* provides comprehensive monographs that link to supporting evidence and references, which makes it a very useful resource for researching a topic in detail. The off-label drug use section is well-researched, with linked references.

Caution: pharmacists rely on the data in the drug information resource at their practice site, but when drug information is updated, there can be a lag time until the PI and the drug's monograph include the update (especially printed versions). Pharmacists may need to check multiple sources to confirm they are retrieving the most current content.

SUMMARY OF GENERAL DRUG INFORMATION RESOURCES

REFERENCE	FORMATS	DESCRIPTION
American Hospital Formulary Service (AHFS) ahfsdruginformation.com An ASHP product	AHFS Drug Information: Book	Collection of drug monographs for medications available in the U.S.
	AHFS DI Essentials: Part of AHFS CDI (below)	Select drug monographs from AHFS Drug Information reformatted for point-of-care decision making; expands on therapeutic evidence and includes additional information (e.g., patient counseling).
	AHFS Clinical Drug Information (AHFS CDI): Online and Mobile App	AHFS Drug Information and AHFS DI Essentials databases, plus real-time updates (e.g., drug shortages, FDA safety alerts).
Clinical Pharmacology (powered by ClinicalKey) clinicalkey.com/pharmacology	Online and Mobile App	Drug information (e.g., monographs for Rx and OTC drugs, natural products and investigational drugs) provided by Clinical Pharmacology with real-time updates (e.g., drug safety changes) and point-of-care solutions supported by ClinicalKey.
Epocrates/Epocrates + epocrates.com	Online and Mobile App	Free with registration; drug information plus guideline summaries. Epocrates + (fee required) expands into evidence-based disease management and includes sections on natural products, lab and diagnostic information and ICD-10 coding (for billing purposes).
Facts & Comparisons eAnswers wolterskluwer.com/en/solutions/lexicomp/facts-and-comparisons	Online	Collection of databases; includes drug monographs, comparative drug charts and other unique resources (e.g., search drugs based on a specific adverse reaction).
Lexicomp wolterskluwer.com/en/solutions/lexicomp	Drug Information Handbook: Book	Drug monographs organized alphabetically; includes useful appendices (e.g., drug class comparisons, equivalent dosing charts).
	Online and Mobile App	Multiple clinical databases beyond drug information monographs depending on subscription level purchased (see the Unique Features and Locating Specific Types of Information tables).
Micromedex merative.com/clinical-decision-support	Online and Mobile App	Multiple clinical databases beyond drug information monographs (see the Unique Features and Locating Specific Types of Information tables).
Prescriber's Digital Reference (*mobile*PDR) pdr.net/mobilepdr/	Online and Mobile App	Free with registration; includes information for drugs, vaccines and biologics. Detail is more than the drug's PI, and includes practical information, such as where injections can be given, and time to reach clinical effect.
PubChem (NLM) pubchem.ncbi.nlm.nih.gov	Online	Free from the National Library of Medicine (NLM). Includes information on chemical properties and structures, general drug information (including toxicity and safety), and links to many other resources.
Drugs.com drugs.com	Online and Mobile App	Free for professionals and consumers; drug information is primarily sourced from other products, including AHFS Drug Information, Micromedex and Cerner Multum.
RxList rxlist.com	Online	Free for professionals and consumers; drug information is primarily sourced from other products, including the FDA, Cerner Multum and First Databank, Inc.

UNIQUE FEATURES OF COMMON DRUG INFORMATION RESOURCES

The table below describes some of the popular features of general drug information resources that are useful in daily practice and commonly accessed by pharmacists. Many online databases link to external sites that have public access (e.g., *Lexicomp* includes vaccine monographs and immunization schedules and provides links to the CDC website).

REFERENCE	Off-Label Uses	IV Drug Compatibility	Drug/Pill Identification	Natural Products	Drug Class Comparisons	Pricing	International Drug Names
AHFS/AHFS CDI	✓	✓					✓ (via USP Dictionary of USAN and International Drug Names)
Clinical Pharmacology	✓	✓ (via Trissel's*)	✓	✓	✓	✓	✓ (via Index Nominum)
Drugs.com	✓		✓	✓	✓	✓	✓
Epocrates/ Epocrates +	✓		✓	✓ (Epocrates +)	✓	✓	
Facts & Comparisons eAnswers	✓	✓ (via Trissel's*)	✓	✓	✓		✓ (via Martindale)
Lexicomp	✓	✓ (via Trissel's*)	✓	✓	✓	✓	✓ (via Martindale)
Micromedex	✓	✓ (via Trissel's*)	✓	✓	✓	✓ (RED BOOK)	✓ (via Martindale, Index Nominum and others)
mobilePDR			✓		✓		

*Data from Trissel's 2 Clinical Pharmaceutics Database

Pharmacist's Letter

Pharmacist's Letter does not contain traditional drug monographs, but is a valuable resource that provides evidence-based drug information. The same company provides similar products called *Prescriber's Letter* and *Pharmacy Technician's Letter*. Subscribers receive a monthly newsletter with short summaries on new or updated drug information, and have online access to helpful practice tools, including:

- New drug approvals, drug withdrawals, new dosage forms and first-time generics
- Charts (e.g., drug class comparisons, disease-state treatment summaries)
- Patient education summaries and patient flyers
- Continuing education (CE)
- Training materials for technicians and intern pharmacists

OTC DRUG INFORMATION

OTC, or nonprescription drugs, are considered safe and effective for self-diagnosed conditions by the general public, have adequate written directions for self-use, and do not require physician supervision. A prescription is not needed to purchase OTC products.

LABELING REQUIREMENTS FOR OTC DRUGS

The labeling on prescription drugs is written for healthcare providers. The labeling on OTC drugs is written for patients who may not have medical training. The language needs to be written in a manner that a layperson can understand, in order to be able to use the drug safely and for its intended purpose. The package labeling information for OTC drugs is in the Drug Facts Panel (see figure to the right) and must include:

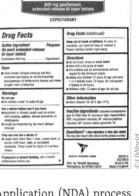

- The active ingredients, including the amount in each dosage unit and the purpose

- The uses (simpler word than indications) for the product

- Specific warnings, including when the drug should not be used (e.g., kidney disease), and when it is appropriate to consult with a doctor or pharmacist

- Side effects, and substances or activities to avoid

- Dosage instructions

- The inactive ingredients

OTC Drug Approval

There are two methods that a manufacturer can use to market an OTC product: the New Drug Application (NDA) process and the OTC Monograph process. The NDA approval process for prescription drugs is managed through the FDA's Center for Drug Evaluation and Research (CDER). OTC drugs can go through the same drug approval process, or the manufacturer can opt to stick to the standards in the OTC monograph for the therapeutic drug class. The monograph for the class will cover the acceptable ingredients, doses, formulations, and labeling, plus study data on the drug's safety and efficacy.

OTC drugs that have gone through the NDA approval process become FDA-approved drugs. The OTC drug labeling can be found on the FDA website through Drugs@FDA, and will be listed in common general drug information resources (e.g., Lexicomp, Micromedex). The labeling for OTC drugs does not need to be a separate document, but can be the container itself, as long as the items specified above are included.

PRACTICE GUIDELINES

Major medical groups and organizations publish practice guidelines to promote evidence-based treatment of conditions. Commonly used guidelines (and the organizations that publish them) should be known for the NAPLEX (see Study Tip Gal).

LOCATING GUIDELINES FOR COMMON CONDITIONS

ANTICOAGULATION
Guidelines from the American College of Chest Physicians (known as CHEST guidelines):

    Stroke Prevention in Atrial Fibrillation
    Venous Thromboembolism

CARDIOVASCULAR DISEASES
Guidelines from the American College of Cardiology/American Heart Association (ACC/AHA):

    Acute Coronary Syndromes
    Atrial Fibrillation
    Heart Failure
    High Cholesterol
    Hypertension

DIABETES
American Association of Clinical Endocrinologists (AACE)
American Diabetes Association (ADA)

INFECTIOUS DISEASES
Infectious Diseases Society of America (IDSA)
HIV/AIDS: US Dept. of Health and Human Services (clinicalinfo.hiv.gov)
Sexually Transmitted Infections: Centers for Disease Control (CDC)

ONCOLOGY
American Society of Clinical Oncology (ASCO)
National Comprehensive Cancer Network (NCCN)

PEDIATRICS
The American Academy of Pediatrics (AAP)

PREGNANCY/WOMEN'S HEALTH
The American College of Obstetricians and Gynecologists (ACOG)

PSYCHIATRIC CONDITIONS
American Psychiatric Association (APA) Diagnostic and Statistical Manual of Mental disorders, 5th Edition (DSM-5)

PULMONARY CONDITIONS
Asthma: Global Initiative for Asthma (GINA)
COPD: Global Initiative for Chronic Obstructive Lung Disease (GOLD)

RENAL DISEASE
Kidney Disease Improving Global Outcomes (KDIGO)

VACCINES
Advisory Committee on Immunization Practices (ACIP)
Centers for Disease Control (CDC)

LOCATING SPECIFIC TYPES OF INFORMATION

The table below highlights select specialty references that may be encountered on the licensure exam. General drug information resources described previously (e.g., *Lexicomp* and *Micromedex*) provide some of the same information.

SPECIALTY REFERENCES BY TOPIC

ADVERSE REACTIONS

FDAble: FDA searchable database of adverse reactions caused by medicines, vaccines, devices, tobacco products, dietary supplements

- MedWatch: FDA's Adverse Event Reporting System (FAERS)
- Vaccine Adverse Event Reporting System (VAERS)
- Manufacturer and User Facility Device Experience (MAUDE)
- Safety Reporting Portal

COMPOUNDING AND PHARMACEUTICS

Allen's The Art, Science, and Technology of Pharmaceutical Compounding

Safety Data Sheets (SDS), previously called Material Safety Data Sheets (MSDS)

Merck Index *Online* (a database of monographs for chemicals, drugs, and biologicals

Remington: The Science and Practice of Pharmacy

USP Compounding Compendium:

- USP 795: Non-Sterile Preparations
- USP 797: Sterile Preparations
- USP 800: Hazardous Drugs - Handling in Healthcare Settings
- USP-NF: monographs for drug substances, dosage forms, compounded preparations and excipients

ASHP's Extemporaneous Formulations for Pediatric, Geriatric, and Special Needs Patients

Handbook of Pharmaceutical Excipients

International Journal of Pharmaceutical Compounding

DRUG INTERACTIONS

Most general drug information resources

DRUG PRICING

RED BOOK (Micromedex)

Medi-Span Price Rx

DRUG SHORTAGES

ASHP Current Drug Shortages

FDA Drug Shortages

CDC Current Vaccine Shortages & Delays

American Hospital Formulary Service Clinical Drug Information (AHFS CDI)

DRUG SUBSTITUTION

FDA's Orange Book: Approved Drug Products with Therapeutic Equivalence Evaluations

FDA's Purple Book: Lists of Licensed Biological Products with Reference Product Exclusivity and Biosimilarity or Interchangeability Evaluations

GERIATRICS

American Geriatrics Society (AGS) Beers Criteria for Potentially Inappropriate Medication Use in Older Adults

Geriatric Lexi-Drugs (Lexicomp)

IMMUNIZATIONS (ADULT AND PEDIATRIC)

CDC Advisory Committee on Immunization Practices (ACIP)

- Updates published in the Morbidity and Mortality Weekly Report (MMWR)

CDC Pink Book: Epidemiology and Prevention of Vaccine-Preventable Diseases

Immunize.org

Vaccines, Blood & Biologics (FDA)

INFECTIOUS DISEASES

Infectious Diseases Society of America (IDSA) Practice Guidelines

Sanford Guide to Antimicrobial Therapy

Human Immunodeficiency Virus (HIV)

HIVInfo.NIH.gov from the US Dept. of Health and Human Services

Sanford Guide to HIV/AIDS Therapy

Johns Hopkins ABX and HIV Guides

Travel Medicine

World Health Organization (WHO)

CDC

- Yellow Book: Health Information for International Travel
- Travelers' Health: resources for travelers and healthcare professionals

International Society of Travel Medicine (ISTM)

INTERNATIONAL DRUG INFORMATION

Index Nominum: International Drug Directory

Martindale: The Complete Drug Reference

USP Dictionary of United States Adopted Names (USAN) and International Drug Names

European Drug Index

INVESTIGATIONAL DRUGS

Clinicaltrials.gov (NIH)

IV DRUG COMPATIBILITY AND STABILITY

ASHP's Handbook on Injectable Drugs

King Guide to Parenteral Admixtures

Trissel's 2 Clinical Pharmaceutics Database

SPECIALTY REFERENCES BY TOPIC (CONTINUED)

MEDICATION SAFETY

FDA MedWatch (report adverse events and medication errors)

Institute for Safe Medication Practices (ISMP)

■ Report medication errors to the ISMP Medication Errors Reporting Program (ISMP MERP)

NIOSH List of Antineoplastic (Chemotherapy) and Other Hazardous Drugs in Healthcare Settings

Crediblemeds.org (QT Drugs Lists)

FDA:

■ Drug and Biologic Recalls

■ Drug Safety Label Changes database

■ Medication Guides

■ Drug Communications and Safety Alerts

NATURAL PRODUCTS/ALTERNATIVE MEDICINE

NatMed (formerly Natural Medicines, a database provided by Therapeutic Research Center)

Dietary Supplements Label Database (NIH)

USP Dietary Supplements Compendium

PEDIATRICS

NeoFax and Pediatrics (Micromedex)

Pediatric & Neonatal Lexi-Drugs (Lexicomp)

Red Book: Report of the Committee on Infectious Diseases (AAP)

The Harriet Lane Handbook

American Academy of Pediatrics (AAP)

Pediatric Pharmacy Association (PPA) Key Potentially Inappropriate Drugs in Pediatrics: The KIDs List

ASHP's Pediatric Injectable Drugs (The Teddy Bear Book)

Nelson Textbook of Pediatrics

PHARMACOLOGY

Goodman and Gilman's The Pharmacological Basis of Therapeutics

Katzung's Basic and Clinical Pharmacology

PREGNANCY AND LACTATION

Briggs' Drugs in Pregnancy and Lactation

CDC: Medications during Pregnancy/Breastfeeding

Hale's Medications and Mothers' Milk

LactMed (NLM)

MotherToBaby

POISONING AND TOXICOLOGY

Lexi-Tox (Lexicomp)

Micromedex Tox & Drug Product Lookup (previously POISINDEX)

Goldfrank's Toxicologic Emergencies

State Poison Control Center

The American Association of Poison Control Centers

REGULATORY AND BUSINESS DEVELOPMENT

FDA Center for Drug Evaluation and Research (CDER)

Pink Sheet

THERAPEUTICS AND DISEASE MANAGEMENT

DiPiro's Pharmacotherapy: A Pathophysiologic Approach

Handbook of Nonprescription Drugs: An Interactive Approach to Self-Care (OTC)

Koda-Kimble's Applied Therapeutics: The Clinical Use of Drugs

The Merck Manual

UpToDate

CDC: Diseases & Conditions

Harrison's Principles of Internal Medicine

Medscape

VETERINARY

Plumb's Veterinary Drugs

SELECTING THE CORRECT "COLOR" DRUG REFERENCE

A number of important references are referred to by a color (see Study Tip Gal on next page). One of the more frequently accessed resources is the FDA's *Orange Book*, available online at accessdata.fda.gov/scripts/cder/ob/. This resource is used to determine if a generic substitution of a branded product is acceptable based on an AB rating, which indicates therapeutic equivalence to the brand.

Below is an example of the methylphenidate extended-release tablet entry from the online *Orange Book* indicating therapeutic equivalence to *Concerta*.

Mkt. Status	Active Ingredient	Proprietary Name	Appl No	Dosage Form	Route	Strength	TE Code	RLD	RS	Applicant Holder
RX	METHYLPHENIDATE HYDROCHLORIDE	CONCERTA	N021121	TABLET, EXTENDED RELEASE	ORAL	18MG	AB	RLD		JANSSEN PHARMACEUTICALS INC
RX	METHYLPHENIDATE HYDROCHLORIDE	CONCERTA	N021121	TABLET, EXTENDED RELEASE	ORAL	27MG	AB	RLD		JANSSEN PHARMACEUTICALS INC
RX	METHYLPHENIDATE HYDROCHLORIDE	CONCERTA	N021121	TABLET, EXTENDED RELEASE	ORAL	36MG	AB	RLD		JANSSEN PHARMACEUTICALS INC
RX	METHYLPHENIDATE HYDROCHLORIDE	CONCERTA	N021121	TABLET, EXTENDED RELEASE	ORAL	54MG	AB	RLD	RS	JANSSEN PHARMACEUTICALS INC

"COLOR" DRUG REFERENCES

Orange Book (FDA)
List of approved drugs that can be interchanged with generics based on therapeutic equivalence.

Pink Book (CDC)
Information on epidemiology and vaccine-preventable diseases.

Pink Sheet (Pharma Intelligence)
News reports on regulatory, legislative, legal and business developments.

Purple Book (FDA)
List of biological drug products, including biosimilars.

Red Book, Pharmacy
Drug pricing information.

Red Book, Pediatrics (AAP)
Summaries of pediatric infectious diseases, antimicrobial treatment and vaccinations.

Yellow Book (CDC)
Information on the health risks of international travel, required vaccines and prophylaxis medications.

Green Book (FDA)
Information on approved animal drug products.

LOCATING CLINICAL STUDY DATA AND RESEARCH SUMMARIES

Pharmacists use several databases to search for published studies, systematic reviews, meta-analyses and review articles. Searches can be done using Medical Subject Headings (MeSH) terms, which are used to group articles with the same content. Two of the more common databases are:

- *PubMed:* accesses MEDLINE (journal articles in medicine, nursing, dentistry, veterinary medicine, life sciences and more) and is a free service available from the NLM (ncbi.nlm.nih.gov/pubmed/).

- *Cochrane Library:* provides evidence-based information to guide clinical decision making. The database of Cochrane Systematic Reviews contains > 7,500 reviews [e.g., *Diagnostic Tests for Autism Spectrum Disorder (ASD) in Preschool Children*]. This important work is supported by government funds and donations, with no cost for users. It can be accessed at cochranelibrary.com.

CONSUMER RESOURCES

Pharmacists should be able to recommend reputable websites for patient-friendly information on medical conditions and drug treatment.

- The CDC (cdc.gov) has a symptom checker and provides information on infectious diseases, immunizations and travelers' health.

- *Drugs.com* (drugs.com) and *RxList* (rxlist.com) provide drug monographs and other information (see earlier descriptions in the General Drug Information Resources section).

- *Mayo Clinic* (mayoclinic.org) provides comprehensive patient information for diseases, symptoms, tests and procedures, and drugs and supplements.

- *MedlinePlus* (medlineplus.gov/, from the NLM) has sections on health topics, drugs and supplements, health-related videos, lab tests and a medical encyclopedia with images.

- *WebMD* (webmd.com) covers diseases, healthy living, pregnancy, prescription and OTC drug information, plus it has a pill identifier and interaction checker.

- FDA For Consumers website (fda.gov/consumers) provides comprehensive information on drugs (including recalls), food products, medical devices, vaccines, tobacco products and other topics that fall under the FDA's jurisdiction. Content can be selected by audience type (e.g., women, children or minority health).

- *MyHealthfinder* (health.gov/myhealthfinder, from the U.S. Department of Health and Human Services) has a mission to encourage healthy living through various topics (e.g., how to eat in a healthy manner, types of physical activity).

- *SafeMedication* (safemedication.com, from ASHP) includes medication tips and tools and a searchable database of patient-focused drug monographs, pulled from AHFS.

CHAPTER CONTENT

CONTENT LEGEND

= Study
Tip Gal

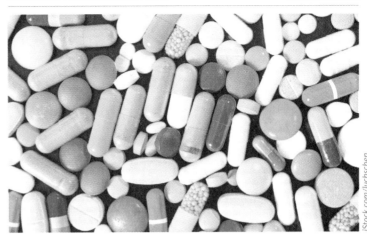

iStock.com/luchschen

CHAPTER 6

DRUG FORMULATIONS & PATIENT COUNSELING

DRUG FORMULATION CONSIDERATIONS

Compressed tablets are the most common formulation type and the least expensive to manufacture. Capsules are also relatively inexpensive to make. If a pharmaceutical company develops a drug in another formulation, the cost will be higher, and there must be a patient group that would benefit from the new formulation. For example, methylphenidate 10 mg immediate-release tablets cost ~$1.00 per tablet. The branded patch, *Daytrana,* is ~$18 per patch. The higher-priced formulation is beneficial in a child who can't swallow tablets or doesn't want to take doses during the day while at school.

It is helpful to recall drug formulation types by asking two questions:

1. Who uses this drug (e.g., which condition/patient population)?

2. Is there a reason to have this type of formulation for this patient population?

These questions can be useful on the exam when unsure if a particular formulation exists.

EXAMPLE: OLANZAPINE

Olanzapine is an antipsychotic that has various formulation options: immediate-release (IR) tablet, orally disintegrating tablet (ODT), short-acting injection and long-acting injection.

Who uses this drug?

People with schizophrenia, bipolar disorder or some type of psychosis.

Why are different formulations beneficial?

Patients with schizophrenia often discontinue their antipsychotics. A long-acting injection can improve adherence. ODTs dissolve quickly in the mouth; they are useful to prevent the patient from hiding the medication in the mouth ("cheeking") and then spitting it out when no one is watching. The likelihood of "cheeking" is further reduced by giving a drink of water after the ODT. The short-acting injection works quickly and is useful for acute agitation.

EXAMPLE: ONDANSETRON

Ondansetron is a 5-HT3 receptor antagonist (5-HT3 RA) used to prevent or treat nausea. It is available in various formulations: IR tablet, oral solution, ODT, oral film and short-acting injection.

Who uses this drug?

Patients receiving emetogenic drugs (e.g., chemotherapy), post-surgical patients or patients with any condition that causes nausea/vomiting.

Why are different formulations beneficial?

Oral medications will not be very effective when a patient is vomiting; an injection would be useful in this case if the patient is in a medical setting. An ODT or oral film can be useful for nausea without vomiting. Dysphagia (difficulty swallowing) is common in patients receiving chemotherapy and with other conditions (e.g., post-stroke, elderly). It would be difficult to swallow tablets with painful esophageal ulcers, strictures or tumors. An oral solution would be preferred in many of these cases. Though tablets can sometimes be crushed and put down a nasogastric (NG) tube, oral solutions are typically preferred when giving medications via NG tube.

Another 5-HT3 RA, granisetron, comes in a long-acting patch (*Sancuso*) that prevents chemotherapy-induced nausea for up to seven days. The patch is applied before the chemotherapy to allow time for the drug to be absorbed through the skin.

ORAL FORMULATIONS

The majority of solid tablets and capsules are designed to be swallowed whole. These can be short-acting or long-acting formulations. Other oral medications include liquids (mainly solutions and suspensions), ODTs, chewable tablets, sublingual tablets/films and granules/powders. See the table below for a summary of oral formulations and their common uses.

FORMULATION	EXAMPLES	REASONS FOR USE
Long-acting oral tablets/capsules	*Concerta* – methylphenidate *Detrol LA* – tolterodine The following suffixes indicate a long-acting formulation: XL, XR, ER, LA, SR, CR, CRT, SA, TR, "cont" (for controlled release); other products may have 24, timecaps or sprinkles in the name. **Osmotic Controlled-Release Oral Delivery System (OROS)** *Concerta, Cardura XL, Procardia XL, Delzicol* and other long-acting medications use an OROS delivery system. Water from the gut is absorbed into the delivery system by osmosis, which increases the pressure inside and forces the drug out through a small opening. The tablet/capsule shell may be visible in the patient's stool (called a ghost tablet/capsule), but the drug has been released (important counseling point). There are several types of OROS formulations. For example, *Concerta* has an outer layer that allows for fast drug delivery, followed by an extended-release.	Drugs may be designed to release slowly to avoid nausea or to provide a long duration of action. Providing a smooth level of drug release over time reduces high "peaks," which reduces side effects (e.g., less drug hitting the "wrong" receptor) and provides a safe level of drug over the dosing interval. Patients must be counseled to not crush or chew any drug that is a long-acting formulation (including ER opioids). It could release all the medication at once, and a fatal dose could be released. Some long-acting capsules (e.g., *Xtampza ER*) can be opened and the contents sprinkled on certain foods. The capsule contents should not be crushed or chewed. Always consult package labeling, as not all formulations have been studied in this way. ISMP's "Do Not Crush List" is a useful resource for drugs that should not be crushed. There are a few long-acting formulations that should not be crushed but can be cut on the score line (e.g., *Toprol XL*, carbidopa/levodopa ER).
Liquid oral suspensions	*Augmentin* – amoxicillin/clavulanate *Tylenol Children's* – acetaminophen, for children	Useful in patients with swallowing difficulty or who are unable to follow directions (e.g., infants and young children, adults with altered mental status, animals). Liquid medications can be administered in the side of the mouth using a dropper, and most can be administered via a feeding tube. Suspensions must be shaken to redisperse the medication prior to administration. Shaking is not required for solutions, as the drug is evenly distributed in the solvent.
Liquid oral solutions	*Constulose* – lactulose, for hepatic encephalopathy *Neurontin* – gabapentin, for neuropathic pain *Rapamune* – sirolimus, for prevention of rejection after organ transplant	

FORMULATION	EXAMPLES	REASONS FOR USE
Chewable tablets	*Singulair* – montelukast *Lamictal* – lamotrigine	Primarily used for children who are unable to swallow tablets. A few chewable products are used by adults. Chewable calcium products are popular because calcium tablets are large and hard for many people to swallow. Lanthanum carbonate (*Fosrenol*) is a phosphate binder that must be chewed for the drug to bind phosphate in the gut.
Lozenges/troches for drug administration to the oral mucosa	Clotrimazole, for oral thrush *Cepacol* – benzocaine/menthol, for sore throat	Used to treat a condition in the oral mucosa; the drug is held in the mouth while the troche slowly dissolves.
Orally disintegrating tablets (ODTs) Placed on the tongue and disintegrates rapidly in saliva (i.e., drinking liquid is not needed) Films that dissolve in the mouth are similar to ODTs	*Lamictal ODT* – lamotrigine, for seizures *Nurtec* - rimegepant, for migraines *Remeron SolTab* – mirtazapine, for depression *Zyprexa Zydis* – olanzapine, for schizophrenia Ondansetron – for nausea, dysphagia	An ODT may be helpful when a patient cannot swallow tablets/capsules due to dysphagia (difficulty swallowing). Paralysis of the throat muscles from stroke is the most common cause. Other causes of dysphagia include: esophagitis, esophageal tumors, ↓ LES pressure/reflux, facial swelling from an allergic reaction and conditions that worsen motor function, including Parkinson disease. Children are often unable to swallow tablets or capsules. Nausea can make it difficult to tolerate anything orally. If vomiting is present or expected, a non-oral route should be used (e.g., a suppository). Non-adherence: ODTs dissolve quickly, which can help prevent "cheeking" (i.e., hiding the drug in the mouth for later disposal).
Sublingual (SL) or buccal delivery with a tablet, film, powder or spray	*Edluar* – zolpidem SL tablet Nitroglycerin SL tablet *Subsys, Fentora* – various fentanyl formulations	SL and buccal formulations have the same benefits as ODTs. With SL/buccal absorption, the onset of action is faster than with a tablet or capsule that is swallowed; the drug is readily absorbed into the venous circulation at the administration site (e.g., under the tongue). Less drug is lost to gut degradation and first-pass metabolism.
Granules, powders or capsules that can be opened and sprinkled into soft food or water**	**Sprinkled on Applesauce** *Adderall XR* – dextroamphetamine/amphetamine ER *Coreg CR* – carvedilol *Dexilant* – dexlansoprazole *Focalin XR* – dexmethylphenidate *Namenda XR* – memantine *Nexium* – esomeprazole *Ritalin LA* – methylphenidate **Other Specific Instructions** *Cambia* – diclofenac powder, in water *Creon* and other pancreatic enzyme products – pancrelipase, on soft food with a low pH (applesauce, pureed pears or banana) *Depakote Sprinkles* – valproic acid, on soft food Potassium chloride ER capsules – on applesauce or pudding *Questran, Questran Light* – cholestyramine, in 2-6 oz water or non-carbonated liquid *Singulair* – montelukast granules, in 5 mL of baby formula or breast milk or in a spoonful of applesauce, carrots, rice or ice cream *Vyvanse* – lisdexamfetamine, in water, yogurt or orange juice	These formulations are primarily for pediatric or geriatric patients who have difficulty swallowing. An oral medication may be given via NG tube rather than converting to IV administration. Some medications are not available in an IV formulation. Instruct the patient on the following: ■ Do not chew any long-acting pellets or beads that are emptied out from a capsule. ■ If capsule contents are mixed in food or liquid, do not let the mixture sit too long (take within the time directed). Use a small amount of food or liquid; the entire mixture should be ingested to ensure the full dose is taken. ■ Do not add to anything warm or hot (the contents will dissolve too quickly). **Always refer to the product labeling for instructions; not all capsule medications should be opened and administered (refer to long-acting capsules section earlier in this table). Medications should only be mixed in the specific foods/liquids that were studied, because the pH of the food/liquid could be critical. Many medications have specific instructions for oral vs. NG tube administration.

RISKS OF SWEETENERS

Formulations that are exposed to taste buds (e.g., ODTs) often contain sweeteners (e.g., aspartame, saccharin), which are generally well-tolerated but can be problematic for some people. Sorbitol metabolism produces gas, cramping and bloating in sensitive patients, including those with irritable bowel syndrome. Phenylalanine is found in the sweetener aspartame, which is used in many ODT, chewable and granule medication formulations. It is a dangerous sweetener for those with phenylketonuria (PKU), a genetic defect in which the enzyme that degrades phenylalanine is absent. Lactose is the most commonly used excipient in drug formulations. It may be an issue in patients with lactose intolerance. Additional sweeteners and excipients are reviewed in the Nonsterile Compounding chapter.

ODT AND ORAL FILM COUNSELING

- Orally disintegrating tablets: do not attempt to push the tablets through foil backing as they are friable (i.e., easily broken/ crumbled). With dry hands, peel back the foil of one blister and remove the tablet.

- Place tablet (or film) on the tongue; it will dissolve in seconds. Once dissolved, you may swallow with saliva. Administration with liquid is not necessary. Wash hands after administration.

SELECT MEDICATIONS IN UNIQUE FORMULATIONS

Medications are increasingly offered in new, unique formulations (e.g., *Onzetra Xsail*, a nasal powder for migraine, or *Cotempla XR-ODT*, a long-acting ODT for ADHD). These formulations are reviewed in the disease state chapters of this book. The following sections summarize commonly encountered unique formulations, including example products and general counseling information. More specific counseling points for drugs that are available in these formulations can be found in the individual disease state chapters.

INJECTIONS

Injections can be given by various routes, including intradermal, subcutaneous, intramuscular (for short- or long-acting effects) and intravenous (see examples in the table below). Injections that patients give themselves are almost always given by SC injection. IM injections use a longer needle and generally hurt more (due to muscle soreness). *EpiPen* is an IM injection that is given in the thigh for acute need (e.g., bronchoconstriction, wheezing); see the Drug Allergies & Adverse Drug Reactions chapter for details.

FORMULATION	EXAMPLES	REASONS FOR USE
Subcutaneous (SC) injections that patients can mostly self-administer	*Enbrel* - etanercept, for rheumatoid arthritis and other autoimmune conditions *Forteo* - teriparatide, for osteoporosis *Imitrex* – sumatriptan, for acute migraine (abortive treatment) Insulins, GLP-1 agonists – see Diabetes chapter *Lovenox* - enoxaparin, for anticoagulation Naloxone – for opioid overdose reversal *Otrexup* - methotrexate, for rheumatoid arthritis	SC administration is used for rapid effect (e.g., for pain or opioid overdose), for drugs that would degrade or not be absorbed if given by oral administration (e.g., enoxaparin, etanercept) or when oral administration is not tolerated (e.g., due to vomiting).
Long-acting intramuscular (IM) injections	*Abilify Maintena* – aripiprazole *Haldol Decanoate*– haloperidol decanoate *Invega Sustenna, Invega Trinza* – paliperidone *Lupron Depot* – leuprolide *Risperdal Consta* – risperidone *Zyprexa Relprevv* – olanzapine	Various drugs come as long-acting injections to improve adherence (such as antipsychotics) or to ↓ the need for more frequent (painful) injections.
Intravenous (IV) injections	Many acute care drugs	Bypasses the oral route for patients who are intubated or sedated; fast response (can quickly achieve desired concentrations); avoids loss of drug due to N/V.

Injectable Medication Counseling

STEP 1	STEP 2	STEP 3	STEP 4	STEP 5
Wash hands	Prepare injection	Select and clean injection site	Inject	Discard syringes, pen needles or entire assembly in sharps container

©UWorld
LCosmo/stock.adobe.com
iStock.com/ZernLiew

- Inject at least 1 inch away from the previous injection site.
- Never use the same needle more than once.
- Some injections "click" when the needle enters the skin and/or "click" when the injection is complete.
- With single-use devices, discard the needle or entire assembly (with attached needle) in a sharps container.
- Do not rub the skin near anticoagulant injections (e.g., enoxaparin, fondaparinux); rubbing can cause severe bruising.
- Do not use any device to heat up cold injections; let the injection sit at room temperature for ~20 minutes.
- Liquids can degrade; if a solution is discolored or contains particles, do not use. Do not use beyond the expiration date.

Biologics and Biosimilars

Biologic medications are those isolated form natural sources and include vaccines, blood and blood components, gene therapies and recombinant proteins. Monoclonal antibodies ("-mAbs") are a type of biologic; they are injectable proteins used to treat many diseases (e.g., cancer, autoimmune conditions). Most monoclonal antibodies can cause injection reactions and require premedication (e.g., acetaminophen and diphenhydramine) to prevent severe symptoms. Select drugs require administration in a healthcare setting under medical supervision to monitor for reactions (e.g., omalizumab).

Regardless of the condition being treated, biologics have similar counseling points for storage and handling. Proteins can easily denature (break apart) if handled incorrectly. Patients should be instructed not to shake the medication, and to avoid exposing the drug to extreme temperatures (hot or cold). Many of these drugs should be stored in the refrigerator prior to use; if refrigeration is needed, they should be slowly brought to room temperature prior to injecting (injecting cold drug is painful).

Many biologics (including mAbs) also have approved biosimilars, which are biologic drugs that are structurally similar to the original/reference biologic drug with no clinically meaningful difference in safety and efficacy. They are essentially a "generic" for a biologic, though true generics are not possible due to the complexity of the compounds. Biosimilars can be recognized by the inclusion of a 4-letter code at the end of their name (e.g., adalimumab-bwwd, pegfilgrastim-pbbk). The 4-letter code does not signify anything specific, simply that the drug is a biosimilar. Biosimilars require the same special handling as the original biologic.

PATCHES

Patch Administration Sites

Most patches (e.g., *Catapres-TTS*, fentanyl transdermal) can be applied to one or more of these common application sites:

- Chest (upper)
- Back (upper and lower)
- Upper arm (on the part facing out)
- Flanks (sides of the body, abdomen level)

Exelon is applied to the same sites, but not the flanks. *Butrans* is applied to the same sites, except rather than the sides of the body near the abdomen, it is applied to the sides of the body, level to the chest. Some pain patches (e.g., *Flector*, *Lidoderm*, *Salonpas* and *Qutenza*) treat local pain, and are applied over the painful area.

The patches in the figures below have unusual application sites. *Daytrana* is applied on the hip, alternating right and left hips daily. *Transderm Scop* is applied behind the ear, at least four hours before needed, alternating ears every 72 hours. Never apply patches with estrogen on the breasts, or testosterone on the scrotum (testicles and surrounding area). Patches can irritate the skin; sites where the patch is placed, with the exception of the topical pain patches, should be alternated.

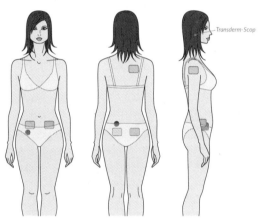

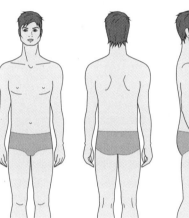
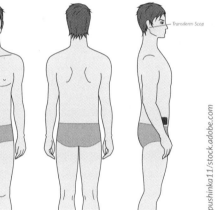

pushinka11/stock.adobe.com

Xulane (back, abdomen, arm or buttock)
Daytrana (hip)
Oxytrol (abdomen, hip or buttock)

Vivelle-Dot (lower abdomen or buttock)
Transderm-Scop (behind the ear)

Daytrana (hip)
Transderm-Scop (behind the ear)

PATCH FREQUENCY

Twice Daily
Diclofenac

Daily
Methylphenidate *(Daytrana)*: QAM, 2 hours prior to school

Nicotine *(NicoDerm CQ)*

Rivastigmine *(Exelon)*

Rotigotine *(Neupro)*

Selegiline *(Emsam)*

Testosterone *(Androderm)*: nightly, not on scrotum

Daily (With Special Instructions)
Lidocaine *(Lidoderm)*: 1-3 patches (as needed), on for 12 hours, off for 12 hours

Nitroglycerin: on for 12-14 hours, then off for 10-12 hours

Every 72 Hours
Fentanyl: Q72H, if it wears off after 48 hours, change to Q48H

Scopolamine *(Transderm Scop)*: Q72H, PRN

Twice Weekly
Estradiol* *(Alora, Vivelle-Dot)*

Oxybutynin *(Oxytrol)*

Weekly
Donepezil *(Adlarity)*

Buprenorphine *(Butrans)*

Clonidine *(Catapres-TTS)*

Estradiol* *(Climara)*

Estradiol/Levonorgestrel

Ethinyl estradiol/norelgestromin *(Xulane, Zafemy)* and ethinyl estradiol/levonorgestrel *(Twirla)*: weekly for 3 weeks, off for 1 week

Estradiol patches may be used on continuous or cyclic (3 weeks on, 1 week off) schedules at the frequency listed above.

Patch Counseling

QUESTION	RESPONSE
Can I cut the patch into pieces?	■ Usually no, except *Lidoderm* and *Qutenza*, which are designed to be cut and applied over the painful regions.
Can the patch be exposed to heat from an electric blanket, heating pad or body temperature > 38°C (> 100.4°F)?	■ Avoid heat exposure with most patches. Heat causes rapid absorption of the medication from the patch, resulting in toxicity. With fentanyl and buprenorphine, this can be quickly toxic (fatal).
The patch is bothering my skin. What can I do?	■ Never apply to skin that is irritated. ■ Alternate the application site. ■ The skin should not be shaved shortly before applying; shaving is irritating to the skin. If needed, cut the hair short with scissors. A topical steroid, such as hydrocortisone, can be applied after the patch is removed.
Which patches need to be removed prior to an MRI?	■ Patches containing metal (e.g., aluminum) need to be removed prior to an MRI or the metal will burn the skin: ❑ Clonidine *(Catapres-TTS)* ❑ Rotigotine *(Neupro)* ❑ Scopolamine *(Transderm Scop)* ❑ Testosterone *(Androderm)* ■ Patches containing the same medication (e.g., generics) may vary in metal content between different manufacturers. It is widely recommended that estradiol patches (e.g., *Alora*, generic estradiol) be removed prior to an MRI. Other patches with variable recommendations include nitroglycerin, oxybutynin, diclofenac, nicotine and fentanyl. Always verify the labeling for a specific product.
Can the patch be covered with tape if it will not stick or falls off?	■ Most patches cannot be covered with tape. A few patches can be taped around the edges. ■ Fentanyl and buprenorphine *(Butrans)* can be covered only with the permitted adhesive film dressings, *Bioclusive* or *Tegaderm*. ■ *Catapres-TTS* comes with its own adhesive cover, which goes over the patch to hold it in place. ■ Never apply patches to skin that is oily. ■ When applied, patches have to be smoothed out on the skin, and then pressed down for a number of seconds, usually 10-30 seconds.
Where is the patch applied?	■ Common application sites include the upper chest or upper/sides of the back (below the neck), upper thigh or upper outer arm; select patches have unique application sites (see previous page). Always verify with product labeling.
How do I dispose of used patches?	■ In most cases, remove and fold the patch to press adhesive surfaces together for disposal. Used drugs should be disposed of according to the manufacturer's instructions, such as throwing it away in a lidded container. ■ Some highly potent narcotic patches (e.g., fentanyl, *Butrans*) and *Daytrana* can be fatal if ingested after removal, especially for a child or pet. For these drugs, the FDA and/or manufacturer may recommend flushing the used patch down the toilet to remove it from the home immediately.
Where is the drug located?	■ The drug can be in a raised pouch, a reservoir (containing a gel or a semi-solid form) or directly incorporated into the adhesive of the patch (the side that adheres to the patient's skin).

TOPICALS

Medications applied to the skin can be used for both local effects or systemic effects throughout the body.

Topical medications used for their local effects have decreased systemic side effects and generally provide faster relief. This includes creams, ointments, gels and solutions. Common conditions treated topically include muscle/joint pain or inflammation, cold sores, acne, eczema or other skin rashes, mild skin infections and hair loss.

Examples of topical medications used for their localized effect include:

■ *Voltaren* – diclofenac gel, treats pain near the skin surface

■ Mupirocin ointment, treats some skin infections

Topical medications used for systemic effects (i.e., transdermal administration) can be used as an alternative to injections. Patches are a unique type of topical medication (discussed earlier) that are usually used for systemic effects. Another example includes testosterone gel *(Fortesta)*, which is used for hypogonadism/testosterone deficiency.

NASAL SPRAYS

The nasal route has a <u>faster onset</u> than the oral route and is <u>useful for acute conditions</u> that should be treated quickly, including pain. Nasal sprays <u>bypass</u> gut absorption and <u>first-pass metabolism</u>; some <u>proteins</u> that would get <u>destroyed in the gut</u> (e.g., calcitonin) can be given nasally. Patients with certain conditions may absorb a drug better nasally vs. orally (e.g., patients lacking intrinsic factor needed for oral absorption of vitamin B12). Examples of nasal sprays include:

- *Imitrex* – sumatriptan, fast onset, alternative to injection
- *Afrin* – oxymetazoline
- *Flonase Allergy Relief* – fluticasone

Afrin and *Flonase* are used primarily to treat <u>localized</u> nasal symptoms.

Nasal Spray Counseling

Before use
- <u>Shake</u> the bottle <u>gently</u> and remove the cap.
- <u>Prime</u> the pump before first use or when you have not used it recently (7 – 14 days on average).
- <u>Blow</u> your <u>nose</u> to clear your nostrils.

Using the spray
- <u>Close one nostril</u> (using your finger, see below) and insert the nasal applicator into the other nostril.
- Start to <u>breathe in</u> through your <u>nose</u>, and <u>press</u> firmly and quickly <u>down</u> once on the applicator to release the spray.

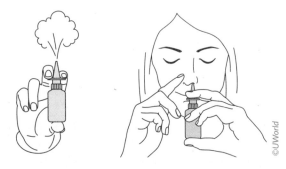

- <u>Breathe out</u> through your <u>mouth</u>.
- If a second spray is needed (in the same nostril or in the other nostril), repeat the above steps.
- Wipe the nasal applicator with a clean tissue and replace the cap.
- Use the bottle for the <u>labeled number of sprays</u> then discard, even if it is not completely empty.
- <u>Do not blow your nose</u> right after using the nasal spray.

EYE AND EAR DROPS

Eye drops and ear drops are used for <u>local effects</u>. <u>Eye drops</u> must be <u>sterile</u> (to prevent infection) and close to the <u>pH of the body</u> (to avoid pain upon administration). The ear is less sensitive, so ear drops have less stringent requirements. Because of this, <u>eye drops</u> can be <u>administered in the ear</u>, but <u>ear drops</u> can <u>never</u> be administered <u>in the eye</u>.

Eye Drop Counseling

- Wash your hands before and after using eye drops.
- Before you open the bottle, <u>shake it a few times</u>. <u>Gels</u> should be inverted and <u>shaken once</u> prior to use (to help the medication reach the tip).
- Bend your neck back so that you are <u>looking up</u>. Use one finger to <u>pull down your lower eyelid</u>. It is helpful, at least initially, to use a mirror.
- <u>Without</u> letting the tip of the bottle <u>touch your eye</u> or eyelid, release one drop of the medication by either squeezing the bottle or tapping on the bottom of the bottle. The drop should go into the space <u>between</u> your <u>eye</u> and your <u>lower eyelid</u>. If you squeeze in more than one drop, you are wasting medication.
- After you squeeze the drop of medication into your eye, <u>close your eye</u>. <u>Press a finger between your eye and the top of your nose</u> for at least <u>one minute</u> so more of the medication stays in your eye and you are less likely to have side effects. Blot extra solution from the eyelid with a tissue.
- If you need to use more than one eye drop:
  - ❏ If there are two drops of the same medication being given at the same time, wait five minutes between drops (do not administer two drops at once).
  - ❏ <u>Wait</u> at least <u>5 – 10 minutes</u> to put a <u>second medication</u> in the same eye. If administering a gel, wait <u>10 minutes</u>.
- If the eye drop contains a <u>preservative</u> called <u>benzalkonium chloride (BAK)</u> and you wear soft contact lenses, <u>remove lenses prior to administration and wait 15 minutes</u> to reinsert them.

Ear Drop Counseling

- If cold, gently shake the bottle or roll it in your hands for 1 – 2 minutes to warm the solution. Do not drop cold medication into the ear, as discomfort and dizziness can occur.
- Lie down or tilt the head so that the <u>affected ear faces up</u>.
- Gently pull the earlobe <u>up</u> and <u>back</u> for <u>adults</u> to straighten the ear canal. Pull <u>down</u> and <u>back</u> for <u>children < 3 years</u> (see image on next page).

- Administer the prescribed number of drops into the ear canal. Keep the ear facing up for about five minutes to allow the medication to coat the ear canal.

- Do not touch the dropper tip to any surface. To clean, wipe with a clean tissue.

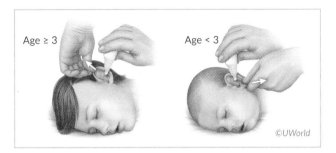

Age ≥ 3   Age < 3
©UWorld

RECTAL MEDICATIONS

Medications given rectally, such as suppositories and enemas, are used either for localized treatment (e.g., constipation, hemorrhoids) or for systemic treatment (e.g., diazepam rectal gel for acute seizures). Suppositories can also be used when the patient is NPO (i.e., nothing by mouth) and systemic treatment is needed (e.g., acetaminophen for pain or fever in an infant). Examples of common rectal medications include:

- *Rowasa* - mesalamine enema, treats local disease (distal ulcerative colitis)

- *Pedia-Lax* - glycerin suppository, treats constipation (stool is in rectum)

- *FeverAll* - acetaminophen suppository, treats pain/fever

Rectal Medication Counseling

All rectal products
- For best results, empty the bowel immediately before use.

Enemas
- Remove the bottle from the pouch and shake well. Remove the protective sheath from the applicator tip. Hold the bottle at the neck to prevent any of the medication from being discharged.

- Best results are obtained by lying on the left side with the left leg extended and the right leg flexed forward for balance. Gently insert the medication or applicator tip into the rectum, pointed slightly toward the navel to prevent damage to the rectal wall.

- Grasp the bottle firmly, and then tilt slightly so that the nozzle is aimed towards the back; squeeze slowly to instill the medication. Steady hand pressure will discharge most of the medication. After administering, withdraw and discard the bottle.

- Remain in position for at least 30 minutes, or preferably all night for maximum benefit.

Suppositories
- Detach one suppository from the strip. Remove the foil wrapper carefully while holding the suppository upright. Do not handle the suppository too much; heat from your hands and body can cause it to melt.

- Insert the suppository, with the pointed end first, completely into your rectum, using gentle pressure. Lubricating gel can be put on the suppository if needed.

- For best results, keep the suppository in your rectum for at least 1 – 3 hours.

VAGINAL MEDICATIONS

Medications administered vaginally can be used for local or systemic effects. Formulations given vaginally include suppositories, creams, ointments, inserts and tablets.

INHALATIONS

Inhaled medications provide immediate (rescue) and long-lasting (maintenance) benefits in lung disorders (e.g., asthma, COPD). The drug is delivered directly to the lungs, which minimizes systemic toxicities. Instructions for use are dependent on the type of device and the medication (see the Asthma, Chronic Obstructive Pulmonary Disease and Cystic Fibrosis chapters for details).

PATIENT COMMUNICATION

Counseling patients on safe and effective medication use is an essential role of pharmacists. Good communication skills are therefore essential for pharmacists, and are linked to patient satisfaction and trust.

HEALTH LITERACY

Pharmacists provide valuable information to patients, but the effort is wasted if the information is not understood. Health literacy is the degree to which individuals are able to obtain, process and understand basic health and medication information to make appropriate health decisions (e.g., being able to correctly interpret a prescription label). Health literacy is different than simply being able to read or being well educated.

Low health literacy is linked to poor health outcomes. It can be an issue for any patient but is more common in the elderly, minority populations, those with lower income, poor health and limited English proficiency. A person's health literacy is dependent on age, communication skills, knowledge, experience and culture. Only about 12% of adults have proficient health literacy.

Do not make assumptions about a patient's health literacy. Approach <u>all patients</u> as if they may not understand the health information presented. Health literacy can be assessed using measurement tools, such as those published by the Agency for Healthcare Research and Quality (AHRQ).

PATIENT COUNSELING

This section reviews best practices for patient counseling and common counseling points for most drugs.

Effective Communication and Education Strategies

- Use <u>non-medical language</u> ("layman's" language) that patients can understand (see the Counseling Language section). Example: say "tired" instead of "fatigued" or "high blood pressure" instead of "hypertension."

- Ask <u>open-ended questions</u> that require more than a "yes" or "no" answer. Example: "what questions can I answer about your medication today?" instead of "do you have questions?"

- Avoid leading questions. Example: "what about your high blood pressure concerns you?" instead of "are you concerned about the side effects from the high blood pressure medication?"

- Confirm understanding. Ask the patient to <u>repeat the information</u> or ask what they would tell their spouse or friend about the new medication.

- Use different communication strategies (<u>verbal, written, visual aids</u>) to enhance understanding. Ask the patient how they prefer to receive the information.

- Use active listening. Clarifying or summarizing what the patient has said is helpful and gives the patient an opportunity to offer correction.

- Speak clearly, make eye contact, introduce yourself and refer to patients by their name. Avoid "sweetie," "dear" and other similar terms.

Missed Doses

- Most medications follow this <u>general rule</u> for when a dose is missed:
  - If you miss a dose, take it <u>as soon as you remember</u>. If it is almost time for your next dose, skip the missed dose and take the next dose at your regularly scheduled time. Do <u>not</u> take <u>two doses at the same time</u> unless instructed by your healthcare provider.

- Exceptions that do not follow these instructions are discussed in the individual chapters. This includes:
  - High-risk drugs (e.g., anticoagulants, transplant medications)
  - Oral contraceptives
  - Drugs that must be taken at <u>specific times</u> (e.g., <u>phosphate binders, pancreatic enzymes</u> and prandial <u>insulin</u> that must be taken before a meal)

Medication Storage

Most medications can be <u>stored</u> in any <u>cool, dry place</u> (e.g., a medicine cabinet, not in a bathroom to avoid steam/humidity). Medications that require unique storage (e.g., in a refrigerator, in the original container) are highlighted throughout the individual disease state chapters.

Adherence Counseling and Monitoring

Pharmacists often review <u>refill histories</u> of medications to understand how a patient is actually using their medication at home. If the <u>medication is used to prevent/control a disease, nonadherence</u> can imply that the patient does not <u>understand</u> how to use their medication, the importance of their medication (common with conditions that have limited symptoms, such as hypertension), is experiencing <u>side effects</u> or requires <u>assistance in remembering</u> to take the drug (e.g., pill boxes or refill reminders).

If the <u>medication is used as needed</u> for acute symptoms (e.g., a rescue inhaler), a refill history can reveal how well the patient's condition is <u>controlled</u>. Infrequent use of a rescue/as needed medication means that the patient is not having symptoms frequently, whereas <u>frequent use</u> can imply that the patient is suffering from <u>symptoms</u> or <u>not using the medication correctly</u>.

When assessing adherence, remember to evaluate the reason for the drug first. Then use a refill history (and patient reports) to better understand what issues may be impacting medication use (see the following Case Scenario).

Counseling on adherence can be challenging; use of <u>motivational interviewing techniques</u> can help the pharmacist to better understand the patient and their individual needs. Motivational interviewing is a <u>counseling approach</u> that focuses on the <u>patient's priorities</u> to help facilitate change. Asking <u>open-ended questions</u>, employing empathy and reserving judgments will help to build patient relationships.

CASE SCENARIO

PK is a 43-year-old male who comes to the pharmacy today (11/14) for a refill of his medications. Upon reviewing his chart, the pharmacist sees the following refill history:

Last Fill	Rx	Medication	Sig	Quantity	Refills
10/24	64255	Sertraline 50 mg	Take one tablet by mouth daily for anxiety	30	1
10/24	64301	Lorazepam 1 mg	Take one tablet by mouth daily as needed for anxiety	30	1
10/1	64255	Sertraline 50 mg	Take one tablet by mouth daily for anxiety	30	2
10/1	64301	Lorazepam 1 mg	Take one tablet by mouth daily as needed for anxiety	30	2
9/12	64255	Sertraline 50 mg	Take one tablet by mouth daily for anxiety	30	3
9/12	64301	Lorazepam 1 mg	Take one tablet by mouth daily as needed for anxiety	30	3

Based on the instructions and your understanding of these medications, what is the purpose of each medication?
Sertraline is being used for maintenance/control of anxiety and lorazepam is being used as needed for acute symptoms of anxiety.

How long should each fill last, if used as instructed?
Each fill of sertraline (30 tablets) should last 30 days.
Each fill of lorazepam (30 tablets) should last at least 30 days, but longer if PK's anxiety is well controlled.

What does the refill history tell you?
PK is likely using both medications in the same way, as he is getting refills of both medications consistently at the same time. He may not be aware that his lorazepam should be used only when needed for symptoms, and that his sertraline should be taken daily (regardless of symptoms).

Furthermore, his refills do not appear to be lasting a full month; he may be taking both medications more frequently than prescribed. A discussion with PK is warranted to determine why these trends have occurred and if he understands how these medications should be taken. Open-ended, non-judgmental questions should be used to best evaluate his understanding.

COUNSELING LANGUAGE

Key counseling points for medications are presented in individual chapters throughout this course book, in simplified lists for easier learning. When counseling a patient, layman's language should be used for a better understanding. In the following table you will find example language that can be used when counseling a patient on common drug-related issues.

PATIENT COUNSELING	LANGUAGE TO USE
Allergy/anaphylaxis	Seek immediate medical help if you develop symptoms of a severe allergic reaction: severe rash with itching, redness or swelling, swelling in your face, lips, tongue or throat, wheezing or trouble breathing, or severe dizziness.
Anticholinergic effects	This medication can cause dry mouth, constipation, difficulty urinating, dry eyes and blurred vision. For select anticholinergic medications, include: this medication can make you feel drowsy.
Avoid grapefruit	Avoid eating grapefruit or drinking grapefruit juice while using this medication. Grapefruit can lead to higher levels of the medication in your blood, which will increase side effects.
Avoid in pregnancy (teratogenic)	This medication can cause birth defects if taken during pregnancy. Women who are pregnant or planning to become pregnant must not use this medication. Effective contraception is required.
Bleeding/bruising	This medication can cause bleeding, such as nosebleeds, bleeding gums and bruising. If you develop serious symptoms, such as coughing up blood or vomit that looks like coffee grounds, dark, tarry-looking stool, or bleeding in unusual places, such as blood in the urine or very large bruises, contact your prescriber immediately. Over-the-counter pain medications and natural products can increase bleeding risk. Talk to your pharmacist before taking any new medications.
Blood clot	This medication can increase the risk of a blood clot, which can be serious. Seek immediate medical help if you have symptoms of a clot. This can occur in your limbs, with symptoms such as swelling, redness or warmth in the lower leg (around the calf muscle) or arm. A blood clot in a lung or the heart can cause chest pain and trouble breathing. A clot in the brain (a stroke) can cause sudden confusion, numbness/weakness on one side of the body, trouble speaking or loss of consciousness.
Body fluid discoloration	This medication can change the color of your urine, saliva and sweat, and may stain clothing. This is not harmful. Some drugs can stain contact lenses.

PATIENT COUNSELING	LANGUAGE TO USE
Cancer	You are more likely to develop certain types of cancers while taking this medication, including skin cancer. Protect your skin from the sun. Use a broad-spectrum sunscreen, with an SPF of at least 30. Follow the recommendations you are given for cancer screenings.
Constipation	This medication can cause constipation. A laxative or stool softener can be helpful. Drink plenty of water, exercise regularly and eat food with fiber such as fruits, vegetables and grains.
Contains phenylalanine – do not use in phenylketonuria (PKU)	This medication contains an artificial sweetener called phenylalanine. People with phenylketonuria (PKU) should not use products that contain phenylalanine.
Decreased heart rate	This medication can decrease heart rate, which can cause dizziness. When you rise from a sitting or lying position, move slowly and carefully to prevent a fall. You may be instructed to monitor your heart rate.
Delirium	This medication can cause confused thinking and unusual behaviors. Contact your healthcare provider if this develops.
Dehydration	This medication can cause dehydration. Symptoms include dry mouth, increased thirst, less frequent urination, dizziness, headache and dry skin. If you develop severe symptoms, such as a rapid breathing and dark-colored urine, contact your healthcare provider immediately. Dehydration in an infant is dangerous. Symptoms can include a sunken soft spot of the head (called a fontanelle), no tears (i.e., when crying), lethargy and listlessness. Products like *Pedialyte* and *Enfalyte* can be used to replace fluids and minerals, such as sodium and potassium. Severe dehydration can require emergency medical treatment.
Depression/psychosis (also see suicidal ideation)	This medication can worsen or cause changes to your mood, including suicidal thoughts and behaviors. In some cases, your thoughts can become strange or psychotic. Notify your healthcare provider right away if your mood or behavior worsens.
Diarrhea	This medication can cause diarrhea. Drink fluids with electrolytes to prevent dehydration. Contact a healthcare provider if symptoms do not improve after a few days or if any of the following are present: age < 6 months, pregnancy, high fever (> 101°F), severe abdominal pain or blood in the stool.
Dizziness	This medication can cause dizziness, which is more likely to occur when you rise from a sitting or lying position. Rise slowly and carefully to prevent a fall.
Drowsiness	This medication can make you feel tired. Use caution when driving, operating machinery or performing other hazardous activities. Alcohol, sleeping pills, pain medications, antihistamines, antidepressants and other medications that cause drowsiness can make this side effect worse, which could be dangerous.
Drug interactions due to binding	This medication can bind to other medications and food, which can change the drug's absorption. Separate antacids, multivitamins/minerals, iron, magnesium, calcium, dairy products and calcium-rich foods from medications that can bind.
Drug interactions due to high gastric pH	This medication uses the acid in your stomach to be absorbed. If you are taking other medications to lower the acid in your stomach, such as heartburn medication, this medication will not work well. Talk to your pharmacist before taking medications to lower stomach acid.
Dry mouth	This medication can cause or worsen dry mouth. Sucking on sugarless hard candy or ice chips, sipping water or chewing sugarless gum can help. With dry mouth, it is especially important to keep your teeth clean to prevent cavities. Over-the-counter saliva substitutes can be helpful.
Dyspepsia	This medication can cause indigestion. Symptoms can include bloating, upset stomach, nausea, burping or heartburn. Taking the medication with food can be helpful. If the symptoms do not improve or worsen, contact your healthcare provider.
Edema	This medication can cause fluid and water to accumulate and cause swelling, especially in the ankles and legs. If you have heart disease, discuss the use of this medication with your healthcare provider, and monitor your weight.
Eye damage	Tell your healthcare provider immediately if you develop any eye pain or vision changes, such as seeing halos or having blurry vision.
Ghost tablet in stool	The tablet that contains this medication can pass into the stool. If there is a tablet in your stool, it is nothing to worry about; it is an empty tablet.
Gingival hyperplasia	This medication can cause swelling and growth of the gums around your teeth. Brush and floss often, and see your dentist for regular cleanings.
Heart failure	This medication can cause or worsen heart failure. Contact your healthcare provider if you develop symptoms, including trouble breathing, shortness of breath, rapid weight gain or swelling in the legs, ankles and feet.
Hyperglycemia	This medication can cause high blood sugar. Symptoms include more frequent urination and increased thirst and hunger. Check your blood sugar if you have a glucose meter. Tell your healthcare provider if you develop symptoms of high blood sugar.

PATIENT COUNSELING	LANGUAGE TO USE
Hyperthyroidism	This medication can change how your thyroid gland works. Tell your healthcare provider if you develop symptoms of an overactive thyroid, including increased sensitivity to heat, unexplained weight loss, thinning hair, unusual sweating, nervousness, irritability or restlessness. Tests can be ordered to check your thyroid function.
Hypoglycemia	This medication can cause low blood sugar. Symptoms can include dizziness, irritability, shakiness, sweating, hunger, confusion, fast heart rate and blurred vision. Check your blood sugar, if able, and eat or drink something with sugar, such as a ½ cup of orange juice or regular soda, 1 cup of milk, 1 tablespoon of honey or 3-4 glucose tablets or gel.
Hypothyroidism	This medication can lower the amount of thyroid hormone you produce. Tell your healthcare provider if you develop symptoms of low thyroid, including feeling tired or cold, weight gain, constipation or hair loss. Tests can be ordered to check your thyroid function.
Increased blood pressure	This medication can increase blood pressure. Monitor blood pressure as directed by your healthcare provider, especially if you have hypertension.
Increased heart rate	This medication can increase heart rate, which can cause dizziness. When you rise from a sitting or lying position, move slowly and carefully to prevent a fall. You may be instructed to monitor your heart rate.
Infection	This medication can lower your body's ability to fight infections. Avoid contact with people who are sick. Regular handwashing is one of the best ways to remove germs and avoid getting sick.
Injection site reaction	The spot where you inject this medication can become red, swollen, painful and itchy. If the area looks especially worrisome or is very painful, let your healthcare provider know.
Insomnia	This medication can cause difficulty sleeping. To improve your sleep, keep a regular sleep schedule and keep the bedroom dark, comfortable and quiet.
Lactic acidosis	This medication can cause a buildup of acid in the blood. Get immediate medical help if you feel very weak or tired, have unusual muscle pain, trouble breathing and/or stomach pain with nausea and vomiting.
Liver damage	This medication can damage the liver. Get medical help if you develop any of the following: yellowing of the white part of your eyes, yellowing of your skin, dark-colored urine, light-colored stool or bad stomach pain and nausea.
Lung damage	This medication can damage the lungs. Get medical help if you develop any of the following: severe/persistent cough, shortness of breath, chest pain or breathing that is difficult or painful.
Many drug interactions	There are many medications that can interact with this drug. Check with your healthcare provider or pharmacist before starting any new medications, including over-the-counter medications, vitamins and/or herbal products.
MedGuide required	This MedGuide contains important information about your medication. Take the MedGuide home and read it carefully so you understand the medication, and how to use it as safely as possible.
Muscle damage	This medication can cause muscle damage. If you develop unusual muscle pain, tenderness or weakness, or if you are urinating less than usual, get medical help.
Nausea	This medication can make you feel nauseous. Taking the medication with food and a glass of water can be helpful.
Nephrotoxicity	This medication can cause problems with the kidneys. Contact your prescriber right away if you have little or no urination, blood in the urine, swelling in your feet or ankles or rapid weight gain.
Orthostasis	This medication can cause the blood pressure to drop when you stand up, which can cause dizziness and light-headedness. This can cause falls and injuries. It is important to get up slowly when lying down or sitting, and to hold onto the bed rail or a strong tabletop until you feel steady.
Pancreatitis	This medication can damage the pancreas. If you are nauseous and have sharp pain in the upper abdomen that feels like it's radiating to your back, get medical help.
Paresthesia	This medication can cause a feeling of "pins and needles" in the legs, hands and feet. It is usually harmless.
Peripheral neuropathy	This medication can cause the nerves in your legs, feet, arms and/or fingers to become damaged. If you develop tingling, stabbing pain or numbness, such as in your feet, contact your prescriber.
Photosensitivity	This medication can cause your skin to be more sensitive to the sun. Stay out of the sun during midday hours, use sun-protective clothing and broad-spectrum sunscreen with an SPF of at least 30.
Priapism	If you develop a prolonged and painful erection that lasts more than four hours, stop using this medication and get medical help right away to avoid permanent damage to the penis.
QT prolongation	This medication can cause a condition called "QT prolongation," which makes the heartbeat too fast and not regular. This can cause dizziness and sudden fainting. If this happens, get immediate medical help. Check with your pharmacist before taking any new medications; other medications can make this more likely.

PATIENT COUNSELING	LANGUAGE TO USE
Rash	Mild rash: this drug can cause a mild rash. If it is itchy, taking 25 or 50 mg of diphenhydramine (*Benadryl*) should help. Severe rash: this medication can cause a severe rash that begins with a fever and flu-like symptoms, followed by a bright red rash. This is an allergic reaction that requires immediate medical help. Some medications can cause both a mild and severe rash.
Reduces ADEK absorption	This medication can block the amount of fat-soluble vitamins (A, D, E, K) that your body absorbs. Take a multivitamin at a different time of day than this medication.
Remove patch before an MRI	Some brands of this patch contain metal, which will burn your skin during an MRI. Remove the patch before an MRI.
Serotonin syndrome	This medication increases the level of serotonin in your blood. If it is taken with other over-the-counter or prescription medications that also increase serotonin, toxicity can occur. Seek urgent medical help if you feel dizzy, shaky, agitated, feverish and have a racing heartbeat.
Sexual dysfunction	This medication can cause sexual problems, including (select counseling point based on medication-specific side effects): ■ Decreased libido: low sexual drive/interest. ■ Ejaculation difficulties: anorgasmia (no ejaculation) or retrograde ejaculation (a "dry orgasm" or very little ejaculate during orgasm). ■ Erectile dysfunction (impotence): difficulty getting or maintaining an erection.
Stomach bleeding (especially for NSAIDs)	This medication can cause stomach bleeding. If your stools are black or tarry-looking, or if you are coughing or vomiting up blood that looks like coffee grounds, contact your healthcare provider immediately.
Subcutaneous injection	This medication is injected under the skin with a very short needle. Before injecting, wash your hands. Rotate where you inject, and do not inject into skin that is injured, tender or bruised.
Suicidal ideation (also see depression/psychosis)	This medication can increase the risk of having suicidal thoughts. Contact your prescriber right away if you notice symptoms of depression, unusual behavior, changes in mood or thoughts of hurting yourself.
Urinary tract infection	This medication increases the risk of a urinary tract infection. Contact your prescriber if you experience burning when you urinate, or if you need to go to the bathroom more often, and suddenly. The urine can also be darker than usual.
Vision changes	This medication can cause vision changes. Tell your healthcare provider if you notice that colors seem different, if there are halos around lights or if your vision becomes blurry.

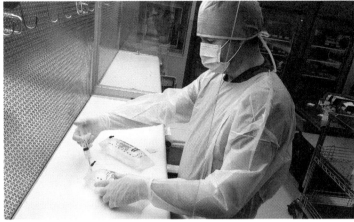

©Michael J. Freudiger

CHAPTER 7

INTRAVENOUS MEDICATION PRINCIPLES

BACKGROUND

Enteral administration [through the gastrointestinal (GI) tract] is the preferred route for drug delivery. When the enteral route is not feasible, a parenteral route (outside of the GI tract) is used. Common routes for parenteral drug administration include intravenous (IV), intramuscular or subcutaneous routes. Other parenteral routes are used for specific purposes, including intra-articular (into the joint) and intrathecal (into the space under the arachnoid membrane of the spinal cord). The intrathecal route is often used by anesthesiologists and for some chemotherapy, but intrathecal administration of select drugs is contraindicated (e.g., intrathecal vincristine is fatal).

IV DRUG DELIVERY

Oral medications require gut dissolution and absorption, which takes time. Common reasons for using a parenteral (IV) route of administration include:

- In hospitalized patients who are NPO (nothing by mouth) or when the gut needs to be bypassed (e.g., surgery, malabsorption).

- Drugs with poor oral bioavailability (e.g., vancomycin, which is only used orally for *C. difficile* treatment).

- When fast (stat) onset is required (e.g., critical situation, such as using a vasopressor to quickly raise cardiac output).

This chapter focuses on the aspects of intravenous administration that are important to the pharmacist, including venous access (IV lines), compatibility and stability issues and administration requirements.

CONTENT LEGEND

 = Key Drug Guy

PHYSIOCHEMICAL CONSIDERATIONS

OSMOLARITY AND TONICITY

Osmolarity and tonicity are related terms; both are used to express the solute concentration in solution. Osmolarity reflects all solutes per liter of solution and tonicity reflects the pressure gradient (and potential fluid shifts) created by solutes that do not cross biological membranes (e.g., the vasculature). Both osmolarity and tonicity can impact intravenous drug administration.

Osmolarity of Intravenous Formulations

Saline concentrations greater than 0.9% (osmolarity ~308 mOsm/L) are referred to as hypertonic. Hypertonic saline (commonly 3% or 23.4%) has various uses in the acute care setting, such as treating hyponatremia (3%) or preparing parenteral nutrition (23.4%). However, hypertonic saline injections can be fatal if given erroneously. When administered into a peripheral vein (see section on Peripheral Lines), the high concentration of solutes relative to the concentration in the blood will cause water to move out of the red blood cells (RBCs) in an attempt to dilute the solute concentration. This will cause the RBCs to become shriveled and dysfunctional.

To avoid adverse outcomes, hypertonic saline is often restricted to the pharmacy and only dispensed for administration in areas of the hospital where safety can be monitored (e.g., a critical care unit).

When a preparation has a lower osmolarity than blood (i.e., it is hypotonic), the RBCs will absorb fluid. This can cause hemolysis (i.e., the RBCs will burst), which can be fatal.

In general, ½NS (0.45%), which has an osmolarity of 154 mOsm/L, is the lowest saline concentration that should be administered intravenously alone. Lower saline concentrations, such as ¼NS (0.225%), can be administered with other fluids that will increase the total osmolarity, such as 5% dextrose. Osmolarity is discussed in more detail in the Calculations II chapter.

pH

The blood has a slightly alkaline pH of 7.35 – 7.45. The body uses the carbonic acid-bicarbonate buffer system to resist changes in pH:

- When the blood becomes more basic, the pH rises. Hydrogen ions (protons) will be released from carbonic acid, which causes the pH of the blood to lower.
- When the blood becomes more acidic, the pH falls. Hydrogen ions get picked up (more bicarbonate binds with protons), which causes the pH of the blood to rise.

There are two other buffer systems that resist changes in pH; the phosphate buffer system and the protein buffer system.

Drugs that are administered intravenously must be formulated to keep the pH within a narrow range to avoid damaging the veins and other tissues. A buffer system (similar to those in the body) may be needed to maintain normal pH.

The pH also impacts the stability of the drug in solution. See the Calculations IV chapter for more discussion on pH.

VENOUS CATHETERS

A catheter is a piece of plastic tubing that is inserted into the body to put fluids in or take them out (e.g., a urinary catheter). A catheter inserted into a vein is called a venous catheter and is used for fluid and drug delivery. A venous catheter is called a line, and the patient is said to have IV access. Lines come in two primary types: peripheral and central.

PERIPHERAL LINES

Percutaneous means through the skin and peripheral refers to locations away from the body's central compartment, such as the arms and legs. Most IV drugs can be delivered through percutaneous, peripheral venous catheters that are inserted into smaller veins. Common veins used for peripheral venous catheters are the cephalic vein in the arm, metacarpal veins in the hands, and the saphenous vein near the ankle.

Peripheral lines are simpler and less expensive to insert than central lines, but they have limitations. Administering drugs into smaller veins can cause phlebitis (vein irritation), venous thrombosis (clots) and interstitial fluid extravasation (when the catheter becomes dislodged from the vein and the infusion contents enter surrounding tissue).

CENTRAL LINES

A central line empties into a larger vein and the contents are quickly diluted. Central lines provide secure, long-term vascular (i.e., blood vessel) access and are required for the administration of:

- Highly concentrated drugs (e.g., potassium chloride > 10 mEq/100 mL)
- Long-term antibiotics (e.g., to treat osteomyelitis)
- Toxic drugs that would cause severe phlebitis or tissue damage [e.g., chemotherapy, especially with vesicants (see next column)] if given peripherally
- Drugs with a pH that is not close to blood pH (7.35 – 7.45)
- Drugs with high osmolarity (i.e., > ~900 mOsmol/L), such as parenteral nutrition

Central lines are sometimes used for patients with collapsed veins due to IV drug use. Additional benefits with a central line include the ability to administer higher volumes and use faster infusion rates.

Central Line Placement

To be considered a central venous catheter, also called a central line, the catheter tip must be located in a large vessel (e.g., superior vena cava, inferior vena cava). The catheter can reach one of these locations by being inserted into a proximal central vein or a peripheral vein. A line inserted in a proximal central vein can be placed in the internal jugular vein (near the top of the chest), subclavian vein (under the collarbone) or femoral vein (in the groin). These are in close proximity to the large vessels and do not require long catheters. Dialysis catheters are placed in this manner.

Peripherally inserted central catheters (PICC) are inserted by placing the line into a peripheral vein and advancing (pushing) the catheter through the vein until the tip ends in the superior vena cava (where the infusion contents will be released).

Central line placement is confirmed with an X-ray to confirm that the tip has reached the right location. A PICC empties into the superior vena cava from a line placed into a peripheral vein (see figure below).

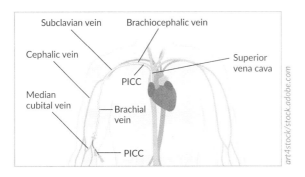

Vesicants are Safer with a Central Line

A vesicant is a drug that will cause severe tissue damage if the catheter tip comes out of the vein, allowing the drug to seep into the surrounding tissues (i.e., extravasate). Vesicants are preferentially administered through a central line because the line is less likely to become dislodged from the vein. Vesicants include vasopressors (e.g., dopamine, norepinephrine), anthracyclines (e.g., doxorubicin), vinca alkaloids (e.g., vincristine, vinblastine), digoxin, foscarnet, nafcillin, mannitol, mitomycin and promethazine.

PROMETHAZINE CAN CAUSE SEVERE TISSUE INJURY

Some hospitals have removed it from formulary due to this risk.

IM administration is preferred, but this also has a risk of tissue injury; intra-arterial or SC routes should not be used.

If using IV: dilute the drug, limit the dose and monitor the patient.

INCOMPATIBILITIES

Incompatible means that substances are unsuitable for use together. The end result could be a physical (e.g., color change, precipitation) or chemical (e.g., drug degradation) incompatibility. When substances deemed incompatible are used together, it can lead to safety concerns for the patient.

CHEMICAL INCOMPATIBILITY

Chemical incompatibility causes drug degradation or toxicity due to a hydrolysis, oxidation or decomposition reaction. These reactions are discussed in more detail in the Basic Science Concepts chapter.

PHYSICAL INCOMPATIBILITY

Physical incompatibilities occur between a drug and one of the following:

- The container (e.g., polyvinyl chloride containers)
- The diluent (solution) (e.g., dextrose or saline)
- Another drug

Container Incompatibility

DEHP from the Container

The majority of polyvinyl chloride (PVC) containers use diethylhexyl phthalate (DEHP) as a "plasticizer" to make the plastic bag more flexible. DEHP can leach from the container into the solution. DEHP is toxic and can harm the liver and, possibly, male fertility.

Container Absorption/Adsorption

Absorption occurs when drug moves into the PVC container, and adsorption occurs when drug adheres (or "sticks") to the container; either will reduce the drug's concentration.

Alternative (Non-PVC) Containers

Drugs that have leaching or absorption/adsorption issues with PVC containers can be placed in polyolefin, polypropylene or glass containers (although glass is heavy and can break). See the Key Drugs Guy on the following page for drugs that should not be placed in PVC containers.

Insulin and PVC Containers

Insulin adsorbs to PVC. Clinicians adjust the rate of insulin infusions to obtain blood glucose control, regardless of the type of IV container and tubing used. It might be useful to know that insulin does adsorb to PVC for testing purposes.

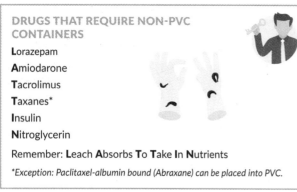

DRUGS THAT REQUIRE NON-PVC CONTAINERS

Lorazepam

Amiodarone

Tacrolimus

Taxanes*

Insulin

Nitroglycerin

Remember: **L**each **A**bsorbs **T**o **T**ake **I**n **N**utrients

*Exception: Paclitaxel-albumin bound (Abraxane) can be placed into PVC.

iStock.com/grivina, VikiVector

Diluent Incompatibility

When drugs are diluted in solution for IV administration, they are commonly placed into a small volume (e.g., 100 mL or less) IV bag that contains 5% dextrose (D5W) or 0.9% sodium chloride (normal saline, NS). For most drugs, either solution is acceptable, but some drugs cannot be put into dextrose, and others cannot be put into saline (see Key Drugs Guy below). These drugs may also be compatible with sterile water, but that would be for reconstitution (e.g., for a drug that comes as a powder) and not for diluting in large volumes for infusion into a patient.

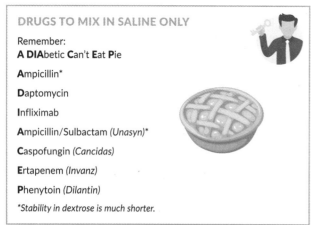

DRUGS TO MIX IN SALINE ONLY

Remember:
A DIAbetic **C**an't **E**at **P**ie

Ampicillin*

Daptomycin

Infliximab

Ampicillin/Sulbactam (*Unasyn*)*

Caspofungin (*Cancidas*)

Ertapenem (*Invanz*)

Phenytoin (*Dilantin*)

*Stability in dextrose is much shorter.

iStock.com/Naddiya

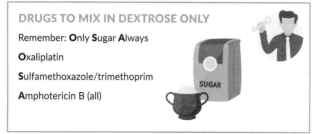

DRUGS TO MIX IN DEXTROSE ONLY

Remember: **O**nly **S**ugar **A**lways

Oxaliplatin

Sulfamethoxazole/trimethoprim

Amphotericin B (all)

GreenSkyStudio/stock.adobe.com

Drug-Drug Incompatibility

Hospitalized patients are usually receiving IV fluids with multiple IV medications. To minimize the number of inserted peripheral and central lines, infusion bags are often joined together in a Y-site and administered in the same line.

Y-Site Administration: Mixing Drugs in the Line

A Y-site describes the shape that forms when lines (from different IV containers) are joined prior to entering the patient. Often, the large (1 liter) container is the patient's fluids and the smaller IV bag [called an IV piggyback (IVPB)] contains the drugs. Since the drugs mix together briefly in the common portion of the IV tubing, it is important that the drugs and solutions are compatible with Y-site administration.

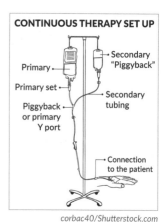

CONTINUOUS THERAPY SET UP

Primary

Primary set

Piggyback or primary Y port

Secondary "Piggyback"

Secondary tubing

Connection to the patient

corbac40/Shutterstock.com

Additive Compatibility: Mixing Drugs in the Same Container

Additive compatibility needs to be confirmed when putting multiple drugs together in the same container or syringe. Drugs mixed in the same container will be in contact for a longer period of time (compared to Y-site administration), so compatibility may differ. Additive compatibility and Y-site compatibility are often listed separately in drug references.

HIGH-RISK INCOMPATIBILITIES

A dangerous example of incompatibility involves ceftriaxone and calcium. Ceftriaxone cannot be mixed with any calcium-containing solutions due to the risk of precipitates. Lactated Ringer's, a common IV fluid, contains calcium and cannot be mixed with ceftriaxone, including Y-site administration. This combination must be avoided in all age groups; neonates have the highest risk for lethal effects.

Calcium and phosphate can form a deadly precipitate in intravenous fluids. The Calculations III chapter discusses methods to prevent calcium-phosphate precipitation when preparing parenteral nutrition.

Information regarding incompatibilities is extensive. Many commonly used drugs (e.g., heparin, IV quinolones, piperacillin/tazobactam, caspofungin, amphotericin B, sodium bicarbonate) are incompatible with other commonly used drugs.

The pharmacist is the primary resource for compatibility questions; reputable resources are required. The primary resources include _ASHP Injectable Drug Information_, _Trissel's 2 Clinical Pharmaceutics Database_, the _King Guide to Parenteral Admixtures_ (commonly called _King's_) and the drug's package insert. Some drug information databases use the IV compatibility information from _Trissel's_ (see Drug References chapter). Recent concerns regarding compatibility issues can also be found in _Pharmacy Practice News_ and _Hospital Pharmacy_. The next section provides an example of how these resources are used in practice.

> ### _BEWARE!_
>
> **Mixing Together Can Be Fatal**
>
> Risk of precipitates→ emboli→ fatality
>
> Calcium & Ceftriaxone*
>
> Calcium & Phosphate**
>
> *_Lactated Ringer's contains calcium._
> **_When calcium and phosphate are both put into parenteral nutrition, methods must be used to reduce the risk of a precipitate._

REFERENCE TABLE INTERPRETATION

The tables shown in this section are similar to tables used to check drug compatibility. The reference drug is listed at the top of the table (cefepime, in the example below) and the drug tested with it for compatibility issues is listed in the row below (gentamicin). A pharmacist can check whether cefepime can be mixed with gentamicin in the same container. The table below reports that cefepime and gentamicin are incompatible (I in the last column) when mixed together in either D5W or NS, at the concentrations listed. In addition to the C/I rating, the remarks (e.g., "cloudiness") include that a precipitate had formed.

Cefepime

DRUG	MFR	CONC/L	MFR	CONC/L	TEST SOLN	REMARKS	REF	C/I
Gentamicin	ES	1.2 g	BR	40 g	D5W, NS	Cloudiness forms in 18 hr at room temp	588	I

C = compatible; I = incompatible

In this next example, a pharmacist can check if cefepime can be given in the same line when gentamicin is infusing (Y-site administration). The pharmacist will find that cefepime and gentamicin are compatible for Y-site administration at the concentrations listed, indicated by the "C" in the far right column and by the remarks.

Cefepime

DRUG	MFR	CONC	MFR	CONC	REMARKS	REF	C/I
Gentamicin	ES	6 mg/mL	BMS	120 mg/mL	Physically compatible with less than 10% cefepime loss. Gentamicin was not tested.	2212	C

C = compatible; I = incompatible
Y-Site Injection Compatibility (1:1 Mixture)

FILTERS

Filters can be required during drug compounding, administration or both. In-line filters (attached to the IV tubing) are used to administer drugs that have a risk of particulates, precipitates, crystals, contaminants or entrapped air in the final solution. The size of the filter required is determined by the size of the particles to be removed. The majority of drugs which require filters use a 0.22 micron filter (1 micron = 1/1,000 mm). Another common filter size is 1.2 micron, which is used for parenteral nutrition to catch calcium-phosphate particulates, and injectable lipid emulsions (e.g., *Intralipid*). Some drugs come packaged with the required filter. Large molecule drugs, including many liposomal formulations of chemotherapy drugs, must not be filtered due to the size of the drug particle.

If compounding IV medications packaged in glass ampules, filter needles or filter straws are used when withdrawing the solution from the ampule to prevent glass particulates from entering the IV bag; a filter may also be required in the line during administration.

COMMON DRUGS WITH FILTER REQUIREMENTS

KEY DRUGS

My **GAL Is PAT**
who has a **MaP**

Golimumab

Amphotericin B (lipid formulations)*

Lipids-1.2 micron

Isavuconazonium

Phenytoin**

Amiodarone

Taxanes
(cabazitaxel and conventional paclitaxel)

Mannitol ≥ 20%

Parenteral nutrition-1.2 micron

*Larger pore size filter required; prepare using a 5 micron filter
**Phenytoin requires a filter when administered by continuous infusion; a filter is not required for IV push

Others:

Abatacept

Albumin (select products)

Antithymocyte globulin

Infliximab

iStock.com/littlemissk
belokrylowa/stock.adobe.com

TEMPERATURE & STABILITY

A drug that is "stable" will be stable only at select concentrations, for a certain time, at a certain temperature and with a certain degree of light exposure.

Time in Solution

Solutions decompose faster than solid (e.g., powder) formulations. The likelihood of a chemical reaction that would degrade the drug increases with time. Compatibility concerns due to longer infusion times have become an important issue with antibiotic extended infusions (e.g., piperacillin/tazobactam). The same drug is commonly used with shorter infusions, without stability issues. The longer infusion period is used to increase time above the minimum inhibitory concentration (T > MIC) in order to more effectively kill the target pathogens. The higher T > MIC is beneficial, but the longer infusion times result in more compatibility issues and drug interactions.

Temperature

Higher temperatures speed up chemical reactions and break down proteins. The majority of IV drugs are refrigerated in order to permit longer stability (i.e., a longer period until the expiration or beyond-use date). There are exceptions; for example, because furosemide and phenytoin crystallize if kept cold, they are stored at room temperature. See the Key Drugs Guy below for IV drugs that are kept at room temperature.

DO NOT REFRIGERATE

KEY DRUGS

Remember:
Dear **S**weet **P**harmacist,
Freezing **M**akes **M**e **E**dgy!

Dexmedetomidine*

Sulfamethoxazole/Trimethoprim

Phenytoin – crystallizes

Furosemide – crystallizes*

Metronidazole

Moxifloxacin

Enoxaparin

*Optional: diluted dexmedetomidine and furosemide can be kept cold.

Others:

Acetaminophen

Acyclovir – crystallizes

Deferoxamine – precipitates

Levetiracetam

Pentamidine –crystallizes

Valproate

iStock.com/hendart, igorshi

Light Exposure

Light exposure causes photo-degradation, which destroys some drugs, and in some cases, increases a drug's toxicity (e.g., nitroprusside). Many medications should be protected from light during storage to avoid degradation. Some medications are supplied in amber (light-protected) vials, and others are stored in the original packaging (foil overwrap or box) until needed. A small number of drugs are so light-sensitive that they require protection from light during administration. Pharmacy staff dispense these medications with a light-protective cover. In some cases, light-protective tubing (generally amber-colored) is needed. See the Key Drugs Guy on the right for a list of photosensitive drugs that require light protection during administration.

PROTECT FROM LIGHT DURING ADMINISTRATION

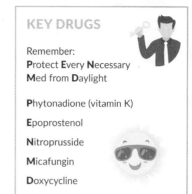

KEY DRUGS

Remember:
Protect **E**very **N**ecessary **M**ed from **D**aylight

Phytonadione (vitamin K)

Epoprostenol

Nitroprusside

Micafungin

Doxycycline

Others:

Amphotericin B Deoxycholate

Anthracyclines

Dacarbazine (if extravasates, protect exposed tissues from light)

Pentamidine

iStock.com/Teploleta

Do Not Shake/Agitate

Agitation destroys some drugs, including hormones and other proteins. Drugs that are easily destroyed/damaged should not be shaken during compounding or transport, and can not be transported via pneumatic tube systems. Examples include:

- Protein/blood products, such as albumin, immune globulins, monoclonal antibodies and insulins (note: some manufacturers allow insulin to be transported via pneumatic tube one time)
- Products that foam, such as alteplase, etanercept (Enbrel), rasburicase or caspofungin; these drugs should only be swirled when reconstituting, do not shake; wait for the foam to dissolve
- Vaccines that have been reconstituted, such as varicella zoster virus vaccine
- Emulsions, such as propofol and injectable lipid emulsions

Check Solutions for Color Changes

Most intravenous medications are clear and colorless. In some cases, discoloration can be of little or no consequence. However, in most cases, discoloration indicates oxidation or another type of decomposition.

DRUG	DO NOT USE WITH COLOR CHANGE	NOTES
Chlorpromazine	Darker than slight yellow	Slight yellow: potency retained, okay to use
Dacarbazine	Pink	
Dobutamine		Oxidation turns the solution slightly pink, but potency is not lost
Dopamine	Darker than slight yellow	Slight yellow: potency retained, okay to use
Epinephrine	Pink, then brown	
Isoproterenol	Pink or darker	Damaged by air, light, heat
Morphine	Dark	
Nitroprusside	Orange → brown → blue	Blue indicates nearly complete dissociation to cyanide
Norepinephrine	Pink or darker	
Tigecycline	Green/black	Normal color: yellow/orange

IV Drugs that Come as Colored Solutions

DRUG	COLOR OF IV FLUID		SKIN AND SECRETIONS DISCOLORATION
Anthracyclines (e.g., doxorubicin)	Red		Sweat and urine
Rifampin	Red		Saliva, urine, sweat and tears
Mitoxantrone	Blue		Skin, eyes, urine
Methotrexate	Yellow		None
Multivitamins for Infusion (MVI)	Yellow		None
Tigecycline	Yellow/Orange		Teeth (if used during teeth development)
IV Iron, various	Brown		Urine

iStock.com/LisLud

Check Solutions for Particulates

The clinician (or the patient if using a self-injectable) should always check parenteral solutions for particulate matter. If particulates are present, the drug should be discarded.

Select Guidelines/References

ASHP Injectable Drug Information, 2023 Ed. American Society of Health-System Pharmacists. 2023.

King Guide to Parenteral Admixtures. https://www.kingguide.com/online.html (accessed 2023 Nov 29).

CONTENT LEGEND

= Study Tip Gal   = Required Formula

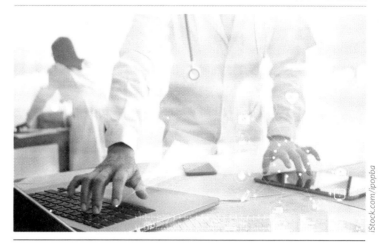
iStock.com/ipopba

CHAPTER 8
ANSWERING CASE-BASED EXAM QUESTIONS

BACKGROUND

Increased use of electronic health records (EHRs) provides pharmacists with greater access to patient-specific information, including labs, test results and progress notes from other healthcare providers. Pharmacists must be prepared to effectively use all of this information to make decisions about drug therapy.

Questions on the NAPLEX are presented mainly in a case-based format. Some of the information provided in the case will be needed to correctly answer the questions. The goal is to assess whether the pharmacist can make the best choices for a specific patient vs. simply recalling facts. This better reflects the role of pharmacists in healthcare today.

This chapter reviews the patient medical record and discusses how to use the information to correctly answer case-based questions on the exam. Practice the techniques discussed in the UWorld RxPrep QBank.

THE PATIENT MEDICAL RECORD

ELECTRONIC HEALTH RECORDS

The patient medical record (PMR) provides complete documentation of a patient's medical history at a particular institution. The PMR can be referred to as the "medical record" or the "patient chart." These terms are from the era of paper records when all of the patient's medical information was gathered into ring binders. Paper charts have been phased out in most healthcare settings and replaced by EHRs, which improve accuracy and efficiency.

The EHR is quicker and easier to review. For example, if a patient is admitted to the hospital with an elevated SCr, the EHR provides current and previous lab results (by selecting a date range that can go back years in time) which are used to determine if this is a new or an old finding, and what recent workup has been completed. Procedures with results recorded on paper or faxed records from another facility can be quickly scanned into the EHR. EHRs allow providers to have immediate access to information when they are off-site. Some community pharmacies have access to EHRs of affiliated clinics.

When the EHR is linked to Computerized Prescriber Order Entry (CPOE) and electronic prescribing (e-prescribing), the problem of illegible handwriting is eliminated. The CPOE system can be designed to present only formulary drugs with proper dosing as options. As a result, pharmacists spend less time clarifying orders or changing to a formulary drug. Clinical decision support (CDS) tools can be built into the order entry process. Examples include order sets, pathways, limited drop-down menus that reflect the preferred drug/s, drug interaction and dose checking alerts. Refer to the Medication Safety & Quality Improvement chapter for additional information.

The Health Insurance Portability and Accountability Act of 1996 (HIPAA) requires security protections for all individually identifiable health information, called protected health information (PHI). These protections apply to both paper records and electronic records. For electronic records, access is limited with PINs and passwords. The information is encrypted, and there is an "audit trail" to track access. Security can still be breached; individuals can access medical records for patients they are not involved with, an employee can forget to log out or the system can be hacked. All personnel using the EHR are responsible for security. Education on security must be continual, and the software must be continuously evaluated for breaches. As part of the HIPAA requirements, patients have a right to access their own medical records kept in either paper or electronic formats.

SECTIONS OF THE PATIENT MEDICAL RECORD

The first additions to the patient medical record (PMR) (paper or EHR) are the patient's demographic data (including insurance information), admission sheet, a service agreement form ("this is what I am having done at this facility"), a page describing the patient's rights (a Joint Commission requirement) and an advance directive. An advance directive documents the patient's wishes concerning medical treatment if they are unable to make decisions on their own behalf. Allergies may be here or listed in a separate area of the medical record.

Certain religious groups will refuse blood transfusions and blood products, which will need to be documented in the PMR. Blood products primarily involve albumin and immune globulins, but some patients will refuse drugs buffered in blood (*Epogen/Procrit*, *Kogenate* - used for hemophilia), natural clotting factors/tissue adhesives/interferons and a few other uncommon products. A few vaccines contain porcine-derived gelatin as a stabilizer. Most religious groups consider this use acceptable, but a specific patient may not.

Other forms or sections in the PMR include progress notes, the vital signs record, laboratory tests, monitoring records used for some medications (e.g., warfarin to track the INR history), medication administration records and procedure records, including the diagnostic and operating room (OR) records. At the end of the hospital stay, the planning and discharge forms are added to the EHR.

When documenting information in the PMR, it is important to avoid abbreviations that could be interpreted to mean something else. The list of "Do Not Use" abbreviations should be easily available (refer to the Medication Safety & Quality Improvement chapter).

REQUIREMENTS FOR REIMBURSEMENT: DOCUMENTATION AND QUALITY OF CARE

Pharmacists are involved with many patient care activities and frequently make verbal patient care recommendations. While verbal recommendations may be effective, they are not part of the PMR and do not allow the information to be shared with other healthcare providers involved in the patient's care who are not present at that time. Interventions require documentation for reimbursement since the quality of the care is (increasingly) tied to the payment. Departments of pharmacy should have policies in place that describe the authority of pharmacists to document in the PMR, what activities will be documented and the proper format for documentation. Some activities that pharmacists document in the PMR include patient counseling, medication histories, consultations (e.g., pharmacokinetics, anticoagulation) and dosage adjustments. Documenting in the PMR is critical to establishing pharmacists as central members of the healthcare team.

The Centers for Medicare and Medicaid Services (CMS) provides health insurance to many Americans. CMS is directly involved with quality measurements and cost control. CMS has penalties for poor care and incentives for quality care. Two areas in which the penalties are steep are the rate of hospital-acquired infections and the hospital's readmission rate. These measures are chosen because they are expensive and are often, but not always, avoidable.

The Joint Commission, the Pharmacy Quality Alliance (PQA) and the Agency for Healthcare Research and Quality (AHRQ) are involved in setting the criteria to measure the quality of care. The PQA quality measurements focus on medications. Specific goals include increasing adherence, avoiding unnecessary or unsafe medications (such as high-risk medications in the elderly) and increasing the use of medications indicated for certain conditions.

Medicare is the federal health insurance program for people ≥ 65 years old, < 65 with disability and all ages with end stage renal disease (ESRD).

The prescription drug benefit under Medicare is called Part D.

Part A covers the hospital visit and Part B covers medical costs, such as doctor visits and some vaccines.

Medicaid provides health insurance for all ages with very low income (< 133% of the federal poverty level). Medicaid is a federal and state program. A senior who qualifies for both Medicare and Medicaid has "dual coverage."

THE SOAP NOTE FORMAT

A progress note records a patient encounter. One common method of organizing a progress note is the SOAP format, which organizes the information into four parts: Subjective, Objective, Assessment and Plan (SOAP). Prior to the use of SOAP notes, it was difficult to understand patient chart entries because the format was not standardized. Pharmacists may write SOAP notes to document their activities and read the SOAP notes of others while providing patient care. An example SOAP note from an EHR is included at the end of this chapter.

SUBJECTIVE

The 1st section in a SOAP note is the subjective information recorded from the patient. It is the patient's narrative of their symptoms. Only the relevant information is recorded. The person conducting the interview should use open-ended and direct questions while avoiding closed-ended and leading questions. For example, the leading question: "You always take your blood pressure pills, right?" is not likely to get a useful response. Phrasing the question in a direct manner that is worded to avoid a "yes or no" response will be more useful: "In a typical week, about how many mornings do you forget to take your blood pressure pills?"

The subjective section contains:

- A one-line Chief Complaint (CC). This is the specific reason the patient is being seen today, such as "I've had a stabbing pain in my right hip for three days."

- A detailed history of present illness (HPI). The HPI contains the onset and duration of the complaint, the quality and severity (e.g., a numerical pain rating), any modifying factors that reduce or aggravate the condition, treatments that have been tried and the effect of the treatment.

- A detailed past medical history (PMH) with social history (alcohol, tobacco and illicit drug use), family history (first-degree relatives only – parents and siblings), allergies and patient-reported medication use. Medications include

prescriptions, over-the-counter (OTC) drugs, vitamins and natural products. Information on start date and last refill is important when recording medication information.

OBJECTIVE

The 2nd section in a SOAP note is the objective information obtained by the clinician, either through observation or analysis. This includes:

- Vital signs (respiration rate, heart rate, blood pressure and temperature). Note that on the top of the sample EHR at the end of this chapter, the vitals are recorded at the top of the page, but vital signs are objective data.

- Other measurements (e.g., height and weight), physical findings, diagnostic tests performed (e.g., ECG, chest X-ray, urinalysis) and laboratory results go into this section.

- The medication list if it is obtained from a source other than the patient (e.g., recording information from prescription bottles or calling another pharmacy) because it was objectively verified.

Critical results are lab values significantly outside the reference range. Since these can indicate a life-threatening situation, they must be reported to a healthcare provider and addressed quickly. This is a Joint Commission National Patient Safety Goal.

Units of Measure

It is important to document measurements according to the policies of the institution. Documentation is generally done in metric system units (e.g., kg, cm). Recording weights and heights with incorrect units (150 pounds vs. 150 kg) can have fatal consequences in terms of dosing medications. Refer to the Calculations chapters to practice common height and weight conversions.

In the U.S., temperatures are still frequently recorded in degrees Fahrenheit and may need to be converted to degrees Celsius. The route that the temperature was taken should be recorded (i.e., rectal, oral, axillary, tympanic). Temperatures taken rectally or orally are more accurate than if taken by axillary (under the arm) or tympanic (in the ear) methods.

Temperature Conversions

$°C = (°F - 32)/1.8$	$°F = (°C \times 1.8) + 32$

CASE SCENARIO

A patient presented with a temperature of 101.6°F. What is this temperature in degrees Celsius? Round to the nearest TENTH.

$$°C = \frac{(101.6°F - 32)}{1.8} = 38.7°C$$

SELECT DRUGS AND CONDITIONS THAT ALTER VITAL SIGNS

Make note of drugs that cause "↓ HR" or "↑ BP" while studying. On the exam, you might be asked about the possible cause of an abnormal vital sign. The table below is not all-inclusive; some conditions have variable effects on vital signs depending on severity (e.g., infection, withdrawal, poisoning). This information will be covered in more detail in the individual disease state chapters.

VITAL SIGN	INCREASED	DECREASED
Blood Pressure (BP)	"Hypertension" **Drugs** See Key Drugs Guy in Hypertension chapter **Conditions** ■ Renal insufficiency/failure ■ Pregnancy ■ Excess salt intake ■ Obesity ■ Adrenal tumors	"Hypotension" **Drugs** ■ Antihypertensives ■ Vasodilators ■ Opioids ■ Benzodiazepines ■ Anesthetics ■ Phosphodiesterase inhibitors **Conditions** ■ Anaphylaxis ■ Blood loss ■ Infection (esp. sepsis) ■ Dehydration (orthostatic hypotension)
Heart Rate (HR)	"Tachycardia" **Drugs** ■ Stimulants (ADHD, weight loss drugs) ■ Decongestants ■ Beta-agonists (esp. overuse) ■ Theophylline (esp. in toxicity) ■ Anticholinergics (tricyclics, antihistamines) ■ Bupropion ■ Antipsychotics ■ Excess caffeine/nicotine, illicit drug use ■ Vasodilators (e.g., nitrates, hydralazine, dihydropyridine CCBs) cause reflex tachycardia **Conditions** ■ Some arrhythmias (e.g., atrial fibrillation, ventricular tachycardia) ■ Hyperthyroidism ■ Anemia ■ Dehydration ■ Anxiety, stress, pain ■ Hypoglycemia ■ Infection ■ Drug withdrawal ■ Serotonin syndrome	"Bradycardia" **Drugs** ■ Beta-blockers ■ Non-dihydropyridine CCBs ■ Digoxin ■ Clonidine, guanfacine ■ Antiarrhythmics (esp. Class III) ■ Opioids ■ Sedatives ■ Anesthetics ■ Neuromuscular blockers ■ Acetylcholinesterase inhibitors **Conditions** ■ Some arrhythmias (sinus bradycardia) ■ Hypothyroidism
Respiratory Rate (RR)	"Tachypnea" **Drugs** ■ Stimulants **Conditions** ■ Asthma and COPD (esp. when poorly controlled) ■ Anxiety, stress ■ Ketoacidosis ■ Pneumonia	"Respiratory depression" **Drugs** ■ Opioids ■ Sedatives **Conditions** ■ Hypothyroidism
Temperature (Temp)	"Hyperthermia" **Drugs** ■ Inhaled anesthetics (malignant hyperthermia) ■ Antipsychotics (neuroleptic malignant syndrome) ■ Topiramate **Conditions** ■ Fever ■ Hyperthyroidism (esp. thyroid storm) ■ Trauma ■ Cancer ■ Serotonin syndrome	"Hypothermia" **Conditions** ■ Exposure to cold ■ Hypothyroidism (esp. myxedema coma) ■ Hypoglycemia

ASSESSMENT

The 3rd section is the assessment. This is the provider's thought process of possible causes of the current situation. Many conditions present with similar signs and symptoms; the assessment will often include a differential diagnosis, which is a list of possible diagnoses that could explain the patient's current signs and symptoms. Each diagnosis on the list will be investigated.

PLAN

The 4th section is the plan. This is how the problem/s will be addressed. The plan should be as specific as possible. Labs might be ordered, the patient might require diagnostic exams, referrals may be requested or the patient may require education (e.g., suspected nonadherence, poor device technique, nutritional education or smoking cessation support). If there is a differential diagnosis, there will be multiple steps in the plan to eliminate ("rule out") some of the possible conditions. Patients often have many medical problems that must be addressed, and they may be vastly different from the complaint that prompted the patient to seek medical attention.

MILITARY TIME

In all medical records, including the SOAP note, time is recorded with a 24-hour clock, rather than splitting the day into two 12-hour segments (AM/PM). The 24-hour clock is called "military time." The day begins at midnight, which is called 24:00 (pronounced "twenty-four hundred").

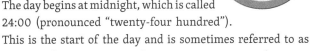

This is the start of the day and is sometimes referred to as 00:00. After 12:00 noon the time continues on the same number scale for the rest of the day: 1:00 PM is 13:00, 2:00 PM is 14:00, and so on. The last minute of the day is 23:59, then 24:00 (midnight), and then the next day begins. Some clocks are labeled for military time (see image).

To convert military time back to 12-hour segments (AM/PM), simply subtract 12 from any number ≥ 13 (e.g., 16:00 = 4 pm, because 16 – 12 = 4).

ANSWERING CASE-BASED QUESTIONS ON THE EXAM

Pharmacists caring for patients (or taking the NAPLEX) are often faced with complex medication regimens. In order to provide the best care possible, a systematic approach to the assessment of the treatment plan and medication regimen is warranted.

IDENTIFYING MEDICATION THERAPY PROBLEMS

Pharmacists should assess for medication therapy problems, intervene when appropriate and document the intervention/s in the PMR as policy permits. Cases on the exam will require the same type of systematic assessment to identify risks to the patient and potential solutions to problems.

Pharmacists develop a process for thoroughly identifying medication problems. One method is shown below (see Study Tip Gal). Ask yourself each question listed: Are there any therapeutic duplications? Are there any drug interactions? You may not be able to answer every question with the information provided. Strong mastery of the material (e.g., brand or generic name identification, drug interactions, guideline recommendations) is essential. The Case Scenario below illustrates how you could be asked several different types of questions about a case.

HOW TO LOOK FOR MEDICATION PROBLEMS IN A PATIENT CASE

Review the case for the following medication problems:

- Untreated medical condition
- Medications used without an indication
- Improper drug selection
- Dose that is too low or high
- Therapeutic duplication
- Lack of patient understanding about medication
- Drug allergy
- Drug interaction
- Improper use of medication
- Failure to receive medication
- Adverse drug reaction
- Nonadherence

Practice reviewing cases until it becomes routine to check for each of these problems, every time. This is essential for a pharmacist.

CASE SCENARIO

A new patient transfers the following prescriptions to a community pharmacy on December 15th: *Benicar* 20 mg daily, *Zocor* 20 mg daily, *Stribild* 1 daily (last refilled November 1st) and *Avapro* 150 mg TID. All are written for a 30-day supply.

Identify the potential problems (see Study Tip Gal above):

- Therapeutic duplication: two ARBs
- Drug interaction: cobicistat is contraindicated with simvastatin
- Dose too high: *Avapro* should be dosed once daily
- Potential nonadherence: *Stribild* should be refilled every 30 days

MATCHING DRUGS TO MEDICAL PROBLEMS

How will you determine whether there are untreated medical conditions, drugs without an indication or duplications of therapy? Pharmacists are skilled at matching up medical problems and drugs as a quick way to assess this.

CASE SCENARIO

Match the medications to the condition being treated. Some conditions may require more than one medication.

Past Medical History	Medications	Past Medical History	Medications
Hypertension	Keflex	Hypertension ⟶	Hydrochlorothiazide
Arthritis	Synthroid	Arthritis ⟶	Meloxicam
Depression	Hydrochlorothiazide	Depression ⟶	Cymbalta
Cellulitis	Renova cream	Cellulitis ⟶	Keflex
Diabetes	Ambien	Diabetes	?
	Meloxicam	? Insomnia	Ambien
	Cymbalta	? Hypothyroidism	Synthroid
		? Acne	Renova cream

■ There are several medications without a documented indication in the patient's past medical history. The pharmacist should interview the patient and/or review labs/vitals (PRN) to determine if these medications are still required or were possibly prescribed in error. It is very common for the medical record to be incomplete or incorrect, but pharmacists must ensure that medications are used properly.

■ There is one condition (diabetes) that is not being treated with a medication. Many patients are able to control type 2 diabetes with diet alone, which might be the case. A review of the labs (blood glucose, A1C) would help answer this question. Again, notice that mastery of brand/generic names is critical.

QUESTIONS ABOUT THE MEDICATION PROFILE

Use the Case Scenario below to answer questions about the medication profile.

CASE SCENARIO

The pharmacist is filling new prescriptions for a patient with the following home medication list:

Advair
Clozapine
Roflumilast
Depakote ER
Dutasteride
Fenofibrate
Hyzaar
ProAir
Spiriva
Tamsulosin

Based on the medication profile, which group of medical problems does this patient have?

A. Asthma, glaucoma and gout
B. Atrial fibrillation, depression and schizophrenia
C. Hypertriglyceridemia, migraine and Parkinson disease
D. BPH, COPD and hypertension
E. Seizures, diabetes and anemia

One of the new prescriptions is for Flomax. This is a duplication of therapy with which of the patient's current medications?

A. Advair
B. Roflumilast
C. Dutasteride
D. Hyzaar
E. Tamsulosin

The patient's labs reveal an increased ammonia level. Which of the home medications is most likely responsible?

A. Advair
B. Clozapine
C. Depakote ER
D. Spiriva
E. Tamsulosin

Answers:

d, e, c

RECOMMENDING DRUG THERAPY

Some exam questions will ask you to make a drug therapy recommendation. This requires strong knowledge of guidelines and indications/contraindications for drugs. Read the question and answer choices first, before extensively evaluating the case. After you read the question, you should be able to quickly determine what information you need from the case.

CASE SCENARIO

A patient has a past medical history of type 2 diabetes and is not taking any medications. Which of the following medications should be recommended to treat the patient's diabetes?

- A. *Glucophage XR*
- B. *Actos*
- C. Januvia
- D. *Glucotrol*
- E. Regular insulin given by IV infusion

How will you decide which answer to pick? Here is the correct approach to the question:

- Metformin is a recommended first-line medication, along with lifestyle modifications, for type 2 diabetes. It is very likely the correct answer, but the question may be testing something more advanced than a simple recall of the recommended first-line medication. Before selecting metformin, make sure it is a safe choice in this specific patient and that nothing was missed in the case that would make another choice better:

  ❏ Insulin is one of the answer choices. Could this patient have hyperglycemia hyperosmolar state (HHS) or diabetic ketoacidosis (DKA), which would require an insulin infusion? Read the HPI. Look for signs, symptoms and labs that help (e.g., very high blood glucose, altered mental status, extreme dehydration; refer to the Diabetes chapter).

  ❏ Metformin should not be started if eGFR is < 45 mL/min/1.73 m^2. If eGFR is not provided, calculate the patient's CrCl and use this as an eGFR estimate. Metformin may not be safe for this patient.

  ❏ Check the progress notes and other information provided. Metformin should not be used within 48 hours of receiving IV iodinated contrast media.

If the patient does not require an insulin infusion to treat DKA or HHS, and there are no contraindications or safety concerns with metformin, select it as the correct answer choice. If metformin is not a safe choice, use a similar process to determine which of the other choices is best for this patient.

EXAMPLE ELECTRONIC HEALTH RECORD SOAP NOTE

JB (MRN: JB747114): SOAP Note for 9/25
Date of birth: 10/24/XXXX
Allergies: NKDA

VS

Height:	Weight:	BMI	Blood Pressure	Pulse	Resp Rate	Oral Temp:
67 in	88.6 kg	30.5 kg/m²	154/92 mmHg	80 bpm	12 rpm	36.6 °C

CC "I feel limp."

S JB is a 40 y/o female who presents with a 3-month history of increasing fatigue. She first noticed that she felt tired when working long hours at work but has been working her usual 8 hours a day for the past 2 months and has not regained her energy. She described her fatigue as "feeling limp." It is present throughout the day and is worse with significant exertion (e.g., walking > 3-4 blocks or going up stairs). She has tried sleeping up to 10 hours/night (increased from 8 hours/night), and it has not helped. She is concerned that there is something seriously wrong, as she is usually full of energy and her family and friends are starting to ask if she is sick. She has not been able to exercise, which she usually enjoys. She has gained about 2.7-3.2 kgs in the last few months, which she attributes to inactivity due to fatigue. Her husband states that she has "always" snored quite loudly. Her menses are regular on timing, heavy flow for 1-2 days, then lighter for another 2-3 days. The pattern is unchanged from before the onset of her fatigue. Her last menstrual period was one week ago.

Denies: chest pain, shortness of breath, abdominal pain, N/V/D, changes in her stool, fever, chills, night sweats and changes in mood.

She reports a history of GERD, HTN, heart murmur and depression. She states that she takes her medications regularly "except the one for her blood pressure because she doesn't feel like her pressure is high."

Her reported medications include *Pepcid AC* 10 mg PO BID, chlorthalidone 25 mg PO Daily, *Zoloft* 100 mg Daily and *Caltrate + D3* 600 mg BID.

O Well-appearing Black female in no acute distress.

SKIN: not pale, no rashes

NECK: no thyromegaly or thyroid nodules

NODES: no cervical, axillary or inguinal lymphadenopathy

CHEST: clear to auscultation and percussion bilaterally

CV: RRR, 2/6 systolic ejection murmur heard best at the LLSB that radiates to the apex, no S3 or S4

ABD: normal active bowel sounds, no hepatosplenomegaly by palpation or percussion, no abdominal tenderness

EXT: no edema, pulses normal

A Recent onset of fatigue with no obvious inciting event. Hypothyroidism is possible given her weight gain, though this may have occurred from her inactivity. Anemia is possible, though her menstrual periods have not lengthened or increased, and there are no other apparent sources of blood loss. A recent menses makes pregnancy unlikely. Given her history of snoring, sleep apnea is possible, but her history of snoring over many years is not entirely consistent with her more recent onset of fatigue. She does not seem to have a recurrence of her depression since she has no new symptoms. She does not have symptoms of infection, nor has her murmur changed, so subacute bacterial endocarditis is unlikely. BP is elevated, and she has been noncompliant with prescribed therapy for HTN.

P #1. Check TSH to rule out hypothyroidism

#2. Check CBC to rule out anemia

#3. If the above are unremarkable, consider a sleep study to rule out sleep apnea

#4. Pharmacy consult for medication adherence

#5. Follow-up visit in 1 week to discuss test results and further workup

Select Guidelines/References
American Society of Health-System Pharmacists. ASHP Guidelines on Pharmacist-Conducted Patient Education and Counseling. *Am J Health-Syst Pharm.* 1997;54:431-4.

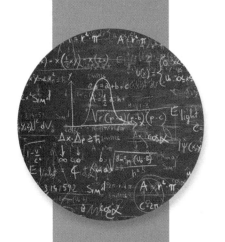 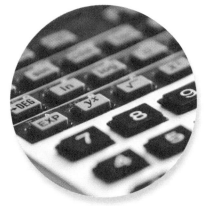 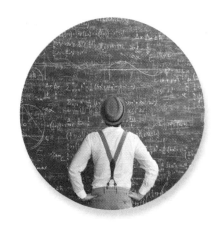

CALCULATIONS

CONTENTS

> This chapter covers basic math concepts that must be mastered for NAPLEX. These topics may be a review for some, but they are the foundation for solving more complex problems in later chapters.

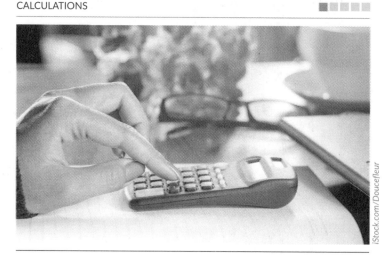

iStock.com/Doucefleur

CHAPTER 9

CALCULATIONS I: MATH BASICS

STUDYING CALCULATIONS

Calculations account for about 14% of the questions on the NAPLEX. The best approach is to study math early, practice it often and mix up the content from the Calculations chapters in the QBank. For example, if you are finished studying the Calculations I, II and III chapters, create tests for yourself in the QBank that include all three chapters. It is also beneficial to mix math with clinical topics in the QBank. When you get close to your exam, you should be able to create mixed tests from any chapters in the QBank and perform well.

ASSESSING READINESS FOR MATH

You are ready to tackle calculations on the NAPLEX when:

✔ All of the math concepts in this course book have been mastered.

✔ All formulas on the Required Formulas Sheet have been memorized and can be quickly recalled in response to a problem.

✔ Each calculations QBank (including biostatistics and pharmacokinetics) has been reviewed multiple times and math mistakes have been remediated.

✔ Each math problem can be completed in ~1.6 minutes (1 minute and 36 seconds). This is the average pace required to complete all questions on the NAPLEX in 6 hours.

Track and monitor your progress on Calculations with the Reports tab in the QBank.

EQUIVALENT MEASUREMENTS

Drugs can be measured in different ways:

- Weight [e.g., grams (g), milligrams (mg), micrograms (mcg), nanograms (ng)]

- Volume [e.g., liters (L), milliliters (mL)]

- Concentration

    ❏ Amount of drug in a given volume of diluent (e.g., mcg/mL, mg/dL, mEq/L), which includes <u>percentage strength</u> (g in 100 mL, g in 100 g or mL in 100 mL), <u>ratio strength</u> and <u>parts per million</u> (see Calculations II chapter).

<u>Common conversions must be known</u> by pharmacists (see <u>Study Tip Gal</u> below); they may or may not be provided on the exam. <u>Actual or approximate conversions can be used</u> for calculations on the exam; both will result in the <u>same answer</u> when rounding instructions provided in the question are followed. If a <u>specific conversion is provided</u> in the question, always <u>use it</u> (see problem #2).

1. **A prescription reads: "take 2 tsp PO Q6H x 7 days." How many milliliters must be dispensed to complete 7 days of therapy?**

$$2 \text{ tsp} \times \frac{5 \text{ mL}}{1 \text{ tsp}} = 10 \text{ mL per dose}$$

$$\frac{10 \text{ mL}}{\text{dose}} \times \frac{4 \text{ doses}}{\text{day}} \times 7 \text{ days} = 280 \text{ mL}$$

2. **If 1 ounce = 30 mL, how many milliliters of sterile water will remain after 50 mL are used from a 16 ounce bottle?**

$$16 \text{ oz} \times \frac{30 \text{ mL}}{1 \text{ oz}} = 480 \text{ mL bottle of sterile water}$$

480 mL – 50 mL = 430 mL of sterile water will remain

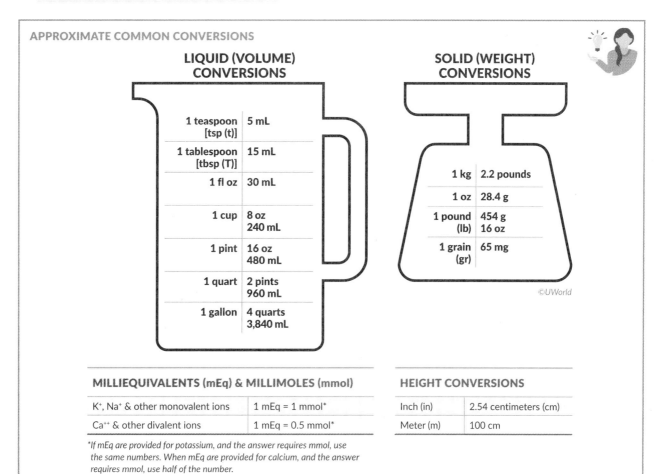

APPROXIMATE COMMON CONVERSIONS

LIQUID (VOLUME) CONVERSIONS

1 teaspoon [tsp (t)]	5 mL
1 tablespoon [tbsp (T)]	15 mL
1 fl oz	30 mL
1 cup	8 oz / 240 mL
1 pint	16 oz / 480 mL
1 quart	2 pints / 960 mL
1 gallon	4 quarts / 3,840 mL

SOLID (WEIGHT) CONVERSIONS

1 kg	2.2 pounds
1 oz	28.4 g
1 pound (lb)	454 g / 16 oz
1 grain (gr)	65 mg

©UWorld

MILLIEQUIVALENTS (mEq) & MILLIMOLES (mmol)

K$^+$, Na$^+$ & other monovalent ions	1 mEq = 1 mmol*
Ca^{++} & other divalent ions	1 mEq = 0.5 mmol*

*If mEq are provided for potassium, and the answer requires mmol, use the same numbers. When mEq are provided for calcium, and the answer requires mmol, use half of the number.

HEIGHT CONVERSIONS

Inch (in)	2.54 centimeters (cm)
Meter (m)	100 cm

ROUNDING

Rounding final answers correctly is very important on the NAPLEX (see Study Tip Gal).

HOW TO ROUND ON THE EXAM

- Underline the number to the right of what is being rounded. If rounding to the nearest whole number, underline the 4 in this example: 347.4̲8

- Look at the number that is underlined and apply one of these rules:
  - ❏ If the underlined number is 5, 6, 7, 8, or 9, round up.
  - ❏ If the underlined number is 0, 1, 2, 3, or 4, round down.

- 347.48 rounded to the nearest whole number is 347.
  - ❏ **Round only once on the last step in the calculation.***

These standard rounding rules do not apply to certain Biostatistics calculations (e.g., number needed to treat or harm) and instances when a pharmacist cannot dispense a partial vial or syringe. This will be clear in the phrasing of the question.

Use the calculator's memory or parentheses function on the exam for the intermediate steps. In the UWorld RxPrep course book, some intermediate steps (that do not affect the final answer) have been rounded for simplicity and space.

---

3. **A pediatric patient is receiving 5.25 mL of drug every 4 hours. How many milliliters will be required for the entire day? Round to the nearest whole number.**

   5.25 mL (per dose) × 6 times/day = 31.5 mL
   Round to the nearest whole number = 32 mL

---

4. **A patient requires 410.9 mg of a drug daily. The daily dose will be divided for BID administration. How many milligrams will the patient receive BID? Round to the nearest whole number.**

   410.9 mg daily/2 times per day = 205.45 mg BID
   Round to the nearest whole number = 205 mg BID

   What if the problem said "round to the nearest tenth?" The correct answer would then be 205.5 mg. Rounding to the nearest tenth is the same as rounding to one decimal place.

---

5. **Enoxaparin 56.5 mg was ordered for a patient. The hospital rounds enoxaparin doses to the nearest 10 mg. What dose should be dispensed?**

   Correct answer: 60 mg. Rounding to the nearest 10 mg is different than rounding to the nearest tenth.

---

6. **A patient is 5'2" tall. What is her height in centimeters? Round to the nearest whole number.**

   $$5 \text{ feet} \times \frac{12 \text{ inches}}{1 \text{ foot}} = 60 \text{ inches} + 2 \text{ inches} = 62 \text{ inches}$$

   $$62 \text{ inches} \times \frac{2.54 \text{ cm}}{1 \text{ inch}} = \begin{array}{l} 157.48 \text{ cm} \\ \text{Round to the nearest whole number} = 157 \text{ cm} \end{array}$$

Watch for products that cannot be split. You cannot dispense part of an insulin vial or part of a *Byetta* pen to a patient, so <u>rounding to the nearest vial or pen</u> would be required, as illustrated in the Case Scenario below.

CASE SCENARIO

A patient takes *Novolog* 16 units TID before meals. How many vials of *Novolog* should be dispensed for a 30-day supply?

Answer: The patient takes 48 units per day or 1,440 units per month. Since each vial of *Novolog* contains 1,000 units, the patient requires two vials for a 30-day supply.

PROPORTIONS AND DIMENSIONAL ANALYSIS

These methods are very important for the math that pharmacists do routinely. Dimensional analysis, individual proportion calculations, or a combination of the two are acceptable. When performed correctly, <u>both methods provide the same answer</u>.

PROPORTIONS

Proportions are two fractions (ratios) that are set equal to each other. One variable is unknown and labeled "X." When setting up <u>proportions</u>, make sure that the <u>units for the numerators match to each other</u> and the <u>units for the denominators match to each other</u> or make sure the items in the left fraction match and the items in the right fraction match (see <u>Study Tip Gal</u> and problem #7 for an example).

DIMENSIONAL ANALYSIS

Dimensional analysis allows multiple proportion calculations to be completed quickly. Diagonal units that are the same can be crossed out ("canceled out"), leaving the desired units. The numbers can be plugged into the calculator exactly as written.

SETTING UP PROPORTIONS

Two methods of matching:

Match both numerators and both denominators:
Every item in the left numerator (drug, route, units) must match to every item in the right numerator (except the values of the numbers).

Every item in the left denominator must match to every item in the right denominator (except the values of the numbers).

Match numerator and denominator of each fraction: Items in the left fraction (numerator and denominator) must match, and items in the right fraction (numerator and denominator) must match (except the value of the numbers).

Carefully review problem #7 to see how both methods provide the same answer.

---

7. **A patient weighs 176 pounds. What is the patient's weight in kilograms?**

Method 1: Proportion. Solve for X by multiplying diagonally and then dividing. Set up in either of the two ways shown.

$$\frac{176 \text{ lbs}}{X \text{ (kg)}} = \frac{2.2 \text{ lbs}}{1 \text{ kg}} \qquad X = 80 \text{ kg}$$

or

$$\frac{176 \text{ lbs}}{2.2 \text{ lbs}} = \frac{X \text{ (kg)}}{1 \text{ kg}} \qquad X = 80 \text{ kg}$$

Method 2: Dimensional analysis. Cancel out the same units diagonally, leaving the desired units.

$$176 \cancel{\text{ lbs}} \times \frac{1 \text{ (kg)}}{2.2 \cancel{\text{ lbs}}} = 80 \text{ kg}$$

Notice that there is an equal sign (=) between the fractions in a proportion and a multiplication symbol (×) between the fractions in dimensional analysis.

CONVERTING COMMON UNITS

LARGER → SMALLER VOLUME

Liters (L) → milliliters (mL)

8. How many milliliters are in 5 liters?

Method 1: Proportion

$$\frac{5\,L}{X\,mL} = \frac{1\,L}{1,000\,mL} \qquad X = 5,000\,mL$$

or

Method 2: Dimensional analysis

$$5\,L \times \frac{1,000\,mL}{1\,L} = 5,000\,\boxed{mL}$$

SMALLER → LARGER VOLUME

Milliliters (mL) → deciliters (dL)

9. How many deciliters are equal to 200 milliliters?

$$200\,mL \times \frac{1\,dL}{100\,mL} = 2\,\boxed{dL}$$

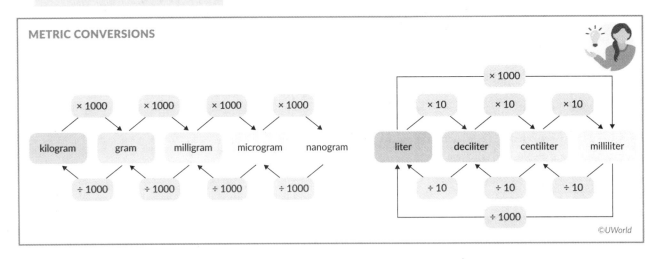

METRIC CONVERSIONS

LARGER → SMALLER WEIGHT

Kilograms (kg) → grams (g) → milligrams (mg) → micrograms (mcg) → nanograms (ng)

10. How many nanograms are equal to 5 kg?

This example requires 4 separate proportions or dimensional analysis (shown).

$$5\,kg \times \frac{1,000\,g}{1\,kg} \times \frac{1,000\,mg}{1\,g} \times \frac{1,000\,mcg}{1\,mg} \times \frac{1,000\,ng}{1\,mcg} = 5\ trillion\,\boxed{ng}\,(or\ 5 \times 10^{12}\ ng)$$

SMALLER → LARGER WEIGHT

Nanograms (ng) → micrograms (mcg) → milligrams (mg) → grams (g) → kilograms (kg)

11. How many grams are equal to 50,000,000 nanograms?

$$50,000,000\,ng \times \frac{1\,mcg}{1,000\,ng} \times \frac{1\,mg}{1,000\,mcg} \times \frac{1\,g}{1,000\,mg} = 0.05\,\boxed{g}$$

When dimensional analysis is presented from this point forward, the strike through lines will be omitted for readability.

CALCULATIONS INVOLVING PRESCRIPTIONS

Interpretation of prescriptions (including common prescription abbreviations), orders and compounding instructions will be necessary on the exam.

12. **A pharmacist receives this prescription for hydrocodone/acetaminophen. How many tablets should be dispensed?**

    A. 6 tablets

    B. 8 tablets

    C. 12 tablets

    D. 16 tablets

    E. 24 tablets

    The correct answer is (C). The dispense quantity is indicated and consistent with the "not to exceed" instructions.

> **John Smith, MD**
> 123 Anywhere Street
> Anytown, USA 00000
> Phone: (555) 555-5555
> DEA # AS1234563
>
> Name _Mary Smith_   DOB _May 15, XXXX_
> Address _177 Green Street_   Date _August 23, XXXX_
>
> *Touch Rx symbol, color will disappear then reappear.*
>
> **Rx**   Hydrocodone/Acetaminophen 5/325 mg #12
>   Sig: i-ii tabs PO q 4-6 hrs prn pain X 2 days. NTE 6/d.
>
> SUBSTITUTION PERMISSABLE _____   DO NOT SUBSTITUTE _____
>
> ✔ DO NOT REFILL ___ REFILL___ TIMES | SIGNATURE OF PRESCRIBER _John Smith_
>
> Prescription is void if more than one controlled substance is written per blank.
> Security Features. Details on Back.

©UWorld

13. **How many milliliters of *Mylanta* suspension are contained in each dose of the prescription below? Round to the nearest whole number.**

PRESCRIPTION	QUANTITY
Belladonna Tincture	10 mL
Phenobarbital	60 mL
Mylanta susp. qs. ad	120 mL
Sig. 5 mL BID	

The total prescription is 120 mL; 10 mL belladonna, 60 mL of phenobarbital, and that leaves 50 mL for the *Mylanta*.

$$\frac{50 \text{ mL } Mylanta}{120 \text{ mL total Rx}} = \frac{X \text{ mL } Mylanta}{5 \text{ mL total Rx dose}} \quad X = 2.08, \text{ or 2 mL } Mylanta \text{ per dose}$$

14. **A pharmacist receives a prescription for "*Vigamox* 0.5%. Dispense 3 mL. 1 gtt tid ou x 7d." How many drops will the patient use per day?**

    A. 1 drop

    B. 2 drops

    C. 3 drops

    D. 6 drops

    E. 21 drops

The correct answer is (D). Abbreviations commonly used on prescriptions must be known. In this case, "gtt" refers to "drop" and "ou" refers to "each eye." The instructions for this prescription read "Instill 1 <u>drop</u> in <u>each eye</u> three times per day." Refer to the Common Conditions of the Eyes & Ears chapter for additional abbreviations used for eye and ear prescriptions.

15. A 7-year-old male child (48 pounds) presents to the urgent care clinic with a fever of 102°F, and nausea/vomiting that started the previous day. He will receive an acetaminophen 5 grain suppository for the fever. A pharmacist receives a prescription for the suppository with the instructions: Use 1 PR Q4-6H PRN temperature > 102°F. How many milligrams per kilogram (mg/kg) will the child receive per dose? Round to the nearest whole number.

$$5 \text{ grains} \times \frac{65 \text{ mg}}{1 \text{ grain}} = 325 \text{ mg per suppository}$$

$$48 \text{ lbs} \times \frac{1 \text{ kg}}{2.2 \text{ lbs}} = \sim21.8182 \text{ kg}$$

Note: if a proportion is used to solve the step above, the repeating decimals must be addressed. It is best to use the calculator's memory or parentheses function on the exam so that all decimals can be carried forward to the next step. Round only once on the last step.

325 mg/21.8182 kg = ~14.896 mg/kg, round to 15 mg/kg

Some pharmacists may have learned the "actual" milligram to grain conversion of 64.8 mg per grain vs the approximate conversion of 65 mg per grain. Both conversions provide the <u>same answer</u> when rounded to the nearest whole number.

---

16. A pharmacist received this sulfamethoxazole/trimethoprim prescription and dispensed 3 oz to the patient. How many days of therapy will the patient be short? Use 30 mL for 1 fluid ounce.

   A. 1
   B. 3
   C. 9
   D. 10
   E. 90

The correct answer is (A).

5 mL (per dose) x 2 times/day x 10 days = 100 mL

Quantity dispensed: 3 oz x 30 mL/oz = 90 mL dispensed

Difference: 100 mL – 90 mL = 10 mL, which is 1 day of therapy

A common mistake is selecting answer (D). The patient will be 10 mL short, but the question asked for "days of therapy." Each tsp (t) is 5 mL. The patient must take 2 tsp (t) daily (or 10 mL), so will be one day short for his prescribed course of therapy.

Jane Smith, MD
555 Anywhere St.
Anytown, USA
(111)111-1111
DEA: AS1234563

Name John Doe   Date February 1, 20XX
Address 123 State St   DOB May 5, XXXX

℞

SMX/TMP 200-5 mg/5mL
Sig: 1 tsp PO BID x 10 days, until all taken.

❏ Do Not Substitute   Refill __0__ Times

Quantity   Units
❏ 1-24
❏ 25-49
❏ 50-74
❏ 75-100
❏ 101-150
❏ 151 and over

Jane Smith
Physician Signature

Prescription is void if more than one controlled substance is written per blank.

©UWorld

17. **A pharmacist has tablets that contain 0.25 mg of levothyroxine per tablet. The tablets will be crushed and mixed with glycerol and water to prepare a prescription for a child weighing 36 pounds. How many levothyroxine tablets will be needed to compound the following prescription?**

PRESCRIPTION	QUANTITY
Levothyroxine Liq.	0.1 mg/mL
Disp.	60 mL
Sig. 0.01 mg per kg PO BID	

$$60 \text{ mL total Rx} \times \frac{0.1 \text{ mg levo}}{\text{mL}} = 6 \text{ mg of levothyroxine needed}$$

$$6 \text{ mg levo} \times \frac{1 \text{ tab}}{0.25 \text{ mg levo}} = 24 \text{ tabs of levothyroxine needed}$$

The first step can also be performed as a proportion. <u>If the proportion is set up correctly, the answers will be the same.</u>

$$\frac{0.1 \text{ mg levo}}{1 \text{ mL}} = \frac{X \text{ mg levo}}{60 \text{ mL}} \quad X = 6 \text{ mg of levothyroxine needed}$$

$$6 \text{ mg levo} \times \frac{1 \text{ tab}}{0.25 \text{ mg levo}} = 24 \text{ tabs of levothyroxine needed}$$

Or, it can be solved by <u>dimensional analysis</u>. Notice that the <u>child's weight is not needed</u> to solve the problem.

$$\frac{1 \text{ tab levo}}{0.25 \text{ mg levo}} \times \frac{0.1 \text{ mg levo}}{\text{mL}} \times 60 \text{ mL total Rx} = 24 \text{ tabs of levothyroxine needed}$$

---

18. **How many milligrams of codeine will be contained in each capsule?**

PRESCRIPTION	QUANTITY
Codeine Sulfate	0.6 g
Guaifenesin	1.2 g
Caffeine	0.15 g
M. ft. caps. no. 24	
Sig. One capsule TID PRN cough	

Begin by converting to the units requested in the answer (mg).

$$0.6 \text{ g codeine} \times \frac{1{,}000 \text{ mg}}{1 \text{ g}} = 600 \text{ mg of codeine for the total prescription}$$

The abbreviation "M. ft." means "<u>mix and make</u>." In this case, all of the ingredients will be combined and used to make 24 capsules.

$$\frac{600 \text{ mg codeine total}}{24 \text{ caps}} = 25 \text{ mg of codeine/capsule}$$

After solving the problem, read the question again to be certain the question was answered with the correct units (mg of codeine per capsule).

19. How many grains of aspirin will be contained in each capsule? Round to the nearest tenth.

PRESCRIPTION	QUANTITY
Aspirin	6 g
Phenacetin	3.2 g
Caffeine	0.48 g
M. ft. no. 20 caps	
Sig. One capsule Q6H PRN pain	

$$6 \text{ g aspirin} \times \frac{1{,}000 \text{ mg}}{1 \text{ g}} \times \frac{1 \text{ grain}}{65 \text{ mg}} = 92.3 \text{ grains}$$

We have 92.3 grains of aspirin that will be divided into 20 capsules.

$$\frac{92.3 \text{ grains}}{20 \text{ capsules}} = 4.6 \text{ grains/capsule}$$

After solving the problem, read the question again to be certain the question was answered with the correct units (grains per capsule).

---

20. A 45 milliliter nasal spray delivers 20 sprays per milliliter of solution. Each spray contains 1.5 mg of active drug. How many milligrams of drug are contained in the 45 mL package?

First, calculate the amount of drug per mL.

$$\frac{1.5 \text{ mg drug}}{\text{spray}} \times \frac{20 \text{ sprays}}{\text{mL}} = 30 \text{ mg/mL}$$

Then, solve for milligrams of drug in 45 mL.

$$\frac{30 \text{ mg}}{\text{mL}} = \frac{X \text{ mg}}{45 \text{ mL}} \quad X = 1{,}350 \text{ mg}$$

---

21. A metered-dose inhaler provides 90 micrograms of albuterol sulfate with each inhalation. The canister provides 200 inhalations. If the patient uses the entire canister, how many total milligrams will the patient have received?

$$200 \text{ inhalations} \times \frac{90 \text{ mcg}}{\text{inhalation}} \times \frac{1 \text{ mg}}{1{,}000 \text{ mcg}} = 18 \text{ mg}$$

22. Digoxin injection is supplied in ampules of 500 mcg per 2 mL. How many milliliters must a nurse administer to provide a dose of 0.2 mg?

Method 1: Two steps using a proportion.

First, convert micrograms to milligrams.

$$500 \text{ mcg} \times \frac{1 \text{ mg}}{1{,}000 \text{ mcg}} = 0.5 \text{ mg}$$

Then, use a proportion to calculate the number of milliliters for a 0.2 mg dose.

$$\frac{0.5 \text{ mg digoxin}}{2 \text{ mL}} = \frac{0.2 \text{ mg digoxin}}{X \text{ mL}} \quad X = 0.8 \text{ mL}$$

Method 2: Dimensional analysis.

$$0.2 \text{ mg} \times \frac{1{,}000 \text{ mcg}}{1 \text{ mg}} \times \frac{2 \text{ mL}}{500 \text{ mcg}} = 0.8 \text{ mL}$$

---

23. If one 10 mL vial contains 0.05 g of diltiazem, how many milliliters should be administered to provide a 25 mg dose of diltiazem?

Method 1: Two steps using a proportion.

First, convert grams to milligrams. It is usually best practice to convert to the units required for the answer when beginning the problem.

$$0.05 \text{ g diltiazem} \times \frac{1{,}000 \text{ mg}}{1 \text{ g}} = 50 \text{ mg}$$

Next, calculate the number of milliliters for a 25 mg dose.

$$\frac{50 \text{ mg}}{10 \text{ mL}} = \frac{25 \text{ mg}}{X \text{ mL}} \quad X = 5 \text{ mL}$$

Method 2: Dimensional analysis.

$$25 \text{ mg dose} \times \frac{1 \text{ g}}{1{,}000 \text{ mg}} \times \frac{10 \text{ mL}}{0.05 \text{ g}} = 5 \text{ mL}$$

CONVERTING FROM ONE DRUG TO ANOTHER

Another common application for proportions is converting from one drug and dose to another drug and dose. Common conversions that pharmacists perform are shown (see Key Drugs Guy). These common drug-dose conversions can also be found on the UWorld RxPrep Required Formulas Sheet.

24. **The pharmacist is consulted to convert a patient from prednisone 10 mg PO BID to an equivalent dose of oral dexamethasone given once daily. What is the equivalent daily dose? Prednisone 5 mg = dexamethasone 0.75 mg.**

$$\frac{20 \text{ mg prednisone}}{X \text{ mg dexamethasone}} = \frac{5 \text{ mg prednisone}}{0.75 \text{ mg dexamethasone}} \quad X = 3 \text{ mg of dexamethasone daily}$$

Notice that the numerators match each other (drug name and units) and the denominators match each other. For the exam, the equivalencies (e.g., prednisone 5 mg = dexamethasone 0.75 mg) must be memorized (see the Systemic Steroids & Autoimmune Conditions chapter for steroid equivalencies).

RATIOS

A ratio is a comparison between two numbers. Ratios can be used to describe how ingredients should be mixed. If compounding instructions state "mix petrolatum and lanolin in a 3:1 ratio," it means 3 parts of petrolatum should be mixed with 1 part of lanolin. The pharmacist needs to know the weight of one part in order to calculate the weight of the other or the weight of the final mixture. The ratio is usually converted to a fraction (e.g., 3:1 = 3/1) for use in math.

25. **How many grams of bacitracin and nystatin are required to prepare 150 g of a 2:3 topical bacitracin:nystatin ointment?**

Since the total weight is provided (150 g) and the total number of parts can be calculated (2 parts + 3 parts = 5 total parts), the value of 1 part can be determined using a proportion.

$$\frac{5 \text{ total parts}}{150 \text{ g}} = \frac{1 \text{ part}}{X \text{ g}} \quad X = 30 \text{ g per 1 part}$$

$$2 \text{ parts bacitracin} \times \frac{30 \text{ grams}}{1 \text{ part}} = 60 \text{ g bacitracin}$$

$$3 \text{ parts nystatin} \times \frac{30 \text{ grams}}{1 \text{ part}} = 90 \text{ g nystatin}$$

RATIO RELATIONSHIPS

$$4:8 = \frac{4}{8} = \frac{1}{2} \quad \text{Or, 1 part to 2 parts}$$

Add the weights to confirm that they match the total weight:

60 g bacitracin + 90 g nystatin = 150 g of 2:3 bacitracin:nystatin ointment

DECIMALS AND PERCENTAGE CONVERSION

To convert a <u>decimal to a percentage</u>, <u>multiply</u> the decimal by 100.

To convert a <u>percentage to a decimal</u>, <u>divide</u> the percentage by 100.

26. **HT is a 16-year-old female who complains of weakness, fatigue and heavy menstrual periods. She is diagnosed with anemia. HT takes ferrous sulfate 220 mg once daily. How many milligrams of elemental iron does HT receive from the supplement? Ferrous sulfate is 20% elemental iron.**

    Divide the percentage by 100: 20%/100 = 0.2

    Multiply the total amount of ferrous sulfate by 0.2 to determine the amount of elemental iron in mg:

    220 mg x 0.2 = 44 mg elemental iron

SQUARING A NUMBER

27. **Calculate 3.5^2.**

    Either method will provide the answer:

    Method 1: Multiply the number by itself:

    3.5 x 3.5 = 12.25

    Method 2: Use the x^2 key on the calculator:

    1. Enter the number to square on the calculator: 3.5
    2. Hit the x^2 key
    3. This will provide the same answer: 12.25

EXPONENTS

28. **Calculate 2^4.**

    1. Enter the first number on the calculator (in this example, enter 2)
    2. Hit the x^y key
    3. Enter the exponent (in this example, enter 4)
    4. This will provide the answer; in this example, the answer is 16

ORDER OF OPERATIONS

Math calculations that involve more than one function need to be completed in a specified order (see Study Tip Gal). The order is brackets (first), then parentheses, then exponents, then multiplication and division (left to right), then addition and subtraction (left to right). In fractions, the fraction bar is a grouping symbol; the entire numerator and the entire denominator are calculated before dividing the denominator into the numerator.

Phenytoin requires a specific formula to calculate the corrected drug level when the albumin is low (< 3.5 g/dL). Refer to the Seizures/Epilepsy chapter for additional discussion. The order of operations must be followed in order to get the correct result.

FOLLOW THE RULES OF MATH

Brackets → Parentheses (and other grouping symbols) → Exponents → Multiplication and Division → Addition and Subtraction

Remember: **B-PEMDAS**

Billy, **Pl**ease **E**at **M**om's **D**elicious **A**pple **S**trudel

---

29. **SJ is a female patient in the internal medicine unit receiving treatment following a motor vehicle accident. Her medications include lorazepam, morphine and phenytoin. Her serum albumin is 1.8 g/dL and her phenytoin level is 9.6 mcg/mL. Her CrCl is 61 mL/min. Calculate SJ's corrected phenytoin level (in mcg/mL) using the formula provided. Round to the nearest one decimal place.**

$$\text{Phenytoin corrected (mcg/mL)} = \frac{\text{Total phenytoin measured}}{(0.2 \times \text{albumin}) + 0.1}^{\dagger}$$

† *Use serum phenytoin in mcg/mL (same as mg/L) and albumin in g/dL (standard units in the U.S.) in the corrected phenytoin formula. The units are not intended to cancel out.*

$$\text{Phenytoin corrected} = \frac{9.6}{(0.2 \times 1.8) + 0.1} = \begin{array}{l} \text{~20.8696 mcg/mL} \\ \text{Round to the nearest one decimal place = 20.9 mcg/mL} \end{array}$$

1. Do the math inside parentheses first: 0.2 x 1.8 = 0.36

2. Add 0.1 to the answer: 0.36 + 0.1 = 0.46

3. Divide 9.6 by the answer: 9.6 divided by 0.46 = 20.9 (per rounding instructions provided)

READY TO SUBMIT YOUR ANSWER?

Not so fast. Do a double check first!

Ask yourself these questions to avoid common mistakes:

- Does the answer match the question?
  - ❏ Re-read the question. Did you solve for the right thing? Remember, many problems on the exam require more than one step.
- Is the answer in the correct units? This is a common mistake. The problem may have been done correctly, but one more step is required to convert the answer to the specified units.
- Is the answer rounded correctly? The rounding instructions must be followed to get the problems right on the exam.
- Does the answer make sense?
  - ❏ If the problem asks how many liters of fluid a patient will receive in one day, 20,000 liters is unlikely to be the right answer. It does not make sense.

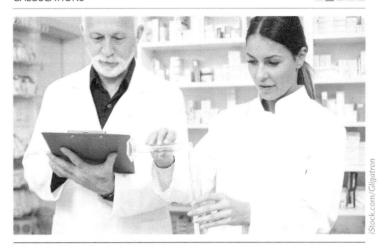

iStock.com/Gligatron

CHAPTER 10

CALCULATIONS II: COMPOUNDING

PERCENTAGE STRENGTH

Drug concentrations can be expressed in many ways, but they are a ratio of the amount of an ingredient to the total amount of the product. A percent is the number of parts in 100. Percents are often written as decimals or fractions (e.g., 25% = 0.25 = 25/100). The types of percentage concentrations are defined as follows:

- Percent weight-in-volume (% w/v) is expressed as g/100 mL (a solid mixed into a liquid). This applies to common IV fluids (see Study Tip Gal on the next page).

- Percent volume-in-volume (% v/v) is expressed as mL/100 mL (a liquid mixed into a liquid).

- Percent weight-in-weight (% w/w) is expressed as g/100 g (a solid mixed into a solid).

---

1. **How many grams of NaCl are in 1 liter of normal saline (NS)?**

    Normal saline contains 0.9 g NaCl per 100 mL of solution (see Study Tip Gal on the next page). Percentage strength problems are solved with simple proportions (reviewed in detail in Calculations I).

$$\frac{0.9\ g}{100\ mL} = \frac{X\ g}{1{,}000\ mL} \qquad X = 9\ g$$

2. **How many grams of NaCl are in 500 mL of 1/2NS? Round to the nearest hundredth.**

   Since NS is 0.9% NaCl, 1/2NS is 0.45%.

   $$\frac{0.45\ g}{100\ mL} = \frac{X\ g}{500\ mL} \qquad X = 2.25\ g$$

3. **How many grams of dextrose are in 250 mL of D5W? Round to the nearest tenth.**

   $$\frac{5\ g}{100\ mL} = \frac{X\ g}{250\ mL} \qquad X = 12.5\ g$$

4. **How many milligrams of triamcinolone should be used in preparing the following prescription? Round to the nearest whole number.**

PRESCRIPTION	QUANTITY
Triamcinolone (w/v)	5%
Glycerin qs	60 mL
Sig. Two drops in right ear once daily	

   $$\frac{5\ g}{100\ mL} = \frac{X\ g}{60\ mL} \qquad X = 3\ g,\ or\ 3{,}000\ mg$$

5. **A prescription reads as follows: "Prepare a 3% w/w coal tar preparation; qs with petrolatum to 150 grams." How many grams of petrolatum are required to compound the prescription? Round to the nearest tenth.**

   $$\frac{3\ g\ coal\ tar}{100\ g\ preparation} = \frac{X\ g\ coal\ tar}{150\ g\ preparation} \qquad X = 4.5\ g\ coal\ tar$$

   150 g (total weight of preparation) – 4.5 g (coal tar) = 145.5 g petrolatum

6. **A pharmacist is compounding a vancomycin oral suspension. The master formulation record says to reconstitute a 5 g vial of vancomycin powder for injection with 50 mL of sterile water, then dilute with sterile water to 200 mL. What is the final percentage strength of the compounded product (w/v)?**

   $$\frac{5\ g}{200\ mL} = \frac{X\ g}{100\ mL} \qquad X = 2.5\ g,\ which\ is\ 2.5\%$$

7. **If 1,250 grams of a mixture contains 80 grams of a drug, what is the percentage strength (w/w) of the mixture? Round to the nearest tenth.**

   $$\frac{80\ g}{1{,}250\ g} = \frac{X\ g}{100\ g} \qquad X = 6.4\ g,\ which\ is\ 6.4\%$$

8. **A mouth rinse contains 1/12% (w/v) of chlorhexidine gluconate. How many grams of chlorhexidine gluconate should be used to prepare 18 liters of mouth rinse? Round to the nearest whole number.**

    First, convert 1/12% to a decimal. 1/12% = 0.083 g per 100 mL (w/v).

    Next, convert L to mL. 18 L x 1,000 mL/L = 18,000 mL.

    Then, solve for grams of chlorhexidine gluconate needed.

    $$\frac{0.083\ g}{100\ mL} = \frac{X\ g}{18,000\ mL} \qquad X = 14.94\ g, \text{ rounded to } 15\ g$$

9. **SS is a 79-year-old female with dry mouth and dry eyes from Sjögren's syndrome. She is picking up the prescription below. What is the maximum milligrams of pilocarpine she will receive per day?**

PRESCRIPTION	QUANTITY
Pilocarpine	1% (w/v)
Sodium chloride qs ad	15 mL
Sig: 2 gtts (0.05 mL/gtt) po TID prn up to 5 days for dry mouth	

    First, calculate the amount of pilocarpine in the prescription.

    $$\frac{1\ g}{100\ mL} = \frac{X\ g}{15\ mL} \qquad X = 0.15\ g$$

    Then, convert to mg since the problem asks for mg of pilocarpine.

    $$0.15\ g \ \times\ \frac{1,000\ mg}{1\ g} = 150\ mg \text{ of pilocarpine}$$

    The patient will receive up to 3 doses per day (0.1 mL x 3 = 0.3 mL). Calculate the amount of pilocarpine in 0.3 mL.

    $$\frac{150\ mg\ pilocarpine}{15\ mL} = \frac{X\ mg}{0.3\ mL} \qquad X = 3\ mg\ pilocarpine$$

10. **A pharmacist dissolves 6 tablets. Each tablet contains 250 mg of metronidazole. The pharmacist will put the drug into a liquid base to prepare 60 mL of a topical solution. What is the percentage strength (w/v) of metronidazole in the prescription? Round to the nearest tenth.**

    $$6\ tablets\ \times\ \frac{250\ mg}{1\ tab} = 1,500\ mg, \text{ or } 1.5\ g\ metronidazole$$

    $$\frac{1.5\ g}{60\ mL} = \frac{X\ g}{100\ mL} \qquad X = 2.5\ g, \text{ which is } 2.5\%\ w/v$$

11. **If 12 grams of lanolin are combined with 2 grams of white wax and 36 grams of petrolatum to make an ointment, what is the percentage strength (w/w) of lanolin in the ointment?**

    $$\frac{12\ g\ lanolin}{50\ g\ ointment} = \frac{X\ g}{100\ g} \qquad X = 24\%\ w/w$$

12. **A pharmacist adds 5.3 grams of hydrocortisone to 150 grams of a 2.5% hydrocortisone ointment. What is the percentage (w/w) of hydrocortisone in the finished product? Round to the nearest whole number.**

    First, determine the amount of hydrocortisone (HC) in the current product.

    $$\frac{2.5 \text{ g HC}}{100 \text{ g ointment}} = \frac{X \text{ g HC}}{150 \text{ g ointment}} \qquad X = 3.75 \text{ g HC}$$

    5.3 grams of HC is being added to the existing product, which contains 3.75 g of HC: 5.3 g + 3.75 g = 9.05 g.

    Next, find the percent concentration of the final product (5.3 g + 150 g = 155.3 g).

    $$\frac{9.05 \text{ g HC}}{155.3 \text{ g ointment}} = \frac{X \text{ g HC}}{100 \text{ g ointment}} \qquad X = 5.8274 \text{ g, rounded to 6\% w/w}$$

---

13. **How many milliliters of hydrocortisone liquid (40 mg/mL) will be needed to prepare 30 grams of a 0.25% cream (w/w)? Round to the nearest hundredth.**

    First, calculate the amount of hydrocortisone needed in the final product.

    $$\frac{0.25 \text{ g}}{100 \text{ g}} = \frac{X \text{ g}}{30 \text{ g}} \qquad X = 0.075 \text{ g or 75 mg}$$

    Then, solve for mL of hydrocortisone liquid needed.

    $$\frac{40 \text{ mg}}{\text{mL}} = \frac{75 \text{ mg}}{X \text{ mL}} \qquad X = 1.875 \text{ mL, rounded to 1.88 mL}$$

    After solving the problem, read the question again to be certain the question was answered with the correct units (mL).

---

14. **What is the percentage strength of imiquimod in the following prescription? Round to the nearest hundredth.**

PRESCRIPTION	QUANTITY
Imiquimod 5% cream	15 g
Xylocaine	20 g
Hydrophilic ointment	25 g

    First, calculate the amount of imiquimod (5%) in the prescription.

    $$\frac{5 \text{ g}}{100 \text{ g}} \times 15 \text{ g} = 0.75 \text{ grams of imiquimod}$$

    The total weight of the prescription is 60 g (15 g + 20 g + 25 g).

    $$\frac{0.75 \text{ g}}{60 \text{ g}} = \frac{X \text{ g}}{100 \text{ g}} \qquad X = 1.25 \text{ g, which is 1.25\% w/w}$$

RATIO STRENGTH

The concentration of a weak solution can be expressed as a ratio strength. It is denoted as one unit of solute contained in the total amount of the solution or mixture (e.g., 1:500). Ratio strength is another way of presenting a percentage strength. This makes sense because percentages are ratios of parts per hundred.

In clinical practice, ratio strengths have been associated with medication errors. The FDA now requires removal of ratio strengths from the labeling of injectable drug products with only one active ingredient (e.g., epinephrine, isoproterenol). Ratio strength is still commonly used in compounding.

> ### SHORTCUT FOR RATIO STRENGTH
>
> Most multi-step calculations will require converting ratio strength to percentage strength. If a ratio strength is presented in a problem, convert it to a percentage strength and convert it back if needed.
>
> - Ratio strength → Percentage strength
>   - ❏ % strength = 100 / ratio strength
> - Percentage strength → Ratio strength
>   - ❏ Ratio strength = 100 / % strength

---

15. **Express 0.04% as a ratio strength.**

$$\frac{0.04}{100} = \frac{1 \text{ part}}{X \text{ parts}} \qquad X = 2{,}500. \text{ Ratio strength is 1:2,500}$$

Convert back to 0.04% by taking 1/2,500 x 100 or simply 100/2,500. Try it.

On the exam there will be instructions for how to enter your answer. Usually you will enter the numbers after the colon in the ratio strength (e.g., for this problem, you would enter 2500). The instructions could read "Calculate the ratio strength. Enter only the numbers after the colon, as shown here with Xs: 1:XXX."

---

16. **Express 1:4,000 as a percentage strength.**

$$\frac{1 \text{ part}}{4{,}000 \text{ parts}} = \frac{X}{100} \qquad X = 0.025, \text{ which is } 0.025\%$$

Problem #16 can be done using the shortcut in the box above for converting between ratio and percentage strength:

Percentage strength = 100 / 4,000 = 0.025%

---

17. **There are 50 mg of drug in 50 mL of solution. Express the concentration as a ratio strength.**

First, convert 50 mg to grams. 50 mg x 1 g/1,000 mg = 0.05 g

Then, calculate grams per 100 mL.

$$\frac{0.05 \text{ g}}{50 \text{ mL}} = \frac{X \text{ g}}{100 \text{ mL}} \qquad X = 0.1 \text{ g}$$

Now solve for ratio strength.

$$\frac{0.1 \text{ g}}{100 \text{ mL}} = \frac{1 \text{ part}}{X \text{ parts}} \qquad X = 1{,}000, \text{ or } 1{:}1{,}000$$

18. How many milligrams of iodine should be used in compounding the following prescription?

ITEM	QUANTITY
Iodine	1:400
Hydrophilic ointment qs ad	10 g
Sig. Apply as directed.	

First, convert the ratio strength to a percentage strength.

$$\frac{1 \text{ part}}{400 \text{ parts}} = \frac{X \text{ g}}{100 \text{ g}} \qquad X = 0.25\% \text{ w/w}$$

Then, determine how much iodine will be needed for the prescription.

$$\frac{0.25 \text{ g}}{100 \text{ g}} = \frac{X \text{ g}}{10 \text{ g}} \qquad X = 0.025 \text{ g, or } 25 \text{ mg}$$

Or, solve another way:

1:400 means 1 g in 400 g of ointment.

$$\frac{1 \text{ g}}{400 \text{ g}} = \frac{X \text{ g}}{10 \text{ g}} \qquad X = 0.025 \text{ g, or } 25 \text{ mg}$$

---

19. A 10 mL mixture contains 0.25 mL of active drug. Express the concentration as a percentage strength (v/v) and a ratio strength.

First, find out how much drug is in 100 mL.

$$\frac{0.25 \text{ mL drug}}{10 \text{ mL}} = \frac{X \text{ mL drug}}{100 \text{ mL}} \qquad X = 2.5 \text{ mL, or } 2.5\% \text{ (v/v)}$$

Now solve for ratio strength.

$$\frac{2.5 \text{ mL drug}}{100 \text{ mL}} = \frac{1 \text{ part}}{X \text{ parts}} \qquad X = 40; \text{ or } 1:40$$

---

20. What is the concentration, in ratio strength, of a trituration made by combining 150 mg of albuterol sulfate and 4.05 grams of lactose?

First, add up the total weight of the prescription.

$$0.150 \text{ g} + 4.05 \text{ g} = 4.2 \text{ g}$$

Now solve for ratio strength.

$$\frac{0.150 \text{ g}}{4.2 \text{ g}} = \frac{1 \text{ part}}{X \text{ parts}} \qquad X = 28, \text{ or } 1:28$$

Refer to the Compounding chapters for discussion of trituration and other compounding terminology.

PARTS PER MILLION

Parts per million (PPM) and parts per billion (PPB) are used to express the strength of very dilute solutions. They are defined as the number of parts of the drug per 1 million (or 1 billion) parts of the whole. The same designations are used as for percentage strength (% w/w, % w/v and % v/v).

SHORTCUT FOR PARTS PER MILLION

- PPM → Percentage strength
  - ❑ Move the decimal left 4 places
- Percentage strength → PPM
  - ❑ Move the decimal right 4 places

21. Express 0.00022% (w/v) as PPM. Round to the nearest tenth.

$$\frac{0.00022 \text{ g}}{100 \text{ mL}} = \frac{X \text{ parts}}{1{,}000{,}000} \qquad X = 2.2 \text{ PPM}$$

22. Express 30 PPM of copper in solution as a percentage.

$$\frac{30 \text{ parts}}{1{,}000{,}000} = \frac{X \text{ g}}{100 \text{ mL}} \qquad X = 0.003\%$$

23. Express 5 PPM of iron in water as a percentage.

$$\frac{5 \text{ parts}}{1{,}000{,}000} = \frac{X \text{ g}}{100 \text{ mL}} \qquad X = 0.0005\%$$

24. A patient's blood contains 0.085 PPM of selenium. How many micrograms of selenium does the patient's blood contain if the blood volume is 6 liters?

$$\frac{0.085 \text{ parts}}{1{,}000{,}000} = \frac{X \text{ g}}{6{,}000 \text{ mL}} \qquad X = 0.00051 \text{ g, or } 510 \text{ mcg}$$

25. A sample of an intravenous solution is found to contain 0.4 PPM of DEHP. How much of the solution, in milliliters, will contain 50 micrograms of DEHP?

$$\frac{0.4 \text{ parts}}{1{,}000{,}000} = \frac{0.00005 \text{ g}}{X \text{ mL}} \qquad X = 125 \text{ mL}$$

If asked to express something in PPB (parts per billion), divide by 1,000,000,000 (9 zeros).

SPECIFIC GRAVITY

Specific gravity (SG) is the ratio of the density of a substance to the density of water. SG can be important for calculating doses of IV medications, in compounding and in interpreting a urinalysis. <u>Water has a specific gravity of 1; 1 g water = 1 mL water.</u> Substances with a SG < 1 are lighter than water and those with SG > 1 are heavier than water.

$$SG = \frac{\text{weight of substance (g)}}{\text{weight of equal volume of water (g)}} \quad \text{or more simply:} \quad SG = \frac{g}{mL}$$

26. **What is the specific gravity of 150 mL of glycerin weighing 165 grams? Round to the nearest tenth.**

$$SG = \frac{165\ g}{150\ mL} \qquad SG = 1.1$$

Check the answer: 150 mL x 1.1 = 165 g

27. **What is the weight of 750 mL of concentrated acetic acid (SG = 1.2)?**

$$1.2 = \frac{X\ g}{750\ mL} \qquad X = 900\ g$$

Check the answer: 900 g/750 mL = 1.2

28. **How many milliliters of polysorbate 80 (SG = 1.08) are needed to prepare a prescription that includes 48 grams of the surfactant/emulsifier (polysorbate)? Round to the nearest hundredth.**

$$1.08 = \frac{48\ g}{X\ mL} \qquad X = 44.44\ mL$$

29. **What is the specific gravity of 30 mL of a liquid weighing 23,400 milligrams? Round to the nearest hundredth.**

$$SG = \frac{23.4\ g}{30\ mL} \qquad SG = 0.78$$

30. **What is the weight of 0.5 L of polyethylene glycol 400 (SG = 1.13)?**

$$1.13 = \frac{X\ g}{500\ mL} \qquad X = 565\ grams$$

31. **Nitroglycerin has a specific gravity of 1.59. How much would 1 quart weigh in grams? Use 1 quart = 946 mL. Round to the nearest whole number.**

$$1.59 = \frac{X\ g}{946\ mL} \qquad X = 1,504\ g$$

Check the answer: 1,504 g/946 mL = 1.59

Note that the SG is <u>equivalent</u> to the <u>density in g/mL (with units)</u>. If asked for the density in the above problem, the answer would be 1.59 g/mL.

DILUTION AND CONCENTRATION

Q1C1

This formula can be used to change the strength or quantity. Q1C1 is used when the problem deals with two concentrations. Be careful: the units on each side must match and one or more may need to be changed, such as mg to gram, or vice-versa.

Q1 x C1 = Q2 x C2	
Q1 = old quantity	Q2 = new quantity
C1 = old concentration	C2 = new concentration

0% AND 100%

If the prescription calls for an ingredient that is pure, the concentration is 100%.

A diluent (e.g., petrolatum, lanolin, alcohol, ointment base, inert base, lactose, *Aquaphor)* does not contain any drug – the concentration of the diluent is 0%.

---

32. A pharmacist has an order for parenteral nutrition that includes 550 mL of D70%. The pharmacist checks the supplies and finds the closest strength he has available is D50%. How many milliliters of D50% will provide an equivalent energy requirement?

550 mL x 70% = Q2 x 50%

Q2 = 770 mL of D50%

---

33. How many grams of petrolatum (diluent) should be added to 250 grams of a 20% ichthammol ointment to make a 7% ichthammol ointment? Round to the nearest tenth.

Note the difference from the previous problem. In this example, the problem asks how much diluent should be added to make the final weight.

250 g x 20% = Q2 x 7%

Q2 = 714.3 g of 7% ichthammol ointment

Read the question again to be certain about what is being asked. Since the question did not ask how much of the 7% ointment can be prepared, but rather how much diluent is required, an additional step is needed:

714.3 g total weight - 250 g (already present) = 464.3 g petrolatum required

---

34. A patient has been receiving 200 mL of an enteral mixture that contains 432 mOsm/L. The pharmacist will reduce the contents to 278 mOsm/L. How many milliliters of bacteriostatic water should be added to the bag? Round to the nearest mL.

200 mL x 432 mOsm/L = Q2 x 278 mOsm/L   X = 311 mL

Q2 = 311 mL of the 278 mOsm/L enteral mixture can be prepared

There are 200 mL in the original bag. The final volume will be 311 mL.

311 mL - 200 mL = 111 mL of bacteriostatic water

35. **If 1 gallon of a 20% (w/v) solution is evaporated to a solution with a 50% (w/v) strength, what will be the new volume (in milliliters)? Round to the nearest 100 mL.**

    3,840 mL × 20% = Q2 × 50%

    Q2 = 1,536 mL, rounded to the nearest 100 mL = 1,500 mL

    The final answer will be the same if the actual conversion for gallon to milliliters is used.

36. **Using 20 grams of a 9% boric acid ointment base, the pharmacist will manufacture a 5% ointment. How much diluent is required?**

    20 g × 9% = Q2 × 5%

    Q2 = 36 g of the 5% ointment can be prepared

    36 g total weight – 20 g (already present) = 16 g diluent required

ALLIGATION

Alligation is used to obtain a new strength (percentage) that is between two strengths the pharmacist has in stock. It is used when the problem deals with <u>three concentrations</u>.

37. **A pharmacist is asked to prepare 80 grams of a 12.5% ichthammol ointment with 16% and 12% ichthammol ointments that she has in stock. How many grams of the 16% and 12% ointment are required?**

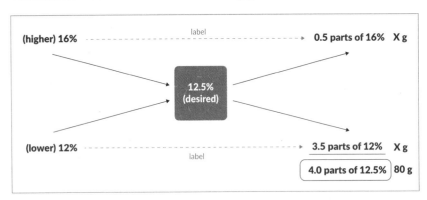

Setting Up An Alligation

- High goes high: write the higher concentration at the top left.
- Low goes low: write the lower concentration on the lower left.
- Write the desired concentration in the middle.
- Subtract diagonally along the X lines to obtain the number of parts. Write the absolute number (no negative sign) on the right side of the X.
  - ❑ 16% – 12.5% = 3.5 parts
  - ❑ 12% – 12.5% = 0.5 parts
- Label horizontally along the dashed lines; the starting concentrations are carried across.
- For some problems, it will be necessary to add up the total number of parts (as shown).

Divide the total weight (80 g) by the number of parts to get the weight per part.

$$\frac{80\ g}{4\ parts} = 20\ grams\ per\ part$$

Take the amount per part (20 g) and multiply it by the parts from each of the concentrations (from the high, and from the low).

$$0.5\ parts\ of\ 16\% \times \frac{20\ g}{part} = 10\ g\ of\ the\ 16\%\ ichthammol\ ointment$$

$$3.5\ parts\ of\ 12\% \times \frac{20\ g}{part} = 70\ g\ of\ the\ 12\%\ ichthammol\ ointment$$

When the two quantities are mixed together, the pharmacist will have 80 g of a 12.5% ichthammol ointment.

38. **A pharmacist is asked to prepare 1 gallon of tincture containing 5.5% iodine. The pharmacy has 3% iodine tincture and 8.5% iodine tincture in stock. How many milliliters of the 3% and 8.5% iodine tincture should be used? (Use 1 gallon = 3,785 mL)**

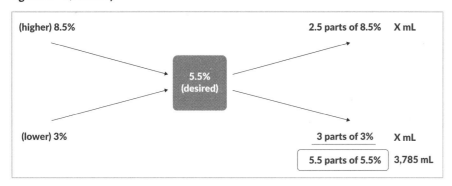

Divide the total volume (3,785 mL) by the number of parts to obtain the volume per part.

$$\frac{3{,}785 \text{ mL}}{5.5 \text{ parts}} = 688.2 \text{ mL per part}$$

$$2.5 \text{ parts} \times \frac{688.2 \text{ mL}}{\text{part}} = 1{,}720 \text{ mL of the 8.5\% iodine tincture}$$

$$3 \text{ parts} \times \frac{688.2 \text{ mL}}{\text{part}} = 2{,}065 \text{ mL of the 3\% iodine tincture}$$

The end product provides 3,785 mL of a 5.5% iodine tincture. Alligation can also be used when the final volume is not known, as shown in the next problem.

---

39. **A hospice pharmacist receives a prescription for 1% morphine sulfate oral solution. She has a 120 mL bottle of morphine sulfate labeled 20 mg/5 mL and a 240 mL bottle of morphine sulfate labeled 100 mg/5 mL. How much of the 100 mg/5 mL product must be mixed with the contents of the 20 mg/5 mL morphine sulfate bottle to prepare the desired percentage strength for the patient?**

First determine the percentage strengths of the two available products.

$$20 \text{ mg/5 mL} \quad \frac{0.02 \text{ g}}{5 \text{ mL}} = \frac{X \text{ g}}{100 \text{ mL}} \quad X = 0.4\% \qquad 100 \text{ mg/5 mL} \quad \frac{0.1 \text{ g}}{5 \text{ mL}} = \frac{X \text{ g}}{100 \text{ mL}} \quad X = 2\%$$

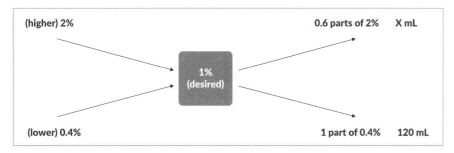

In this case, we do not know the final volume of the product, but we know the proper ratio of the parts (0.6:1).

$$\frac{1 \text{ part of 0.4\% morphine}}{0.6 \text{ parts of 2\% morphine}} = \frac{120 \text{ mL of 0.4\% morphine}}{X \text{ mL of 2\% morphine}} \quad X = 72 \text{ mL of 2\% morphine sulfate}$$

72 mL of 2% (100 mg/5 mL) morphine sulfate must be added to the 120 mL of 0.4% (20 mg/5 mL) morphine sulfate to get a 1% solution. Ultimately, 192 mL of 1% product can be prepared, but the alligation must be solved to determine that.

40. **A pharmacist must prepare 100 grams of a 50% hydrocortisone powder using the 25% and 75% powders that she has in stock. How much of each is required?**

Since the desired strength is exactly in the middle of the strengths available, divide the desired quantity in half:

100 g / 2 = 50 grams. Use 50 g of the 75% and 50 g of the 25% to prepare 100 g of a 50% powder.

DILUTION AND CONCENTRATION EXTRA CREDIT

How many milliliters of sargramostim 500 mcg/mL must be diluted with 250 mL of normal saline to prepare a concentration of 20 mcg/mL?

The final volume is not 250 mL. When the final volume is unknown, you cannot use simple Q1C1. Two methods to solve this problem are shown: the algebraic method (below) and alligation (below, right; which is set up like #39 with unknown final volume). Notice in the alligation, the normal saline is labeled "0 mcg/mL." It is serving as a diluent here. Normal saline contains 0 mcg/mL of sargramostim.

$$Q1C1 + Q2C2 = (Q1+Q2)(C3)$$

$$250 \text{ mL } (0 \text{ mcg/mL}) + X \text{ mL } (500 \text{ mcg/mL}) = (250 \text{ mL} + X \text{ mL})(20 \text{ mcg/mL})$$

$$0 + 500X = 5{,}000 + 20X$$

$$480X = 5{,}000$$

$$X = 10.417 \text{ mL}$$

Solve in reverse to check yourself:

$$500 \text{ mcg/mL} = X \text{ mcg}/10.417 \text{ mL}$$

$$X = 5{,}208.5 \text{ mcg}$$

$$\text{Total volume} = 10.417 \text{ mL} + 250 \text{ mL} = 260.417 \text{ mL}$$

500 mcg/mL ⟶ 20 parts of 500 mcg/mL   X mL
     20 mcg/mL
0 mcg/mL (NS) ⟶ 480 parts of 0 mcg/mL (NS)   250 mL

$$\frac{20 \text{ parts } 500 \text{ mcg/mL}}{480 \text{ parts } 0 \text{ mcg/mL (NS)}} = \frac{X \text{ mL}}{250 \text{ mL}} \qquad X = 10.417 \text{ mL}$$

OSMOLARITY

The total number of particles in a given solution is directly proportional to its osmotic pressure. The particles are usually measured in milliosmoles. Osmolarity is the measure of total number of particles (or solutes) per liter of solution, defined as osmoles/liter (Osmol/L) or, more commonly as milliosmoles/liter (mOsmol/L). Solutes can be either ionic (such as NaCl, which dissociates into two solutes in solution, Na^+ and Cl^-) or non-ionic (which do not dissociate, such as glucose and urea).

Since the volume of water changes according to temperature, the term osmolality (mOsmol/kg) is used in clinical practice; it is independent of temperature. When solute concentrations are very low, osmolarity and osmolality are similar.

Milliosmole calculation problems differ from osmolarity calculation problems in that osmolarity will always need to be normalized to a volume of 1 liter. Math problems usually use osmolarity. The compounds and dissociation particles shown in the table should be known for the exam.

COMPOUND	# OF DISSOCIATION PARTICLES
Dextrose	1
Mannitol	
Potassium chloride (KCl)	2
Sodium chloride (NaCl)	
Sodium acetate ($NaC_2H_3O_2$)	
Magnesium sulfate ($MgSO_4$)	
Calcium chloride ($CaCl_2$)	3
Sodium citrate ($Na_3C_6H_5O_7$)	4

$$mOsmol/L = \frac{\text{Wt of substance (g/L)}}{\text{MW (g/mole)}} \times \text{(\# of particles)} \times 1{,}000$$

Step 1. Add up the number of particles into which the compound dissociates.

Step 2. Calculate the number of grams of the compound present in 1 L.

Step 3. Use the molecular weight (MW) to solve the problem.

Milliosmole calculations do not normalize to 1 liter.

---

41. **What is the osmolarity, in mOsmol/L, of normal saline (0.9% NaCl)? MW = 58.5 g/mol. Round to the nearest whole number.**

NaCl dissociates into 2 particles; Na^+ and Cl^-.

Calculate the number of grams of the compound (NaCl) present in 1 L.

$$\frac{0.9\ g}{100\ mL} = \frac{X\ g}{1{,}000\ mL} \qquad X = 9\ g$$

Use the molecular weight to solve for mOsmol/L.

$$mOsmol/L = \frac{9\ g/L}{58.5\ g/mol} \times 2 \times 1{,}000 = 308\ mOsmol/L$$

---

42. **What is the osmolarity, in mOsmol/L, of D5W? MW = 198 g/mol. Round to the nearest tenth.**

Dextrose does not dissociate and is counted as 1 particle.

$$\frac{5\ g}{100\ mL} = \frac{X\ g}{1{,}000\ mL} \qquad X = 50\ g$$

Use the molecular weight to solve for mOsmol/L.

$$mOsmol/L = \frac{50\ g/L}{198\ g/mol} \times 1 \times 1{,}000 = 252.5\ mOsmol/L$$

---

43. **How many milliosmoles of $CaCl_2$ (MW = 111 g/mol) are represented in 150 mL of a 10% (w/v) calcium chloride solution? Round to the nearest whole number.**

$$\frac{10\ g}{100\ mL} = \frac{X\ g}{150\ mL} \qquad X = 15\ g$$

$$mOsmol = \frac{15\ g}{111\ g/mol} \times 3 \times 1{,}000 = 405\ mOsmol$$

Note that the problem is asking for milliosmoles and not osmolarity. The answer is in milliosmoles and not mOsmol/L. It is not normalized to 1 liter.

44. **A solution contains 373 mg Na ions per liter. How many milliosmoles are represented in the solution? MW = 23 g/mol. Round to the nearest tenth.**

First, convert the units to match the formula.

$$\frac{373 \text{ mg Na}}{\text{L}} \times \frac{1 \text{ g}}{1,000 \text{ mg}} = 0.373 \text{ g/L}$$

$$\text{mOsmol} = \frac{0.373 \text{ g/L}}{23 \text{ g/mol}} \times 1 \times 1,000 = 16.2 \text{ mOsmol}$$

The problem asks for milliosmoles and not osmolarity. Since the problem provides the amount of Na ions in 1 liter, the numerical answer is the same (mOsmol or mOsmol/L).

45. **How many grams of potassium chloride are needed to make 200 mL of a solution containing 250 mOsmol/L? Round to the nearest hundredth. K (MW = 39 g/mol), Cl (MW = 35.5 g/mol)**

First calculate the MW of KCl.

$$\text{MW of KCl} = \text{MW of K} + \text{MW of Cl} = 39 + 35.5 = 74.5$$

$$250 \text{ mOsmol/L} = \frac{X}{74.5} \times 2 \times 1,000 \qquad X = 9.31 \text{ g/L}$$

$$\frac{9.31 \text{ g}}{1,000 \text{ mL}} = \frac{X \text{ g}}{200 \text{ mL}} \qquad X = 1.86 \text{ g}$$

You may be provided with the molecular weight on the exam or asked to calculate it.

46. **A solution contains 200 mg of Ca ions per liter. How many milliosmoles are represented in the solution? MW = 40 g/mol.**

$$\text{mOsmol} = \frac{0.2 \text{ g/L}}{40 \text{ g/mol}} \times 1 \times 1,000 = 5 \text{ mOsmol}$$

The problem is asking for milliosmoles and not osmolarity. The answer is in milliosmoles and not mOsmol/L. It is not normalized to 1 liter.

47. **Calculate the osmolar concentration, in milliosmoles, represented by 1 liter of a 10% (w/v) solution of anhydrous dextrose (MW = 180 g/mol) in water. Round to the nearest one decimal place.**

$$\frac{10 \text{ g}}{100 \text{ mL}} = \frac{X \text{ g}}{1,000 \text{ mL}} \qquad X = 100 \text{ g}$$

$$\text{mOsmol} = \frac{100 \text{ g/L}}{180 \text{ g/mol}} \times 1 \times 1,000 = 555.6 \text{ mOsmol}$$

The problem asks for milliosmoles and not osmolarity. Since the problem asks for mOsmol of dextrose in 1 liter, the numerical answer is the same (mOsmol or mOsmol/L).

48. A patient was ordered 1 liter of D5NS with 20 mEq of KCl for dehydration. How many milliosmoles are in 1 liter of this fluid (MW dextrose = 198 g/mol, Na = 23 g/mol, K = 39 g/mol, Cl = 35.5 g/mol)? Round to the nearest whole number.

First, solve for the osmolarity of the dextrose component.

$$\frac{5 \text{ g dextrose}}{100 \text{ mL}} \times \frac{X \text{ g}}{1{,}000 \text{ mL}} = 50 \text{ g/L}$$

$$\text{mOsmol} = \frac{50 \text{ g/L}}{198 \text{ g/mol}} \times 1 \times 1{,}000 = 252.5252 \text{ mOsmol/L}$$

Next, solve for the osmolarity of the NS component.

$$\frac{0.9 \text{ g NaCl}}{100 \text{ mL}} \times \frac{X \text{ g}}{1{,}000 \text{ mL}} = 9 \text{ g/L}$$

$$\text{mOsmol} = \frac{9 \text{ g/L}}{58.5 \text{ g/mol}} \times 2 \times 1{,}000 = 307.6922 \text{ mOsmol/L}$$

Then, solve for the osmolarity of the KCl component, using the milliequivalent formula (reviewed later in this chapter).

$$20 \text{ mEq} = \frac{X \text{ mg} \times 1}{74.5} = 1{,}490 \text{ mg} = 1.49 \text{ g}$$

$$\text{mOsmol} = \frac{1.49 \text{ g/L}}{74.5 \text{ g/mol}} \times 2 \times 1{,}000 = 40 \text{ mOsmol/L}$$

The final step is to add the three components together to find the total osmolarity.

$$252.5252 \text{ mOsmol/L dextrose} + 307.6922 \text{ mOsmol/L NaCl} + 40 \text{ mOsmol/L KCl} = 600.217 \text{ mOsmol/L, or } 600 \text{ mOsmol/L}$$

ISOTONICITY

When discussing osmotic pressure gradients between fluids, the term tonicity is used; solutions can be isotonic (osmolality is the same as blood, which is ~300 mOsmol/kg), hypotonic or hypertonic. When solutions are prepared, they need to <u>match the tonicity of the body fluid</u> as closely as possible. If the osmolality is higher in one cellular compartment, it will cause water to move from the lower to the higher concentration of solutes. If a parenteral nutrition (PN) solution is injected with a higher osmolality than blood, fluid will flow into the vein, resulting in edema, inflammation, phlebitis and possible thrombosis. Isotonicity is desired when preparing eye drops and nasal solutions.

Since isotonicity is related to the number of particles in solution, the <u>dissociation factor</u> (or ionization), symbolized by the letter i, is determined for the compound (drug). Non-ionic compounds do not dissociate and will have a dissociation factor, i, of one. The table shows the dissociation factors (i) based on the percentage that dissociates into ions; for example, a dissociation factor of 1.8 means that 80% of the compound will dissociate in a weak solution.

NUMBER OF DISSOCIATED IONS	DISSOCIATION FACTOR (OR IONIZATION) i
1	1
2	1.8
3	2.6
4	3.4
5	4.2

(+ 0.8 between each successive value)

As mentioned previously, body fluids are isotonic, having an osmotic pressure equivalent to 0.9% sodium chloride. When making a medication to place into a body fluid, the drug provides solutes to the solvent and needs to be accounted for in the prescription in order to avoid making the prescription hypertonic. The relationship between the amount of drug that produces a particular osmolarity and the amount of sodium chloride that produces the same osmolarity is called the sodium chloride equivalent, or "E value" for short. This is the formula for calculating the E value of a compound:

$$E = \frac{(58.5)(i)}{(MW \text{ of drug})(1.8)}$$

The "E value" formula takes into account the molecular weight of NaCl (58.5) and the dissociation factor of 1.8 since normal saline is around 80% ionized, adding 0.8 for each additional ion beyond 1 into which the drug dissociates. The compound being prepared is compared to NaCl because NaCl is the major determinant of the isotonicity of body fluid.

Once the "E value" is determined, the following steps outline the process of doing isotonicity problems:

Step 1. Calculate the total amount of NaCl needed to make the final product/prescription isotonic by multiplying 0.9% NS by the desired volume of the prescription.

Step 2. Calculate the amount of NaCl represented by the drug. To do this, multiply the total drug amount (in milligrams or grams) by the "E value."

Step 3. Subtract step 2 from step 1 to determine the total amount of NaCl needed to prepare an isotonic prescription.

---

49. Calculate the E value for mannitol (MW = 182 g/mol). Round to the nearest hundredth.

$$\frac{(58.5)(i)}{(MW \text{ of drug})(1.8)} = \frac{58.5\,(1)}{182\,(1.8)} = 0.18$$

---

50. The E value for ephedrine sulfate is 0.23. How many grams of sodium chloride are needed to compound the following prescription? Round to 3 decimal places.

PRESCRIPTION	QUANTITY
Ephedrine sulfate	0.4 g
Sodium chloride	qs
Purified water qs	30 mL
Make isotonic soln.	
Sig. Use 2 drops in each nostril as directed.	

Step 1. Determine how much NaCl would make the product isotonic.

$$\frac{0.9\,g}{100\,mL} = \frac{X}{30\,mL} \qquad X = 0.27\,g$$

Step 2. Determine amount of sodium chloride represented from ephedrine sulfate.

0.4 g × 0.23 ("E value") = 0.092 g of sodium chloride

Step 3. Subtract step 2 from step 1.

0.27 g - 0.092 g = 0.178 g of NaCl are needed to make an isotonic solution

51. Calculate the E value for potassium iodide, which dissociates into 2 particles (MW = 166 g/mol). Round to two decimal places.

$$\frac{(58.5)(i)}{(MW\ of\ drug)(1.8)} = \frac{58.5\ (1.8)}{166\ (1.8)} = 0.35$$

52. Physostigmine salicylate (MW = 413 g/mol) is a 2-ion electrolyte, dissociating 80% in a given concentration (i.e., use a dissociation factor of 1.8). Calculate its sodium chloride equivalent. Round to two decimal places.

$$\frac{(58.5)(i)}{(MW\ of\ drug)(1.8)} = \frac{58.5\ (1.8)}{413\ (1.8)} = 0.14$$

53. The pharmacist receives an order for 10 mL of tobramycin 1% ophthalmic solution. He has tobramycin 40 mg/mL solution. Tobramycin does not dissociate and has a MW of 468 g/mol. Find the E value for tobramycin and determine how many milligrams of NaCl are needed to make the solution isotonic.

$$\frac{(58.5)(i)}{(MW\ of\ drug)(1.8)} = \frac{58.5\ (1)}{468\ (1.8)} = 0.07,\ \text{which is the "E value" for tobramycin}$$

The "E value" for tobramycin is 0.07. The prescription asks for 10 mL of 1% solution.

Step 1. Determine how much NaCl would make the product isotonic (if that is all you were using).

$$\frac{0.9\ g}{100\ mL} = \frac{X}{10\ mL} \qquad X = 0.09\ g,\ or\ 90\ mg$$

Step 2. Determine amount of sodium chloride represented from tobramycin.

$$\frac{1\ g}{100\ mL} = \frac{X}{10\ mL} \qquad X = 0.1\ g,\ or\ 100\ mg$$

100 mg × 0.07 ("E value") = 7 mg of sodium chloride

Step 3. Subtract step 2 from step 1. You are using tobramycin, so you do not need all the NaCl. Subtract out the equivalent amount of tonicity provided by the tobramycin, which is 7 mg.

90 mg − 7 mg = 83 mg (83 mg additional sodium chloride is needed to make an isotonic solution)

MOLES AND MILLIMOLES

A mole (mol) is the molecular weight of a substance in grams, or g/mole. A millimole (mmol) is 1/1,000 of the molecular weight in grams, or 1/1,000 of a mole. For monovalent species, the numeric value of the milliequivalent and millimole are identical.

$$mols = \frac{g}{MW} \qquad or \qquad mmols = \frac{mg}{MW}$$

54. How many moles of anhydrous magnesium sulfate (MW = 120.4 g/mol) are present in 250 grams of the substance? Round to the nearest hundredth.

$$mols = \frac{250\ g}{120.4} = 2.076,\ or\ 2.08\ mols$$

55. How many moles are equivalent to 875 milligrams of aluminum acetate (MW = 204 g/mol)? Round to 3 decimal places.

First, convert 875 mg to grams.

$$875 \text{ mg} \times \frac{1 \text{ g}}{1{,}000 \text{ mg}} = 0.875 \text{ g}$$

Next, solve for mols.

$$\text{mols} = \frac{0.875 \text{ g}}{204} = 0.004 \text{ mols}$$

---

56. How many millimoles of sodium phosphate (MW = 138 g/mol) are present in 90 g of the substance? Round to the nearest whole number.

$$\text{mmols} = \frac{90{,}000 \text{ mg}}{138} = 652 \text{ mmols}$$

Or, solve another way:

$$\frac{90 \text{ g}}{138} = 0.652 \text{ mols, which is } 652 \text{ mmols}$$

---

57. How many moles are equivalent to 45 grams of potassium carbonate (MW = 138 g/mol)? Round to the nearest thousandth.

$$\text{mols} = \frac{45 \text{ g}}{138} = 0.326 \text{ mols}$$

---

58. How many millimoles of calcium chloride (MW = 147 g/mol) are represented in 147 mL of a 10% (w/v) calcium chloride solution?

Step 1: Calculate the amount (g) of $CaCl_2$ in 147 mL of 10% $CaCl_2$ solution.

$$\frac{10 \text{ g}}{100 \text{ mL}} = \frac{X \text{ g}}{147 \text{ mL}} \qquad X = 14.7 \text{ g}$$

Step 2: Calculate the mols of $CaCl_2$ in 147 mL of 10% $CaCl_2$ solution.

$$\text{mols} = \frac{14.7 \text{ g}}{147} = 0.1 \text{ mol}$$

Step 3: Solve the problem by converting moles to millimoles.

$$0.1 \text{ mol} \times 1{,}000 = 100 \text{ mmols}$$

---

59. How many milligrams of sodium chloride (MW = 58.5 g/mol) represent 0.25 mmol? Do not round the answer.

$$0.25 \text{ mmols} = \frac{X \text{ mg}}{58.5} \qquad X = 14.625 \text{ mg}$$

60. **How many grams of sodium chloride (MW = 58.5 g/mol) should be used to prepare this solution? Do not round the answer.**

PRESCRIPTION	QUANTITY
Methylprednisolone	0.5 g
NaCl solution	60 mL

Each 5 mL should contain 0.6 mmols of NaCl

First, determine how many mmols of NaCl will be in 60 mL of the compounded preparation.

$$\frac{0.6 \text{ mmols}}{5 \text{ mL}} = \frac{X \text{ mmols}}{60 \text{ mL}} \qquad X = 7.2 \text{ mmols NaCl}$$

Next, use the total mmols of NaCl to calculate grams of NaCl.

$$7.2 \text{ mmols} = \frac{X \text{ mg}}{58.5} \qquad X = 421.2 \text{ mg or } 0.4212 \text{ g NaCl}$$

MILLIEQUIVALENTS

Drugs can be expressed in solution in different ways:

- Milliosmoles refers to the number of particles in solution.
- Millimoles refers to the molecular weight (MW).
- Milliequivalents (mEq) represent the amount, in milligrams (mg), of a solute equal to 1/1,000 of its gram equivalent weight, taking into account the valence of the ions. Like osmolarity, the quantity of particles is important – but so is the electrical charge. Milliequivalents refers to the chemical activity of an electrolyte and is related to the total number of ionic charges in solution and considers the valence (charge) of each ion.

To count the valence, divide the compound into its positive and negative components, and then count the number of either the positive or the negative charges. For a given compound, the milliequivalents of cations equals that of anions. Some common compounds and their valences are listed in the table to the right. A comparison of valence and dissociation particles is presented in the Study Tip Gal on the next page. Remember, there are a lot of chelation drug interactions with "divalent" cations (calcium, magnesium and iron). Use that interaction to remember which compounds have a valence of 2.

COMPOUND	VALENCE
Ammonium chloride (NH_4Cl)	
Potassium chloride (KCl)	
Potassium gluconate ($KC_6H_{11}O_7$)	
Sodium acetate ($NaC_2H_3O_2$)	1
Sodium bicarbonate ($NaHCO_3$)	
Sodium chloride (NaCl)	
Calcium carbonate ($CaCO_3$)	
Calcium chloride ($CaCl_2$)	
Ferrous sulfate ($FeSO_4$)	2
Lithium carbonate (Li_2CO_3)	
Magnesium sulfate ($MgSO_4$)	

$$mEq = \frac{mg \times valence}{MW} \qquad or \qquad mEq = mmols \times valence$$

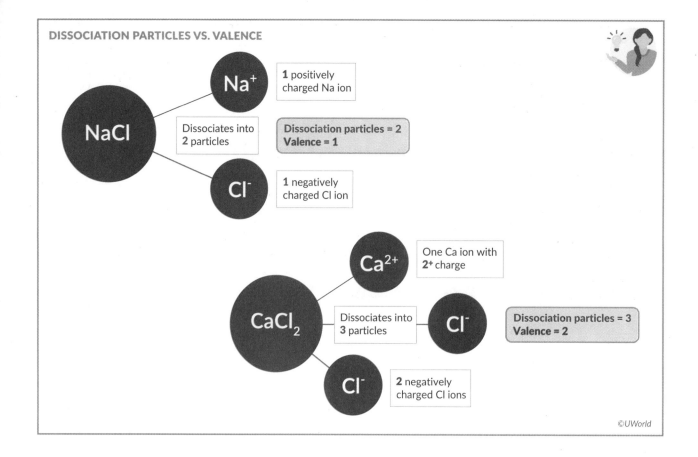

DISSOCIATION PARTICLES VS. VALENCE

©UWorld

---

61. A 20 mL vial is labeled potassium chloride (2 mEq/mL). How many grams of potassium chloride (MW = 74.5 g/mol) are present? Round to the nearest hundredth.

$$20 \text{ mL} \times \frac{2 \text{ mEq}}{\text{mL}} = 40 \text{ mEq KCl total}$$

$$40 \text{ mEq} = \frac{\text{mg} \times 1}{74.5} = 2{,}980 \text{ mg, which is } 2.98 \text{ g}$$

If asked to convert <u>KCl liquid to tablets</u> or vice versa, use a simple proportion since <u>KCl 10% = 20 mEq/15 mL</u> (see Required Formulas Sheet). For example, if someone is using *Klor-Con* 20 mEq BID, the total daily dose is 40 mEq. Convert to KCl 10%, as follows:

$$\frac{40 \text{ mEq}}{X \text{ mL}} = \frac{20 \text{ mEq}}{15 \text{ mL}} \qquad X = 30 \text{ mL of KCl 10\% liquid (15 mL PO BID) is equal to Klor-Con 40 mEq (20 mEq PO BID)}$$

---

62. How many milliequivalents of potassium chloride are present in a 12 mL dose of a 10% (w/v) potassium chloride (MW = 74.5 g/mol) elixir? Round to 1 decimal place.

$$\frac{10 \text{ g}}{100 \text{ mL}} = \frac{X \text{ g}}{12 \text{ mL}} \qquad X = 1.2 \text{ g, or } 1{,}200 \text{ mg}$$

$$\text{mEq} = \frac{1{,}200 \text{ mg} \times 1}{74.5} = 16.1 \text{ mEq}$$

63. **Calculate the milliequivalents of a standard ammonium chloride (MW = 53.5 g/mol) 21.4 mg/mL sterile solution in a 500 mL container.**

$$\frac{21.4 \text{ mg}}{\text{mL}} \times 500 \text{ mL} = 10,700 \text{ mg}$$

$$\text{mEq} = \frac{10,700 \text{ mg} \times 1}{53.5} = 200 \text{ mEq}$$

64. **How many milliequivalents of MgSO₄ (MW = 120.4 g/mol) are represented in 1 gram of anhydrous magnesium sulfate? Round to the nearest tenth.**

$$\text{mEq} = \frac{1,000 \text{ mg} \times 2}{120.4} = 16.6 \text{ mEq}$$

65. **How many milliequivalents of sodium are in a 50 mL vial of 8.4% sodium bicarbonate (MW = 84 g/mol)?**

$$\frac{8.4 \text{ g}}{100 \text{ mL}} = \frac{X \text{ g}}{50 \text{ mL}} \qquad X = 4.2 \text{ g, or } 4,200 \text{ mg}$$

$$\text{mEq} = \frac{4,200 \text{ mg} \times 1}{84} = 50 \text{ mEq}$$

66. **A 74-year-old male takes *Lithobid* (lithium carbonate, Li₂CO₃) 450 mg PO BID, but reports difficulty swallowing the capsules. How many milliliters of lithium citrate syrup provide an equivalent daily dose of lithium? Round to the nearest whole number. (MW of lithium carbonate = 74 g/mol)**

The problem can be solved with the milliequivalent formula if the MW is provided. The valence of lithium carbonate is 2 (2 positively charged lithium ions and carbonate, which carries a negative 2 charge).

$$\text{mEq} = \frac{900 \text{ mg} \times 2}{74} = 24.324 \text{ mEq of Li ion per day}$$

Refer to the <u>Required Formulas Sheet</u> for the conversion between lithium salts:

$$\frac{24.324 \text{ mEq Li ion}}{X \text{ mL}} = \frac{8 \text{ mEq Li ion}}{5 \text{ mL lithium citrate syrup}} \qquad X = 15 \text{ mL of lithium citrate per day}$$

Alternative method:

$$\frac{900 \text{ mg Li}_2\text{CO}_3}{X \text{ mEq}} = \frac{300 \text{ mg Li}_2\text{CO}_3}{8 \text{ mEq}} \qquad X = 24 \text{ mEq Li ion per day}$$

$$\frac{24 \text{ mEq Li ion}}{X \text{ mL}} = \frac{8 \text{ mEq Li ion}}{5 \text{ mL lithium citrate syrup}} \qquad X = 15 \text{ mL of lithium citrate per day}$$

CONTENT LEGEND

= Study
Tip Gal

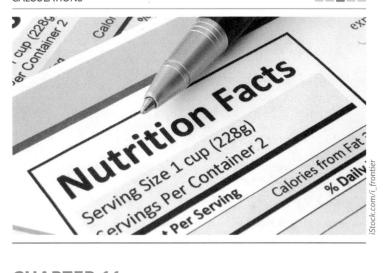

iStock.com/i_frontier

CHAPTER 11

CALCULATIONS III: PARENTERAL & ENTERAL NUTRITION

BACKGROUND

When a patient cannot eat enough to stay healthy, nutrition support may be required. Examples include patients with stroke, cancer, GI disorders (e.g., bowel obstruction, Crohn's disease, ulcerative colitis) or patients in a coma. Enteral nutrition (EN) uses the GI tract to deliver all or part of a patient's caloric needs (e.g., eating food orally or delivering a formula via a feeding tube into the stomach or intestine). Parenteral nutrition (PN), also referred to as total parenteral nutrition (TPN), delivers calories into a vein through a peripheral or central line. When the GI tract is working, enteral nutrition is preferred; it is most physiologic, has fewer complications and is generally less expensive. Parenteral nutrition can be used when the GI tract is not functioning, or in patients who cannot maintain nutritional status enterally.

CALORIE SOURCES

A calorie is a measurement of the energy, or heat, it takes to raise the temperature of 1 gram of water by 1°C. Calories are associated with nutrition because humans obtain energy from the food they consume orally or from EN/PN. Calories are provided by these 3 components: carbohydrates, fat and protein (called macronutrients).

A calorie is a very small unit, and these are therefore measured in kilocalories, or kcals, where 1,000 calories = 1 kcal. It is common to find the term "calories" used interchangeably for kcals. For example, the "Nutrition Facts" box on the side of a container of Honey Nut Cheerios® states that a ¾ cup serving of the cereal provides 110 Calories. Precisely, this is 110 kcals. Looking at the box, the word "Calories" is written with a capital "C" which is sometimes used to indicate kcals, versus a lower case "c." For pharmacy calculations, "calories" or "Calories" are meant to refer to kilocalories, or kcals.

PARENTERAL NUTRITION

Compared to EN, PN is more <u>invasive, less physiologic</u> and has a higher risk of complications (e.g., infection and thrombosis). PN may be indicated when the patient is not able to absorb adequate nutrition via the GI tract for <u>> 5 days</u>. Conditions that often require PN include bowel obstruction, ileus, severe diarrhea, radiation enteritis and untreatable malabsorption.

There are 2 types of PN admixtures. Both types contain sterile water for injection, electrolytes, vitamins and minerals.

- <u>2-in-1 formulations</u> contain <u>two macronutrients (dextrose and amino acids)</u> in one container. Lipids are infused separately, if needed.

- <u>3-in-1 formulations</u> contain <u>three macronutrients (dextrose, amino acids and lipids)</u> in one container. 3-in-1 formulations are also called total nutrient admixture (TNA) or "all-in-one" formulations.

PN admixtures are <u>compounded sterile products (CSPs)</u> and their preparation must comply with <u>USP Chapter 797</u> requirements. They are also classified as <u>high-alert</u> medications by the Institute for Safe Medication Practices (ISMP). Many large hospitals use automated compounding devices to combine the ingredients into a single container, but <u>multi-chamber bags</u> can be purchased for convenience. Two-chamber premixed PN products have an amino acid solution in one chamber and a dextrose solution in another chamber. The seal between the chambers is broken before administration to mix the solutions together. Three-chamber options (with lipid emulsion in the third chamber) are also available. *Clinimix* is one of the commonly used multi-chamber products. *Clinimix-E* products contain electrolytes.

If the PN is expected to be used short-term (< 1 week), peripheral administration may be possible, but has a high risk of phlebitis (inflammation of the vein) and vein damage. <u>Central line</u> placement allows for a higher osmolarity and wider variation in pH. Common types of central lines include <u>peripherally inserted central catheters ("PICC" lines)</u>, Hickman, Broviac, Groshong and others. Administration of <u>PN requires a filter due to the risk of a precipitate</u>.

Each patient's fluid, kcal, protein and lipid requirements, plus the initial electrolyte, vitamin and trace element requirements will be determined. PN requires careful monitoring, including assessing the degree of glucose intolerance and the risk of refeeding syndrome, which is an intracellular loss of electrolytes, particularly phosphate, that causes serious complications.

DETERMINING FLUID NEEDS

Fluid requirements are determined first when designing a PN regimen. Enough fluid needs to be given to maintain adequate hydration, but not too much to cause accumulation. Daily fluid needs can be calculated using this formula:

> When weight > 20 kg: 1,500 mL + (20 mL)(weight in kg* – 20)

Total body weight (the patient's weight on the scale) is used for most PN calculations, unless the question specifies otherwise.

Some institutions estimate adult fluid requirements using a general guideline of 30 – 40 mL/kg/day. The PN and fluid volume should be tailored to the patient. If the patient has problems with fluid accumulation (e.g., heart failure or renal dysfunction), the amount of fluid provided should be reduced. Fluid volume from medications, including intravenous piggybacks (IVPBs), should be included in the calculation of the overall volume the patient is receiving.

1. **GG is a 57-year-old female admitted to the hospital with bowel obstruction. She will be NPO for the next 5 – 7 days. The decision was made to start PN therapy. She weighs 65 kg. Her SCr is 1.3 mg/dL. Calculate GG's daily fluid requirements.**

   1,500 mL + (20 mL) (65 - 20) = 2,400 mL/day

2. **A 76-year-old, 154-pound patient is NPO and needs hydration. She is afebrile and does not have heart failure, renal disease or ascites. What volume of fluid should the patient receive per day?**

   1,500 mL + (20 mL) (70 - 20) = 2,500 mL/day

DETERMINING CALORIC NEEDS

Basal Energy Expenditure

The basal energy expenditure (BEE), otherwise referred to as the basal metabolic rate (BMR), is the energy expenditure in the resting state, exclusive of eating and activity. It is estimated differently in male and female adults using the Harris-Benedict equations below. Most pharmacists do not memorize these equations; they will likely be provided on the exam.

> BEE (males): 66.47 + 13.75 (weight in kg*) + 5 (height in cm) – 6.76 (age in years)
>
> BEE (females): 655.1 + 9.6 (weight in kg*) + 1.85 (height in cm) – 4.68 (age in years)

Total body weight (the patient's weight on the scale) is used for most PN calculations, unless the question specifies otherwise.

Total Energy Expenditure

Total energy expenditure (TEE; or total daily expenditure, TDE) is a measure of BEE plus excess metabolic demands as a result of stress, the thermal effects of feeding and energy expenditure from activity. Once the BEE is calculated, calculate the TEE by taking the BEE calories and multiplying by the appropriate activity factor and stress factor. This will increase the calories required. Energy requirements are increased 12% with each degree of fever over 37°C.

> TEE = BEE x activity factor x stress factor

The activity factor is either 1.2 if confined to bed (non-ambulatory), or 1.3 if out of bed (ambulatory). Commonly used stress factors are listed in the table. The formula for BEE and patient-specific stress factors are likely to be provided if needed on the exam.

STATE OF STRESS	STRESS FACTOR
Minor surgery	1.2
Infection	1.4
Major trauma, sepsis, burns up to 30% BSA	1.5
Burns over 30% BSA	1.5–2

---

3. **Using the Harris-Benedict equation, calculate the basal energy expenditure for a 66-year-old male with major trauma (stress factor 1.5). He weighs 174 pounds and is 5'10". Activity factor is 1.2. Round to the nearest whole number.**

   Height = 70 inches x 2.54 cm/inch = 177.8 cm. Weight = 174 pounds x 1 kg/2.2 pounds = 79.0909 kg.

   BEE (males): 66.47 + 13.75 (weight in kg) + 5 (height in cm) – 6.76 (age in years)

   > BEE = 66.47 + (13.75 x 79.0909) + (5 x 177.8) – (6.76 x 66)

   > BEE = 66.47 + 1,087.5 + 889 – 446.16 = 1,596.81, or 1,597 kcal/day

   The stress factor is not needed in this calculation, because you were asked to calculate BEE only. The BEE can be estimated using 15 – 25 kcal/kg/day (adults). It may be helpful to check the calculation with this estimate and see if the numbers are close. In this case, an estimation using 20 kcal/kg/day would provide 1,582 kcal/day (very close to 1,597 kcal/day as above).

---

4. **Calculate the total energy expenditure for a major trauma patient (stress factor is 1.5, activity factor is 1.2) who is a 66-year-old male, weighing 174 pounds and measuring 5'10" in height. (Use the BEE calculated from the patient in the previous problem.) Round to the nearest whole number.**

   TEE = BEE x activity factor x stress factor. BEE was calculated above.

   > TEE = 1,597 kcal/day x 1.2 x 1.5 = 2,875 kcal/day

5. **A 25-year-old female major trauma patient survives surgery and is recovering in the surgical intensive care unit. The medical team wants to start PN therapy. She is 122 pounds, 5'7" with some mild renal impairment. Calculate her BEE using the Harris-Benedict equation and her TEE (stress factor = 1.7 and activity factor = 1.2). Round each to the nearest whole number.**

Height = 67 inches x 2.54 cm/inch = 170.18 cm. Weight = 122 pounds x 1 kg/2.2 pounds = 55.4545 kg.

BEE (females): 655.1 + 9.6 (weight in kg) + 1.85 (height in cm) – 4.68 (age in years)

$$BEE = 655.1 + (9.6 \times 55.4545) + (1.85 \times 170.18) - (4.68 \times 25)$$

$$BEE = 655.1 + 532.3632 + 314.833 - 117 = 1{,}385.2962, \text{ or } 1{,}385 \text{ kcal/day}$$

TEE = BEE x activity factor x stress factor

$$TEE = 1{,}385 \text{ kcal/day} \times 1.2 \times 1.7 = 2{,}825 \text{ kcal/day}$$

Once the total caloric needs are determined, the calories provided from each macronutrient can be calculated using the conversions shown in the Study Tip Gal below.

CALORIES PROVIDED FROM MACRONUTRIENTS

USUAL DIET*			EN FORMULAS*		PN FORMULAS	
Carbs	Bread, Rice....	4 kcal/gram	Corn syrup solids, cornstarch, sucrose....	Premixed solutions that contain carbohydrates, fat and protein. See Enteral Nutrition at the end of this chapter. Examples of EN formulas: *Ensure, Osmolite, Jevity, Glucerna* and others	Dextrose Monohydrate	3.4 kcal/gram
					Glycerol/Glycerin**	4.3 kcal/gram
Fat	Butter, Oil....	9 kcal/gram	Borage oil, canola oil, corn oil....		Injectable Lipid Emulsion (ILE) 10%	1.1 kcal/mL
					Injectable Lipid Emulsion (ILE) 20% (*Intralipid, Smoflipid*)	2 kcal/mL
					Injectable Lipid Emulsion (ILE) 30%	3 kcal/mL
Protein	Fish, Meat....	4 kcal/gram	Casein, soy, whey....		Amino Acid Solutions (*Aminosyn, FreAmine*, others)	4 kcal/gram

*The diet and enteral formula components shown are common examples; there are others.
**Glycerol may be used to decrease hyperglycemia; more commonly, the dextrose load is decreased or the insulin dose is increased.

PROTEIN

Protein is used either to repair or build muscle cells or as a source of energy. Protein in enteral intake is present in various forms, and in PN as the constituent amino acids. Because critically ill patients are catabolic (protein breakdown occurs faster than synthesis), many clinicians prefer to use "protein sparing" techniques in this population. This means that most or all of the TEE calories are provided by dextrose and fat. If adequate energy is provided by carbohydrates and fat, the protein may be "spared" and can be used by muscle (although the protein calories may not end up in the intended location). If "protein sparing" is used, the energy required by the patient will come from only the dextrose and lipids, which are the "non-protein calories" (NPC). Overall, whether to include the calories from protein in the total calories provided by a PN regimen is controversial.

Protein from food, enteral nutrition formulas or parenteral amino acid solutions provides 4 kcal/gram. The typical protein requirement for a non-stressed, ambulatory patient is 0.8 – 1 g/kg/day. The weight to use to calculate the protein requirement will likely be specified (if needed) in an exam scenario. Some prescribers order protein based on the patient's ideal body weight (IBW). Protein requirements increase if the patient is placed under stress, which is defined by the illness severity. The more severely ill, the greater the protein requirements will be. In patients with a high degree of metabolic stress the protein requirements can be as high as 2 g/kg/day.

CONDITION	PROTEIN REQUIREMENTS
Ambulatory, non-hospitalized (non-stressed)	0.8–1 g/kg/day
Hospitalized or malnourished	1.2–2 g/kg/day

6. **MK is a 62-year-old female who has been admitted with enteritis and pneumonia. She has a history of Crohn's disease and COPD. Her IBW is 54.7 kg. The staff gastroenterologist has ordered PN therapy with 1.5 g/kg IBW/day of protein. How many grams of protein will MK receive per day? Round to the nearest whole number.**

> 54.7 kg × 1.5 g/kg IBW/day = 82 g protein/day

7. **PP is a 46-year-old male who weighs 207 pounds. He is admitted for bowel resection surgery. Post surgery, he is to be started on PN therapy. The physician wants the patient to receive 1.3 g/kg/day of protein. Calculate his protein requirement. Round to the nearest whole number.**

First, convert pounds to kg: 207 pounds x 1 kg/2.2 pounds = 94.1 kg.

Then, calculate the protein requirement.

> 94.1 kg × 1.3 g/kg/day = 122 g protein/day

NITROGEN BALANCE

Grams of Nitrogen from Protein

Nitrogen is released during protein catabolism and is mainly excreted as urea in the urine. Nitrogen balance is the difference between the body's nitrogen gains and losses. While grams of protein are calculated in a nutritional plan, grams of nitrogen are used as an expression of the amount of protein received by the patient. There is 1 g of nitrogen (N) for each 6.25 g of protein. To calculate the grams of nitrogen in a certain weight of protein, divide the protein grams by 6.25.

$$\text{Nitrogen intake} = \frac{\text{grams of protein intake}}{6.25}$$

8. **A patient is receiving PN containing 540 mL of 12.5% amino acids per day. How many grams of nitrogen is the patient receiving? Round to the nearest tenth.**

$$\frac{12.5 \text{ g}}{100 \text{ mL}} = \frac{X \text{ g}}{540 \text{ mL}} \qquad X = 67.5 \text{ g of protein}$$

$$\frac{67.5 \text{ g of protein}}{6.25} = 10.8 \text{ g of nitrogen}$$

Non-Protein Calories to Nitrogen Ratio

The non-protein calorie to nitrogen ratio (NPC:N) is calculated as follows:

- First, calculate the grams of nitrogen supplied per day (1 g N = 6.25 g of protein).

- Then, divide the total non-protein calories (dextrose + lipids) by the grams of nitrogen.

Desirable NPC:N ratios are:

- 80:1 in the most severely stressed patients

- 100:1 in severely stressed patients

- 150:1 in an unstressed patient

9. **A patient is receiving PN containing 480 mL of dextrose 50% and 50 grams of amino acids plus electrolytes. Calculate the non-protein calories to nitrogen ratio for this patient.**

    First, calculate the nitrogen intake.

    $$\text{Nitrogen} = \frac{50 \text{ g of protein}}{6.25} = 8 \text{ g}$$

    Next, calculate the non-protein calories.

    $$\frac{50 \text{ g dextrose}}{100 \text{ mL}} = \frac{X \text{ g}}{480 \text{ mL}} \quad X = 240 \text{ g dextrose}$$

    $$240 \text{ g dextrose} \times \frac{3.4 \text{ kcal dextrose}}{1 \text{ g}} = 816 \text{ kcal of dextrose}$$

    Then, set up the NPC:N ratio.

    NPC:N ratio is 816:8, or 102:1

AMINO ACID CALCULATIONS

Amino acids are the protein source in PN. Amino acids come in stock preparations of 5%, 8.5%, 10%, 15% and others. They all provide 4 kcal/gram. Branded amino acid solutions commonly used for PN include *Aminosyn, FreAmine, Travasol, TrophAmine* and *Clinisol*.

---

10. **If the pharmacy stocks *Aminosyn* 8.5%, how many milliliters will be needed to provide 108 grams of protein? Round to the nearest whole number.**

    $$\frac{8.5 \text{ g}}{100 \text{ mL}} = \frac{108 \text{ g}}{X \text{ mL}} \quad X = 1{,}270.58, \text{ or } 1{,}271 \text{ mL}$$

---

11. **How many calories are provided by 108 grams of protein?**

    $$\frac{4 \text{ kcal}}{g} \times 108 \text{ g} = 432 \text{ kcal of protein}$$

---

12. **The pharmacy stocks *FreAmine* 10%. A patient requires 122 grams of protein per day. How many milliliters of *FreAmine* will the patient need?**

    $$\frac{10 \text{ g}}{100 \text{ mL}} = \frac{122 \text{ g}}{X \text{ mL}} \quad X = 1{,}220 \text{ mL}$$

13. JR is a 55-year-old male (weight 189 pounds) who is confined to bed (activity factor 1.2) due to his current infection (stress factor 1.5). JR requires 1.4 g/kg/day of protein and the pharmacy stocks *Aminosyn* 8.5%. Calculate the amount of *Aminosyn*, in milliliters, JR should receive. Round to the nearest whole number.

First, convert weight to kg: 189 pounds x 1 kg/2.2 pounds = 85.90 kg.

Next, calculate the protein requirement: 1.4 g/kg/day x 85.9090 kg = 120.27 g/day.

Then, calculate the amount of *Aminosyn* (mL) needed. Note that the activity factor and stress factor are not required to calculate the protein requirement.

$$\frac{8.5\ g}{100\ mL} = \frac{120.27\ g}{X\ mL} \qquad X = 1{,}414.97,\ or\ 1{,}415\ mL$$

14. JR is receiving 97 grams of protein in an *Aminosyn* 8.5% solution on day 8 of his hospitalization. How many calories are provided by this amount of protein?

$$\frac{4\ kcal}{g} \times 97\ g = 388\ kcal\ of\ protein$$

15. A PN order is written to include 800 mL of 10% amino acid solution. The pharmacy only has 15% amino acid solution in stock. Using the 15% amino acid solution instead, how many milliliters should be added to the PN bag? Round to the nearest whole number.

First, calculate the grams of protein that would be provided with the 10% solution.

$$\frac{10\ g}{100\ mL} = \frac{X\ g}{800\ mL} \qquad X = 80\ g$$

Next, calculate how much of the 15% amino acid solution will supply 80 grams of protein.

$$\frac{15\ g}{100\ mL} = \frac{80\ g}{X\ mL} \qquad X = 533\ mL$$

CARBOHYDRATES

Glucose is the <u>primary energy source</u>. Unless a patient purchases glucose tablets or gel, carbohydrates are consumed as simple sugars, such as fruit juice, or complex "starchy" sugars, such as legumes and grains. These are hydrolyzed by the gut into the monosaccharides fructose, galactose and glucose, which are absorbed. The liver converts the first two into glucose, and excess glucose is stored as glycogen.

<u>Carbohydrates from food or in enteral nutrition formulas provide 4 kcal/gram</u>. In PN, <u>dextrose monohydrate</u> provides the <u>carbohydrate source</u>. This is the isomer of glucose (D-glucose) which can be metabolized for energy. The <u>dextrose in PN provides 3.4 kcal/gram</u>. Occasionally, glycerol is used as an alternative to dextrose in patients with impaired insulin secretion. Glycerol provides 4.3 kcal/gram and comes premixed with amino acids.

The usual distribution of non-protein calories is 70 – 85% as carbohydrate (dextrose) and 15 – 30% as fat (lipids). Dextrose comes in concentrations of 5%, 10%, 20%, 30%, 50%, 70% and others. The higher concentrations are used for PN. When calculating the dextrose, do not exceed 4 mg/kg/min (some use 7 g/kg/day). These are conservative estimates of the maximum amount of dextrose that the liver can handle.

16. Using 50% dextrose in water, how many milliliters are required to fulfill a PN order for 405 grams of dextrose?

$$\frac{50\ g}{100\ mL} = \frac{405\ g}{X\ mL} = 810\ mL$$

17. **DF, a 44-year-old male, is receiving 1,235 mL of D30W, 1,010 mL of *FreAmine* 8.5%, 200 mL of *Intralipid* 20% and 50 mL of electrolytes/minerals in his PN. How many calories from dextrose is DF receiving from the PN? Round to the nearest whole number.**

$$\frac{30\ g}{100\ mL} \times \frac{1{,}235\ mL}{day} \times \frac{3.4\ kcal}{g} = 1{,}260\ kcal/day$$

18. **A pharmacist mixed 200 mL D20% with 100 mL D5%. What is the percentage strength of dextrose in the final bag?**

The 200 mL bag has 40 g of dextrose (20 g/100 mL x 200 mL).

The 100 mL bag has 5 g of dextrose. There are a total of 45 g of dextrose in the bag.

$$\frac{45\ g}{300\ mL} = \frac{X\ g}{100\ mL} \quad X = 15\ g;\ the\ percentage\ strength\ is\ 15\%$$

19. **If a 50% dextrose injection provides 170 kcal in each 100 mL, how many milliliters of a 70% dextrose injection would provide the same caloric value? Round to the nearest tenth.**

There are several ways to solve this problem. Option 1:

$$\frac{70\ g}{100\ mL} = \frac{50\ g}{X\ mL} = 71.4\ mL$$

Option 2:

$$\frac{100\ mL}{70\ g} \times \frac{1\ g}{3.4\ kcal} \times 170\ kcal = 71.4\ mL$$

Option 3: since the calories are from 50% dextrose and the pharmacist is using 70% dextrose, the Q1C1 (dilution and concentration) method can be used (see the Calculations II chapter):

$$100\ mL \times 50\% = Q2 \times 70\%$$

$$Q2 = 71.4\ mL$$

20. **AH is receiving 640 mL of D50W in her PN. How many calories does this provide?**

$$\frac{50\ g}{100\ mL} \times \frac{640\ mL}{day} \times \frac{3.4\ kcal}{g} = 1{,}088\ kcal$$

21. **A PN order is written for 500 mL of 50% dextrose. The pharmacy only has D70W in stock. How many milliliters of D70W should be added to the PN bag? Round to the nearest whole number.**

First, calculate the grams of dextrose needed for the PN as written.

$$\frac{50\ g}{100\ mL} = \frac{X\ g}{500\ mL} \quad X = 250\ g$$

Next, calculate how much of the 70% dextrose solution provides 250 grams of dextrose.

$$\frac{70\ g}{100\ mL} = \frac{250\ g}{X\ mL} \quad X = 357\ mL\ of\ D70W$$

FAT

Fats, or lipids, are used by the body for energy and various critical functions. Fats are an essential component of cell membranes, serve as a solvent for fat-soluble vitamins, and play a role in hormone production and activity, as well as in cell signaling. In food and EN formulas, fat is provided as four types: saturated, *trans*, monounsaturated and polyunsaturated. Each of these provides 9 kcal/gram. In PN, injectable lipid emulsion (ILE) is the fat source. Fat calories in PN are not measured in kcal/gram; they are measured in kcal/mL due to the caloric contribution provided by the egg phospholipid and glycerol components in the ILE. A 10% ILE provides 1.1 kcal/mL, 20% provides 2 kcal/mL and 30% provides 3 kcal/mL.

Non-protein calories are comprised of 70 – 85% carbohydrate (dextrose) and 15 – 30% fat (lipids). Lipids are available as 10%, 20% or 30% emulsions, with brand names *Intralipid* (all concentrations) and *Smoflipid* (20% only); *Smoflipid* contains 4 oils, while traditional ILE contains only soybean oil, so they are not interchangeable. ISMP has received numerous reports of mix-ups between them.

Lipids do not need to be given daily; if a patient has high triglycerides, lipid administration may be reduced to three times per week or once weekly. If lipids are given once weekly, divide the total calories by 7 to determine the daily amount of fat the patient receives. Due to the risk of infection, the recommended hang time limit for ILE is 12 hours when infused alone. However, an admixture containing fat emulsion, such as a TNA, may be administered over 24 hours. Lipid emulsions cannot be filtered through 0.22 micron filters; 1.2 micron filters are commonly used for lipids.

Some medications are formulated in a lipid emulsion (propofol and clevidipine) that provides fat calories. If a patient is receiving PN along with one or both of these medications, the calorie contribution from the medication must be considered. Refer to the Acute & Critical Care Medicine and Hypertension chapters for further discussion.

22. **A patient is receiving 500 mL of 10% lipids. How many calories is the patient receiving from the lipids? Round to the nearest whole number.**

$$\frac{1.1 \text{ kcal}}{\text{mL}} = \frac{X \text{ kcal}}{500 \text{ mL}} \quad X = 550 \text{ kcal}$$

23. **The total energy expenditure (TEE) for a critically ill patient is 2,435 kcal/day. The patient is receiving 1,446 kcal from dextrose and 810 kcal from protein. In this critical care unit, clinicians do not include protein calories in the TEE estimation. How many kcal should be provided by the lipids?**

As stated in the problem, at this institution TEE refers to the non-protein calories.

2,435 kcal (total non-protein) – 1,446 kcal (dextrose) = 989 kcal remaining from lipids

24. **Using 20% *Smoflipid*, how many milliliters are required to meet 989 calories? Round to the nearest whole number.**

$$\frac{2 \text{ kcal}}{\text{mL}} = \frac{989 \text{ kcal}}{X \text{ mL}} \quad X = 495 \text{ mL}$$

25. **A patient is receiving 660 mL of 10% *Intralipid* on Saturdays along with his normal daily PN therapy of 1,420 mL of D20W, 450 mL *Aminosyn* 15%, and 30 mL of electrolytes. What is the daily amount of calories provided by the lipids? Round to the nearest whole number.**

$$\frac{1.1 \text{ kcal}}{\text{mL}} = \frac{X \text{ kcal}}{660 \text{ mL}} \quad X = 726 \text{ kcal/week. Divide by 7 to get kcal/day} = 104 \text{ kcal/day}$$

26. **A patient is receiving 180 mL of 30% lipids. How many calories is the patient receiving from the lipids?**

$$\frac{3 \text{ kcal}}{\text{mL}} = \frac{X \text{ kcal}}{180 \text{ mL}} \quad X = 540 \text{ kcal}$$

27. **A PN order calls for 475 calories to be provided by lipids. The pharmacy has 10% lipid emulsion in stock. How many milliliters should be administered to the patient? Round to the nearest whole number.**

$$\frac{1.1 \text{ kcal}}{\text{mL}} = \frac{475 \text{ kcal}}{X \text{ mL}} \qquad X = 432 \text{ mL}$$

ELECTROLYTES

Electrolytes in the PN must be individualized to the patient's needs. Electrolytes include sodium, potassium, phosphate, chloride and calcium. More or less of an electrolyte may be needed based on the patient's conditions (e.g., renal disease).

SODIUM

Sodium is the principal <u>extracellular</u> cation. Sodium may need to be reduced in renal dysfunction or cardiovascular disease, including hypertension. Sodium chloride (NaCl) comes in many concentrations, such as 0.9% (normal saline, or NS), 0.45% (½NS) and others. Sodium chloride 23.4% is used for PN preparation and contains 4 mEq/mL of sodium. Hypertonic saline (greater than 0.9%) is dangerous if used incorrectly and is discussed in the Medication Safety & Quality Improvement chapter.

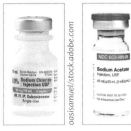

Sodium can be added to PN as either sodium <u>chloride</u>, sodium <u>acetate</u>, sodium <u>phosphate</u> or a combination of these. If <u>acidosis</u> is present, <u>sodium acetate</u> should be used; sodium acetate is converted to sodium bicarbonate and may help correct the acidosis.

28. **The pharmacist is going to add 80 mEq of sodium to the PN; half will be given as sodium acetate (2 mEq/mL) and half as sodium chloride (4 mEq/mL). How many milliliters of sodium chloride will be needed?**

40 mEq will be provided by the NaCl.

$$\frac{4 \text{ mEq}}{\text{mL}} = \frac{40 \text{ mEq}}{X \text{ mL}} \qquad X = 10 \text{ mL}$$

29. **The pharmacist is making PN that needs to contain 80 mEq of sodium and 45 mEq of acetate. The available pharmacy stock solutions include sodium chloride (4 mEq/mL of sodium) and sodium acetate (2 mEq/mL of sodium). The final volume of the PN will be 2.5 liters to be infused at 100 mL/hr. What quantity, in milliliters, of each stock solution should be added to the PN to meet the requirements? Round to the nearest hundredth.**

First, calculate the volume of sodium acetate needed (since acetate can only be provided by sodium acetate and sodium will also be provided by this solution).

$$\frac{2 \text{ mEq}}{\text{mL}} = \frac{45 \text{ mEq}}{X \text{ mL}} \qquad X = 22.5 \text{ mL of sodium acetate}$$

Next, determine how many mEq of sodium are supplied by 22.5 mL sodium acetate.

$$\frac{2 \text{ mEq}}{\text{mL}} \times 22.5 \text{ mL sodium acetate} = 45 \text{ mEq of sodium}$$

So, 45 mEq (22.5 mL) of sodium acetate supplies 45 mEq of acetate and 45 mEq of sodium. How many mEq of sodium are left to be provided by the sodium chloride?

80 mEq Na total – 45 mEq Na from Na Acetate = 35 mEq of sodium still needed from NaCl

Calculate the volume of sodium chloride that will supply the remaining sodium (35 mEq).

$$\frac{4 \text{ mEq}}{\text{mL}} = \frac{35 \text{ mEq}}{X \text{ mL}} \qquad X = 8.75 \text{ mL of sodium chloride}$$

30. **A 2 liter PN solution is to contain 60 mEq of sodium and 30 mEq of acetate. The pharmacy has in stock sodium chloride (4 mEq/mL) and sodium acetate (2 mEq/mL). What quantity, in milliliters, of each solution should be added to the PN? Round to the nearest tenth.**

First, calculate the amount of sodium acetate needed.

$$\frac{2 \text{ mEq}}{\text{mL}} = \frac{30 \text{ mEq}}{X \text{ mL}} \qquad X = 15 \text{ mL of sodium acetate}$$

This amount (15 mL of sodium acetate) supplies 30 mEq of sodium (15 mL x 2 mEq/mL = 30 mEq). The additional amount of sodium required is 30 mEq from NaCl (60 mEq – 30 mEq).

Now, calculate the amount of sodium chloride needed.

$$\frac{4 \text{ mEq}}{\text{mL}} = \frac{30 \text{ mEq}}{X \text{ mL}} \qquad X = 7.5 \text{ mL of NaCl}$$

POTASSIUM

Potassium is the principal intracellular cation. Potassium may need to be reduced in renal or cardiovascular disease. Potassium can be provided by potassium chloride (KCl), potassium phosphate (KPhos, KPO4), potassium acetate or a combination of these. The normal range for serum potassium is 3.5 – 5 mEq/L.

PHOSPHATE

Phosphorus (or phosphate, PO4) is present in DNA, cell membranes and ATP. It acts as an acid-base buffer and is vital in bone metabolism. Phosphate can be provided by sodium phosphate (NaPO4) or potassium phosphate (KPhos, KPO4). The two forms do not provide equivalent amounts of phosphate. The PN order should be written in mmol of phosphate, followed by the type of salt form (potassium or sodium). Phosphate will often need to be reduced in renal disease.

31. **The pharmacist has calculated that a patient requires 30 mmol of phosphate and 80 mEq of potassium. The pharmacy has stock solutions of potassium phosphate (3 mmol of phosphate with 4.4 mEq of potassium/mL) and potassium chloride (2 mEq K/mL). How many milliliters each of potassium phosphate and potassium chloride will be required to meet the patient's needs?**

First, calculate the volume of potassium phosphate required (since phosphate can only be provided by KPO4 and potassium will also be provided by this solution).

$$\frac{3 \text{ mmol phosphate}}{\text{mL}} = \frac{30 \text{ mmol phosphate}}{X \text{ mL}} \qquad X = 10 \text{ mL KPO4}$$

Each mL of the potassium phosphate (KPO4) supplies 4.4 mEq of potassium. Calculate the amount of potassium the patient will receive from the 10 mL of KPO4.

10 mL x 4.4 mEq/mL = 44 mEq potassium from KPO4

The remaining potassium will be provided by KCl.

80 mEq K required – 44 mEq K (from KPO4) = 36 mEq to be obtained from KCl

$$\frac{2 \text{ mEq K}}{\text{mL}} = \frac{36 \text{ mEq K}}{X \text{ mL}} \qquad X = 18 \text{ mL KCl}$$

The patient requires 10 mL of potassium phosphate and 18 mL of potassium chloride.

CALCIUM

Calcium is important for many functions, including cardiac conduction, muscle contraction and bone homeostasis. The normal serum calcium level is 8.5 – 10.5 mg/dL. Almost half of serum calcium is bound to albumin. Low albumin will lead to a measured serum calcium concentration that is falsely low. If albumin is low (< 3.5 g/dL), the calcium level must be corrected with the equation below prior to determining the calcium needs in the PN or providing calcium replacement in any manner:

$$Ca_{corrected} \text{ (mg/dL)} = calcium_{reported(serum)} + [(4.0 - albumin) \times (0.8)] \,^{\dagger}$$

†Use serum calcium in mg/dL and albumin in g/dL (standard units in the U.S.) in the corrected calcium formula

32. Calculate the corrected calcium value for a patient with the following reported lab values:

LAB	REFERENCE RANGE	RESULT
Calcium (mg/dL)	8.5–10.5	7.6
Albumin (g/dL)	3.5–5	1.5

$$Ca_{corrected} = 7.6 + [(4.0 - 1.5) \times (0.8)] = 9.6 \text{ mg/dL}$$

The corrected calcium provides a more accurate estimate of the patient's true serum calcium level (i.e., what it would be if the albumin was normal). In this example, the patient's corrected calcium is within the reference range for the lab.

33. A patient is to receive 8 mEq of calcium. The pharmacy has calcium gluconate 10% in stock which provides 0.465 mEq/mL. How many milliliters of calcium gluconate should be added to the PN? Round to the nearest whole number.

$$8 \text{ mEq Ca} \times \frac{1 \text{ mL}}{0.465 \text{ mEq Ca}} = 17.2, \text{ or } 17 \text{ mL calcium gluconate}$$

Calcium and Phosphate Solubility

Phosphate and calcium can bind together and precipitate, which can cause a pulmonary embolus. This can be fatal. The following steps can help reduce the risk of a calcium-phosphate precipitate:

- Choose calcium gluconate over calcium chloride ($CaCl_2$) because it has a lower risk of precipitation with phosphates. Calcium gluconate has a lower dissociation constant than calcium chloride, leaving less free calcium available in solution to bind phosphates.

- Add phosphate first (after the dextrose and amino acids), followed by other PN components, agitate the solution, then add calcium near the end to take advantage of the maximum volume of the PN formulation.

- The calcium and phosphate added together (units must be the same to do this) should not exceed 45 mEq/L.

  ❏ Automated PN compounding software may use a calcium phosphate solubility curve to assess risk. Generally, when calcium and phosphate concentrations are plotted on the X- and Y-axis of the solubility graph, the lines should meet below the curve. Values that plot above the curve indicate a risk for precipitation.

- Maintain a proper pH (lower pH = less risk of precipitation) and refrigerate the bag once prepared. When temperature increases, more calcium and phosphate dissociate in solution and precipitation risk increases.

34. A patient is receiving 30 mmol of phosphate and 8 mEq of calcium. The volume of the PN is 2,000 mL. There are 2 mEq PO4/mmol. Confirm that the sum of the calcium and phosphorus does not exceed 45 mEq/L.

First, calculate the mEq of phosphate.

$$\frac{2 \text{ mEq PO4}}{\text{mmol}} \times 30 \text{ mmol PO4} = 60 \text{ mEq phosphate}$$

Then, add the phosphate and calcium mEq together. 60 mEq phosphate + 8 mEq calcium = 68 mEq.

Read the question again. Has it been answered? The volume of the PN is 2,000 mL, or 2 L. Calculate the mEq per liter.

68 mEq/2 L = 34 mEq/L, which is less than 45 mEq/L.

OTHER ADDITIVES

Multivitamins and trace elements are usually added to the PN formula. Insulin and histamine-2 receptor antagonists (H2RAs) are occasionally added. Adding any other IV medications to the PN is generally discouraged, because the entire PN would be wasted if a medication was discontinued or changed during the day.

MULTIVITAMINS

There are 4 fat-soluble vitamins (A, D, E, K) and 9 water-soluble vitamins (thiamine, riboflavin, niacin, pantothenic acid, pyridoxine, ascorbic acid, folic acid, cyanocobalamin, biotin) in the standard MVI-13 mixture. The MVI-12 mixture does not contain vitamin K since certain patients may need less or more of this vitamin. If a patient on PN therapy is taking warfarin, the INR must be monitored.

TRACE ELEMENTS

The standard mix includes zinc, copper, chromium and manganese (and possibly selenium). Manganese and copper should be withheld in severe liver disease. Chromium, molybdenum and selenium should be withheld in severe renal disease. Iron is not routinely given in PN.

INSULIN

Because of the large carbohydrate component of PN, insulin may be required (even in patients without diabetes). Half the sliding scale requirement from the previous day (or less) can be added to the PN as regular insulin to safely control blood glucose. This can be supplemented by SC insulin as needed. PN formulas are often titrated on and off (e.g., started at less than the goal rate and not abruptly stopped) to facilitate physiologic glucose regulation.

ENTERAL NUTRITION

EN, which provides nutrients via the GI tract, is the preferred method of feeding for patients who cannot meet their nutritional needs through voluntary oral intake. Several advantages of EN over PN include lower cost, it uses the gut (which prevents atrophy and other problems) and it has a lower risk of complications (less infections, less hyperglycemia, reduced risk of cholelithiasis and cholestasis). EN is sometimes administered through a feeding tube (see section on following page).

Example EN formulas include *Ensure, Osmolite, Jevity, Glucerna, Novasource* and many others. Some are specialized for certain types of patients (e.g., *Nepro* is a renal formula, *Glucerna* is for patients with diabetes), and some can be purchased OTC for meal replacement or those needing additional calories.

FEEDING TUBES

- A tube from the nose to the stomach is called a <u>nasogastric (NG)</u>, or nasoenteral, tube.

- A tube that goes through the skin into the stomach is called a <u>gastrostomy, or percutaneous endoscopic gastrostomy (PEG or G) tube</u>.

- A tube into the small intestine is called a <u>jejunostomy, or percutaneous endoscopic jejunostomy (PEJ or J) tube</u>.

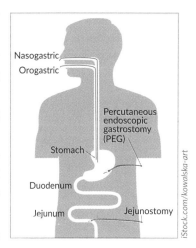

<u>NG tubes are often used</u>, primarily for short-term enteral nutrition administration. For longer-term, or if the stomach cannot be used, tubes are placed further down the GI tract. Tube feedings can range from providing adjunctive support to providing complete nutrition support.

The most common risk associated with tube feeding is aspiration, which can lead to pneumonia. Tube feeds do not, by themselves, provide enough water. Water is given in addition to the tube feeds. If fluid intake is inadequate, it will be uncomfortable for the patient and put them at risk for complications, including hypernatremia.

DRUG ADMINISTRATION VIA FEEDING TUBES

Drug administration through a feeding tube is an important part of patient care but can be prone to errors. Medications should never be added directly to the EN formula, and oral dosage forms (solid and liquid) are not always compatible with tube administration. Drug physical and chemical changes (e.g., from crushing and diluting an oral tablet), alterations in absorption, or interactions with nutrients (see below) can reduce the effect or increase the toxicity of a drug. Additionally, improper administration can cause blockage of the feeding tube. It is prudent to always consult package labeling for product-specific information, but in general, the following types of drugs <u>should not</u> be crushed and administered via a feeding tube:

- Enteric-coated products

- Delayed- or extended-release products

- Sublingual or buccal formulations

- Hazardous drugs (e.g., chemotherapeutics, hormones, teratogens)

Drug-Nutrient Interactions

The general rule for preventing drug/enteral feeding interactions is to <u>hold the feedings 1 hour before and 1 – 2 hours after</u> drug administration.

- <u>Warfarin</u>: many enteral products bind warfarin, resulting in low INRs and the need for dose adjustments. <u>Hold tube feeds one hour before and one hour after warfarin</u> administration. EN formulas contain varying amounts of vitamin K, which can complicate warfarin dosing in some patients.

- <u>Tetracyclines, quinolones and levothyroxine</u>: will <u>chelate</u> with polyvalent cations, including calcium, magnesium and iron, which reduces drug bioavailability; <u>separate</u> from tube feeds.

- <u>Ciprofloxacin</u>: the oral suspension is not compatible with tube feeds because the oil-based suspension adheres to the tube. <u>Immediate-release tablets</u> are used instead; <u>crush and mix</u> with water, and flush the line with water before and after administration.

- <u>Phenytoin</u> (*Dilantin* suspension): <u>levels are reduced</u> when the drug binds to the feeding solution, leading to less free drug availability and subtherapeutic levels; <u>separate</u> tube feeds by 2 hours.

Patient Case (For Questions 35 – 37)

WT is a patient starting enteral nutrition therapy. She has a past medical history significant for type 2 diabetes. She will be started on *Glucerna* ready-to-drink vanilla shakes. See the Nutrition Facts label provided.

35. What percent of calories will WT receive from the protein component? Round to the nearest whole number.

First, calculate the amount of calories provided by the protein component.

$$19.6 \text{ g protein} \times \frac{4 \text{ kcal}}{g} = 78.4 \text{ kcal}$$

Next, find the percentage of protein calories.

$$\frac{78.4 \text{ kcal}}{356 \text{ kcal}} \times 100 = 22\%$$

36. How many calories will WT receive from the fat component of one (8 fl oz) shake? Round to the nearest whole number.

$$17.8 \text{ g} \times \frac{9 \text{ kcal}}{g} = 160.2, \text{ or } 160 \text{ kcal}$$

Nutrition Facts	
Serving Size	8 fl oz (237 mL)
Amount Per Serving	
Calories	**356 kcal**
Total Fat 17.8 g	
Protein 19.6 g	
Total Carbohydrate 31.5 g	
Dietary Fiber	3.8 g
L-Carnitine	51 mg
Taurine	40 mg
m-Inositol	205 mg
Vitamin A	
Viamin C	
Iron	

37. What percent of calories are derived from the fat component? Round to the nearest whole number.

$$\frac{160.2 \text{ kcal}}{356 \text{ kcal}} \times 100 = 45\%$$

Patient Case (For Questions 38 – 40)

JB is a patient receiving *Osmolite* (a high-protein, low-residue enteral nutrition formula) through a PEG tube. See the Nutrition Facts label provided.

38. How many calories will JB receive from the carbohydrate component if he receives 4 fl oz? Round to the nearest whole number.

First, calculate the total calories from carbohydrates in one carton (8 fl oz).

$$37.4 \text{ g carbohydrate} \times \frac{4 \text{ kcal}}{g} = 149.6 \text{ kcal from 8 fl oz}$$

The question asks about calories in 4 fl oz (½ carton).

$$\frac{149.6 \text{ kcal}}{2} = 74.8, \text{ or } 75 \text{ kcal from 4 fl oz}$$

Nutrition Facts	
Serving Size	8 fl oz (237 mL)
Amount Per Serving	
Calories	**285 kcal**
Total Fat 9.2 g	
Protein 13.2 g	
Total Carbohydrate 37.4 g	
L-Carnitine	36 mg
Taurine	36 mg
Vitamin A	
Viamin C	
Iron	

39. **What percent of calories will JB receive from the carbohydrate component? Round to the nearest whole number.**

First, calculate the amount of calories from the carbohydrate component.

$$37.4 \text{ g carbohydrate} \times \frac{4 \text{ kcal}}{g} = 149.6 \text{ kcal}$$

Next, find the percentage of carbohydrate calories.

$$\frac{149.6 \text{ kcal}}{285 \text{ kcal}} \times 100 = 52.49, \text{ or } 52\%$$

40. **The nurse was administering one carton (8 fl oz) of *Osmolite* to JB when she accidentally spilled 2 fl oz on the floor. The remaining amount in the carton was accurately delivered to the patient. How many calories did he actually receive? Do not round the answer.**

$$\frac{8 \text{ fl oz}}{285 \text{ kcal}} = \frac{6 \text{ fl oz}}{X \text{ kcal}} \qquad X = 213.75 \text{ kcal}$$

ADDITIONAL PN PRACTICE

Use the following PN order to answer questions 41 – 42:

Parenteral Nutrition Order Form

Macronutrients 2-in-1	Directions (2-in-1 PN)
Premixed:	Infuse: ☒ Daily ☐ _____ times weekly
☐ **Clinimix (5/15)** Amino acids 5% / Dextrose 15%	Select rate or volume:
☐ **Clinimix (5/15) with electrolytes** Amino acids 5% / Dextrose 15%	Rate: ☒ Continuous infusion _75_ mL/hr
☐ **Clinimix (4.25/10)** Amino acids 4.25% / Dextrose 10%	☐ 12-hour infusion _____ mL/hr
☒ **Clinimix (4.25/10) with electrolytes** Amino acids 4.25% / Dextrose 10%	Volume (liters/day): ☐ 1 ☐ 2 ☐ Other _____

©UWorld

41. **How many calories will the PN provide from protein each day? Round to the nearest whole number.**

Using the rate specified on the PN order form, calculate how many milliliters of PN the patient will receive each day.

$$75 \text{ mL/hr} \times 24 \text{ hrs} = 1,800 \text{ mL/day}$$

Then use the percentage strength of protein from the product ordered to calculate kcals/day from protein.

$$\frac{4.25 \text{ g protein}}{100 \text{ mL}} \times \frac{4 \text{ kcal}}{\text{g protein}} \times \frac{1,800 \text{ mL}}{\text{day}} = 306 \text{ kcal/day from protein}$$

42. **How many calories will the PN provide from carbohydrates each day? Round to the nearest whole number.**

$$\frac{10 \text{ g}}{100 \text{ mL}} \times \frac{3.4 \text{ kcal}}{\text{g}} \times \frac{1,800 \text{ mL}}{\text{day}} = 612 \text{ kcal from carbohydrates}$$

43. How many liters of this PN should be ordered to provide 1,420 kcals per day? Round to the nearest whole number.

Parenteral Nutrition Order Form

Macronutrients 2-in-1

Premixed:
☐ **Clinimix (5/15)**   Amino acids 5% / Dextrose 15%
☒ **Clinimix (5/15) with electrolytes**   Amino acids 5% / Dextrose 15%
☐ **Clinimix (4.25/10)**   Amino acids 4.25% / Dextrose 10%
☐ **Clinimix (4.25/10) with electrolytes**   Amino acids 4.25% / Dextrose 10%

Directions (2-in-1 PN)

Infuse: ☒ Daily   ☐ _____ times weekly

Select rate or volume:

Rate:

☐ Continuous infusion _____ mL/hr

☐ 12-hour infusion _____ mL/hr

Volume (liters/day):

☐ 1   ☐ 2   ☐ Other _____

First, calculate how many kcals/L the PN provides.

Protein

$$\frac{5\text{ g protein}}{100\text{ mL}} = \frac{X\text{ g}}{1{,}000\text{ mL}} \qquad X = 50\text{ g protein/L}$$

$$\frac{50\text{ g protein}}{L} \times \frac{4\text{ kcal}}{g} = 200\text{ kcal protein/L}$$

Dextrose

$$\frac{15\text{ g dextrose}}{100\text{ mL}} = \frac{X\text{ g}}{1{,}000\text{ mL}} \qquad X = 150\text{ g dextrose/L}$$

$$\frac{150\text{ g dextrose}}{L} \times \frac{3.4\text{ kcal}}{g} = 510\text{ kcal dextrose/L}$$

Total

200 kcal/L protein + 510 kcal/L dextrose = 710 kcal/L for PN

Now determine how many liters will provide 1,420 kcals.

$$\frac{710\text{ kcals}}{L} = \frac{1{,}420\text{ kcals}}{X\text{ L}} \qquad X = 2\text{ L}$$

---

44. How many calories will this PN provide per day? Round to the nearest whole number.

Parenteral Nutrition Order Form

Macronutrients 2-in-1

Premixed:
☒ **Clinimix (5/20)**   Amino acids 5% / Dextrose 20%
☐ **Clinimix (5/20) with electrolytes**   Amino acids 5% / Dextrose 20%
☐ **Clinimix (4.25/5)**   Amino acids 4.25% / Dextrose 5%
☐ **Clinimix (4.25/5) with electrolytes**   Amino acids 4.25% / Dextrose 5%

Directions (2-in-1 PN)

Infuse: ☒ Daily   ☐ _____ times weekly

Select rate or volume:

Rate:

☐ Continuous infusion _____ mL/hr

☐ 12-hour infusion _____ mL/hr

Volume (liters/day):

☐ 1   ☐ 2   ☒ Other _1.5_

Question 44 continued on next page.

$$\frac{5\ g}{100\ mL} \times \frac{4\ kcal}{g} \times \frac{1,500\ mL}{day} = 300\ kcal/day\ from\ protein$$

$$\frac{20\ g}{100\ mL} \times \frac{3.4\ kcal}{g} \times \frac{1,500\ mL}{day} = 1,020\ kcal/day\ from\ dextrose$$

300 kcal/day protein + 1,020 kcal/day dextrose = 1,320 kcal per day

---

45. **TE is a 35-year-old female who is receiving PN therapy with 325 grams of dextrose, 85 grams of amino acids and 300 mL of 10% lipids. What percentage of total calories is provided by the protein content? Round to the nearest whole number.**

First, calculate the calories from all sources; dextrose, amino acids and lipids.

Dextrose

$$\frac{3.4\ kcal}{g} \times 325\ g = 1,105\ kcal\ of\ dextrose$$

Protein

$$\frac{4\ kcal}{g} \times 85\ g = 340\ kcal\ of\ protein$$

Lipids

$$\frac{1.1\ kcal}{mL} \times 300\ mL = 330\ kcal\ of\ fat$$

Then, add up the total calories from all the sources. 1,105 + 340 + 330 = 1,775 kcal

Finally, calculate the percent of calories from protein.

$$\frac{340\ kcal}{1,775\ kcal} \times 100 = 19\%$$

Use the following PN order to answer questions 46 – 54:

ITEM	QUANTITY	ITEM	QUANTITY
Dextrose 70%	250 g	Calcium	12 mEq
Amino acids	50 g	MVI-12	5 mL
Sodium chloride (M.W. 58.5)	44 mEq	Trace elements-5	1 mL
Sodium acetate (M.W. 82)	20 mEq	Vitamin K-1	0.5 mg
Potassium	40 mEq	Famotidine	10 mg
Magnesium sulfate	12 mEq	Regular insulin	20 units
Phosphate	18 mmol	Sterile water qs ad	960 mL

---

46. **How many milliliters of dextrose 70% should be added to the PN? Round to the nearest whole number.**

$$\frac{70\ g}{100\ mL} = \frac{250\ g}{X\ mL} \qquad X = 357\ mL\ of\ dextrose\ 70\%$$

47. **Using potassium phosphate (3 mmol of phosphate and 4.4 mEq of potassium/mL) vials in stock, calculate the amount of potassium phosphate that should be added to the PN to meet the phosphate requirement.**

$$\frac{3 \text{ mmol phosphate}}{\text{mL}} = \frac{18 \text{ mmol phosphate}}{X \text{ mL}} \qquad X = 6 \text{ mL potassium phosphate}$$

48. **If the pharmacist adds 6 mL of potassium phosphate (3 mmol/mL of phosphate and 4.4 mEq/mL of potassium) to the 2-in-1 product, how much potassium chloride (2 mEq/mL), in milliliters, should be added to fulfill the order? Round to the nearest tenth.**

    First, calculate the amount of K already added to the PN in the form of potassium phosphate.

    $$\frac{4.4 \text{ mEq K}}{\text{mL}} \times 6 \text{ mL} = 26.4 \text{ mEq K}$$

    Total K needed is 40 mEq. 40 mEq − 26.4 mEq = 13.6 mEq still needed from KCl.

    $$\frac{2 \text{ mEq K}}{\text{mL}} = \frac{13.6 \text{ mEq K}}{X \text{ mL}} \qquad X = 6.8 \text{ mL KCl}$$

49. **The pharmacy has calcium gluconate 10% (0.465 mEq/mL) in stock. How many milliliters of calcium gluconate 10% should be added to the PN? Round to the nearest whole number.**

    $$\frac{0.465 \text{ mEq Ca}}{\text{mL}} = \frac{12 \text{ mEq Ca}}{X \text{ mL}} \qquad X = 25.8, \text{ or } 26 \text{ mL calcium gluconate 10\%}$$

50. **The PN calls for 18 mmol of phosphate and 12 mEq of calcium (provided by 26 mL of calcium gluconate 10%, as calculated in the previous problem) in a volume of 960 mL. There are 2 mEq PO4/mmol. Confirm that the sum of the calcium and phosphorus do not exceed 45 mEq/L.**

    First, calculate the mEq of phosphate.

    $$\frac{2 \text{ mEq PO4}}{\text{mmol}} \times 18 \text{ mmol PO4} = 36 \text{ mEq phosphate}$$

    Then, add up the milliequivalents of phosphate and calcium. 36 mEq phosphate + 12 mEq calcium = 48 mEq.

    The volume of the PN is 960 mL, or 0.96 L. Calculate the mEq per liter.

    48 mEq/0.96 L = 50 mEq/L, which is greater than 45 mEq/L

    When the sum of calcium and phosphate milliequivalents exceeds 45 mEq/L, there is a risk of precipitation (see previous discussion of Calcium and Phosphate Solubility in this chapter). The pharmacist should contact the prescriber to amend the order.

51. **Calculate the amount of magnesium sulfate (4 mEq/mL) that should be added to the PN.**

    $$\frac{4 \text{ mEq}}{\text{mL}} = \frac{12 \text{ mEq}}{X \text{ mL}} \qquad X = 3 \text{ mL magnesium sulfate}$$

52. What percentage of the total calories from the PN are represented by the protein component? Round to the nearest whole number.

First, calculate the total calories.

Dextrose

$$\frac{3.4 \text{ kcal dextrose}}{g} \times 250 \text{ g dextrose} = 850 \text{ kcal of dextrose}$$

Protein

$$\frac{4 \text{ kcal protein}}{g} \times 50 \text{ g protein} = 200 \text{ kcal of protein}$$

Total calories = 850 + 200 = 1,050 kcal. Now, calculate the percent of calories from protein.

$$\frac{200 \text{ kcal}}{1{,}050 \text{ kcal}} \times 100 = 19\%$$

Questions 53 – 54 require knowledge of milliequivalents from the Calculations II chapter.

53. How many milliliters of 23.4% sodium chloride should be added to the PN?

$$44 \text{ mEq} = \frac{X \text{ mg} \times 1}{58.5} \qquad X = 2{,}574 \text{ mg, or } 2.574 \text{ g}$$

$$\frac{23.4 \text{ g}}{100 \text{ mL}} = \frac{2.574 \text{ g}}{X \text{ mL}} \qquad X = 11 \text{ mL of } 23.4\% \text{ NaCl}$$

This concentration of NaCl is hypertonic and is a high-alert drug due to heightened risk of patient harm when dosed incorrectly. Refer to the Medication Safety & Quality Improvement chapter.

---

54. Calculate the amount of 16.4% sodium acetate that should be added to the PN.

$$20 \text{ mEq} = \frac{X \text{ mg} \times 1}{82} \qquad X = 1{,}640 \text{ mg, or } 1.64 \text{ g}$$

$$\frac{16.4 \text{ g}}{100 \text{ mL}} = \frac{1.64 \text{ g}}{X \text{ mL}} \qquad X = 10 \text{ mL of } 16.4\% \text{ sodium acetate}$$

CONTENT LEGEND

☀ = Study Tip Gal

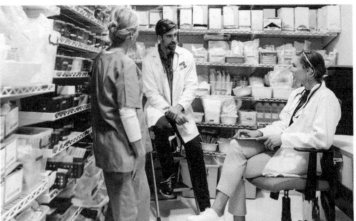
iStock.com/jacoblund

CHAPTER 12
CALCULATIONS IV: CLINICAL

BODY MASS INDEX

Overweight and obesity are health problems associated with increased morbidity from hypertension, dyslipidemia, diabetes, coronary heart disease, stroke, gallbladder disease, osteoarthritis and other conditions. Higher body weights are also associated with increases in all-cause mortality. Body mass index (BMI) is a measure of body fat based on height and weight that applies to adult men and women. BMI is a useful measure of body fat, but the BMI can over-estimate body fat in persons who are muscular, and can under-estimate body fat in frail elderly persons and others who have lost muscle mass. Waist circumference is used concurrently with BMI. If most of the fat is around the waist, there is higher disease risk. High risk is defined as a waist size > 35 inches for women or > 40 inches for men. Underweight can be a problem if a person is fighting a disease such as a frail, hospitalized patient with an infection.

BMI (in kg/m^2) should be calculated as follows:

$$BMI\ (kg/m^2) = \frac{weight\ (kg)}{[height\ (m)]^2}$$

Alternatively, BMI can be calculated with weight in pounds and height in inches using a conversion factor to convert to units of kg/m^2:

$$BMI\ (kg/m^2) = \frac{weight\ (pounds)}{[height\ (in)]^2} \times 703\ (to\ convert\ to\ kg/m^2)$$

BMI CLASSIFICATIONS

BMI (kg/m²)	CLASSIFICATION
< 18.5	Underweight
18.5 – 24.9	Normal weight
25 – 29.9	Overweight
≥ 30	Obese

1. **A male patient comes to the pharmacy and tells the pharmacist he is 6'7" tall and 250 pounds. His waist circumference is 43 inches. Calculate his BMI. Round to the nearest whole number. Is the patient underweight, normal weight, overweight or obese?**

   - Convert weight to kg: 250 pounds x 1 kg/2.2 lbs = 113.6363 kg

   - Convert height to cm: 6'7" = 79 inches x 2.54 cm/inch = 200.66 cm

   $$200.66 \text{ cm} \times \frac{1 \text{ m}}{100 \text{ cm}} = 2.0066 \text{ m}$$

   $$\text{BMI (kg/m}^2) = \frac{113.6363 \text{ kg}}{(2.0066 \text{ m})^2} = 28.2 \text{ kg/m}^2\text{, rounded to 28, overweight}$$

   Because of the rounding specifications in the question, the answer is the same regardless of the formula used. Expect the same on the exam.

2. **Calculate the BMI for a male who is 6' tall and weighs 198 lbs. Round to the nearest whole number. Is the patient underweight, normal weight, overweight or obese?**

   $$\text{BMI (kg/m}^2) = \frac{198 \text{ pounds}}{(72 \text{ in})^2} \times 703 = 26.85 \text{ kg/m}^2\text{, rounded to 27, overweight}$$

   Because of the rounding specifications in the question, the answer is the same regardless of the formula used. Expect the same on the exam.

BODY WEIGHT

There are three potential measures of body weight for a patient: actual (or total) body weight, ideal body weight and adjusted body weight. In pharmacy, weights are used to calculate drug doses, flow rates, creatinine clearance and more. The weight that should be used for each type of calculation (in an individual patient) is not always the same.

ACTUAL BODY WEIGHT OR TOTAL BODY WEIGHT

Actual body weight or total body weight (TBW) is the weight of the patient when weighed on a scale.

IDEAL BODY WEIGHT

Ideal body weight (IBW) is the healthy (ideal) weight for a person.

IBW (males) = 50 kg + (2.3 kg)(number of inches over 5 feet)

IBW (females) = 45.5 kg + (2.3 kg)(number of inches over 5 feet)

There are alternate methods of calculating IBW in children and adults < 5 feet.

ADJUSTED BODY WEIGHT

Adjusted body weight is calculated when patients are obese or overweight.

$$\text{AdjBW}_{0.4} = \text{IBW} + 0.4(\text{TBW} - \text{IBW})$$

Adult doses are generally the same for all patients (e.g., lisinopril 10 mg daily). Weight-based (mg/kg) dosing is common in pediatrics and is recommended for some medications in adult patients. Total body weight is used for weight-based dosing of most drugs in adults, but there are exceptions. Some drugs with a narrow therapeutic index (e.g., aminophylline, theophylline) are dosed based on IBW to avoid toxicity. Some drugs (e.g., enoxaparin, vancomycin) are dosed based on total body weight (even if a patient is obese) because of the results of clinical trials. Dosing drugs in obesity is challenging because there is a risk of underdosing (when standard doses are used) and overdosing (when dosing based on total body weight). In clinical practice, consult primary literature for the best dosing strategy in obese patients. Refer to the Study Tip Gal on the next page for guidance on selecting the correct weight for drug dosing (mg/kg).

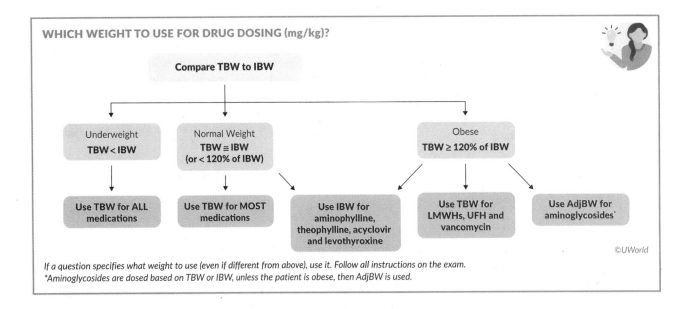

WHICH WEIGHT TO USE FOR DRUG DOSING (mg/kg)?

Compare TBW to IBW

Underweight
TBW < IBW

Normal Weight
TBW ≅ IBW
(or < 120% of IBW)

Obese
TBW ≥ 120% of IBW

Use TBW for ALL medications

Use TBW for MOST medications

Use IBW for aminophylline, theophylline, acyclovir and levothyroxine

Use TBW for LMWHs, UFH and vancomycin

Use AdjBW for aminoglycosides*

©UWorld

If a question specifies what weight to use (even if different from above), use it. Follow all instructions on the exam.
*Aminoglycosides are dosed based on TBW or IBW, unless the patient is obese, then AdjBW is used.

---

3. A female patient is to receive 5 mg/kg/day of theophylline. The patient is 5'7" and weighs 243 pounds. Calculate the daily theophylline dose the patient should receive.

$$\text{Total Body Weight} = 243 \text{ lb} \times \frac{1 \text{ kg}}{2.2 \text{ lbs}} = 110.4545 \text{ kg}$$

$$\text{IBW (female)} = 45.5 \text{ kg} + (2.3 \times 7 \text{ in}) = 61.6 \text{ kg}$$

$$\% \text{ above IBW} = \frac{110.4545 \text{ kg}}{61.6 \text{ kg}} = \sim 1.8, \text{ she is 180\% of her IBW or 80\% above her IBW}$$

Refer to the Study Tip Gal to determine which weight to use to dose the theophylline. This patient is obese. Theophylline, aminophylline, acyclovir and levothyroxine are narrow therapeutic index drugs. They are dosed on IBW in normal weight and obese patients for safety.

$$\text{Theophylline } 5 \text{ mg/kg} \times 61.6 \text{ kg} = 308 \text{ mg}$$

---

4. A 34-year-old male (height 6'7", weight 287 pounds) is hospitalized after a motor vehicle accident. He develops a *Pseudomonas aeruginosa* infection. The physician orders tobramycin 2 mg/kg IV Q8H. Calculate the tobramycin dose. Round to the nearest 10 milligrams.

$$\text{Total Body Weight} = 287 \text{ lb} \times \frac{1 \text{ kg}}{2.2 \text{ lbs}} = 130.4545 \text{ kg}$$

$$\text{IBW (male)} = 50 \text{ kg} + (2.3 \times 19 \text{ in}) = 93.7 \text{ kg}$$

$$\% \text{ above IBW} = \frac{130.4545 \text{ kg}}{93.7 \text{ kg}} = 1.39, \text{ he is 139\% of his IBW or 39\% above his IBW}$$

Refer to the Study Tip Gal to determine which weight to use to dose the aminoglycoside. This patient is obese. Aminoglycosides are dosed using adjusted body weight in obese patients.

$$\text{AdjBW}_{0.4} = 93.7 + 0.4(130.4545 - 93.7) = 108.4 \text{ kg}$$

$$\text{Tobramycin } 2 \text{ mg/kg} \times 108.4 \text{ kg} = 216.8 \text{ mg, round to 220 mg IV Q8H}$$

HEIGHT IN INCHES

In the U.S., heights are generally presented in feet and inches vs using the metric system.

- Example 1: A patient is 5 feet 6 inches tall (often written 5'6"). How many inches tall is the patient?
  - ❏ 1 ft = 12 inches, so 5 ft = 60 inches
  - ❏ Next, add the additional 6 inches
  - ❏ 5'6" = 66 inches
  - ❏ For IBW calculation: patient is 6 inches over 5 feet
- Example 2: A patient is 6'3". How many inches tall is this patient?
  - ❏ 6 ft x 12 inches/ft = 72 inches
  - ❏ Next, add the additional 3 inches
  - ❏ 6'3" = 75 inches
  - ❏ For IBW calculation: patient is 15 inches over 5 feet

FLOW RATES

Intravenous (IV) infusions or continuous infusions are commonly used to deliver medications in different settings, including hospitals. Flow rates are used to specify the volume or amount of drug a patient will receive over a given period of time. An order can specify the flow rate in many ways. Some examples include: milliliters per hour, milligrams per hour, mcg/kg/min or as the total time to administer the entire volume of the infusion (e.g., give over 8 hours). Sometimes flow rates are expressed in drops/min, which is discussed later in this chapter.

Flow rate problems can be performed with proportions or dimensional analysis. Principles of each are reviewed in Calculations I. Some of the following problems will be illustrated using both methods, but not all. Feel free to use either method.

5. **A patient will receive 400 mg of a drug in a 250 mL IV bag. The rate of drug administration is 375 mcg per minute. Calculate the flow rate in milliliters per hour. Round to the nearest whole number.**

   The order specifies the rate of administration as 375 mcg/min. Many infusion pumps are set to deliver a certain volume of fluid per unit of time (e.g., mL/hr). This requires a conversion.

   Dimensional analysis works well for flow rate problems. Here are the steps:

   1. The 1st fraction is the drug concentration. Since you are solving for mL/hr, milliliters needs to be in the numerator.
   2. The 2nd fraction converts the drug weight from milligrams to micrograms.
   3. The 3rd fraction is the rate of drug administration.
   4. The 4th fraction converts minutes to hours.
   5. This combines the individual steps into one calculation. If using dimensional analysis, make sure that all <u>units cancel out</u> to leave the correct units:

   $$\frac{250\ mL}{400\ mg} \times \frac{1\ mg}{1{,}000\ mcg} \times \frac{375\ mcg}{min} \times \frac{60\ min}{1\ hr} = 14\ mL/hr$$

   Flow rates depend on the <u>dose</u> of the medication and the <u>concentration</u> available. If the concentration of the medication is 400 mg/250 mL (in the example above), then the IV needs to run at 14 mL/hr to deliver 375 mcg/min.

   If the pharmacy prepared a more concentrated product (e.g., 800 mg/250 mL, or twice as concentrated), then the IV will only need to run at 7 mL/hr to deliver the same dose. See math below:

   $$\frac{250\ mL}{800\ mg} \times \frac{1\ mg}{1{,}000\ mcg} \times \frac{375\ mcg}{min} \times \frac{60\ min}{1\ hr} = 7\ mL/hr$$

6. **The pharmacist has an order for heparin 25,000 units in 250 mL D5W to infuse at 1,000 units/hour. The pharmacy has the following premixed heparin bags in stock: 25,000 units in 500 mL ½ NS, 10,000 units in 250 mL D5W, and 25,000 units in 250 mL D5W. What should the infusion rate be set at in mL/hour?**

   The pharmacy has the heparin concentration that was ordered. First, calculate the concentration (units per mL).

   $$\frac{25{,}000\ units}{250\ mL} = 100\ units/mL$$

   Next use the concentration to convert the infusion rate from units/hour to mL/hr.

   $$\frac{1{,}000\ units}{1\ hr} \times \frac{1\ mL}{100\ units} = 10\ mL/hr$$

   Since 1,000 units/hour must be delivered to the patient and there are 100 units in each mL, the pump should be programmed for an infusion rate of 10 mL/hr.

Question 6 continued on next page

A second way to solve flow rate problems is using dimensional analysis:

$$\frac{250 \text{ mL}}{25,000 \text{ units}} \times \frac{1,000 \text{ units}}{1 \text{ hr}} = 10 \text{ mL/hr}$$

Another way to solve these problems is to use a proportion:

$$\frac{25,000 \text{ units}}{250 \text{ mL}} = \frac{1,000 \text{ units}}{X \text{ mL}} \qquad X = 10 \text{ mL (10 mL/hr since we need to administer 1,000 units in 1 hour)}$$

Try solving the problems in this section both ways and decide which you prefer.

---

7. If 200 mg of drug are added to a 500 mL bag, what rate of flow, in milliliters per hour, will deliver 500 mcg of drug per hour? Round to the nearest hundredth.

$$200 \text{ mg} \times \frac{1,000 \text{ mcg}}{1 \text{ mg}} = 200,000 \text{ mcg}$$

$$\frac{200,000 \text{ mcg}}{500 \text{ mL}} = \frac{500 \text{ mcg}}{X} \qquad X = 1.25 \text{ mL/hour}$$

---

8. A nurse is hanging a 4% lidocaine drip for a patient. If the dose ordered is 6 mg/min, how many hours will a 250 mL bag last? Round to the nearest whole number.

$$\frac{4 \text{ g}}{100 \text{ mL}} = \frac{X \text{ g}}{250 \text{ mL}} \qquad X = 10 \text{ g or 10,000 mg}$$

$$\frac{6 \text{ mg}}{\text{min}} = \frac{10,000 \text{ mg}}{X \text{ min}} \qquad X = 1,666.67 \text{ minutes}$$

Convert minutes to hours = 27.777 hrs, or 28 hrs

Or, solve another way:

$$\frac{1 \text{ hr}}{60 \text{ min}} \times \frac{1 \text{ min}}{6 \text{ mg}} \times \frac{1,000 \text{ mg}}{1 \text{ g}} \times \frac{4 \text{ g}}{100 \text{ mL}} \times 250 \text{ mL} = 27.777 \text{ hrs, or 28 hrs}$$

---

9. A 68 kg patient is receiving a drug in a standard concentration of 400 mg/250 mL of ½ NS running at 15 mL/hr. Calculate the dose in mcg/kg/min. Round to the nearest hundredth.

$$\frac{15 \text{ mL}}{\text{hr}} \times \frac{400 \text{ mg}}{250 \text{ mL}} = 24 \text{ mg/hr}$$

$$\frac{24 \text{ mg}}{\text{hr}} \times \frac{1,000 \text{ mcg}}{1 \text{ mg}} = 24,000 \text{ mcg/hr}$$

$$\frac{24,000 \text{ mcg}}{\text{hr}} \times \frac{1 \text{ hr}}{60 \text{ min}} = 400 \text{ mcg/min}$$

$$\frac{400 \text{ mcg/min}}{68 \text{ kg}} = 5.88 \text{ mcg/kg/min}$$

Or, solve another way:

$$\frac{15 \text{ mL}}{1 \text{ hr}} \times \frac{400 \text{ mg}}{250 \text{ mL}} \times \frac{1,000 \text{ mcg}}{1 \text{ mg}} \times \frac{1 \text{ hr}}{60 \text{ min}} \div 68 \text{ kg} = 5.88 \text{ mcg/kg/min}$$

10. The pharmacist has an order for heparin 25,000 units in 250 mL D5W to infuse at 1,000 units/hour. How many hours will it take to infuse the entire bag?

$$25{,}000 \text{ units} \times \frac{1 \text{ hr}}{1{,}000 \text{ units}} = 25 \text{ hrs}$$

11. If 50 mg of drug are added to a 500 mL bag, what rate of flow, in milliliters per hour, will deliver 5 mg of drug per hour?

$$\frac{500 \text{ mL}}{50 \text{ mg}} \times \frac{5 \text{ mg}}{\text{hr}} = 50 \text{ mL/hour}$$

12. A patient is to receive *Keppra* at a rate of 5 mg/min. The pharmacy has a 5 mL *Keppra* vial (100 mg/mL) which will be diluted in 100 mL of NS. What is the *Keppra* infusion rate, in mL/min? Do not include the volume of the 5 mL additive.

First, calculate the amount of *Keppra* in the vial.

$$\frac{100 \text{ mg}}{\text{mL}} = \frac{X \text{ mg}}{5 \text{ mL}} \qquad X = 500 \text{ mg}$$

Then, solve for the answer in mL/min.

$$\frac{100 \text{ mL}}{500 \text{ mg}} \times \frac{5 \text{ mg}}{\text{min}} = 1 \text{ mL/min}$$

FINAL VOLUME OF COMPOUNDED IV SOLUTIONS

Why does problem #12 say "do not include the volume of the 5 mL additive"? Because the answer might be different (depending on the rounding instructions) if you used 100 mL vs 105 mL for the final volume.

- Exam scenarios:
  - ❏ Explicit instructions (e.g., #12).
  - ❏ Language stating that a specific volume is "added to" some volume of a fluid (e.g., #22).
  - ❏ Rounding instructions are such that either method will yield the correct answer or volumes of additives are not provided.
  - ❏ Language stating that a specific volume is added "to make 1 liter" or "for a final volume of 1 L."

This can be handled in many ways in clinical practice, but institutions should have clear policies to avoid medication errors.

13. A patient is to receive 600,000 units of penicillin G potassium in 100 mL D5W. A vial of penicillin G potassium 1,000,000 units is available. The manufacturer states that when 4.6 mL of diluent is added, a 200,000 units/mL solution will result. How many milliliters of reconstituted solution should be withdrawn and added to the bag of D5W?

$$\frac{200{,}000 \text{ units}}{\text{mL}} = \frac{600{,}000 \text{ units}}{X \text{ mL}} \qquad X = 3 \text{ mL}$$

14. A patient is to receive *Flagyl* at a rate of 12.5 mg/min. The pharmacy has a 5 mL (100 mg/mL) *Flagyl* injection vial to be diluted in 100 mL of NS. How much drug in milligrams will the patient receive over 20 minutes?

$$\frac{12.5 \text{ mg}}{\text{min}} \times 20 \text{ minutes} = 250 \text{ mg}$$

15. A physician has ordered 2 grams of cefotetan to be added to 100 mL NS for a 56-year-old female with an anaerobic infection. Using a reconstituted injection containing 154 mg/mL, how many milliliters should be added to prepare the order? Round to the nearest whole number.

$$2{,}000 \text{ mg} \times \frac{1 \text{ mL}}{154 \text{ mg}} = 13 \text{ mL}$$

16. **JY is a 58-year-old male hospitalized for a total knee replacement. He was given unfractionated heparin and developed heparin-induced thrombocytopenia (HIT). Argatroban was ordered at a dose of 2 mcg/kg/min. The pharmacy mixes a concentration of 100 mg argatroban in 250 mL of D5W. JY weighs 187 lbs. At what rate (mL/hour) should the nurse infuse argatroban to provide the desired dose? Round to the nearest whole number.**

First, determine the amount of drug needed based on the body weight provided.

$$2 \text{ mcg/kg/min} \quad \times \quad 85 \text{ kg} \quad = \quad 170 \text{ mcg/min}$$

Then, calculate mL/hr.

$$\frac{250 \text{ mL}}{100 \text{ mg}} \times \frac{1 \text{ mg}}{1{,}000 \text{ mcg}} \times \frac{170 \text{ mcg}}{\text{min}} \times \frac{60 \text{ min}}{\text{hr}} = 25.5 \text{ mL/hr, rounded to 26 mL/hr}$$

17. **A 165-pound patient is to receive 250 mL of a dopamine drip at a rate of 17 mcg/kg/min. The pharmacy has dopamine premixed in a concentration of 3.2 mg/mL in D5W. Calculate the infusion rate in mL/minute. Round to the nearest tenth.**

Step 1: Calculate amount of drug in the 250 mL.

$$\frac{3.2 \text{ mg}}{\text{mL}} \times 250 \text{ mL} = 800 \text{ mg}$$

Step 2: Calculate amount of drug the patient needs per minute.

$$\frac{17 \text{ mcg}}{\text{kg/min}} \times \frac{1 \text{ kg}}{2.2 \text{ lbs}} \times 165 \text{ lbs} = 1{,}275 \text{ mcg/min or 1.275 mg/min}$$

Step 3: Solve for milliliters per minute.

$$\frac{250 \text{ mL}}{800 \text{ mg}} \times \frac{1.275 \text{ mg}}{\text{min}} = 0.398 \text{ mL/min, or 0.4 mL/min}$$

18. **An order is written for phenytoin IV. A loading dose of 15 mg/kg is to be infused at 0.5 mg/kg/min for a 33-pound child. The pharmacy has phenytoin injection solution 50 mg/mL in a 5 mL vial in stock. The pharmacist will put the dose into 50 mL NS. Over how many minutes should the dose be administered? Round to the nearest whole number.**

First, calculate the child's body weight in kg.

$$33 \text{ lbs} \times \frac{1 \text{ kg}}{2.2 \text{ lbs}} = 15 \text{ kg}$$

Next, find the dose the child will receive.

$$\frac{15 \text{ mg}}{\text{kg}} \times 15 \text{ kg} = 225 \text{ mg}$$

Then, calculate the time it will take to infuse this amount of drug at the given rate.

$$0.5 \text{ mg/kg/min} \times 15 \text{ kg} = 7.5 \text{ mg/min}$$

$$\frac{1 \text{ min}}{7.5 \text{ mg}} \times 225 \text{ mg} = 30 \text{ minutes}$$

DROP FACTOR

IV tubing is set to deliver a certain number of <u>drops per minute (gtts/min)</u>. There are various types of IV tubing and each has a hollow plastic chamber called a drip chamber. The number of drops per minute can be counted by looking at the drip chamber. It is important to know how big the drops are to calibrate the tubing in terms of drops/mL. This is called the <u>drop factor</u>. Calculating flow rates from a drop factor is not as common with the prevalence of programmable "smart" pumps. It is a good skill to know for situations when a programmable pump is not available (or fails) and as a "double check."

19. A physician orders an IV infusion of D5W 1 liter to be delivered over 8 hours. The IV infusion set delivers 15 drops/mL. How many drops/min will the patient receive? Round to the nearest whole number.

$$\frac{15 \text{ drops}}{1 \text{ mL}} \times \frac{1{,}000 \text{ mL}}{8 \text{ hr}} \times \frac{1 \text{ hr}}{60 \text{ min}} = 31.25 \text{ drops/min, rounded to 31 drops/min}$$

20. A physician orders 15 units of regular insulin in 1 liter of D5W to be given over 10 hours. What is the infusion rate, in drops/minute, if the IV set delivers 15 drops/mL? Do not include the insulin volume in the calculation.

$$\frac{15 \text{ drops}}{\text{mL}} \times \frac{1{,}000 \text{ mL}}{10 \text{ hrs}} \times \frac{1 \text{ hr}}{60 \text{ min}} = 25 \text{ drops/min}$$

21. The pharmacy has insulin vials containing 100 units of insulin/mL. A physician orders 15 units of regular insulin in 1 liter of D5W to be given over 10 hours. How many units of insulin will the patient receive each hour if the IV set delivers 15 drops/mL? Do not round the answer.

$$\frac{15 \text{ units}}{10 \text{ hrs}} = \frac{X \text{ units}}{1 \text{ hr}} \qquad X = 1.5 \text{ units/hr}$$

22. An order is written for 10 mL of a 10% calcium chloride injection and 10 mL of multivitamin injection (MVI) to be added to 500 mL of D5W. The infusion is to be administered over 6 hours. The IV set delivers 15 drops/mL. What should be the rate of flow in drops/minute to deliver this infusion? Round to the nearest whole number.

Total volume of the infusion = 500 mL (D5W) + 10 mL ($CaCl_2$) + 10 mL (MVI) = 520 mL

$$\frac{15 \text{ drops}}{\text{mL}} \times \frac{520 \text{ mL}}{6 \text{ hr}} \times \frac{1 \text{ hr}}{60 \text{ min}} = 21.6666, \text{ rounded to 22 drops/min}$$

23. RS is a 45-year-old male, 5'5", 168 pounds, hospitalized with a diabetic foot infection. The pharmacist prepared a 500 mL bag of D5W containing 1 gram of vancomycin to be infused over 4 hours using a 20 gtts/mL IV tubing set. How many milligrams of vancomycin will the patient receive each minute? Round to the nearest tenth.

$$\frac{1{,}000 \text{ mg vanco}}{4 \text{ hrs}} \times \frac{1 \text{ hr}}{60 \text{ min}} = 4.166 \text{ mg/min, rounded to 4.2 mg/min}$$

Notice that the patient's height and weight are not needed to solve this problem.

24. A patient is to receive 1.5 liters of NS running at 45 gtts/min using a 15 gtts/mL IV tubing set. Calculate the total infusion time in hours. Round to the nearest tenth.

$$\frac{15 \text{ gtts}}{1 \text{ mL}} = \frac{45 \text{ gtts}}{X \text{ mL}} \qquad X = 3 \text{ mL}$$

$$\frac{3 \text{ mL}}{\text{min}} = \frac{1{,}500 \text{ mL}}{X \text{ min}} \qquad X = 500 \text{ min}$$

$$500 \text{ min} \times \frac{1 \text{ hr}}{60 \text{ min}} = 8.3 \text{ hrs}$$

25. The 8 AM medications scheduled for a patient include *Tygacil* dosed at 6 mg/kg. The patient weighs 142 pounds. The nurse has *Tygacil* labeled 500 mg/50 mL NS. The dose will be administered over thirty minutes. The IV tubing in the unit delivers 15 drops per milliliter. What is the correct rate of flow in drops per minute? Round to the nearest drop.

$$\frac{142 \text{ pounds}}{2.2 \text{ pounds/kg}} \times \frac{6 \text{ mg}}{\text{kg}} = 387.27 \text{ mg required dose}$$

$$387.27 \text{ mg} \times \frac{50 \text{ mL}}{500 \text{ mg}} = 38.727 \text{ mL}$$

$$\frac{38.727 \text{ mL}}{30 \text{ min}} \times \frac{15 \text{ drops}}{\text{mL}} = 19.36 \text{ drops/min, rounded to 19 drops/min for 30 minutes}$$

RENAL FUNCTION AND CREATININE CLEARANCE ESTIMATION

Creatinine is a break-down product produced when muscle tissue makes energy. The normal range for serum creatinine is approximately 0.6 – 1.3 mg/dL. If kidney function declines and creatinine cannot be cleared (excreted), the creatinine level will increase in the blood and the creatinine clearance (CrCl) will decrease. This tells us that the concentration of drugs that are renally cleared will also increase and a dose reduction may be required. Sometimes the serum creatinine can appear normal even when renal function is compromised (e.g., in the elderly). Refer to the Lab Values & Drug Monitoring and Renal Disease chapters.

Patients should be assessed for dehydration when the serum creatinine is elevated. Dehydration can cause both the serum creatinine (SCr) and the blood urea nitrogen (BUN) to increase. A BUN:SCr ratio > 20:1 indicates dehydration. Correcting the dehydration will reduce both BUN and SCr, and can prevent or treat acute renal failure. Signs of dehydration should also be assessed and these can include decreased urine output, tachycardia, tachypnea, dry skin/mouth/mucous membranes, skin tenting (skin does not bounce back when pinched into a fold) and possibly fever. Dehydration is usually caused by diarrhea, vomiting and/or a lack of adequate fluid intake.

26. Looking at the laboratory values below, make an assessment of the patient's hydration status.

	PATIENT'S VALUE	REFERENCE RANGE
BUN	54 mg/dL	7–20 mg/dL
Creatinine	1.8 mg/dL	0.6–1.3 mg/dL

A. The patient appears to be well hydrated.

B. The patient appears to be too hydrated.

C. The patient is not experiencing dehydration.

D. The patient is experiencing dehydration.

E. The patient is experiencing fluid accumulation.

The correct answer is (D). The patient's BUN:SCr ratio is 54/1.8 = 30:1. Since 30:1 > 20:1, the BUN is disproportionately elevated relative to the creatinine, indicating that the patient is dehydrated.

27. **NK is receiving a furosemide infusion at 5 mg/hr. The nurse notices her urine output has decreased in the last hour. Laboratory values are drawn and the patient has a SCr of 1.5 mg/dL and a BUN of 26 mg/dL. The nurse wants to know if she should stop the furosemide infusion due to the patient becoming dehydrated. What is the correct assessment of the patient's hydration status?**

    A. The patient appears to be too hydrated given the laboratory results.

    B. The patient is not experiencing dehydration given the laboratory results.

    C. The patient is experiencing dehydration and may need to be started on fluids.

    D. The patient has objective information indicating dehydration but the patient needs to be assessed subjectively as well.

    E. None of the above are correct.

The correct answer is (B). The BUN:SCr ratio is 26/1.5 = 17.3:1, which is < 20:1. Continue to monitor the patient.

THE COCKCROFT-GAULT EQUATION

This formula is used by pharmacists to estimate renal function. It is <u>not reliable</u> in very <u>young children, ESRD</u> patients or when <u>renal function is fluctuating</u> rapidly. There are different methods used to estimate renal function in these circumstances. <u>The Cockcroft-Gault equation should be known, as it is commonly used in practice.</u>

$$\text{CrCl (mL/min)} = \frac{140 - (\text{age of patient})}{72 \times \text{SCr}} \times \text{weight in kg (} \times 0.85 \text{ if female)}$$

Use age in years, weight in kg and SCr in mg/dL (same as mmol/L) in the Cockcroft-Gault equation

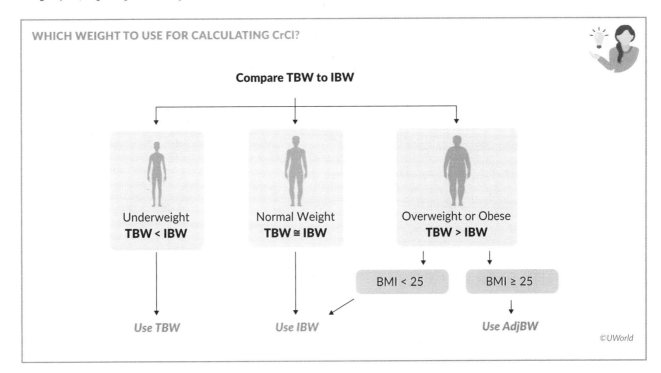

The CrCl is used to renally adjust most necessary medications [some medications are adjusted based on eGFR (e.g., metformin, SGLT2 inhibitors)]. The proper weight to use in the Cockcroft-Gault equation <u>will not always be the same</u> weight used to calculate a weight-based (mg/kg) dose. The following examples illustrate this point.

28. **A 64-year-old female patient (height 5'5", weight 205 pounds) is hospitalized with a nosocomial pneumonia which is responding to treatment. Her current antibiotic medications include ciprofloxacin, *Primaxin* and vancomycin. Her morning laboratory values include: K 4 mEq/L, BUN 60 mg/dL, SCr 2.7 mg/dL and glucose 222 mg/dL. Based on the renal dosage recommendations from the package labeling below, what is the correct dose of *Primaxin* for this patient?**

CrCl	≥ 90 mL/min	60–89 mL/min	30–59 mL/min	15–29 mL/min
Primaxin Dose	1,000 mg IV Q8H	500 mg IV Q6H	500 mg IV Q8H	500 mg IV Q12H

Use the Study Tip Gal to determine which weight to use to calculate CrCl.

Total Body Weight = 93.1818 kg

$$IBW = 45.5 \text{ kg} + (2.3 \times 5 \text{ in}) = 57 \text{ kg}$$

$$BMI = \frac{205 \text{ lbs}}{(65 \text{ inches})^2} \times 703 = 34.1 \text{ kg/m}^2, \text{ obese}$$

Because her BMI is ≥ 25, adjusted body weight should be calculated:

$$AdjBW_{0.4} = 57 + 0.4 (93.1818 - 57) = 71.47 \text{ kg}$$

Then, use adjusted body weight in the Cockcroft-Gault equation:

$$CrCl = \frac{140 - 64}{72 \times 2.7} \times 71.47 (0.85) = 23.75 \text{ mL/min}$$

The correct dose of *Primaxin* is 500 mg IV Q12H.

29. **Levofloxacin, dosing per pharmacy, is ordered for an 87-year-old female patient (height 5'4", weight 103 pounds). Her labs include BUN 22 mg/dL and SCr 1 mg/dL. Choose the correct dosing regimen based on the renal dosage adjustments from the package labeling below.**

CrCl	≥ 50 mL/min	20–49 mL/min	< 20 mL/min
Levofloxacin Dose	500 mg Q24 hours	250 mg Q24 hours	250 mg Q48 hours

First, determine which weight to use in calculating the CrCl.

Total Body Weight = 46.8181 kg

$$IBW = 45.5 \text{ kg} + (2.3 \times 4 \text{ in}) = 54.7 \text{ kg}$$

Use total body weight for calculating CrCl since the patient's total body weight is less than her IBW.

$$CrCl = \frac{140 - 87}{72 \times 1} \times 46.8181 \text{ kg} (\times 0.85) = 29 \text{ mL/min}$$

The correct dose of levofloxacin is 250 mg Q24H.

30. A 50-year-old male (height 6'1", weight 177 pounds) has HIV and is being started on tenofovir disoproxil fumarate, emtricitabine and efavirenz therapy. His laboratory values include K 4.4 mEq/L, BUN 40 mg/dL, SCr 1.8 mg/dL, and CD4 count of 455 cells/mm³. Using the renal dosage recommendations from the package labeling below, what is the correct dose of tenofovir for this patient?

CrCl	≥ 50 mL/min	30–49 mL/min	10–29 mL/min	< 10 mL/min
Tenofovir Dose	300 mg daily	300 mg Q48 hours	300 mg Q72-96 hours	300 mg weekly

First, determine which weight to use in calculating the CrCl.

Total Body Weight = 80.4545 kg

IBW = 50 kg + (2.3 × 13 in) = 79.9, or 80 kg

The IBW is almost the same as the actual weight. Either weight will yield a similar CrCl.

Next, calculate the CrCl.

$$CrCl = \frac{140 - 50}{72 \times 1.8} \times 80 \, kg = 55 \, mL/min$$

The dose of tenofovir should be 300 mg daily.

ACID-BASE AND ARTERIAL BLOOD GASES

pH

The pH refers to the acidity or basicity of a solution. As a solution becomes more acidic (the concentration of protons increases), the pH decreases. Conversely, when the concentration of protons decrease, the pH increases and the solution is more basic, or alkaline. Pure water is neutral at a pH of 7, and blood, with a pH of 7.4, is slightly alkaline. Stomach acid has a pH of ~2, and is therefore acidic, with many protons in solution.

ARTERIAL BLOOD GASES

The acid-base status of a patient can be determined with an arterial blood gas (ABG). The primary buffering system of the body is the bicarbonate/carbonic acid system. The kidneys help to maintain a neutral pH by controlling bicarbonate (HCO3) reabsorption and elimination. Bicarbonate acts as a buffer and a base. The lungs help maintain a neutral pH by controlling carbonic acid (which is directly proportional to the partial pressure of carbon dioxide or pCO2) retained or released from the body. Carbon dioxide acts as a buffer and an acid. Alterations from the normal values lead to acid-base disorders. Diet and cellular metabolism lead to a large production of hydrogen ions (protons) that need to be excreted to maintain acid-base balance. ABGs are presented as follows in a written chart note:

ABG: pH/pCO2/pO2/HCO3/O2 Sat

INTERPRETING ABGs

- Step #1: Is it an acidosis or alkalosis?
  - ❏ ↓ pH = acidosis
  - ❏ ↑ pH = alkalosis
- Step #2: What other values are abnormal?
  - ❏ Respiratory: ↓ CO2 = alkalosis   ↑ CO2 = acidosis
  - ❏ Metabolic: ↑ HCO3 = alkalosis   ↓ HCO3 = acidosis
- Step #3: Which of the abnormal values in Step #2 matches with the pH in Step #1?
  - ❏ Example: ↓ pH, ↑ CO2 and normal HCO3
  - ❏ pH = acidosis and ↑ CO2 = acidosis; this is a respiratory acidosis
- Step #4: What if both CO2 and HCO3 are abnormal?
  - ❏ Usually only one of the values will match the pH, the other will go in the opposite direction as expected from the pH. This is called compensation.
  - ❏ Example: ↓ pH, ↓ CO2 and ↓ HCO3
  - ❏ ↓ pH = acidosis, ↓ HCO3 = acidosis and ↓ CO2 = alkalosis; this is a metabolic acidosis with some degree of respiratory compensation

An acid-base disorder that leads to a pH < 7.35 is called an acidosis. If the disorder leads to a pH > 7.45, it is called an alkalosis. These disorders are further classified as either metabolic or respiratory in origin. The primary disturbance in a metabolic acid-base disorder is the plasma HCO3 concentration. A metabolic acidosis is characterized primarily by a decrease in plasma HCO3 concentration. In a metabolic alkalosis, the plasma HCO3 concentration is increased. Metabolic acidosis may be associated with an increase in the anion gap. The primary disturbance in a respiratory acid-base disorder is pCO2. In respiratory acidosis, the pCO2 is elevated and in respiratory alkalosis, the pCO2 is decreased. Each disturbance has a compensatory (secondary) response that attempts to correct the imbalance toward normal and keep the pH neutral (see Study Tip Gal on previous page for the steps to interpret ABGs).

ABG PARAMETER	REFERENCE RANGE
pH	7.35 – 7.45
pCO2	35 – 45 mmHg
pO2	80 – 100 mmHg
HCO3	22 – 26 mEq/L
O2 Sat	> 95%

Reference ranges for an arterial sample. Bicarbonate reported on ABG is a calculated value and the reference range will differ from a venous sample.

31. **A baby sitter brings a 7-year-old boy to the Emergency Department. He is unarousable. Labs are ordered and an ABG is drawn. The ABG results are as follows: 6.72/40/89/12/94%. What acid-base disorder does the child have?**

    Based on the pH, this is an acidosis. The pCO2 is normal and the HCO3 is decreased (low bicarbonate indicates acidosis). This is a metabolic acidosis.

32. **An elderly female is admitted to the hospital after a motor vehicle accident. She suffered a head injury and is in the ICU. An ABG is obtained and the results are as follows: 8.25/29/97/26/98%. What acid-base disorder does the patient have?**

    Based on the pH, this is an alkalosis. The pCO2 is decreased (low pCO2 indicates alkalosis) and the HCO3 is normal. This is a respiratory alkalosis.

ANION GAP

When a patient is experiencing metabolic acidosis, it is common to calculate an anion gap. The anion gap is the difference in the measured cations and the measured anions in the blood. An anion gap assists in determining the cause of the acidosis. A mnemonic to remember the causes of a gap acidosis is CUTE DIMPLES [cyanide, uremia, toluene, ethanol (alcoholic ketoacidosis), diabetic ketoacidosis, isoniazid, methanol, propylene glycol, lactic acidosis, ethylene glycol, salicylates]. The anion gap is considered high if it is > 12 mEq/L (meaning the patient has a gap acidosis). The anion gap can be low, which is less common. A non-gap acidosis is caused by other factors, mainly hyperchloremic acidosis. Anion gap is calculated with this formula, using the values from the basic metabolic panel (venous sample).

> Anion gap (AG) = Na – Cl – HCO3

33. **A patient in the ICU has recently developed an acidosis. Using the laboratory parameters below, calculate the patient's anion gap.**

Na	139
Cl	101
K	4.6
HCO3	19
SCr	1.6
BUN	38

    Anion Gap = 139 – 101 – 19 = 19; therefore, the patient has a positive anion gap acidosis

34. SJ was recently admitted to the ICU with a pH of 7.27. Below is her laboratory data. Calculate SJ's anion gap.

144	95	68	
3.22	21	2.1	414

The stick diagram method of presenting a basic metabolic panel (BMP) and complete blood count (CBC) is presented in the Lab Values & Drug Monitoring chapter

Anion Gap = 144 - 95 - 21 = 28; therefore, SJ has a positive anion gap acidosis

BUFFER SYSTEMS AND IONIZATION

Buffer systems help to reduce the impact of too few or too many hydrogen ions in body fluids. These hydrogen ions could cause harm, including degrading some drugs, destabilizing proteins, inhibiting cellular functions and, with too much of a change outside of the narrow range, cells die and death can occur. Therefore, buffers minimize fluctuations in pH so that harm is avoided. Buffer systems are common in the body and are composed of either a weak acid and salt of the acid (e.g., acetic acid and sodium acetate), or a weak base and salt of the base (e.g., ammonium hydroxide and ammonium chloride). An <u>acid</u> is a compound that dissociates, <u>releasing (donating) protons into solution</u>. Once the proton is released, the compound is now a conjugate base, or its salt form. For example, HCl in solution is an acid and dissociates (giving up the proton) into H^+ and Cl^-. A <u>base picks up, or binds, the proton</u>. For example, NH_3 is a base that can pick up a proton and become NH_4^+.

Acid-base reactions are equilibrium reactions; there is drug moving back and forth between the acid and base state. The pH and the pKa are used to determine if the drug is acting as an acid or a base. When the pH = pKa, the molar concentration of the salt form and the molar concentration of the acid form of the buffer acid-base pair will be equal: 50% of the buffer will be in salt form and 50% in acid form. Notice that the percentage of buffer in the acid form when added to the percentage of buffer in the salt form will equal 100%. <u>When the pH = pKa, this is the point at which half the compound is not protonated (ionized), and half is protonated (un-ionized)</u>.

A 'strong' acid or base means 100% dissociation and a 'weak' acid or base means very limited dissociation. Any time a pKa is provided, it refers to the acid form losing protons to give to the base, or salt, form.

If the 'pKb' is provided, think 'base' simply because of the definitions of the two terms.

<u>If the pH > pKa, more of the acid is ionized</u>, and more of the conjugate base is un-ionized.

<u>If the pH = pKa, the ionized and un-ionized forms are equal</u>.

<u>If the pH < pKa, more of the acid is un-ionized</u>, and more of the conjugate base is ionized.

The percentage of drug in the ionized versus un-ionized state is important because <u>an ionized drug is soluble but cannot easily cross lipid membranes. An un-ionized drug is not soluble but can cross the membranes and reach the proper receptor site. Most drugs are weak acids</u>. They are soluble, and can pick up a proton to cross the lipid layer.

Most drug molecules are weak acids (or weak bases). These molecules can exist in either the un-ionized or the ionized state, and the degree of ionization depends on the dissociation constant (Ka) of the drug and the pH of the environment. This leads to the <u>Henderson-Hasselbalch</u> equation, also known as the buffer equation, <u>which is used to solve for the pH</u>.

THE pH OF A SOLUTION

Weak Acid Formula

$$pH = pK_a + \log\left[\frac{salt}{acid}\right]$$

Weak Base Formulas

$$pH = (pK_{w^*} - pK_b) + \log\left[\frac{base}{salt}\right] \quad or \quad pH = pK_a + \log\left[\frac{base}{salt}\right]$$

*where pKw = 14

CALCULATING THE LOG OF A NUMBER

35. Calculate log (1/0.5). Round to the nearest tenth.

$$\log\left[\frac{1}{0.5}\right]$$

1. If there is a division, solve the division first: 1/0.5 = 2.

2. The number 2 will be on the calculator screen. Solve for log[2] by hitting the $\log_{10}$ or log key.

   Some hand-held and on-screen calculators may require you to press the log key first, followed by "2" to solve this problem.

3. In this example, the answer is 0.3 (rounded to the nearest tenth).

Some calculators have parenthesis that allow you to enter the calculation as written in the problem, rather than performing each step separately. Practice these steps until you are familiar with them.

---

36. What is the pH of a solution prepared to be 0.5 M sodium citrate and 0.05 M citric acid (pKa for citric acid = 3.13)? Round to the nearest hundredth.

$$pH = pK_a + \log\left[\frac{salt}{acid}\right]$$

$$pH = 3.13 + \log\left[\frac{0.5M}{0.05M}\right]$$

$$pH = 3.13 + \log[10]$$

$$pH = 3.13 + 1$$

$$pH = 4.13$$

---

37. What is the pH of a solution prepared to be 0.4 M ammonia and 0.04 M ammonium chloride (pKb for ammonia = 4.76)? Round to the nearest hundredth.

$$pH = (pK_w - pK_b) + \log\left[\frac{base}{salt}\right]$$

$$pH = (14 - 4.76) + \log\left[\frac{0.4}{0.04}\right]$$

$$pH = 9.24 + \log[10]$$

$$pH = 9.24 + 1$$

$$pH = 10.24$$

38. **What is the pH of a buffer solution containing 0.5 M acetic acid and 1 M sodium acetate in 1 liter of solution (pKa for acetic acid = 4.76)? Round to the nearest hundredth.**

$$pH = pK_a + \log\left[\frac{salt}{acid}\right]$$

$$pH = 4.76 + \log\left[\frac{1}{0.5}\right]$$

$$pH = 4.76 + \log[2]$$

$$pH = 4.76 + 0.301$$

$$pH = 5.06$$

39. **A buffer solution is prepared using 0.3 mole of a weakly basic drug and an unknown quantity of its salt (pKa of the drug = 10.1). The final solution has a pH of 8.99. How much of the salt was used? Round to the nearest hundredth.**

$$pH = pK_a + \log\left[\frac{base}{salt}\right]$$

$$8.99 = 10.1 + \log\left[\frac{0.3}{X}\right]$$

$$8.99 - 10.1 = \log\left[\frac{0.3}{X}\right]$$

$$10^{-1.11} = \frac{0.3}{X}$$

$$X = 3.86 \text{ mole of the salt}$$

PERCENTAGE OF DRUG IONIZATION IN A SOLUTION

The Henderson-Hasselbalch equation can be modified to calculate the percent of ionization of a drug. Since the pH is a measurement of the hydrogen ions (protons) in the solution, the percent ionization is the percentage of the drug in the solution that has deprotonated.

To calculate the % ionization of a weak acid:

$$\% \text{ ionization} = \frac{100}{1+10^{(pKa-pH)}}$$

To calculate the % ionization of a weak base:

$$\% \text{ ionization} = \frac{100}{1+10^{(pH-pKa)}}$$

---

40. **What is the percent ionization of amitriptyline, a weak base with a pKa = 9.4, at a physiologic pH of 7.4?**

Use the weak base formula:

$$\% \text{ ionization} = \frac{100}{1+10^{(pH-pKa)}}$$

$$\% \text{ ionization} = \frac{100}{1+10^{(7.4-9.4)}}$$

$$\% \text{ ionization} = \frac{100}{1+10^{(-2)}}$$

$$\% \text{ ionization} = \frac{100}{1.01}$$

$$\% \text{ ionization} = 99\%$$

---

41. **What is the percent ionization of naproxen, a weak acid with a pKa of 4.2, in the stomach at a pH of 3? Round to the nearest whole number.**

Use the weak acid formula:

$$\% \text{ ionization} = \frac{100}{1+10^{(pKa-pH)}}$$

$$\% \text{ ionization} = \frac{100}{16.85}$$

$$\% \text{ ionization} = 6\%$$

DRUG CONVERSIONS

CALCIUM SALT CONVERSIONS

Calcium carbonate (Oscal, Tums) has acid-dependent absorption and should be taken with meals. Calcium carbonate is a dense form of calcium and contains 40% elemental calcium. A tablet that advertises 500 mg of elemental calcium weighs 1,250 mg. If 1,250 mg is multiplied by 0.40 (which is 40%), it will yield 500 mg elemental calcium.

Calcium citrate (Citracal) has acid-independent absorption and can be taken with or without food. Calcium citrate is less dense and contains 21% elemental calcium. A tablet that advertises 315 mg calcium weighs 1,500 mg. If 1,500 mg is multiplied by 0.21 (or 21%), it will yield 315 mg elemental calcium. This is why the larger calcium citrate tablets provide less elemental calcium per tablet. They may be preferred if the gut fluid is basic, rather than acidic.

Calcium acetate is used as a phosphate binder and not for calcium replacement. Though the capsules contain 25% elemental calcium, absorption from this formulation is poor. Calcium carbonate and citrate are most commonly used for calcium replacement. See the Osteoporosis, Menopause & Testosterone Use chapter for further details.

42. **A patient is taking 3 calcium citrate tablets daily (one tablet, TID). Each weighs 1,500 mg total (non-elemental) weight. She wishes to trade her calcium tablets for the carbonate form. If she is going to use 1,250 mg carbonate tablets (by weight), how many tablets will she need to take to provide the same total daily dose of elemental calcium?**

1,500 mg/tablet x 3 tablets/day x 0.21 = 945 mg elemental calcium daily

Each of the carbonate tablets (1,250 mg x 0.4) has 500 mg elemental calcium per tablet.

$$\frac{945 \text{ mg elemental calcium}}{X \text{ tablets}} = \frac{500 \text{ mg elemental calcium}}{1 \text{ tablet}} \qquad X = 1.89 \text{ tablets}$$

She would need to take 2 tablets daily to provide a similar dose. Calcium absorption increases with lower doses, so this patient should be instructed to take one tablet with the morning meal and one with the evening meal.

AMINOPHYLLINE TO THEOPHYLLINE

Aminophylline and theophylline are narrow therapeutic index drugs. They are dosed using IBW in normal weight and obese patients for safety (see Body Weight section at the beginning of this chapter). Conversions between aminophylline and theophylline must be known for the exam. To convert aminophylline to theophylline, remember "ATM":

- **A**minophylline to **T**heophylline: **M**ultiply by 0.8
- Theophylline to Aminophylline: Divide by 0.8

43. **A physician writes an order for aminophylline 500 mg IV, dosed at 0.5 mg per kg per hour for a female patient (185 pounds, 5'1"). There is only theophylline in stock. How many milligrams of theophylline will the patient receive per hour? Round to the nearest whole number.**

IBW (female) = 45.5 kg + (2.3 x 1 in) = 47.8 kg

$$\frac{0.5 \text{ mg aminophylline}}{kg/hr} \times 47.8 \text{ kg} = 23.9 \text{ mg/hr aminophylline}$$

The aminophylline dose must now be converted to theophylline.

23.9 mg/hr aminophylline x 0.8 = 19.12 mg/hr, rounded to the nearest whole number = 19 mg/hr of theophylline

After solving the problem, read the question again to be certain the question was answered with the correct units (mg per hour of theophylline).

ABSOLUTE NEUTROPHIL COUNT

Neutrophils are our body's main defense against infection. The lower a patient's neutrophil count, the more susceptible that patient is to infection (see table below). The Clozapine REMS Program is designed to reduce the risk of severe clozapine-induced neutropenia; clozapine cannot be refilled if the ANC is < 1,000 cells/mm³. A neutropenic patient should be monitored for signs of infection, including fever, shaking, general weakness or flu-like symptoms. Precautions to reduce infection risk, such as proper hand-washing and avoiding others with infection, should be followed. Further information is available in the Lab Values & Drug Monitoring chapter.

ANC (CELLS/MM³)	DEFINITION
2,200 – 8,000	Normal
< 1,000	Neutropenia (at risk for infection)
< 500	Severe neutropenia
< 100	Profound neutropenia

CALCULATING THE ANC

Multiply the WBC (in total cells/mm³) by the percentage of neutrophils (the segs plus the bands) and divide by 100. Neutrophils can be labeled polymorphonuclear cells (PMNs or polys) or segmented neutrophils (segs) on a lab report.

ANC (cells/mm³) = WBC (cells/mm³) x [(% segs + % bands)/100]

44. **A patient is being seen at the oncology clinic today after her first round of chemotherapy one week ago. A CBC with differential is ordered and reported back as WBC = 14.8 x 10³ cells/mm³, segs 10% and bands 11%. Calculate this patient's ANC.**

WBC = 14,800 cells/mm³, Segs = 10% Bands = 11%

ANC = 14,800 x [(10% + 11%)/100] = 14,800 x 0.21 = 3,108 cells/mm³

The WBC is reported as "14.8 x 10³ cells/mm³," which is equal to 14,800 cells/mm³. Use the full number in the formula.

45. **A patient is taking clozapine and is at the clinic for a routine visit. Today's labs include WBC = 4,300 cells/mm³ with 48% segs and 2% bands. Calculate this patient's ANC.**

WBC = 4,300 cells/mm³, Segs = 48% Bands = 2%

ANC = 4,300 x [(48% + 2%)/100] = 4,300 x 0.5 = 2,150 cells/mm³

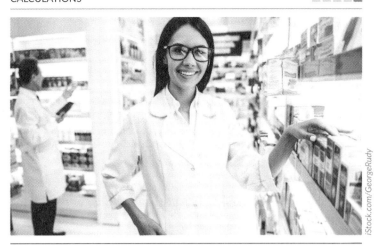

iStock.com/GeorgeRudy

CHAPTER 13

CALCULATIONS V: EXAM-STYLE MATH PRACTICE

PRACTICE WHAT YOU'VE LEARNED

After all of the math concepts in Calculations I – IV have been mastered, test yourself with this exam-style math practice. Put all of your notes and formula sheets away. Grab a calculator and some scrap paper. <u>Time yourself</u> to finish the following 30 questions in ≤ 50 minutes. An answer key with detailed explanations follows.

TOOLS YOU WILL NEED

■ Pen or Pencil

■ Scrap paper

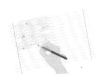

■ Calculator
(use yours or an online scientific calculator)

EXAM-STYLE MATH PRACTICE

1. A pharmacist receives a prescription for a 1.5% (w/w) hydrocortisone cream using cold cream as the base. She will use hydrocortisone injection (100 mg/mL, SG 1.5) to prepare the prescription because she has no hydrocortisone powder in stock. How many grams of cold cream are required to compound 60 grams of the preparation? Round to the nearest one decimal place.

2. How many milliliters of a 1:2,500 (w/v) solution of aluminum acetate can be made from 100 mL of a 0.2% solution?

3. A pharmacist will prepare an amoxicillin suspension to provide a 1600 mg daily dose for a child with an otitis media infection. The dose will be divided BID. To prepare amoxicillin 200 mg/5 mL, the pharmacist should add 76 mL of water to the powder for a final volume of 100 mL. The pharmacist mistakenly adds too much water and finds that the final volume is 110 mL. The pharmacy has no other bottles of amoxicillin, so the pharmacist will dispense the bottle with the extra water added. How many milliliters should the patient take twice daily to receive the correct dose? Round to the nearest whole number.

4. What is the ratio strength (w/v) of 50 mL containing a 1:20 (w/v) ammonia solution diluted to 1 liter?

5. A pharmacist receives an order for sodium chloride 4 mEq/kg/day for a patient who weighs 165 pounds. Using ½NS, how many liters will the patient require per day? Round to the nearest tenth. (M.W. of Na = 23, M.W. of Cl = 35.5)

6. How many milligrams of aminophylline will Mr. Kelly receive per day based on the order in the profile? Round to the nearest whole number.

PATIENT PROFILE

Patient Name:	Mike Kelly
Address:	65 Laney Road
Age:	22 **Sex:** M
Allergies:	NKDA

DIAGNOSES

Asthma
Allergies

MEDICATIONS

Date	Prescriber	Drug/Strength/Sig
8/23	Sanchez	*Singulair* 10 mg 1 tablet in the evening daily
8/23	Sanchez	*Qvar Redihaler* 1 puff (40 mcg) BID
9/29	Williams	Methylprednisolone 40 mg IV Q12H
9/29	Williams	Aminophylline 0.5 mg/kg/hr
9/29	Williams	D5½NS at 80 mL/hr
9/29	Williams	Albuterol nebulization 2.5 mg Q6H

LAB/DIAGNOSTIC TESTS

Test	Normal Value	Date: 1/7	Date: 3/23	Date: 9/29
			Results	
Weight		155 pounds	156 pounds	160 pounds
Height		5'9"		5'9"
WBC	4,000–11,000 cells/mm³	12,000		11,225
K	3.5–5 mEq/L	3.7	4.1	3.6
Glu	65–99 mg/dL	101		142

7. A patient is receiving D5½NS with potassium chloride at 20 drops/min. After 10 hours, the patient has received a total of 40 mEq of potassium chloride using tubing that delivers 15 drops/mL. What is the percentage concentration of potassium chloride in the patient's IV fluid? Round to 2 decimal places. (M.W. of K = 39, M.W. of Cl = 36)

8. An order is written for a dopamine drip in the ICU. The order reads: "Start dopamine drip at 3 mcg/kg/min, titrate by 5 mcg/kg/min Q5 minutes to achieve SBP > 100 mmHg. Page the critical care resident for additional orders if maximum dose of 20 mcg/kg/min is reached." The patient weighs 165 pounds and the ICU stocks premixed dopamine drips (400 mg/250 mL) in the automated dispensing cabinet (ADC). What rate (mL/hr) should the dopamine drip be started at? Round to the nearest whole number.

9. A 46-year-old female with radiation enteritis is receiving 1,800 kcal from her parenteral nutrition. The solution contains amino acids, dextrose and electrolytes. There are 84.5 grams of protein in the PN and it is running at 85 mL/hour over 24 hours. What is the final concentration of dextrose in the PN solution? Express the answer as a percentage. Round to the nearest whole number.

10. ML is a 165-pound male receiving a premixed dopamine drip (400 mg/250 mL) in the ICU. The order states that the drip can be titrated to a maximum dose of 20 mcg/kg/min. What is the maximum rate (mL/hr) at which the drip can be run? Round to the nearest whole number.

11. A pharmacist in an oncology clinic receives the following prescription for a patient with Hodgkin's lymphoma: "Prednisone 40 mg/m²/day PO on days 1-14." The patient is 5'1" and weighs 116 pounds. The hospital uses the following formula for BSA (m²) = 0.007184 x height(cm)$^{0.725}$ x weight(kg)$^{0.425}$. How many 20 mg prednisone tablets should be dispensed to the patient?

12. A nephrologist is treating a patient with hyponatremia. She estimates the patient's sodium deficit to be 210 mEq. How many milliliters of normal saline (M.W. Na = 23, M.W. Cl = 35.5) will be required to replace the deficit?

13. A pharmacy technician is asked to compound three 500 mL doses of 5% albumin. How many 50 mL vials of 25% albumin will be required?

14. A patient is to receive a potassium acetate infusion prepared by adding 9 mL of 39.2% potassium acetate $(KC_2H_3O_2)$ to 0.45% NS to make 1 liter. The patient is to receive the potassium acetate at 5 mEq/hr. What rate (mL/hr) will provide this dose? Round to the nearest whole number. (M.W. of K = 39, M.W of $C_2H_3O_2$ = 59)

15. An intravenous infusion contains 2 mL of a 1:1,000 (w/v) solution of epinephrine and 250 mL of D5W. At what flow rate (mL/min) should the infusion be administered to provide 0.3 mcg/kg/min of epinephrine to an 80 kg patient? Round to the nearest whole number.

16. A cough syrup contains 4 grams of brompheniramine maleate per liter. How many milligrams are contained in one teaspoonful of the elixir?

17. A patient is to receive acyclovir 5 mg/kg every 8 hours for an acute outbreak of herpes zoster. What daily dose, in milligrams, should a 110-pound female receive?

Use the following case to answer questions 18 – 20:

PATIENT PROFILE

Patient Name:	Helene Gudot					
Address:	1365 Stephens Avenue					
Age:	64	**Sex:**	F	**Height:** 5'5"	**Weight:**	135 pounds
Allergies:	Bactrim					

DIAGNOSES

Type 2 Diabetes	Dyslipidemia
Hypertension	Heart Failure

MEDICATIONS

Date	Prescriber	Drug/Strength/Sig
12/10	Marks	Metformin 1 gram BID
12/10	Marks	Regular insulin sliding scale per protocol
12/11	Marks	Lantus 10 units SC QHS
12/12	Ventrakhan	D51/4NS + 20 mEq KCl at 75 mL/hr
12/12	King	Coreg 6.25 mg BID
12/13	Marks	D51/2NS + 10 mEq KCl at 60 mL/hr
12/13	Marks	Lasix 40 mg IV Q12H
12/13	Ventrakhan	Altace 5 mg BID

LAB/DIAGNOSTIC TESTS

Test	Normal Value	Results Date: 12/13	Date: 12/12	Date: 12/11
WBC	4,000-11,000 cells/mm^3	10.7	10.1	12.2
Na	135-146 mEq/L	139	142	145
K	3.5-5.3 mEq/L	4.3	4.1	3.3
Cl	98-110 mEq/L	104	105	101
HCO3	22-28 mEq/L	26	26	25
BUN	7-25 mg/dL	23	26	28
Creatinine	0.6-1.2 mg/dL	1.1	1.3	1.4
Glu	65-99 mg/dL	180 @ 0700	140 @ 0700	260 @ 0700
Glu	65-99 mg/dL	280 @ 1100	280 @ 1100	320 @ 1100
Glu	65-99 mg/dL	220 @ 1700	300 @ 1700	280 @ 1700
Glu	65-99 mg/dL	100 @ 2100	220 @ 2100	220 @ 2100

18. Mrs. Gudot uses the following regular insulin sliding scale: "take 1 unit of insulin SC for every 20 mg/dL of blood sugar > 160 mg/dL." How many units of sliding scale insulin should have been administered on December 12th?

19. The pharmacist is asked to convert several of Mrs. Gudot's labs to different units so her case can be compared to a published case report. Convert her serum potassium (M.W. of potassium = 39) on December 13th to mg/dL. Round to the nearest tenth.

20. Convert Mrs. Gudot's serum sodium level on December 11th to mmol/L. Round to the nearest whole number. (M.W. of Na = 23)

21. A patient received 4 mg of IV morphine. What is an equivalent dose of oral hydromorphone? Round to the nearest whole number. (10 mg of IV morphine is equivalent to 7.5 mg of oral hydromorphone)

22. If 200 capsules contain 500 mg of an active ingredient, how many milligrams of the active ingredient will 76 capsules contain?

23. If phenobarbital elixir contains 18.2 mg of phenobarbital per 5 mL, how many grams of phenobarbital would be used in preparing a pint of the elixir? Round to the nearest tenth.

24. **How many calories will the patient receive each day from the following PN order? Round to the nearest whole number.**

┌───┐

Parenteral Nutrition Order Form

Macronutrients 2-in-1

Premixed:

☐ **Clinimix (5/15)**
  Amino acids 5% / Dextrose 15%

☒ **Clinimix (5/15) with electrolytes**
  Amino acids 5% / Dextrose 15%

☐ **Clinimix (4.25/10)**
  Amino acids 4.25% / Dextrose 10%

☐ **Clinimix (4.25/10) with electrolytes**
  Amino acids 4.25% / Dextrose 10%

Directions (2-in-1 PN)

Infuse: ☒ Daily   ☐ _____ times weekly

Select rate or volume:

Rate:
☒ Continuous infusion __60__ mL/hr

☐ 12-hour infusion _____ mL/hr

Volume (liters/day):
☐ 1   ☐ 2   ☐ Other _____

└───┘

©UWorld

25. **A penicillin V 250 mg tablet equals 400,000 units of penicillin activity. A patient is taking penicillin V 500 mg tablets QID for 7 days. How much penicillin activity, in units, will this patient receive in the total prescription?**

26. **Oral potassium chloride 20% solution contains 40 mEq of potassium per 15 milliliters of solution. A patient needs 25 mEq of potassium daily. How many milliliters of 20% potassium chloride should the patient take? Round to the nearest tenth.**

27. **The pharmacist reviews Ms. Hoydt's *Lovenox* order and labs in the profile. At this hospital, pharmacists have the authority to make renal dosage adjustments per package labeling when necessary. What is the correct *Lovenox* dose for Ms. Hoydt?**

PATIENT PROFILE

Patient Name:	Carolyn Hoydt					
Address:	13 Windgate Road					
Age:	37	Sex:	F	Height: 5'6"	Weight:	175 pounds
Allergies:	NKDA					

DIAGNOSES

DVT confirmed by ultrasound

MEDICATIONS

Date	Prescriber	Drug/Strength/Sig
7/5	Langston	Ortho Tri-Cyclen 1 PO daily
7/5	Langston	Centrum 1 PO daily
11/15	Mason	Lovenox 1 mg/kg SC Q12H
11/15	Mason	D5½NS @ 70 mL/hr

LAB/DIAGNOSTIC TESTS

Test	Normal Value	Results Date: 7/5	Date: 11/15	Date:
Na	135-146 mEq/L	136	142	
K	3.5-5.3 mEq/L	3.5	5.2	
Cl	98-110 mEq/L	109	105	
HCO3	22-28 mEq/L	25	26	
BUN	7-25 mg/dL	10	22	
Creatinine	0.6-1.2 mg/dL	0.7	1.4	
Glu	65-99 mg/dL	100	120	
Hgb	12-16 g/dL	12	13.6	
Hct	36-46%	37	41	

A. 175 mg SC Q12H

B. 175 mg SC once daily

C. 80 mg SC once daily

D. 80 mg SC Q12H

E. 60 mg SC Q12H

28. The pharmacist reviews the order for IV *Bactrim* and the labs for Mr. Ross in the profile. What dose should Mr. Ross receive given the renal dosage recommendations below?

CrCl	> 30 mL/min	15–30 mL/min	< 15 mL/min
Sulfamethoxazole/ Trimethoprim (SMX/TMP)	No dosage adjustment required	Administer 50% of the recommended dose	Use is not recommended

---

PATIENT PROFILE

Patient Name:	Jeremy Ross						
Address:	22 Harris Lane						
Age:	41	**Sex:**	M	**Height:**	6'1"	**Weight:**	70 kg
Allergies:	NKDA						

DIAGNOSES

Depression	Dyslipidemia
HIV	

MEDICATIONS

Date	Prescriber	Drug/Strength/Sig
5/5	Sangler	Nicotine patch 21 mg/day – apply 1 patch daily
5/5	Sangler	*Stribild* 1 tablet daily
6/15	Sangler	*Celexa* 20 mg 1 tablet daily
11/15	Mason	*Lipitor* 10 mg 1 tablet daily
12/1	Hern	*Bactrim* 20 mg TMP/kg/day IV divided Q6H

LAB/DIAGNOSTIC TESTS

Test	Normal Value	Results Date: 12/1	Results Date: 5/5	
WBC	4,000-11,000 cells/mm³	10.7	9.5	
CD4	800–1,100 cells/mm³	187	226	
Na	135-146 mEq/L	139	142	
K	3.5-5.3 mEq/L	3.7	4.1	
Cl	98-110 mEq/L	109	105	
HCO3	22-28 mEq/L	24	26	
BUN	7-25 mg/dL	7	9	
Creatinine	0.6-1.2 mg/dL	0.6	0.8	
Glu	65-99 mg/dL	120	136	

A. 1400 mg TMP IV Q6H

B. 700 mg TMP IV Q6H

C. 400 mg TMP IV Q12H

D. 350 mg TMP IV Q6H

E. Mr. Ross should not receive *Bactrim*

---

29. MH is a 72-year-old male patient hospitalized with decompensated heart failure and fever. Cultures are positive for aspergillosis. MH weighs 110 kg and will receive 0.25 mg/kg per day of amphotericin B (reconstituted and diluted to 0.1 mg/mL) by IV infusion. How many milliliters of amphotericin solution are required to deliver the daily dose?

---

30. What is the pH of a solution containing 0.2 mole of a weakly basic drug and 0.02 mole of its salt per liter of solution (pKa of the drug = 9.36)? Round to the nearest hundredth.

ANSWER KEY AND EXPLANATIONS

1. **First, calculate the grams of hydrocortisone required for the prescription.**

$$\frac{1.5\ g}{100\ g} = \frac{X\ g}{60\ g} \qquad X = 0.9 \text{ grams of hydrocortisone required}$$

Calculate the volume of hydrocortisone injection required.

$$\frac{100\ mg}{1\ mL} = \frac{900\ mg}{X\ mL} \qquad X = 9\ mL$$

Calculate the weight of 9 mL of hydrocortisone injection using the SG provided.

$$1.5 = \frac{X\ g}{9\ mL} \qquad X = 13.5 \text{ grams (weight of hydrocortisone injection)}$$

Calculate the grams of cold cream required.

$$60\ g \text{ final product} \quad - \quad 13.5\ g \text{ (weight of hydrocortisone)} \quad = \quad 46.5\ g \text{ of cold cream}$$

2. **Both concentrations must be in the same units to use the $Q_1C_1 = Q_2C_2$ formula. So, 1:2,500 must be converted to a percentage strength first.**

$$\frac{1\ part}{2,500\ parts} = \frac{X\ g}{100\ mL} \qquad X = 0.04\ g, \text{ or } 0.04\%$$

Now use the formula.

$$100\ mL \quad \times \quad 0.2\% \quad = \quad Q_2 \quad \times \quad 0.04\%$$

$$Q_2 = 500\ mL$$

3. **Two methods to solve this calculation are shown:**

$$\frac{200\ mg}{5\ mL} = \frac{X\ mg}{100\ mL} \qquad X = 4,000\ mg \qquad\qquad \frac{4,000\ mg}{110\ mL} = \frac{X\ mg}{mL} \qquad X = 36.36\ mg/mL$$

$$\frac{4,000\ mg}{110\ mL} = \frac{800\ mg}{X\ mL} \qquad X = 22\ mL \qquad\qquad \frac{36.36\ mg}{1\ mL} = \frac{800\ mg}{X\ mL} \qquad X = 22\ mL$$

4. **First, convert 1:20 to a percentage strength.**

$$\frac{1\ part}{20\ parts} = \frac{X\ g}{100\ mL} \qquad X = 5\ g, \text{ or } 5\%$$

$$50\ mL \quad \times \quad 5\% \quad = \quad 1,000\ mL \quad \times \quad C_2$$

$$C_2 \quad = \quad 0.25\%$$

$$\text{Convert } 0.25\% \text{ to ratio strength} \quad = \quad 1:400$$

5.

$$\frac{4 \text{ mEq}}{\text{kg}} \times 75 \text{ kg} = 300 \text{ mEq/day}$$

$$300 \text{ mEq} = \frac{X \text{ mg} \times 1}{58.5} = 17{,}550 \text{ mg, or } 17.55 \text{ g}$$

$$\frac{0.45 \text{ g}}{100 \text{ mL}} = \frac{17.55 \text{ g}}{X \text{ mL}} \qquad X = 3{,}900 \text{ mL or } 3.9 \text{ L}$$

---

6. Aminophylline is dosed based on IBW.

$$\text{IBW (male)} = 50 \text{ kg} + (2.3 \times 9 \text{ in}) = 70.7 \text{ kg}$$

$$\text{Aminophylline } 0.5 \text{ mg/kg/hr} \times 70.7 \text{ kg} \times 24 \text{ hrs} = 848.4 \text{ mg/day, round to } 848 \text{ mg/day}$$

7.

$$40 \text{ mEq} = \frac{X \text{ mg} \times 1}{75} = 3{,}000 \text{ mg, or } 3 \text{ g of KCl have been given in 10 hours}$$

$$\frac{20 \text{ drops}}{\text{min}} \times \frac{60 \text{ min}}{1 \text{ hr}} \times 10 \text{ hrs} = 12{,}000 \text{ drops infused in 10 hours}$$

$$\frac{15 \text{ drops}}{\text{mL}} = \frac{12{,}000 \text{ drops}}{X \text{ mL}} \qquad X = 800 \text{ mL have infused in 10 hours}$$

$$\frac{3 \text{ g KCl}}{800 \text{ mL}} = \frac{X \text{ g}}{100 \text{ mL}} \qquad X = 0.375 \text{ g, or } 0.38\%$$

8.

$$3 \text{ mcg/kg/min} \times 75 \text{ kg} = 225 \text{ mcg/min}$$

$$\frac{250 \text{ mL}}{400 \text{ mg}} \times \frac{1 \text{ mg}}{1000 \text{ mcg}} \times \frac{225 \text{ mcg}}{\text{min}} \times \frac{60 \text{ min}}{1 \text{ hr}} = 8.4 \text{ mL/hr, or } 8 \text{ mL/hr}$$

---

9. First, calculate the calories from dextrose by subtracting out the protein component.

$$84.5 \text{ g} \times \frac{4 \text{ kcal}}{\text{g}} = 338 \text{ kcal}$$

$$1{,}800 \text{ kcal} - 338 \text{ kcal of protein} = 1{,}462 \text{ kcal from dextrose}$$

Next, calculate the grams of dextrose in this PN.

$$1{,}462 \text{ kcal} \times \frac{1 \text{ g}}{3.4 \text{ kcal}} = 430 \text{ grams of dextrose}$$

Then, calculate the final concentration. This requires calculating the total volume the patient is receiving.

$$\frac{85 \text{ mL}}{\text{hr}} \times 24 \text{ hours} = 2{,}040 \text{ mL}$$

$$\frac{430 \text{ g dextrose}}{2{,}040 \text{ mL}} = \frac{X \text{ g}}{100 \text{ mL}} \qquad X = 21\%$$

10.

$$20 \text{ mcg/kg/min} \quad \times \quad 75 \text{ kg} \quad = \quad 1500 \text{ mcg/min}$$

$$\frac{250 \text{ mL}}{400 \text{ mg}} \times \frac{1 \text{ mg}}{1000 \text{ mcg}} \times \frac{1500 \text{ mcg}}{\text{min}} \times \frac{60 \text{ min}}{1 \text{ hr}} = \begin{array}{l} 56.25 \text{ mL/hr – max rate per order} \\ \text{Round to the nearest whole number = 56 mL/hr} \end{array}$$

11.

$$\text{BSA (m}^2) = 0.007184 \times (154.94)^{0.725} \times (52.7272)^{0.425} = 1.5 \text{ m}^2$$

$$40 \text{ mg/m}^2\text{/day} \times 1.5 \text{ m}^2 = 60 \text{ mg/day}$$

Refer to the Oncology chapter for a discussion of BSA.

The patient will take 60 mg of prednisone (three 20 mg tablets) per day for 14 days. The pharmacist should dispense 42 of the 20 mg prednisone tablets.

12.

$$210 \text{ mEq} = \frac{\text{mg} \times 1}{58.5} \quad 12{,}285 \text{ mg or } 12.285 \text{ g}$$

$$\frac{0.9 \text{ g}}{100 \text{ mL}} = \frac{12.285 \text{ g}}{X \text{ mL}} \quad X = 1{,}365 \text{ mL of NS are required}$$

13.

$$\frac{5 \text{ g}}{100 \text{ mL}} = \frac{X \text{ g}}{500 \text{ mL}} \quad X = 25 \text{ g, or } 75 \text{ g for the three required doses}$$

$$\frac{25 \text{ g}}{100 \text{ mL}} = \frac{X \text{ g}}{50 \text{ mL}} \quad X = 12.5 \text{ g per 50 mL vial}$$

$$75 \text{ g required} \times \frac{1 \text{ vial}}{12.5 \text{ g}} \quad X = 6 \text{ vials of 25\% albumin required}$$

14.

$$\frac{39.2 \text{ g}}{100 \text{ mL}} = \frac{X \text{ g}}{9 \text{ mL}} \quad X = 3.528 \text{ g or } 3{,}528 \text{ mg}$$

$$X \text{ mEq} = \frac{3{,}528 \text{ mg} \times 1}{98} = 36 \text{ mEq}$$

$$\frac{1{,}000 \text{ mL}}{36 \text{ mEq}} \times \frac{5 \text{ mEq}}{\text{hr}} = 138.88 \text{ mL/hr, or } 139 \text{ mL/hr}$$

15.

1:1,000 ratio strength = 0.1% (w/v)

$$\frac{0.1\ g}{100\ mL} = \frac{X\ g}{2\ mL} \qquad X = 0.002\ g,\ or\ 2\ mg$$

The patient is 80 kg x 0.3 mcg/kg/min = 24 mcg/min

$$\frac{252\ mL}{2\ mg} \times \frac{1\ mg}{1,000\ mcg} \times \frac{24\ mcg}{min} = 3\ mL/min$$

---

16. First, convert grams to milligrams.

$$4\ g \times \frac{1000\ mg}{1\ g} = 4,000\ mg\ per\ 1\ liter$$

1 L = 1,000 mL

1 teaspoonful = 5 mL

Next, solve using a proportion.

$$\frac{4,000\ mg}{1,000\ mL} = \frac{X\ mg}{5\ mL} \qquad X = 20\ mg$$

---

17. Begin by converting the patient's weight in pounds (lbs) to kilograms (kg).

$$110\ pounds \times \frac{1\ kg}{2.2\ pounds} = 50\ kg$$

Acyclovir should be dosed based on IBW in normal weight or obese patients [refer to Which Weight to Use for Drug Dosing (mg/kg) in Calculations IV]. Since no height is provided in the question, the only option is to use the weight provided. An adult female weighing 110 pounds is likely very close to IBW.

$$\frac{5\ mg}{1\ kg} = \frac{X\ mg}{50\ kg} \qquad X = 250\ mg/dose \times 3\ doses/day = 750\ mg/day$$

18.

140 mg/dL = no insulin

280 mg/dL – 160 mg/dL = 120 mg/dL; 120 mg/dL / 20 mg/dL = 6 units

300 mg/dL – 160 mg/dL = 140 mg/dL / 20 mg/dL = 7 units

220 mg/dL – 160 mg/dL = 60 mg/dL / 20 mg/dL = 3 units

Total sliding scale units for December 12th = 6 + 7 + 3 = 16 units

---

19.

$$4.3\ mEq = \frac{X\ mg \times 1}{39} \qquad X = 167.7\ mg$$

4.3 mEq = 167.7 mg. The patient's serum potassium is reported as 4.3 mEq/L, which equals 167.7 mg/L.

$$\frac{167.7\ mg}{1\ L} \times \frac{1\ L}{10\ dL} = 16.8\ mg/dL$$

20.

$$145 \text{ mEq} \quad = \quad \frac{X \text{ mg} \times 1}{23} \qquad X = 3{,}335 \text{ mg}$$

$$X \text{ mmols} \quad = \quad \frac{3{,}335 \text{ mg}}{23} \qquad X = 145 \text{ mmols, therefore } 145 \text{ mEq/L} = 145 \text{ mmol/L for sodium}$$

Note that mmols = mEq in this problem. For Na and K, the mmol and mEq are the same; 1 mmol = 1 mEq.

21.

$$\frac{4 \text{ mg IV morphine}}{X \text{ mg oral hydromorphone}} \quad = \quad \frac{10 \text{ mg IV morphine}}{7.5 \text{ mg oral hydromorphone}} \qquad X = 3 \text{ mg oral hydromorphone}$$

22.

$$\frac{200 \text{ caps}}{500 \text{ mg}} \quad = \quad \frac{76 \text{ caps}}{X \text{ mg}} \qquad X = 190 \text{ mg}$$

---

23. First, convert milligrams to grams.

$$18.2 \text{ mg} \quad \times \quad \frac{1 \text{ g}}{1{,}000 \text{ mg}} \quad = \quad 0.0182 \text{ g}$$

Use a proportion to calculate the grams needed for 1 pint.

$$\frac{0.0182 \text{ g}}{5 \text{ mL}} \quad = \quad \frac{X \text{ g}}{480 \text{ mL}} \qquad X = 1.7 \text{ g}$$

Because of the rounding specifications in the question, the answer is the same regardless of the pint conversion used. Expect the same on the exam.

---

24. First, calculate how many milliliters of PN the patient will receive in 24 hours based on the rate ordered:

$$60 \text{ mL/hr} \times 24 \text{ hours} \quad = \quad 1{,}440 \text{ mL/day}$$

Use the percentage strength of dextrose from the product ordered to calculate the calories from dextrose:

$$\frac{3.4 \text{ kcal}}{g} \quad \times \quad \frac{15 \text{ g}}{100 \text{ mL}} \quad \times \quad 1{,}440 \text{ mL} \quad = \quad 734.4 \text{ kcal from dextrose}$$

Use the percentage strength of amino acids from the product ordered to calculate the calories from protein:

$$\frac{4 \text{ kcal}}{g} \quad \times \quad \frac{5 \text{ g}}{100 \text{ mL}} \quad \times \quad 1{,}440 \text{ mL} \quad = \quad 288 \text{ kcal from protein}$$

Since no lipids were ordered, add the dextrose and protein calories to get the total calories:

$$734.4 \text{ kcals} + 288 \text{ kcals} \quad = \quad 1{,}022.4, \text{ or } 1{,}022 \text{ kcals/day}$$

25. If 250 mg contains 400,000 units, then 500 mg contains 800,000 units. The patient is taking 4 tablets daily, for 7 days (or 28 total tablets), at 800,000 units each.

$$\frac{800{,}000 \text{ units}}{1 \text{ tab}} = \frac{X \text{ units}}{28 \text{ tabs}} \qquad X = 22{,}400{,}000 \text{ units}$$

26.

$$\frac{40 \text{ mEq K}}{15 \text{ mL}} = \frac{25 \text{ mEq K}}{X \text{ mL}} \qquad X = 9.375, \text{ or } 9.4 \text{ mL}$$

27. The correct answer is (D). Total body weight is used to determine the weight-based dose of LMWHs. Since the patient's BMI is 28.3 kg/m² (overweight), her adjusted body weight is used in the Cockcroft-Gault equation to calculate CrCl. Her CrCl is 58.5 mL/min (well above the threshold of 30 mL/min, for changing the dosing interval of *Lovenox* to once daily).

28. The correct answer is (D). Mr. Ross is of normal weight per BMI (BMI = 20.4 kg/m²). His *Bactrim* dose will be calculated with his total body weight (20 mg TMP/kg/day x 70 kg = 1400 mg TMP/day or 350 mg TMP Q6H for normal renal function). His TBW is less than his IBW, so his CrCl should be calculated with his TBW and is ~160 ml/min. Renal dose adjustments will not be needed for any medications at this level of CrCl.

29. Begin by calculating the total daily dose (mg) for this patient.

$$\frac{0.25 \text{ mg}}{1 \text{ kg}} = \frac{X \text{ mg}}{110 \text{ kg}} \qquad X = 27.5 \text{ mg daily}$$

Calculate the volume of reconstituted amphotericin B solution needed per day.

$$\frac{27.5 \text{ mg}}{X \text{ mL}} = \frac{0.1 \text{ mg}}{1 \text{ mL}} \qquad X = 275 \text{ mL}$$

30.

$$pH = pK_a + \log\left[\frac{base}{salt}\right]$$

$$pH = 9.36 + \log\left[\frac{0.2}{0.02}\right]$$

$$pH = 9.36 + 1$$

$$pH = 10.36$$

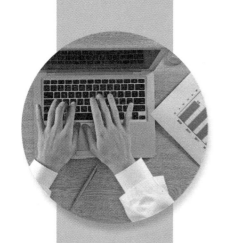
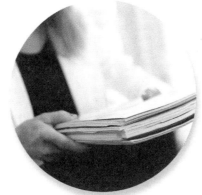
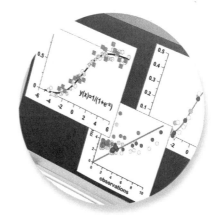

BIOSTATISTICS

CONTENTS

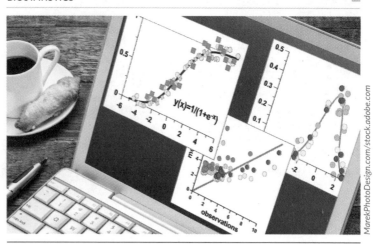

Marek PhotoDesign.com/stock.adobe.com

CHAPTER 14

BIOSTATISTICS

PURPOSE OF BIOSTATISTICS

Statistics involves the collection and analysis of all types of data, from the average number of cars on a freeway to the blood pressure reduction expected from a calcium channel blocker. When statistics are used to understand the effects of a drug or medical procedure on people and animals, the statistical analysis is called biostatistical analysis, or simply, biostatistics.

A basic understanding of biostatistics is required to interpret studies in medical and pharmacy journals, such as the *New England Journal of Medicine* or *Pharmacotherapy*. Simple formulas and definitions, described here, prepare the reader to interpret most journal articles and feel confident tackling common practice-based situations, such as:

A physician asks if a patient should be switched from standard of care treatment to a new drug based on the relative risk reduction reported in a clinical trial.

A patient taking warfarin wants to know if he should switch to Xarelto because he saw a commercial claiming that "it prevents DVT or PE in 98% of patients."

STEPS TO JOURNAL PUBLICATION

The path to publication for the classic type of research study is shown in the figure on the next page. A study manuscript (description of the research, with results) can be submitted for publication in a professional, peer-reviewed journal. The editor of the journal selects potential publications and sends them to experts in the topic area for peer review. Peer review is intended to assess the research design and methods, the value of the results and conclusions to the field of study, how well the manuscript is written, and whether it is appropriate for the readership of the journal. The reviewers make a recommendation to the editor to either accept the article (usually with revisions) or reject it. Data that contradicts a previous recommendation, or presents new information, can change treatment guidelines.

CONTENT LEGEND

Study Tip Gal   = Required Formula

BEGIN with a RESEARCH QUESTION

 DESIGN the **STUDY**

ENROLL the **SUBJECTS**

COLLECT the **DATA**

ANALYZE the **DATA**

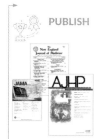 **PUBLISH**

Write a null hypothesis to answer the research question, such as: New drug is not as effective as current drug.	Is it randomized, placebo-controlled, a case-control or other type of study?	Assign to a treatment group or control group, or identify subjects belonging to a cohort or other group.	Prospectively (going into the future for a set period of time) or retrospectively (looking back in time using medical records).	Enter the data into statistical software; assess the results (e.g., risk reductions, confidence intervals).	

©UWorld   iStock.com/dilyanah

ORGANIZATION OF A PUBLISHED CLINICAL TRIAL

A published clinical trial begins with an abstract that provides a brief summary of the article. The introduction to the study comes next, which includes background information, such as disease history and prevalence, and the research hypothesis. This is followed by the study methods, which describe the variables and outcomes, and the statistical methods used to analyze the data.

The results section includes figures, tables and graphs. A reader needs to interpret basic statistics and common graphs in order to understand the study results. The researchers conclude the article with an interpretation of the results and the implications for current practice.

TYPES OF STUDY DATA

When data points, or values, are collected during a study, they can be analyzed to determine the degree of difference between groups, or some other type of association. The statistical tests used to perform the analysis depend on the type of data.

CONTINUOUS DATA

Continuous data has a logical order with values that continuously increase (or decrease) by the same amount (e.g., a HR of 120 BPM is twice as fast as a HR of 60 BPM). The two types of continuous data are interval data and ratio data. The difference between them is that interval data has no meaningful zero (zero does not equal none) and ratio data has a meaningful zero (zero equals none). The Celsius temperature scale is an example of interval data because it has no meaningful zero (0°C does not mean no temperature; it is the freezing point of water). Heart rate is an example of ratio data; a HR of 0 BPM is cardiac arrest (zero equals none; the heart is not beating).

DISCRETE (CATEGORICAL) DATA

The two types of discrete data, nominal and ordinal, have categories, and are sometimes called categorical data. Nominal and name are derived from the same word; with nominal data, subjects are sorted into arbitrary categories (names), such as male or female (0 = male, 1 = female or 0 = female, 1 = male). It is sometimes described as "yes/no" data. Ordinal comes from the word order; ordinal data is ranked and has a logical order, such as a pain scale. In contrast to continuous data, ordinal scale categories do not increase by the same amount; a pain scale rating of 4 is worse than a pain scale rating of 2, but it does not mean that there is twice as much pain.

CONTINUOUS DATA		DISCRETE (CATEGORICAL) DATA	
Data is provided by some type of measurement which has unlimited options (theoretically) of continuous values		Data fits into a limited number of categories	
RATIO DATA	**INTERVAL DATA**	**NOMINAL DATA**	**ORDINAL DATA**
Equal difference between values, with a true, meaningful zero (0 = NONE)	Equal difference between values, but without a meaningful zero (0 ≠ NONE)	Categories are in an arbitrary order *Order of categories does not matter*	Categories are ranked in a logical order, but the difference between categories is not equal *Order of categories matters*
Examples: age, height, weight, time, blood pressure	**Examples:** Celsius and Fahrenheit temperature scales	**Examples:** gender, ethnicity, marital status, mortality	**Examples:** NYHA Functional Class I-IV; 0-10 pain scale
Ordered, Equal	Ordered, Equal	No Set Order	Ordered, Ranked

SUMMARIZING THE DATA

MEASURES OF CENTRAL TENDENCY

Descriptive statistics provide simple summaries of the data. The typical descriptive values are called the <u>measures of central tendency</u>, and include the mean, the median and the mode (see <u>Study Tip Gal</u> below for mean, median and mode calculation examples).

- <u>Mean</u>: the <u>average</u> value; it is calculated by <u>adding up</u> the values and <u>dividing the sum</u> by the <u>number of values</u>. The mean is preferred for <u>continuous data</u> that is <u>normally distributed</u> (described below).

- <u>Median</u>: the value <u>in the middle</u> when the values are arranged from <u>lowest to highest</u>. When there are <u>two</u> center values (as with an even number of values), <u>take the average</u> of the two center values. The median is preferred for <u>ordinal data</u> or <u>continuous data</u> that is <u>skewed</u> (not normally distributed).

- <u>Mode</u>: the value that occurs <u>most frequently</u>. The mode is preferred for <u>nominal data</u>.

SPREAD (VARIABILITY) OF DATA

Two common methods of describing the variability, or spread, in data are the range and the standard deviation (SD).

- <u>Range</u>: the difference between the highest and lowest values.

- <u>Standard deviation (SD)</u>: indicates <u>how spread out</u> the data is, and to what degree the data is dispersed <u>away from the mean</u> (i.e., spread out over a smaller or larger range). A large number of data values close to the mean has a smaller SD. Data that is <u>highly dispersed</u> has a <u>larger SD</u>.

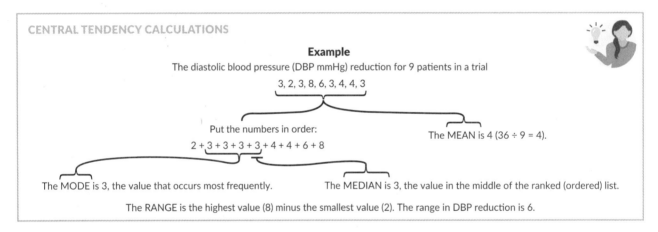

CENTRAL TENDENCY CALCULATIONS

Example

The diastolic blood pressure (DBP mmHg) reduction for 9 patients in a trial

3, 2, 3, 8, 6, 3, 4, 4, 3

Put the numbers in order:

2 + 3 + 3 + 3 + 3 + 4 + 4 + 6 + 8

The MEAN is 4 (36 ÷ 9 = 4).

The MODE is 3, the value that occurs most frequently.

The MEDIAN is 3, the value in the middle of the ranked (ordered) list.

The RANGE is the highest value (8) minus the smallest value (2). The range in DBP reduction is 6.

GAUSSIAN (NORMAL) DISTRIBUTIONS

<u>Large sample sets</u> of <u>continuous data</u> tend to form a <u>Gaussian</u>, or "<u>normal</u>" (bell-shaped), distribution (see the figure at the top of the next page). For example, if a researcher collects 5,000 blood pressure measurements (continuous data) from Idaho residents and plots the values, the graph would form a normal distribution.

Characteristics of a Gaussian Distribution

When the distribution of data is <u>normal</u>, the curve is <u>symmetrical</u> (even on both sides), with most of the values closer to the middle. <u>Half of the values</u> are on the <u>left side</u> of the curve, and <u>half of the values</u> are on the <u>right side</u>. A small number of values are in the <u>tails</u>. When data is normally distributed:

- The <u>mean, median</u> and <u>mode</u> are the <u>same</u> value, and are at the center point of the curve.

- <u>68% of the values</u> fall within <u>1 SD</u> of the mean and <u>95% of the values</u> fall within <u>2 SDs</u> of the mean.

Normal Distribution Shapes

The examples to the right show how the curve of normally distributed data changes based on the spread (or range) of the data. The curve gets taller and skinnier as the range of data narrows. The curve gets shorter and wider as the range of data widens (or is more spread out).

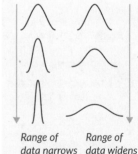

Range of data narrows   *Range of data widens*

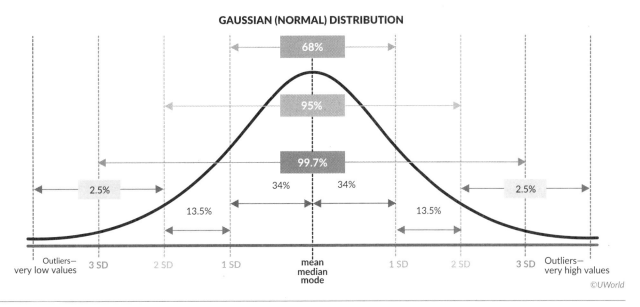

GAUSSIAN (NORMAL) DISTRIBUTION

©UWorld

SKEWED DISTRIBUTIONS

Data that are skewed do not have the characteristics of a normal distribution; the curve is not symmetrical, 68% of the values do not fall within 1 SD from the mean, and the mean, median and mode are not the same value. This usually occurs when the number of values (sample size) is small and/or there are outliers in the data.

Outliers (Extreme Values)

An outlier is an extreme value, either very low or very high, compared to the norm. For example, if a study reports the mean weight of included adult patients as 90 kg, then a patient in the same study with a weight of 40 kg or 186 kg is an outlier. When there are a small number of values, an outlier has a large impact on the mean and the data becomes skewed. In this case, the median is a better measure of central tendency. In the examples to the right, the median is right in the middle of the data and is not affected by outliers.

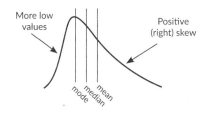

The distortion of the central tendency caused by outliers is decreased by collecting more values; as the number of values increases, the effect of outliers on the mean decreases.

Skew Refers to the Direction of the Tail

Data is skewed towards outliers. When there are more low values in a data set and the outliers are the high values, data is skewed to the right (positive skew). When there are more high values in the data set and the outliers are the low values, the data is skewed to the left (negative skew).

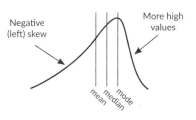

DEPENDENT AND INDEPENDENT VARIABLES

A variable in a study is any data point or characteristic that can be measured or counted. Examples include age, gender, blood pressure or pain. Variables can be clinical endpoints such as death, stroke, hospitalization or an adverse event, or they can be intermediate (or surrogate) endpoints used to assess an outcome, such as measuring serum creatinine to assess the degree of renal impairment.

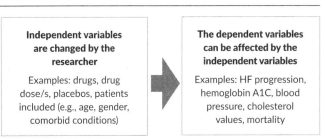

Independent variables are changed by the researcher	The dependent variables can be affected by the independent variables
Examples: drugs, drug dose/s, placebos, patients included (e.g., age, gender, comorbid conditions)	Examples: HF progression, hemoglobin A1C, blood pressure, cholesterol values, mortality

An independent variable is changed (manipulated) by the researcher in order to determine whether it has an effect on the dependent variable (the outcome). Independent variables are the characteristics of the subject groups (treatment and control) selected for inclusion (e.g., age, gender, presence or absence of hypertension, diabetes or other comorbid conditions), or any other characteristic that could have an effect on the dependent variable.

TESTING THE HYPOTHESIS FOR SIGNIFICANCE

If a drug or device manufacturer wants to sell their product and make money, they will want research data that demonstrates that their product is <u>significantly better</u> than (or <u>superior</u> to) the current treatment or a placebo (no treatment). To show significance, the trial needs to demonstrate that the <u>null hypothesis</u> is not true and should be rejected, and the <u>alternative hypothesis</u> can be accepted. The null hypothesis and alternative hypothesis are always complementary; when one is accepted, the other is rejected.

THE NULL HYPOTHESIS AND ALTERNATIVE HYPOTHESIS

Null means none or no; a <u>null hypothesis</u> (H_0) states that there is <u>no statistically significant difference</u> between groups. A researcher who is studying a drug versus a placebo would write a null hypothesis that states that there is no difference in efficacy between the drug and the placebo (drug efficacy = placebo efficacy). The <u>null hypothesis</u> is what the researcher <u>tries to disprove</u> or <u>reject</u>.

The <u>alternative hypothesis</u> (H_A) states that there is a <u>statistically significant difference</u> between the groups (drug efficacy ≠ placebo efficacy). The <u>alternative hypothesis</u> is what the researcher hopes to <u>prove</u> or <u>accept</u>.

ALPHA LEVEL: THE STANDARD FOR SIGNIFICANCE

When investigators design a study, they select a maximum permissible <u>error margin</u>, called <u>alpha (α)</u>. Alpha is the threshold for rejecting the null hypothesis. In medical research, alpha is <u>commonly set at 5% (or 0.05)</u>. A smaller alpha value can be chosen (e.g., 1%, or 0.01), but this requires more data, more subjects (which means more expense) and/or a larger treatment effect.

ALPHA CORRELATES WITH THE VALUES IN THE TAILS WHEN DATA HAS A NORMAL DISTRIBUTION

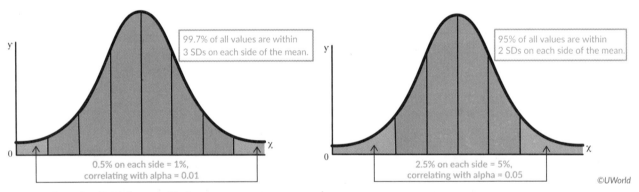

99.7% of all values are within 3 SDs on each side of the mean.

0.5% on each side = 1%, correlating with alpha = 0.01

95% of all values are within 2 SDs on each side of the mean.

2.5% on each side = 5%, correlating with alpha = 0.05

©UWorld

Comparing the P-Value to Alpha

Once the alpha value is determined, statistical tests are performed to compare the data, and a p-value is calculated. The <u>p-value</u> is <u>compared to alpha</u>. If alpha is set at 0.05 and the <u>p-value is less than</u> 0.05, the <u>null hypothesis is rejected</u>, and the result is termed <u>statistically significant</u>. If the p-value is greater than or equal to alpha (p ≥ 0.05), the study has failed to reject the null hypothesis, and the result is not statistically significant.

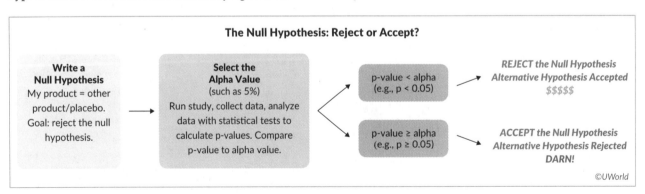

The Null Hypothesis: Reject or Accept?

Write a Null Hypothesis
My product = other product/placebo.
Goal: reject the null hypothesis.

Select the Alpha Value (such as 5%)
Run study, collect data, analyze data with statistical tests to calculate p-values. Compare p-value to alpha value.

p-value < alpha (e.g., p < 0.05)

p-value ≥ alpha (e.g., p ≥ 0.05)

REJECT the Null Hypothesis
Alternative Hypothesis Accepted
$$$$$

ACCEPT the Null Hypothesis
Alternative Hypothesis Rejected
DARN!

©UWorld

CONFIDENCE INTERVALS

A <u>confidence interval (CI)</u> provides the same information about <u>significance</u> as the p-value, plus the <u>precision</u> of the result. Alpha and the CI in a study will correlate with each other.

$$CI = 1 - \alpha$$

If alpha is <u>0.05</u>, the study reports <u>95% CIs</u>; an <u>alpha of 0.01</u> corresponds to a <u>CI of 99%</u>. The relationship between alpha, the p-value and the CI is described in the table here and in the figure on the previous page.

ALPHA	P-VALUE	MEANING	
0.05	≥ 0.05	Not statistically significant	
0.05	< 0.05	95% probability (confidence) that the conclusion is correct; less than 5% chance it's not.	Statistically Significant
0.01	< 0.01	99% probability (confidence) that the conclusion is correct; less than 1% chance it's not.	Statistically Significant
0.001	< 0.001	99.9% probability (confidence) that the conclusion is correct; less than 0.1% chance it's not.	

INTERPRETING CONFIDENCE INTERVALS

- **The values in the CI range are used to determine whether significance has been reached**
- **Determining statistical significance using the CI alone (without a p-value) is required for the exam**

COMPARING DIFFERENCE DATA (MEANS)
- Difference data is based on subtraction [e.g., the difference in Δ FEV1 between roflumilast and placebo (below) was 38 (46 − 8 = 38)]
- The result is statistically significant if the CI range does not include zero (e.g., zero is not present in the range of values); for example:
  - ❑ The 95% CI for the difference in Δ FEV1 (18-58 mL) does not include zero → the result is statistically significant
  - ❑ The 95% CI for the difference in Δ FEV1/FVC (-0.26-0.89%) includes zero → the result is not statistically significant

LUNG FUNCTION	DRUG* (N = 745)	PLACEBO (N = 745)	DIFFERENCE (95% CI)
Δ FEV1 (mL)	46	8	38 (18-58)
Δ FEV1/FVC (%)	0.314	0.001	0.313 (-0.26-0.89)

*Roflumilast

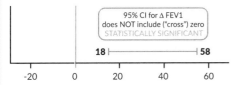

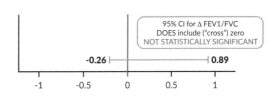

COMPARING RATIO DATA (RELATIVE RISK, ODDS RATIO, HAZARD RATIO)
- Ratio data is based on division [e.g., the ratio of severe exacerbations between roflumilast and placebo (below) was 0.92 (0.11/0.12 = 0.92)]
- The result is statistically significant if the CI range does not include one (e.g., one is not present in the range of values); for example:
  - ❑ The 95% CI for the relative risk of severe exacerbations (0.61-1.29) includes one → the result is not statistically significant
  - ❑ The 95% CI for the relative risk of moderate exacerbations (0.72-0.99) does not include one → the result is statistically significant

EXACERBATIONS*	DRUG** (N = 745)	PLACEBO (N = 745)	RELATIVE RISK (95% CI)
Severe	0.11	0.12	0.92 (0.61-1.29)
Moderate	0.94	1.11	0.85 (0.72-0.99)

*Mean rate, per patient per year
**Roflumilast

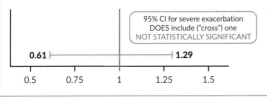

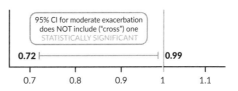

©UWorld

Confidence Intervals and Estimation (Extent and Variability in the Data)

The goal of the majority of medical research is to use the study results to promote the procedure or drug for use in the general population of patients with the same medical condition. Clinicians need to understand how their patients would benefit. The CI includes the treatment effect and the range; both are helpful in estimating the effect on others.

A CI can be written in slightly different formats. For example, a study comparing metoprolol to placebo finds a 12% absolute risk reduction (ARR) in heart failure progression, with a 95% CI range of 6 – 35%. This can be written as ARR 12% (95% CI 6% – 35%) or as decimals, with commas in the range, such as ARR 0.12 (0.95 CI 0.06, 0.35). The CI indicates that you are 95% confident that the true value of the ARR for the general (or true) population lies somewhere within the range of 6% – 35%, with some values as low as 6% and others as high as 35%.

A narrow CI range implies high precision, and a wide CI range implies poor precision. If the reported CI range was 4% – 68%, the true value would still be within the range, but where? The range is wider, and therefore less precise. Cardiologists who interpret the results for their patients would not know whether to expect a result closer to 4% or 68%. A large range correlates to a large dispersion in the data. A narrower range is preferable.

In some studies, specific patient types will cause a wider distribution in data. For example, fibrates are used to lower triglyceride levels; they cause a greater reduction in patients with higher triglycerides. The consideration of where the patient is likely to fall within the range will become part of the assessment of the individual's baseline risk.

TYPE I AND TYPE II ERRORS

Consider what would happen if a drug manufacturer developed and marketed a new drug as better for heart failure than the standard of care, when in fact the new, expensive drug has similar benefits to the old drug (it is not better at all). The null hypothesis stated that the new drug and the old drug are equal. The statistical tests found a significant benefit with the new drug, and the null hypothesis was rejected when it should have been accepted.

Type I Errors: False-Positives

In the scenario described above, the conclusion was wrong and a type I error was made. The alternative hypothesis was accepted and the null hypothesis was rejected in error. The probability, or risk, of making a type I error is determined by alpha and it relates to the confidence interval.

$$CI = 1 - \alpha \text{ (type I error)}$$

When alpha is 0.05 and a study result is reported with $p < 0.05$, it is statistically significant and the probability of a type I error (making the wrong conclusion) is $\leq 5\%$. You are 95% confident (0.95 = 1 – 0.05) that your result is correct and not due to chance.

Type II Errors: False-Negatives

The probability of a type II error, denoted as beta (β), occurs when the null hypothesis is accepted when it should have been rejected. Beta is set by the investigators during the design of a study. It is typically set at 0.1 or 0.2, meaning the risk of a type II error is 10% or 20%. The risk of a type II error increases if the sample size is too small. To decrease this risk, a power analysis is performed to determine the sample size needed to detect a true difference between groups.

Study Power

Power is the probability that a test will reject the null hypothesis correctly (i.e., the power to avoid a type II error). Power = 1 – β. As the power increases, the chance of a type II error decreases. Power is determined by the number of outcome values collected, the difference in outcome rates between the groups, and the significance (alpha) level. If beta is set at 0.2, the study has 80% power (there is a 20% chance of missing a true difference and making a type II error). If beta is set at 0.1, the study has 90% power. A larger sample size is needed to increase study power and decrease the risk of a type II error.

	H₀ ACCEPTED	H₀ REJECTED
H₀ is TRUE (NO difference between groups)	Correct Conclusion	Type I Error Committed FALSE POSITIVE
H₀ is FALSE (There IS a difference between groups)	Type II Error Committed FALSE NEGATIVE	Correct Conclusion

H₀ = the null hypothesis

RISK

In healthcare, risk refers to the probability of an event (how likely it is to occur) when an intervention, such as a drug, is given. The lack of intervention is measured as the effect in the placebo (or control) group.

RELATIVE RISK (OR RISK RATIO)

The relative risk (RR) is the ratio of risk in the exposed group (treatment) divided by risk in the control group.

RR Formula

$$\text{Risk} = \frac{\text{Number of subjects in group with an unfavorable event}}{\text{Total number of subjects in group}}$$

$$\text{RR} = \frac{\text{Risk in treatment group}}{\text{Risk in control group}}$$

RR Calculation

A placebo-controlled study was performed to evaluate whether metoprolol reduces disease progression in patients with heart failure (HF). A total of 10,111 patients were enrolled and followed for 12 months. What is the relative risk of HF progression in the metoprolol-treated group versus the placebo group?

Calculate the risk of HF progression in each group. Then calculate RR.

	METOPROLOL N = 5,123	CONTROL N = 4,988
HF progression	823	1,397

Metoprolol Risk	Control Risk
$\frac{823}{5,123} = 0.16$	$\frac{1,397}{4,988} = 0.28$

$$\text{RR} = \frac{0.16}{0.28} = 0.57 \times 100 = 57\%$$

Answer can be expressed as a decimal or a percentage; the exam question will specify with instructions

RR Interpretation

RR = 1 (or 100%) implies no difference in risk of the outcome between the groups.

RR > 1 (or 100%) implies greater risk of the outcome in the treatment group.

RR < 1 (or 100%) implies lower risk (reduced risk) of the outcome in the treatment group.

In the metoprolol study, the RR of HF progression was 57%. Patients treated with metoprolol were 57% as likely to have progression of disease as placebo-treated patients.

INTERPRETING THE RELATIVE RISK (RR)

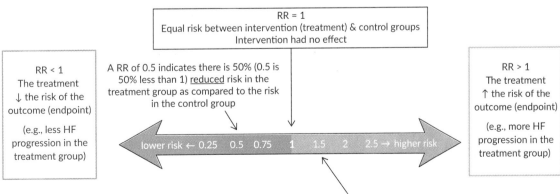

RELATIVE RISK REDUCTION

The RR calculation determines whether there is less risk (RR < 1) or more risk (RR > 1). The relative risk reduction (RRR) is calculated after the RR and indicates how much the risk is reduced in the treatment group compared to the control group.

RRR Formula

$$RRR = \frac{(\% \text{ risk in control group} - \% \text{ risk in treatment group})}{\% \text{ risk in the control group}}$$

or

$$1 - RR^*$$

Decimals or percentages may be used for risks

*Must use decimal form of RR

RRR Calculation

Using the risks previously calculated for HF progression in the treatment and control groups (metoprolol: 16% and placebo: 28%), calculate the RRR of HF progression.

$$RRR = \frac{(28\% - 16\%)}{28\%} = 0.43$$

or

$$RRR = 1 - 0.57 = 0.43$$

Answer can be expressed as a decimal or percentage; the exam question will specify with instructions

RRR Interpretation

The RRR is 43%. Metoprolol-treated patients were 43% less likely to have HF progression than placebo-treated patients.

INTERPRETING THE RELATIVE RISK REDUCTION (RRR)

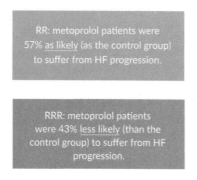

RR: metoprolol patients were 57% as likely (as the control group) to suffer from HF progression.

RRR: metoprolol patients were 43% less likely (than the control group) to suffer from HF progression.

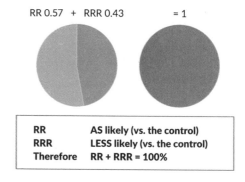

RR 0.57 + RRR 0.43   = 1

RR	AS likely (vs. the control)
RRR	LESS likely (vs. the control)
Therefore	RR + RRR = 100%

©UWorld

ABSOLUTE RISK REDUCTION

A clinician is listening to a presentation on a drug. The drug manufacturer representative reports that the drug causes 48% less nausea than the standard treatment. The result sounds great; the clinician asks the pharmaceutical representative: what is the absolute risk reduction (ARR)?

The RR and RRR provide relative (proportional) differences in risk between the treatment group and the control group; they have no meaning in terms of absolute risk.

Absolute risk reduction is more useful because it includes the reduction in risk and the incidence rate of the outcome. If the risk of nausea is reduced, but the risk was small to begin with (perhaps the drug caused very little nausea), the large risk reduction has little practical benefit.

It is best if a study reports both ARR and RRR, and for clinicians to understand how to interpret the risk for their patients. If the ARR is not reported, it is possible that the risk reduction, in terms of a decrease in absolute risk, is minimal.

ARR Formula

$$ARR = (\% \text{ risk in control group}) - (\% \text{ risk in treatment group})$$

ARR Calculation

Using the risks previously calculated for HF progression in the metoprolol study, calculate the ARR of HF progression.

Metoprolol Risk		Control Risk	
$\dfrac{823}{5{,}123}$	= 0.16	$\dfrac{1{,}397}{4{,}988}$	= 0.28

ARR = 0.28 − 0.16 = 0.12 × 100 = 12%

Answer can be expressed as a decimal or a percentage; the exam question will specify with instructions

ARR Interpretation

The ARR is 12%, meaning 12 out of every 100 patients benefit from the treatment. Said another way, for every 100 patients treated with metoprolol, 12 fewer patients will have HF progression.

An additional benefit of calculating the ARR is to be able to use the inverse of the ARR to determine the number needed to treat (NNT) and number needed to harm (NNH). These concepts are discussed next.

INTERPRETING THE ABSOLUTE RISK REDUCTION (ARR)

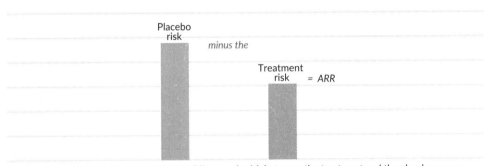

The absolute risk reduction is the true difference in risk between the treatment and the placebo groups.
Said another way, the ARR is the net effect (benefit) beyond the effect obtained from a placebo.

©UWorld

NUMBER NEEDED TO TREAT OR HARM

NNT and NNH help clinicians answer the question: how many patients need to receive the drug for one patient to get benefit (NNT) or harm (NNH)? This information, taken into consideration with the patient's individual risk, helps guide decisions.

NUMBER NEEDED TO TREAT

NNT is the number of patients who need to be treated for a certain period of time (e.g., one year) in order for one patient to benefit (e.g., avoid HF progression).

NNT Formula

$$NNT = \frac{1}{(\text{risk in control group}) - (\text{risk in treatment group})^*} \quad \text{or} \quad \frac{1}{ARR^*}$$

*Risk and ARR are expressed as decimals

NNT Calculation

The ARR in the metoprolol study was 12%. The duration of the study period was one year. Calculate the number of patients that need to be treated with metoprolol for one year in order to prevent one case of HF progression.

$$NNT = \frac{1}{0.12} = 8.3, \text{ rounded up to } 9^*$$

*Numbers greater than a whole number are rounded up

NNT Interpretation

For every 9 patients who receive metoprolol for one year, HF progression is prevented in one patient.

NUMBER NEEDED TO HARM

NNH is the number of patients who need to be treated for a certain period of time in order for one patient to experience harm.

NNT and NNH are calculated with the same formula (see the NNT formula on the previous page). There are two differences:

1. NNT is rounded up, and NNH is rounded down (see Study Tip Gal).

2. The absolute value of the ARR is used with NNH, as shown in the following example.

NNH Calculation

A study evaluated the efficacy of clopidogrel versus placebo, both given in addition to aspirin, in reducing the risk of cardiovascular death, MI and stroke. The study reported a 3.9% risk of major bleeding in the treatment group and a 2.8% risk of major bleeding in the control group.

ARR = 2.8% – 3.9% = –1.1%; the absolute value is the difference between the two groups. There is a 1.1% higher risk of major bleeding in the treatment group.

$$NNH = \frac{1}{0.011} = 90.9, \text{ rounded down to } 90^*$$

*Numbers greater than a whole number are rounded down

NNH Interpretation

One additional case of major bleeding is expected to occur for every 90 patients taking clopidogrel instead of placebo.

ODDS RATIO AND HAZARD RATIO

ODDS RATIO

Odds are the probability that an event will occur versus the probability that it will not occur. Case-control studies, described in the Types of Medical Studies section, are not suitable for relative risk calculations. In case-control studies, the odds ratio is used to estimate the risk of unfavorable events associated with a treatment or intervention.

Case-control studies enroll patients who have a clinical outcome or disease that has already occurred (e.g., lung cancer). The patient medical charts are reviewed retrospectively (in the past) to search for possible exposures (e.g., smoking) that increased the risk of the clinical outcome or disease. In this case, the odds ratio (OR) is used to calculate the odds of an outcome occurring with an exposure, compared to the odds of the outcome occurring without the exposure. ORs are used most commonly with case-control studies but can be used in cohort and cross-sectional studies.

OR Formula

EXPOSURE/TREATMENT	OUTCOME PRESENT	OUTCOME ABSENT
Present	A	B
Absent	C	D

$$OR = \frac{AD}{BC}$$

A = # that have the outcome, with exposure

B = # without the outcome, with exposure

C = # that have the outcome, without exposure

D = # without the outcome, without exposure

OR Calculation

A case-control study was conducted to assess the risk of falls with fracture (outcome) associated with serotonergic antidepressant (AD) use (exposure) among a cohort of Chinese females ≥ 65 years old. Cases were matched with 33,000 controls (1:4, by age, sex and cohort entry date).

EXPOSURE/ TREATMENT	FALLS W/ FRACTURE (CASES)	FALLS W/O FRACTURE (CONTROLS)
Serotonergic AD-YES	4,991	18,270
Serotonergic AD-NO	3,259	14,730

$AD = 4,991 \times 14,730 = 73,517,430$

$BC = 18,270 \times 3,259 = 59,541,930$

$$OR = \frac{73,517,430}{59,541,930} = 1.23$$

Conclusion: serotonergic ADs are associated with a 23% increased risk of falls with fracture (see OR and HR Interpretation below).

HAZARD RATIO

In a survival analysis (e.g. analysis of death or disease progression), instead of using "risk," a hazard rate is used. A hazard rate is the rate at which an unfavorable event occurs within a short period of time. Similar to RR, the hazard ratio (HR) is the ratio between the hazard rate in the treatment group and the hazard rate in the control group.

HR Formula

$$HR = \frac{\text{Hazard rate in the treatment group}}{\text{Hazard rate in the control group}}$$

HR Calculation

A placebo-controlled study was performed to evaluate whether niacin, when added to intensive statin therapy, reduces cardiovascular risk in patients with established cardiovascular disease. The primary endpoint was the first event of the composite endpoint (death from coronary heart disease, nonfatal myocardial infarction, ischemic stroke, hospitalization for an acute coronary syndrome or coronary or cerebral revascularization). A total of 3,414 patients were enrolled and followed for three years.

Calculate the hazard ratio.

	NIACIN N = 1,718	PLACEBO N = 1,696
Primary endpoint	282	274

Niacin Hazard Rate	Control Hazard Rate
$\dfrac{282}{1,718} = 0.16$	$\dfrac{274}{1,696} = 0.16$

$$HR = \frac{0.16}{0.16} = 1 \times 100 = 100\%$$

Answer can be expressed as a decimal or a percentage; the exam question will specify with instructions

Conclusion: there is no benefit to cardiovascular risk when adding niacin to intensive statin therapy (see OR and HR Interpretation below).

OR AND HR INTERPRETATION

OR and HR are interpreted in a similar way to RR:

OR or HR = 1: the event rate is the same in the treatment and control arms. There is no advantage to the treatment.

OR or HR > 1: the event rate in the treatment group is higher than the event rate in the control group; for example, a HR of 2 for an outcome of death indicates that there are twice as many deaths in the treatment group.

OR or HR < 1: the event rate in the treatment group is lower than the event rate in the control group; for example, a HR of 0.5 for an outcome of death indicates that there are half as many deaths in the treatment group.

PRIMARY AND COMPOSITE ENDPOINTS

The primary endpoint is the main (primary) result that is measured to see if the treatment had a significant benefit. In the metoprolol trial, the primary endpoint was HF progression.

A composite endpoint combines multiple individual endpoints into one measurement. This is attractive to researchers, as combining several endpoints increases the likelihood of reaching a statistically significant benefit with a smaller, less costly trial.

When a composite endpoint is used, each individual endpoint gets counted toward the same (composite) outcome.

Primary Endpoints (distinct and separate)	Composite Endpoint (combined into one)
Death from cardiovascular causes	Death from cardiovascular causes
or	and
Nonfatal stroke	Nonfatal stroke
or	and
Nonfatal MI	Nonfatal MI

COMPOSITE ENDPOINTS: CAUTION

All endpoints in a composite must be similar in magnitude and have similar, meaningful importance to the patient. For example, the composite endpoint of blood pressure reduction should not be included with heart attack and stroke reduction. The FDA requires each individual endpoint to be measured and reported when a composite endpoint is used. When assessing a composite measurement, it is important to use the composite endpoint value, rather than adding together the values for the individual endpoints. The value of the sum of the individual endpoints may not equal the value of the composite endpoint, since a patient can have more than one non-fatal endpoint during a trial.

TYPES OF STATISTICAL TESTS

The next step following data collection (and calculation of risks, RR, ARR, HR, etc.) is to analyze the data to check if differences between the treatment and control groups are statistically significant or if there is an association or relationship in the data. Selecting the correct test to analyze the data depends on the type of data and the outcomes measured.

CONTINUOUS DATA

With continuous data, the type of test used to determine statistical significance depends on the distribution of data (discussed previously). If it is normally distributed, parametric methods are appropriate. If the data is not normally distributed, nonparametric methods are appropriate.

T-Tests

This is a parametric method used when the endpoint has continuous data and the data is normally distributed. When data from a single sample group is compared with known data from the general population, a one-sample t-test is performed. If a single sample group is used for a pre-/post-measurement (i.e., the patient serves as their own control), a paired t-test is appropriate.

A student t-test is used when the study has two independent samples: the treatment and the control groups. For example, a study comparing the reduction in hemoglobin A1C values between metformin and placebo would use an independent or unpaired student t-test.

Analysis of Variance

Analysis of variance (ANOVA), or the F-test, is used to test for statistical significance when using continuous data with 3 or more samples, or groups.

DISCRETE (CATEGORICAL) DATA

Chi-Square Test

For nominal or ordinal data, a chi-square test is used to determine statistical significance between treatment groups. For example, if a study assesses the difference in mortality (nominal data) between two groups, or pain scores based on a pain scale (ordinal data), a chi-square test could be used.

SELECTING A TEST TO ANALYZE THE DATA

NUMBER OF GROUPS	TYPE OF DATA		
	Continuous		Discrete/Categorical
	PARAMETRIC TESTS (data has normal distribution)	**NON-PARAMETRIC TESTS** (data has skewed distribution)	
1	One-sample t-test	Sign test	Chi-square test
1 (with before & after measures)	Dependent/paired t-test	Wilcoxon Signed-Rank test	Wilcoxon Signed-Rank test
2 (treatment & control)	Independent/unpaired student t-test	Mann-Whitney (Wilcoxon Rank-Sum) test	Chi-square test or Fisher's exact test Mann-Whitney (Wilcoxon Rank-Sum) test (may be preferred for ordinal data)
≥ 3	ANOVA (or F-test)	Kruskal-Wallis test	Kruskal-Wallis test

EXAMPLES OF TEST TYPE SELECTION

Example 1

A study is performed to assess the safety and efficacy of ketamine-dexmedetomidine (KD) versus ketamine-propofol (KP) for sedation in patients after coronary artery bypass graft surgery.

ENDPOINT (MEAN VALUES)	KD	KP
Fentanyl dose, mcg	41.94 ± 20.43	152.8 ± 51.2
Weaning/extubation time, min	374.05 ± 20.25	445.23 ± 21.7

Measurements of dose and time are both continuous data. The trial has two independent samples, or groups (KD and KP). An appropriate test is an independent/unpaired student t-test. If the trial included a third group, ANOVA would be used.

Example 2

An emergency medical team wants to see if there is a statistically significant difference in death due to multiple drug overdose with at least one opioid taken, versus no opioid taken. Which test can determine a statistically significant difference in death?

ENDPOINT	YES OPIOID N = 250	NO OPIOID N = 150
Death (n, %)	52 (20.8%)	35 (23.3%)

The variable (dead or alive) is nominal. The chi-square test is used to test for significance when there are two groups.

CORRELATION AND REGRESSION

CORRELATION

Correlation is a statistical technique that is used to determine if one variable (such as number of days hospitalized) changes, or is related to, another variable (such as incidence of hospital-acquired infection). When the independent variable (number of hospital days) causes the dependent variable (infections) to increase, the direction of the correlation is positive (increases to the right). When the independent variable causes the dependent variable to decrease, the direction of the correlation is negative (decreases to the right).

Different types of data require different tests for correlation. Spearman's rank-order correlation, referred to as Rho, is used to test correlation with ordinal, ranked data. The primary test used for continuous data is the Pearson's correlation coefficient, denoted as r, which is a calculated score that indicates the strength and direction of the relationship between two variables. The values range from –1 to +1, and are described in the figure on the next page.

It is not possible to conclude from a correlation analysis that the change in a variable causes the change in another variable. A correlation, whether positive or negative, does not prove a causal relationship.

TESTING FOR CORRELATION WITH THE PEARSON CORRELATION COEFFICIENT

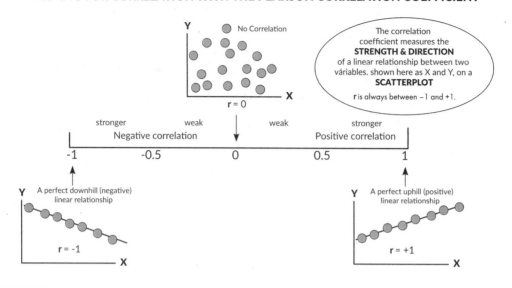

©UWorld

REGRESSION

Regression is used to describe the relationship between a dependent variable and one or more independent (or explanatory) variables, or how much the value of the dependent variable changes when the independent variables changes. Regression is common in observational studies where researchers need to assess multiple independent variables or need to control for many confounding factors. There are three typical types of regressions: 1) linear, for continuous data, 2) logistic, for categorical data, and 3) Cox regression, for categorical data in a survival analysis.

SENSITIVITY AND SPECIFICITY

Lab and diagnostic tests are used to screen for and diagnose medical conditions. Interpreting sensitivity and specificity correctly is required to answer these two questions concerning the validity of lab or diagnostic test results:

- If the result is positive, what is the likelihood of having the disease?
- If the result is negative, what is the likelihood of not having the disease?

SENSITIVITY, THE TRUE POSITIVE

Sensitivity describes how effectively a test identifies patients with the condition. The higher the sensitivity, the better; a test with 100% sensitivity will be positive in all patients with the condition. Sensitivity is calculated from the number of patients who test positive, out of those who actually have the condition (sensitivity is the percentage of "true-positive" results).

SPECIFICITY, THE TRUE NEGATIVE

Specificity describes how effectively a test identifies patients without the condition. The higher the specificity the better; a test with 100% specificity will be negative in all patients without the condition. Specificity is calculated from the number who test negative, out of those who actually do not have the condition (specificity is the percentage of "true-negative" results).

Sensitivity and Specificity Formula

TEST RESULT	HAVE CONDITION	NO CONDITION
Positive	A	B
Negative	C	D
Total	A + C	B + D

$$\text{Sensitivity} = \frac{A}{A + C} \times 100$$

$$\text{Specificity} = \frac{D}{B + D} \times 100$$

A = # that have the condition, with a positive test result
B = # without the condition, with a positive test result
C = # that have the condition, with a negative test result
D = # without the condition, with a negative test result

Sensitivity and Specificity Calculation and Interpretation

The tables below show how sensitivity and specificity is calculated for two lab tests used in the diagnosis of rheumatoid arthritis (RA), cyclic citrulline peptide (CCP) and rheumatoid factor (RF). Based on study data, CCP has a sensitivity of 98% and a specificity of 98% for RA, while RF has a sensitivity of 28% and a specificity of 87%.

Using the RF lab test as an example, a sensitivity of 28% means that only 28% of patients with the condition will have a positive RF result; the test is negative in 72% of patients with the disease (and the diagnosis can be missed). A specificity of 87% means that the test is negative in 87% of patients without the disease; but 13% of patients without the disease can test positive (potentially causing an incorrect diagnosis).

CCP RESULTS	HAVE CONDITION	NO CONDITION
Positive	A = 147	B = 9
Negative	C = 3	D = 441
Total	A + C = 150	B + D = 450
Sensitivity	147/150 x 100 = 98%	
Specificity		441/450 x 100 = 98%

RF RESULTS	HAVE CONDITION	NO CONDITION
Positive	A = 21	B = 26
Negative	C = 54	D = 174
Total	A + C = 75	B + D = 200
Sensitivity	21/75 x 100 = 28%	
Specificity		174/200 x 100 = 87%

Sensitivity and Specificity Application

If an elderly female patient with swollen finger joints is referred to a rheumatologist and lab tests reveal a positive CCP and a positive RF, the positive CCP indicates a very strong likelihood that the patient has RA because it has high sensitivity and specificity (98%). If the RF is positive and the CCP is negative, the rheumatologist would consider the possibility of other autoimmune/inflammatory conditions that could be contributing to swollen joints because of the low sensitivity of RF (28%).

INTENTION-TO-TREAT AND PER PROTOCOL ANALYSIS

Data from clinical trials can be analyzed in two different ways; intention-to-treat or per protocol. Intention-to-treat analysis includes data for all patients originally allocated to each treatment group (active and control) even if the patient did not complete the trial according to the study protocol (e.g., due to non-compliance, protocol violations or study withdrawal). This method provides a conservative (real-world) estimate of the treatment effect. A per protocol analysis is conducted for the subset of the trial population who completed the study according to the protocol (or at least without any major protocol violations). This method can provide an optimistic estimate of treatment effect since it is limited to the subset of patients who were adherent to the protocol.

NONINFERIORITY AND EQUIVALENCE TRIAL DESIGNS

The standard design of most trials is to establish that a treatment is superior to another treatment; the researcher wishes to show that the new drug is better than the old drug or a placebo. Perhaps a new treatment is developed that is less expensive or less toxic than the standard of care. Researchers would hope to demonstrate that the new drug is roughly equivalent, or at least not inferior, to the standard of care. Two types of trials are used for this purpose: equivalence and non-inferiority trials.

Equivalence trials attempt to demonstrate that the new treatment has roughly the same effect as the old (or reference) treatment. These trials test for effect in two directions, for higher or lower effectiveness, which is called a two-way margin. Non-inferiority trials attempt to demonstrate that the new treatment is no worse than the current standard based on the predefined non-inferiority (delta) margin. The delta margin is the minimal difference in effect between the two groups that is considered clinically acceptable based on previous research.

FOREST PLOTS AND CONFIDENCE INTERVALS

Forest plots are graphs that have a "forest" of lines. Forest plots can be used for a single study in which individual endpoints are pooled (gathered together) into a composite endpoint (see figure labeled Pogue, et al. below). More commonly, forest plots are used when the results from multiple studies are pooled into a single study, such as with a meta-analysis (see first figure below on comparing difference data).

Forest plots provide CIs for difference data or ratio data. Interpreting forest plots correctly can help identify whether a statistically significant benefit has been reached. When interpreting statistical significance using a forest plot:

- The boxes show the effect estimate. In a meta-analysis, the size of the box correlates with the size of the effect from the single study shown. Diamonds (at the bottom of the forest plot) represent pooled results from multiple studies.

- The horizontal lines through the boxes illustrate the length of the confidence interval for that particular endpoint (in a single study) or for the particular study (in a meta-analysis). The longer the line, the wider the interval, and the less reliable the study results. The width of the diamond in a meta-analysis serves the same purpose.

- The vertical solid line is the line of no effect; a significant benefit has been reached when data falls to the left of the line; data to the right of the line indicates significant harm. The vertical line is set at zero for difference data and at one for ratio data.

COMPARING DIFFERENCE DATA

The study shown to the right (a meta-analysis) uses a forest plot to display the difference in all-cause mortality risk for each individual study, and the pooled result of the studies. Recall for difference data, a result is not statistically significant if the confidence interval crosses zero, so the vertical line (line of no difference) is set at zero. Examples:

- 1st study (PEARL): shows a statistically significant benefit; the data point, plus the entire confidence interval, is to the left of the vertical line and does not cross zero.

- 2nd study (PEONY): the result is not statistically significant; the confidence interval crosses zero.

- 3rd study (PINK): shows a statistically significant harmful outcome; the data point, plus the entire confidence interval, is all to the right of the vertical line and does not cross zero.

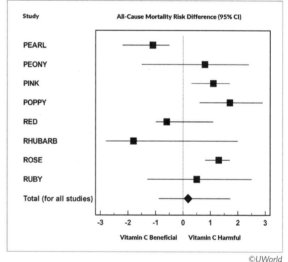

©UWorld

COMPARING RATIO DATA

The study shown to the right (by Pogue, et al.) uses a forest plot to show the results of a composite endpoint reported as ratio data, in this case hazard ratio. Recall for ratio data, the result is not statistically significant if the confidence interval crosses one, so the vertical line (line of no difference) is set at one. Examples:

- Primary composite endpoint: a statistically significant benefit was shown with treatment; the CI (0.7 – 0.99) does not cross one (and the horizontal line representing the CI does not touch or cross the vertical line at one).

- CV death: shows no statistically significant benefit (or harm); the CI (0.92 – 1.83) crosses one (and the horizontal line representing the CI crosses the vertical line at one).

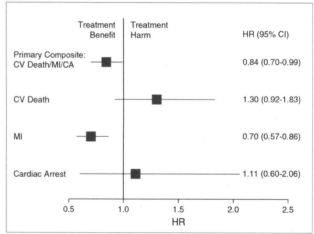

Pogue, et al. PLoS One 2012; 7(4): e34785.

TYPES OF MEDICAL STUDIES

Evidence-based medicine (EBM), which is largely guideline and protocol-driven, is the foundation of practice and most patient care recommendations are based on valid study data. The type of study that a researcher chooses is a major factor in determining the quality of the study data and the clinical value or impact. The pyramid figure to the right depicts the reliability of each of the major study types.

Common types of studies include:

- Case-control studies: retrospective comparisons of cases (patients with a disease) and controls (patients without a disease).

- Cohort studies: retrospective or prospective comparisons of patients with an exposure to those without an exposure.

- Randomized controlled trials: prospective comparison of patients who were randomly assigned to groups.

- Meta-analyses: analyzes the results of multiple studies.

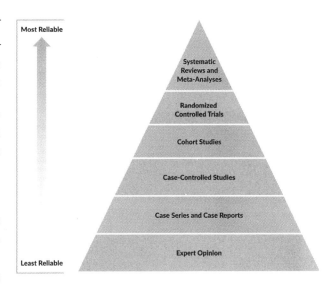

Most Reliable

- Systematic Reviews and Meta-Analyses
- Randomized Controlled Trials
- Cohort Studies
- Case-Controlled Studies
- Case Series and Case Reports
- Expert Opinion

Least Reliable

Each type of study has benefits and limitations. The table below describes the various study types and provides an example of each study.

STUDY TYPE, BENEFITS AND LIMITATIONS	STUDY TYPE EXAMPLE
CASE-CONTROL STUDY Compares patients with a disease (cases) to those without the disease (controls). The outcome of the cases and controls is already known, but the researcher looks back in time (retrospectively) to see if a relationship exists between the disease (outcome) and various risk factors. **Benefits** Data is easy to get from medical records. Good for looking at outcomes when the intervention is unethical (e.g., exposing patients to a pesticide to test an association with cancer; cases that occurred are used instead). Less expensive than a RCT. **Limitations** Cause and effect cannot reliably be determined (associations may be proven to be non-existent).	***Predictors of surgical site infection after open lower extremity bypass (LEB) revascularization.*** **Methods** Data was pulled from 35 hospitals for all patients who had LEB during a 3-year period. Cases of surgical site infection (SSI) were identified and compared to those who did not develop an SSI (controls). An odds ratio (OR) was calculated for various risk factors that might increase SSI risk. **Statistical Data** Renal failure OR: 4.35 (95% CI 3.45-5.47; $p < 0.001$). Hypertension OR: 4.29 (95% CI 2.74-6.72; $p < 0.001$). BMI ≥ 25 kg/m^2 OR: 1.78 (95% CI 1.23-2.57; $p = 0.002$). **Conclusion** Renal failure, hypertension and BMI ≥ 25 kg/m^2 were all associated with an increased risk of SSI.
COHORT STUDY Compares outcomes of a group of patients exposed and not exposed to a treatment; the researcher follows both groups prospectively (in the future) or retrospectively (less common) to see if they develop the outcome. **Benefits** Good for looking at outcomes when the intervention would be unethical. **Limitations** More time-consuming and expensive than a retrospective study. Can be influenced by confounders, which are other factors that affect the outcome (e.g., smoking, lipid levels).	***Statin use and cognitive function in adults with type 1 diabetes.*** **Methods** Patients with type 1 diabetes who were taking statins (exposed) were compared to those not taking statins (not exposed) and followed for 7-12 years to see if statin use was associated with cognitive impairment (outcome). **Statistical Data** Statin use and odds of cognitive impairment OR: 4.84 (95% CI 1.63-14.44; $p = 0.005$). **Conclusion** In type 1 diabetes, patients taking statins were more likely to develop cognitive impairment compared to those who did not take statins.

STUDY TYPE, BENEFITS AND LIMITATIONS	STUDY TYPE EXAMPLE
CROSS-SECTIONAL SURVEY Estimates the relationship between variables and outcomes (prevalence) at one particular time (cross-section) in a defined population. **Benefits** Can identify associations that need further study (hypothesis-generating). **Limitations** Does not determine causality (further studies needed if association found).	***Association of selective serotonin reuptake inhibitors and bone mineral density (BMD) in elderly women.*** **Methods** A cross-sectional analysis of 250 elderly women (defined population) from August 2010 to April 2015 (time period) was performed. Data was collected retrospectively for two groups: SSRI users (variable) and SSRI nonusers (variable) to compare the prevalence of low BMD. **Statistical Data** No difference in the prevalence of low BMD at the femoral neck (p = 0.887) or the spine (p = 0.275). **Conclusion** There was no difference in the prevalence of low BMD between elderly women on SSRIs and not on SSRIs.
CASE REPORT AND CASE SERIES Describes an adverse reaction or a unique condition that appears in a <u>single patient (case report)</u> or a <u>few patients (case series)</u>. The outcome of the case in each of these is already known. A case series is more reliable than a case report. **Benefits** Can identify new diseases, drug side effects or potential uses. Generates hypotheses that can be tested with other study designs. **Limitations** Conclusions cannot be drawn from a single or few cases.	***Tardive oculogyric crisis during treatment with clozapine: report of three cases.*** **Methods** A psychiatrist identified three cases of patients at his center who experienced the adverse effect, wrote it up, and it was printed in a medical journal. **Statistical Data** No statistical validity; risk cannot be compared to the general population as there is no control. **Conclusion** The findings of oculogyric crisis in patients treated with clozapine are interesting but do not provide important information on prevalence.
RANDOMIZED CONTROLLED TRIAL (RCT) Compares an experimental treatment to a control (placebo or existing treatment) to determine which is better. Subjects with the desired characteristics (inclusion criteria) are carefully selected, and patients with characteristics that may influence the outcome are excluded (exclusion criteria). Patients are <u>randomized</u> (have an <u>equal chance</u> of being assigned to the treatment or control group) and sometimes <u>blinded</u> (unaware if they are receiving treatment or control). Common types of blinding designs include: ■ <u>Double</u>-blind: both the <u>patient</u> and the <u>investigator</u> are unaware of the treatment assignment. ■ <u>Single</u>-blind: the <u>patient is unaware</u> of the treatment assignment, but the investigator knows. ■ <u>Open label</u> (or unblinded): <u>all parties know</u> which <u>treatment</u> is being given to the patient. **Benefits** Preferred study type to determine cause and effect or superiority. Less potential for bias. **Limitations** Time-consuming and expensive. May not reflect real-life scenarios (when rigorous exclusion criteria are used).	***Angiotensin-neprilysin inhibition versus enalapril in heart failure (PARADIGM-HF study).*** **Methods** Patients with heart failure were randomized in a double-blind manner to receive a new drug (angiotensin-neprilysin inhibitor) or the current standard of care (enalapril). The effectiveness of the treatments was measured as a primary composite outcome of death from cardiovascular causes or hospitalization for heart failure. **Statistical Data** Primary outcome HR: 0.8 (95% CI 0.73-0.87, p < 0.001). **Conclusion** The new drug demonstrated a statistically significant benefit in reducing death from cardiovascular causes or hospitalizations due to heart failure. The null hypothesis (that there was no difference between the two arms) was rejected.
PARALLEL RCT Subjects are randomized to the treatment or control arm for the entire study.	The PARADIGM-HF study (discussed above) is an example of a parallel study design and is the most common type of RCT.

STUDY TYPE, BENEFITS AND LIMITATIONS	STUDY TYPE EXAMPLE

CROSSOVER RCT
Patients are randomized to one of two sequential treatments:

Group 1 – receive treatment A first, then crossover (change) to treatment B.

Group 2 – receive treatment B first, then crossover (change) to treatment A.

Benefits
Patients serve as their own control; this minimizes the effects from confounders.

Limitations
A washout period is needed to minimize the influence of the first drug during the second treatment.

Crossover comparison of timolol and latanoprost in chronic primary angle-closure glaucoma.

Methods
Patients with chronic primary angle-closure glaucoma were randomized after surgery to latanoprost or timolol. Three months after treatment with the first drug, the second drug was substituted. Intraocular pressure (IOP) was recorded before starting and at 3 and 7 months in both groups.

Statistical Data
Decrease in IOP from baseline was 8.2 ± 2 mmHg with latanoprost ($p < 0.001$) and 6.1 ± 1.7 mmHg with timolol ($p = 0.01$).

Conclusion
Latanoprost was associated with a greater decrease in IOP from baseline than timolol.

FACTORIAL DESIGN
Randomizes to more than the usual two groups to test a number of experimental conditions.

Benefits
Evaluates multiple interventions (multiple drugs or dosing regimens) in a single experiment.

Limitations
With each arm added, more subjects are needed to have adequate power.

Prednisolone or pentoxifylline for alcoholic hepatitis.

Methods
A 2-by-2 factorial design was used to evaluate the effect of prednisolone or pentoxifylline on 28-day mortality in patients with alcoholic hepatitis. Patients were randomized to 1 of 4 groups: prednisolone (PR)-pentoxifylline (PE), PR-placebo, PE-placebo, or placebo-placebo.

Statistical Data
Pentoxifylline (PE-PR and PE-placebo groups) OR: 1.04 (95% CI 0.77-1.49; $p = 0.69$).

Prednisolone (PR-placebo) OR: 0.72 (95% CI 0.52-1.01; $p = 0.06$).

Conclusion
Pentoxifylline (alone or in combination with prednisolone) and prednisolone alone did not reduce mortality in patients with alcoholic hepatitis.

META-ANALYSIS
Combines results from multiple studies in order to develop a conclusion that has greater statistical power than is possible from the individual smaller studies.

Benefits
Smaller studies can be pooled instead of performing a large, expensive study. See previous forest plot explanation for how data can be presented.

Limitations
Studies may not be uniform (size, inclusion and exclusion criteria, etc). Validity can be compromised if lower quality studies are weighted equally to higher quality studies.

Antioxidants for chronic kidney disease (CKD).

Methods
The authors searched the PubMed database to locate studies investigating the use of antioxidants in people with CKD. Ten studies were identified, and the results were pooled to determine whether antioxidants had an effect on cardiovascular disease and mortality in patients with CKD.

Statistical Data
Antioxidant use and cardiovascular disease RR: 0.78 (95% CI 0.52-1.18; $p = 0.24$).

All-cause mortality RR: 0.93 (95% CI 0.76-1.14; $p = 0.48$).

Conclusion
Antioxidant use did not reduce cardiovascular disease or mortality in CKD patients.

SYSTEMATIC REVIEW ARTICLE
Summary of the clinical literature that focuses on a specific topic or question (e.g., treatment options for a condition). Begins with a question followed by a literature search, then the information is summarized, and sometimes includes a meta-analysis to synthesize results.

Benefits
Inexpensive (studies already exist).

The evolving treatment landscape of advanced renal cell carcinoma (RCC) in patients progressing after VEGF inhibition.

Methods
It is still unclear which patients benefit most from VEGF and mTOR inhibitors and the ideal sequence, timing and duration of therapy. The review wanted to define the appropriate treatment sequence after first-line treatment failure.

Statistical Data
No statistical tests reported.

Conclusion
There are no predictive biomarkers that determine the best therapy for the right patient or the best sequence of treatment. More studies are needed.

PHARMACOECONOMICS

BACKGROUND

Healthcare costs in the United States rank among the highest of all industrialized countries. In 2017, total healthcare expenditures reached $3.5 trillion, which translates to an average of $10,739 per person, or about 17.9% of the national gross domestic product. The increasing costs have highlighted the need to understand how limited resources can be used most effectively and efficiently in the care of individual patients and society as a whole. It is necessary to scientifically evaluate the value (i.e., costs vs. outcomes) of interventions such as medical procedures or drugs.

DEFINITIONS

Pharmacoeconomics is a collection of descriptive and analytic techniques for evaluating pharmaceutical interventions (e.g., drugs, devices, procedures) in the healthcare system. Pharmacoeconomic research identifies, measures and compares the costs (direct, indirect and intangible) and the consequences (clinical, economic and humanistic) of pharmaceutical products and services.

Various research methods can be used to determine the impact of the pharmaceutical product or service. These methods include cost-effectiveness analysis, cost-minimization analysis, cost-utility analysis and cost-benefit analysis. The term "pharmacoeconomics" is sometimes referred to as "outcomes research," but they are not the same thing. Pharmacoeconomic methods are specific to assessing the costs and consequences of pharmaceutical products and services. Outcomes research represents a broader research discipline that attempts to identify, measure and evaluate the end result of healthcare services.

Healthcare providers, payers and other decision makers use these methods to evaluate and compare the total costs and consequences of pharmaceutical products and services. The results of pharmacoeconomic analyses can vary significantly based on the point of view of the analyst; the study perspective is critical for interpretation. What may be viewed as good value for society or for the patient may not be deemed as such from an institutional or provider perspective (e.g., the costs of lost productivity due to illness are critically important to a patient or employer, but perhaps less so to a health plan).

Pharmacoeconomic analyses provide useful supplemental evidence to traditional efficacy and safety endpoints. They help translate important clinical benefits into economic and patient-centered terms, and can assist providers and payers in determining where, or if, a drug fits into the treatment paradigm for a specific condition. Pharmacoeconomic studies serve to guide optimal healthcare resource allocation in a standardized and evidence-based manner.

The ECHO model (Economic, Clinical and Humanistic Outcomes) provides a broad evaluative framework to assess the outcomes associated with diseases and treatments.

- Economic outcomes: include direct, indirect and intangible costs of the drug compared to a medical intervention.

- Clinical outcomes: include medical events that occur as a result of the treatment or intervention.

- Humanistic Outcomes: include consequences of the disease or treatment as reported by the patient or caregiver (e.g., patient satisfaction, quality of life).

MEDICAL COST CATEGORIES: DIRECT, INDIRECT AND INTANGIBLE

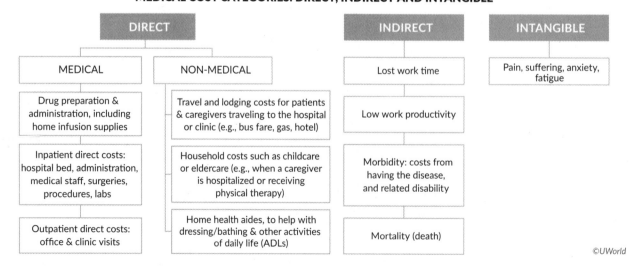

©UWorld

AVERAGE AND INCREMENTAL COST-EFFECTIVENESS RATIOS

The results of a pharmacoeconomic analysis are commonly expressed in terms of a cost ratio, representing the costs incurred to achieve a particular outcome [e.g., cost per case cured, cost per treatment success, cost per quality-adjusted life year (QALY) gained]. Two fundamental cost ratios are commonly used to communicate results of a pharmacoeconomic analysis.

Average Cost-Effectiveness Ratios

Average cost-effectiveness ratios reflect the cost per outcome of one treatment independent of other treatment alternatives. For example, if a treatment costs $50 to generate successful outcomes in two patients, the average cost-effectiveness ratio is $25/treatment success ($50/2 successfully treated patients).

Incremental Cost-Effectiveness Ratios

Incremental cost-effectiveness ratios represent the change in costs and outcomes when two treatment alternatives are compared. An incremental cost-effectiveness ratio is calculated when evaluating costs and outcomes between competing alternatives, and represents the additional costs required to produce an additional unit of effect. It is calculated as shown to the right, where C is for costs and E is for effects.

$$\text{Incremental Cost Ratio} = \frac{(C_2 - C_1)}{(E_2 - E_1)}$$

- Example: if spending $200 on Drug A results in 5 treatment successes while spending $300 on Drug B results in 7 treatment successes, what is the incremental cost ratio?

$$\text{Incremental Cost Ratio} = \frac{(\$300 - \$200)}{(7 - 5)} = \frac{\$100}{2} = \$50$$

Conclusion: Drug B costs $50 more relative to Drug A for each additional treatment success.

PHARMACOECONOMIC METHODOLOGIES

Cost-Minimization Analysis

Cost-minimization analysis (CMA) is used when two or more interventions have demonstrated equivalence in outcomes, and the costs of each intervention are being compared. CMA measures and compares the input costs of treatment alternatives that have equivalent outcomes. This determination of equivalence is a key consideration in adopting this methodology. Ideally, evidence exists to support the clinical equivalence of the alternatives. In some instances, assumptions are made in the absence of relevant evidence.

For example, two ACE inhibitors, captopril and lisinopril, are considered therapeutically equivalent in the literature, but the acquisition cost (the price paid for the drug) and administrative costs may be different (captopril is administered TID and lisinopril is administered once daily). A CMA looks at "minimizing costs" when multiple drugs have equal efficacy and tolerability. Another example of CMA is looking at the same drug regimen given in two different settings (e.g., hospital versus home health care). CMA is considered the easiest analysis to perform, but use of this method is limited given its ability to compare only alternatives with demonstrated equivalent outcomes.

Cost-Benefit Analysis

Cost-benefit analysis (CBA) is a systematic process for calculating and comparing benefits and costs of an intervention in terms of monetary units (dollars). CBA consists of identifying all the benefits from an intervention and converting them into dollars in the year that they will occur. The costs associated with the intervention are identified, allocated to the year when they occur, and then discounted back to their present day value. Given that all other factors remain constant, the program with the largest present day value of benefits minus costs is the best economic value. In CBA, it can be difficult to assign a dollar amount to a benefit (e.g., measuring the benefit of patient quality of life, which is difficult to quantify, and assigning a dollar value to it). One advantage to using CBA is the ability to determine if the benefits of the intervention exceed the costs of implementation. CBA can also be used to compare multiple programs for similar or unrelated outcomes, as long as the outcome measures can be converted to dollars.

Cost-Effectiveness Analysis

Cost-effectiveness analysis (CEA) is used to compare the clinical effects of two or more interventions to the respective costs. The resources associated with the intervention are usually measured in dollars, and clinical outcomes are usually measured in natural health units (e.g., LDL values in mg/dL, % clinical cures, length of stay). The main advantage of this method is that the outcomes are easier to quantify when compared to other analyses, and clinicians are familiar with these types of outcomes since they are similar to outcomes seen in clinical trials and practice. CEA is the most common pharmacoeconomic methodology seen in biomedical literature.

A disadvantage of CEA is the inability to directly compare different types of outcomes. For example, one cannot compare the cost-effectiveness of implementing a diabetes program with implementing an asthma program where the outcome units are different (e.g., blood glucose values versus asthma exacerbations). It is also difficult to combine two or more outcomes into one value of measurement (e.g., comparing one chemotherapeutic agent that prolongs survival, but has significant side effects, to another chemotherapeutic agent that has less effect on prolonging survival but fewer side effects).

Cost-Utility Analysis

Cost-utility analysis (CUA) is a specialized form of CEA that includes a quality-of-life component of morbidity assessments, using common health indices such as quality-adjusted life years (QALYs) and disability-adjusted life years (DALYs). CEA can measure the quantity of life (years gained) but not the "quality" or "utility" of those years. In CUA, the intervention outcome is measured in terms of QALYs gained. QALY takes into account both the quality (morbidity) and the quantity (mortality) of life gained.

CUA measures outcomes based on years of life that are adjusted by utility weights, which range from 1 for "perfect health" to 0 for "dead." These weights can take into account patient and society preferences for specific health states. There is no consensus on the measurement, since both patient and society preferences can vary based on culture. An advantage of CUA is that different types of outcomes, and diseases with multiple outcomes of interest, can be compared (unlike CEA which can only compare one common unit).

Four Basic Pharmacoeconomic Methodologies

METHODOLOGY	COST MEASUREMENT UNIT	OUTCOME UNIT
Cost-minimization analysis	Dollars	Demonstrated or assumed to be equivalent in comparative groups
Cost-benefit analysis	Dollars	Dollars
Cost-effectiveness analysis	Dollars	Natural units (e.g., life-years gained, mmHg blood pressure, % at treatment goal)
Cost-utility analysis	Dollars	Quality-adjusted-life year (QALY) or other utilities

HEALTH-RELATED QUALITY OF LIFE

Health-related quality of life (HRQOL) refers to the effects of a disease and its treatment on an individual's function and well-being, as perceived by that individual. It is commonly included under a broad umbrella of assessments known as patient-reported outcomes (PROs). HRQOL is comprised of several important domains, including physical and mental functioning, role functioning, vitality, social functioning and general health perceptions.

HRQOL assessments can provide important patient-centered information related to the effects of a disease or treatment on patient functioning and well-being. These assessments are typically developed as either general (or generic) health status instruments that can be used across a number of disease areas (e.g., the SF-36 Health Survey can be used for asthma, diabetes and other conditions) or disease-specific measures applicable to a limited disease population (e.g., the Asthma Quality of Life Questionnaire). Prior to their use in practice, it is critical that the reliability and validity of HRQOL assessments in specific patient populations has been documented.

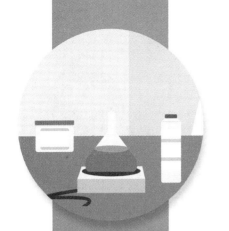
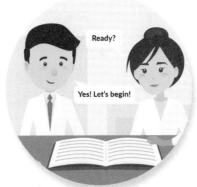
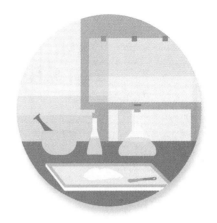

COMPOUNDING & HAZARDOUS DRUGS

CONTENTS

CONTENT LEGEND

☀ = Study Tip Gal 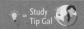   ⚏ = Required Formula

---

CHAPTER 15
NONSTERILE COMPOUNDING

INTRODUCTION TO COMPOUNDING

Compounding is the process of combining or altering ingredients to create a medication. A traditional compounded drug is prepared for an individual patient based on a prescription. Compounded drugs meet unique needs and are not FDA-approved. The dose or formulation cannot be commercially available as a manufactured product.

TYPES OF COMPOUNDING

Depending on where in the body the drug is intended to be delivered, drugs are compounded as either nonsterile or sterile preparations. These compounds can be categorized further as either nonhazardous or hazardous (see Study Tip Gal on next page) based on the drug within the compound (e.g., the drug causes cancer or reproductive toxicity).

COMPOUNDING STANDARDS AND RESOURCES

U.S. Pharmacopeia
The U.S. Pharmacopeia (USP) sets the standards for compounding. Information is divided into chapters; chapters numbered below 1,000 are required and chapters numbered 1,000 and above are informational. USP chapters related to compounding include:

- USP 795 – Nonsterile Preparations
- USP 797 – Sterile Preparations
- USP 800 – Hazardous Drugs – Handling in Healthcare Settings

The USP chapters are considered to be the minimum acceptable standards by the FDA, state boards of pharmacy and the Joint Commission. USP standards apply to all who engage in compounding (e.g., pharmacy staff, nurses, physicians) in any practice setting (e.g., hospitals, clinics, pharmacies, veterinary offices).

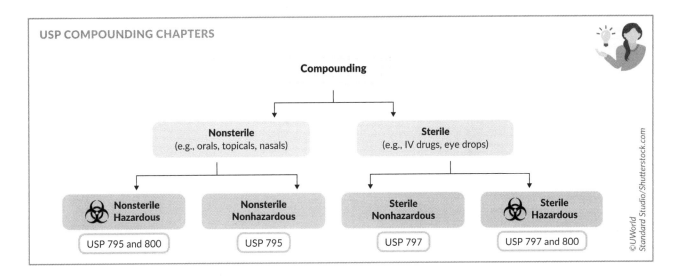

NONSTERILE COMPOUNDING

Compounded nonsterile preparations (CNSPs) include those administered <u>orally</u>, via <u>tube</u> (e.g., gastric tube), <u>rectally</u>, <u>vaginally, topically, nasally or in the ear</u> (unless the eardrum is perforated).

Nonsterile compounding is primarily used to:

- Prepare a <u>dose or formulation</u> that is <u>not commercially available</u>, such as:
  - Changing a solid tablet to a liquid for a patient who cannot swallow the tablet
  - Diluting a 10% ointment to 5%
- <u>Avoid an excipient</u> (e.g., gluten or red dye)
- <u>Add a flavor</u> to make a medication more palatable (e.g., a cherry-flavored suspension for a child)

Splitting tablets, repackaging or reconstituting a manufactured product (according to the manufacturer's labeling) are not considered compounding. Use of compounding kits, which contain pre-measured ingredients for a compounded product, is considered compounding.

SPACE REQUIREMENTS

Nonsterile compounding can be performed in ambient air (<u>room air</u>), but must be <u>separated from the dispensing part</u> of the pharmacy. The nonsterile compounding space must be <u>specifically designated</u>.

Adequate space with shelving and storage is needed to avoid mix-ups of ingredients, containers and other equipment. All ingredients, equipment and containers must be <u>stored off the floor</u>. The space must be clean and well-lit, and should not be carpeted. Heating, ventilation and air conditioning systems must be controlled to avoid drug deterioration. <u>Temperature</u> should be monitored <u>daily (or continuously)</u>. A spill kit must be readily available and personnel trained on use.

Adequate plumbing is required and a clean, easily accessible <u>sink</u> with hot and cold water. <u>Purified water</u>, distilled water or reverse osmosis water are needed for <u>rinsing equipment</u> and <u>utensils</u>.

COMPOUNDING PERSONNEL

There must be a <u>designated person</u> (or people) responsible and accountable for overseeing the performance and operation of the compounding facility and personnel (i.e., staff) involved.

TRAINING

Personnel must have proper <u>training</u>, with <u>documentation</u>, for each type of compounding they perform.

Training, with demonstrated <u>proficiency</u> in certain core competencies, must be completed <u>initially</u> and <u>every 12 months</u>. Core competencies include <u>hand hygiene, garbing</u>, cleaning/sanitizing, use of equipment, measuring and mixing, and documentation of the compounding process.

GARBING

Personal hygiene and garb are needed to reduce the risk of contaminating CNSPs. A compounder must remove any jewelry, personal garments (e.g., hats) and headphones to maintain cleanliness, and they must <u>notify the designated person</u> if they have any <u>concerns for contamination</u> (e.g., upper respiratory infection, rash, conjunctivitis).

When entering the compounding area, the compounder must complete <u>hand hygiene</u> with <u>soap and water</u> for ≥ 30 seconds. <u>Gloves</u> are <u>required</u>; other garb will be determined by the facility and type of compounding being performed.

EQUIPMENT

Equipment should be kept clean, in proper working order and free from contamination, and must be <u>calibrated</u> regularly to <u>confirm accuracy</u>. For some types of equipment, the calibration can be frequent (e.g., electronic balances are calibrated routinely before use). Complex equipment can require calibration by an outside expert.

Equipment should be made of material that does not react with the compounding ingredients (e.g., <u>metal spatulas</u> should <u>not</u> be used with compounds containing <u>metal ions</u>).

All <u>measurements</u> should be made in the <u>metric system</u>.

WEIGHING EQUIPMENT

Balances

There are two types of balances used to weigh ingredients. The older balance is the <u>Class III torsion balance</u> (sometimes called a <u>Class A balance</u>). This type of balance is still used, though less commonly than the electronic balance [see "Torsion Balances" box for a description and the <u>minimum weighable quantity (MWQ)</u> calculation].

The top-loading <u>electronic balance</u> (called an <u>analytical balance</u> or a <u>scale</u>) is used most commonly.

- This type of balance is simple to use and has <u>higher sensitivity</u> (i.e., can weigh with more precision, including very small amounts). It is not necessary to calculate the MWQ with an electronic balance.

- The compounder must place a weigh boat or glassine paper on the scale, then "<u>tare</u>" or "<u>zero out</u>" the balance. This ensures that <u>only the ingredients</u> are weighed and the container or paper used to hold the ingredients is not included in the weight.

With either balance, the <u>material</u> to be <u>weighed</u> (e.g., powder) should <u>never</u> be <u>placed directly on the balance</u>. Material should be placed on a <u>weigh boat</u> (a shallow dish made of plastic or other material) or on <u>glassine weighing paper</u>, which is coated to reduce moisture penetration.

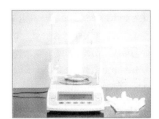

Electronic balance
KuLouKu/Shutterstock.com

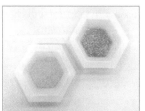

Weigh boats
Artur Wnorowski/Shutterstock.com

TORSION BALANCES

<u>Class III (Class A) torsion balances</u> have internal weights, which are used to weigh quantities ≤ 1 gram. When weighing > 1 gram, external weights (see picture) are placed on one pan and the substance to be weighed is placed on the other. The external weights must be handled with forceps (pincers) to avoid getting oil from the skin on the weights.

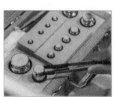

tonaquatic/stock.adobe.com

Torsion balances have a <u>sensitivity requirement</u> (SR) that is most often 6 mg, meaning 6 mg can be added or removed before the dial moves 1 division.

The <u>minimum weighable quantity</u> (MWQ), or the minimum amount that can be weighed, is calculated based on the SR and <u>acceptable error rate</u> (typically <u>0.05 or 5%</u>):

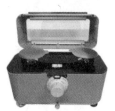

Torsion balance
©UWorld

MWQ	=	SR / acceptable error rate (0.05 or 5%)

MWQ = 6 mg / 0.05 = 120 mg

MEASURING VOLUME

Pharmacists use various equipment to measure the <u>volume</u> of ingredients, and nurses and patients use some of the same equipment to administer medication.

Cylindrical and Conical Graduates

Graduates, which are a type of equipment with <u>lines</u> on the glass that are used to <u>measure volume</u>, include graduated cylinders, conical (cone-shaped) graduates, beakers and graduated medication containers.

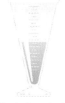

Conical graduate

A <u>graduated cylinder</u> has the <u>same diameter</u> from the <u>top to the bottom</u> of the container and provides <u>more accurate</u> measurements than conical graduates or beakers, which have wide mouths (makes it easier to stir mixtures with a <u>glass stirring rod</u>). The <u>wider</u> the <u>mouth</u>, the <u>lower</u> the <u>accuracy</u>.

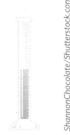

Graduated cylinder

ShannonChocolate/Shutterstock.com

Some important points about measuring volume using graduates include:

- Measuring volumes that are smaller than <u>20%</u> of the graduate's <u>capacity</u> can cause a measuring <u>error</u>.
  - For example, measuring 5 mL in a 100 mL graduate has a higher risk of error than measuring 87 mL in a 100 mL graduate. A smaller graduate (no larger than 25 mL) is required to measure 5 mL.

- To <u>read the volume</u> in a graduate, place it on a flat surface and view the height of the liquid in the cylinder at <u>eye level</u>.

- The liquid can curve downward from both sides, especially with viscous liquids. This curve is called the meniscus.

- The measurement is read at the bottom of the meniscus, at the center (see image).

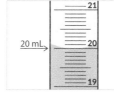

Measure at the bottom of the meniscus, at eye level. This contains 20 mL.
©UWorld

Syringes

Oral syringes and hypodermic (injection) syringes (also called parenteral syringes) can be used for measuring volume in nonsterile compounding.

- Syringes are most accurate for measuring small volumes, and are especially useful for measuring viscous (thick) liquids, such as glycerin and mineral oil.

- Oral syringes are useful for compounded medications that are drawn up into patient-specific doses (i.e., unit dose) for administration into the mouth (e.g., children, animals), through a feeding tube (e.g., a nasogastric tube) or to deliver small amounts of topical preparations.

  ❏ Safety measures must be in place to prevent oral medications from being given by the wrong route.

  ❏ Clearly label oral syringes by placing a "For Oral Use Only" sticker over the syringe cap.

Pipettes and Droppers

Pipettes are thin plastic or glass tubes used to measure small volumes and release liquid in drops (can be referred to as droppers).

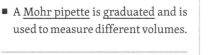

Mohr pipette (graduated)
chromatos/Shutterstock.com

- A volumetric pipette draws up a set volume only.

- A Mohr pipette is graduated and is used to measure different volumes.

GRINDING, MIXING AND TRANSFERRING EQUIPMENT

Mortars and Pestles

Mortars and pestles are used to grind substances into a finer consistency, and a mortar can be used to stir and mix small amounts of ingredients. The mortar is the bowl, and the pestle is the blunt, heavy stick. A compounding pharmacy needs at least one glass and one Wedgwood or porcelain mortar and pestle.

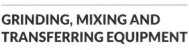

Disposable pipette
Paket/Shutterstock.com

- Glass mortars are used for liquids and for mixing compounds that are oily or can stain.

- Wedgwood mortars have a rough surface and are preferred for grinding dry crystals and hard powders.

- Porcelain mortars have a smooth surface and are preferred for blending powders and pulverizing gummy consistencies.

Types of Mortar and Pestles

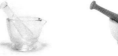

Glass
aSculptor/ stock.adobe.com

Wedgwood
Sponner/ Shutterstock.com

Porcelain
akepong srichaichana/ Shutterstock.com

Spatulas

Spatulas are used to mix and transfer ingredients from one place (such as an ointment slab) to another place (such as a container). The flat part of the blade can be used to flatten and grind down ingredients, and to pack preparations such as ointments into containers. Spatulas are made of stainless steel, plastic or hard rubber. Stainless steel and disposable plastic spatulas are used commonly. The type of spatula used depends on what ingredients are being transferred or mixed.

- A steel (metal) spatula would not be used if making a mixture that contains metallic ions.

- A rubber spatula is used to handle corrosive material.

Ointment Slabs

Ingredients are mixed into ointments on a compounding (or ointment) slab, which is a flat board made of porcelain or glass.

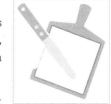

Slab and spatula
moe/stock.adobe.com

- Ointment slabs are used as a work surface for other purposes besides making ointments since the material is hard and non-reactive. For example, an ointment slab can be used to form pills (in which case it can be referred to as a pill tile) and for rolling out suppositories.

- Disposable parchment ointment pads can be used as a work surface if the water content of the mixture will not cause the paper to tear.

- Mixtures that have a higher water content than an ointment, such as a cream, can be mixed on an ointment slab if the mixture will hold its shape (and not flow off the slab). Otherwise, different equipment can be used to hold the preparation, such as a mortar bowl or a beaker.

Powder Sieves

Sieves are sifters similar to those used in baking.

- After a powder has been ground fine, it is sifted in order to ensure a uniform particle size.

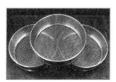

Sieves
Claudio Caridi/stock.adobe.com

ELECTRIC MIXING EQUIPMENT

Mixing can be performed manually or with electric mixing equipment, which speeds up the process. <u>Ointment mills</u>, <u>homogenizers</u> and <u>grinders</u> are types of electronic mixing equipment.

Ointment Mills

An <u>ointment mill</u> draws the ointment (or another semi-solid preparation) between rollers that <u>grind</u> and <u>homogenize</u> (i.e., make smooth and <u>uniform</u>) the ingredients.

Homogenizers

A <u>homogenizer</u> (also called an <u>electric mortar and pestle</u>) can be used to mix ointments, creams or other semi-solid preparations.

- The homogenizer is similar to a blender, but more powerful. Homogenizers can be small and hand-held.

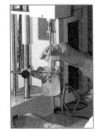

Homogenizer
defun/stock.adobe.com

Grinders

Electric grinders are similar to coffee bean grinders. In fact, coffee bean grinders are used in some pharmacies. When used for compounding, they must be dedicated for compounding use only. A grinder is useful for <u>grinding hard tablets</u> into a <u>rough powder</u>. The powder will need further manipulation to produce a fine powder.

HEATING DEVICES

Hot Plates

Hot plates provide direct heat to soften and melt ingredients and to hasten chemical reactions.

- A <u>water bath</u> is helpful when the temperature needs to be <u>carefully controlled</u>. The water bath protects the ingredients from overheating and burning.
  - The ingredients to be melted will be <u>in a container</u> (e.g., a beaker) that is <u>placed into</u> a <u>larger container</u> filled with <u>water</u>.
  - The water in the outer container separates the inner container from the direct heat source, to prevent burning.

- A <u>hot plate</u> with a <u>magnetic stirrer</u> can save time by continuously stirring ingredients to dissolve and mix them.
  - The stirrer has a <u>rotating magnet</u> under the ceramic plate, which causes the <u>stir bar</u> (placed inside the glass) to spin and stir the components.

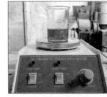

Hot plate with a stir bar in the glass. A magnet inside the hot plate moves the stir bar.
Andri wahyudi/Shutterstock.com

Microwave ovens

Microwaves heat quickly; be careful that the heat is applied uniformly as some microwaves provide uneven heat.

MOLDS

Reusable or disposable <u>molds</u> are used to prepare tablets, lozenges, troches and suppositories.

- Soft delivery vehicles (e.g., suppositories, lozenges) are often dispensed in <u>disposable</u> plastic <u>molds</u> to keep the product in the correct shape. <u>Refrigeration</u> also helps soft products retain shape.

A <u>tablet press</u> (or tablet mold) is two plastic or metal plates used to compress damp powder into tablets.

TUBE SEALERS

Tube sealers heat and squeeze the ends of tubes shut; the end will look similar to the crimped end of a toothpaste tube.

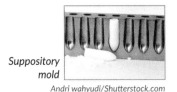

Suppository mold
Andri wahyudi/Shutterstock.com

Lozenge mold
Cuhle-Fotos/Shutterstock.com

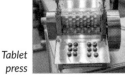

Tablet press
Itsanan/Shutterstock.com

Tube sealer (sealed at bottom)
Katy Pack/Shutterstock.com

CAPSULES AND CAPSULE MACHINES

Capsules can be <u>soft gels</u> or <u>hard shells</u>, which are more commonly used for compounding. The shells are made of <u>gelatin</u>, an animal product which is <u>pork-derived</u>, or from <u>hypromellose</u> or a similar <u>plant</u>-derived product. A capsule-filling machine is a device that holds the capsule bodies upright, to allow for powder to be placed inside, then the caps are placed over the capsule bodies to close the capsules.

COMPOUNDING INGREDIENTS

All medications, whether compounded or not, include the drug/s (called the <u>active pharmaceutical ingredients</u>, or <u>APIs</u>) and the <u>excipients</u>. Excipients do not produce therapeutic effect, but are needed to make the dosage form stable, functional and, with some oral dosage forms, palatable.

INGREDIENT QUALITY

High-quality ingredients ensure the purity and safety of the formulation. Ingredients should be listed in the <u>USP National Formulary (USP-NF)</u> and come from an FDA-registered facility.

MISSING EXPIRATION DATE

Ingredients degrade, and expiration dates are important to ensure that the product retains potency and is non-toxic. If there is an ingredient without an expiration date, the pharmacist will assign a conservative (cautious) date that is no more than 3 years from the date of receipt (the day the pharmacy received the item).

COMMON EXCIPIENTS

SURFACTANTS

Surfactant is a contraction of the words surface active agent. Surfactants lower the surface tension between two ingredients (or phases) in a preparation to make them more miscible (i.e., easier to mix together).

For example, an oil and vinegar salad dressing has an oil phase that will become dispersed in the water phase (the vinegar) when shaken. The dressing will quickly settle back into the two distinct phases because the "tension" between the two surfaces is high and the oil and water will repel each other. A surfactant added to the salad dressing will lower the tension between the two surfaces, and keep the phases from quickly separating.

Surfactants are amphiphilic; they are both hydrophilic (on one side) and hydrophobic (on the other side). In the case of oil and water, the oil will interact with the lipophilic (i.e., lipid-loving) end of the surfactant, and the water will interact with the hydrophilic (i.e., water-loving) end of the surfactant.

Types of Surfactants

Surfactants have many uses in compounding. For example, adding a surfactant to a suspension leads to delivery of a more consistent dose by keeping the drug dispersed for longer. Surfactants also make it easier to grind particles to a smaller size, and to mix ingredients. Surfactants are called by a variety of names, depending on the use or the type of preparation, as described below.

Wetting Agents/Levigating Agents

Wetting agents, also called levigating agents, are substances that reduce the surface tension between a liquid and a solid. Levigation is a technique used to grind particles (i.e., make particles smaller) with a small amount of liquid (i.e., the wetting agent) in which the powder is insoluble. This creates a paste that can be incorporated into an ointment or suspension. Mineral oil is a common levigating agent for lipophilic (oil-soluble) compounds, and glycerin or propylene glycol are used for aqueous (water-soluble) compounds.

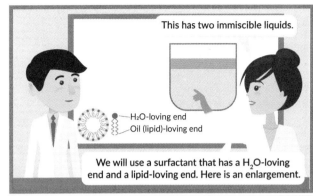

H₂O-loving end
Oil (lipid)-loving end

We will use a surfactant that has a H₂O-loving end and a lipid-loving end. Here is an enlargement.

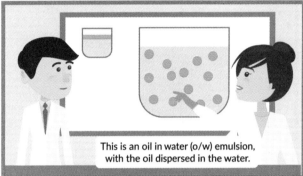

This is an oil in water (o/w) emulsion, with the oil dispersed in the water.

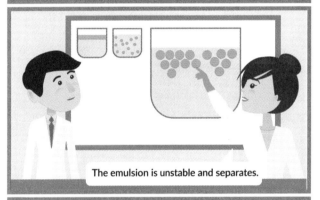

The emulsion is unstable and separates.

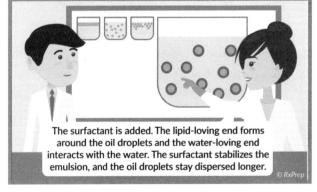

The surfactant is added. The lipid-loving end forms around the oil droplets and the water-loving end interacts with the water. The surfactant stabilizes the emulsion, and the oil droplets stay dispersed longer.

© RxPrep

Suspending Agents

A suspension is a solid dispersed in a liquid (e.g., amoxicillin powder does not dissolve in water, and is delivered as a suspension). Suspending agents are added to suspensions to help keep the solid particles from settling. Suspending agents do not keep suspensions separated for long, and suspensions must be shaken to redisperse the solid prior to use. Suspending agents can also be called dispersants (or dispersing agents) or plasticizers, where plasticizer means that it will make the preparation easier to shape or mold. Sorbitol can be used as a plasticizer for gelatin capsules.

COMMERCIALLY AVAILABLE SUSPENDING AGENTS

Ora-Plus:
- Composed of a gel-like structure that keeps drug particles suspended and prevents settling
- Slightly acidic to prevent drug degradation through oxidation
- Bland taste; must be combined with *Ora-Sweet* for flavor

Ora-Sweet:
- Similar to simple syrup
- Provides flavor to *Ora-Plus*

Ora-Blend is a commercially available combination of *Ora-Plus* and *Ora-Sweet*

Ora-Sweet and *Ora-Blend* are available in sugar-free formulations sweetened with saccharin (*Ora-Sweet SF, Ora-Blend SF*)

Foaming Agents

A major use of surfactants in manufacturing is in detergents and soaps; they contain a foaming agent that helps foam form, which reduces the surface tension between dirt (often lipophilic) and water during the cleaning process. In nonsterile compounding, anti-foaming agents are more commonly used (e.g., simethicone).

Glycols and Gels

The commonly used products polyethylene glycol (PEG) and poloxamer, by itself or as the P in PLO gel (described later), are both delivery vehicles and surfactants. They have both hydrophilic and hydrophobic parts, which makes them useful for a variety of preparations. Glycols and gels are discussed in more detail in the following tables

Emulsifiers

An emulsion is a mixture of two or more liquids which are not able to be blended together (immiscible), such as water droplets dispersed in oil, or oil droplets dispersed in water. Emulsifiers are added to an emulsion to help keep the liquid droplets dispersed throughout the liquid vehicle. This helps prevent the two liquids from separating. Emulsifiers can also be called emulgents.

The Hydrophilic-Lipophilic Balance

Selecting the right surfactant to make an emulsion is important to keep the liquid droplets adequately dispersed.

A primary consideration in selecting the surfactant is whether the emulsion is a water-in-oil (w/o) emulsion or an oil-in-water (o/w) emulsion.

- The taste of w/o formulations is not palatable; they are primarily used topically.
- Oral products are typically o/w formulations.

The hydrophilic-lipophilic balance (HLB) number determines the type of surfactant required to make an emulsion (see Study Tip Gal).

THE HLB NUMBER

The HLB scale range is 0 – 20. The midpoint is 10.

Surfactants with a low HLB number (< 10) are more lipid-soluble and are used for water-in-oil (w/o) emulsions.

Surfactants with a high HLB number (> 10) are more water-soluble and are used for oil-in-water (o/w) emulsions.

Lower HLB #   10   Higher HLB #

0 ←————————————————————→ 20

More Lipid Soluble (w/o)   More H_2O Soluble (o/w)

The following table has examples of surfactants and their HLB values. In the table, PEG 400 and *Tween 85* have HLB values greater than 10, and would be possible options for forming an o/w emulsion. The HLB values that are less than 10 (e.g., *Span 65*) would be possible options for forming a w/o emulsion.

Examples of Surfactants and their HLB Values

COMMERCIAL NAME	CHEMICAL NAME	HLB VALUE
Glyceryl monostearate	Glyceryl monostearate	3.8
PEG 400 monooleate	Polyoxyethylene monooleate	11.4
Span 65	Sorbitan tristearate	2.1
Tween 81	Polyoxyethylene sorbitan monooleate	10
Tween 85	Polyoxyethylene sorbitan trioleate	11

OTHER EXCIPIENTS

EXCIPIENT	PURPOSE AND NOTES	SELECT EXAMPLES
Binders *ahasoft2000 © 123RF.com*	Binders allow the contents of a tablet to stick together while permitting the contents to be released once ingested. They can provide stability and strength.	Acacia Starch paste Sucrose syrup Compressible sugar (e.g., *Nu-Tab*)
Diluents and fillers *iStock.com/Anna_zabella*	Diluents (to make something more dilute) and fillers (to bulk up a small amount) add size to very small dosages. In liquids, the diluent helps dissolve or suspend the drug and facilitates disintegration, which is required for absorption (see disintegrants below).	**Tablets/capsules:** Sugars: Lactose, Mannitol, Sorbitol; Starches; Calcium salts; Cellulose powder **Liquids:** Water, Glycerin, Alcohol **Topicals:** Petrolatum, Mineral oil, Lanolin
Disintegrants *ahasoft2000 © 123RF.com*	Disintegrants facilitate the breakup of a tablet after oral administration. Oral products have to be dissolved in order to be absorbed in the small intestine, where most drugs are absorbed. Alginates and cellulose absorb water, causing the tablet to swell and release its contents.	Alginic acid Cellulose products Starches
Flavorings and coloring agents *Olzas/Shutterstock.com*	Flavorings and coloring agents make the product look and taste better. Salty or sweet tastes mask a bitter flavor. Mint and spices mask poor flavor. Acids (such as citric acid) enhance fruit flavors.	**Sweeteners:** Non-caloric, artificial: Aspartame, Saccharin, Sucralose; Glycerin; Dextrose; Sugar alcohols (e.g., mannitol, sorbitol, xylitol); Stevia **Coloring agents:** D&C Red No. 3; Yellow No. 6; Caramel; Ferric oxide (red)
Lubricants *sulit.photos/Shutterstock.com*	Lubricants and anti-adherents prevent ingredients from sticking to each other and to equipment. This can be useful for tablet molds and punches, suppository molds and for capsule filling. Can be called glidants or anti-adherents. Glidants improve powder flowability by reducing interparticle friction.	Magnesium stearate, calcium stearate, stearic acid PEG Glycerin Mineral oil Talc
Preservatives Sodium Benzoate Potassium Sorbate *sulit.photos/Shutterstock.com*	Preservatives slow or prevent microorganism growth. They are required in most preparations except if sterile and used immediately or if packaged as single-use preparations. Ophthalmic (eye) preparations in multi-dose containers need a preservative. Do not use preservatives in neonates. Alcohols and acids are often used as preservatives. Preservatives commonly have "benz," "cetyl," "phenyl/ol" or "parabens" in the name.	Chlorhexidine [also used as an antiseptic in surgical scrubs to eliminate or reduce microorganisms (*Hibiclens*) and as a dental rinse (*Peridex*)] Povidone iodine (used as a topical antiseptic and as a preservative in some ophthalmics) Sodium benzoate/benzoic acid, benzalkonium chloride, benzyl alcohol Sorbic acid/potassium sorbate Methyl/ethyl/propyl parabens EDTA Thimerosal (contains mercury, used in some vaccines) Cetylpyridinium chloride

EXCIPIENT	PURPOSE AND NOTES	SELECT EXAMPLES
Buffers *iStock.com/Cathal Stadler*	Buffers keep the pH within a certain range, which can improve stability and solubility and decrease irritation to sensitive tissues in the body. Ionized compounds are more polar, which makes them more water-soluble. The pKa determines how much of a compound is ionized when placed into a solution with a set pH. The pH of a buffer system can be calculated with the Henderson-Hasselbalch equation (see the Calculations IV chapter).	**Buffers used to maintain acidic pH:** Hydrochloric acid Acetic acid/sodium acetate Citric acid/sodium citrate **Buffers used to maintain alkaline pH:** Sodium hydroxide Boric acid/sodium borate Sodium bicarbonate/sodium carbonate **Buffers used to maintain neutral pH:** Sodium biphosphate/sodium phosphate Potassium phosphate/metaphosphate
Adsorbents	Adsorbents keep powders dry and prevent hydrolysis reactions.	Magnesium oxide/carbonate, kaolin
Anti-foaming agents	Anti-foaming agents break up and inhibit the formation of foams.	Simethicone, dimethicone
Coatings (regular)	Coatings prevent degradation due to oxygen, light and moisture, and mask unpalatable taste. Enteric coatings prevent drug degradation in the stomach for drugs that can be destroyed by stomach acid.	Shellac, gelatin, gluten (food grade) Cellulose acetate phthalate
Gelling (thickening) agents	Gelling agents increase the viscosity of a substance; can stabilize the mixture. Gelatin, cellulose and bentonite are used commonly; they swell when mixed with water.	Agar, alginates, various gums [guar, xanthan, acacia (a natural gum)], gelatins, bentonite (a type of clay), cellulose, starches, cetyl alcohol, magnesium aluminum silicate, poloxamer (pluronic) gels, polyvinyl alcohol (eye lubricant), sorbitol
Humectants	Prevent preparations from becoming dry and brittle; when put into emollients, humectants draw water into the skin to moisturize.	Glycerin or glycerol, propylene glycol, PEG, lecithin, hyaluronic acid

SOLVENTS

Hydrophilic Solvents

SOLVENTS	PURPOSE AND NOTES	SELECT EXAMPLES
Water Distilled Water H₂O *ggw/stock.adobe.com*	Water is commonly used as a solvent, as a delivery vehicle and for cleaning equipment and tools. As a delivery vehicle, water is used for oral liquid formulations (e.g., solutions, suspensions, emulsions), topicals (e.g., creams, lotions) and in all types of injectable medications.	USP specifies that purified water must be used in compounding, unless otherwise specified. Purified water has been treated to remove chemicals and contaminants. Types of purification include distillation, deionization, reverse osmosis and carbon filtration. Distilled water is used for reconstitution [i.e., adding water to lyophilized (freeze-dried) powder] to prepare oral suspensions and in nonsterile compounding preparations. Potable water (drinking/tap water) is safe to drink and used for hand washing.
Sterile Water Sterile Water for Inj., USP *Burlingham/Shutterstock.com*	For preparation and reconstitution of sterile drugs.	Sterile water for injection (SWFI) must be free of bacterial endotoxins (pyrogens) produced by microorganisms that inhabit water. Bacteriostatic water for injection: SWFI with antimicrobial preservatives. Sterile water for irrigation: sterile water packaged in large containers for washing, rinsing and dilution of products used for irrigating body cavities, wounds, urinary catheters or surgical drainage tubes.
Alcohols BD ALCOHOL SWAB *Mohd Syis Zulkipli/Shutterstock.com*	Alcohols have high miscibility (mixes easily) with water and can be used to dissolve solutes that would be insoluble in water alone. Isopropyl alcohols (IPAs) are used as disinfectants on equipment or on skin (e.g., on an alcohol swab for skin disinfection prior to a needle stick). They can be used as solvents when compounding topicals.	Benzyl alcohol: used as a solvent, preservative and for the aroma (fragrance). Alcohol USP: ethanol (grain alcohol, ethyl alcohol or drinking alcohol). IPA 70%: preferred disinfectant for sterile compounding equipment.
Glycols	Glycols have a low freezing point, a high boiling point and are water-soluble. Polyethylene glycol (PEG) has low toxicity and low systemic absorption. It is used as a surfactant, solvent, plasticizer, suppository base, ointment base, humectant, lubricant and troche base. It is water-soluble and water-miscible. When PEG is linked to a protein drug (pegylated), such as PEG-filgrastim, it increases the half-life.	Polyethylene glycol (PEG): PEGs are numbered based on the molecular weight. PEG 400 is used commonly in compounding and PEG 3350 is used as a laxative. Polybase is a PEG mixture used as a suppository base. It is a good delivery vehicle and slides out of molds without the need for a lubricant. It is also a good emulsifier. Glycerin Propylene glycol: used in small quantities as a solvent (large quantities are toxic)

Hydrophobic Solvents

SOLVENTS	PURPOSE AND NOTES	SELECT EXAMPLES
Oils and Fats Oils are hydrocarbon liquids derived from plants, animals or petroleum [i.e., petrolatum (Vaseline petroleum jelly)]. Oils are immiscible in water; they are hydrophobic, lipophilic compounds.	Oils are used as delivery vehicles, for therapeutic or nutritional use, and some are used as scents or flavorings.	Mineral oil: derived from petroleum, and is the ingredient in baby oil Almond, borage, canola, castor, coconut Omega-3 (alpha-linolenic fatty acids, DHA/EPA) Omega-6 (gamma-linoleic fatty acids)

EMOLLIENTS (MOISTURIZERS)

An emollient refers to a product that <u>softens and soothes the skin</u>. <u>Ointments</u> are best for <u>extremely dry skin</u> and <u>thick skin</u>, such as on elbows and feet. <u>Creams</u> are usually best for <u>normal and dry skin</u>. <u>Lotions</u> have the <u>most water</u>, and are best for <u>oily skin</u>. <u>Humectants</u> are put into many emollient formulations to pull in water from the atmosphere to moisturize the skin. They can be sticky-feeling, and are combined with more soothing ingredients.

<u>Occlusive</u> ointments, including <u>petroleum jelly</u> (i.e., <u>white petrolatum</u>), <u>theobroma</u> oil (i.e., <u>cocoa butter</u>), beeswax, paraffin and other <u>waxes</u> form a protective <u>barrier</u> to <u>prevent the loss of water</u> molecules from the top layer of the skin (epidermis). USP separates ointments into four groups (see below). Some contain water and some do not, which is important in determining the BUD.

EMOLLIENT	PURPOSE AND NOTES	SELECT EXAMPLES
Ointments Defined as semisolids, with <u>0–20% water</u>, hydrocarbons, waxes and/or polyols (compounds with multiple OH groups) Separated into four groups (see below)	Provide a barrier to water loss from the skin and are used as vehicles for topical drug delivery	<u>Petrolatum</u>, lanolin, mineral oil *Polybase* *Aquaphor* *Aquabase*
1. Hydrocarbon Bases	Called "<u>oleaginous</u>" ointments (i.e., oil-containing, <u>no water</u>); good for drug delivery and forming a protective barrier, hard to wash off/greasy	White ointment, white <u>petrolatum</u> (e.g., *Vaseline* <u>petroleum jelly</u>)
2. Absorption Bases	Can be used to form water-in-oil emulsions	Hydrophilic petrolatum, lanolin
3. Water-Removable Bases	Hydrophilic, oil-in-water emulsions. Per USP, more correctly called creams; more easily diluted, and easier to wash off the skin.	Hydrophilic ointment
4. Water-Soluble Bases	Do not contain petrolatum; per USP, are more correctly called gels.	Polyethylene glycol ointment
Creams <u>20-50% water</u> (more than ointments)	Creams are semi-solid preparations that have a soft, spreadable consistency. Most creams are <u>water-in-oil or oil-in-water emulsions</u>. Water-in-oil creams feel more greasy.	*Lipoderm* cream *Eucerin* *Cetaphil*
Lotions <u>Contain the most water</u> (more water than creams) More fluid – lotions are sometimes poured from a container, which is not feasible with creams.	Lotions can be aqueous or hydroalcoholic, with a small amount of <u>alcohol</u> added to <u>solubilize</u> ingredients, or to hasten evaporation of the solvent from the skin	*Versabase* lotion
Gels Semisolid preparations of small inorganic particles or large organic molecules interpenetrated by a liquid.	Gels can be used to administer medications by various routes, including topical, oral, intranasal, vaginal and rectal. <u>Gelling agents</u> are added to increase the viscosity and thicken the product. Aqueous solutions of poloxamers are <u>liquid when refrigerated</u> and form a <u>gel at room temperature</u>. PLO gel is used often because of this property; compounds are easily mixed into the liquid (when taken from the refrigerator), which then forms a gel when stored at room temperature. This works well for <u>transdermal</u> drug delivery, especially for animals (e.g., application to a dog's ear).	<u>Poloxamer (Pluronic) Lecithin Organogel (PLO) gel</u> <u>Poloxamers</u> contain a <u>hydrophobic</u> chain of polyoxypropylene with two <u>hydrophilic</u> chains of polyoxyethylene. This means poloxamer gel can be used for hydrophobic or hydrophilic drug delivery.
Pastes	Pastes contain powder in an ointment base	Zinc oxide paste, used for diaper rash; zinc oxide is a desiccant (draws water from the baby's bottom).
Suppository bases Made of various fats and glycols	Suppository bases have to stay intact for insertion and melt once inserted. Cocoa butter used to be a common base for suppositories, but it melts easily. Newer bases are now more popular.	*Polybase*, cocoa butter (theobroma oil), <u>hydrogenated vegetable oils</u> (palm, palm kernel, and coconut oils), <u>PEG</u> polymers, glycerinated <u>gelatin</u>

EXCIPIENTS TO AVOID IN SOME PATIENTS

EXCIPIENT	AVOID IN	ALTERNATIVE
Alcohol Used as a solvent	Children	Select an alternative solvent; see excipient table
Aspartame (contains **phenylalanine**) Used as a sweetener	Phenylketonuria (PKU), as these patients are not able to metabolize phenylalanine	Select an alternative sweetener; see excipient table
Gelatin Made from animal (e.g., cows, pigs) collagen and used to form capsule shells	Vegetarians and vegans or anyone who wishes to avoid animal products	Hypromellose capsule shells, which are made from cellulose and are vegan (no meat or dairy) and vegetarian (no meat)
Gluten Used as a starch (filler). Gluten is in wheat, barley and rye. Gluten as a starch in drugs is primarily from wheat.	Celiac disease or anyone who wishes to avoid gluten	Starch from non-gluten sources (e.g., corn, potato, tapioca)
Lactose Used as a sweetener, to compress tablets and as a filler/diluent	Lactose intolerance or lactose allergy	Select an alternative depending on the purpose; see excipient table
Preservatives	Neonates	Use preservative-free formulations.
Sorbitol Used as a sweetener	Irritable bowel syndrome (IBS); sorbitol can cause GI distress	Select an alternative sweetener; see excipient table
Sucrose (table sugar) Used as a sweetener and coating	Diabetes: depending on amount used, can increase blood glucose	Select an alternative sweetener; see excipient table
Xylitol Used as a sweetener.	Dogs; can cause xylitol toxicosis (hypoglycemia and hepatotoxicity) Humans that have GI upset with xylitol use	Select an alternative sweetener; see excipient table

NONSTERILE COMPOUNDING PREPARATION

Before compounding, the pharmacist will need to evaluate the prescription and determine if it is appropriate for the patient, and whether the proposed formulation is reasonable (e.g., likely to have acceptable stability and palatability).

When ready to compound, the initial steps will be similar for most formulations, such as calibrating equipment and weighing ingredients. The final steps will be similar, and include packaging and performing quality control (QC). What changes most are the steps in between, which depend on the type of formulation being prepared.

Always review the Safety Data Sheets (SDS) for each bulk ingredient to determine safety procedures, including the recommended personal protective equipment (PPE).

INITIAL STEPS

1. Calculate the quantities needed for each component.
2. Gather all ingredients, containers and equipment.
3. Wash equipment, if needed, and calibrate.
4. Perform hand hygiene and garb.

COMPOUNDING STEPS

Make the product according to the master formulation record (see section at end of chapter).

- Most formulations will require common techniques, such as trituration, levigation and geometric dilution (discussed on the next page).
- Other steps are unique to the formulation type, such as calculating the density factor to make suppositories.

COMPLETION STEPS

1. Document all compounding steps, ingredients and other details in the compounding record (see section at end of chapter).

2. Package the product and apply the container label and any needed auxiliary labels.

3. Perform QC: validate the weight, check the product for mixing adequacy, color, clarity, odor, consistency and pH. Enter the measurements and observations in the compounding record.

4. Counsel the patient. If any subsequent adverse drug reactions (ADRs) are reported, they should be recorded according the facility's standard operating procedures.

PREPARING POWDERS

Powders are fine particles of a solid. A dose of medication can be given as a dry powder (put into liquid or a small amount of soft food) for someone who is not able to swallow capsules or tablets (e.g., a child), or powders can be used to prepare tablets, capsules, inhalations, suspensions, ointments, creams and other topicals. Powders often include excipients, such as:

- Glidant/lubricant to improve the flowability of a powder: magnesium stearate.
- Surfactant to neutralize the static charge and keep the powder from floating away: sodium lauryl sulfate.

REDUCING PARTICLE SIZE

When making a compound with dry ingredients, the goal is to make an evenly-distributed mixture with fine powder. The compounder usually starts with coarse granules or tablets that need to be finely ground into smaller particles (0.1 – 10 microns). This can be accomplished with comminution, which means to reduce particle size by grinding, crushing, milling, vibrating or other process (manual or mechanical).

After the powder has been ground, it is placed into a sieve (sifter) and stirred with a sieve brush or a plastic spatula to force the particles through the mesh, which ensures that the particle size is uniform. A high mesh size has many wires that make many holes; only a fine powder will get through the mesh. The sieve number is based on the number of holes per inch (e.g., #100 sieve has 100 openings/inch).

Three Main Methods of Comminution

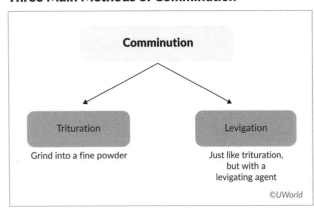

- Trituration: a general term that means "mix thoroughly" (or make the product homogenous). Pharmacists most commonly associate trituration with grinding tablets with a mortar and pestle until a fine powder is achieved, but the term can describe liquids (e.g., triturating an emulsion by shaking it).

- Levigation and spatulation:
  - ❑ Levigation involves triturating the powder with a mortar and pestle and incorporating a small amount of liquid (a levigating agent or wetting agent) to help with the grinding process and create a uniform paste.
  - ❑ Spatulation is similar to levigation, but performed on an ointment slab with a spatula (not with a mortar and pestle).

- Pulverization by intervention is used for crystalline powders that will not crush easily. The crystals are dissolved with an intervening solvent and mixed until the solvent evaporates. When the powder recrystallizes, the particles are finer.

MIXING INGREDIENTS

GEOMETRIC DILUTION

Geometric dilution is a method of mixing ingredients to ensure that ingredients are evenly distributed in a diluent or delivery vehicle. A small amount of the drug is mixed into an equal amount of the diluent. After the initial small amount is thoroughly mixed, another equal amount of the ingredients is mixed in. This is repeated until all the ingredients are mixed together. Geometric dilution can be used with dry powder ingredients alone, or when making a paste. When using multiple ingredients, begin with the ingredient that has the smallest quantity, followed by the ingredient with the next smallest quantity, and up until each has been added.

MELTING POINT ORDER

Heat is sometimes used when compounding to help facilitate mixing. If melting ingredients, melt the ingredient with the highest melting point before adding the ingredient/s with lower melting points (i.e., line up the ingredients from highest to lowest melting temperature and melt in that order). This prevents exposing substances with low melting points to higher temperatures than necessary.

Eutectic Mixtures

A eutectic mixture means that the combination of the ingredients will melt at a lower temperature than either of the individual component's melting temperatures.

Eutectic mixtures can create difficulty during compounding.

- If a pharmacist is not aware that the components form a eutectic mixture, the temperature on the hot plate can be set too high and the mixture can burn.

- If the components are solid powders at room temperature, the mixture of the powders can melt and become sticky, ruining the dry preparation. An adsorbent powder can be used to keep the powder dry.

DOSAGE FORMS

SOLUTIONS, SUSPENSIONS AND EMULSIONS

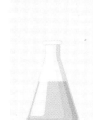

A **SOLUTION** is a solute dissolved in a solvent (such as sodium chloride dissolved in water).

Solutions are homogenous (i.e., consistent, uniform throughout). If the solute concentration is too high, it can lead to unwanted precipitation (see below).

Solutions are usually for oral use. Lotions are topical solutions.

TYPES OF SOLUTIONS:

- Syrups are oral solutions with sucrose, other sugars or artificial sugars.

- Elixirs are sweet hydroalcoholic solutions used for drugs that would be insoluble in a purely aqueous formulation. Hydroalcohol is a mixture of alcohol and water.

- Tinctures are plant or animal extracts dissolved in alcohol or hydroalcohol.

- Spirits are alcohols or hydroalcohols of volatile, aromatic compounds such as camphor. Volatile means the compound vaporizes (evaporates) easily.

A **SUSPENSION** is a solid dispersed in a liquid. It is a two-phase heterogeneous (i.e., not uniform) mixture.

A wetting agent/levigating agent is a type of surfactant used to incorporate an insoluble drug into a liquid, which makes a suspension.

An **EMULSION** is a liquid dispersed in a liquid. It is a two-phase heterogeneous mixture. Emulsions are oil-in-water (oil droplets in an aqueous vehicle) or water-in-oil.*

An emulsifier is a type of surfactant that is used to reduce the surface tension between two liquids and prevent them from separating.

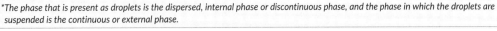

*The phase that is present as droplets is the dispersed, internal phase or discontinuous phase, and the phase in which the droplets are suspended is the continuous or external phase.

PRECIPITATION/SEDIMENTATION is when the dispersed phase settles (clumps) together. The process of a solid settling on the bottom of a container is sedimentation.

This can happen with suspensions and emulsions, and less commonly with solutions. Shake or gently roll to redisperse.

GraphicsRF.com/Shutterstock.com

HOW TO PREPARE SOLUTIONS

Gather ingredients. Reduce the particle size of the solid drug to a fine powder. Dissolve the solute in the solvent. The dissolution rate can be used to determine the time it will take for the solute to dissolve (calculated using Fick's First Law of Diffusion). A larger surface area (i.e., smaller particles), stirring the preparation and using heat will increase the dissolution rate.

Add any required excipients (e.g., a buffer to resist changes in pH, a preservative to protect against bacterial growth, flavorings, sweeteners or coloring agents). Package the solution and apply a BUD and appropriate auxiliary labels.

HOW TO PREPARE SUSPENSIONS

Gather ingredients. Reduce the particle size of the solid drug to a fine powder. Wet the powder, and levigate to form a paste. Continue to add liquid in portions. Add a surfactant to help keep the suspension dispersed. Transfer the mixture into a conical graduate or the container in which it will be dispensed and add a quantity of water sufficient to make (QS) the final volume.

Add any required excipients (e.g., a preservative to protect against bacterial growth, flavorings, sweeteners or coloring agents). Package the suspension and apply a BUD. Will need to be redispersed (i.e., shaken) prior to use.

HOW TO PREPARE EMULSIONS

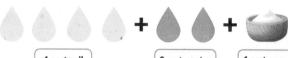

| 4 parts oil | + | 2 parts water | + | 1 part gum (e.g., acacia) |

Emulsions can be made by either the Continental or English gum method, mixing oil, water, and an emulsifier (gum) in a 4:2:1 ratio.

Continental (dry gum) method:
1. Levigate the gum with oil.
2. Add the water all at once.
3. Triturate by shaking in a bottle or mixing in a mortar until a cracking sound is heard and mixture is creamy white.
4. Add other ingredients by dissolving them first in solution and QS with water up to the final volume.
5. Homogenize (with a homogenizer machine).

English (wet gum) method:
1. Triturate the gum with water to form a mucilage (thick and sticky like mucus).
2. Add oil slowly while shaking or mixing.
3. Add other ingredients as in the dry gum method.

Hint: *It rains a lot in England (wet), and the oil is added slowly because you cannot drive too fast in the rain. The continent is dry, and you can add the water quickly (all at once).*

iStock.com/Anna_zabella

TABLETS

There are many types of tablets, including molded tablets, sublingual tablets, buccal tablets, orally disintegrating tablets, chewable tablets, effervescent tablets and compressed tablets. The molded tablet is the most common tablet type made in compounding, and the compressed tablet is the most common type made in manufacturing.

Tablets contain the active drug and excipients, including diluents, binders, disintegrants, lubricants, coloring agents and flavoring agents.

HOW TO PREPARE MOLDED TABLETS

Triturate the dry ingredients and mix by geometric dilution. Add alcohol and/or water to moisten the powder. The powder mixture should have a pasty consistency, which can be molded into tablets (using tablet molds), and allowed to dry. Coloring and a coating may be added.

CAPSULES

Capsules are soluble shells of gelatin (an animal product) or hypromellose (a vegetable product), which are filled with the active drug, diluents and other excipients. Hard-shell capsules are used most commonly in compounding, and are filled with powders. Soft-shell capsules are used mostly for oils. Glycerol and sorbitol are used as plasticizers to make the capsules less brittle and more flexible.

HOW TO PREPARE CAPSULES

Triturate the dry ingredients and geometrically mix with the fillers/other excipients. The powder is put into the capsules by either hand filling (also known as the "punch method") or by using a capsule-filling machine.

Hand filling: the powder is placed on powder paper or an ointment slab. The pile of powder is smoothed with a spatula to a height about a third of the length of the capsule. The open end of the capsule is repeatedly "punched" into the pile of powder until the capsule is filled. When the base is filled, it is fitted with the cap.

Manual capsule-filling machine: these are small devices that help the pharmacist quickly load 50, 100 or 300 capsules. Plates help sort the capsule bodies and hold them upright and in place. The powder is put above the capsules on to a plastic

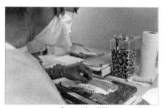

Capsule-filling machine
felipe caparros/Shutterstock.com

sheet where a plastic spreader is used to move the powder into the capsules. A comb or tamper and a spreader are used repeatedly until the powder is packed into the capsules. Then, the caps are put over the capsule bodies.

If filling capsules with liquid instead of powder, the liquids are added to upright capsule bodies with a pipette or dropper.

LOZENGES/TROCHES

Lozenges (or troches) can be hard or soft tablets that slowly dissolve in the mouth, or chewable tablets that are easily chewed and swallowed. Lozenges/troches are generally used to deliver a medication that acts locally in the mouth. A commercially available example is a clotrimazole troche for treatment of oral thrush.

A lozenge contains the active drug in a base of:

- Sucrose or syrup for hard lozenges
- Polyethylene glycol (PEG) for soft lozenges
- Glycerin or gelatin for chewable lozenges

Flavoring agents and coloring agents may be added. The base is melted, mixed with the API and excipients, placed into a mold and allowed to cool back into a solid.

TOPICAL FORMULATIONS

Creams, lotions, ointments, pastes and gels are delivery vehicles (see Emollients section). Lotions contain a lot of water, so they can be delivered in pumps. Creams and ointments are packaged in tubes and tubs.

> **HOW TO PREPARE OINTMENTS**
>
> Powders should be triturated well, using a levigating agent. The levigating agent must be miscible with the base. The powder will be mixed into the ointment base, using geometric dilution.
>
> Certain ointments will require heat in order to mix the components together well. This is called the fusion method. Always use the lowest temperature possible to prevent undesired chemical reactions (see previous section on Melting Point Order). A water bath used to heat the ointment components will help prevent over-heating.

SUPPOSITORIES

A suppository base is either oil-soluble (oleaginous) or water-soluble. Oil-soluble bases include cocoa butter and hydrogenated vegetable oils (palm, palm kernel and coconut oils). Water-soluble bases include PEG polymers and glycerinated gelatin.

- If a drug powder is added to a base, the powder should be triturated to a fine consistency.

- If the preparation softens or melts easily, such as with cocoa butter, the molds will need to be stored in the refrigerator to make the suppository hard and easier to insert.

> **HOW TO PREPARE SUPPOSITORIES**
>
> There are three methods to prepare a suppository:
>
> Hand molding can be used when only a few suppositories are being prepared. When using a cocoa butter base, the cocoa butter is grated and then mixed with the drug/s in a mortar and pestle or on a pill tile with a spatula. The mass is rolled into a cylinder then cut into pieces. A tip is formed on one end to make insertion easier.
>
> In the commonly-used fusion molding method, the base is gently heated, the ingredients are added, the mixture is poured into room temperature molds, and left to harden. If the base is poured into a cold mold, the suppository can crack and split. If the suppository does not harden, the molds can be refrigerated. Often, the suppositories are dispensed in the mold to prevent damage.
>
> In the compression molding method, the pharmacist will need to know the weight of each mold, and the drug's density factor. The amount of base required to fill each mold is calculated, the base is grated, mixed with the drug and put into a cold compression mold.
>
> Lubricants can be applied to the mold so the suppositories can be removed more easily, but it must be opposite of the suppository base in terms of solubility. The goal is to reduce friction. For example: glycerin or propylene glycol (both water-soluble) are good lubricants for molds containing suppositories made with oil-soluble bases, while mineral oil or vegetable oil spray (oil-soluble) are good lubricants for molds containing suppositories made with water-soluble bases.

STABILITY AND DEGRADATION

USP defines stability as the extent to which a product retains, within specified limits, and throughout its period of storage and use (i.e., the shelf-life), the same properties and characteristics it possessed at the time it was made. The stability of compounded products can be easily compromised if they are not prepared or stored properly. This can be recognized by changes in texture, color or odor or development of precipitates. Drug degradation and incompatibility are discussed in more detail in the Basic Science Concepts and Intravenous Medication Principles chapters.

SELECTING THE BEYOND-USE DATE FOR NONSTERILE PREPARATIONS

The beyond-use date (BUD) is the date or time after which the compounded product must not be used. The BUD is based on how susceptible the compounded nonsterile preparation is to microbial contamination and degradation. This is determined by the formulation of the product and the water activity (Aw), which can be thought of as the available water to support microbial growth and hydrolysis. An aqueous preparation (e.g., gel, cream, solution) has an $Aw \geq 0.60$. These have a higher risk of contamination/degradation and are assigned a shorter BUD. Nonaqueous preparations (e.g., tablet, suppository, ointment) have an $Aw < 0.60$, and a lower risk of contamination/degradation, with a longer BUD.

The Study Tip Gal provides the default BUDs for CNSPs that are packaged per USP 795 standards.

BEYOND-USE DATES FOR NONSTERILE COMPOUNDED PRODUCTS

FORMULATION	BEYOND-USE DATE
Aqueous dosage forms (Aw ≥ 0.6)	
Nonpreserved aqueous dosage forms	14 days Store in refrigerator
Preserved aqueous dosage forms	35 days
Nonaqeuous dosage forms (Aw < 0.6)	
Oral liquids	90 days
Other nonaqueous dosage forms	180 days

Beyond-Use Date Examples

PREPARATION	FORMULATION	MAXIMUM BUD
Cream (oil in water emulsion, petrolatum free), with preservative (Aw 0.968)	Preserved aqueous	35 days
Oral suspension (water-based), without preservative (Aw 0.992)	Nonpreserved aqueous	14 days, refrigerated
Ointment (in petrolatum) (Aw 0.396)	Nonaqueous (other)	180 days
Foam, without preservative (Aw 0.983)	Nonpreserved aqueous	14 days, refrigerated
Lip balm (Aw 0.181)	Nonaqueous (other)	180 days
Gelatin-based lozenge (Aw 0.332)	Nonaqueous (other)	180 days
Suppository (in an oleaginous base) (Aw 0.385)	Nonaqueous (other)	180 days
Powder for inhalation (Aw 0.402)	Nonaqueous (other)	180 days
Nasal spray, with preservative (Aw 0.991)	Preserved aqueous	35 days

Beyond-Use Date Exceptions

Individual products may have shorter stability and/or different storage requirements which will override USP-provided defaults. Specific exceptions include:

- If any ingredient expires before the BUD, use the earlier expiration date.
- BUDs can be extended to a maximum of 180 days if stability data is obtained that determines the drug is stable for a longer period.

Unit-Dose Repackaging

A unit-dose refers to a package that contains one dose of a medication. Unit-dose preparations can come from the manufacturer or a repackaging company, or a pharmacy can repackage multi-dose containers into unit-dose packages.

Unit-dose repackaging is not compounding, but shares some commonalities, including the assignment of a BUD. BUDs for repackaged drugs should be the manufacturer's expiration date from the original container or 6 months from the repackaging date, whichever is earlier.

QUALITY ASSURANCE

A quality assurance (QA) plan outlines the steps and actions that ensure proper standards are maintained. It includes the Standard Operating Procedures (SOPs), which are itemized steps on how to perform routine and expected tasks. The QA plan must be reviewed at least every 12 months by the designated person.

The QA program should include periodic testing of the finished compounded preparations. A pharmacy may do some QA testing in-house (e.g., confirming weight and consistency) and outsource others (e.g., sending products out to another company for sterility or stability testing).

QA records need to include the names of the compounding staff, including their job orientation and training records.

EVALUATION AND LABELING

Before a compound is dispensed to a patient, there must be a visual inspection (with documentation) to make sure the CNSP looks as intended.

Every CNSP must be labeled clearly with an internal identification number, the active ingredients (and amounts), the BUD and storage information, the dosage form and the total volume. Certain formulations may need additional auxiliary labels, such as "shake well," "refrigerate" or "for external use only."

DOCUMENTATION

Two very important records that each compounded product must have are the master formulation record and the compounding record. The master formulation record (or master formula) is the recipe that is followed to compound a preparation. The compounding record (or log) is the log book of all products made at the pharmacy (see example images on the following pages).

The compounding record must be detailed enough that another trained person can replicate the steps involved in the preparation, evaluate if the procedure was correct and trace the origin of all components.

PATIENT COUNSELING

Counseling for the patient or caregiver about the proper use of a compounded product should be provided, as is required for any prescription drug. ADRs resulting from a compounded product should be reported to the pharmacy and documented per the facility's standard operating procedures. Depending on the reaction, further action may be necessary (e.g., reporting serious events and suspect drugs to the FDA).

Master Formulation Record #3755
IBUPROFEN 200 mg SUPPOSITORIES

Formula:

Ibuprofen 200 mg Suppositories

Strength:	200 mg	**Quantity:**	10

Equipment:	Balance, mortar and pestle, strainer, hot plate, molds, spatula

Ingredients:	**Quantity:**
Ibuprofen powder USP	0.2 gm
SilicaGel	0.02 gm
Base MBK (Fatty Acid Base)	Calculate

Procedure:

Note: calculations should be made to make an excess amount of 10% of the amount needed.

1. Calculate and weigh ingredients to prepare 10 ibuprofen 200 mg suppositories in the blue mold which is calibrated to 1.28 gm of *Base MBK* per suppository. Use the Suppository, General Formula worksheet.

2. Melt *Base MBK* at 50 degrees C using a hot water bath.

3. Using a mortar and pestle, triturate ibuprofen and *SilicaGel* together to a fine powder.

4. Sift the powder from Step 3 into the melted *Base MBK* while stirring. The use of a strainer helps to ensure small particle size.

5. Turn off heat and stir until mixture looks consistently suspended.

6. Pour into molds (may use a large bore syringe if available) and allow to cool to room temperature.

7. Package in universal sleeve and label.

Recommended Beyond-Use Date:	180 days (per USP-NF)
Recommended Storage/ Auxiliary Labels:	Refrigerate
Quality control and physical description:	White, smooth suppositories

Notes:

MASTER FORMULATION RECORD

Compound's official or assigned name

Strength or activity

Dosage form

Ingredients, with amounts

Calculations, if appropriate

Instructions for preparation (including a description of compounding steps, equipment and supplies)

Recommended BUD (with reference source)

Storage requirements

Physical description of the final product

Container closure system

Labeling requirements

Quality control procedures and expected results

What you SHOULD do

Formula # 3755

Raindrop Compounding Pharmacy
COMPOUNDING RECORD

PRODUCT

Drug Name and Strength	Use/Dosage Form	Quantity	Control/Rx #	Date
Ibuprofen 200 mg	Suppositories	#10	37-865	4-10-24

INGREDIENTS

Ingredient	NDC or Manufacturer #	QTY	LOT	EXP
Ibuprofen powder USP	IB100-25, Spectrum	2 g	A3472-19	3/27
Silica gel	S1935, Spectrum	0.2 g	S1008-19	12/26
MBK base	30-156, PCCA	12.8 g	1234-18	2/26
Disposable supp molds	Apothecary			

COMPOUNDING DETAILS

Calculations:	Ibuprofen 0.2 g x 10 = 2 g, Silica 0.02 g x 10 = 0.2 g, MBK base 1.28 g x 10 = 12.8 g
QC Weight:	1.5 g, smooth uniform surface, even color
Description:	1.5 g white suppositories
Beyond-Use Date:	9/10/24
Storage:	refrigerate

Weighed by: Dacy L

Prepared by: Dacy L

COMPOUNDING RECORD

Compound's official or assigned name

Strength or activity

Dosage form

Date of preparation (and time, if needed)

Internal identification number

Ingredients (including manufacturers/sources, lot numbers and expiration dates) and quantities

Staff involved in compounding

Total quantity compounded

Assigned BUD and storage requirements

Calculations

Physical description of final product

Results of quality control procedures

What you DID

©UWorld

CONTENT LEGEND

 = Study Tip Gal

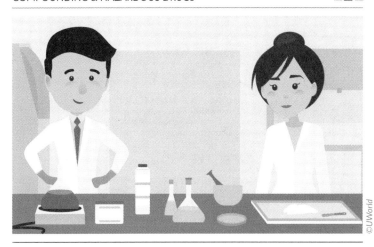

CHAPTER 16
STERILE COMPOUNDING

STERILE COMPOUNDING

Drugs administered into any body site that is not typically exposed to the outside environment (e.g., blood, bladder cavity, lungs) or is highly susceptible to infection (e.g., eyes) must be prepared using sterile techniques. This ensures that the compound will be free of microorganisms (e.g., bacteria, viruses, fungi) and contaminants (e.g., glass shards, precipitates, particles).

Sterile compounding includes combining, admixing, reconstituting, diluting or repackaging/altering a drug or bulk substance in order to create a sterile preparation.

Sterile compounding is used to prepare:

- Injections, including intravenous (IV), intramuscular (IM), subcutaneous (SC, SQ) and intrathecal drugs
- Eye drops
- Irrigations (liquid "washes" that go into a body cavity)
- Pulmonary inhalations (does not include nasal inhalations)
- Baths and soaks for live tissues/organs
- Implants

Minimum acceptable standards for sterile compounding are set by the U.S. Pharmacopeia (USP) in chapter 797. These standards apply to any person who prepares sterile compounds in any setting, for humans or animals. To adequately prepare for the chapter discussion, review the acronyms and terminology used by USP, which are provided in the Study Tip Gal on the following page.

INTERPRETING USP TERMINOLOGY

ACRONYM	MEANING	COMMON TERMS
CSPs	Compounded sterile product	IV or other drugs that require sterile manipulation
SVP	Small volume parenteral	IV bag or container with a volume ≤ 100 mL
LVP	Large volume parenteral	IV bag or container with a volume > 100 mL
PPE	Personal protective equipment	Garb (e.g., gown, gloves, mask); "don" means to put on, "doff" is to take off
PEC	Primary engineering control	Sterile hood that provides ISO 5 air for sterile compounding
LAFW	Laminar airflow workbench	A type of open-front sterile hood (PEC); air flow in one direction (i.e., unidirectional)
SEC	Secondary engineering control	The room containing ISO 7 air where the sterile hood (PEC) is located; also called the buffer room
SCA	Segregated compounding area	Designated space that contains an ISO 5 sterile hood (PEC) but is not part of a cleanroom suite; air in the designated space (i.e., room air) is not ISO-rated
CAI	Compounding aseptic isolator	A type of closed-front ISO 5 sterile hood (PEC) used for nonhazardous drug compounding; sometimes referred to as a "glovebox"
RABS	Restricted access barrier system	Any closed-front ISO 5 sterile hood (includes CAIs); sometimes referred to as a "glovebox"

SPACE REQUIREMENTS

There are greater (and stricter) compounding space requirements for sterile compounding than nonsterile compounding. This chapter focuses on the requirements for nonhazardous sterile compounding; the following chapter (Compounding with Hazardous Drugs) will focus on both nonsterile and sterile hazardous drug compounding.

PHYSICAL SPACE BASICS

Surfaces of ceilings, walls, floors, fixtures, shelving, counters and cabinets must be smooth, impervious, and free from cracks and crevices to make them easy to clean and disinfect. Stainless steel equipment is often used. Objects that shed particles (e.g., cardboard boxes) should not be brought into the sterile compounding space.

AIR QUALITY

ISO Ratings

Clean air in the compounding area reduces the risk of contamination. The International Standards Organization (ISO) sets the standards for air quality, which is determined by the number and size of particles per volume of air (see table below). The lower the particle count, the cleaner the air. Ambient (room) air is not rated; if it were, most room air would be about ISO 9.

In critical areas that are closest to exposed sterile drugs and containers [i.e., inside the sterile hood (PEC)], the air quality must be at least ISO 5. This means that there are no more than 3,520 particles per cubic meter. Particles are included in this count if they are 0.5 microns (micrometers) or larger.

The farther away from the PEC, the dirtier the air. The buffer area (the SEC, which contains PECs) must be at least ISO 7. The anteroom (the room adjacent to the SEC where hand washing and garbing occurs) must be at least ISO 8 if it opens into a positive-pressure buffer area (i.e., used for nonhazardous sterile compounding).

COMPOUNDING AREA	ISO RATING	PARTICLES/M³
Primary engineering control (PEC, called the sterile hood or isolator/"glovebox")	5	3,520
Not applicable (ISO 6 is not used for pharmacy spaces)	6	35,200
Secondary engineering control (SEC, called the buffer room or buffer area)	7	352,000
Anteroom	7 or 8*	3,520,000

*ISO 8 is acceptable if the anteroom opens into a positive-pressure buffer room (i.e., for nonhazardous sterile compounding), but cleaner air (ISO 7) can be used; ISO 7 is required for an anteroom that opens into a negative-pressure buffer room (i.e., hazardous drug compounding).

Air Changes

Air in spaces used for compounding can be contaminated and needs to be regularly replaced. The air changes per hour (ACPH) is the number of times (per hour) that the air is replaced in the room. For a room with ISO 7 air (e.g., the SEC), there must be at least 30 ACPH. For a room with ISO 8 air, there must be at least 20 ACPH.

Air Pressure

In addition to the ISO air quality, the air pressure in a space relative to the adjacent space is important.

The air pressure inside the PEC and SEC are both positive for nonhazardous drug compounding. Positive air pressure helps protect the compounded sterile products (CSPs) from contamination.

TYPES OF STERILE COMPOUNDING AREAS

- Cleanroom suite: one or more sterile hoods (ISO 5 PECs) inside an ISO 7 buffer room (SEC) that is entered through an adjacent anteroom.

- Segregated compounding area (SCA) with an ISO 5 PEC: a sterile hood, often an isolator ("glovebox") with a closed front, located in a segregated space with unclassified air.

PRIMARY ENGINEERING CONTROL

The PEC provides an ISO 5 environment for sterile compounding. In most pharmacies, the way to achieve ISO 5 air is by using a sterile hood. In other industries and larger hospital pharmacies, whole rooms may have ISO 5 air.

High-Efficiency Particulate Air Filters

High-efficiency particulate air (HEPA) filters remove particles when the air runs through the filter. HEPA filters are > 99.97% efficient in removing particles as small as 0.3 microns wide, including bacteria, viruses, fungi and dust.

Inside a PEC, a HEPA filter provides the clean ISO 5 air for compounding. The space in front of the HEPA filter is called the direct compounding area (DCA), and the air coming directly out of the HEPA filter is called the first air (see the Study Tip Gal on the following page). The HEPA filter must be recertified by a specialist every 6 months and anytime a PEC has been moved.

Types of PECs

- A laminar airflow workbench (LAFW) is an open-front PEC where air flows in unidirectional lines from the HEPA filter, typically from the back of the hood, known as horizontal laminar airflow (see image). Positive-pressure laminar airflow keeps the cleaner air in the PEC from mixing with the dirtier air in the buffer room and keeps particles from colliding with each other and landing on the DCA surface or CSPs.

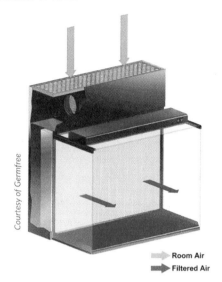

Courtesy of Germfree

⟶ Room Air
⟶ Filtered Air

Horizontal laminar airflow

- A compounding aseptic isolator (CAI) is a closed-front PEC that can be located in a buffer room (SEC), but is often located in a segregated compounding area (SCA). The closed front keeps the unclassified room air around it from mixing with the clean ISO 5 air inside the PEC. It is commonly referred to as a "glovebox" because the pharmacist or technician inserts their hands through the ports on the front into gloves that reside within the PEC.

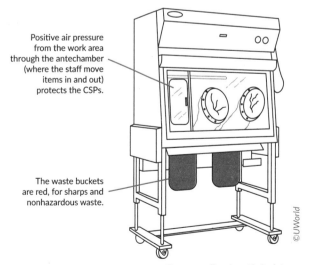

Positive air pressure from the work area through the antechamber (where the staff move items in and out) protects the CSPs.

The waste buckets are red, for sharps and nonhazardous waste.

©UWorld

Compounding Aseptic Isolator

AIR QUALITY INSIDE THE PEC

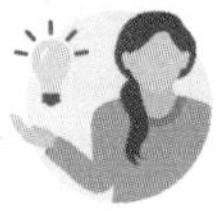

The Direct Compounding Area and First Air

The PEC provides ISO 5 air quality for sterile compounding. The air coming directly out of the HEPA filter is called the first air, which is cleaner than the rest of the air in the sterile hood. To prevent contamination of CSPs during compounding, the injection port of the container and the syringe needle must be kept in the first air (see image).

- Do not obstruct first air, especially the area where the needle enters the vial or ampule.
- Do not block airflow from the HEPA filter with hands or supplies.
- Place items correctly inside the PEC to avoid creating turbulence, which can lead to contamination of the CSPs.

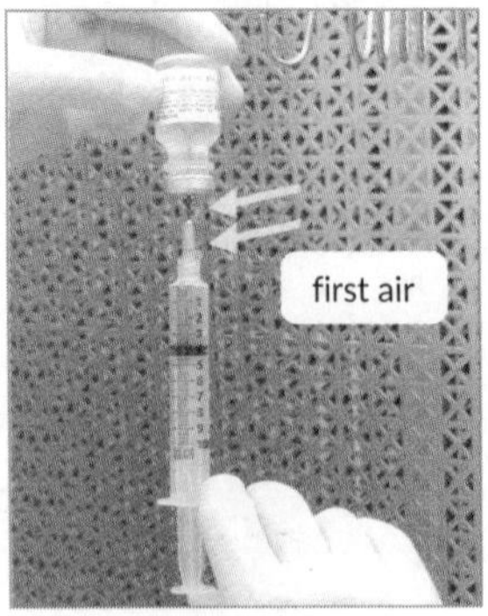

Richard Fincher/Shutterstock.com

Most contamination to CSPs comes from the compounding staff, largely from inadequate hand hygiene and garbing; correct technique is essential, and is described later in this chapter.

SECONDARY ENGINEERING CONTROL

The SEC is the room that contains the PEC or multiple PECs. The SEC is commonly called the buffer area or buffer room because it provides a "buffer" of relatively clean air (ISO 7) around the PEC (ISO 5).

ANTEROOM

The anteroom (sometimes called the ante-area) connects the rest of the pharmacy to the buffer room (SEC). It contains a sink, cabinets and benches to facilitate garbing and preparation for compounding. Running down the center of the anteroom is a large visible line called the line of demarcation, which separates the room into clean and dirty sections. The side closest to the other areas of the pharmacy is considered to be the dirty side of the anteroom. This is where hair and face covers are donned. The side of the anteroom closest to the buffer room is considered to be the clean side. Shoe covers must be applied one at a time while stepping over the demarcation line, placing the covered shoe on the clean side. Handwashing and donning of the gown occur on the clean side of the anteroom.

SEGREGATED COMPOUNDING AREA

An SCA is an option when a cleanroom is not able to be installed. It is a designated area with unclassified air; it does not have a buffer area or anteroom, and can only be used for certain CSPs.

Segregated means kept apart from other areas of the pharmacy (e.g., the corner of the pharmacy) to minimize interruptions, contamination and noise. There must be a visible, defined perimeter around an SCA, and it cannot be located adjacent to food preparation, warehouses, restrooms, or windows/doors that connect to the outdoors or areas of high traffic flow (e.g., not near the pharmacy pick-up area).

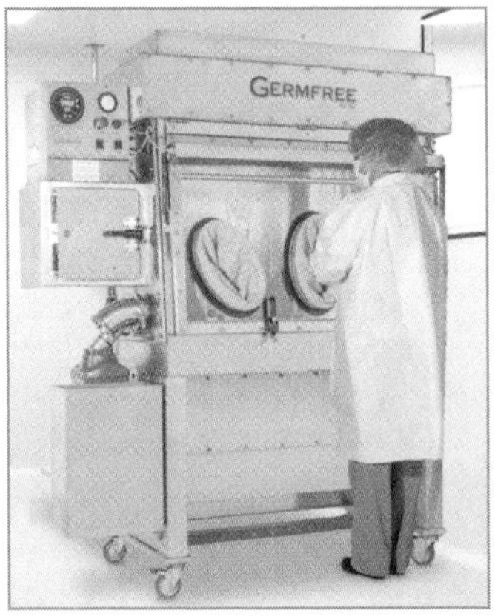

©UWorld

CAI in a Segregated Compounding Area

SCAs are useful for satellite pharmacies that are a distance away from the main pharmacy in a large hospital, for infusion centers, clinics and small hospitals.

STERILE COMPOUNDING CLEANROOM

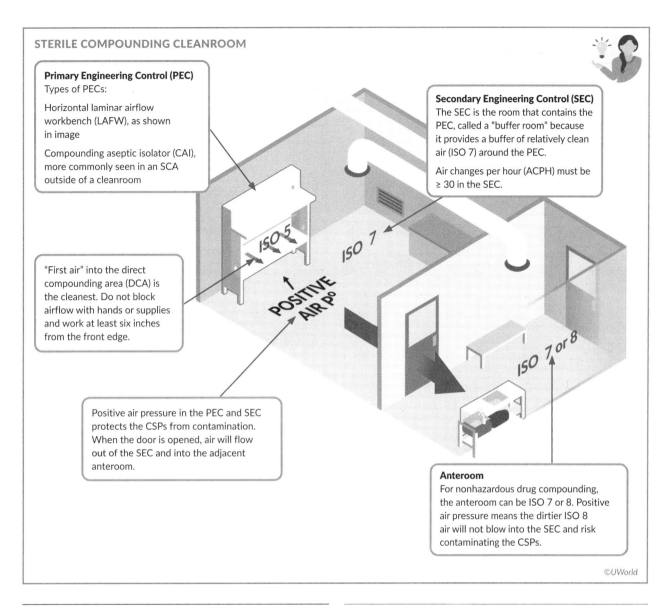

Primary Engineering Control (PEC)
Types of PECs:

Horizontal laminar airflow workbench (LAFW), as shown in image

Compounding aseptic isolator (CAI), more commonly seen in an SCA outside of a cleanroom

Secondary Engineering Control (SEC)
The SEC is the room that contains the PEC, called a "buffer room" because it provides a buffer of relatively clean air (ISO 7) around the PEC.

Air changes per hour (ACPH) must be ≥ 30 in the SEC.

"First air" into the direct compounding area (DCA) is the cleanest. Do not block airflow with hands or supplies and work at least six inches from the front edge.

Positive air pressure in the PEC and SEC protects the CSPs from contamination. When the door is opened, air will flow out of the SEC and into the adjacent anteroom.

Anteroom
For nonhazardous drug compounding, the anteroom can be ISO 7 or 8. Positive air pressure means the dirtier ISO 8 air will not blow into the SEC and risk contaminating the CSPs.

ISO 5

ISO 7

ISO 7 or 8

POSITIVE AIR P°

©UWorld

PERSONNEL TRAINING AND TESTING

Each facility is required to have a designated person who is responsible for training and oversight of compounding personnel (i.e., staff). Any person who compounds or has direct oversight of compounders must have proper training, and all training must be documented, including:

- Initial training, where knowledge and competency of compounding sterile products must be demonstrated before performing any job functions independently.

- Continuous (ongoing) training, which must be completed at least every 12 months.

Other personnel with less direct/frequent contact with compounding space or materials (e.g., technician who restocks the sterile compounding area) must have training outlined in the Standard Operating Procedures (SOP) for the facility.

ASEPTIC PROCEDURES

Staff must demonstrate that they can follow adequate aseptic procedures for each of these items prior to independently compounding sterile products:

- Hand hygiene
- Garbing and gloving technique
- Cleaning and disinfecting procedures for the sterile space and equipment
- Sterile drug preparation

Adequate aseptic technique in hand hygiene, garbing and gloving is demonstrated by passing a garbing competency evaluation, which is completed ≥ 3 times and includes visual observation of procedures and the gloved fingertip test.

Adequate aseptic technique in sterile drug preparation is demonstrated by passing the media-fill test and surface sampling.

Both the gloved fingertip test and the media-fill test must be completed by a compounder initially, then every 6 months (if compounding only category 1 and 2 CSPs) or every 3 months (if compounding category 3 CSPs). CSP compounding categories are discussed later in this chapter.

GLOVED FINGERTIP TEST

To complete the test, the evaluator collects a gloved sample from each hand of the compounder by rolling the pads of the fingers and thumb over a surface which contains microbial growth agar [e.g., tryptic soy agar (TSA)]. If microorganisms are present, they will use the TSA as a food source and replicate.

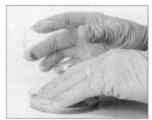

Courtesy of Bio-Med QC, LLC
Gloved Fingertip Test

The plates are incubated (heated, to facilitate growth) and then inspected for microbial growth after ≥ 7 days, which will be visible as spots on the plates. Spots that form are called colony-forming units (CFUs) and indicate contamination was present on the gloves.

Passing a Gloved Fingertip Test
- After garbing: passing requires three consecutive gloved fingertip samples, taken after garbing, with zero CFUs for both hands.
- After media-fill testing: passing requires at least one sample taken from each hand immediately after completion of the media-fill test, with ≤ 3 CFUs total for both hands.

MEDIA-FILL TEST

The media-fill test is used to determine if a compounder is preparing CSPs in an aseptic manner. It is followed by a gloved fingertip test and surface sampling (discussed later).

To complete the test, the compounder must prepare a compound with aseptic technique using a small IV bag or vial. Tryptic soy broth (TSB) takes the place of the drug in the preparation. TSB is a growth medium used by organisms to replicate. Multiple aseptic manipulations (transfers using the same syringe) are completed and then the product is incubated and checked for bacterial growth. Turbidity (cloudiness) means contamination is present.

Passing a Media-Fill Test

If the liquid stays clear after 14 days of incubation, the compounder passed the test.

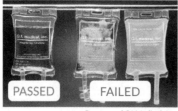

PASSED   FAILED

Courtesy of QI Medical, Inc.
Media Fill Test

ENVIRONMENTAL MONITORING

TEMPERATURE AND HUMIDITY MONITORING

Temperatures and humidity must be kept in the appropriate range; monitoring and documentation on the temperature log sheet must be completed on days when compounding occurs or by using a continuous monitoring device. The SEC (buffer room) should be checked once daily and be maintained at 20°C (68°F), or cooler, with humidity at 60% or less (because excess moisture can lead to bacterial growth).

Temperature in the CSP storage areas (e.g., refrigerator, freezer) should be monitored at least daily. If the temperature is out of range, action must be taken and documented. Temperature monitoring devices must be calibrated at least every 12 months.

AIR AND SURFACE TESTING

In addition to personnel testing with the gloved fingertip test and the media-fill test, there are other tests that are used to ensure that the environment for compounding sterile products is acceptably free of contaminants. This includes:

- Air sampling for contaminants, performed at least every 6 months.
- Surface sampling for contaminants, performed every 30 days for all classified areas and pass-through spaces; areas touched most frequently (e.g., inside the PEC, door handles) should be tested at the end of the compounding shift (dirtiest state), before cleaning and disinfecting.
- Air pressure testing, using a continuous monitoring device, to confirm the correct differential (difference in pressures) between two spaces and ensure that the airflow is unidirectional.

KEEPING THE STERILE COMPOUNDING AREA CLEAN

KEEP THE PEC RUNNING

PECs are preferably kept running at all times to help keep the surfaces clean. If there is a power outage, all compounding must stop, and the PECs will need to be cleaned and disinfected, then sterile 70% isopropyl alcohol (IPA) applied prior to re-initiation of compounding activities. The PEC must be on for at least 30 minutes before compounding can begin.

CLEANING THE PEC

The PEC is cleaned daily and anytime contamination is suspected, and sterile 70% IPA is applied to the work surface throughout the day (every 30 minutes). First, the PEC is cleaned with a detergent, then disinfected (a one-step disinfectant cleaner is also acceptable). Next, 70% IPA is applied. A sporicidal disinfectant is required as well, but less frequently.

Sterile, low-lint wipes are used to clean the PEC. There are wipes that come pre-soaked with the appropriate agent. Alternatively, a spray bottle can be used to wet a dry wipe. Never spray inside the PEC.

PECs are cleaned from top to bottom, back to front (see image). This means that the cleanest areas will be cleaned first, and the dirtiest areas will be cleaned last. Use slightly overlapping, unidirectional strokes rather than circular motions. Use a new side of the wipe for the next area cleaned, and replace used wipes often.

Cleaning a Horizontal Laminar Airflow PEC

This is an example of the order of cleaning for a PEC.

1. Clean the ceiling of the hood, from back to front.

2. Clean the back of the hood (the grill over the HEPA filter), from top to bottom.

3. Clean the IV bar and hooks.

4. Clean the side walls starting from back to front, wiping up and down in a long sweeping motion.

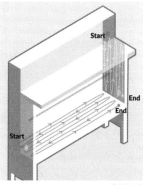

©UWorld

Clean side walls and work surface from back to front in long sweeps.

5. Clean anything kept in the hood [e.g., automated compounding device (used for parenteral nutrition), or other equipment].

6. Clean the bottom surface (the work area) starting from back to front, with a side to side motion.

Do not start compounding until the surfaces have dried.

CLEANING FREQUENCY

Required cleaning frequencies for each site in the cleanroom are shown in the table below. Each site requires cleaning, disinfecting and use of a sporicidal disinfectant.

SITE	CLEANING*	DISINFECTING*	SPORICIDAL DISINFECTANT**
PEC (and equipment inside)	Daily	Daily	Monthly
Pass-through chambers			
Work surfaces outside the PEC			
Floors			
Walls, doors	Monthly	Monthly	
Ceiling			
Storage shelves and bins			
Equipment outside the PEC			

*Daily cleaning and disinfecting are only required on days when compounding occurs.
**For Category 1 and 2 CSPs. Higher frequency needed for Category 3 CSPs.

GARBING FOR STERILE COMPOUNDING

The following pages illustrate how to <u>don garb</u> for <u>sterile compounding</u> in a cleanroom, which should occur in the <u>anteroom</u>. The specific order of garbing should minimize contamination risk (i.e., <u>dirtiest to cleanest</u>), and must be outlined in the facility SOPs. What is shown below is a general approach. Garb required when compounding in a CAI depends on the manufacturer's instructions, but minimally <u>hand hygiene</u> must be performed and <u>sterile, powder-free gloves</u> should be used inside the CAI (placed over the long gloves attached to the isolator).

Minimum garb attire includes <u>head covers</u> (bonnets), facial hair covers, special shoes or <u>shoe covers, gowns</u>, powder-free <u>gloves</u> and <u>face masks</u>. All garb should be low-lint. The staff have to be protected from chemical exposure (some drugs are more toxic than others), and the drug needs to be protected from contamination.

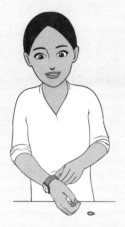 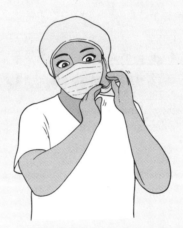 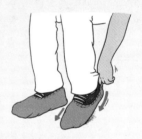

- **Remove** <u>coats, rings, watches,</u> bracelets and <u>makeup</u> before entering the anteroom. <u>Artificial or long nails are not</u> permitted.
- Makeup is not permitted because it sheds.

- Don <u>head and facial hair covers and face masks</u>, then <u>shoe covers while stepping over the line of demarcation</u> that separates the dirty side of the anteroom from the clean side. The anteroom should have a mirror that is used to check that the hair is completely covered. An eye shield is optional.

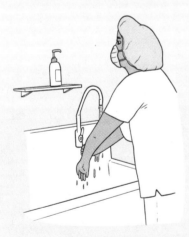 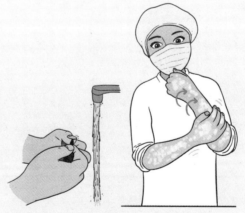 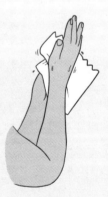

- Perform <u>hand hygiene</u> with <u>soap and warm water</u>. Note: depending on sink placement, this step may come after entering the SEC. In that case, an alcohol-based hand rub should be used before donning garb.

- Under warm water, <u>clean under fingernails</u> to remove debris.
- Working from the <u>fingertips to the elbows</u>, wash for ≥ <u>30 seconds</u>.

- Dry hands and forearms with low-lint disposable towels or wipers.

©UWorld

GARBING FOR STERILE COMPOUNDING continued

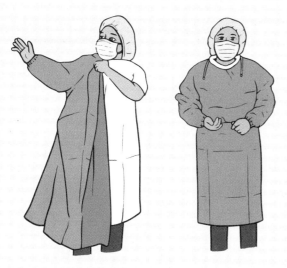

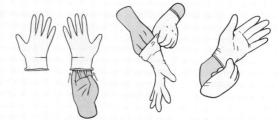

- Enter the buffer area (SEC).

- Apply an alcohol-based surgical hand scrub with persistent antimicrobial activity for the recommended amount of time (per manufacturer) and allow to dry. Chlorhexidine is used frequently, but serious allergic reactions can occur. Another option is povidone-iodine (Betadine), which can be used if there has been an allergic reaction to chlorhexidine.

- Don sterile, powder-free gloves.

- Sanitize the gloves with sterile 70% IPA routinely during compounding and whenever the gloves touch nonsterile surfaces. Do not resume compounding until the alcohol has dried. Continually inspect gloves for tears.

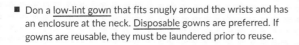

- Don a low-lint gown that fits snugly around the wrists and has an enclosure at the neck. Disposable gowns are preferred. If gowns are reusable, they must be laundered prior to reuse.

- All garb must be used when compounding with an isolator ("glovebox") unless the isolator's manufacturer provides written documentation that garb is not required.

- When the compounding is completed and the compounding personnel leaves the cleanroom/compounding area, all garb except for the gown goes into the disposal container. If the gown is not visibly soiled, it can be taken off and kept on the clean side of the anteroom in order to be re-worn for the current work shift. The gown cannot leave the anteroom if it is going to be re-worn. Hand hygiene is repeated, and all other garb is replaced when re-entering the compounding area.

©UWorld

WHEN TO RE-GARB

- Garb should not be worn outside of the anteroom; if the anteroom has been exited, complete regarbing is required, including hand hygiene.

- If working in an SCA and it is left for any reason, regarbing is required.

EQUIPMENT

COMMON PRODUCTS USED IN STERILE COMPOUNDING

SYRINGES AND NEEDLES

Syringes: <u>hypodermic</u> (parenteral) syringes are commonly used for sterile compounding to <u>transfer</u> drugs and additives from and into sterile containers (e.g., vials, IV bags). Syringes come with cannulas (needles) attached, or the cannula is separate and can be screwed onto the tip of the syringe. Hypodermic syringes are available in many sizes (e.g., 1 mL, 3 mL, 5 mL, 10 mL).

For drawing up medication, use the <u>smallest syringe</u> that can hold the <u>desired amount</u> of solution (for accuracy), but <u>do not</u> use a syringe the <u>exact size</u> of the amount needed (i.e., do not completely fill a syringe because the plunger can easily become dislodged). Select the closest syringe size above the size needed. Do not add two different syringe sizes for a dose.

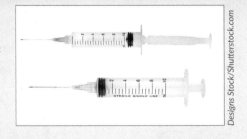

Designs Stock/Shutterstock.com

Needles: <u>recapping</u> needles can lead to <u>needle-stick injuries</u>. In sterile compounding, a needle-stick can <u>injure</u> the staff and cause <u>contamination</u> to the CSPs.

In general, <u>do not recap</u> needles. If the needle must be recapped, it is safer to place the cap on the work surface (rather than holding it) and slip the tip of the needle into the cap, without letting the needle tip touch the work surface.

It is preferable to <u>use syringes with safety features</u>, such as safety shields that cover the needle immediately after use.

Luer Locks: luer locks make <u>secure, leak-free connections</u> between syringes, needles, catheters and IV lines. The ends twist together to form a tight seal (see image). A luer lock can be used during compounding to facilitate mixing or transferring fluids between drug delivery devices or IV sets. A luer lock tip of a syringe is also designed to screw into the luer lock connector on a patient's IV access catheter or onto a needle for patient safety during drug administration.

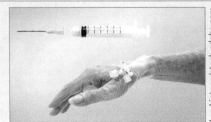

Leo Lintang/stock.adobe.com
PK289/Shutterstock.com

AMPULES AND VIALS

Ampules: ampules are small, sealed glass containers that contain liquid medication. The ampule has a long neck and is broken by snapping the neck at the narrowest part (where the glass is weakest). This can introduce glass particles into the drug solution. A <u>filter needle</u> or <u>filter straw</u> is required when withdrawing liquid from the ampule to remove the glass.

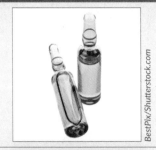

BestPix/Shutterstock.com

Vials that contain liquids: a volume of drug from the vial is drawn up in a syringe, which can then be added to an IV bag.

The compounder will <u>inject a volume of air equal</u> to the <u>volume</u> of drug that is <u>withdrawn</u> to equalize the pressure.

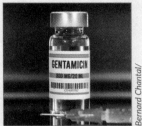

Bernard Chantal/Shutterstock.com

Vials that contain lyophilized or freeze-dried powder: the powder needs to be <u>reconstituted</u> by adding <u>sterile water</u> for injection, bacteriostatic water for injection or a diluent supplied by the manufacturer. Drugs may be commercially available as powders because they are unstable as a solution. The image to the right shows a vial of lyophilized powder before and after reconstitution.

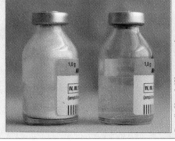

Patrik Slezak/Shutterstock.com

IV BAGS

Small volume parenteral (SVP): IV bags or syringes that contain a small volume (100 mL or less) of fluid. SVPs can contain plain fluid, such as NS or D5W, that can be used as a diluent for a compounded product (i.e., drug is added to the SVP). SVPs can also contain a liquid drug with or without a diluent. SVPs can be compounded in the pharmacy or come in ready-to-use containers from the manufacturer (see section below).

SVPs are often "piggybacked" onto a large volume parenteral (LVP). These are called IV piggybacks (IVPBs). This reduces the need to have multiple lines running into the patient. The drugs will mix together in the tubing so they must be compatible in the IV line.

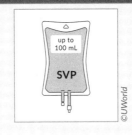

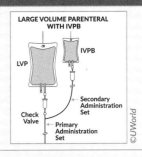

Large volume parenteral (LVP): IV containers that contain more than 100 mL. Liter bags are commonly used to provide fluids, and are available in a variety of formulations: NS, ½NS, D5W, D5½NS, D5NS, Lactated Ringer's (LR) and others used less commonly, including D10NS, D2.5½NS, D5⅓NS, D5¼NS. Parenteral nutrition (PN) for adults is prepared as an LVP.

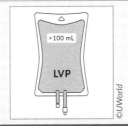

READY-TO-USE STERILE MEDICATIONS

Ready-to-use medications (RTUs): available as prepared IV bags or prefilled syringes. The pharmacy staff opens the outer container and applies the patient label. These are not compounded. The expiration date is provided by the manufacturer, and is on the packaging.

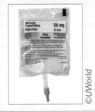

Ready-to-use vial/bag systems (_ADD-Vantage_, _Minibag Plus_, others): vials and bags are supplied together. The vial can be attached to the bags at the bedside by the nurse for immediate use (and is not considered compounding). If the vial is attached in the pharmacy cleanroom (in an ISO 5 hood inside an ISO 7 buffer room), it can be saved for an extended period of time as indicated by the manufacturer on the packaging. This is considered compounding and is subject to USP 797 requirements. Each of the proprietary bag and vial systems are different in design, but all involve an activation step of releasing IV fluid into the drug vial and then returning the reconstituted drug back into the bag.

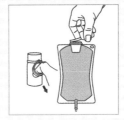
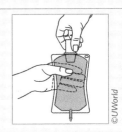

TECHNOLOGY IN STERILE COMPOUNDING

The role of technology in sterile compounding is increasing, with more products available and more organizations supporting the role of technology solutions to improve patient safety. Commonly used automated equipment includes:

- Automated compounding devices (ACDs) that aseptically transfer ingredients into a sterile final container, such as when compounding parenteral nutrition (see image). This replaces the need for manual transfer of ingredients and reduces user error and contamination risk. ACDs should be interfaced with the electronic health record to prevent transcription errors. Other benefits include clinical decision support warnings when a solution has a risk of error (e.g., osmolarity exceeds the maximum limit, solution contents are incompatible).

- IV workflow management systems (IVWMS), also called IV room assisted workflow technology, that automate the preparation, verification, tracking and documentation of

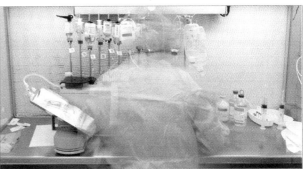

HERRNDORFF_ images/stock.adobe.com

CSPs. IVWMS include technology to identify medications for compounding through barcode scanning, as well as photo capture or measurement of specific gravity or density for CSP verification.

- IV robots used to compound solutions with a high volume of use and/or products that require large batch preparations.

WORKFLOW FOR CSP PREPARATION

- Review the order (must be performed by a pharmacist).
- Gather and inspect all materials.
- Clean hood. Place only needed items in the hood.
- Prepare CSPs with aseptic technique.
- Properly dispose of syringes and needles into the sharps container (see the Medication Safety & Quality Improvement chapter).
- Visually inspect all finished CSPs.
- Complete terminal sterilization and/or sterility testing, if appropriate.

SETTING UP ITEMS IN THE STERILE HOOD

Only required items should be placed in the hood. No paper, pens, labels, calculators or trays.

- All components (e.g., outer wrapping for a sterile syringe or IV bag) should be wiped off with 70% IPA to remove contaminants and dust prior to being brought into the PEC.
- All work within the PEC must be performed at least six inches from the front, where there is less chance that ISO 5 air has mingled with ISO 7 air in the buffer room.
- Place all items in the sterile hood side-by-side. Items should not be within six inches of the back of the hood.
- Nothing should be between the sterile objects and the HEPA filter in a horizontal airflow hood or above the sterile objects in a vertical airflow hood.
- Sterile syringes and other equipment are individually wrapped, and must be opened along the seal (not torn open) inside the PEC to avoid shedding (i.e., release of particles) in the sterile space. Do not touch sterile components (e.g., syringe tip or plunger), even with gloved hands.
- Move waste out of the PEC shortly after it is created; do not let it accumulate inside the sterile hood.

TRANSFERRING SOLUTIONS

- Swab the rubber top of the vial (or ampule neck) and port on the IV bag with 70% IPA, and wait for it to air-dry; do not blow on or wave over it to dry it faster.
- Drug powders are reconstituted into a liquid by introducing a diluent such as sterile water for injection, bacteriostatic water for injection (which is sterile) or a diluent provided by the manufacturer. In some cases, saline or dextrose are used for dilution.
- Prior to withdrawing any liquid from a vial (i.e., containing diluent or drug), inject a volume of air equal to the volume of fluid to be removed.

- Puncture the rubber top of the vial with the needle, bevel up and at a 45-degree angle. Then bring the syringe straight up to a 90-degree angle while the needle penetrates the stopper; press the syringe down so that the needle is inserted into the vial. Depress the plunger of the syringe, emptying the air into the vial. Invert the vial with the attached syringe. Draw up the amount of liquid required. Withdraw the needle from the vial. In the case of a multi-dose vial, the rubber cap will close, sealing the contents of the vial.
- The volume of solution drawn into a syringe is measured at the point of contact between the rubber piston and the side of the syringe barrel.
- Coring occurs when a small piece of rubber from the stopper is aspirated into the needle, and is put into the solution in the vial. The rubber piece can get injected into a patient. Look for small cored pieces floating near the top of the solution during the visual inspection of the CSP.
- If the medication is in a glass ampule, open the ampule by snapping the neck away from you. Tilt the ampule, then withdraw the fluid using a filter straw or filter needle to remove any glass particles that may have fallen into the ampule. The needle must be changed before injecting the syringe contents into an IV bag to avoid introducing glass or particles into the bag. A standard needle could be used to withdraw the drug from the ampule, as long as it is then replaced with a filter device before the drug is pushed out of the syringe.

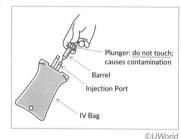

Plunger: do not touch; causes contamination
Barrel
Injection Port
IV Bag

©UWorld

- Inject solutions from the syringe into the IV bag via the injection port.

VISUAL INSPECTION

- The supervising pharmacist should verify that the correct volume of product is in the syringe before compounding continues. This is the safest method because the pharmacist can see the actual volume in the syringe. The "syringe pull-back method" is when the pharmacist verifies the volume in an empty syringe after the compounding is completed; the technician "pulls-back" the plunger of the syringe to the volume of product that was added into the IV admixture and places the empty syringe next to the vial. This method relies on memory and is not recommended.
- Finished CSPs are visually inspected immediately after preparation, against a dark background, for particulates, cored pieces, precipitates and cloudiness. The container should be lightly squeezed to check for leakage.

STERILITY TESTING

Sterility is the absence of viable microorganisms. After a sterile compound has been made, sterility testing can be performed to ensure the absence of contamination. Testing for sterility is required for certain categories of CSPs (see Establishing Beyond-Use Dates section).

STERILIZATION

Terminal sterilization is required for CSPs that are compounded with any nonsterile ingredients. Terminal sterilization methods include steam sterilization (with an autoclave), dry-heat sterilization (depyrogenation) and filtration.

Do not use heat on heat-sensitive drugs (e.g., proteins, including hormones and insulin). CSPs that are heat-labile can be sterilized with filtration using a sterile 0.22-micron filter. The filter will remove microorganisms larger than 0.22 microns, including bacteria, viruses, yeast and fungi.

If filtering is used, the manufacturer of the filter might require a test for filter integrity, such as the bubble-point test. This test determines the pressure required to see "bubbles" out of a filter.

PYROGEN (BACTERIAL ENDOTOXIN) TESTING

Endotoxins, a type of pyrogen, are produced by both gram-positive and gram-negative bacteria and fungi. Endotoxins from gram-negative bacteria are more potent and represent a serious threat to patient safety. Pyrogens can come from using equipment (such as glassware and utensils) washed with tap water. To avoid this issue, glassware and utensils should be rinsed with sterile water and depyrogenated using dry-heat (steam) sterilization with an autoclave.

Any CSPs made from nonsterile components must be tested for endotoxins.

ESTABLISHING BEYOND-USE DATES

USP categorizes CSPs by the risk of contamination, which is based on the conditions they are made in, aseptic processing, ingredients and equipment used, whether sterility testing is performed and the storage conditions. A sterile product that is contaminated with microorganisms or any other type of contaminant can cause severe illness and death.

The risk levels are category 1, 2 and 3, with category 1 having a higher risk of contamination than category 3. These risk levels are then used to determine an appropriate beyond-use date (BUD), which is the date or time after which the CSP should not be used.

CATEGORY 1 STERILE COMPOUNDING

Category 1 CSPs are those prepared in an ISO 5 PEC that is placed in a segregated compounding area (SCA), which has unclassified air. Because these have a higher risk for contamination, they require shorter BUDs compared to Category 2 or 3 CSPs, and no sterility testing is required. The BUD for a CSP made in an SCA is ≤ 12 hours at controlled room temperature, or ≤ 24 hours if refrigerated.

CATEGORY 2 STERILE COMPOUNDING

Category 2 CSPs are made in a cleanroom suite (i.e., an ISO 5 PEC located in an ISO 7 SEC). They can have longer BUDs compared to Category 1 CSPs. Sterility testing may be required based on the BUD assignment (i.e., a longer BUD can be assigned if sterility testing was performed).

CATEGORY 3 STERILE COMPOUNDING

Category 3 CSPs must be made in accordance with specific requirements, which allows them to be assigned longer BUDs, up to a maximum of 180 days. Some of these requirements include sterility testing, endotoxin testing (when applicable), frequent environmental monitoring and personnel qualifications.

STERILE COMPOUNDING FOR EMERGENCIES

The requirements described in this chapter for compounding sterile products, including putting on protective garb and cleaning the PEC, take time.

In certain circumstances, IV drugs are needed immediately, with no time for aseptic preparation, such as in an ambulance or during a code blue when quick action is needed to save a life. This is emergency use (also called immediate-use), and because the drug has been prepared for that patient under suboptimal conditions for sterility, the CSP will have a very short BUD of 4 hours, after which the drug can no longer be used and must be discarded.

DETERMINING THE BEYOND-USE DATE BASED ON CSP CATEGORY

The <u>BUD</u> is determined by the <u>CSP category</u> and the <u>stability/expiration date of the individual ingredients</u>, whichever is shorter.

Each category of CSP has a <u>maximum BUD limit</u> (see Study Tip Gal), but the specific BUD will vary based on preparation conditions (e.g., aseptic preparation versus terminal sterilization), storage conditions, sterility testing and other criteria. A CSP stored in a colder temperature (e.g., refrigerator, freezer) or that underwent sterility testing will generally have a longer BUD.

BEYOND-USE DATES FOR COMPOUNDED STERILE PRODUCTS

CSP CATEGORY	ENVIRONMENT	ROOM TEMP BUD LIMIT*	REFRIGERATED BUD LIMIT*	FROZEN BUD LIMIT*
Immediate-use	Uncontrolled (no PEC)	4 hours (for any storage condition)		
Category 1	ISO 5 PEC in SCA	12 hours	24 hours	N/A
Category 2	ISO 5 PEC in cleanroom	1-45 days	4-60 days	45-90 days
Category 3	ISO 5 PEC in cleanroom with additional requirements	60-90 days	90-120 days	120-180 days

*Temperatures should be kept as follows: controlled room temperature 20 to 25°C, refrigerator 2 to 8°C, freezer -25 to -10°C.

BUDs for Single-Dose Containers (SDC) and Multi-Dose Containers (MDC)

The BUDs in the table below are for the vials, bags, bottles, syringes and ampules that contain the ingredients that are being put into CSPs. For example, a single-dose 1 gram vial of vancomycin, once opened, can be used for up to 12 hours if the vial was opened in and remains in the PEC, which has ISO 5 air.

DOSE	BUD
SDC – vial, bag, bottle, syringe, inside an ISO 5 environment	Up to 12 hours from puncture or opening
SDC – ampule, inside or outside an ISO 5 environment	Any unused contents left in the ampule cannot be stored and must be discarded
MDC - inside or outside an ISO 5 environment	Up to 28 days from puncture or opening

DOCUMENTATION

INTERNAL RECORDS

Sterile compounding records can include the master formulation record and the compounding record, similar to nonsterile compounding (see the Nonsterile Compounding chapter). However, these are only required in certain situations and the requirements are different.

- The <u>master formulation record</u> is needed for CSPs prepared for <u>more than one patient</u> or from <u>nonsterile ingredients</u>.

- The <u>compounding record</u> is needed for <u>Category 1, 2 and 3 CSPs</u>, as well as for any <u>immediate-use CSPs</u> prepared for <u>more than one patient</u>. The prescription or medication order can serve as the compounding record. If a CSP is prepared for more than one patient or from nonsterile ingredients, the vendor, lot number and expiration date for each component must be recorded in the compounding record.

LABEL REQUIREMENTS

CSP labels (i.e., the information on the immediate container) must have the <u>names</u> and <u>amounts or concentrations of ingredients</u>, the total volume, the <u>BUD</u>, the dosage form, the <u>route of administration</u>, the <u>storage</u> requirements, an internal identification number (e.g., order number, barcode) and other information for safe use.

<u>Auxiliary labels</u> should be placed on CSPs that require <u>special handling</u> (e.g., if a filter or light protection is required, if the CSP should not be refrigerated).

<u>High-alert medications</u> (defined by ISMP) are drugs that have a high risk of causing significant patient harm when used incorrectly. Appropriate <u>warning labels</u> such as "Contains Potassium" or "Warning: Paralyzing Agent" should be used.

CSP QUALITY ASSURANCE

Each compounding facility must have established quality assurance (QA) and quality control (QC) programs documented in their SOPs. QA ensures that the compounding process is consistent in meeting quality standards, whereas QC includes the sampling, testing and documentation of results that ensures each CSP has met quality standards. The QA and QC plans should minimally include:

- Adherence to procedures
- Error prevention and detection
- Evaluation of complaints
- Investigations and corrective actions

If a problem has been identified or a medication error or safety issue has occurred, a root cause analysis should be initiated as soon as possible (discussed in the Medication Safety & Quality Improvement chapter). A failure mode and effects analysis of new techniques can help to identify problems with new procedures in advance.

RECALLS

When CSPs are dispensed before receiving the results of their sterility tests, there must be a written procedure in place to take appropriate action if the finalized testing shows that the CSP did not meet specifications. These actions include immediate notification of the prescriber, recall of any dispensed CSPs, quarantine of remaining stock and investigation of other lots that could be affected.

If the CPS fails sterility testing, there should be an investigation of aseptic technique, environmental control and other sterility assurance measures to determine the source of contamination and improve the methods or processes.

PHYSIOCHEMICAL CONSIDERATIONS

Human blood and body tissues have an osmotic pressure (number of particles in solution) equivalent to 0.9% sodium chloride (which is considered isotonic) and a pH of 7.35 – 7.45. The body has natural buffer systems in place to help maintain this pH (see the Intravenous Medication Principles chapter for details).

Most CSPs, including IV solutions and ophthalmic products, should be isotonic to human blood, contain a similar number of particles in solution and have a pH that is close to neutral (pH of 7). Isotonicity is discussed further in the Calculations II chapter.

Compounded preparations that require a narrow pH range will need a buffer system that can resist changes in pH. Buffer systems, similar to the buffer systems in the body, consist of an acid and its salt. For example, acetic acid is used with sodium acetate, its salt, in a common buffer system:

- Acetic acid serves as the proton donor to decrease the pH.
- Sodium acetate serves as the proton acceptor, to increase the pH.

In the Calculations IV chapter, the Henderson-Hasselbalch equation is used to calculate the pH of a solution when the molar (M) concentrations of the buffer components are provided. A variation of the Henderson-Hasselbalch can be used to determine the amount of buffer required.

Select Guidelines/References

United States Pharmacopeia (2022). General Chapter 797. Pharmaceutical Compounding—Sterile Preparations. USP-NF. Rockville, MD: United States Pharmacopeia. DOI: https://doi.org/10.31003/USPNF_M99925_06_01

Institute for Safe Medication Practices (ISMP). ISMP Guidelines for Sterile Compounding and the Safe Use of Sterile Compounding Technology. ISMP; 2022.

CHAPTER CONTENT

CONTENT LEGEND

 = Study Tip Gal   = Key Drug Guy

©UWorld

CHAPTER 17

COMPOUNDING WITH HAZARDOUS DRUGS

HAZARDOUS DRUGS

Hazardous drugs (HDs) can cause toxicity to the healthcare workers who handle them in any manner, including when unloading drugs in the receiving dock, stocking shelves, preparing drugs in the pharmacy, administering drugs to a patient and obtaining and cleaning up body fluids that contain HD residues.

HDs require workspaces, equipment, devices and procedures that are designed to reduce exposure (e.g., dermal absorption, mucosal absorption, inhalation) of the drug to the staff. The standards for handling HDs are set by the U.S. Pharmacopeia (USP) in chapter 800. These are in addition to the requirements for nonsterile compounding (outlined in USP chapter 795) or sterile compounding (outlined in USP chapter 797). The Nonsterile Compounding and Sterile Compounding chapters in this course book should be reviewed prior to this chapter.

THE NATIONAL INSTITUTE FOR OCCUPATIONAL SAFETY AND HEALTH (NIOSH)

The National Institute for Occupational Safety and Health (NIOSH) determines which drugs are hazardous. NIOSH keeps a list of all HDs called the *NIOSH List of Antineoplastic and Other Hazardous Drugs in Healthcare Settings* (see Key Drugs Guy on the following page). A drug is considered hazardous if it is:

- Carcinogenic (cancer-causing)

- Teratogenic (causes congenital abnormalities) or associated with other developmental toxicity

- Toxic to reproduction (e.g., causes infertility)

- Genotoxic (damages DNA, which can cause cancer)

- Toxic to organs at low doses

- Similar in structure or toxicity profile to a drug previously determined to be hazardous

---

SELECT HAZARDOUS KEY DRUGS ON THE NIOSH LIST

Antineoplastic Drugs (Chemotherapeutics)

Non-Antineoplastic Hazardous Drugs:

5 Alpha-Reductase Inhibitors (for BPH)
Dutasteride, finasteride

Abortifacients
Mifepristone, misoprostol

Anticoagulants
Warfarin

Antivirals
Cidofovir, ganciclovir, valganciclovir

Antiseizure Medications
Carbamazepine, oxcarbazepine, fosphenytoin, phenytoin, topiramate, valproate

Benzodiazepines
Clonazepam, temazepam

Dyslipidemia Medications
Lomitapide

Heart Failure Medications
Spironolactone

Hepatitis Medications
Ribavirin

PAH Medications
Ambrisentan, bosentan, macitentan, riociguat

Retinoic Acid Derivatives
Tretinoin

SSRIs
Paroxetine

Thionamides (for Hyperthyroidism)
Methimazole, propylthiouracil

Transplant Medications
Cyclosporine, mycophenolate, tacrolimus, sirolimus

Treatment for Autoimmune Conditions
Acitretin, azathioprine, fingolimod, leflunomide, teriflunomide

Hormonal Agents
Androgens (e.g., testosterone)

Estrogens (e.g., estradiol)

Oxytocin

Progestins (e.g., medroxyprogesterone)

SERD/SERMs (e.g., fulvestrant, raloxifene, tamoxifen)

Uliprristal

SAFETY DATA SHEETS (SDS)

Safety Data Sheets (SDS, previously called MSDS) are a series of safety documents required by the Occupational Safety and Health Administration (OSHA) to be accessible to all employees who are working with hazardous materials, including drugs. Each HD has its own document that provides guidance on drug-specific safety information, including:

- Personal protective equipment (PPE)
- First aid procedures
- Spill clean-up procedures

HAZARD COMMUNICATION PROGRAM

Each facility must have a designated person who is responsible for creating Standard Operating Procedures (SOPs) focused on worker safety during all aspects of HD handling. This hazard communication program includes a written plan that details implementation of HD safety procedures, proper training of personnel, competency assessment and maintaining all required HD documentation. Pharmacies must maintain a list of all HDs stocked, and the list must be reviewed every 12 months or whenever a new drug or dosage form is stocked or used. Prior to handling any HDs, both men and women with reproductive capability must confirm in writing that they understand the risks associated with handling HDs.

ASSESSING RISK

The USP 800 requirements for safe handling of HDs are extensive, but some activities and drugs are not as risky as others. Some examples of lower-risk activities include counting and packaging tablets. A pharmacy can conduct an Assessment of Risk (AoR) to avoid having to follow all USP 800 requirements for drugs that will be dispensed without manipulation.

As part of the AoR, SOPs must be developed, which include actions to limit staff exposure, such as:

- Putting HDs in distinctive shelf bins to alert staff
- Wearing chemotherapy gloves when handling HDs
- Dedicating a counting tray and spatula for counting HDs and decontaminating both after use
- Placing prepared HD containers into a sealable plastic bag

If any manipulation of the low-risk HD is required (e.g., using powder to prepare a solution, cutting tablets in half, adding a vial of HD to a large volume fluid), USP 800 requirements must be followed. If no AoR is conducted, the pharmacy must follow the full USP 800 requirements. AoR documents must be reviewed at least every 12 months.

SPACE REQUIREMENTS FOR HAZARDOUS DRUG COMPOUNDING

PHYSICAL SPACE BASICS

Hoods and buffer rooms used for compounding HDs include the word containment:

- Containment-primary engineering control (C-PEC)
- Containment-secondary engineering control (C-SEC)
- Containment-segregated compounding area (C-SCA)
- Compounding aseptic containment isolator (CACI)

<u>Containment</u> is required to keep hazardous drugs, particles and vapors <u>contained within the space</u> due to toxicity risk. All spaces should have <u>negative air pressure</u> to protect the worker from being exposed to the HDs they are working with (see section on air handling).

C-PECs for Hazardous Drug Compounding

Both <u>sterile and nonsterile hazardous</u> compounds must be prepared in an ISO 5 <u>C-PEC</u> that is located in a <u>C-SEC or C-SCA</u>. Types of C-PECs are listed below.

- <u>Biological safety cabinets (BSCs)</u> have unidirectional air flow (e.g., <u>vertical laminar airflow</u>, where air flows downwards from the HEPA filter at the top of the hood). For <u>sterile</u> HD compounding, the BSC must be <u>Class II</u> (most common) or Class III.

- <u>Containment ventilated enclosures (CVEs)</u> are powder containment hoods with HEPA-filtered air and negative air pressure used for <u>nonsterile</u> compounding only.

- <u>Compounding aseptic containment isolators (CACIs)</u> are closed-front C-PECs (commonly called "gloveboxes") that can be located in a buffer room (C-SEC), but are often located in a C-SCA (see image).

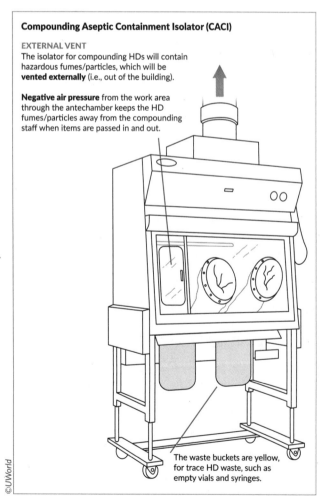

Compounding Aseptic Containment Isolator (CACI)

EXTERNAL VENT
The isolator for compounding HDs will contain hazardous fumes/particles, which will be **vented externally** (i.e., out of the building).

Negative air pressure from the work area through the antechamber keeps the HD fumes/particles away from the compounding staff when items are passed in and out.

The waste buckets are yellow, for trace HD waste, such as empty vials and syringes.

Compounding Aseptic Containment Isolator

Nonsterile and Sterile HD Compounding in the Same Space

While it is preferable to keep <u>nonsterile</u> and <u>sterile</u> compounding space <u>separate</u>, an <u>exception</u> can be made if these requirements are met:

- The <u>C-SEC maintains ISO 7</u> air even when it is being used for nonsterile HD compounding.

- If there are <u>separate sterile and nonsterile C-PECs</u> in the same C-SEC, they must be kept at least <u>1 meter apart</u>.

- Particle-generating activity, such as working with powders, cannot be performed when any sterile compounding is being performed in the same C-SEC.

- Occasional nonsterile HD compounding can be completed in a sterile C-PEC, but it must be properly decontaminated, cleaned and disinfected before compounding sterile HDs.

AIR HANDLING

Negative Air Pressure

C-PECs, C-SECs and <u>C-SCAs</u> must have <u>negative air pressure</u>. This means that the air pressure inside the space is lower than the air pressure outside the space. The negative pressure will cause the air inside the space (which is potentially contaminated) to not flow outwards into the non-contaminated areas.

- Negative air pressure in the C-PEC causes the air flowing in (e.g., from the HEPA filter at the top of the hood) to flow away from the person who is standing at the front of the hood, and then to flow out of the C-PEC through the external exhaust at the top of the hood.

- Negative air pressure in the C-SEC keeps air from flowing into the anteroom (where hand washing and garbing occurs). It is removed through the room exhaust.

- The anteroom will have positive air pressure. For HD compounding, the negative pressure in the C-SEC will pull air from the anteroom into the C-SEC, so the air in the <u>anteroom</u> must be maintained at <u>ISO 7</u> (same as the C-SEC) to prevent dirtier air from co-mingling (and potentially contaminating the sterile products).

Air Changes

Air in spaces used for HD compounding can become contaminated and needs to be replaced regularly. The <u>air changes per hour (ACPH)</u> is the <u>number of times</u> (per hour) that the <u>air is replaced</u> in the room.

- In a space where <u>nonsterile HDs</u> are compounded there must be at least <u>12 ACPH</u>.

- In a <u>sterile C-SEC</u> there must be at least <u>30 ACPH</u> (same as for any sterile compounding).

- In a <u>C-SCA</u> there must be at least <u>12 ACPH</u>.

External Exhaust

Air that has been contaminated with HDs must be externally exhausted. This means that the air is moved out of the space (from the C-PEC, the C-SEC or the C-SCA) and cannot be recirculated and returned to the room. It is sent outside of the building and takes any contamination out with it.

Redundant HEPA Filters Instead of External Exhaust

Community pharmacies that prepare HDs can be located in areas that would not welcome contaminated air (e.g., a busy park, a residential neighborhood).

An alternative option to an external exhaust (for nonsterile HD compounding only) is to use redundant HEPA filters, where air is passed through two or more HEPA filters in a series before returning to the compounding space.

HAZARDOUS DRUG STORAGE

HDs must be stored separately from non-HDs. They should be stored in a room with external ventilation and negative-pressure, with at least 12 ACPH. Select HDs may be stored with non-HDs (e.g., non-antineoplastic HDs, antineoplastic HDs in final dosage forms) if defined in the written AoR.

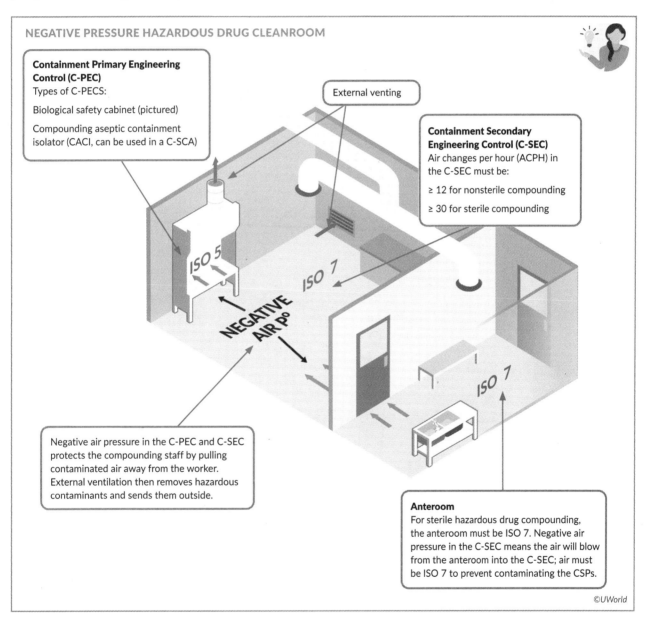

NEGATIVE PRESSURE HAZARDOUS DRUG CLEANROOM

Containment Primary Engineering Control (C-PEC)
Types of C-PECS:

Biological safety cabinet (pictured)

Compounding aseptic containment isolator (CACI, can be used in a C-SCA)

External venting

Containment Secondary Engineering Control (C-SEC)
Air changes per hour (ACPH) in the C-SEC must be:

≥ 12 for nonsterile compounding

≥ 30 for sterile compounding

ISO 5

ISO 7

ISO 7

NEGATIVE AIR P°

Negative air pressure in the C-PEC and C-SEC protects the compounding staff by pulling contaminated air away from the worker. External ventilation then removes hazardous contaminants and sends them outside.

Anteroom
For sterile hazardous drug compounding, the anteroom must be ISO 7. Negative air pressure in the C-SEC means the air will blow from the anteroom into the C-SEC; air must be ISO 7 to prevent contaminating the CSPs.

©UWorld

GARB FOR HAZARDOUS DRUGS

Appropriate personal protective equipment (PPE) must be worn during each activity involving HDs: receiving, storage, transporting, compounding (sterile and nonsterile), administration, sanitization and spill control. This can include hair and shoe covers, respiratory protection or a face mask (for sterile compounding), and chemotherapy gowns and gloves. It can also include more advanced eye/face and respiratory protection if there is a risk of spills or splashes.

Garb required for HD compounding is described in the image below. Garb for compounding is donned in the anteroom. The order in which the garb should be donned is from dirtiest to cleanest.

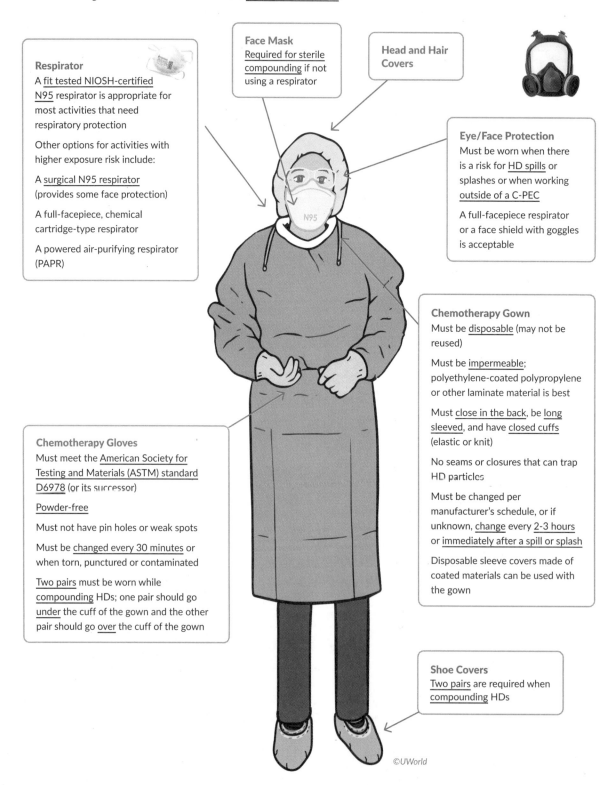

Respirator

A fit tested NIOSH-certified N95 respirator is appropriate for most activities that need respiratory protection

Other options for activities with higher exposure risk include:

A surgical N95 respirator (provides some face protection)

A full-facepiece, chemical cartridge-type respirator

A powered air-purifying respirator (PAPR)

Face Mask
Required for sterile compounding if not using a respirator

Head and Hair Covers

Eye/Face Protection
Must be worn when there is a risk for HD spills or splashes or when working outside of a C-PEC

A full-facepiece respirator or a face shield with goggles is acceptable

Chemotherapy Gown
Must be disposable (may not be reused)

Must be impermeable; polyethylene-coated polypropylene or other laminate material is best

Must close in the back, be long sleeved, and have closed cuffs (elastic or knit)

No seams or closures that can trap HD particles

Must be changed per manufacturer's schedule, or if unknown, change every 2-3 hours or immediately after a spill or splash

Disposable sleeve covers made of coated materials can be used with the gown

Chemotherapy Gloves
Must meet the American Society for Testing and Materials (ASTM) standard D6978 (or its successor)

Powder-free

Must not have pin holes or weak spots

Must be changed every 30 minutes or when torn, punctured or contaminated

Two pairs must be worn while compounding HDs; one pair should go under the cuff of the gown and the other pair should go over the cuff of the gown

Shoe Covers
Two pairs are required when compounding HDs

©UWorld

RESPIRATORY PROTECTION

A fit-tested, NIOSH-certified <u>N95 respirator</u> is sufficient for most HD compounding, but does not provide adequate protection against gases, vapors or direct liquid splashes. A <u>surgical N95 respirator</u> adds some protection against splashes and droplets.

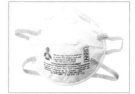

N95 respirator mask
sasapanchenko/stock.adobe.com

Additional respiratory protection is needed in situations with direct HD exposure, including when cleaning up <u>large HD spills</u>, sanitizing the <u>undertray of a C-PEC</u>, or if there is a known or suspected airborne exposure to HD powders or vapors. For any of these situations, one of the following should be worn:

- A fit-tested respirator mask with attached gas canisters (a "gas mask"); see picture below on the left.

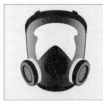 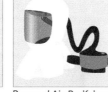

Respirator mask with gas canisters   *Powered Air-Purifying Respirator (PAPR)*

© CDC.gov

- A powered air-purifying respirator (PAPR) that blows air through the filter to the user (see picture above on the right). PAPRs are easier to breathe through than the gas mask type but require a fully charged battery to work properly. They use the same filters as gas masks.

GARB FOR ADMINISTRATION

Appropriate PPE must be worn when <u>administering</u> HDs. <u>Two pairs of chemotherapy gloves</u> are required when administering antineoplastic <u>HDs</u> and performing any manipulation of HDs (e.g., crushing tablets). A <u>single pair</u> of gloves can be used for handling <u>intact tablets or capsules</u>. A chemotherapy <u>gown</u> is required when administering <u>injectable HDs</u> and recommended when administering other HDs (e.g., oral).

If there is a risk of spills/splashes (e.g., administration of an irrigation), face and eye protection should be worn.

GARB FOR RECEIVING, STORAGE AND TRANSPORT

When HDs are unpacked and are not contained in plastic, the staff member should wear an elastomeric half-mask, with a multi-gas cartridge and P100-filter, until assessment of the packaging integrity ensures that no breakage or spillage

occurred during transport. <u>A single pair of chemotherapy gloves</u> can be used for HD <u>receiving and storage</u>.

When HDs need to be transported, they must be properly labeled and packaged to minimize the risk of spillage or breakage. <u>Pneumatic tube</u> systems <u>cannot</u> be used to transport any <u>liquid HDs</u> or <u>any antineoplastics</u> because of the potential for breakage and contamination.

HAZARDOUS DRUG EQUIPMENT AND PREPARATION

<u>Equipment</u> used for HD compounding, including routine equipment such as counting trays and spatulas, should be <u>dedicated</u> for HD preparation and <u>sanitized</u> after use, or they should be <u>disposable</u> (i.e., single use only). Equipment that cannot be thoroughly sanitized (e.g., automated counting or packaging machines) should not be used for HDs as any residue could contaminate other drugs.

Pharmacy and nursing staff should <u>avoid manipulating</u> oral HDs. If a liquid formulation of the drug is available, it should be used. If manipulation is required (e.g., crushing tablets, opening capsules) it should be done in a C-PEC. If this is not feasible, PPE must be worn and manipulation should be done in a plastic bag to contain any dust or particles.

When compounding with HDs, <u>air should not be injected into a vial</u> (as you generally would in sterile compounding). Positive pressure in the vial can cause the HD to spray out around the needle, contaminating the workspace and endangering personnel. Instead, the <u>negative-pressure technique</u> or a <u>closed-system transfer device (CSTD)</u> should be used.

NEGATIVE-PRESSURE TECHNIQUE

First, pull the plunger back to fill the syringe with a volume of air equal to the volume of drug to be removed. Insert the needle into the vial, invert the vial and pull on the plunger. This will create a vacuum that pulls the drug out of the vial and into the syringe. This should be done in small increments, pausing to allow the air to move out of the syringe and into the vial, until the desired volume of drug has been drawn up.

CLOSED-SYSTEM TRANSFER DEVICES

CSTDs are vial transfer systems that offer an additional level of protection against HD exposure. They have a <u>built-in valve</u> that <u>equalizes</u> the <u>air pressure</u> when fluid is added or withdrawn from the vial.

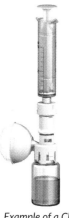

Example of a Closed System Transfer Device

CSTDs should be used to transfer HDs whenever possible as they keep the HDs contained within the device. CSTDs reduce leaks and spills when withdrawing solutions from vials, injecting solutions into IV bags, reconstituting dried powders into solutions and during syringe to syringe transfers. CSTDs are recommended when compounding HDs and required for administering antineoplastics.

LABEL REQUIREMENTS

All hazardous preparations must have a label that reads "Chemotherapy – dispose of properly" or something similar. Any special handling precaution should also be clearly stated on the label.

HAZARDOUS DRUG DISPOSAL

All PPE worn when handling HDs is considered contaminated with trace amounts. The outer chemotherapy gloves worn during compounding are discarded in a yellow trace chemotherapy waste bin located inside the C-PEC or put in a sealable bag if discarding outside the C-PEC. Remove the outer glove before handling and labeling the compounded preparation. The rest of the garb (e.g., chemotherapy gown, shoe covers) must be taken off before exiting the negative-pressure area (the C-SEC or C-SCA) and thrown away in the yellow trace chemotherapy waste bin.

All trace hazardous waste (i.e., empty vials, empty syringes, empty IV bags, IV tubes) is thrown away in a yellow container, which will be destroyed by incineration (burning) at a waste facility.

Bulk hazardous waste, which includes unused or partially empty IV bags, syringes and vials, are thrown away in a black container, which will be incinerated at a waste facility.

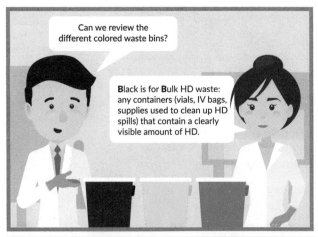

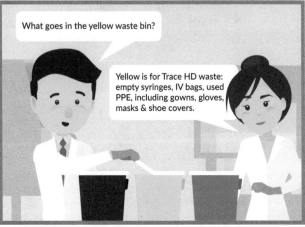

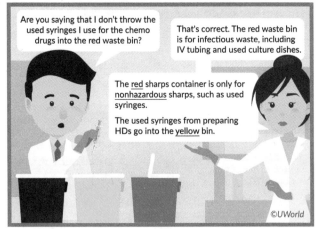

HAZARDOUS DRUG COMPOUNDING CLEANING SPECIFICS

SANITIZATION

All areas and equipment used for handling HDs must be sanitized, which includes deactivating, decontaminating and cleaning, at least once daily. Sterile compounding areas and equipment must be disinfected as a final step. It is important to perform the sanitizing steps in the correct order; if the disinfecting step is completed before the deactivating step, it will spread the HD residue.

DEACTIVATION

Make compound inert/inactive
Peroxide or sodium hypochlorite (2% bleach)

DECONTAMINATION

Remove HD residue
Alcohol, water, peroxide or sodium hypochlorite (2% bleach)

CLEANING

Remove dirt and microbial contamination
Germicidal detergent

DISINFECTION
(Sterile Compounding Only)

Destroy microorganisms
EPA-registered disinfectant or 70% isopropyl alcohol

---

*EPA = Environmental Protection Agency

Wetted wipes should be used for the sanitizing agents instead of a spray bottle, because directly spraying onto the surfaces and equipment can cause HD residue to aerosolize and spread to other areas.

There are several commercially available kits which simplify the sanitization process, including multi-purpose agents that combine deactivation and decontamination (such as *Peridox RTU)*. Bleach or peroxide can be used for both steps. Bleach can cause corrosion on stainless steel surfaces, including the surfaces of C-PECs. To prevent corrosion, neutralize the bleach by wiping surfaces afterwards with sodium thiosulfate, sterile alcohol, sterile water or a germicidal detergent.

All workers performing these activities must wear appropriate PPE, including two pairs of chemotherapy gloves and a disposable, impermeable gown. Advanced respiratory protection (e.g., fit-tested respirator mask, PAPR) is needed when deactivating, decontaminating and cleaning underneath the work surface of a C-PEC (see previous section on respiratory protection).

SURFACE SAMPLING

Pharmacies involved in HD compounding should perform wipe sampling of all compounding surfaces initially and at least every 6 months to ensure that hazardous residue is adequately contained. Areas in the C-PEC, C-SEC and anteroom should be tested for contamination.

HAZARDOUS DRUG SPILLS

HD spills must be cleaned up immediately. Depending on the facility, all of the compounding staff can be trained to handle HD spills or the facility can have a trained spill response team. There must be a designated person who oversees training and compliance for handling HD spills, and SOPs must be developed to both prevent HD spills and to direct cleanup of HD spills. The Safety Data Sheet (SDS) for the HD should be consulted for guidance on spill clean-up procedures.

Establish the Who, What and When

- Who refers to the staff who will respond to assist people exposed to the spill and clean up the spill. If HD exposure has occurred, emergency medical help will be needed.
- What refers to the rapid assessment of the situation to determine if additional help will be needed.
- When refers to the need to clean up HD spills immediately.

Managing the Spill

- Spill kits for HDs must be kept in areas where HDs are prepared, stored and administered. The spill kits must be available immediately wherever HDs travel, which is where they can spill.
- Quickly limit access to the area, and post warning signs around the perimeter of the spill. Pregnant women should not be involved with any clean-up activities and should immediately leave the area.
- The warning sign should state *Caution: Hazardous Spill, Proceed with Care!* or something similar.

Spill Kit Contents

- Protective gown, latex gloves (minimally), N95 respirator mask plus goggles with side shields
- HD waste bag, scoop and scraper to get spill waste into the waste bag, chemo pads to absorb hazardous liquid
- HD spill report exposure form to document HD exposure

Procedure for Cleaning up a Spill

Open the spill kit. The PPE should be donned immediately to protect the staff cleaning up the spill.

- Put <u>ASTM D6978 (chemotherapy)-rated gloves</u> on first (these are the type used for HD compounding), then the heavy-duty gloves over top. The heavy-duty gloves protect the hands from broken glass.

- Clean up large amounts of spilled drug and broken glass.
  - ❏ Never use a brush to clean up broken glass and powder that is contaminated with HDs. Brushes can cause particles to become airborne.

- Cover any liquid with an absorbent spill pad.

- Decontaminate the surfaces on which the HD has spilled, moving from the area of lesser contamination to areas of greater contamination to avoid spreading the hazard.

- If wetted wipes are not available, pour the decontamination solution on the pads. Do not spray.

- Put trash into a hazardous waste bag, and seal. This is <u>bulk hazardous waste</u>, which is discarded in the <u>black</u> bulk hazardous <u>waste bin</u> (see Disposal section).

After the Spill is Cleaned

- Doff (remove) garb and perform hand hygiene.
- Decontaminate the respirator and replace the cartridges.
- Replace the spill kit.

DRUG EXPOSURE

The most urgent action to take when a staff member has an exposure, whether the drug is hazardous or not, is to get the <u>drug or chemical off</u> the person <u>as soon as possible</u>. The first 10 to 15 seconds after exposure are critical. Delaying treatment, even for a few seconds, may cause serious injury.

Protocols for emergency procedures should be kept in the pharmacy. Minimal actions to take include:

1. For an exposure to gloves or gown, immediately <u>remove</u> the garb that has the drug on it.

2. Immediately <u>cleanse any affected skin</u> with soap and water.

3. For an eye exposure, flood the affected eye at an eyewash fountain (see image), or with water or an isotonic eyewash, for <u>at least 15 minutes</u>. Depending on the chemical, the time required for flushing can be longer.

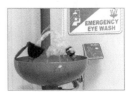

settapong/stock.adobe.com

4. Obtain <u>medical attention</u>, when warranted.

5. Document the exposure in the employee's record.

Select Guidelines/References

United States Pharmacopeia (2023). General Chapter 800. Hazardous Drugs - Handling in Healthcare Settings. USP-NF. Rockville, MD: United States Pharmacopeia. DOI: https://doi.org/10.31003/USPNF_M7808_07_01.

Connor TH, MacKenzie BA, DeBord DG, et al. NIOSH list of antineoplastic and other hazardous drugs in healthcare settings, 2016. U.S. Department of Health and Human Services, Centers for Disease Control and Prevention, National Institute for Occupational Safety and Health, DHHS (NIOSH) Publication Number 2016-161 (Supersedes 2014-138).

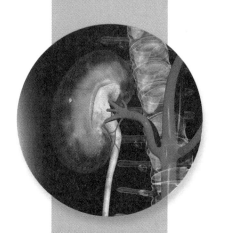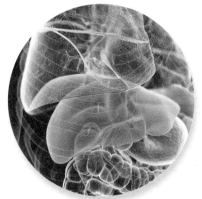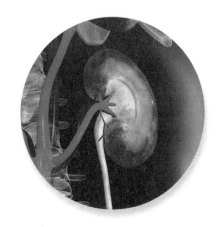

RENAL & LIVER DISEASE

CONTENTS

DEFINITIONS

Acute Kidney Injury (AKI)
A sudden loss of kidney function. Often reversible (temporary) but can be permanent if the precipitating condition is not corrected. Can be drug-induced; a common cause is dehydration (can present with a BUN:SCr ratio > 20:1 plus decreased urine output, dry mucus membranes and tachycardia).

Chronic Kidney Disease (CKD)
A progressive loss of kidney function over months or years. The degree of kidney function is assessed based on the glomerular filtration rate (GFR) or creatinine clearance (CrCl) and by how much albumin is in the urine.

Kidney Failure [End-Stage Renal Disease (ESRD)]
Total and permanent kidney failure. Fluid and waste accumulates. Dialysis (or transplant) is needed to perform the functions of the kidneys.

CONTENT LEGEND

 = Study Tip Gal    = Key Drug Guy

---

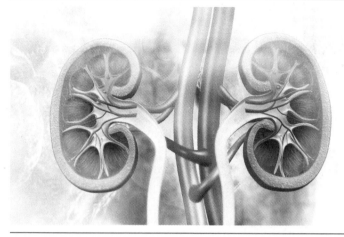

crystal light/Shutterstock.com

CHAPTER 18
RENAL DISEASE

BACKGROUND

Approximately 35 million U.S. adults (more than one in seven) have chronic kidney disease (CKD). The risk is highest in African Americans, Hispanic Americans, American Indians and Asians. The most common causes are diabetes and hypertension; controlling blood glucose and blood pressure can prevent renal damage and delay progression to end-stage renal disease (ESRD).

Less common causes of CKD include polycystic kidney disease, some types of infections (e.g., HIV, hepatitis B and C), renal artery stenosis (a narrowed or blocked artery that prevents blood flow to the kidney) and certain medications.

Pharmacists should assess the degree of kidney impairment in patients with CKD to ensure safe and effective medication dosing. They can recognize and recommend treatment for related disorders, such as anemia, hypertension, acid-base and electrolyte disturbances and disorders of bone and mineral metabolism (e.g., management of parathyroid hormone, phosphate, calcium and vitamin D levels).

RENAL PHYSIOLOGY

The nephron is the functional unit of the kidney. Its primary function is to control the concentration of sodium and water. The nephrons reabsorb what is needed back into the blood, and the remainder is excreted in the urine. This regulates blood volume, and in turn, blood pressure and pH. The major parts of the nephron include Bowman's capsule, the glomerulus, the proximal tubule, the loop of Henle, the distal convoluted tubule and the collecting duct (see the figure on the following page). There are roughly one million nephrons in each kidney.

GLOMERULUS

The afferent arteriole delivers blood into the glomerulus, a large filtering unit that is located within Bowman's capsule. Substances with a molecular weight < 40,000 daltons, including most drugs, pass through the glomerular capillaries into the filtrate (inside the lumen of the nephron) and are excreted in the urine. If the glomerulus is healthy, larger substances (e.g., proteins and protein-bound drugs) are not filtered and stay in the blood (exiting the nephron via the efferent arteriole). If the glomerulus is damaged, some albumin passes into the urine. The amount of albumin in the urine is used, along with the glomerular filtration rate (GFR), to assess the severity of kidney disease (also called nephropathy). This is discussed later in the chapter.

PROXIMAL TUBULE

Proximal means "close to." The proximal tubule is closest to Bowman's capsule (the entry point of the nephron). Much of the sodium (Na), chloride (Cl), calcium (Ca) and water that was initially filtered out of the blood is reabsorbed back into the bloodstream here. Blood pH is regulated by the exchange of hydrogen and bicarbonate ions. Medications that work here include the sodium-glucose cotransporter 2 (SGLT2) inhibitors (see the Diabetes chapter for details).

LOOP OF HENLE

As filtrate moves down the loop of Henle (the descending limb), water is reabsorbed into the blood, but Na and Cl ions are not, which ↑ the concentration of Na and Cl in the filtrate. As the filtrate moves up the loop of Henle (the ascending limb), Na and Cl ions are reabsorbed back into the blood, but water is not, unless antidiuretic hormone (ADH or vasopressin) is present. In the presence of ADH, water will be reabsorbed into the blood in the ascending limb; less water is then excreted in the urine (anti-diuresis).

The ascending limb of the loop of Henle is the site of reabsorption for about 25% of the filtered Na. When loop diuretics inhibit the Na-K pump in the thick ascending limb of the loop of Henle, less Na is reabsorbed back into the blood. There is a significant ↑ in the concentration of Na in the filtrate, causing less water to be subsequently reabsorbed (more water stays in the filtrate and is excreted in the urine along with Na). By blocking the pump, loop diuretics also cause less Ca reabsorption back into the blood, leading to Ca depletion. Long-term use of loop diuretics can decrease bone density because of this.

DISTAL CONVOLUTED TUBULE

Distal means "farther away." The distal convoluted tubule is the farthest point away from entry into the nephron. It is

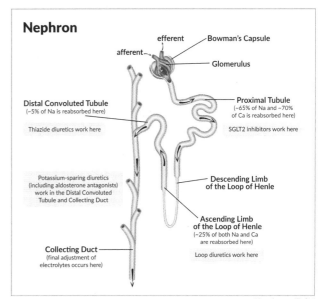

Nephron

efferent — Bowman's Capsule
afferent
— Glomerulus

Distal Convoluted Tubule
(~5% of Na is reabsorbed here)

Thiazide diuretics work here

Proximal Tubule
(~65% of Na and ~70% of Ca is reabsorbed here)

SGLT2 inhibitors work here

Potassium-sparing diuretics
(including aldosterone antagonists)
work in the Distal Convoluted
Tubule and Collecting Duct

Descending Limb
of the Loop of Henle

Ascending Limb
of the Loop of Henle
(~25% of both Na and Ca
are reabsorbed here)

Collecting Duct
(final adjustment of
electrolytes occurs here)

Loop diuretics work here

iStock.com/TefiM

involved in regulating potassium (K), Na, Ca and pH. Thiazide diuretics inhibit the Na-Cl pump in the distal convoluted tubule. Only about 5% of Na is reabsorbed at this point, making thiazides weaker diuretics than loops. Thiazides ↑ Ca reabsorption in the distal convoluted tubule. Unlike loop diuretics, the long-term use of thiazide diuretics has a protective effect on bones.

COLLECTING DUCT

The collecting duct is a network of tubules and ducts that connect the nephrons in each kidney to a ureter. The urine filtrate passes from the ureters into the bladder and then out of the body via the urethra (see figure at right). The collecting duct is involved with water and electrolyte balance, which is affected by levels of

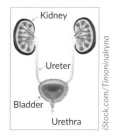

Kidney

Ureter

Bladder

Urethra

iStock.com/Timoninalryna

ADH and aldosterone. Potassium-sparing diuretics, including aldosterone antagonists (e.g., spironolactone, eplerenone), work in the distal convoluted tubule and collecting duct to ultimately ↓ Na and water reabsorption and ↑ K retention.

DRUG-INDUCED NEPHROTOXICITY

Drug-induced nephrotoxicity (or renal toxicity) is linked to numerous medications (see Key Drugs Guy on the next page); it can be acute and reversible if the medication is stopped, but it can also be irreversible and progress to CKD. It is especially common in the hospital setting and contributes to morbidity and mortality. Risk factors include ↓ renal blood flow [e.g., due to dehydration or hypotension (sometimes drug-induced), preexisting kidney disease, chronic or acute heart failure], ↑ age, use of multiple nephrotoxic medications at the same time and frequent use or large doses of nephrotoxic medications.

SELECT DRUGS THAT CAUSE NEPHROTOXICITY

Aminoglycosides	NSAIDs
Amphotericin B	Polymyxins
Cisplatin	Radiographic contrast dye**
Cyclosporine	
Loop diuretics*	Tacrolimus
	Vancomycin

Associated with acute kidney injury due to excessive volume loss.
***Sometimes called contrast media or contrast agent; used during imaging tests (e.g., angiography, MRI, CT).*

ESTIMATING KIDNEY FUNCTION

Two common laboratory markers used to estimate kidney function are blood urea nitrogen (BUN) and serum creatinine (SCr). BUN measures the amount of nitrogen in the blood that comes from urea, a waste product of protein metabolism. Because urea is excreted by the kidneys, as kidney function declines, BUN increases. BUN is not used alone to estimate kidney function because other factors besides renal impairment can increase the BUN (primarily dehydration).

Creatinine, a waste product of muscle metabolism, is mostly filtered by the glomerulus and is easily measured. As kidney function decreases, SCr increases (similar to BUN). The normal range of SCr is ~0.6 – 1.3 mg/dL. Any creatinine that is not filtered is secreted into the nephron tubules. The amount secreted increases as renal function declines and less creatinine is filtered (a compensatory mechanism); because of this, the initial decline in kidney function may not be accurately represented by creatinine levels.

CREATININE CLEARANCE

The Cockcroft-Gault equation for CrCl is most commonly used to estimate kidney function when dosing medications. The accuracy of creatinine-based estimation equations is decreased when a patient has very low muscle mass, which is often the case in frail elderly patients (low muscle mass = low SCr). This can lead to an overestimation of CrCl and inappropriate drug dosing for the patient's true kidney function.

Obesity, liver disease, pregnancy, high muscle mass and other conditions associated with abnormal muscle turnover can affect the estimation of kidney function using measured SCr. The Cockcroft-Gault equation is not preferable in very young children, in kidney failure or in unstable renal function (e.g., SCr is fluctuating or changing over a short period of time).

Drug dosing recommendations are generally based on CrCl (using the Cockcroft-Gault equation). A few specific drugs use GFR for dosing recommendations, including the SGLT2 inhibitors and metformin.

CrCl vs. GFR

CrCl

- Cockcroft-Gault equation

$$\text{CrCl (mL/min)} = \frac{140 - (\text{patient age})}{72 \times \text{SCr}} \times \text{weight (kg)} \times 0.85 \text{ (if female)}$$

- Use actual body weight if less than IBW, use IBW if normal weight, use adjusted body weight if overweight (by BMI)*

- Medication contraindications and dosing adjustments are typically based on CrCl calculated using the Cockcroft-Gault equation

GFR

- Not commonly calculated by pharmacists, but may be reported with a basic metabolic panel (BMP)

- CKD-EPI and MDRD equations are used

- Used for staging kidney disease and for dosing select drugs (e.g., metformin, SGLT2 inhibitors)

- For the exam, if GFR is not provided, CrCl provides an estimate to determine drug contraindications and dosing adjustments

See the Calculations IV chapter for more information on weights and CrCl.

GFR AND ALBUMINURIA FOR EVALUATING KIDNEY DISEASE

GFR [or estimated GFR (eGFR)] is calculated using the Modification of Diet in Renal Disease (MDRD) and Chronic Kidney Disease Epidemiology Collaboration (CKD-EPI) equations. Albumin is the primary protein that is measured in the urine to assess kidney disease; albuminuria is sometimes referred to as proteinuria.

CKD Criteria

The Kidney Disease Improving Global Outcomes (KDIGO) guidelines recommend using the GFR and degree of albuminuria (level of albumin present in the urine), along with the cause of CKD, to evaluate the severity of renal impairment (see the two tables on the following page).

The criteria for confirming CKD includes either:

- eGFR < 60 mL/min/1.73 m² (this is less than half the normal value of 125 mL/min/1.73 m² expected with healthy kidneys)

- Albuminuria (a marker of kidney damage) equivalent to urine albumin excretion rate (AER) ≥ 30 mg/24 hours or urine albumin-to-creatinine ratio (UACR) ≥ 30 mg/g.

Decreased eGFR or albuminuria must have occurred for greater than 3 months to be considered CKD (as opposed to an acute kidney injury).

GFR Categories

GFR (mL/min/1.73 m²)	TERMS	GFR CATEGORY	CKD STAGE
≥ 90 + kidney damage*	Normal or high	G1	Stage 1
60-89 + kidney damage*	Mild decrease	G2	Stage 2
45-59	Mild to moderate decrease	G3a	Stage 3
30-44	Moderate to severe decrease	G3b	Stage 3
15-29	Severe decrease	G4	Stage 4
< 15 or dialysis dependent	Kidney failure	G5	Stage 5

Example markers of kidney damage include a history of kidney transplant, structural abnormalities on imaging, or presence of albuminuria.

Degree of Albuminuria

ACR (mg/g) or AER (mg/24 hr)	TERMS	ALBUMINURIA CATEGORY
< 30	Normal to mild increase (previously called normoalbuminuria)	A1
30-300	Moderate increase (previously called microalbuminuria)	A2
> 300	Severe increase (previously called macroalbuminuria)	A3

ACR: albumin to creatinine ratio; AER: albumin excretion rate

---

DELAYING PROGRESSION OF CHRONIC KIDNEY DISEASE

Guidelines (e.g., KDIGO, ADA) provide treatment recommendations to delay CKD progression, typically in the setting of comorbid hypertension and/or diabetes (the two most common causes of CKD); however, the treatments discussed below may also be appropriate for patients with albuminuria due to other etiologies.

HYPERTENSION

The KDIGO Blood Pressure in CKD Guideline recommends a target SBP < 120 mmHg (if tolerated) for those with hypertension and CKD. This is lower than < 130/80 mmHg, which is the ACC/AHA recommended target for the general population with hypertension.

An ACE inhibitor or ARB is first line for patients with CKD and hypertension (see Study Tip Gal).

After starting an ACE inhibitor or ARB, the baseline SCr can ↑ up to 30%. This is expected, and treatment should not be stopped. If SCr ↑ by > 30%, treatment should be discontinued (and the patient referred to a nephrologist).

ACE inhibitors and ARBs should never be used together due to the risk of hyperkalemia. Patients should also be counseled to avoid potassium supplements and salt substitutes (with potassium chloride).

Changes in blood pressure, serum creatinine and potassium should be monitored 2 – 4 weeks after initiating an ACE inhibitor or ARB. If possible (e.g., potassium is normal, SCr increased < 30%), the dose of the ACE inhibitor or ARB should be maximized.

ACE INHIBITORS AND ARBs FOR ALBUMINURIA

Who?
Recommended in patients with hypertension and albuminuria

Why?
To prevent kidney disease progression

How?
Inhibit renin-angiotensin-aldosterone system (RAAS), causing efferent arteriolar dilation

What?
Reduce pressure in the glomerulus, decrease albuminuria and delay progression to ESRD

DIABETES

The KDIGO Guideline for Diabetes Management in CKD recommends treatment with a sodium-glucose cotransporter 2 (SGLT2) inhibitor (if eGFR ≥ 20 mL/min/1.73 m²).

Select SGLT2 inhibitors (e.g., canagliflozin, dapagliflozin, empagliflozin, sotagliflozin) have demonstrated a reduction in cardiovascular events and/or CKD progression. If the patient is unable to use these medications or requires additional glycemic control, a glucagon-like peptide 1 (GLP-1) receptor agonist is recommended.

Finerenone, a nonsteroidal mineralocorticoid receptor antagonist, is indicated to ↓ CKD progression and cardiovascular risks; it can be added to an SGLT2 inhibitor and maximally-tolerated dose of an ACE inhibitor or ARB in patients with an eGFR ≥ 25 mL/min/1.73 m², albuminuria and normal potassium levels.

MODIFYING DRUG THERAPY

Common scenarios related to medications and kidney disease include:

- The drug is eliminated through the kidneys.
  - The <u>dose</u> may require <u>reduction</u> and/or the dosing <u>interval</u> is <u>extended</u> to <u>avoid accumulation and side effects/toxicity</u>. Some drugs are <u>contraindicated</u> at a specific level of kidney impairment because <u>accumulation</u> is <u>unsafe</u> (e.g., increased bleeding risk with some anticoagulants).
- The drug can directly <u>cause or worsen kidney disease</u> (it is nephrotoxic).
- The drug becomes <u>less effective</u> as kidney function declines (e.g., thiazide diuretics, nitrofurantoin).
- The drug's side effects may be more significant due to reduced kidney function (e.g., hyperkalemia with aldosterone receptor antagonists).

Remember the basic principles of medication dosing in patients with impaired renal function. <u>Dose adjustments</u> may be necessary when CrCl is <u>≤ 60 mL/min</u>; when CrCl is <u>≤ 30 mL/min</u>, additional adjustments may be needed or the drug may be <u>contraindicated</u> (see <u>Key Drugs Guys</u> below).

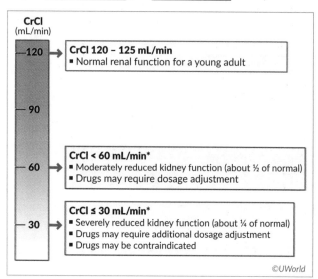

Check package labeling for individual drug requirements.

SELECT DRUGS THAT REQUIRE ↓ DOSE OR ↑ INTERVAL IN CKD

KEY DRUGS

Anti-Infectives
Aminoglycosides
(↑ dosing interval primarily)

Beta-lactam antibiotics
[except antistaphylococcal penicillins (nafcillin, oxacillin) and ceftriaxone]

Fluconazole

Quinolones (except moxifloxacin)

Vancomycin

Cardiovascular Drugs
LMWHs (enoxaparin)

Rivaroxaban* (for AF)

Apixaban* (for AF)

Dabigatran* (for AF)

Gastrointestinal Drugs
H2RAs (famotidine, ranitidine)

Metoclopramide

Other
Bisphosphonates*

Lithium

Others:

Anti-Infectives
Amphotericin B
Anti-tuberculosis medications (ethambutol, pyrazinamide)
Antivirals (acyclovir, valacyclovir, ganciclovir, valganciclovir, oseltamivir)
Aztreonam
NRTIs, including tenofovir
Polymyxins
Sulfamethoxazole/ Trimethoprim

Cardiovascular Drugs
Antiarrhythmics (digoxin, disopyramide, dofetilide, procainamide, sotalol*)
Statins (pravastatin, rosuvastatin)

Pain/Gout Drugs
Allopurinol
Colchicine
Gabapentin, pregabalin
Morphine and codeine
Tramadol

Others
Cyclosporine
Tacrolimus
Topiramate

Medication has indication-specific recommendations.

SELECT DRUGS THAT ARE CONTRAINDICATED IN CKD

KEY DRUGS

CrCl < 60 mL/min
Nitrofurantoin

CrCl < 50 mL/min
Tenofovir disoproxil fumarate containing products
(e.g., *Complera, Delstrigo, Stribild**, Symfi*)

Voriconazole IV
(due to the vehicle)

CrCl < 30 mL/min
Tenofovir alafenamide containing products (e.g., *Biktarvy, Descovy, Genvoya, Odefsey, Symtuza*)

NSAIDs

Dabigatran* (for DVT/PE)

eGFR < 30 mL/min/1.73 m²
Metformin***

Other**
Meperidine

Rivaroxaban*

SGLT2 inhibitors*

Others:

CrCl < 30 mL/min
Avanafil
Bisphosphonates*
Duloxetine
Fondaparinux
Potassium-sparing diuretics
Tadalafil*
Tramadol ER

Others**
Dofetilide
Edoxaban
Glyburide
Sotalol* (*Betapace AF*)

* Medication has indication-specific recommendations.
** For treated patients; do not start treatment if CrCl < 70 mL/min.
*** For treated patients; do not start treatment if eGFR ≤ 45 mL/min/1.73 m².
**** Not specified or another CrCl cut-off is used.

COMPLICATIONS OF CHRONIC KIDNEY DISEASE

See the figure illustrating the common complications of chronic kidney disease (exam studies should focus on the treatments).

CKD MINERAL AND BONE DISORDER

CKD mineral and bone disorder (CKD-MBD) is common in patients with renal impairment and affects almost all patients receiving dialysis. CKD-MBD is associated with fractures, cardiovascular disease and ↑ mortality. Patients with advanced kidney disease require monitoring of parathyroid hormone (PTH), phosphorus (phosphate, PO4), Ca and vitamin D levels.

Hyperphosphatemia

Hyperphosphatemia contributes to chronically elevated PTH levels (secondary hyperparathyroidism) and must be treated to prevent bone disease and fractures. Treatment is initially focused on restricting dietary phosphate (e.g., avoiding dairy products, cola, chocolate and nuts). As CKD progresses, phosphate binders are often required. Phosphate binders block the absorption of dietary PO4 by binding to it in the intestine. They are taken just prior to (or at the start of) each meal. If a dose is missed (and the food is absorbed), the phosphate binder should be skipped, and the patient should resume normal dosing at the next meal or snack. There are three types of phosphate binders: 1) aluminum-based, 2) calcium-based and 3) aluminum-free, calcium-free. Ferric citrate is systemically absorbed, while the other aluminum-free, calcium-free products are not.

Tenapanor (Xphozah), a sodium/hydrogen exchanger 3 inhibitor, may be considered for patients on dialysis with an inadequate response to phosphate binders or those unable to tolerate them.

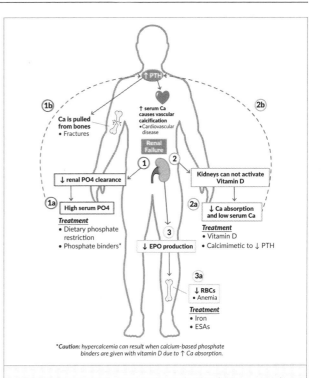

Caution: hypercalcemia can result when calcium-based phosphate binders are given with vitamin D due to ↑ Ca absorption.

The interactions of Ca, PO4 and vitamin D in CKD are complex. **1)** PO4 levels increase (because the kidneys cannot eliminate excess PO4 absorbed from the diet). **2)** Vitamin D can not be activated by the kidney, causing dietary calcium absorption to decrease. Both high PO4 **(1a)** and low Ca **(2a)** cause increased release of PTH **(1b, 2b)**. In a patient with healthy kidneys, PTH would cause the kidneys to increase Ca reabsorption, but in CKD this is not possible so Ca is pulled from the bones, leading to bone demineralization and increased fractures. Normally, when Ca levels return to normal, PTH release is shut down, but the chronically high PO4 levels continue to stimulate PTH release and hypercalcemia can persist, causing calcification and cardiovascular disease. **3)** In CKD, the kidneys produce less erythropoietin (EPO), resulting in decreased RBC production **(3a)** in the bone marrow and subsequent anemia.

Phosphate Binders

DRUG	DOSE	SAFETY/SIDE EFFECTS/MONITORING
Aluminum-based		
Aluminum hydroxide Suspension	300-600 mg PO TID with meals	**SIDE EFFECTS** Aluminum intoxication (can cause CNS and bone toxicity, including confusion and seizures), osteomalacia, constipation, nausea **MONITORING** Ca, PO4, PTH, s/sx of aluminum toxicity **NOTES** Treatment duration limited to 4 weeks

DRUG	DOSE	SAFETY/SIDE EFFECTS/MONITORING
Calcium-based		
Calcium acetate *(Calphron, Phoslyra*)* Tablet, capsule, solution	1,334 mg PO TID with meals, titrate based on PO4 levels	**SIDE EFFECTS** Hypercalcemia, constipation, nausea **MONITORING** Ca, PO4, PTH
Calcium carbonate *(Tums, others)* Tablet, chewable tablet	500 mg PO TID with meals (can vary with formulation used), titrate based on PO4 levels Total daily dose of elemental calcium should be ≤ 2,000 mg (from diet and supplements)	**NOTES** Calcium acetate binds more dietary phosphorus on an elemental calcium basis compared to calcium carbonate Hypercalcemia is especially problematic with concomitant use of vitamin D (due to increased calcium absorption)
Aluminum-free, calcium-free: no aluminum accumulation, less hypercalcemia, but more expensive than calcium-based products.		
Sucroferric oxyhydroxide *(Velphoro)* Chewable tablet	500 mg PO TID with meals, titrate based on PO4 levels	**WARNINGS** Iron absorption occurs with ferric citrate; dosage reduction of IV iron may be necessary; store out of reach of children to prevent accidental overdose **SIDE EFFECTS** Diarrhea, discolored (black) feces, constipation (ferric citrate) **MONITORING** PO4, PTH, iron/ferritin/TSAT (only with ferric citrate)
Ferric citrate *(Auryxia)* Tablet	2 tablets (420 mg) PO TID with meals, titrate based on PO4 levels	
Lanthanum carbonate *(Fosrenol)* Chewable tablet, powder	500 mg PO TID with meals, titrate based on PO4 levels Must chew tablet thoroughly to reduce risk of severe GI adverse effects Use powder if unable to chew tablets	**CONTRAINDICATIONS** GI obstruction, fecal impaction, ileus **WARNINGS** GI perforation **SIDE EFFECTS** Nausea/vomiting, diarrhea, constipation, abdominal pain **MONITORING** Ca, PO4, PTH
Sevelamer carbonate *(Renvela)* Tablet, powder **Sevelamer hydrochloride** *(Renagel)* Tablet	800-1,600 mg PO TID with meals, titrate based on PO4 levels	**CONTRAINDICATIONS** Bowel obstruction **WARNINGS** Can reduce dietary absorption of vitamins D, E, K and folic acid; consider vitamin supplementation Tablets can cause dysphagia and get stuck in the esophagus; consider using powder if swallowing difficulty is present **SIDE EFFECTS** Nausea/vomiting/diarrhea (all ~20%), dyspepsia, constipation, abdominal pain, flatulence, metabolic acidosis (with sevelamer hydrochloride) **MONITORING** Ca, PO4, HCO3, Cl, PTH **NOTES** Can lower total cholesterol and LDL by 15-30%; sevelamer carbonate can maintain bicarbonate concentrations

Brand discontinued but name still used in practice

Phosphate Binder Drug Interactions

- Phosphate binders are designed to "bind," and some phosphate binders contain polyvalent cations (e.g., calcium, iron, aluminum) that can chelate other drugs. Because of this, phosphate binders can have many drug interactions. It is especially important to separate the administration of phosphate binders from levothyroxine, quinolones and tetracyclines.

Vitamin D Deficiency & Secondary Hyperparathyroidism

Vitamin D deficiency occurs when the <u>kidney</u> is <u>unable</u> to hydroxylate vitamin D to its final <u>active form, 1,25-dihydroxy vitamin D</u>. Vitamin D deficiency worsens bone disease (by contributing to hypocalcemia and subsequent <u>elevations in PTH</u>), impairs immunity and increases the risk of cardiovascular disease.

Vitamin D has two primary forms: <u>vitamin D3</u> (or <u>cholecalciferol</u>), which is synthesized in the <u>skin</u> after exposure to <u>ultraviolet light</u> (e.g., the sun), and <u>vitamin D2</u> (or <u>ergocalciferol</u>), which is produced from plant sterols and is the <u>primary dietary source</u> of vitamin D. Supplementation with oral ergocalciferol or cholecalciferol may be necessary, especially in patients with early CKD (e.g., stage 3 and 4).

The <u>vitamin D analogs</u> should be reserved for the later stages of CKD (e.g., stages 4 and 5) with severe and progressive hyperparathyroidism; they can ↑ <u>calcium absorption</u> from the gut, ↑ serum calcium concentrations and <u>inhibit PTH secretion</u>. Calcitriol *(Rocaltrol)* is the <u>active form of vitamin D3</u>. Newer vitamin D analogs, such as paricalcitol and doxercalciferol, are alternatives that cause less hypercalcemia than calcitriol.

PTH release can also be inhibited by increasing the sensitivity of the calcium receptor on the parathyroid gland. <u>Cinacalcet</u> *(Sensipar)* is a "calcimimetic" which mimics the actions of calcium on the parathyroid gland and causes a further <u>reduction in PTH</u>. It is only used in dialysis patients.

Vitamin D Analogs and Calcimimetics

DRUG	DOSING	SAFETY/SIDE EFFECTS/MONITORING
Vitamin D analogs		
Calcitriol *(Rocaltrol)* Capsule, solution, injection	CKD: 0.25-0.5 mcg PO daily Dialysis: 0.25-1 mcg PO daily or 0.5-4 mcg IV 3x weekly	**CONTRAINDICATIONS** Hypercalcemia, vitamin D toxicity **WARNINGS** <u>Hypercalcemia</u> **SIDE EFFECTS** Hyperphosphatemia, N/V/D **MONITORING** <u>Ca</u>, PO4, PTH, 25-hydroxy vitamin D (calcifediol) **NOTES** Take with food or shortly after a meal to ↓ GI upset (calcitriol) Calcifediol is a prodrug of calcitriol
Calcifediol *(Rayaldee)* ER capsule	CKD Stage 3 or 4: 30-60 mcg PO QHS	
Doxercalciferol *(Hectorol)* Capsule, injection	CKD: 1-3.5 mcg PO daily Dialysis: 10-20 mcg PO 3x weekly or 4-6 mcg IV 3x weekly	
Paricalcitol *(Zemplar)* Capsule, injection	CKD: 1-2 mcg PO daily or 2-4 mcg PO 3x weekly Dialysis: 2.8-7 mcg IV 3x weekly	
Calcimimetics		
Cinacalcet (Sensipar)	Dialysis: 30-180 mg PO daily with food Take tablet whole, do not crush or chew	**CONTRAINDICATIONS** Hypocalcemia **WARNINGS** <u>Hypocalcemia</u> (use caution in patients with history of seizure and/or QT prolongation), GI bleeding, decreased bone turnover **SIDE EFFECTS** N/V/D, HA, anorexia, constipation, weakness, myalgia, URTIs **MONITORING** Ca, PO4, PTH
Etelcalcetide *(Parsabiv)*	Dialysis: 2.5-15 mg IV 3x weekly	**WARNINGS** <u>Hypocalcemia</u>, worsening HF, GI bleeding, decreased bone turnover **SIDE EFFECTS** <u>Muscle spasms</u>, paresthesia, N/V/D **MONITORING** Ca, PO4, PTH

ANEMIA OF CKD

Anemia is defined as a hemoglobin (Hgb) level < 13 g/dL. It is common in CKD and is due to a combination of factors. The primary problem is a lack of erythropoietin (EPO), which is normally produced by the kidneys and travels to the bone marrow to stimulate the production of red blood cells (RBCs). RBCs (which contain Hgb) are released into the blood where they transport oxygen. As kidney function declines, EPO production decreases. This leads to ↓ Hgb levels and symptoms of anemia (e.g., fatigue, pale skin).

Erythropoiesis-stimulating agents (ESAs) work like EPO to produce more RBCs and can prevent the need for blood transfusions. ESAs include epoetin alfa (*Procrit, Epogen, Retacrit*) and the longer-acting formulation darbepoetin alfa (*Aranesp*). ESAs have risks, including elevated blood pressure and thrombosis. They should only be used when the Hgb is < 10 g/dL and the dose should be held or discontinued if the Hgb exceeds 11 g/dL, as the risk for thromboembolic disease (DVT, PE, MI, stroke) is ↑ with higher Hgb levels.

ESAs are only effective if adequate iron is available to make Hgb. It is important to assess an iron panel (iron, ferritin and TSAT) and provide supplementation to prevent iron deficiency. Intravenous (IV) iron is given at the dialysis center. See the Anemia chapter for more information on identifying different types of anemia and use of ESAs and IV iron.

Daprodustat (*Jesduvroq*) is an oral ESA indicated for CKD patients who have been receiving dialysis for at least four months. It increases EPO levels and has a similar boxed warning and target Hgb levels as the parenteral ESAs.

HYPERKALEMIA

A normal potassium level is 3.5 – 5 mEq/L. Hyperkalemia can be defined as a potassium level > 5.3 or > 5.5 mEq/L (ranges vary), though clinicians will be concerned with any level > 5 mEq/L.

Potassium is the most abundant intracellular cation and is essential for life. Humans obtain potassium through the diet from many foods, including meats, beans and fruits. Normal daily intake through the GI tract is about 1 mEq/kg/day.

Excess potassium intake is excreted, primarily via the kidneys and partially via the gut. Renal potassium excretion is increased by the hormone aldosterone, diuretics (loops > thiazides), a high urine flow (via osmotic diuresis) and by negatively charged ions in the distal tubule (e.g., bicarbonate).

High dietary potassium intake does not typically cause hyperkalemia unless there is significant renal damage. With normal kidney function, the acute rise in potassium from a meal would be offset by the release of insulin, which causes potassium to shift into the cells.

The most common cause of hyperkalemia is decreased renal excretion due to kidney failure. The risk can be increased with a high dietary potassium intake or use of drugs that interfere with potassium excretion (see Key Drugs Guy).

Patients with diabetes are at a higher risk for hyperkalemia, as insulin deficiency reduces the ability to shift potassium into the cells, and many patients with diabetes take ACE inhibitors or ARBs (which ↑ potassium). Hospitalized patients are at a higher risk of hyperkalemia than outpatients, primarily due to the concurrent use of drugs and IV solutions containing potassium. Rarely, acute hyperkalemia can be due to tumor lysis, rhabdomyolysis or succinylcholine administration.

A patient with an ↑ potassium level may be asymptomatic. When symptoms are present, they can include muscle weakness, bradycardia and fatal arrhythmias. If the potassium is high and/or the heart rate/rhythm is abnormal, the patient is usually monitored with an ECG. The risk for severe, negative outcomes ↑ as the potassium level ↑.

SELECT DRUGS THAT RAISE POTASSIUM LEVELS

KEY DRUGS

ACE inhibitors

Aliskiren

ARBs

Canagliflozin

Drospirenone-containing COCs

Potassium-containing IV fluids (including parenteral nutrition)

Potassium-sparing diuretics (e.g., triamterene, spironolactone)

Potassium supplements

Sulfamethoxazole/ Trimethoprim

Transplant drugs (cyclosporine, tacrolimus)

Others:

Glycopyrrolate

Heparin (chronic use)

NSAIDs

Pentamidine

Treatment of Hyperkalemia

All potassium sources must be discontinued. If hyperkalemia is severe, there is an urgent clinical need to stabilize the myocardial cells (to prevent arrhythmias, this is done first), rapidly shift potassium intracellularly and induce elimination from the body.

The Study Tip Gal below lists the medication options for management of hyperkalemia. Several medications move potassium from the extracellular to the intracellular compartment. One or more of these methods are used in severe hyperkalemia. These drugs work quickly, but they do not lower total body potassium. Interventions to enhance potassium elimination take longer to reduce potassium and are only used alone in less severe situations; they are mostly used in combination with a drug that shifts potassium intracellularly.

STEPS FOR TREATING SEVERE HYPERKALEMIA

MECHANISM	INTERVENTION	ROUTE OF ADMINISTRATION	ONSET	NOTES
Stabilize the heart Prevent arrhythmias	Calcium gluconate (preferred) Calcium chloride	IV	1-2 minutes	Does not decrease potassium. Stabilizes myocardial cells to prevent arrhythmias.
Move it Shift K intracellularly	Regular insulin + Dextrose	IV	30 minutes	Insulin and dextrose are co-administered to prevent hypoglycemia. Give insulin alone if blood glucose is ≥ 250 mg/dL.
	Sodium bicarbonate	IV		Used when metabolic acidosis is present.
	Albuterol	Nebulized		Monitor for tachycardia and chest pain.
Remove it Eliminate K from the body	Loop diuretics	IV	5 minutes	Eliminates K in the urine. Monitor volume status.
	Sodium polystyrene sulfonate	Oral or rectal	2-24 hours	Binds K in the GI tract. Due to adverse effects (GI necrosis), used for emergency situations only. Oral may take hours to days to work. Rectal route has a faster onset and can be used in acute (emergency) treatment, though less effective than oral.
	Patiromer	Oral	~7 hours	Binds K in the GI tract. Delayed onset limits use in life-threatening emergencies.
	Sodium zirconium cyclosilicate	Oral	1 hour	Binds K in the GI tract. Potassium binder with fastest onset of action; may be preferred for emergency situations.
	Hemodialysis		Immediate, once started	Removes K from the blood. It takes several hours to set up/complete dialysis. Other methods are generally used in conjunction.

Potassium Binders (Non-Absorbed Cation Exchange Resins)

DRUG	DOSE	SAFETY/SIDE EFFECTS/MONITORING
Sodium polystyrene sulfonate (SPS, *Kayexalate**) Powder, oral suspension, rectal suspension	Oral: 15 grams 1-4 times/day Rectal: 30-50 grams Q6H	**WARNINGS** Electrolyte disturbances (hypernatremia, hypokalemia, hypomagnesemia, hypocalcemia), fecal impaction, GI necrosis (↑ risk when administered with sorbitol; do not use together) **SIDE EFFECTS** N/V, constipation or diarrhea **MONITORING** K, Mg, Na, Ca **NOTES** Can bind other oral medications (check for drug interactions and separate administration) Do not mix oral products with fruit juices containing K Due to the risk of GI necrosis, limit use to specific situations (e.g., life-threatening hyperkalemia and other therapies to remove potassium are not available or possible)
Patiromer *(Veltassa)* Powder for oral suspension	8.4 grams PO once daily; max dose 25.2 grams once daily	**WARNINGS** Can worsen GI motility, hypomagnesemia **SIDE EFFECTS** Constipation, nausea, diarrhea **MONITORING** K, Mg **NOTES** Binds to many oral drugs; separate by at least 3 hours before or 3 hours after Delayed onset of action limits the use in life-threatening hyperkalemia Store powder in the refrigerator (must be used within 3 months if stored at room temperature)
Sodium zirconium cyclosilicate *(Lokelma)* Powder for oral suspension	10 g PO TID for up to 48 hours, then 10 g once daily	**WARNINGS** Can worsen GI motility, edema, contains sodium (may need to adjust dietary sodium intake) **SIDE EFFECTS** Peripheral edema **NOTES** Can bind other drugs; separate by at least 2 hours before or 2 hours after Generally the preferred potassium binder due to fastest onset of action Store at room temperature

*Brand discontinued but name still used in practice.

METABOLIC ACIDOSIS

The ability of the kidney to reabsorb bicarbonate decreases as CKD progresses. This can result in the development of metabolic acidosis. In the ambulatory care setting, treatment of metabolic acidosis is initiated when the serum bicarbonate concentration is < 22 mEq/L. Drugs to replace bicarbonate include:

- Sodium bicarbonate
  - ❏ Sodium load can cause fluid retention.
  - ❏ Monitor sodium level and use caution in patients with hypertension or cardiovascular disease.
- Sodium citrate/citric acid solution *(Cytra-2, Oracit)*
  - ❏ Monitor sodium level.
  - ❏ Metabolized to bicarbonate by the liver; may not be effective in patients with liver failure.

DIALYSIS

If CKD progresses to failure (stage 5 disease), dialysis is required in all patients who do not receive a kidney transplant. The two primary types of dialysis are hemodialysis (HD) and peritoneal dialysis (PD). In HD, the patient's blood is pumped to the dialyzer (dialysis machine) and runs through a semipermeable dialysis filter, which, using a concentration gradient, removes waste products, electrolytes and excess fluid. HD is a 3 – 4 hour process, several times per week (usually three times). Patients who do HD at home can do it more frequently (e.g., 5 – 6 times per week).

In PD, a dialysis solution (usually containing glucose) is pumped into the peritoneal cavity (the abdominal cavity surrounding the internal organs). The peritoneal membrane acts as the semipermeable membrane (i.e., as the dialyzer). The solution is left in the abdomen to "dwell" for a period of time to allow for waste product and electrolyte exchange, then is drained. This cycle is repeated throughout the day, every day. PD is performed by the patient at home.

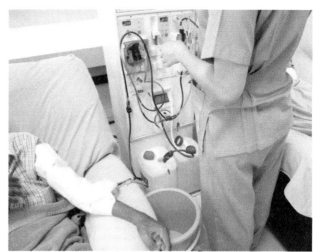

khawfangenvi16/Shutterstock.com

FACTORS AFFECTING DRUG REMOVAL DURING DIALYSIS

When a patient receives dialysis, the pharmacist must consider the amount of medication cleared during dialysis in order to recommend the correct dose and interval. Medications that are removed during dialysis (including many antibiotics) must be given after dialysis or may require a supplemental dose following dialysis. Drug removal during dialysis depends primarily on the factors below.

FACTOR	EFFECT
Drug Characteristic	
Molecular weight/size	Smaller molecules are more readily removed by dialysis
Volume of distribution	Drugs with a large Vd are less likely to be removed by dialysis
Protein-binding	Highly protein-bound drugs are less likely to be removed by dialysis
Dialysis Factors	
Membrane	High-flux (large pore size) and high-efficiency (large surface area) HD filters remove more substances than conventional/low-flux filters
Blood flow rate	Higher dialysis blood flow rates increase drug removal over a given time interval

Select Guidelines/References

Kidney Disease: Improving Global Outcomes (KDIGO) CKD Work Group. KDIGO 2012 Clinical Practice Guideline for the Evaluation and Management of Chronic Kidney Disease. *Kidney Int.*, Suppl. 2013;3:1-150.

Kidney Disease: Improving Global Outcomes (KDIGO) Blood Pressure Work Group. KDIGO 2021 Clinical Practice Guideline for the Management of Blood Pressure in Chronic Kidney Disease. *Kidney Int.* 2021;99(3S):S1-S87.

Kidney Disease: Improving Global Outcomes (KDIGO) Diabetes Work Group. KDIGO 2022 Clinical Practice Guideline for Diabetes Management in Chronic Kidney Disease. *Kidney Int.* 2022;102(5S):S1-S127.

Inferior Vena Cava — Aorta

Hepatic Artery

Portal Vein

Gallbladder

Common Bile Duct

iStock.com/blueringmedia

CHAPTER 19

HEPATITIS & LIVER DISEASE

HEPATITIS

BACKGROUND

Hepatitis means <u>inflammation of the liver</u>. Hepatitis viruses are the most common cause, but alcohol, certain drugs, autoimmune diseases and other viruses/infections can also cause hepatitis. Viruses that damage the liver include hepatitis A through E (most cases of viral hepatitis are caused by hepatitis A, B or C), herpes viruses, cytomegalovirus, Epstein-Barr virus and adenoviruses. Symptoms and treatment differ depending on the cause of hepatitis and extent of liver damage. Many patients with hepatitis B and C do not know they are infected.

HEPATITIS A, B AND C

The <u>Study Tip Gal</u> on the following page provides a comparison of hepatitis A, B and C viruses. Hepatitis A virus (HAV) usually causes an <u>acute, self-limiting illness</u>. Transmission occurs primarily via the <u>fecal-oral</u> route, due to either <u>improper handwashing</u> after exposure to an infected person or ingestion of <u>contaminated food/water</u>. Symptoms are generally mild and non-specific.

Hepatitis B virus (HBV) and hepatitis C virus (HCV) can cause <u>acute illness</u> and can lead to <u>chronic infection, cirrhosis, liver cancer, liver failure and death</u>. Transmission occurs from contact with infectious <u>blood</u> and/or other <u>body fluids</u> (e.g., having sex with an infected person, sharing contaminated needles to inject drugs, perinatal transmission from a mother to her newborn).

A one-time screening for HBV and HCV is recommended for anyone ≥ 18 years of age. Periodic, repeat screening is recommended for those with enhanced risk. Pregnant women should be screened for HBV and HCV with each pregnancy. <u>HBV vaccination</u> is also recommended for <u>all adults</u> (see the Immunizations chapter for details).

CONTENT LEGEND

 Study Tip Gal

 Key Drug Guy

COMPARISON OF HEPATITIS VIRUSES

	HEPATITIS A	HEPATITIS B	HEPATITIS C
Acute vs. Chronic	Acute only	Both	Both
Transmission	Fecal-oral	Blood, body fluid	Blood
Vaccine	Yes*	Yes*	No
First-Line Treatment	Supportive	PEG-IFN or NRTI (tenofovir or entecavir)	Treatment-naïve: DAA combination
Other Treatments for Select Patients			DAA combination + RBV

DAA = direct-acting antiviral, PEG-IFN = pegylated interferon, RBV = ribavirin
*See Immunizations chapter

DRUG TREATMENT FOR HEPATITIS C

There are <u>six different HCV genotypes</u> (1 – 6) and various subtypes (e.g., 1a, 1b). <u>Treatment</u> is recommended for <u>all patients</u> with acute or chronic HCV; options and duration of therapy depend on the genotype, the presence of cirrhosis and whether the patient has been previously treated. <u>Preferred HCV regimens consist of <u>2 – 3 direct-acting antivirals (DAAs) with different mechanisms</u>, usually for <u>8 – 12 weeks</u>.

Adding ribavirin to DAA therapy is an alternative treatment option (usually for patients with cirrhosis or after treatment failure). <u>Interferon</u> alfa-based regimens have historically been used to treat HCV. However, due to the success of DAAs, they are <u>no longer recommended</u> per HCV guidelines. HCV treatment is typically handled by specialists; healthcare providers should consult the American Association for the Study of Liver Diseases (AASLD) website for the most up-to-date recommendations (www.hcvguidelines.org).

DIRECT-ACTING ANTIVIRALS (DAAs)

DAAs revolutionized the treatment of <u>HCV</u> by eliminating older, poorly-tolerated treatments (e.g., interferon, ribavirin) and offering a <u>cure</u> for most patients. HCV treatment is approached much like HIV, with combination regimens that target different phases of the HCV life cycle (see <u>Study Tip Gal</u> for DAA mechanisms). Many DAAs are available only in combination products.

For <u>treatment-naïve</u> patients without cirrhosis (or with compensated cirrhosis), recommended regimens for <u>all genotypes</u> include:

- <u>Glecaprevir/pibrentasvir</u> *(Mavyret)* for 8 weeks
- <u>Sofosbuvir/velpatasvir</u> *(Epclusa)* for 12 weeks

Other products, including *Harvoni, Vosevi* and *Zepatier,* are recommended for specific genotypes.

DAA MECHANISMS AND REGIMENS

Preferred HCV regimens include 2-3 DAAs with different mechanisms of action (often in one tablet)

MECHANISM	NAME CLUE	EXAMPLES
NS3/4A Protease Inhibitors	–previr P for PI	Gleca*previr* Grazo*previr* Voxila*previr*
NS5A Replication Complex Inhibitors	–asvir A for NS5A	Elb*asvir* Ledip*asvir* Pibrent*asvir* Velpat*asvir*
NS5B Polymerase Inhibitors	–buvir B for NS5B	Sofos*buvir*

Be able to recognize appropriate and inappropriate combinations.

Example:

Velpat*asvir* + sofos*buvir*: preferred regimen combining 2 different MOAs.

Elb*asvir* + ledip*asvir*: two DAAs with the same MOA; should not be used together in a combination regimen.

What do the protease inhibitors used for HIV and HCV have in common? They are taken with food.

Remember: **P**rotease **I**nhibitors & **G**rub (**PIG**) **Take With Food***

*Exception: elbasvir/grazoprevir (Zepatier) for HCV (take without regard to food)

DRUG	DOSING	SAFETY/SIDE EFFECTS/MONITORING
All DAAs		**BOXED WARNING** Risk of reactivating HBV; test all patients for HBV before starting a DAA **WARNINGS** Potentially serious drug interactions (see DAA Drug Interactions on the following page) Rapid ↓ in HCV viral load can improve glucose metabolism in patients with diabetes; hypoglycemia can occur, especially if DAAs are used in combination with insulin or other hypoglycemic drugs (without a dose reduction) **SIDE EFFECTS** Well-tolerated; HA, fatigue, diarrhea, nausea **MONITORING** LFTs (including bilirubin), HCV-RNA
Glecaprevir/pibrentasvir (Mavyret)	3 tablets once daily with food	**CONTRAINDICATIONS** *Mavyret*: moderate-severe hepatic impairment (Child-Pugh class B or C); history of hepatic decompensation; coadministration with rifampin (↓ *Mavyret* serum concentration) or atazanavir (↑ *Mavyret* serum concentration) *Vosevi*: concurrent use with rifampin **WARNINGS** Sofosbuvir-containing regimens: do not use amiodarone with sofosbuvir as serious symptomatic bradycardia has been reported *Mavyret, Vosevi*: rare cases of liver failure (typically in patients with baseline hepatic impairment) **NOTES** Sofosbuvir monotherapy is not effective and not recommended *Sovaldi, Epclusa, Harvoni, Vosevi*: protect from moisture; dispense in original container *Epclusa, Harvoni* and *Vosevi*: avoid or minimize acid-suppressive therapy during treatment (see DAA Drug Interactions)
Sofosbuvir/velpatasvir (Epclusa)	1 tablet daily with or without food	
Sofosbuvir/ledipasvir (Harvoni)	1 tablet daily with or without food	
Sofosbuvir/velpatasvir/ voxilaprevir (Vosevi)	1 tablet daily with food	
Sofosbuvir (Sovaldi)	400 mg daily with or without food	
Elbasvir/grazoprevir (Zepatier)	1 tablet daily with or without food	**CONTRAINDICATIONS** Moderate-severe hepatic impairment (Child-Pugh class B or C); history of hepatic decompensation; use with strong CYP3A4 inducers, OATP1B1/3 inhibitors or efavirenz **WARNINGS** ↑ ALT (> 5x ULN) at or after 8 wks of treatment, rare cases of liver failure **NOTES** Screening for NS5A polymorphism is recommended when treating HCV genotype 1a

DAA DRUG INTERACTIONS

All DAAs have significant drug interaction potential. This summary is not all-inclusive. Consult the package labeling of each drug for additional details.

All DAAs

- Avoid strong inducers of CYP3A4 (e.g., carbamazepine, oxcarbazepine, phenobarbital, phenytoin, rifampin, rifabutin, St. John's wort).
- Most DAAs ↑ statin concentrations and myopathy risk.
- ↓ BG can occur with insulin and other diabetes medications. Monitor BG and ↓ diabetes medication doses as needed.

Mavyret

- Do not use with select statins (atorvastatin, lovastatin, simvastatin), select protease inhibitors (atazanavir, darunavir, lopinavir, ritonavir), cyclosporine (> 100 mg per day) or ethinyl estradiol (> 20 mcg per day).

Epclusa, Harvoni and Vosevi

- Contains sofosbuvir: do not use with amiodarone due to the risk of bradycardia.
- Antacids, H2RAs and PPIs can cause ↓ concentrations of ledipasvir and velpatasvir.
  - ❏ Separate from antacids by four hours.
  - ❏ Take H2RAs at the same time or separated (~12 hours) and use famotidine ≤ 40 mg BID or equivalent.
  - ❏ PPIs are not recommended with Epclusa.

Zepatier

- Do not use with efavirenz, cyclosporine or select protease inhibitors (atazanavir, darunavir, lopinavir, tipranavir) .
- Not recommended with nafcillin, ketoconazole, bosentan, tacrolimus, etravirine, Stribild, Genvoya and modafinil.

RIBAVIRIN

Ribavirin (RBV) is an oral antiviral drug that inhibits replication of RNA and DNA viruses. It can be used for HCV in combination with DAAs, but never as monotherapy.

DRUG	DOSING	SAFETY/SIDE EFFECTS/MONITORING
Ribavirin Capsule, tablet *Virazole* inhalation solution – for RSV	300-600 mg BID, varies based on indication, patient weight and genotype ↑ tolerability if given with food Hgb < 10 g/dL: ↓ dose (avoid if Hgb < 8.5 g/dL) Capsule should not be crushed, chewed, opened or broken	**BOXED WARNINGS** Significant teratogenic effects; monotherapy not effective for HCV; hemolytic anemia (mostly occurs within 1-2 wks of initiation – can worsen cardiac disease and lead to MI; do not use in patients with significant or unstable cardiac disease) **CONTRAINDICATIONS** Pregnancy, women of childbearing age who will not use contraception reliably, male partners of pregnant women, hemoglobinopathies, CrCl < 50 mL/min (capsule), autoimmune hepatitis **SIDE EFFECTS** Fatigue, HA, insomnia, anxiety/mood changes, N/V/D, anorexia, myalgia, hypothyroidism, alopecia **MONITORING** CBC with differential, platelets, electrolytes, LFTs/bili, HCV-RNA, TSH, monthly pregnancy tests **NOTES** Avoid pregnancy in females (including female partners of male-treated patients) during treatment and for 6-9 months after completion; at least 2 reliable forms of effective contraception are required during treatment and the post-treatment follow-up period

Ribavirin Drug Interactions

- Ribavirin can ↑ the hepatotoxic effects of NRTIs; lactic acidosis can occur.
- Zidovudine can ↑ the risk and severity of anemia from ribavirin.

DRUG TREATMENT FOR HEPATITIS B

NUCLEOSIDE/TIDE REVERSE TRANSCRIPTASE INHIBITORS (NRTIs)

NRTIs inhibit HBV replication by inhibiting HBV polymerase, which results in DNA chain termination. The NRTIs listed below can be used as monotherapy for HBV. Prior to starting, all patients should be tested for HIV. Some NRTIs used for HBV have activity against HIV; however, if a patient is co-infected with both HIV and HBV, two NRTIs are recommended to minimize the risk of HIV antiviral resistance.

DRUG	DOSING	SAFETY/SIDE EFFECTS/MONITORING
All HBV NRTIs	CrCl < 50 mL/min: ↓ dose or frequency Exception: *Vemlidy* (see below)	**BOXED WARNINGS** Lactic acidosis and severe hepatomegaly with steatosis, which can be fatal (downgraded from boxed warning to warning for both tenofovir formulations and lamivudine) Exacerbations of HBV can occur upon discontinuation, monitor closely Can cause HIV resistance in HBV patients with unrecognized or untreated HIV infection (downgraded from boxed warning to warning for both tenofovir formulations) See HIV chapter for further information
Tenofovir disoproxil fumarate, TDF *(Viread)* Tablet, oral powder Preferred therapy	300 mg daily	**WARNINGS** ↑ risk with TDF vs. TAF: renal toxicity, including acute renal failure and/or Fanconi syndrome, ↓ bone mineral density **SIDE EFFECTS** Nausea, diarrhea, headache, abdominal pain, fatigue, depression, ↑ LFTs
Tenofovir alafenamide, TAF *(Vemlidy)* Tablet Preferred therapy	25 mg daily with food CrCl < 15 mL/min: not recommended	Lipid abnormalities (↑ risk with TAF) **NOTES** *Viread* tablets and *Vemlidy*: protect from moisture; dispense only in original container *Vemlidy* is approved only for treating HBV; see HIV chapter for tenofovir alafenamide combination products used for HIV
Entecavir *(Baraclude)* Tablet, oral solution Preferred therapy	Treatment-naïve: 0.5 mg daily Lamivudine-experienced or decompensated cirrhosis: 1 mg daily	**SIDE EFFECTS** Ascites, ↑ LFTs, hematuria, nephrotoxicity, hyperglycemia, glycosuria **NOTES** Food reduces AUC by 18-20%; take on an empty stomach (2 hours before or after a meal)
Lamivudine *(Epivir HBV)* Tablet, oral solution	100 mg daily 150 mg BID or 300 mg daily if co-infected with HIV	**BOXED WARNING** Do not use *Epivir HBV* for treatment of HIV (contains lower dose of lamivudine and can result in HIV resistance) **SIDE EFFECTS** Headache, N/V/D, fatigue, insomnia, myalgia, ↑ LFTs, pancreatitis (rare)
Adefovir *(Hepsera)* Tablet	10 mg daily	**BOXED WARNING** Caution in patients with renal impairment or those at risk of renal toxicity (including those using concurrent nephrotoxic drugs or NSAIDs) **SIDE EFFECTS** HA, weakness, abdominal pain, dyspepsia, nephrotoxicity

NRTI Drug Interactions

- Ribavirin can ↑ the hepatotoxic effects of all NRTIs; lactic acidosis can occur.

- Tenofovir formulations: do not use with adefovir due to ↑ risk of virologic failure and side effects.

- Tenofovir alafenamide: do not use with oxcarbazepine, phenytoin, phenobarbital, rifampin and St. John's wort.

- SMX/TMP can ↑ lamivudine levels due to ↓ excretion.

INTERFERON ALFA

Interferons are naturally-produced cytokines that have antiviral, antiproliferative and immunomodulatory effects. The pegylated form of interferon alfa (PEG-IFN-alfa) is approved as monotherapy for the treatment of chronic HBV. PEG-IFN-alfa has polyethylene glycol added, which prolongs the half-life and reduces the dosing to once weekly. Interferon beta formulations are used for the treatment of multiple sclerosis (see the Systemic Steroids & Autoimmune Conditions chapter for additional information). Interferons have toxicities (e.g., flu-like syndrome) and lab abnormalities that limit their use (see table below), however they may be preferred in some patients (instead of NRTIs) because they have a finite treatment course (48 weeks).

DRUG	DOSING	SAFETY/SIDE EFFECTS/MONITORING
Pegylated interferon-alfa-2a (*Pegasys*)	180 mcg SC weekly	**BOXED WARNINGS** Can cause or exacerbate neuropsychiatric, autoimmune, ischemic or infectious disorders **CONTRAINDICATIONS** Autoimmune hepatitis, decompensated liver disease in cirrhotic patients, infants/neonates **WARNINGS** Myelosuppression, cardiovascular events, visual disorders (retinopathy, decrease in vision), endocrine disorders (hypo/hyperthyroidism, hypo/hyperglycemia), pancreatitis, skin reactions **SIDE EFFECTS** CNS effects (fatigue, depression, anxiety, weakness), GI upset, ↑ LFTs (5-10x ULN), mild alopecia Flu-like syndrome (fever, chills, HA, malaise); pre-treat with acetaminophen and an antihistamine **MONITORING** CBC with differential, platelets, LFTs, uric acid, SCr, electrolytes, TGs, thyroid function tests, serum HBV-DNA levels

LIVER DISEASE AND CIRRHOSIS

BACKGROUND

Cirrhosis is advanced fibrosis (scarring) of the liver that is usually irreversible. There are many causes, but the most common in the U.S. are hepatitis C and alcohol consumption. As scar tissue replaces the healthy liver tissue, blood flow through the liver is impaired, leading to numerous complications, including portal hypertension, gastroesophageal varices, ascites and hepatic encephalopathy.

CLINICAL PRESENTATION

Symptoms can include nausea, loss of appetite, vomiting, diarrhea, malaise, pain in the upper right quadrant of the abdomen, yellowed skin and whites of the eyes (jaundice) and darkened urine. Stool can become lighter in color (white or clay-colored) due to decreased bile (from decreased production or a blocked bile duct).

OBJECTIVE CRITERIA

Cirrhosis is definitively diagnosed with a liver biopsy, but certain lab results can suggest cirrhosis or other types of liver damage (see Study Tip Gal). Aspartate aminotransferase (AST) and alanine aminotransferase (ALT) are liver enzymes. The normal range for both is 10 – 40 units/L. In general, the higher the values, the more active (acute) the liver disease or

LAB TESTS FOR LIVER DISEASE

Specific liver function test (LFT) abnormalities can help distinguish between types of liver disease.

Acute liver toxicity, including from drugs
- ↑ AST/ALT

Chronic liver disease (e.g., cirrhosis)
- ↑ AST/ALT, Alk Phos, Tbili, LDH, PT/INR
- ↓ Albumin

Alcoholic liver disease
- ↑ AST > ↑ ALT (AST will be about double the ALT), ↑ gamma-glutamyl transpeptidase (GGT)

Hepatic encephalopathy
- ↑ Ammonia

Jaundice
- ↑ Tbili

inflammation. Clinical signs of liver disease, in addition to ↑ ALT and ↑ AST, include ↓ albumin (protein produced by the liver; normal range 3.5 – 5.5 g/dL), ↑ alkaline phosphatase (Alk Phos or ALP), ↑ total bilirubin (Tbili), ↑ lactate dehydrogenase (LDH), and ↑ prothrombin time (PT) and INR.

A hepatic panel (AST, ALT, Tbili and Alk Phos), also called liver function tests (LFTs), is used to assess acute and chronic liver inflammation/disease, and for baseline and routine monitoring of hepatotoxic drugs. Albumin and PT/INR are markers of synthetic liver function (production ability) and are likely to be altered in chronic liver disease (particularly cirrhosis). Liver disease can be classified as hepatocellular (↑ ALT and ↑ AST), cholestatic (↑ Alk Phos and ↑ Tbili) or mixed (↑ AST, ALT, Alk Phos and Tbili). See the Lab Values & Drug Monitoring chapter for additional information.

ASSESSING SEVERITY OF LIVER DISEASE

The severity of liver disease serves as a predictor of patient survival, surgical outcomes and the risk of complications, such as variceal bleeding. The Child-Turcotte-Pugh (CTP) or Child-Pugh classification system is widely used and online calculators are available. The score ranges from 5 – 15. Class A (mild disease) is defined as a score < 7, class B (moderate disease) is a score of 7 – 9 and class C (severe disease) is a score of 10 – 15. The model for end-stage liver disease (MELD) is another scoring system that ranges from 6 – 40. Higher numbers indicate a greater risk of death within three months. Noninvasive tests are increasingly used to predict fibrosis and cirrhosis.

Unlike drug dosing in renal failure, information to guide drug dosing of hepatically cleared drugs in liver failure is not as widely available. It is becoming more common to see package labeling for medications make specific recommendations based on Child-Pugh class. In general, caution is advised when using hepatically cleared drugs in severe liver disease (class C) and, in select cases, dose adjustment could be necessary. For drugs that are extensively hepatically metabolized, it is best to start at lower doses and titrate to clinical effect.

NATURAL PRODUCTS

Milk thistle, an extract derived from a member of the daisy family, is sometimes used by patients with liver disease. Milk thistle does not appear to be harmful, but there is limited data to demonstrate efficacy. A possible side effect is mild diarrhea and there are concerns for possible drug interactions between milk thistle and DAAs for HCV. Kava and comfrey are known hepatotoxins.

DRUG-INDUCED LIVER INJURY

Many drugs can cause liver damage (see Key Drugs Guy). The primary treatment (in most cases) is to stop the drug. Hepatotoxic drugs are typically discontinued when LFTs are > 3 times the upper limit of normal, but clinical judgment is warranted. Rechallenging with the drug can be considered if clinically necessary. An excellent reference for drug-induced liver injury (DILI) is http://livertox.nih.gov.

Acetaminophen is a known hepatotoxic drug and can cause severe injury if not dosed appropriately. Acetaminophen can still be used by patients with cirrhosis for limited periods of time and at lower dosages (e.g., < 2 grams/day). Patients with alcoholic cirrhosis who are actively drinking and/or malnourished are more susceptible to further liver damage. NSAIDs should be avoided in patients with cirrhosis because these drugs can lead to decompensation, including bleeding.

SELECT DRUGS WITH A BOXED WARNING FOR LIVER DAMAGE

KEY DRUGS

Acetaminophen (high doses, acute or chronic)
Amiodarone
Isoniazid
Ketoconazole
Methotrexate
Nefazodone
Nevirapine
Propylthiouracil
Valproic acid
Zidovudine

Others:
Bosentan
Felbamate
Flutamide
Leflunomide and teriflunomide
Lomitapide
Maraviroc
Tipranavir
Tolcapone

ALCOHOL-ASSOCIATED LIVER DISEASE

Alcohol-associated liver disease (ALD), sometimes called alcoholic liver disease, is a common type of liver disease. Risk increases with the duration and amount of alcohol consumed, and women have a higher risk than men. Chronic alcohol ingestion over a long period of time causes "steatosis" (fatty liver) due to fat deposition in the hepatocytes. This can be reversible and self-limiting (if drinking is stopped) or progress to alcoholic hepatitis, fatty liver (steatohepatitis) or chronic hepatitis with hepatic fibrosis or cirrhosis. Acute alcoholic hepatitis specifically is associated with poor short-term survival.

Chronic consumption of alcohol results in the secretion of pro-inflammatory cytokines (TNF-alpha, IL-6, IL-8), oxidative stress, lipid peroxidation and acetaldehyde toxicity. These factors cause inflammation, apoptosis (cell death) and eventually fibrosis of liver cells. Of all chronic heavy drinkers, ~15 – 20% develop hepatitis or cirrhosis. If the patient stops drinking, the liver can possibly regenerate to some extent.

TREATMENT

The most important part of treatment is <u>alcohol cessation</u>. Maintenance of abstinence is essential to improving outcomes and should include the use of drug treatment to control cravings. <u>Benzodiazepines</u> are often used to control <u>alcohol withdrawal</u> symptoms; gabapentin and carbamazepine may also be used for mild withdrawal. <u>Naltrexone</u> (*Vivitrol*), <u>acamprosate</u> and <u>disulfiram</u> (formerly *Antabuse*) are used to <u>prevent relapses</u>. An alcohol rehabilitation program and a support group whose members share common experiences and problems are extremely helpful in breaking the addiction to alcohol.

Proper nutrition is essential to help the liver recover. Vitamins and trace minerals, including vitamin A, vitamin D, thiamine (vitamin B1), folate, pyridoxine (vitamin B6) and zinc can help reverse malnutrition. <u>Thiamine</u> is used to <u>prevent and treat Wernicke-Korsakoff syndrome</u>. Wernicke's encephalopathy and Korsakoff syndrome are different conditions that are both due to <u>brain damage</u> caused by a <u>lack of vitamin B1</u>.

COMPLICATIONS OF LIVER DISEASE AND CIRRHOSIS

PORTAL HYPERTENSION AND VARICEAL BLEEDING

Fibrotic tissue in the liver causes resistance to blood flow, which increases blood pressure in the portal vein (known as <u>portal hypertension</u>). This can lead to blood backing up and flowing into smaller blood vessels (e.g., in the esophagus), causing them to balloon out. These enlarged vessels, known as <u>esophageal varices</u>, are at risk of breaking open, resulting in bleeding.

Esophageal Varices

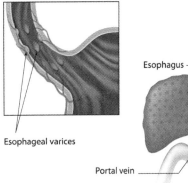
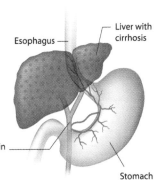

Esophageal varices

Aliia Medical Media/stock.adobe.com

Acute <u>variceal bleeding can be fatal</u>. Patients are stabilized with supportive therapies (e.g., blood transfusions, mechanical ventilation, correction of coagulopathy) and attempts to stop the bleeding and prevent rebleeding. <u>Band ligation</u> (putting a band around the vessel) or <u>sclerotherapy</u> (injecting a solution into the vessel to make it collapse and close) are endoscopic procedures often used for the initial management of bleeding varices. <u>Medications that vasoconstrict the splanchnic (GI) circulation</u> can stop or minimize the bleeding. <u>Octreotide is selective</u> for the splanchnic vessels whereas <u>vasopressin is non-selective</u>.

Surgical interventions can be considered if the patient is not responding to treatment or to prevent future rebleeding episodes. Common surgical procedures include balloon tamponade or transjugular intrahepatic portosystemic shunt (TIPS), in which a stent is placed in the liver to allow blood to flow directly from the portal vein to the hepatic vein (bypassing the scarred liver tissue). Short-term antibiotic prophylaxis (ceftriaxone or ciprofloxacin for up to 7 days) should be given to cirrhotic patients with a variceal bleed to reduce bacterial infections and mortality. <u>Non-selective beta-blockers</u> can be used for primary and secondary <u>prevention</u> of variceal bleeding (see next page).

Vasoconstricting Medications for Bleeding Varices

DRUG	DOSING	SAFETY/SIDE EFFECTS/MONITORING
Octreotide (Sandostatin, *Sandostatin LAR Depot*) Analog of somatostatin (inhibits vasodilatory hormones)	Bolus: 25-100 mcg <u>IV</u> (usual 50 mcg), can repeat in 1 hr if hemorrhage not controlled Continuous infusion: 25-50 mcg/hr x 2-5 days	**SIDE EFFECTS** <u>Bradycardia, cholelithiasis, biliary sludge</u>, fatigue, HA, hyperglycemia, hypoglycemia (highest risk in type 1 diabetes), hypothyroidism, N/V/D, abdominal pain, dizziness, flatulence, constipation, injection site pain, URTIs **MONITORING** Blood glucose, HR, ECG
Vasopressin (*Vasostrict*) <u>Antidiuretic hormone analog</u> Not first line (usually used with nitroglycerin IV to prevent myocardial ischemia)	Infusion: 0.2-0.4 units/min IV (max 0.8 units/min), max duration 24 hours	**SIDE EFFECTS** Atrial fibrillation, myocardial ischemia, ↓ HR, ↓ cardiac output, ↑ BP **MONITORING** BP, HR, ECG, fluid balance

Non-Selective Beta-Blockers for Portal Hypertension

The non-selective beta-blockers (NSBBs) nadolol and propranolol are used for primary and secondary prevention of variceal bleeding. NSBBs decrease cardiac output (via beta-1 blockade) and cause splanchnic vasoconstriction (via beta-2 blockade and unopposed alpha activity); this reduces portal venous inflow, resulting in decreased portal pressure. NSBBs are titrated to the maximally tolerated dose (target HR 55 – 60 BPM, SBP ≥ 90 mmHg) and continued indefinitely.

Carvedilol is an NSBB that has an added mechanism via its alpha-1 blocking effects (i.e., causes vasodilation within the intrahepatic circulation which decreases vascular resistance) that further reduces portal pressure. The AASLD guidelines support the use of carvedilol for the primary prevention of variceal bleeding.

DRUG	DOSING	SAFETY/SIDE EFFECTS/MONITORING
Nadolol (*Corgard*)	Initial: 20-40 mg PO daily	Refer to the Hypertension chapter for a complete review of beta-blockers **BOXED WARNING** Do not withdraw beta-blockers abruptly (particularly in patients with CAD/IHD); gradually taper dose over 1-2 wks to avoid acute tachycardia, hypertension and/or ischemia **CONTRAINDICATIONS** Severe bradycardia; 2nd or 3rd degree AV block or sick sinus syndrome (unless a permanent pacemaker is in place); overt cardiac failure or cardiogenic shock; bronchial asthma **WARNINGS** Use caution in patients with diabetes: can worsen hypoglycemia and mask hypoglycemic symptoms (see Diabetes chapter)
Propranolol (*Inderal LA,* **_Inderal XL,_** *InnoPran XL, Hemangeol)*	Initial: 20 mg PO BID	Use caution with bronchospastic diseases (e.g., asthma, COPD) Use caution with Raynaud's/other peripheral vascular diseases (requires slow dose titration) and pheochromocytoma (requires adequate alpha-blockade first) Can mask signs of hyperthyroidism (e.g., tachycardia) **SIDE EFFECTS** Bradycardia, hypotension, CNS effects (e.g., fatigue, dizziness, depression), impotence, cold extremities (can exacerbate Raynaud's) **MONITORING** HR (↓ dose if symptomatic bradycardia), BP **NOTES** Propranolol has high lipid solubility (lipophilic) and crosses the blood-brain barrier; it is associated with more CNS side effects
Carvedilol (*Coreg*)	Initial: 6.25mg PO daily in 1-2 divided doses	Same as for nadolol and propranolol plus: **CONTRAINDICATIONS** Severe hepatic impairment **WARNING** Intraoperative floppy iris syndrome has occurred in cataract surgery patients who were on or were previously treated with an alpha-1 blocker **SIDE EFFECTS** Edema, weight gain **NOTES** Take carvedilol with food to ↓ the rate of absorption and the risk of orthostatic hypotension

HEPATIC ENCEPHALOPATHY

Hepatic encephalopathy (HE) is caused by acute or chronic hepatic insufficiency. Symptoms include musty odor of the breath and/or urine, changes in thinking, confusion, forgetfulness, drowsiness, disorientation, mood changes, poor concentration, worsening handwriting, flapping hand tremor (asterixis), sluggish movements and risk of coma.

The symptoms of HE result from an accumulation of gut-derived nitrogenous substances in the blood (such as ammonia, glutamate). These substances would normally be cleared by the liver, but when the liver is not functioning properly, blood is shunted through collateral vessels that empty directly into the circulation instead.

Treatment includes identifying and treating precipitating factors and reducing blood ammonia levels through diet (by limiting the amount of animal protein) and drug therapy.

Daily protein intake should be 1.2 – 1.5 g/kg. Vegetable and dairy sources of protein are preferred to animal sources due to the lower calorie to nitrogen ratio. If protein supplementation is required, branched-chain amino acids (e.g., leucine, isoleucine, valine) are recommended.

Drug therapy consists of nonabsorbable disaccharides (e.g., lactulose) and antibiotics (e.g., rifaximin, neomycin). Lactulose is first line for both acute and chronic (prevention) therapy. It works by converting ammonia produced by intestinal bacteria to ammonium, which is polar and therefore cannot readily diffuse into the blood. Lactulose also enhances diffusion of ammonia into the colon for excretion. Antibiotics work by inhibiting the activity of urease-producing bacteria, which decreases ammonia production. Rifaximin can be considered for add-on treatment.

DRUG	DOSING	SAFETY/SIDE EFFECTS/MONITORING
Lactulose (Enulose, Constulose, Generlac, Kristalose) Oral solution and packet	Treatment: 30-45 mL (20-30 grams) PO every hour until stool evacuation; then 30-45 mL PO 3-4 times/day, titrated to produce 2-3 soft bowel movements daily Enema: Q4-6H PRN Prevention: 30-45 mL PO 3-4 times/day, titrated to produce 2-3 soft bowel movements daily	**CONTRAINDICATIONS** Low galactose diet **SIDE EFFECTS** Flatulence, diarrhea, dyspepsia, abdominal discomfort, dehydration, hypernatremia, hypokalemia **MONITORING** Mental status, bowel movements, ammonia, fluid status, electrolytes
Rifaximin (Xifaxan) Tablet	Treatment or prevention: 400 mg PO Q8H or 550 mg PO BID	**SIDE EFFECTS** Peripheral edema, dizziness, fatigue, nausea, ascites, headache **MONITORING** Mental status, ammonia
Neomycin	4-12 grams daily divided Q4-6H x 5-6 days	**BOXED WARNINGS** Neurotoxicity (hearing loss, vertigo, ataxia); nephrotoxicity (particularly in renal impairment or with concurrent use of other nephrotoxic drugs); can cause neuromuscular blockade and respiratory paralysis, especially when given soon after anesthesia or with muscle relaxants **SIDE EFFECTS** GI upset, irritation/soreness of mouth/rectal area **MONITORING** Mental status, renal function, hearing, ammonia

ASCITES

Ascites is <u>fluid accumulation</u> within the <u>peritoneal space</u> that can lead to the development of spontaneous bacterial peritonitis (SBP) and hepatorenal syndrome (HRS). There are many treatment approaches to managing ascites, which are chosen based on the severity; all patients with <u>cirrhosis and ascites</u> should be considered for liver <u>transplantation</u>.

Patients with ascites due to portal hypertension should <u>restrict dietary sodium intake</u> to < 2 grams/day, avoid sodium-retaining medications (including NSAIDs) and use diuretics to increase fluid loss. Restriction of fluid is recommended only in patients with moderate or severe hyponatremia (serum Na ≤ 125 mEq/L).

Diuretic therapy for ascites can be initiated with either <u>spironolactone monotherapy</u> or a <u>combination of furosemide and spironolactone. Furosemide by itself is ineffective.</u> Spironolactone is initiated at a single daily dose of 50 – 100 mg and increased to a maximum of 400 mg per day. When used in combination, the drugs should be titrated to a maximal weight loss of 0.5 kg/day; if possible, a <u>ratio of 40 mg furosemide to 100 mg spironolactone</u> should be used to <u>maintain potassium balance</u>.

The spironolactone oral suspension (*CaroSpir*) is not therapeutically equivalent to oral tablets (*Aldactone*). The approved *CaroSpir* dose for treating edema associated

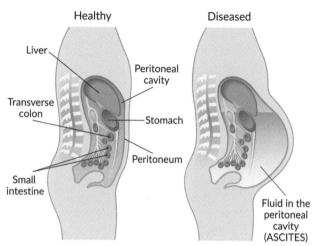

Healthy   Diseased

Liver — Peritoneal cavity — Transverse colon — Stomach — Peritoneum — Small intestine — Fluid in the peritoneal cavity (ASCITES)

rob3000/stock.adobe.com

with cirrhosis is 75 mg (15 mL) in single or divided doses (see Chronic Heart Failure and Hypertension chapters for additional information).

In severe cases, abdominal <u>paracentesis</u> is needed to directly remove ascitic fluid. Large-volume paracentesis (removal of > 5 L) is associated with significant fluid shifts, and the addition of <u>albumin</u> (6 – 8 grams per liter of fluid removed) is recommended to prevent paracentesis-induced circulatory dysfunction and progression to hepatorenal syndrome.

SPONTANEOUS BACTERIAL PERITONITIS

<u>Spontaneous bacterial peritonitis (SBP)</u> is an <u>acute infection</u> of the <u>ascitic fluid</u>. Diagnosis is guided by cell and microbiologic analysis. Targeting streptococci and enteric gram-negative pathogens with <u>ceftriaxone</u> (or an equivalent) for 5 – 7 days is recommended. The addition of albumin (1.5 grams/kg of body weight on day 1 and 1 gram/kg on day 3) can improve survival in some patients. Patients who have survived an episode of SBP should receive <u>secondary prophylaxis</u> with oral <u>ciprofloxacin</u> or <u>sulfamethoxazole/trimethoprim</u>.

HEPATORENAL SYNDROME

Hepatorenal syndrome (HRS) is the development of renal failure in patients with advanced cirrhosis. It occurs as a result of renal vasoconstriction, mediated by activation of the renin-angiotensin-aldosterone system (RAAS) and the sympathetic nervous system (SNS) through a feedback mechanism known as hepatorenal reflex. Prevention of HRS is critical given the high mortality rate and difficulty in managing this patient population. This can be accomplished by appropriately treating the various stages and complications of cirrhosis, preventing possible precipitating factors (e.g., gastrointestinal bleeding, avoiding large-volume paracentesis without albumin), and avoiding nephrotoxins and renal hypoperfusion.

HRS can be treated with vasoconstrictors such as terlipressin or norepinephrine, in combination with albumin. Terlipressin (*Terlivaz*) is a vasopressin analog approved for the treatment of HRS. Of note, the use of vasoconstrictors requires close monitoring in an intensive care unit setting. When this is not possible, HRS can be treated with a combination of albumin, octreotide and midodrine.

RENAL & LIVER DISEASE

KEY COUNSELING POINTS

See the Drug Formulations and Patient Counseling chapter for counseling language/layman's terminology.

ALL DIRECT-ACTING ANTIVIRALS

- Many drug interactions.

MAVYRET

- Take with food.

RIBAVIRIN

- Avoid in pregnancy (teratogenic), including in male partners of pregnant women.
- Can cause hemolytic anemia.

NRTIs

- Can cause lactic acidosis.
- *Epivir HBV* tablets and oral solution are not interchangeable with the *Epivir* tablets and solution used in HIV (which have higher doses).
- Take entecavir on an empty stomach.

BETA-BLOCKERS

- Do not abruptly discontinue without consulting your healthcare provider.

Select Guidelines/References

American Association of Liver Diseases-Infectious Diseases Society of America (AASLD-IDSA) HCV Guidance: Recommendations for Testing, Managing, and Treating Hepatitis C. www.hcvguidelines.org (accessed 2023 Dec 19).

Update on Prevention, Diagnosis, and Treatment of Chronic Hepatitis B: AASLD 2018 Hepatitis B Guidance. *Hepatology.* 2018;67(4):1560-1599.

Diagnosis and Treatment of Alcohol-Associated Liver Diseases: 2019 Practice Guidance From the American Association for the Study of Liver Diseases. *Hepatology.* 2020;71(1):306-333.

Diagnosis, Evaluation, and Management of Ascites, Spontaneous Bacterial Peritonitis and Hepatorenal Syndrome: 2021 Practice Guidance by the American Association for the Study of Liver Diseases. *Hepatology.* 2021;74(2):1014-1048.

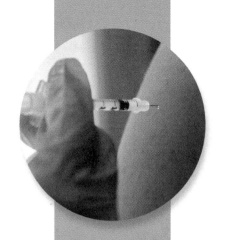
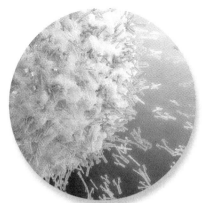
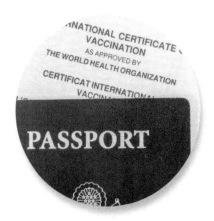

IMMUNIZATIONS & TRAVELERS

CONTENTS

CHAPTER CONTENT

CONTENT LEGEND

 = Study Tip Gal

 = Key Drug Guy

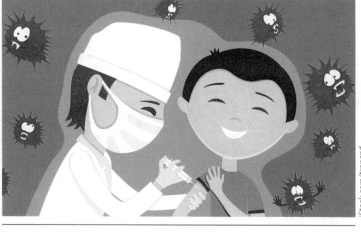

iStock.com/tronand

CHAPTER 20

IMMUNIZATIONS

BACKGROUND

Vaccines prevent patients from acquiring serious or potentially fatal diseases. Childhood diseases that used to be common (e.g., diphtheria, meningitis, polio, tetanus) are now rare because children are vaccinated or are protected by herd immunity (when vaccinated people protect the unvaccinated, making them less likely to become infected). If vaccination rates drop below 85% – 95%, vaccine-preventable diseases can become more prevalent and result in outbreaks.

VACCINE RESOURCES

- The FDA approves the indication for a vaccine based on the demonstrated safety and efficacy.

- The Advisory Committee on Immunization Practices (ACIP) provides the recommendations for vaccine administration in children and adults (i.e., who gets what vaccine and when).

- The Centers for Disease Control and Prevention (CDC) approves the ACIP recommendations and publishes them in the CDC's Morbidity and Mortality Weekly Report (MMWR) and The Pink Book (Epidemiology and Prevention of Vaccine-Preventable Diseases).

- Immunize.org provides vaccine information and education materials for healthcare professionals.

Reliable Vaccine Information for Patients

Vaccine Information Statements (VISs) are prepared by the CDC for each vaccine to explain their benefits and risks. Federal law requires that a VIS be handed to the patient (or parent) before a vaccination is administered. VISs can be found on the CDC website and Immunize.org.

VACCINES AND AUTISM

Some people believe that vaccines cause autism. The causes of autism are not fully understood, but there is no evidence that autism is caused by vaccines. Parents often first notice the behaviors of autism at an age when most childhood vaccine series are near completion (e.g., 18 – 24 months).

Thimerosal, a mercury-containing preservative used in some vaccines, was alleged to be contributing to the increase in autism since mercury has been linked to some brain disorders. There is no evidence that thimerosal poses a risk for autism. Thimerosal was removed from childhood vaccines in 2001, and the rates of autism have continued to increase. Thimerosal is contained in some multidose flu vaccines; parents may request a single-dose flu vaccine that does not contain a preservative, or a multidose vaccine without thimerosal.

IMMUNITY

The purpose of the immune system is to distinguish self substances (normal body parts/components) from non-self (foreign) substances, which are called antigens. When an antigen is detected, antibodies are produced to provide immunity and destroy the antigen. Immunoglobulin is the medical term for antibody.

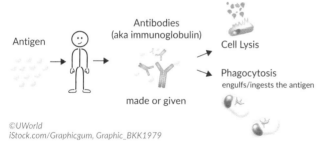

©UWorld
iStock.com/Graphicgum, Graphic_BKK1979

Immunity is acquired actively or passively. Active immunity develops when the person's own immune system produces antibodies to fight an infection or in response to vaccine administration. Passive immunity is acquired when antibodies are provided from someone else (see image to the right).

Active Immunity

When a person's own immune system creates antibodies (in response to a vaccine or infection). Lasts a long time, often a lifetime.

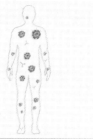

Passive Immunity

Received from someone else, such as receiving immunoglobulins (Ig) that are pooled from other people, or through transfer from a mother to baby.

Mother gives baby a copy of her immunoglobulins before birth. These provide short-term immunity until the child's own antibody production increases.

Intravenous immunoglobulin (IVIG) provides already made antibodies, and can be used for quick immunity after exposure to an antigen. For example, a person who is bitten by a rabid animal will receive the rabies vaccine (which will take time to work) and rabies immunoglobulin, to help the patient fight the rabies organism right away.

MaskaRad/Shutterstock.com
Juliia, Yulia Lazebnaya, grgroup/stock.adobe.com
iStock.com/Tatiana_Stulbo

TYPES OF VACCINES

Live attenuated (weakened) vaccines are produced by modifying a disease-producing ("wild") virus or bacterium; they have the ability to replicate (grow) and produce immunity but usually do not cause illness. Live attenuated vaccines are most similar to the actual disease and produce a strong immune response to the vaccine, but they are contraindicated in immunocompromised and pregnant patients since uncontrolled replication of the pathogen can occur.

Most inactivated vaccines are composed of either killed whole virus or bacterium, or fractions of either. Immunity resulting from an inactivated vaccine can diminish with time and supplemental (booster) doses may be required to increase immunity.

INACTIVATED VACCINES

Inactivated vaccines use the killed version of a wild virus or bacteria that causes the disease. Inactivated vaccines cannot replicate (and cause disease). They are less affected by circulating antibodies than live vaccines.*

Limitation: immunity is not as strong as with live vaccines; boosters may be required for ongoing immunity.

Polysaccharide, Conjugate and Recombinant Vaccines

Target a section of the organism, such as a protein, sugar, or capsid (outer casing).

Polysaccharide Vaccines

Polysaccharide (sugar) molecules are taken from the outside layer of encapsulated bacteria. Polysaccharide vaccines do not produce a good immune response in children < 2 years of age.

Ex: Pneumococcal Polysaccharide Vaccine (Pneumovax 23)

Conjugate Vaccines

Conjugate vaccines use polysaccharide (sugar) molecules from the outside layer of encapsulated bacteria and join the molecules to carrier proteins. Conjugation increases the immune response in infants, and the antibody response to multiple doses of vaccine.

Ex: Pneumococcal Conjugate Vaccine (Prevnar 20), Meningococcal Conjugate Vaccine (e.g., Menveo)

Recombinant Vaccines

A gene segment of a protein from the organism is inserted into the gene of another cell, such as a yeast cell, where it replicates.

Ex: Human Papillomavirus Vaccine (Gardasil 9), Recombinant Influenza Vaccine (Flublok Quadrivalent)

Toxoid Vaccines

The vaccine targets a toxin produced by the disease.

Ex: Diphtheria Toxoid Vaccine, Tetanus Toxoid Vaccine

mRNA Vaccines

The vaccine gives instructions to the body's cells (in the form of mRNA) to produce a protein specific to the pathogen, which then triggers an immune response.

Ex: select COVID-19 Vaccines

LIVE VACCINES

Live vaccines are most similar to the actual disease and provide a strong, long-lasting immune response.

Limitations: 1) Patients who are immunocompromised may not be able to halt replication; vaccination could cause the disease. 2) Circulating antibodies can interfere with vaccine replication.*

See the Key Drugs Guy for a list of common live vaccines.

*See the Live Vaccines and Antibodies section.

COMMON LIVE VACCINES

KEY DRUGS

MMR
Intranasal Influenza
Cholera
Rotavirus
Oral Typhoid
Varicella
Yellow Fever
Remember: **MICRO-VY**

Others:
Tuberculosis (BCG)
Dengue
Smallpox
Ebola

TIMING AND SPACING OF VACCINES

SIMULTANEOUS ADMINISTRATION

Most live and inactivated vaccines can be administered simultaneously (on the same day or at the same visit) without decreasing the antibody response or increasing the risk of adverse reactions (see the Study Tip Gal on the following page). Simultaneous administration of all vaccines for which a child is eligible is very important in childhood vaccination to improve compliance and increase the probability that a child will be fully immunized at the appropriate age. Combination vaccines help accomplish this with less injections.

VACCINES GIVEN IN A SERIES

Increasing the interval between the doses of a vaccine given in a series does not diminish the effectiveness of the vaccine after completion of the series, but it may delay complete protection. Decreasing the interval between doses of a vaccine can interfere with the antibody response and is generally avoided. In a few cases, the interval can be shortened for high-risk patients (e.g., between doses of two different pneumococcal vaccines in an immunocompromised patient).

LIVE VACCINES AND ANTIBODIES

Antibodies, in some blood and IVIG products, can interfere with live vaccine replication and a separation period may be required (see the Study Tip Gal on the following page). This is a concern with live vaccines because replication is required to produce an immune response.

The interval between an antibody-containing product and a measles, mumps and rubella-containing vaccine (MMR) or a varicella-containing vaccine (Varivax or MMRV) is a minimum of 3 months and can be up to 11 months. The specific product and dose determines the separation time.

Maternal antibodies passed from the mother to the baby before birth reduce the infant's response to live vaccines. Most live vaccines are therefore withheld until the child is 12 months of age, when the maternal antibodies will be depleted. An exception is live rotavirus vaccine, which is given to infants. It has been shown to be effective at preventing rotavirus-induced gastroenteritis despite the presence of maternal antibodies.

Inactivated vaccines can be given at any time. Inactivated vaccines are started when an infant is two months old, except for the hepatitis B vaccine series, which is started at birth.

LIVE VACCINES AND THE TB SKIN TEST

The tuberculin skin test (TST), also called a purified protein derivative (PPD) test, can be used to diagnose latent tuberculosis (TB). Live vaccines can cause a false negative TST result. Options to reduce this risk include:

1. Give the live vaccine on the same day as the TST.

2. Wait 4 weeks after a live vaccine to perform the TST.

3. Administer the TST first, wait ≥ 24 hours, then give the live vaccine.

VACCINE TIMING & SPACING

General Rules
- Vaccines can usually be given at the same time (same visit or same day).
- Multiple live vaccines can be given on the same day or (if not given on the same day) spaced 4 weeks apart.*
- If a vaccine series requires > 1 dose, the intervals between doses can be extended without restarting the series, but they should not be shortened in most cases.

Live Vaccines and Antibodies
- MMR and varicella-containing vaccines require separation from antibody-containing products (e.g., blood transfusions, IVIG). The recommended spacing is:
  - ❏ Vaccine → 2 weeks → antibody-containing product
  - ❏ Antibody-containing product → ≥ 3 months → vaccine
- Simultaneous administration of vaccine and antibody (in the form of immunoglobulin) is recommended for post-exposure prophylaxis of certain diseases (e.g., hepatitis A and B, rabies, tetanus).

*Exception: no separation is required for oral rotavirus or typhoid vaccines.

VACCINE ADVERSE REACTIONS

Reactions can range from local (e.g., soreness, redness, itching) to severe and life-threatening (e.g., anaphylaxis). Patients are screened for precautions and contraindications before vaccine administration to reduce the risk of severe reactions (see the Screening Prior to Vaccine Administration section on the following page).

The patient should be monitored for at least 15 minutes after vaccination (to watch for an allergic reaction, syncope, dizziness or falls). Adverse reactions that require some type of assistance should be reported to patient's healthcare provider and the FDA's Vaccine Adverse Event Reporting System (VAERS).

LOCAL REACTIONS

Local reactions occur at or near the injection site. These are common, more so with inactivated vaccines, and include pain, swelling and redness. Rarely, local reactions may be severe.

SYSTEMIC REACTIONS

Systemic reactions are less common than local reactions. They include fever, malaise, myalgia (muscle pain), headache, loss of appetite or a mild illness that has similarities to the disease being prevented, such as a few chickenpox vesicles after receiving the varicella vaccine. Patients who have experienced systemic symptoms after a flu shot might think (incorrectly) that the vaccine caused the flu. The flu shot is an inactivated (killed) vaccine and cannot cause disease.

With live vaccines, mild systemic reactions can occur 3 – 21 days after the vaccine is given (i.e., after an incubation period). Intranasal flu vaccine can replicate in the upper airways (nose and throat) and can cause mild cold-like symptoms, such as a runny nose.

True Allergic Reactions

True allergic reactions are uncommon, and can be caused by the vaccine itself or a component of the vaccine product, such as a stabilizer, preservative or antibiotic (used to inhibit bacterial growth). Minor allergic reactions will resolve quickly and can be treated with diphenhydramine or hydroxyzine. A minor reaction is not a contraindication to future vaccinations.

Severe allergic reactions are very rare (< 1 in 500,000 doses). A severe reaction with anaphylaxis can be life-threatening if not managed correctly (see section on the following page). Anaphylactic reactions are IgE-mediated and occur within 30 – 60 minutes of receiving the vaccine. Symptoms can include urticaria (hives), swelling of the mouth and throat, difficulty breathing, wheezing, abdominal cramping and hypotension or shock.

MANAGEMENT OF SEVERE ALLERGIC REACTIONS

All providers who administer vaccines must have emergency protocols and supplies to treat anaphylaxis. The primary healthcare provider should remain with the patient, assessing airway, breathing, circulation and level of consciousness. A second person should activate the emergency medical system (EMS) by calling 911.

Care should be provided until EMS arrives:

- For adults, administer aqueous epinephrine 1 mg/mL (1:1,000 dilution) intramuscularly, 0.01 mg/kg (maximum dose is 0.5 mg). Most pharmacies use prefilled epinephrine auto-injectors. At least three adult (0.3 mg) auto-injectors should be available. Most adults will require 1 – 3 doses administered every 5 – 15 minutes.

- Diphenhydramine can be given to reduce swelling and pruritus. Oral drugs should not be administered if airway swelling is present due to a risk of choking.

- The patient should be placed in a supine position (flat on the back), unless they have difficulty breathing. Elevating the head will help breathing, but caution must be taken to keep the blood pressure adequate. If the blood pressure is low, elevate the legs only. Monitor the blood pressure and pulse every 5 minutes.

- Provide cardiopulmonary resuscitation (CPR), if necessary. Immunizing pharmacists need current basic life support (BLS) certification.

- Record all vital signs and administered medications.

VACCINE CONTRAINDICATIONS AND PRECAUTIONS

There are specific circumstances when vaccines should not be given. Most precautions are temporary, and the vaccine can be given at a later time. For example, if the patient has a moderate or severe acute illness, vaccine administration should be delayed until it resolves. Mild acute illness is not a precaution, and the vaccine can be administered.

A contraindication is a condition that significantly increases the potential of a serious adverse reaction. Pregnancy and immunosuppression are two important contraindications to the use of live vaccines. Live vaccine administration must be timed carefully in patients who have recently received an antibody-containing blood product, as previously described. A severe or anaphylactic reaction following a vaccine dose is a contraindication to any subsequent doses of the same vaccine.

INVALID CONTRAINDICATIONS TO VACCINATION

Vaccinations may be given, if indicated, in the following situations:

- Mild acute illness (slight fever, mild diarrhea)

- Current antimicrobial treatment (there are some exceptions: see varicella, live influenza and oral typhoid vaccines)

- Previous mild-moderate local skin reaction from a vaccine

- Allergy to penicillin or products not in the vaccine

- Pregnancy (except live vaccines), breastfeeding, premature birth

- Recent tuberculin skin test (see text for timing and spacing with live vaccines only)

- Immunosuppressed person in the household, recent exposure to the disease or convalescence

- Family history of adverse events to the vaccine

SCREENING PRIOR TO VACCINE ADMINISTRATION

Use of a screening form rules out specific contraindications and precautions to the vaccine in adults. A "yes" response to some of these questions will indicate a type of vaccine to use, rather than a contraindication to all formulations (e.g., if a person has an allergy to thimerosal, then a single-dose vial or prefilled syringe may be required to avoid the preservative).

1. Are you sick today?

2. Do you have allergies to medications, food, a vaccine component or latex?

3. Have you ever had a serious reaction after receiving a vaccine?

4. Do you have a long-term health problem caused by heart disease, lung disease, kidney disease, metabolic disease (e.g., diabetes), anemia or other blood disorder?

5. Do you have cancer, leukemia, AIDS or any other immune system problem?

6. Do you take cortisone, prednisone, other steroids, anticancer drugs or have you had radiation treatments?

7. Have you ever had a seizure or nervous system problem?

8. During the past year, have you received a transfusion of blood or blood products, or been given immune (gamma) globulin or an antiviral drug?

9. For patients of child-bearing potential: are you pregnant or do you plan to become pregnant during the next month?

10. Have you received any vaccinations in the past 4 weeks?

Vaccine Contraindications and Precautions

VACCINE	CONTRAINDICATIONS	PRECAUTIONS
All vaccines	Severe allergic reaction (e.g., anaphylaxis) to a vaccine or vaccine component after a previous dose.	Illness: If a child or adult has only a mild illness (such as a cold), vaccines should be given (see the Study Tip Gal on the previous page). Treatment with antibiotics is not a valid reason to delay vaccines. If the person has a moderate or severe acute illness (regardless of antibiotic use) it is reasonable to delay vaccine administration until the condition has improved.
Live vaccines	Pregnancy (do not attempt to become pregnant until 4 weeks after receiving a live vaccine). Immunosuppression (see the Vaccinations for Specific Conditions/Populations chart on the following page).	Recent administration of an antibody-containing blood product (see the section on Live Vaccines and Antibodies).
Diphtheria, tetanus and pertussis vaccines	Pertussis-containing vaccines: encephalopathy (e.g., coma, decreased level of consciousness, prolonged seizures) that is not attributable to another cause within 7 days after receiving a previous pertussis-containing vaccine.	Guillain-Barré syndrome (GBS) within 6 weeks of a previous diphtheria, tetanus and/or pertussis vaccine. For DTaP and Tdap only: infantile spasms, uncontrolled seizures.
Hepatitis B vaccines Human papillomavirus vaccine (HPV)	Hypersensitivity to yeast.	
Influenza vaccines	Live attenuated influenza vaccine (LAIV4): pregnant, immunosuppressed, use of aspirin-containing products (children and adolescents), recent use of influenza antiviral medications (oseltamivir or zanamivir in the past 48 hours, peramivir in the last 5 days or baloxavir in the last 17 days), children age 2-4 years with asthma or a wheezing episode in the last 12 months, close contact with an immunosuppressed person.	All influenza vaccines: history of GBS within 6 weeks of a previous influenza vaccination. LAIV4: asthma in any patient age ≥ 5 years, underlying conditions that predispose to influenza complications (e.g., chronic lung, heart, renal, hepatic, neurologic, hematologic and metabolic disorders, including diabetes).
Recombinant zoster vaccine (RZV)		Pregnancy, breastfeeding: consider delaying vaccination.
Varicella vaccines	History of severe allergic reaction (e.g., anaphylaxis) to gelatin or neomycin.	Use of acyclovir, famciclovir or valacyclovir in the 24 hours before vaccination; avoid these antivirals for 14 days after vaccination.
Rotavirus vaccines	History of intussusception (when part of the intestine slides into an adjacent intestine part, blocking food/fluids).	Chronic gastrointestinal disease.
Yellow fever vaccine	Severe allergic reaction (e.g., anaphylaxis) to eggs.	
Latex present on vial stoppers and in prefilled syringes	Most latex sensitivities are a contact-type allergy, which does not prohibit vaccine administration; if the reaction to latex is severe (e.g., anaphylactic), avoid vaccine products packaged with latex.	

VACCINATIONS FOR SPECIFIC CONDITIONS/POPULATIONS

VACCINATIONS FOR SPECIAL GROUPS*

*An annual influenza vaccine is recommended for all special groups (age ≥ 6 months).

Infants and Children

- 3-dose hepatitis B vaccine started at birth
- RSV monoclonal antibody if mother was not vaccinated during pregnancy
- Other vaccine series start at age 2 months: PCV15 or PCV20, DTaP, Hib, polio, rotavirus
- Live vaccine series generally start at age ≥ 12 months, including: MMR, varicella
- No polysaccharide vaccines before age 2 years

Healthcare Professionals
—including pharmacists, nurses, physicians

- Annual influenza vaccine is usually required by employers
- Hepatitis B, varicella and MMR if there is no demonstrated immunity (by vaccination history or blood test)

Adolescents and Young Adults

- Meningococcal quadrivalent vaccine (MenACWY) (Menveo or MenQuadfi)
  - 2 doses: 1 dose at age 11-12 years and 1 dose at age 16 years
  - First-year college students in residential housing (if not previously vaccinated): 1 dose
- Human papillomavirus vaccine
  - Recommended at age 11-12 years
  - 2 or 3 doses (depending on age at start)
- Tdap: first dose at age 11-12 years

Sickle Cell Disease & Other Causes of Asplenia (Damaged/Missing Spleen)
—the spleen contains T-cells and B-cells; a damaged or missing spleen (e.g., splenectomy) causes a type of immunodeficiency

- *H. influenzae* type b (Hib) vaccine
- Pneumococcal vaccine (age 19-64 years), give one of the following regimens:
  - PCV20 x 1
  - PCV15 x 1, then PPSV23 x 1 ≥ 8 weeks later
- Meningococcal vaccines
  - Meningococcal quadrivalent vaccine (MenACWY) (Menveo or MenQuadfi)
  - Meningococcal serogroup B vaccine (MenB) (Bexsero or Trumenba)

Pregnancy

- Live vaccines are contraindicated
- Inactivated influenza vaccine, given in any trimester
- RSV vaccine (Abrysvo) administered if at weeks 32-36 during RSV season
- Tdap x 1 with each pregnancy (weeks 27-36, optimally)*

*To protect the infant from pertussis; also vaccinate others in close contact with the infant (e.g., father, grandparents, child-care providers), if not up-to-date.

Immunodeficiency
—called altered immunocompetence, immunosuppression or immunocompromise; caused by drugs or conditions**

- Live vaccines are contraindicated
- Pneumococcal vaccine (age 19-64 years), give one of the following regimens:
  - PCV20 x 1
  - PCV15 x 1, then PPSV23 x 1 ≥ 8 weeks later
- Herpes zoster vaccine (Shingrix): age ≥ 19 years, 2 doses, 2-6 months apart
- Additional vaccines for patients with HIV infection
  - Meningococcal quadrivalent vaccine (MenACWY) (Menveo or MenQuadfi)
  - Hepatitis A vaccine
  - Hepatitis B vaccine

Older Adults

- Herpes zoster vaccine (Shingrix): age ≥ 50 years, 2 doses, 2-6 months apart
- Pneumococcal vaccine (age ≥ 65 years), give one of the following regimens:
  - PCV20 x 1
  - PCV15 x 1, then PPSV23 x 1 ≥ 12 months later (or ≥ 8 weeks later if immunocompromised)

**Immunocompromising conditions:
- Chronic renal failure or nephrotic syndrome
- Malignancy
- HIV infection
- Solid organ transplant
- Treatment with immunosuppressive drugs [e.g., chemotherapy, TNF-alpha inhibitors, transplant medications, systemic steroids ≥ 14 days at doses equivalent to ≥ 20 mg (or 2 mg/kg) prednisone daily]

Diabetes

- Pneumococcal vaccine (age 19-64 years), give one of the following regimens:
  - PCV20 x 1
  - PCV15 x 1, then PPSV23 x 1 ≥ 12 months later (or ≥ 8 weeks later if immunocompromised)
- Hepatitis B: age ≥ 60 years (if not previously vaccinated)

VACCINATIONS FOR ADULTS

Influenza

Annually for all patients

Tdap, Td

Tdap x 1 if not received previously, then Td or Tdap every 10 years

Shingles

Shingrix:
All adults age ≥ 50 years or ≥ 19 years if immunosuppressed (or expected to become immunosuppressed)

2-dose series, with second dose given 2-6 months after the first dose (can shorten to 1-2 months if immunosuppressed)

Vaccinate even if patient previously had chickenpox or shingles or received *Zostavax*

Human Papillomavirus (HPV)

Adults ≤ 26 years who did not complete the HPV series*

*Can be given at age 27-45 years based on shared clinical decision making

Meningococcal

Serogroup B (MenB) vaccines *(Bexsero, Trumenba)*: give if complement component deficiency, taking eculizumab or ravulizumab, asplenia, microbiologist with exposure to *Neisseria meningitidis*, serogroup B meningococcal disease outbreak exposure

Quadrivalent conjugate (MenACWY) vaccines *(Menveo, MenQuadfi)*:
same groups as above, plus: HIV, travelers/residents to countries in which the disease is common, military recruits, first-year college students living in residential housing, if not up-to-date

Pneumococcal

Age 19-64 years with a specific medical condition* or age ≥ 65 years (if never received before): PCV20 x 1 or PCV15 x 1 followed by PPSV23 ≥ 12 months later (or ≥ 8 weeks later if immunocompromised)

*Alcohol use disorder, cigarette smoking, diabetes, chronic heart, lung or liver disease, sickle cell disease/asplenia, HIV infection, malignancy, solid organ transplant, chronic renal failure, taking immunosuppressive drugs (e.g., chemotherapy, long-term systemic steroids)

Hepatitis B

If not previously vaccinated, all adults age 19-59 years and patients ≥ 60 years with risk factors, including chronic liver disease, HIV infection, exposure via sexual activity (e.g., men who have sex with men, multiple sex partners), IV drug use, incarcerated, travel to an endemic area, blood exposure (e.g., healthcare personnel, diabetes, dialysis)

Give alone or with hepatitis A vaccine *(Twinrix)*

Hepatitis A

Adults traveling to an endemic area, household members and other close contacts of adopted children newly arriving from countries with moderate-high infection risk, liver disease, hemophilia, men who have sex with men, illicit drug use, people experiencing homelessness, HIV

Give alone or with hepatitis B vaccine *(Twinrix)*

ROUTINE VACCINES

VACCINE	ADMINISTRATION RECOMMENDATIONS	STORAGE/ADMINISTRATION
COVID-19 Vaccines Patients should receive the updated formulations of the vaccine designed to protect against the most likely circulating variants.		
mRNA Vaccines: *Comirnaty* (Pfizer-BioNTech) *Spikevax* (Moderna) Protein Subunit Vaccine: Novavax COVID-19 Vaccine	**Age ≥ 12 Years (Not Moderately or Severely Immunocompromised)** If previously unvaccinated: 1 dose of Moderna or Pfizer-BioNTech or a 2-dose series of Novavax (given at 0 and 3-8 weeks). If previously vaccinated: 1 dose of any vaccine administered at least 8 weeks after the most recent COVID-19 vaccine. **Age < 12 Years or Immunocompromised** Consult the CDC website for guidance on recommended vaccines and schedules for the primary series and subsequent boosters.	Storage varies by product. Give IM.
Diphtheria Toxoid-, Tetanus Toxoid- and acellular Pertussis-Containing Vaccines The pediatric formulations (with the upper-case D, as in DTaP) have 3-5 times more diphtheria component than the adult formulations. The adult formulations have a lower-case d (Tdap or Td).		
DTaP: *Daptacel, Infanrix* DTaP-IPV: *Kinrix, Quadracel* **DTaP-HepB-IPV: *Pediarix*** DTaP-IPV / Hib: *Pentacel* DTaP-IPV-Hib-HepB: *Vaxelis* Td: *Tenivac, TDVax* **Tdap: *Adacel, Boostrix***	**DTaP** A routine childhood vaccine series; 5 doses given at age 2, 4, 6, 15-18 months and 4-6 years. For children younger than 7 years of age. **Td or Tdap** Tdap booster typically given at age 11-12 years. Routine booster given every 10 years in adults. Otherwise recommended for: 1. Pregnant people in the third trimester of each pregnancy (see Vaccinations for Specific Conditions/Populations) to prevent pertussis in infants < 2 months of age. 2. Close contacts of infants younger than age 12 months (e.g., parent, grandparent, child-care provider), if not up-to-date. 3. Healthcare personnel with direct patient contact, if not up-to-date. 4. Wound prophylaxis, if deep or dirty wounds and it has been more than 5 years since the last Td or Tdap dose. Tetanus immunoglobulin (TIG) may be required if no previous tetanus vaccines have been given.	Store in the refrigerator. Do not freeze. Shake the prefilled syringe or vial before use. Give IM.
***Haemophilus influenzae* Type B (Hib)-Containing Vaccines**		
Hib: *ActHIB, Hiberix, PedvaxHIB* DTaP-IPV / Hib: *Pentacel* DTaP-IPV-Hib-HepB: *Vaxelis*	Hib: a routine childhood vaccine series given between ages 2-15 months. *ActHIB* and *Hiberix* are 4-dose series, *PedvaxHIB* is a 3-dose series. Given to adults with asplenia.	Store in the refrigerator. Do not freeze. Shake the prefilled syringe or vial before use. Give IM.

VACCINE	ADMINISTRATION RECOMMENDATIONS	STORAGE/ADMINISTRATION
Hepatitis-Containing Vaccines		
Hepatitis A: *Havrix, Vaqta* **Hepatitis B:** *Engerix-B, Heplisav-B, Recombivax HB, PreHevbrio* *Engerix-B* and *Recombivax HB:* available in pediatric and adult strengths *Heplisav-B* and *PreHevbrio:* for age ≥ 18 years only; do not use in pregnancy High-dose *Recombivax HB* (40 mcg/mL) is indicated for dialysis patients Hepatitis A and B: *Twinrix* **DTaP-HepB-IPV:** *Pediarix* DTaP-IPV-Hib-HepB: *Vaxelis*	**Hepatitis A** Children: a routine childhood vaccine series; 2 doses given at age 12-23 months (minimal interval between doses is 6 months). Adults: men who have sex with men, illicit drug use, <u>chronic liver disease</u>, people experiencing homelessness, HIV infection, travelers to an endemic area, anyone else who wants it. **Hepatitis B** Children: a routine childhood vaccine series started <u>within 24 hours after birth</u>; 3 doses given at age 0, 1-2 and 6-18 months. Adults (if not previously vaccinated): <u>all age 19-59 years or those ≥ 60 years</u> with <u>risk factors</u>, including <u>chronic liver disease, HIV infection, blood exposure</u> (e.g., <u>healthcare workers, dialysis, diabetes</u>), IV drug use, sexual exposure risk (e.g., men who have sex with men, multiple sex partners), incarcerated people, travel to an endemic area. *Engerix-B, Recombivax HB* and *PreHevbrio:* 3-dose series given at months 0, 1 and 6 (can be completed in 4 months if necessary, but may require a booster at 1 year if the series is accelerated). *Heplisav-B:* 2-dose series given at months 0 and 1. **Hepatitis A and B** 3-dose series given at months 0, 1 and 6; can be completed faster if needed prior to travel to high-risk areas.	Store in the refrigerator. Do not freeze. Shake the vial or prefilled syringe before use. Give IM.
Human Papillomavirus Vaccine <u>Prevents cervical</u>, vulvar, vaginal, oropharyngeal, penile and anal <u>cancers</u>, and <u>genital warts</u>.		
HPV9 (9-Valent): *Gardasil 9*	**Age 9-26 Years*** <u>Recommended age: 11-12 years</u> (may be started at age 9**). Use is contraindicated with a severe yeast allergy. **Regimens** If started <u>before age 15</u> → <u>2 doses</u> (at months 0 and 6-12) If started at <u>age 15 or older</u>, or if immunocompromised → <u>3 doses</u> (at months 0, 1-2 and 6)	Store in refrigerator. Do not freeze. Shake the prefilled syringe or vial before use. Give IM. Caution for fainting (although incidence is similar to other vaccines); administer to seated patient and monitor after vaccination.

*Recommended by ACIP for anyone ≤ 26 years, and for some adults age 27-45 years per clinical shared decision making.
**Start at age 9 years in anyone with a history of sexual abuse.

INFLUENZA VACCINES

Influenza (the flu) is one of the <u>most common vaccine-preventable illnesses in the U.S.</u> Influenza A and B are the two types of influenza viruses that cause epidemic disease. Influenza A virus has subtypes based on the two surface antigens, hemagglutinin and neuraminidase. Immunity to the surface antigens reduces the likelihood of infection, and severity of disease if infection occurs.

The <u>influenza vaccine</u> is given <u>annually</u>. The vaccine changes every year to account for antigenic drift, which causes variations in the virus. More dramatic antigenic changes, or shifts, occur approximately every 30 years and can result in the emergence of a novel influenza virus, with the potential to cause a pandemic.

Influenza vaccination helps prevent complications due to influenza illness, which can exacerbate underlying medical conditions (e.g., pulmonary or cardiac disease) and lead to secondary bacterial pneumonia or primary influenza viral pneumonia. Vaccination also reduces hospitalizations and death, which are more common in people with comorbid conditions or those age < 5 years or ≥ 65 years. See the Infectious Diseases III chapter for a discussion on the signs and symptoms of influenza and treatment with antiviral medications. See the <u>Study Tip Gal</u> to the right for important details about influenza vaccines.

INFLUENZA VACCINE TIPS

RECOMMENDED ANNUALLY

All patients age ≥ 6 months, unless contraindicated.

All brand names have **FLU** in the name (e.g., A*flu*ria, **Flu**zone).

SPECIFIC PATIENT CONSIDERATIONS

- **Age 6 months to 8 years (not previously vaccinated)**
  - ❑ Give 2 doses (4 weeks apart).
- **Patients with an egg allergy**
  - ❑ Can receive any age-appropriate influenza vaccine, even if severe allergy symptoms (e.g., wheezing requiring epinephrine). No additional observation period is recommended (beyond the required 15 minutes).
  - ❑ Egg-free products include *Flublok* (approved for age ≥ 18 years only) and *Flucelvax* (approved for age ≥ 6 months).
- **Pregnant patients**
  - ❑ Can receive any age-appropriate inactivated influenza vaccine. Do not administer the live influenza vaccine (*FluMist*).
- **Preferred for patients age ≥ 65 years**
  - ❑ *Fluzone High-Dose, Fluad* or *Flublok.*

VACCINE	ADMINISTRATION RECOMMENDATIONS	STORAGE/ADMINISTRATION
Influenza Vaccines Key differences between <u>quadrivalent</u> vaccines (protect against two influenza A's and two influenza B's) include whether the virus is <u>inactivated</u> (IIV4) or <u>live attenuated</u> (LAIV4), the route (IM, intranasal), the antigen dose or the presence of adjuvant.		
Quadrivalent Inactivated Influenza Vaccines (IIV4) ■ *Afluria* Quadrivalent, **Fluarix** Quadrivalent, **FluLaval** Quadrivalent, **Fluzone** Quadrivalent: approved for age ≥ 6 months ■ **Flucelvax** Quadrivalent (grown in cell culture, ccIIV4, <u>egg-free</u>): approved for age ≥ 6 months ■ *Flublok* Quadrivalent (recombinant inactivated vaccine, RIV4, <u>egg-free</u>): approved for age ≥ 18 years ■ **Fluzone High-Dose** Quadrivalent, **Fluad** Quadrivalent: approved for <u>age ≥ 65 years</u> **Quadrivalent Live Attenuated Influenza Vaccine (LAIV4)** ■ **FluMist** Quadrivalent: approved for <u>healthy people age 2-49 years</u>	**Vaccine Timing** <u>Give vaccine as soon as it is available</u> (preferably before October but individuals should still be vaccinated later in the season). Outbreaks usually peak by February. **Live Attenuated Vaccine** LAIV4 is indicated for healthy patients age 2-49 years. Do <u>not</u> use if <u>pregnant</u> or <u>immunocompromised</u>, or if influenza medications were recently taken (oseltamivir or zanamivir within past 48 hours, peramivir in the past 5 days or baloxavir in the past 17 days). See the previous table with vaccine contraindications and precautions for details.	Store in the refrigerator. Do not freeze. Administer <u>IM except *FluMist* Quadrivalent</u>, which is given intranasally as 0.2 mL, divided between the <u>two nostrils</u>. *Fluzone High-Dose Quadrivalent, Fluad Quadrivalent* and *Flublok Quadrivalent* are preferred in patients age ≥ 65 years. *Afluria Quadrivalent*: can be given with a needle-free jet injector.

VACCINE	ADMINISTRATION RECOMMENDATIONS	STORAGE/ADMINISTRATION
Measles, Mumps and Rubella-Containing Vaccines (Live Attenuated)		
MMR: _M-M-R II_, _Priorix_ **MMRV** (MMR + Varicella): **_ProQuad_**	Children: a routine vaccine series; 2 doses given at age 12-15 months and 4-6 years. _ProQuad_: indicated for patients age 12 months-12 years. Adults: 1 dose if no evidence of immunity. Give 1-2 doses (4 weeks apart), if no evidence of immunity, to: healthcare workers, HIV patients with a CD4 count ≥ 200 cells/mm³ for at least 6 months, nonpregnant patients of childbearing age (if no evidence of immunity to rubella), international travelers, household contacts of immunocompromised people and students in postsecondary educational institutions. Do not use in pregnancy or if immunocompromised. Adults born before 1957 are generally considered immune to measles and mumps.	_M-M-R II_: store in the refrigerator or freezer. _Priorix_: store in the refrigerator. MMRV: store in the freezer (due to the varicella component). Store diluents at room temperature or in the refrigerator. Give SC; _M-M-R II_ and _ProQuad_ may be given IM.
Meningococcal Vaccines Quadrivalent meningococcal conjugate vaccines (MCV4) include serogroups A, C, W and Y (MenACWY). Serogroup B (MenB) is available in a separate vaccine or in combination with A, C, W and Y (i.e., MenABCWY, a pentavalent conjugate vaccine).		
MenACWY **_MenQuadfi_:** for age ≥ 2 years **_Menveo_:** for age 2 months-55 years (can be used in adults age ≥ 56 years, if needed)	**Routine Vaccination** Adolescents: 2-dose series given at age 11-12 years and 16 years. **Special Populations at High Risk** Travelers to certain countries, such as the African meningitis belt. Proof of vaccination is required by Saudi Arabia for travel to the Hajj and Umrah pilgrimages. Age 2 months and older with asplenia/sickle cell disease, HIV infection, complement component deficiencies or use of eculizumab or ravulizumab. Lab workers with _N. meningitidis_ exposure. First-year college students living in residential housing, if not up-to-date. Military recruits. The number of doses and timing (intervals) will depend on age and specific risk. People with ongoing risk of meningococcal disease should be revaccinated every 5 years.	Store in the refrigerator. Do not freeze. Give IM. _Menveo_: both vials (the powder and the liquid) contain vaccine; use only the supplied liquid for reconstitution.
MenB: _Bexsero, Trumenba_ **MenABCWY: _Penbraya_** For age 10-25 years (can administer MenABCWY when vaccination against all serogroups is indicated at the same visit)	**Age ≥ 10 Years at High Risk** Asplenia/sickle cell disease, complement component deficiencies or use of eculizumab or ravulizumab. Lab workers with _N. meningitidis_ exposure. During an outbreak. _Bexsero, Penbraya_: 2 doses (given 1 month apart). _Trumenba_: 2 doses (given 6 months apart). If high risk of meningococcal disease or during an outbreak: give 3 doses (at months 0, 1-2 and 6). **Not at High Risk** Optional for patients age 16-23 years who want the vaccine (if given, the preferred age is 16-18 years).	Store in the refrigerator. Do not freeze. Give IM. _Penbraya_: the prefilled syringe contains MenB and the vial contains MenACWY; use of both components is required.

PNEUMOCOCCAL VACCINES

The bacteria *S. pneumoniae*, referred to as pneumococcus, is the most common cause of otitis media, pneumonia, meningitis and bloodstream infections in children. Adults age 65 years and older and those with certain chronic conditions or altered immunocompetence are also at increased risk of pneumococcal disease. As you learn the pneumococcal vaccine recommendations, keep these key concepts in mind:

- There are two recommended pneumococcal conjugate vaccines, PCV15 *(Vaxneuvance)* and PCV20 *(Prevnar 20)*, and one polysaccharide vaccine, PPSV23 *(Pneumovax 23)*.

- Children age < 5 years receive PCV15 *(Vaxneuvance)* or PCV20 *(Prevnar 20)* as part of routine childhood vaccinations.

  ❏ Young children (< 2 years) should not receive *Pneumovax 23* because they do not produce an adequate antibody response to polysaccharide vaccines.

- Adults should receive either PCV20 *(Prevnar 20)* alone, or PCV15 *(Vaxneuvance)* followed by PPSV23 *(Pneumovax 23)*. The recommended age of administration in adults is based on the presence of underlying medical conditions (see table below).

VACCINE	ADMINISTRATION RECOMMENDATIONS	STORAGE/ADMINISTRATION
Pneumococcal Vaccines		
Conjugate Vaccines: **Prevnar 20 (PCV20)** **Vaxneuvance (PCV15)**	Children: a routine childhood vaccine series; 4 doses of PCV15 or PCV20 given at age 2, 4, 6 and 12-15 months. **Adults (if never received before) age 19-64 years with specific medical conditions (see below) or age ≥ 65 years** PCV20 x 1 or PCV15 x 1 followed by PPSV23 x 1 ≥ 12 months later (PPSV23 may be given ≥ 8 weeks later if immunocompromised) Specific medical conditions: alcohol use disorder, cigarette smoking, diabetes, chronic heart, lung or liver disease, an immunocompromised state [includes sickle cell disease/asplenia, HIV infection, malignancy, solid organ transplant, chronic renal failure, taking immunosuppressive drugs (e.g., chemotherapy, long-term systemic steroids)] **Other Scenarios** Patients who previously received PCV13 or PPSV23: consult the CDC recommendations for guidance on additional pneumococcal vaccine doses that may be recommended.	Store in the refrigerator. Do not freeze. Shake the vial or prefilled syringe prior to use. PCV15, PCV20: give IM. PPSV23: give IM or SC.
Polysaccharide Vaccine: **Pneumovax 23 (PPSV23)**	Children age 2-18 years: indicated after PCV15 or PCV20 series completion in patients with select medical conditions. Adults: indicated after PCV15 (see above).	

VACCINE	ADMINISTRATION RECOMMENDATIONS	STORAGE/ADMINISTRATION
Poliovirus-Containing Vaccines Only inactivated poliovirus vaccine (IPV) is available in the U.S. Oral polio vaccine (live attenuated) may be administered in other countries.		
IPV: *IPOL* DTaP-IPV: *Kinrix, Quadracel* **DTaP-HepB-IPV:** *Pediarix* DTaP-IPV / Hib: *Pentacel* DTaP-IPV-Hib-HepB: *Vaxelis*	A routine childhood vaccine series; 4 doses given at age 2, 4, 6-18 months and 4-6 years.	Store in the refrigerator. Do not freeze. Shake the prefilled syringe or vial before use. IPV: give IM or SC.
Rotavirus Vaccines (Live Attenuated)		
RV1: *Rotarix* RV5: *RotaTeq*	A routine infant vaccine series. Do not initiate the series after age 15 weeks. *Rotarix:* 2 doses at age 2 and 4 months. *RotaTeq:* 3 doses at age 2, 4 and 6 months.	Store in the refrigerator. Do not freeze. Give orally.
Respiratory Syncytial Virus (RSV) Vaccines and Antibodies Prevents RSV-associated lower respiratory tract disease during RSV season in high-risk populations.		
RSV Vaccines: *Abrysvo*, *Arexvy* **RSV Monoclonal Antibodies:** **Nirsevimab** *(Beyfortus)* **Palivizumab** *(Synagis)*	**RSV Vaccine** Pregnant people 32-36 weeks gestation during RSV season (September-January): administer 1 dose of *Abrysvo* to prevent RSV in infants < 6 months old. Adults age ≥ 60 years at increased risk (COPD, asthma, heart failure, kidney or liver disease, diabetes, immunocompromised, residence in a long-term care facility): option (per clinical shared decision making) to administer 1 dose of *Abrysvo* or *Arexvy*. **RSV Monoclonal Antibody** Neonates and infants age < 8 months born during or entering their first RSV season: administer 1 dose of nirsevimab (if mother not vaccinated during pregnancy). Palivizumab is reserved for premature infants and infants at highest risk of hospitalization due to RSV infection (see the Pediatric Conditions chapter).	Store vaccines and antibodies in the refrigerator. Do not freeze. Give IM.
Varicella- and Zoster-Containing Vaccines Varicella virus-containing vaccines are live attenuated vaccines. *Shingrix* is a recombinant (not live) zoster vaccine.		
Varicella Virus Vaccine **(for chickenpox):** *Varivax* **MMRV:** *ProQuad* **Zoster Virus Vaccine** **(for herpes zoster/shingles):** *Shingrix*	*Varivax* A routine childhood vaccine series; 2 doses, given at age 12-15 months and 4-6 years. Any adolescent or adult without evidence of immunity to varicella: give 2 doses. Do not use in pregnancy or if immunocompromised. Some antivirals (e.g., acyclovir, valacyclovir, famciclovir) can interfere with *Varivax* (live vaccine). Stop 24 hours before vaccine administration and do not take for 14 days after vaccination. *Shingrix* All adults age ≥ 50 years or adults age ≥ 19 years who are or will be immunosuppressed: 2 doses given at months 0 and 2-6 (2nd dose may be given at month 1-2 if immunocompromised). Vaccinate even if the patient has previously received *Varivax* or *Zostavax* (live zoster vaccine no longer available) or has a history of zoster infection, since recurrence is possible.	*Varivax* Store vaccine in the freezer. Store the diluent in the refrigerator or at room temperature. Reconstitute immediately upon removal from the freezer and administer within 30 minutes. Do not give if there is a hypersensitivity to gelatin or neomycin. Give SC or IM. *Shingrix* Store vaccine and adjuvant liquid in the refrigerator. Do not freeze. Give IM.

NON-ROUTINE VACCINES

The vaccines in the table below are administered only when there is exposure or risk of exposure to a particular infectious pathogen. For the majority, the risk is incurred when traveling to a high-risk area.

DRUG	ADMINISTRATION RECOMMENDATIONS	STORAGE/ADMINISTRATION
Rabies vaccine: *RabAvert, Imovax Rabies*	Prevention when there is a high risk of exposure (e.g., animal handlers, traveling to a high risk area): 2 doses. Post-exposure (with previous vaccination): 2 doses. Post-exposure (without previous vaccination): 4 doses plus 1 dose of rabies immune globulin (RIG) with the first vaccine dose.	Store in the refrigerator. Reconstitute with the provided diluent. Give IM.
Typhoid vaccine: *Vivotif* (live vaccine) Oral *Typhim Vi* (inactivated polysaccharide vaccine) Injection	To prevent typhoid fever caused by *Salmonella typhi* (see the Travelers chapter for disease information). Oral: take 1 capsule PO on alternate days (days 0, 2, 4 and 6). Complete at least 1 week prior to possible exposure. Give every 5 years if continued risk or exposure. Injection: give 1 dose at least 2 weeks prior to possible exposure. Give every 2 years if continued risk or exposure.	Oral capsules: store in the refrigerator. Take on an empty stomach (1 hour before a meal) with cold or lukewarm water. Injection: store in the refrigerator. Do not freeze. Give IM.
Japanese encephalitis virus vaccine: *Ixiaro*	Give if spending ≥ 1 month in endemic areas during transmission season, especially if travel will include rural areas. Give 2 doses, 28 days apart. Complete at least 1 week prior to potential exposure (see the Travelers chapter for disease information).	Store in the refrigerator. Do not freeze. Give IM.
Tuberculosis Bacille Calmette-Guérin (BCG) vaccine Live vaccine	Not used in the U.S. Given to infants and children in countries with higher TB incidence.	Can cause a positive reaction to the TB skin test (see the Infectious Diseases II chapter).
Dengue vaccine: *Dengvaxia* Live vaccine	Give to people age 9-16 years who have previously tested positive for dengue infection and live in endemic areas. Not indicated for primary prevention. Give 3 doses at months 0, 6 and 12.	Store in the refrigerator. Reconstitute with the provided diluent; swirl, do not shake. Give SC.
Yellow fever vaccine: *YF-VAX* Live vaccine	Give to those who travel to, or live in, areas of risk and to travelers to countries that require vaccination (see the Travelers chapter). Contraindicated with a severe (life-threatening) allergy to eggs or gelatin, immunosuppression, age < 6 months or breastfeeding. Avoid donating blood for 2 weeks after receiving the vaccine. The International Certificate of Vaccination (yellow card) is provided and is valid for 10 years, starting 10 days after vaccination. It may be required to enter endemic areas.	Store in the refrigerator. Reconstitute with the provided diluent; swirl, do not shake. Give SC.
Cholera vaccine: *Vaxchora* Live vaccine	Give to people age 2-64 years who are traveling to an area of active toxigenic *Vibrio cholerae* transmission. Give 1 oral dose ≥ 10 days prior to exposure.	Store the packet for reconstitution in the refrigerator. Dissolve the buffer packet in 100 mL of cold or room temperature water, then add the active component packet; stir for 30 seconds and drink within 30 minutes on an empty stomach.
Smallpox and monkeypox vaccine: *Jynneos* Live vaccine	Give to adults age ≥ 18 years who are at high risk for infection. Give 2 doses, four weeks apart.	Keep frozen. Allow vaccine to thaw and reach room temperature before use. Swirl for at least 30 seconds. Give SC; may be administered intradermally during supply shortages (less volume needed per dose).

STORAGE

Vaccines should be stored on the shelves of refrigerator or freezer units designed for storing biologics (including vaccines); household freezer units or dormitory-style combined refrigerator/freezer units should not be used. Rotate stock, so vaccines and diluents with the earliest expiration date are used first.

Keep vaccines in the original packaging (box) until use; some vaccines require protection from light. Never place vaccines in the doors of the freezer or the refrigerator as the temperature there is unstable.

Measure refrigerator and freezer temperatures (using a buffered temperature probe) and document at least twice each workday (e.g., in the morning and before the end of the workday). Keep temperature logs for 3 years (or longer, as required by individual states).

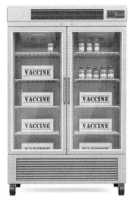

Staff can easily confuse the vaccines within the storage unit. Use labels and separate containers.

VACCINE STORAGE REQUIREMENTS

- Most vaccines are stored in the refrigerator.
- Some vaccines (e.g., varicella, MMRV) should be stored in the freezer.
- M-M-R II is stored either in the refrigerator or freezer.

- Some vaccines require reconstitution before use. The diluents supplied with varicella, MMR and MMRV vaccines can be stored in the refrigerator or at room temperature.
- Reconstituted vaccines should be used shortly after preparation.

ADMINISTRATION

ROUTES OF ADMINISTRATION

IM ONLY	SC ONLY	IM OR SC	INTRANASAL	PO
Most vaccines	Yellow fever, dengue, smallpox and monkeypox*	M-M-R II, MMRV, varicella, PPSV23, IPV	*FluMist* Quadrivalent	Typhoid (*Vivotif*) capsules Oral solutions: cholera and rotavirus

Smallpox and monkeypox vaccine can be administered intradermally, if needed during supply shortages (less volume required per dose).

ADMINISTRATION TECHNIQUE

- Never mix vaccines in the same syringe.
- IM: use a 22 – 25 gauge needle. Inject at a 90-degree angle.
  - Adults: inject into the deltoid muscle above the level of the armpit and below the shoulder joint.
  - Infants: inject into the anterolateral mid-thigh muscle.
  - IM needle length: per ACIP guidelines, a 1 inch needle is acceptable for most adults; for males > 260 pounds or females > 200 pounds, a 1.5 inch needle is recommended.

- SC: use a 23 – 25 gauge, 5/8" needle at a 45-degree angle. Adults: inject into the fatty tissue over the triceps. Infants: inject into the thigh.

IMMUNIZATION INFORMATION SYSTEMS

Immunization information systems are computerized databases that collect vaccination histories and help ensure correct and timely immunizations, especially for children. They are useful for healthcare providers, who can use the registries to obtain the patient's history, produce vaccine records and manage vaccine inventories, among other benefits. They help to identify groups who are not receiving vaccines in order to target outreach efforts. Some systems are able to notify patients if vaccines are needed. Where allowed, pharmacists should strive to report all vaccines administered to their state or local registry.

Select Guidelines/References

CDC Vaccine and Immunization websites: https://www.cdc.gov/vaccines, https://www.cdc.gov/vaccines/hcp/acip-recs/ and https://www.cdc.gov/travel (accessed 2023 Dec 4). The pediatric and adult schedules are updated annually and published in January.

The CDC's Pink Book, Epidemiology and Prevention of Vaccine Preventable Diseases (published every 2 years). https://www.cdc.gov/vaccines/pubs/pinkbook/index.html (accessed 2023 Dec 4).

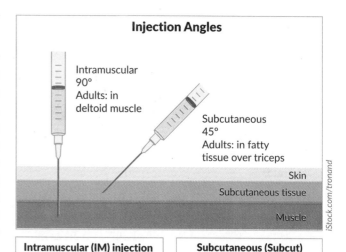

Injection Angles

Intramuscular
90°
Adults: in deltoid muscle

Subcutaneous
45°
Adults: in fatty tissue over triceps

Skin
Subcutaneous tissue
Muscle

iStock.com/tronand

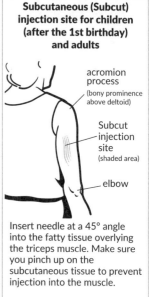

Intramuscular (IM) injection site for children and adults

level of armpit

acromion process
(bony prominence above deltoid)

IM injection site
(shaded area)

elbow

Give in the central and thickest portion of the deltoid muscle – above the level of the armpit and approximately 2-3 fingerbreadths (~2") below the acromion process. See the diagram. To avoid causing an injury, do not inject too high (near the acromion process) or too low.

Subcutaneous (Subcut) injection site for children (after the 1st birthday) and adults

acromion process
(bony prominence above deltoid)

Subcut injection site
(shaded area)

elbow

Insert needle at a 45° angle into the fatty tissue overlying the triceps muscle. Make sure you pinch up on the subcutaneous tissue to prevent injection into the muscle.

© http://www.immunize.org/catg.d/p2020.pdf

CONTENT LEGEND

 = Study Tip Gal

 = Key Drug Guy

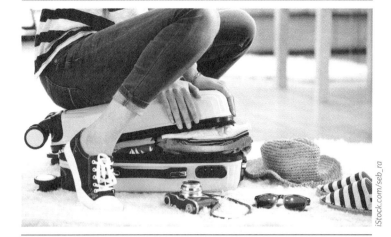

iStock.com/seb_ra

CHAPTER 21
TRAVELERS

BACKGROUND

A traveler's risk for contracting disease is assessed based upon travel duration, destination-specific risks, itinerary and patient-specific health concerns. Pharmacists assist travelers by providing formal advice, travel vaccines, malaria prophylaxis and other medications prior to travel. Consultative services provided by pharmacists can include educational awareness of country-specific risks, and ways to prevent and address them.

Travelers should have a list of their medical conditions and medications (prescription and OTC). Travel vaccinations should be documented on the International Certificate of Vaccination or Prophylaxis (ICVP) card, sometimes called the "yellow card." Prescription medications should be stored in the original prescription containers. Medications and medical supplies should be packed in carry-on luggage.

When preparing a patient for travel, healthcare professionals should consider: 1) diseases spread through food and water, 2) diseases spread through blood and bodily fluids and 3) diseases transmitted by insects. CDC's Health Information for International Travel (the "Yellow Book") is available on the CDC website and contains travel health information, including travel health insurance recommendations. Travel advisories and visa requirements can be checked on the U.S. State Department website.

DISEASES TRANSMITTED THROUGH CONTAMINATED FOOD AND WATER

Contaminated food and water cause many travel-related illnesses. Many international travel destinations (especially developing countries) vary in the availability of clean water, plumbing and refrigeration. These factors can lead to unsafe food handling practices and food and water contamination with fecal matter, leading to an increased risk of illness.

TRAVELERS' DIARRHEA

Travelers' diarrhea (TD) is the most common travel-related illness, occurring in 30 – 70% of travelers, depending on the destination and season. Areas of highest risk include most of Asia, the Middle East, Africa, Mexico and Central and South America. TD presents with acute symptoms ranging from mild cramps and frequent loose stools to severe abdominal pain, fever and vomiting. Severity is determined based on the impact on the patient and can be mild, moderate or severe. The severity also determines the initial treatment (see Study Tip Gal on the following page). If blood is mixed in with the stool, it is classified as dysentery, which is often accompanied by systemic symptoms such as fever. Dysentery is classified as severe.

Symptoms usually begin within 6 – 72 hours if caused by a bacterial or viral pathogen. More than 80% of TD cases are bacterial. The primary pathogen is *E. coli*, followed by *Campylobacter jejuni*, *Shigella* species and *Salmonella* species. Untreated bacterial diarrhea can last 3 – 7 days, and some pathogens can cause invasive infections outside of the GI tract. Persistent TD, defined as diarrhea lasting ≥ 14 days, is more likely to occur with certain bacterial and protozoal pathogens and requires additional testing.

TD Prevention

Safe food and water habits can reduce, but do not eliminate, the risk of TD. The rule "boil it, cook it, peel it or forget it" is helpful when discussing food safety. These food and water precautions can be recommended:

- Eat only food that is cooked and served hot. Avoid food that has been sitting on a buffet.
- Eat raw fruits and vegetables only if washed in clean water or peeled (e.g., oranges).
- Use bottled water or boil for approximately one minute before drinking or using to brush teeth. Avoid ice.
- Eating at well-known restaurants can help reduce risk. Poor hygiene practices can increase the risk of contracting TD.
- Keep hands clean and out of the mouth. Wash hands often with soap and water, especially after using the bathroom and before eating. If soap and water are not available, use an alcohol-based hand sanitizer.

Prophylaxis with bismuth subsalicylate (BSS), the active ingredient of *Pepto-Bismol*, reduces the incidence of TD by ~50%. Do not use BSS in patients with an aspirin allergy, pregnancy, renal insufficiency, gout, ulcer, or anyone taking anticoagulants, probenecid or methotrexate. Taking BSS with aspirin or other salicylates can cause salicylate toxicity. BSS is FDA-approved for OTC use in children ≥ 12 years old, but has been used off-label in younger children (≥ 3 years old) as long as they have had no recent or current viral infections (due to the risk of Reye's syndrome). BSS tablets or liquid can be recommended as prophylaxis in any appropriate traveler.

Antibiotic prophylaxis should not be used by most travelers. It can be used by people who are at high risk of developing complications of TD (e.g., immunosuppressed patients or significant comorbidities) or those with travel for performance reasons (e.g., a professional athlete). If antibiotic prophylaxis is indicated, rifaximin is preferred. Alternatives include azithromycin and rifamycin.

TD Treatment

Hydration (with increased fluid and salt intake) is essential for all TD cases. In an elderly patient with severe diarrhea or any traveler with prolonged watery diarrhea or vomiting, oral rehydration solution is preferred for fluid replacement. The packets are available in pharmacies throughout the world. They are easy to prepare: mix one packet with one liter of boiled, purified water.

Antibiotics are not required for mild cases of TD. OTC anti-diarrheal drugs will reduce the number of bowel movements, allowing travelers to continue their planned itinerary. The primary antimotility drug used for acute diarrhea is loperamide *(Imodium A-D)*. Loperamide decreases the frequency and urgency of bowel movements, making it easier for a person with diarrhea to continue travel activities (e.g., ride on a bus or airplane). The dose is 4 mg after the first loose stool and 2 mg after each subsequent loose stool, up to a maximum dose of 16 mg/day by prescription or 8 mg/day OTC. Loperamide can be used for self-treatment for up to two days. If symptoms remain after 48 hours, a healthcare provider should be seen. It should not be used in children < 2 years old (< 6 years old if OTC) or in patients with bloody diarrhea. See the Constipation & Diarrhea chapter for more information on loperamide.

BSS is another treatment option. The salicylate portion of BSS has antisecretory, anti-diarrheal properties and can reduce stools passed by ~40%. See the Constipation & Diarrhea chapter for specific information on contraindications and side effects, such as black tongue/stools, risk of Reye's syndrome in children and salicylate toxicity.

Compared with BSS, loperamide showed a greater reduction in the number of diarrheal stools passed and has been shown to shorten the duration of acute diarrhea in both children and adults.

DRUGS FOR TRAVELERS' DIARRHEA

Prophylaxis
- Bismuth subsalicylate 524-1050 mg PO 4 times daily (with meals and at bedtime)
- Antibiotics (rifaximin preferred)
  - ❏ Only used if there is a high risk of complications from TD

Treatment
- Mild TD: loperamide or bismuth subsalicylate
- Moderate TD: loperamide ± antibiotics
  - ❏ Azithromycin or a quinolone (if low resistance)
  - ❏ Rifaximin is an alternative
- Severe TD (including dysentery): antibiotics ± loperamide
  - ❏ Azithromycin preferred
  - ❏ Quinolones or rifaximin as alternatives

Antibiotics shorten the duration of moderate-to-severe TD to a little over 24 hours. Azithromycin, quinolones or rifaximin can be used (typically a single-dose regimen), depending on the TD severity and antibiotic resistance patterns. Azithromycin is preferred for severe TD and dysentery. Quinolones, rifaximin or rifamycin can be used for severe TD if no dysentery is present. Rifaximin and rifamycin cannot be used to treat infections in which invasive pathogens (e.g., *Campylobacter jejuni*, *Salmonella* species) are suspected.

TYPHOID FEVER

Typhoid fever is caused by the bacterium *Salmonella typhi*. The disease can be life-threatening. The highest risk areas for contracting typhoid fever include East and Southeast Asia, Africa, the Caribbean and Central and South America.

Humans are the only source for this bacteria. Disease is spread through food or water contaminated by the feces of someone with either an acute infection or from a chronic, asymptomatic carrier. The incubation period of typhoid fever and paratyphoid fever (a similar illness) is 6 – 30 days. Patients present with fatigue and increasing fever over 3 – 4 days. Additional symptoms may include headache, malaise, anorexia, rash and enlargement of the liver and spleen. Intestinal hemorrhage or perforation can occur 2 – 3 weeks later and can be fatal.

Typhoid vaccines are recommended but are only 50 – 80% effective; even vaccinated travelers should follow safe food and water precautions and wash their hands frequently. These precautions are the only prevention method for paratyphoid fever because there is not a vaccine available.

Typhoid vaccines include *Vivotif*, an oral, live-attenuated vaccine, and *Typhim Vi*, an inactivated, intramuscular injection. The oral vaccine regimen should be completed ≥ 1 week prior to travel. It should not be used in children < 6 years old, patients taking antibiotics or in those with an extremely sensitive stomach. The intramuscular vaccine must be given ≥ 2 weeks before the expected exposure and is not recommended for children < 2 years old. Revaccination is recommended every five years for *Vivotif* and every two years for *Typhim Vi* in patients who remain at risk.

CHOLERA

Cholera is a bacterial infection caused by *Vibrio cholerae*. The disease is very rare in the U.S., but still occurs in many places, including Africa, Southeast Asia and Haiti. The infection is often mild or asymptomatic, but in severe cases, it can present with profuse diarrhea and vomiting, and eventual dehydration that can be life-threatening. The most common symptom includes watery diarrhea, which is referred to as "rice-water stools."

In addition to food and water precautions, a live-attenuated vaccine (*Vaxchora*) is recommended for those traveling to a region with active cholera transmission. *Vaxchora* is administered as a single, oral liquid dose at least 10 days before travel and is approved for use in ages 2 through 64 years.

POLIO

Most people in the U.S. received the polio vaccine in childhood, but the virus is not eradicated worldwide. Many countries remain endemic and have had an active spread of poliovirus in the recent past. These include Afghanistan, Myanmar (Burma), Guinea, Laos, Nigeria, Madagascar, Pakistan and Ukraine. The CDC recommends a single lifetime booster dose of inactivated poliovirus vaccine at least four weeks prior to travel for adults who have previously completed a poliovirus vaccine series and who are traveling to regions where poliovirus is circulating. Travelers might be required to show proof of polio vaccination when leaving a polio-infected country.

HEPATITIS A

Hepatitis A is a common vaccine-preventable infection among international travelers. People from developed countries who travel to developing countries are at the highest risk. The infected patient can be asymptomatic or might have symptoms that include fever, malaise, jaundice, nausea and abdominal discomfort that can last up to six months. Vaccination should be considered for travelers visiting areas with high or intermediate risk, though some experts advise vaccination regardless of destination.

TRAVEL VACCINES

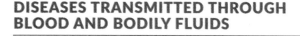

Inactivated Vaccines
Hepatitis A (*Havrix, VAQTA*)

Hepatitis B (*Engerix-B, Heplisav-B, Recombivax HB*)

Hepatitis A/B (*Twinrix*)

Japanese encephalitis (*Ixiaro*)

Meningococcus (*Menveo, MenQuadfi*)

Polio (*IPOL*)

Typhoid-IM (*Typhim Vi*)

Live Vaccines*
Cholera-PO (*Vaxchora*)

Typhoid-PO (*Vivotif*)

Yellow fever-SC (*YF-VAX*)

*Live vaccines are generally avoided in people who are immunocompromised.

DISEASES TRANSMITTED THROUGH BLOOD AND BODILY FLUIDS

HEPATITIS B

Hepatitis B is transmitted through contact with contaminated blood or other body fluids. The risk for travelers who do not participate in high-risk behaviors is low. Hepatitis B has an incubation period of about 90 days. Infection can present as malaise, jaundice, nausea and abdominal discomfort. Chronic infection with Hepatitis B can result in chronic liver disease and liver cancer.

Hepatitis B vaccination is extremely important for travelers who plan to receive medical care, volunteer to provide medical work or have unprotected sexual encounters with new partners. Piercings and tattoos can also transmit the virus and therefore the health risk should be strongly considered if deciding to obtain one. The 3-dose vaccine series takes six months to complete. If a traveler is unable to receive all three doses before departure, administer as many doses as possible before departure and complete the series upon return. In instances of high risk, an accelerated series can be administered; when a 3-dose accelerated series is used, a booster dose is required at one year for long-term immunity.

MENINGOCOCCAL MENINGITIS

Bacterial meningitis involving *N. meningitidis* has a high mortality rate and is a medical emergency. Patients with symptoms of fever, severe and unrelenting headache, nausea, stiff neck (nuchal rigidity) and mental status changes require urgent treatment to avoid the risk of permanent neurological damage and death. Diagnosis is made by a lumbar puncture (LP). See the Infectious Diseases II chapter.

Meningitis is spread by respiratory secretions and is widespread in many parts of the world. Vaccination is recommended for people who travel to or reside in countries where *N. meningitidis* is hyperendemic or epidemic, particularly if spending a long time in contact with the local population. High-risk regions include the meningitis belt of Africa during the dry season (December – June). The government of Saudi Arabia requires the meningococcal vaccine for travel during the annual Hajj and Umrah pilgrimages. Current recommendations include only the quadrivalent vaccines (*Menveo* and *MenQuadfi*) which contain four bacterial types: ACWY. There are no recommendations to use the serogroup B meningococcal vaccines for travelers.

DISEASES TRANSMITTED BY INSECT BITES

Insects that transmit disease are vectors; a vector carries an organism to an individual, causing infection. A reservoir is any place (such as an animal, insect, soil or plant) in which the disease lives and can multiply. The primary insects that transmit infections to travelers are mosquitoes, which transmit Japanese encephalitis, yellow fever, dengue, malaria and Zika virus. The following strategies should be employed to avoid insect bites as much as possible:

- Stay and sleep in screened or air-conditioned rooms and use a bed net, which can be pre-treated with mosquito repellent, such as those listed below.

- Cover exposed skin by wearing long-sleeved shirts, long pants and hats.

- Use proper application of mosquito repellents containing 20% – 50% DEET as the active ingredient on exposed skin. DEET also protects against ticks. Other insect repellents that can be used topically for mosquitoes (but not for ticks) are picaridin, oil of lemon, eucalyptus or IR3535.

- Use permethrin to treat clothing, gear and bed nets but do not apply directly to the skin.

DENGUE

Dengue is transmitted by *Aedes aegypti* and *Aedes albopictus* mosquitoes. In many parts of the tropics and subtropics, dengue is endemic; it occurs every year, usually during a season when mosquito populations are high and rainfall is optimal for breeding. An estimated 75% of infections are asymptomatic, but up to 5% of patients develop severe, life-threatening disease. Severe dengue can include shock, severe bleeding or organ failure. Treatment is supportive, as there are no specific medications to treat dengue infection. *Dengvaxia* is a live-attenuated recombinant vaccine recommended only to those with a past dengue infection. Protection from mosquito bites is essential.

JAPANESE ENCEPHALITIS

The Japanese Encephalitis (JE) virus is transmitted by mosquitoes. Infection is usually asymptomatic, but can develop into encephalitis (swelling around the brain) with rigors, risk of seizures, coma and death. Infection risk is highest in rural agricultural areas. The best prevention is to reduce exposure to mosquitoes. The JE vaccine is sometimes recommended with travel to Asia and parts of the western Pacific. The vaccine *(Ixiaro)* is recommended for travelers who are planning extended exposure to the outdoors (e.g., campers) or who plan to spend at least one month in endemic areas during the JE virus transmission season. There is an accelerated schedule available for those traveling with little notice.

MALARIA

Malaria is transmitted by the Anopheles mosquito. Once in a human host, it multiplies first in the liver and then moves into the red blood cells, multiplying and destroying them. Classic symptoms of malaria include shaking, chills, high fever and flu-like illness; these should not be ignored in a patient with recent travel. Malaria is endemic in Asia, Latin America, North Africa, Eastern Europe and the South Pacific. *Plasmodium vivax* is the most common of four human malaria species *(P. falciparum, P. malariae, P. ovale* and *P. vivax)*. *P. vivax* causes 50% of malaria cases in India and is becoming increasingly resistant to malaria drugs. *P. falciparum* is the most deadly species. About 2,000 cases of malaria are diagnosed in the U.S. annually, mostly in returned travelers. Even with treatment, malaria can be fatal, so prophylactic medications are recommended for travelers to certain regions. The CDC website features maps of malaria presence by country, the species of malaria, and resistance patterns. All of this information is incorporated into the CDC's region-specific prophylaxis medication recommendations. Recommendations can change year-to-year.

Malaria Prophylaxis Regimens

Malaria prophylaxis must be started prior to travel and continue after returning (see following tables for specific requirements). Malaria drugs cause nausea; taking with sufficient water, food or milk decreases nausea.

Quick Starts

DRUG	DOSING	SAFETY/SIDE EFFECTS/NOTES
These medications are initiated just 1-2 days prior to travel, which makes them ideal when traveling with little advance notice		
Doxycycline *(Doryx, Vibramycin)*	Stop: 4 weeks after travel	Causes photosensitivity* **Not used in:**
Also prevents rickettsial infections and leptospirosis; preferred in hiking/ camping	Taken daily	Pregnancy Children < 8 years old (due to tooth development/ discoloration)
Atovaquone/Proguanil *(Malarone)*	Stop: 1 week after travel	**Not used in:** Pregnancy
Good coverage	Taken daily	Breastfeeding Severe renal impairment
Primaquine	Stop: 1 week after travel	**Not used in:**
Most effective drug against *P. vivax*	Taken daily	G6PD deficiency (CDC requires screening prior to use due to risk of hemolytic anemia) Pregnancy Breastfeeding (unless infant is tested for G6PD deficiency)

Daily regimens

Avoid these in pregnancy

Cause nausea; to decrease, take with food, milk or water

*Use broad-spectrum sunscreen (protects against UVA and UVB rays) with Sun Protection Factor (SPF) at least 30, plus water resistant. Other strategies: seek shade, wear protective clothing, avoid mid-day sun.

Advance Starts

	DRUG	DOSING	SAFETY/SIDE EFFECTS/NOTES
	These medications must be started 1-2 weeks prior to travel		
Weekly regimens Safe in children, pregnancy Choice depends on resistance in the region	Chloroquine Resistance issues with *P. falciparum* and *P. vivax*	Start: 1-2 weeks before travel Stop: 4 weeks after travel Taken weekly Patients taking chronic hydroxychloroquine are covered (depending on resistance)	**SIDE EFFECTS** Retinal toxicity/visual changes, exacerbation of psoriasis, serious skin rash (rare), blue-gray skin pigmentation (rare with short-term use) Contraindicated for prophylaxis if underlying retinal or visual changes **Not used in:** Areas of chloroquine or mefloquine resistance
	Mefloquine	Start: ≥ 2 weeks before travel Stop: 4 weeks after travel Taken weekly	**Not used in:** Underlying psychiatric conditions Seizures Arrhythmias Areas of mefloquine resistance
	This medication requires a loading dose starting 3 days before travel		
	Tafenoquine *(Arakoda)* May be used for up to 6 months of continuous dosing	Loading dose: 3 days before travel, taken daily Maintenance dose: 7 days after last dose of loading regimen Taken weekly Terminal dose: single dose after the last dose of the maintenance regimen	**Not used in:** G6PD deficiency (CDC requires screening prior to use due to risk of hemolytic anemia) Pregnancy Breastfeeding (unless infant is tested for G6PD deficiency) Underlying psychiatric conditions

YELLOW FEVER

Yellow fever is caused by a virus and transmitted by mosquitoes found in tropical and subtropical areas in Africa and Central and South America. Reducing mosquito exposure is essential. Most infections are asymptomatic. If symptoms develop, the initial illness presents with influenza-like symptoms. Most patients will improve, but ~15% progress to a more toxic form of the disease with risk of shock, bleeding and organ failure. There is no specific treatment for acute infection except symptomatic relief with fluids, analgesics and antipyretics. Aspirin and other NSAIDs cannot be used due to an increased risk of bleeding.

A live-attenuated vaccine (YF-VAX) is available to prevent yellow fever and stop transmission. After vaccination, patients are provided an ICVP ("yellow card"), which is required as a condition of entry for some countries. The card is valid beginning 10 days after date of vaccination. A single dose of yellow fever vaccine provides life-long protection and is adequate for most travelers. Healthcare providers should review the entry requirements for destination countries, as some countries continue to require a booster vaccine dose every 10 years (per previous guideline recommendations).

The vaccine is contraindicated with hypersensitivity to eggs and in people who are severely immunocompromised. Due to the risks of serious adverse effects, vaccination is recommended only in travelers at a high risk of exposure or who require proof of vaccination to enter a country. Mild adverse effects are common (occurring in 10 – 30% of patients) and include low-grade fever and headache lasting for 5 – 10 days. In rare cases, severe adverse effects occur, such as yellow fever vaccine-associated neurologic disease.

ZIKA VIRUS

The Zika virus is transmitted primarily by the *Aedes* species mosquito. Sexual and possible blood transfusion-associated transmission have been reported. Most Zika virus infections are asymptomatic. Symptomatic infections are generally mild with symptoms consisting of fever, maculopapular rash, arthralgia (joint pain) and conjunctivitis (red eyes).

The most pressing concern with Zika virus arose in 2015 when Brazil observed a marked increase in the number of infants born with microcephaly, a birth defect that can cause significant disability and can be life-threatening in severe cases. Zika virus RNA was subsequently identified in tissues from infants with microcephaly and from fetal losses in women infected during pregnancy. Zika infection during pregnancy can cause birth defects of the brain and eyes, hearing deficits and impaired growth. Reports of Guillain-Barré syndrome, an uncommon sickness of the nervous system, have also increased in areas affected by Zika.

No vaccine is available yet for the Zika virus. Avoiding mosquito bites and using condoms during sexual contact with people with possible Zika virus infection reduces transmission risk.

The CDC recommends against pregnant women traveling to any area with ongoing transmission of Zika virus. Women who are trying to become pregnant should consult with their healthcare provider prior to travel. Men who have a pregnant partner and have traveled to an area with Zika should use condoms or avoid sex during the pregnancy.

ADDITIONAL CONCERNS FOR TRAVELING INDIVIDUALS

VENOUS THROMBOEMBOLISM PREVENTION

Travelers are at increased risk for deep vein thrombosis (DVT) and pulmonary embolism (PE) due to limited movement with long air travel. Wearing compression stockings during long trips reduces risk; these are sold in pharmacies. Travelers should be instructed to stand up, walk and perform lower leg exercises when sitting. Patients should know the symptoms of a DVT and PE and be instructed to seek immediate medical care if suspected. DVT risk factors, symptoms and treatment are discussed in the Anticoagulation chapter.

ALTITUDE SICKNESS AND MOTION SICKNESS

Acute mountain sickness (AMS) occurs when people climb rapidly to a high altitude. It occurs commonly above 8,000 feet and is more likely in individuals who live close to sea level and those who have had the condition previously. Symptoms include dizziness, headache, tachycardia and shortness of breath. The primary prophylactic medication is acetazolamide (Diamox) 125 mg twice daily, started the day before (preferred) or on the day of ascent. Higher doses are used for treatment. This can improve breathing, but is not without side effects (polyuria, photosensitivity, taste alteration, risk of dehydration, urticaria and a possibility of severe skin rashes). Acetazolamide is contraindicated with a sulfa allergy. Sun protection and hydration are recommended. In acute cases of altitude sickness, oxygen, inhaled beta-agonists and dexamethasone are given to reduce cerebral edema.

Motion sickness is common among travelers and is discussed in the Motion Sickness chapter.

THE RETURNED TRAVELER

It is imperative that travelers who are ill upon returning home see a healthcare provider. It is important for patients to communicate travel specifics to the healthcare provider, including the travel itinerary, the trip duration, accommodations (where they stayed), travel activities and any precautions that were taken to reduce infection risk, including vaccination history prior to leaving the U.S.

Some diseases have longer incubation periods and symptoms might not appear for weeks or months. Travelers often return home before their symptoms begin. This can lead to epidemics and the spread of disease from country to country. An example of this is the 2014 outbreak of the Ebola virus in West Africa, the largest Ebola outbreak in history. Ebola is transmitted by direct contact with blood or bodily fluids of a symptomatic person. Symptoms (fever, headache, diarrhea and hemorrhaging) can appear from 2 – 21 days after exposure. Due to the potentially long incubation, an infected person could be asymptomatic when returning to the U.S. and spread the disease before a diagnosis is made. Isolation upon return can reduce transmission.

Another example of this is illustrated by the Zika outbreak discussed previously in this chapter. In 2015, the Zika virus was identified for the first time in the Western hemisphere, with large outbreaks reported in Brazil. Since then, the virus has spread throughout much of the Americas and is still a concern for travelers, especially for those who are pregnant or are planning a pregnancy in the near future.

Select Guidelines/References

Centers for Disease Control (CDC) Center on Travelers Health. Available at http://wwwnc.cdc.gov/travel (accessed 2022 Dec 17).

International Society of Travel Medicine (ISTM), Pharmacist Professional Group of the ISTM. Available at www.istm.org (accessed 2022 Dec 17).

Riddle MS, Connor BA, Beeching, NJ, et al. Guidelines for the prevention and treatment of travelers' diarrhea: a graded expert panel report. J Travel Med 2017; 24(Suppl 1):S63-S80.

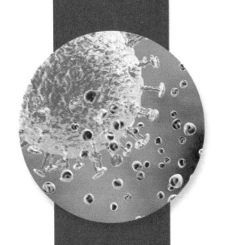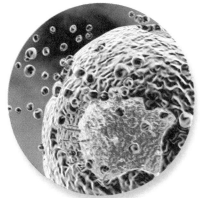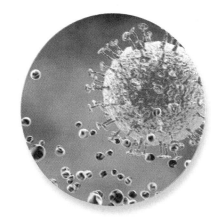

INFECTIOUS DISEASES

CONTENTS

CHAPTER CONTENT

CONTENT LEGEND

 = Study Tip Gal

 = Key Drug Guy

---

iStock.com/AndreasReh

CHAPTER 22

INFECTIOUS DISEASES I: BACKGROUND & ANTIBIOTICS BY DRUG CLASS

BACKGROUND

An infectious disease (ID) is caused by one or more pathogens [viruses, bacteria, fungi, protozoa, parasites and/or infectious proteins (prions)]. Infectious diseases are transmitted through various mechanisms, including physical contact with an infected individual or their body fluids, consuming contaminated food or water or touching contaminated objects. Some conditions are transmitted by airborne droplets and others are spread by a vector (carrier). Transmissible diseases that are spread from <u>person to person</u> are referred to as <u>communicable</u> (i.e., <u>contagious</u>).

HOW TO APPROACH INFECTIOUS DISEASES

Infectious diseases is organized into four chapters:

- ID I covers the principles of infectious diseases and provides summaries of antibacterial drugs by class.

- ID II reviews treatment of specific bacterial infections.

- ID III discusses antifungals, antivirals and select viral infections.

- ID IV reviews prophylaxis and treatment of opportunistic infections in immunocompromised patients.

Three primary factors impact treatment decisions in infectious diseases: the <u>bug</u> (pathogen), the <u>drug</u> (antimicrobial) and the <u>patient</u> (host). Do not be tempted to think of bugs, drugs and infectious diseases as separate sections to memorize; they must be considered together.

HOW DO I START?

- Recognize common organisms and groups of organisms.
- Focus on resistant organisms and the drugs that treat them.
- Learn the basic spectrum of activity for antimicrobial classes.
- Use bolded drugs, underlined information and Study Tip Gals to identify important points.
- Think about how to assess the patient profile on the exam.

ANTIBIOTIC SELECTION

- The <u>presence of an infection</u> is determined by:
  - ❏ Signs and symptoms, including <u>fever, elevated white blood cell count</u> and site-specific symptoms (e.g., dysuria with a urinary tract infection).
  - ❏ Diagnostic findings, such as culture results, X-rays and markers of inflammation (e.g., procalcitonin).

- <u>Antibiotic selection</u> is based on:
  - ❏ The <u>infection site</u> and <u>likely organisms</u> (see image below).
  - ❏ Infection <u>severity</u> and risk of multidrug-resistant (MDR) pathogens (e.g., <u>community-</u> vs. <u>hospital-acquired</u> infections).

- ❏ Antibiotic characteristics, including <u>spectrum of activity</u> and ability to <u>penetrate</u> the <u>site of infection</u> (e.g., antibiotics that are not renally eliminated may not achieve adequate concentrations in the urine).

- ❏ Patient characteristics, including <u>age, body weight, allergies, renal or hepatic function, comorbid</u> conditions, <u>recent antibiotic use, colonization</u> with resistant bacteria, vaccination status, pregnancy status and immune function.

- ❏ Treatment <u>guidelines</u> (e.g., <u>IDSA, CDC</u>), which factor in the criteria above and provide evidence-based recommendations.

Common Bacterial Pathogens for Select Sites of Infection

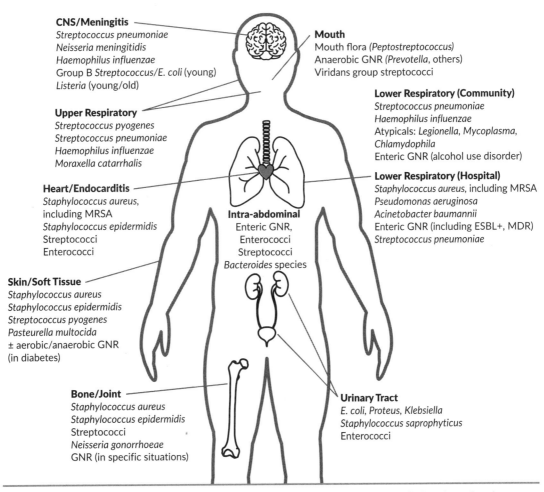

CNS/Meningitis
Streptococcus pneumoniae
Neisseria meningitidis
Haemophilus influenzae
Group B *Streptococcus/E. coli* (young)
Listeria (young/old)

Upper Respiratory
Streptococcus pyogenes
Streptococcus pneumoniae
Haemophilus influenzae
Moraxella catarrhalis

Heart/Endocarditis
Staphylococcus aureus, including MRSA
Staphylococcus epidermidis
Streptococci
Enterococci

Skin/Soft Tissue
Staphylococcus aureus
Staphylococcus epidermidis
Streptococcus pyogenes
Pasteurella multocida
± aerobic/anaerobic GNR (in diabetes)

Bone/Joint
Staphylococcus aureus
Staphylococcus epidermidis
Streptococci
Neisseria gonorrhoeae
GNR (in specific situations)

Mouth
Mouth flora (*Peptostreptococcus*)
Anaerobic GNR (*Prevotella*, others)
Viridans group streptococci

Lower Respiratory (Community)
Streptococcus pneumoniae
Haemophilus influenzae
Atypicals: *Legionella, Mycoplasma, Chlamydophila*
Enteric GNR (alcohol use disorder)

Lower Respiratory (Hospital)
Staphylococcus aureus, including MRSA
Pseudomonas aeruginosa
Acinetobacter baumannii
Enteric GNR (including ESBL+, MDR)
Streptococcus pneumoniae

Intra-abdominal
Enteric GNR,
Enterococci
Streptococci
Bacteroides species

Urinary Tract
E. coli, Proteus, Klebsiella
Staphylococcus saprophyticus
Enterococci

CNS = central nervous system; GNR = gram-negative rods; Enteric GNR = *Proteus, E. coli, Klebsiella, Enterobacter, Serratia*;
ESBL = extended-spectrum beta-lactamase; MDR = multidrug-resistant; MRSA = methicillin-resistant *Staphylococcus aureus*

EMPIRIC TREATMENT

A fluid or tissue sample taken from the infection site (e.g., urine, blood, abscess, wound) is sent to the microbiology lab for Gram stain, culture and susceptibility testing. Antibiotics are often started while awaiting these results (i.e., before the pathogen is identified). This empiric treatment is usually broad-spectrum (covers several types of bacteria) and can be guided by local resistance patterns (e.g., the antibiogram).

ANTIBIOGRAM

An antibiogram is a chart that combines culture data collected from patients at a single institution over a specific time period (usually 1 year). The antibiogram shows susceptibility patterns and can be used to monitor resistance trends over time.

Refer to the example antibiogram below. Bacteria are listed vertically, and drugs are listed horizontally. The numbers inside the table represent the percentage of samples of each isolated organism that were susceptible to the listed drug. The Case Scenario that follows is an example of how an antibiogram is used to select empiric treatment.

Hospital Antibiogram Example (Abridged)

JANUARY-DECEMBER	# OF ISOLATES	PENICILLIN	OXACILLIN	AMPICILLIN	CEFTRIAXONE	CLINDAMYCIN	ERYTHROMYCIN	GENTAMICIN	LEVOFLOXACIN	LINEZOLID	TETRACYCLINE	SMX/TMP	VANCOMYCIN
Gram-Positive Organisms (All Isolates)		REPORTED AS % SUSCEPTIBLE											
Staphylococcus aureus	1360												
MSSA	830	–	100	–	–	88	78	98§	87	100	93	98	100
MRSA	530	–	–	–	–	78	10	92§	15	100	93	92	100
Streptococcus pneumoniae	42	91	–	–	100	–	79	–	97	–	85	80	100
Enterococcus spp.	663	–	–	93	–	–	–	69§	–	99	–	–	100
Enterococcus faecalis	99	–	–	98	–	–	–	62§	–	99	–	–	87
Enterococcus faecium	164	–	–	10	–	–	–	90§	100	99	–	–	15
Urine Isolates													
Enterococcus spp.	153	–	–	79	–	–	–	–	61	100	–	–	81

§Synergy only

CASE SCENARIO

A 77-year-old female is admitted to the ICU from home with confusion, cough, temperature = 101.9°F, respiratory rate = 32 breaths per minute and oxygen saturation = 88% on room air. Her chest X-ray is consistent with pneumonia and a sputum Gram stain shows gram-positive cocci in pairs, which is likely S. pneumoniae. The pharmacist is asked to choose a beta-lactam antibiotic to add to azithromycin for empiric treatment.

After reviewing the institutional antibiogram (see example above), the pharmacist recommends ceftriaxone because local susceptibility patterns demonstrate 100% of S. pneumoniae isolates are susceptible to ceftriaxone, and use of a third-generation cephalosporin is consistent with national guideline recommendations.

GRAM STAIN

A Gram stain of the collected fluid or tissue sample categorizes the organism by stain result and shape (morphology) (see Study Tip Gal on next page) and provides quick, preliminary results (e.g., gram-negative rods). Although it does not identify the exact organism (e.g., Klebsiella pneumoniae), it narrows the list of potential organisms that may be causing the infection, which provides an opportunity to adjust the empiric antibiotic regimen before the species is identified.

- Gram-positive organisms have a thick cell wall and stain dark purple or blue from the crystal violet stain.

- Gram-negative organisms have a thin cell wall and take up the safranin counterstain, resulting in a pink color.

- Atypical organisms do not have a cell wall and do not stain well.

GRAM STAIN FOR SELECT BACTERIAL ORGANISMS

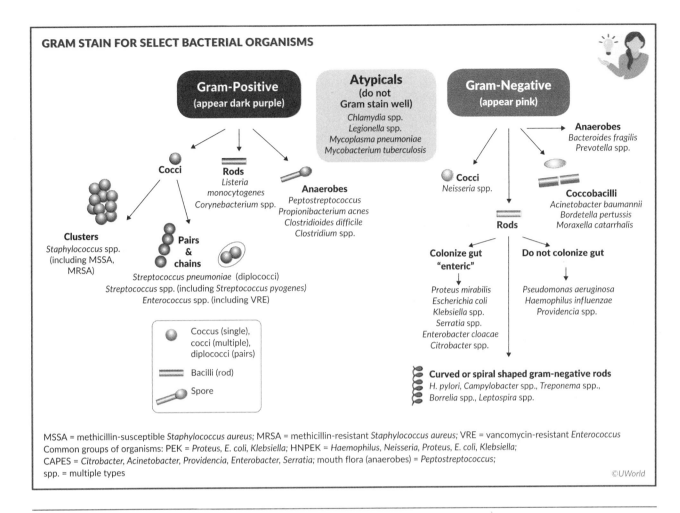

MSSA = methicillin-susceptible *Staphylococcus aureus*; MRSA = methicillin-resistant *Staphylococcus aureus*; VRE = vancomycin-resistant *Enterococcus*
Common groups of organisms: PEK = *Proteus, E. coli, Klebsiella*; HNPEK = *Haemophilus, Neisseria, Proteus, E. coli, Klebsiella*;
CAPES = *Citrobacter, Acinetobacter, Providencia, Enterobacter, Serratia*; mouth flora (anaerobes) = *Peptostreptococcus*;
spp. = multiple types

©UWorld

ANTIBIOTIC STREAMLINING

CULTURE AND SUSCEPTIBILITY

The microbiology lab uses various methods to determine which organism is present in a culture sample. For example, lactose (a sugar) can be used to determine the type of gram-negative bacteria that may be present (e.g., *E. coli* breaks down lactose in a unique way whereas *Pseudomonas* does not).

Staphylococci (gram-positive organisms occurring in clusters) can be differentiated with a coagulase (enzyme) test. *Staphylococcus aureus* is coagulase-positive; other *Staphylococcus* species (e.g., *S. epidermidis*) are sometimes referred to as coagulase-negative staphylococci (CoNS).

Once the organism has been identified, susceptibility testing is performed to determine which antibiotics are active against the particular strain. The bacteria is cultured (grown on an agar plate) and exposed to varying concentrations of select antibiotics.

The lab identifies the minimum concentration of each antibiotic that inhibits bacterial growth, which is called the minimum inhibitory concentration (MIC). The lab compares the MIC to the susceptibility breakpoint, which is the usual drug concentration that inhibits bacterial growth [as determined by the Clinical & Laboratory Standards Institute (CLSI)]. An interpretation is made as to which drugs inhibit growth (and at what concentration) and which drugs do not.

Culture and Susceptibility Report

The culture and susceptibility (C & S) report is usually available within 24 – 72 hours. It lists the organism and provides susceptibility testing results (see Study Tip Gal on the following page). The empiric antibiotics can then be streamlined, which can include discontinuing one or more antibiotics and/or changing to a more narrow-spectrum treatment. MICs are specific to each antibiotic and organism and should not be compared among different antibiotics. An antibiotic marked susceptible (S) should be selected. Drugs listed as intermediate (I) may be effective under specific circumstances (e.g., higher doses, extended infusions), but usually would not be selected over a drug that is reported as susceptible. Drugs listed as resistant (R) should not be selected.

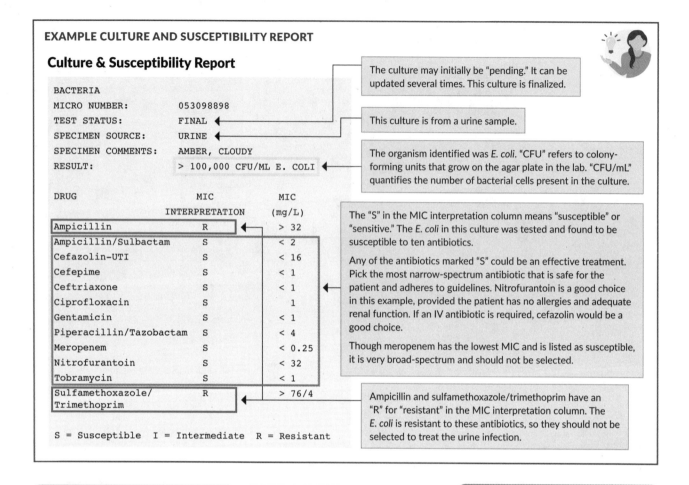

EXAMPLE CULTURE AND SUSCEPTIBILITY REPORT

Culture & Susceptibility Report

```
BACTERIA
MICRO NUMBER:        053098898
TEST STATUS:         FINAL
SPECIMEN SOURCE:     URINE
SPECIMEN COMMENTS:   AMBER, CLOUDY
RESULT:              > 100,000 CFU/ML E. COLI
```

DRUG	MIC INTERPRETATION	MIC (mg/L)
Ampicillin	R	> 32
Ampicillin/Sulbactam	S	< 2
Cefazolin-UTI	S	< 16
Cefepime	S	< 1
Ceftriaxone	S	< 1
Ciprofloxacin	S	1
Gentamicin	S	< 1
Piperacillin/Tazobactam	S	< 4
Meropenem	S	< 0.25
Nitrofurantoin	S	< 32
Tobramycin	S	< 1
Sulfamethoxazole/ Trimethoprim	R	> 76/4

S = Susceptible   I = Intermediate   R = Resistant

The culture may initially be "pending." It can be updated several times. This culture is finalized.

This culture is from a urine sample.

The organism identified was *E. coli*. "CFU" refers to colony-forming units that grow on the agar plate in the lab. "CFU/mL" quantifies the number of bacterial cells present in the culture.

The "S" in the MIC interpretation column means "susceptible" or "sensitive." The *E. coli* in this culture was tested and found to be susceptible to ten antibiotics.

Any of the antibiotics marked "S" could be an effective treatment. Pick the most narrow-spectrum antibiotic that is safe for the patient and adheres to guidelines. Nitrofurantoin is a good choice in this example, provided the patient has no allergies and adequate renal function. If an IV antibiotic is required, cefazolin would be a good choice.

Though meropenem has the lowest MIC and is listed as susceptible, it is very broad-spectrum and should not be selected.

Ampicillin and sulfamethoxazole/trimethoprim have an "R" for "resistant" in the MIC interpretation column. The *E. coli* is resistant to these antibiotics, so they should not be selected to treat the urine infection.

Empiric Treatment

Select empiric treatment based on the likely organisms at the infection site (e.g., lower respiratory tract, CNS, skin/soft tissue).

Is the patient at risk for MRSA? MDR bacteria? If yes, provide coverage.

Use the antibiogram and Gram stain results (if available) to guide the treatment selection.

Streamline

When the C & S results are available, streamline to more narrow-spectrum antibiotics as soon as possible; if > 1 organism is present, try to find one antibiotic that will treat both.

Consider IV to PO conversion if the patient is stable, eating and there is an appropriate oral drug (e.g., that can penetrate the infection site).

Assess the Patient

Monitor for improvement of signs and symptoms. A lack of response can be multifactorial [e.g., inadequate dose, nonadherence, uncontrolled source, resistance, drug interaction, alternative etiology (viral, fungal)].

Determine the duration of treatment; do not continue antibiotics for longer than necessary.

Synergy

An infection could require more than one antibiotic for successful treatment. The effect of two antibiotics can be additive (an effect equal to the sum of the individual drugs) or synergistic (an effect greater than the sum of the individual drugs). For example, aminoglycosides and beta-lactams can be used together synergistically to treat certain invasive gram-positive infections (e.g., infective endocarditis); the beta-lactam breaks down the antibiotic cell wall, allowing the aminoglycoside to reach its intracellular target at safe doses.

ANTIBIOTIC RESISTANCE

Antibiotic resistance is the ability of an organism to multiply in the presence of a drug that normally limits its growth or kills it. The CDC estimates that there are ~2,000,000 infections per year where the causative organism is resistant to the usual treatment. These infections are difficult to treat and often require drugs that are costly and/or toxic.

Common mechanisms of resistance include:

- Intrinsic resistance: the resistance is natural to the organism. For example, E. coli is resistant to vancomycin because this antibiotic is too large to penetrate the cell wall of E. coli.

- Selection pressure: resistance occurs when antibiotics kill susceptible bacteria, leaving behind more resistant strains to multiply. For example, normal GI flora includes Enterococcus. When antibiotics (e.g., vancomycin) eliminate susceptible enterococci, vancomycin-resistant Enterococcus (VRE) can become predominant.

- Acquired resistance: bacterial DNA containing resistant genes can be transferred between species and/or picked up from dead bacterial fragments in the environment.

- Antibiotic degradation: bacterial enzymes break down the antibiotic.
    - Bacteria that produce beta-lactamases break down beta-lactams (e.g., penicillins) before they can bind to their site of activity. Beta-lactamase inhibitors (e.g., clavulanate, sulbactam, tazobactam, avibactam) are combined with some beta-lactams to preserve or increase their spectrum of activity.
    - Extended-spectrum beta-lactamases (ESBLs) are beta-lactamases that can break down all penicillins and most cephalosporins. Because organisms that produce ESBLs can be difficult to eradicate, they are typically treated with carbapenems or newer cephalosporin/beta-lactamase inhibitor combinations.
    - Carbapenem-resistant Enterobacterales (CRE) are MDR gram-negative organisms (e.g., Klebsiella spp., E. coli) that produce enzymes (e.g., carbapenemase) capable of breaking down penicillins, most cephalosporins and carbapenems. CRE infections typically require treatment with a combination of antibiotics that include drugs such as the polymyxins, which have a high risk for toxicity (see the Polymyxins drug table), or ceftazidime/avibactam (Avycaz).

COMMON RESISTANT PATHOGENS

Klebsiella pneumoniae (ESBL, CRE)

Escherichia coli (ESBL, CRE)

Acinetobacter baumannii

Enterococcus faecalis, Enterococcus faecium (VRE)

Staphylococcus aureus (MRSA)

Pseudomonas aeruginosa

Remember: **K**ill **E**ach **A**nd **E**very **S**trong **P**athogen

ESBL = extended-spectrum beta-lactamase
CRE = carbapenem-resistant Enterobacterales
VRE = vancomycin-resistant Enterococcus

CLOSTRIDIOIDES DIFFICILE INFECTION

When an antibiotic kills GI flora (i.e., normal, healthy organisms) along with the targeted pathogens, it can result in an overgrowth of Clostridioides difficile, which can produce toxins that inflame the GI mucosa and lead to a C. difficile infection (CDI).

Symptoms can be mild (loose stools and abdominal cramping) to severe (pseudomembranous colitis that can require colectomy or be fatal). All antibiotics have a warning for the risk of CDI, but the risk is highest with broad-spectrum penicillins and cephalosporins, quinolones, carbapenems, and clindamycin, which has a boxed warning. When appropriate, antibiotics should be streamlined or discontinued to reduce CDI risk.

ANTIMICROBIAL STEWARDSHIP PROGRAMS

Antimicrobial stewardship programs (ASPs) are designed to improve patient safety and outcomes, limit drug resistance, reduce adverse effects and promote cost-effectiveness.

ASPs consist of collaborative teams (e.g., ID physicians, ID pharmacists, microbiology lab staff, infection prevention personnel) that establish antibiotic guidance for their facility. ASPs conduct audits of prescribing habits and provide education to change suboptimal practices and improve care.

Example ASP interventions include: 1) pharmacokinetic monitoring of aminoglycosides and vancomycin, 2) use of clinical decision support software to rapidly identify pathogens and shorten the time to starting effective treatment, 3) authorization for use of select antimicrobials, 4) prospective audit and feedback to prescribers of selected antibiotics and 5) timely transitions from IV to PO antibiotics.

ANTIBIOTIC MECHANISMS OF ACTION

Knowledge of drug mechanisms of action can help distinguish what types of organisms can be treated with a given antibiotic. The target sites of common antibacterials are outlined in the following diagram. Generally, cell wall and cell membrane inhibitors, DNA/RNA inhibitors and aminoglycosides are bactericidal (kill bacteria), while most protein and folic acid synthesis inhibitors are bacteriostatic (inhibit bacterial growth). A detailed description of the mechanism of action for each antibiotic or antibiotic class is included on the following pages.

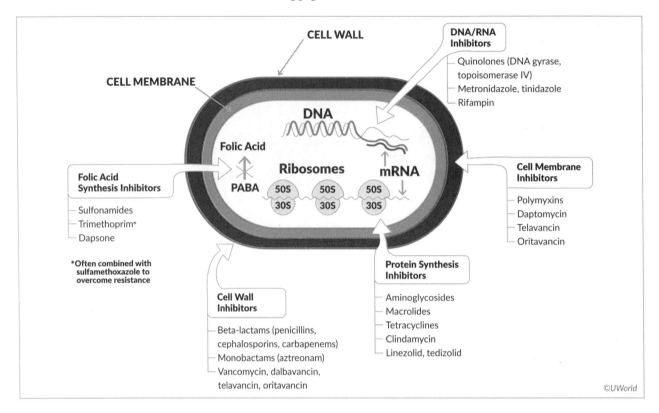

ANTIBIOTIC PHARMACOKINETICS AND PHARMACODYNAMICS

Appropriate selection of an antibiotic regimen requires an understanding of antibiotic pharmacokinetic (PK) principles (absorption, distribution, metabolism and excretion – refer to the Pharmacokinetics chapter) and pharmacodynamic principles (e.g., concentration-dependent or time-dependent killing).

HYDROPHILIC AND LIPOPHILIC DRUGS

Hydrophilicity or lipophilicity of an antibiotic can be used to predict some PK parameters (see figure below).

HYDROPHILIC AGENTS	
Beta-lactams	1) Small volume of distribution → Less tissue penetration
Aminoglycosides	2) Mostly renally eliminated → Drug accumulation and side effects can occur if not dose adjusted
Vancomycin	3) Low intracellular concentrations → Not active against atypical (intracellular) pathogens
Daptomycin	4) Poor bioavailability → IV:PO ratio is not 1:1
Polymyxins	

LIPOPHILIC AGENTS	
Quinolones	1) Large volume of distribution → Better tissue penetration
Macrolides	2) Mostly hepatically metabolized → Potential for hepatotoxicity and drug-drug interactions
Rifampin	3) Achieve higher intracellular concentrations → Active against atypical (intracellular) pathogens
Linezolid	4) Excellent bioavailability → IV:PO ratio is often 1:1
Tetracyclines	

IV = intravenous, PO = oral

DOSE OPTIMIZATION

The pharmacodynamics of select antibiotics are displayed in the figure below. Drugs with concentration-dependent killing (such as aminoglycosides) can be dosed less frequently and in higher doses to maximize the concentration above the MIC. Drugs with time-dependent killing (such as beta-lactams) can be dosed more frequently or each dose can be administered for a longer duration to maximize the time above the MIC. An example is extending the infusion time of beta-lactam antibiotics (e.g., from 30 minutes to 4 hours or administering as a continuous infusion), which has been shown to reduce hospital length of stay, mortality and costs when treating select infections (e.g., pseudomonal pneumonia).

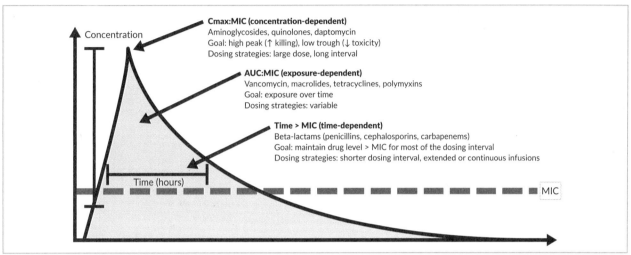

AUC = area under the concentration-time curve, Cmax = maximum plasma concentration, MIC = minimum inhibitory concentration

BETA-LACTAM ANTIBIOTICS

Beta-lactam antibiotics (penicillins, cephalosporins and carbapenems) have a chemical structure that is characterized by a beta-lactam ring (see the Basic Science Concepts chapter). They inhibit bacterial cell wall synthesis by binding to penicillin-binding proteins (PBPs). This prevents the final step of peptidoglycan synthesis in bacterial cell walls.

Penicillins and cephalosporins are available in multiple formulations, including child-friendly oral formulations (e.g., chewable tablets, suspensions) and injectables (e.g., IV, IM). Knowing the oral and injectable products within a penicillin or cephalosporin subcategory (i.e., that have a similar spectrum of activity) can be useful for the exam. Carbapenems are available only in parenteral form.

PENICILLINS

Coverage varies by subgroup of penicillin. As a class, they are not active against MRSA or atypical organisms.

- Natural penicillins are active against gram-positive cocci (streptococci and enterococci, but not staphylococci) and gram-positive anaerobes (mouth flora). They have no appreciable gram-negative activity.

- Antistaphylococcal penicillins cover streptococci and methicillin-susceptible *Staphylococcus aureus* (MSSA), but they lack activity against *Enterococcus*, gram-negative pathogens and anaerobes.

- Aminopenicillins cover streptococci, enterococci and gram-positive anaerobes (mouth flora) plus the gram-negative bacteria *Haemophilus, Neisseria, Proteus* and *E. coli*.

  ❏ Aminopenicillins combined with beta-lactamase inhibitors (e.g., clavulanate, sulbactam) have added activity against MSSA, more resistant strains of gram-negative bacteria [e.g., *Haemophilus, Neisseria, Proteus, E. coli, Klebsiella* (HNPEK)] and gram-negative anaerobes (B. fragilis).

- Extended-spectrum penicillins, combined with a beta-lactamase inhibitor (e.g., piperacillin/tazobactam), have broad-spectrum activity. They cover the same organisms as aminopenicillin/beta-lactamase inhibitor combinations (see above) plus have expanded coverage of other gram-negative bacteria, including *Citrobacter, Acinetobacter, Providencia, Enterobacter, Serratia* (CAPES) and *Pseudomonas*.

Select Penicillins

DRUG	DOSING	SAFETY/SIDE EFFECTS/MONITORING
Natural Penicillins		**BOXED WARNING** Penicillin G benzathine: not for IV use; can cause cardio-respiratory arrest and death
Penicillin V Potassium	PO: 125-500 mg Q6-12H on an empty stomach	
Penicillin G Aqueous (*Pfizerpen*)	IV: 2-4 million units Q4-6H	**CONTRAINDICATIONS** Type 1 hypersensitivity reaction to another penicillin or beta-lactam antibiotic
Penicillin G Benzathine (*Bicillin L-A*)	IM: 1.2-2.4 million units x 1 (frequency varies)	*Augmentin* and *Unasyn*: history of cholestatic jaundice or hepatic dysfunction associated with previous use
Penicillin G Benzathine and Penicillin G Procaine (*Bicillin C-R*)		Severe renal impairment (CrCl < 30 mL/min): do not use amoxicillin/clavulanate extended-release (*Augmentin XR*) or the 875 mg strength
Antistaphylococcal Penicillins		**SIDE EFFECTS**
Dicloxacillin	PO: 125-500 mg Q6H	Seizures (with accumulation when not correctly dose adjusted in renal dysfunction), GI upset, diarrhea, rash (including SJS/TEN), allergic reactions/anaphylaxis, hemolytic anemia (identified with a positive Coombs test), renal failure, ↑ LFTs
Nafcillin	IV/IM: 1-2 grams Q4-6H	
Oxacillin	IV: 250-2,000 mg Q4-6H	**MONITORING** Renal function, symptoms of anaphylaxis with 1st dose, CBC and LFTs with prolonged courses
Aminopenicillins		**NOTES** **Antistaphylococcal Penicillins**
Amoxicillin	PO: dosing varies with formulation	Preferred for MSSA soft tissue, bone and joint, endocarditis and bloodstream infections
Amoxicillin/Clavulanate (*Augmentin, Augmentin ES-600*)	PO: dosing varies with formulation; XR tablet is taken Q12H with food	No renal dose adjustments
Ampicillin	PO: 250-500 mg Q6H on an empty stomach 30 minutes before or 2 hrs after meals	Nafcillin is a vesicant – administration through a central line is preferred; if extravasation occurs, use cold packs and hyaluronidase injections
	IV/IM: 1-2 grams Q4-6H	
Ampicillin/Sulbactam (*Unasyn*)	IV: 1.5-3 grams Q6H	**Aminopenicillins**
Extended-Spectrum Penicillin		Ampicillin PO is rarely used due to poor bioavailability; amoxicillin is preferred if switching from IV ampicillin
Piperacillin/Tazobactam (*Zosyn*)	IV: 3.375 grams Q6H or 4.5 grams Q6-8H	*Augmentin ES-600* suspension: preferred formulation for acute otitis media treatment in children (lower clavulanate concentration and lower risk of diarrhea – see ID II chapter)
	Prolonged or extended infusions: 3.375-4.5 grams IV Q8H (each dose infused over 4 hours)	IV ampicillin and ampicillin/sulbactam is preferably diluted in NS

Penicillin Drug Interactions

- Probenecid can ↑ the levels of beta-lactams by interfering with renal excretion. This combination is sometimes used intentionally in severe infections to ↑ antibiotic levels.

- Penicillins can ↑ the serum concentration of methotrexate.

- Beta-lactams (except nafcillin and dicloxacillin) can enhance the anticoagulant effect of warfarin by inhibiting the production of vitamin K-dependent clotting factors.

- Nafcillin and dicloxacillin (CYP enzyme inducers) can inhibit the anticoagulant effect of warfarin.

KEY FEATURES OF PENICILLINS

CLASS EFFECTS

- All penicillins should be avoided in patients with a beta-lactam allergy

    ❑ Exceptions: treatment of syphilis during pregnancy or in patients with poor compliance/follow-up – desensitize and treat with penicillin G benzathine

- All penicillins increase the risk of seizures if accumulation occurs (e.g., failure to dose adjust in renal dysfunction)

ORAL

Penicillin VK

- A first-line treatment for pharyngitis ("strep throat")

Amoxicillin

- First-line treatment for acute otitis media (pediatric dose: 80-90 mg/kg/day)

- Drug of choice for infective endocarditis prophylaxis before dental procedures (2 grams PO x 1, 30-60 minutes before procedure)

- Used in *H. pylori* treatment regimens*

Amoxicillin/Clavulanate (*Augmentin*)

- First-line treatment for acute otitis media (pediatric dose: 90 mg/kg/day) and bacterial sinusitis (if antibiotics indicated)

- Use the lowest dose of clavulanate to ↓ diarrhea

Dicloxacillin

- Covers MSSA (no MRSA)

- No renal dose adjustments needed

PARENTERAL

Penicillin G Benzathine (*Bicillin L-A*)

- Drug of choice for syphilis (2.4 million units IM x 1)

- Not for IV use; can cause death

Nafcillin and Oxacillin

- See dicloxacillin above

Piperacillin/Tazobactam (*Zosyn*)

- Only penicillin active against *Pseudomonas*

- Extended infusions (4 hours) can be used to maximize T > MIC

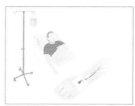

iStock.com/Graphic_BKK1979

*See the Gastroesophageal Reflux Disease (GERD) & Peptic Ulcer Disease (PUD) chapter.

CEPHALOSPORINS

The spectrum of activity varies by cephalosporin "generation." Generally, the gram-negative spectrum increases with each generation. As a class, they are <u>not active against *Enterococcus* spp. or atypical organisms</u>.

- <u>First generation</u>: excellent activity against <u>gram-positive cocci</u> (i.e., streptococci, staphylococci) and preferred when a cephalosporin is used for <u>MSSA</u> infections. They have some activity against the <u>gram-negative rods</u> *Proteus, E. coli* and *Klebsiella* (<u>PEK</u>).

- <u>Second generation</u>: covers staphylococci, more resistant strains of *S. pneumoniae* plus *Haemophilus, Neisseria, Proteus, E. coli* and *Klebsiella* (<u>HNPEK</u>). <u>Cefotetan and cefoxitin</u> have added activity against gram-negative <u>anaerobes (*B. fragilis*)</u>.

- <u>Third generation</u>: there are two groups.

    ❑ Group 1: includes <u>ceftriaxone</u>, cefotaxime and oral drugs (e.g., <u>cefdinir</u>); they cover <u>resistant streptococci</u> (*S. pneumoniae* and viridans group streptococci), staphylococci (MSSA), gram-positive anaerobes and <u>resistant</u> strains of <u>HNPEK</u>.

    ❑ Group 2: includes <u>ceftazidime</u>, which <u>lacks gram-positive activity</u> but covers *Pseudomonas*.

- <u>Fourth generation</u>: only includes <u>cefepime</u>, which has broad gram-negative activity (HNPEK, CAPES and *Pseudomonas*), and gram-positive activity similar to ceftriaxone.

- <u>Fifth generation</u>: only includes <u>ceftaroline</u>, which has gram-negative activity similar to ceftriaxone, but <u>broad gram-positive activity</u>; it is the only beta-lactam that <u>covers MRSA</u>.

- Other cephalosporins:

    ❑ <u>Beta-lactamase inhibitor combinations</u>: ceftazidime/avibactam and ceftolozane/tazobactam have a similar spectrum as ceftazidime but with added activity against <u>MDR gram-negative rods</u>.

    ❑ Siderophore cephalosporin: cefiderocol uses the iron transport system to enter the gram-negative cell wall. It is active against PEK, *Enterobacter* and *Pseudomonas*.

DRUG	DOSING	SAFETY/SIDE EFFECTS/MONITORING
1st Generation		**CONTRAINDICATIONS (CEFTRIAXONE)** Hyperbilirubinemic neonates (causes biliary sludging, kernicterus)
Cefazolin	IV/IM: 1-2 grams Q8H	
Cephalexin	PO: 250-500 mg Q6-12H	Concurrent use with calcium-containing IV products in neonates (see Cephalosporin Drug Interactions)
Cefadroxil	PO: 500-2,000 mg Q12-24H	**WARNINGS**
2nd Generation		Cross-reactivity with penicillin allergy (< 10%, higher risk with 1st generation cephalosporins): do not use in patients with a type 1 hypersensitivity to penicillin (swelling, angioedema, anaphylaxis)
Cefuroxime	PO/IV/IM: 250-1,500 mg Q8-12H	
Cefotetan	IV/IM: 1-2 grams Q12H	Cefotetan can cause a disulfiram-like reaction with alcohol ingestion
Cefoxitin	IV/IM: 1-2 grams Q6-8H	
Cefaclor	PO: 250-500 mg Q8H	**SIDE EFFECTS** Seizures (with accumulation when not correctly dose adjusted in renal dysfunction), GI upset, diarrhea, rash (including SJS/TEN), allergic reactions/anaphylaxis, acute interstitial nephritis, hemolytic anemia (identified with a positive Coombs test), myelosuppression with prolonged use, ↑ LFTs, drug fever
Cefprozil	PO: 250-500 mg Q12-24H	
3rd Generation Group 1		
Cefdinir	PO: 300 mg Q12H or 600 mg daily	
Ceftriaxone	IV/IM: 1-2 grams Q12-24H	**MONITORING** Renal function, signs of anaphylaxis with 1st dose, CBC, LFTs
Cefotaxime*	IV/IM: 1-2 grams Q4-12H	
Cefixime (Suprax)	PO: 400 mg divided Q12-24H	**NOTES** Ceftriaxone: no renal dose adjustments, CNS penetration at high doses (e.g., 2 grams Q12H) when meninges inflamed
Cefpodoxime	PO: 100-400 mg Q12H	
3rd Generation Group 2		Cefixime is available in a chewable tablet
Ceftazidime (Tazicef)	IV/IM: 1-2 grams Q8-12H	Ceftazidime/avibactam: activity against some carbapenem-resistant Enterobacterales (CRE)
4th Generation		
Cefepime	IV/IM: 1-2 grams Q8-12H	Cefiderocol: increase to 2 grams Q6H if CrCl ≥ 120 mL/min
5th Generation		
Ceftaroline fosamil (Teflaro)	IV: 600 mg Q12H	
Cephalosporin Combinations		
Ceftazidime/Avibactam (Avycaz)	IV: 2.5 grams Q8H	
Ceftolozane/Tazobactam (Zerbaxa)	IV: 1.5-3 grams Q8H	
Siderophore Cephalosporin		
Cefiderocol (Fetroja)	IV: 2 grams IV Q8H	

*No longer manufactured in the U.S. A non-FDA approved product is available via importation if needed.

Cephalosporin Drug Interactions

- Insoluble precipitates may form when ceftriaxone is administered in the same line as calcium-containing IV fluids. Simultaneous administration should be avoided in all patients. In adults, these products can be administered at different times of day as long as the IV line is flushed with a compatible fluid between administration of each product. In neonates, concurrent use (including administration at different times of day) is contraindicated.

- Drugs that decrease stomach acid can decrease the bioavailability of some oral cephalosporins. Cefuroxime, cefpodoxime and cefdinir should be separated by two hours from short-acting antacids. H2RAs and PPIs should be avoided.

KEY FEATURES OF CEPHALOSPORINS

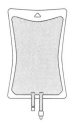

CLASS EFFECTS

- Although the risk of cross-reactivity is low, do not choose a cephalosporin on the exam if the patient has a penicillin allergy (exception: pediatric patients with acute otitis media and a mild penicillin allergy*)

- Risk of seizures if accumulation occurs (e.g., failure to dose adjust in renal dysfunction)

ORAL

1st Generation: Cephalexin

- Common uses: skin infections (MSSA), strep throat

2nd Generation: Cefuroxime

- Common uses: acute otitis media, community-acquired pneumonia (CAP)

3rd Generation: Cefdinir

- Common use: acute otitis media

PARENTERAL

1st Generation: Cefazolin

- Common use: surgical prophylaxis

2nd Generation: Cefotetan and Cefoxitin

- Anaerobic coverage (B. fragilis)

- Common use: surgical prophylaxis (gastrointestinal procedures)

- Cefotetan can cause a disulfiram-like reaction with alcohol ingestion

3rd Generation: Ceftriaxone

- Common uses: CAP, meningitis, spontaneous bacterial peritonitis, pyelonephritis

- No renal dose adjustments

- Do not use in neonates (age 0-28 days)

Ceftazidime (3rd Generation) and Cefepime (4th Generation)

- Active against Pseudomonas

Ceftolozane/Tazobactam and Ceftazidime/Avibactam

- Used for MDR gram-negative organisms (including Pseudomonas)

Ceftaroline

- Only beta-lactam active against MRSA

- Common uses: CAP, skin and soft tissue infections

Delayed-onset reaction (> 48 hours after the first antibiotic dose) appearing as a nonpruritic or mildly pruritic, maculopapular rash, but lacking systemic symptoms (e.g., hives, bronchospasm, anaphylaxis) or other serious reactions (e.g., Stevens-Johnson syndrome).

CARBAPENEMS

Carbapenems are very broad-spectrum antibiotics that are generally <u>reserved for MDR gram-negative</u> infections. They are active against most gram-positive, gram-negative (including <u>ESBL-producing bacteria</u>) and anaerobic pathogens, but provide <u>no coverage</u> of <u>atypical pathogens, MRSA, VRE</u>, *C. difficile* or *Stenotrophomonas*.

<u>Ertapenem is different</u> from other carbapenems as it has <u>no activity against *Pseudomonas, Acinetobacter*</u> or *Enterococcus*. Carbapenem/beta-lactamase inhibitor combinations are typically reserved for highly resistant infections (e.g., CRE) that are unable to be treated with a carbapenem alone.

DRUG	DOSING	SAFETY/SIDE EFFECTS/MONITORING
Meropenem *(Merrem)* Meropenem/Vaborbactam *(Vabomere)*	IV: 500-1,000 mg Q8H IV: 4 grams Q8H	**CONTRAINDICATIONS** Anaphylactic reaction to beta-lactam antibiotics **WARNINGS** <u>Do not use in patients with penicillin allergy</u> (risk of cross-reactivity) CNS adverse effects, including confusion and <u>seizures</u>; higher risk with imipenem/cilastatin, large doses or impaired renal function
Imipenem/Cilastatin *(Primaxin I.V.)* Imipenem/Cilastatin/Relebactam *(Recarbrio)*	IV: 500-1,000 mg Q6-8H IV: 1.25 grams Q6H	**SIDE EFFECTS** Diarrhea, rash/severe skin reaction (DRESS), bone marrow suppression with prolonged use, ↑ LFTs **MONITORING** <u>Renal function</u>, symptoms of anaphylaxis with 1st dose, CBC, LFTs
Ertapenem *(Invanz)* <u>Stable in NS only</u>	IV/IM: 1 gram daily	As above plus: **NOTES** No coverage of *Pseudomonas, Acinetobacter* or *Enterococcus*

Carbapenem Drug Interactions

- Carbapenems can ↓ serum concentrations of valproic acid, leading to a loss of seizure control.
- Use with caution in patients with a history of seizure disorder, or in combination with other drugs known to lower the seizure threshold (e.g., clozapine, quinolones, bupropion, tramadol). See the Seizures/Epilepsy chapter.

CASE SCENARIO

Think of how you would approach a case on the exam in which one of the answer choices is *Invanz* 1 gram IV Q24H. Assess the following, using the underlined information in the carbapenem drug table:

- Allergies: if the patient has a penicillin allergy, there is likely a better answer choice because of the possibility of cross-reactivity.
- Culture and susceptibility: if the culture is growing ESBL-positive *E. coli*, ertapenem may be a good choice. If *Pseudomonas* is growing, ertapenem can be ruled out based on a lack of activity against this pathogen.
- Past medical history and medication profile: if the patient has a history of seizures or takes an antiseizure drug, such as phenytoin, there is likely a better choice than a carbapenem, which can increase the risk for seizures.

KEY FEATURES OF CARBAPENEMS

Class Effects
- All active against ESBL-producing organisms and (except ertapenem) *Pseudomonas*
- Do not use with penicillin allergy
- Seizure risk (with higher doses, failure to dose adjust in renal dysfunction or use of imipenem/cilastatin)

Organisms Not Covered
- Atypicals, VRE, MRSA, *C. difficile, Stenotrophomonas*
- Ert**AP**enem does not cover **PEA**: *Pseudomonas, Enterococcus, Acinetobacter*

Common Uses
- Polymicrobial infections (e.g., severe diabetic foot infection)
- Empiric therapy when resistant organisms are suspected
- ESBL-positive infections
- Resistant *Pseudomonas* or *Acinetobacter* infections (except ertapenem)

All are IV only. Ertapenem must be diluted in normal saline.

MONOBACTAM

AZTREONAM

Aztreonam has a mechanism of action similar to beta-lactams; it inhibits bacterial cell wall synthesis by binding to penicillin-binding proteins (PBPs), which prevents the final step of peptidoglycan synthesis in bacterial cell walls. Aztreonam covers many gram-negative organisms, including *Pseudomonas* and CAPES. It has no gram-positive or anaerobic activity. The monobactam structure makes cross-reactivity with a beta-lactam unlikely, therefore aztreonam is primarily used when a beta-lactam allergy is present.

DRUG	DOSING	SAFETY/SIDE EFFECTS/MONITORING
Aztreonam (*Azactam*) Injection *Cayston* – inhaled, for cystic fibrosis	IV: 500-2,000 mg Q6-12H CrCl < 30 mL/min: dose adjustment required	**SIDE EFFECTS** Similar to penicillins, including rash, N/V/D, ↑ LFTs **NOTES** Can be used with a penicillin allergy

BETA-LACTAM ANTIBIOTICS SPECTRUM OF ACTIVITY SUMMARY

The chart below provides a visual representation of the general spectrum of activity for select beta-lactams and aztreonam. It can be used to identify antibiotics with activity against common pathogens, drugs with unique coverage (e.g., drugs active against *Pseudomonas* or MRSA) or where coverage is lacking (e.g., drugs that do not cover *Enterococcus*).

Drug	\<span\>Gram-Positive Aerobes\</span\> S. aureus (MRSA)	S. aureus (MSSA)	S. pneumoniae	Viridans group streptococci	Enterococcus (not VRE)	\<span\>Gram-Negative Aerobes\</span\> PEK	HNPEK	CAPES	Pseudomonas	Anaerobes Gram-positive (mouth flora)	Gram-negative (*Bacteroides fragilis*)	Atypicals (*Chlamydia, Legionella, Mycoplasma*)
Penicillin			X	X	X					X		
Amoxicillin[a]			X	X	X	X	X	X		X		
Oxacillin / Nafcillin		X	X	X								
Amoxicillin/Clavulanate / Ampicillin/Sulbactam		X	X	X	X	X	X	X		X	X	
Piperacillin/Tazobactam		X	X	X	X	X	X	X	X	X	X	
Cefazolin / Cephalexin		X	X	X		X				X		
Cefuroxime / Cefotetan / Cefoxitin		X	X	X		X	X			X	X	
Ceftriaxone / Ceftazidime		X	X	X		X	X	X	X	X		
Aztreonam						X	X	X	X			
Cefepime		X	X	X		X	X	X	X			
Ceftaroline	X	X	X	X		X	X	X		X		
Ceftazidime/Avibactam[b] / Ceftolozane/Tazobactam[b]		X	X	X		X	X	X	X			
Imipenem/Cilastatin[c] / Meropenem[c]		X	X	X	X	X	X	X	X	X	X	
Ertapenem / Ertapenem[d]		X	X	X		X	X	X		X	X	

[a] No Klebsiella coverage
[b] Must be given with metronidazole for adequate anaerobic coverage
[c] E. faecalis only
[d] No Acinetobacter coverage

MRSA = methicillin-resistant *Staphylococcus aureus*; MSSA = methicillin-susceptible *Staphylococcus aureus*; VRE = vancomycin-resistant *Enterococcus*; PEK = *Proteus, E. coli, Klebsiella*; HNPEK = *Haemophilus, Neisseria, Proteus, E. coli, Klebsiella*; CAPES = *Citrobacter, Acinetobacter, Providencia, Enterobacter, Serratia*; mouth flora = *Peptostreptococcus*

AMINOGLYCOSIDES

Aminoglycosides bind to the ribosome, which interferes with bacterial protein synthesis and results in a defective bacterial cell membrane. They are active against gram-negative bacteria, including _Pseudomonas_ (primarily tobramycin) and are typically used as part of an empiric regimen with other antibiotics (not as monotherapy). Gentamicin and streptomycin are used for synergy, in combination with a beta-lactam or vancomycin, when treating gram-positive infections (e.g., enterococcal endocarditis).

There are two dosing strategies for aminoglycosides; traditional dosing uses lower doses more frequently (e.g., Q8H if renal function is normal). Extended interval dosing uses higher doses (to attain higher peaks) less frequently (e.g., once daily if renal function is normal). With extended interval dosing, there is less accumulation of drug, lower risk of nephrotoxicity and decreased cost. See Study Tip Gal for more on aminoglycosides.

KEY FEATURES OF AMINOGLYCOSIDES

Class Effects
- Kill gram-negative bacteria (including _Pseudomonas_)
- Synergistic for gram-positive organisms (when combined with a beta-lactam or vancomycin)
- Concentration-dependent activity
- Post-antibiotic effect (killing continues after the serum level drops below the MIC)

Risks
- Nephrotoxicity
- Ototoxicity (hearing loss/tinnitus/balance problems); may be irreversible

Dosing Strategy
- Extended-interval dosing takes advantage of the concentration-dependent kinetics → give larger doses less frequently → this gives the kidneys time to recover between doses

DRUG	DOSING	SAFETY/SIDE EFFECTS/MONITORING
Gentamicin IV, IM, ophthalmic, topical	If underweight (< ideal body weight): use total body weight for dosing If normal weight (not obese or underweight): ideal body weight or total body weight can be used for dosing (per institutional protocol)	**BOXED WARNINGS** Nephrotoxicity, ototoxicity (hearing loss, vertigo, ataxia), neuromuscular blockade and respiratory paralysis, avoid with other neurotoxic/nephrotoxic drugs, fetal harm if given in pregnancy
Tobramycin IV, IM, ophthalmic, inhaled Tobramycin inhalation for CF _(Tobi, Tobi Podhaler, Bethkis, Kitabis Pak)_	If obese, use adjusted body weight for dosing (see Notes) **Traditional IV Dosing** Gentamicin and tobramycin: 1-2.5 mg/kg/dose; lower doses are used for gram-positive infections; higher doses are used for gram-negative infections Amikacin: 5-7.5 mg/kg/dose	**WARNINGS** Use caution in patients with impaired renal function, older adults, and those taking other nephrotoxic drugs (amphotericin B, cisplatin, polymyxins, cyclosporine, loop diuretics, NSAIDs, radiocontrast dye, tacrolimus, vancomycin) **MONITORING** Drug levels, renal function, urine output, hearing tests
Amikacin IV, IM	**Renal Dose Adjustments (Traditional Dosing)** CrCl ≥ 60 mL/min: Q8H CrCl 40-60 mL/min: Q12H CrCl 20-40 mL/min: Q24H	Traditional dosing: draw a trough level immediately before (or 30 minutes before) the 4th dose; draw a peak level 30 minutes after the end of the 30-minute infusion for the 4th dose (see table on the following page for target peaks and troughs)
Streptomycin IM	CrCl < 20 mL/min: 1x dose, then dose per levels **Extended Interval IV Dosing (Gentamicin/Tobramycin)** 4-7 mg/kg/dose (commonly 7 mg/kg)	Extended interval dosing: draw a random level per the timing on the nomogram (see example on following page) **NOTES** The clinical definition of obesity varies (but TBW > 120% IBW is commonly used for drug dosing); on the exam, obesity will be
Plazomicin _(Zemdri)_ IV For complicated UTI only (used last line)	Frequency (dosing interval) is determined by a nomogram (see example on following page) but the shortest interval is Q24H if renal function is normal **Other Dosing** Plazomicin 15 mg/kg IV Q24H (dose adjustments required if CrCl < 60 mL/min)	obvious, and may be stated in the question, indicating that adjusted body weight should be used for weight-based dosing (see the Calculations IV chapter for more information)

TRADITIONAL DOSING: TARGET DRUG CONCENTRATIONS

When peak and trough levels are drawn with the 4th aminoglycoside dose (see the Monitoring section of the drug table on the previous page), the levels are compared to the goal peaks and troughs to determine if dose adjustments are needed. Hospitals have protocols that guide dose adjustments. See the Pharmacokinetics chapter for details.

DRUG	PEAK	TROUGH
Gentamicin, gram-positive infection (synergy)	3-4 mcg/mL	< 1 mcg/mL
Gentamicin, gram-negative infection	5-10 mcg/mL	≤ 2 mcg/mL
Tobramycin		
Amikacin	20-30 mcg/mL	< 5 mcg/mL

EXTENDED INTERVAL DOSING NOMOGRAM

With extended interval dosing nomograms, a random level is drawn after the first dose (the timing depends on the nomogram; the Hartford nomogram shown below uses a window of 6 – 14 hours after the start of the infusion). The nomogram is used to plot the patient's level and determine the appropriate dosing interval (see Case Scenario). If the level plots on a line, round up to the next dosing interval to avoid potential toxicity.

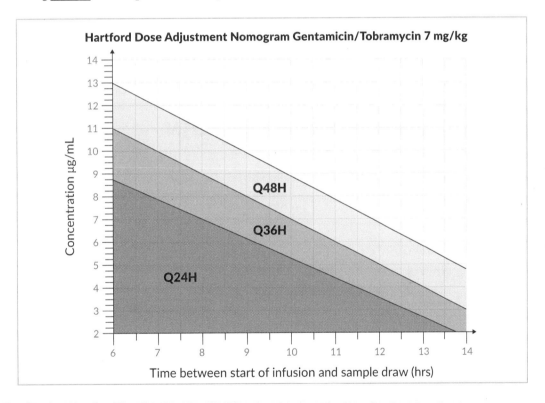

CASE SCENARIO

PR, a 56-year-old hospitalized female (height: 5'4", weight: 79 kg), is prescribed an antibiotic regimen that includes extended-interval tobramycin. The pharmacy aminoglycoside dosing protocol includes the Hartford nomogram method for dosing.

First, calculate the initial tobramycin dose.
- Determine which weight to use: since PR's TBW of 79 kg is > 120% greater than her IBW of 54.7 kg, adjusted body weight should be used. PR's adjusted body weight is 64.4 kg.
- Calculate the initial dose: 7 mg/kg x 64.4 kg = ~450 mg.

Next, determine the frequency of dosing.
- A random tobramycin level drawn 10 hours after the start of the 450 mg infusion is 6 mcg/mL.
- When plotted on the nomogram above, the lines meet in the Q36H dosing section, so her dose should be 450 mg IV Q36H.

QUINOLONES

Quinolones inhibit bacterial DNA topoisomerase IV and DNA gyrase (topoisomerase II). This prevents supercoiling of DNA and promotes breakage of double-stranded DNA. Quinolones have concentration-dependent antibacterial activity and a broad-spectrum of activity against gram-negative, gram-positive and atypical pathogens. Some notable distinctions in the class include:

- Levofloxacin and moxifloxacin are referred to as "respiratory quinolones" due to enhanced coverage of S. pneumoniae and atypical pathogens.

- Ciprofloxacin and levofloxacin have enhanced gram-negative activity, including activity against Pseudomonas.

- Moxifloxacin has enhanced gram-positive and anaerobic activity and can be used alone for polymicrobial infections (e.g., intra-abdominal infections). It is the only quinolone that cannot be used to treat urinary tract infections.

- Delafloxacin is active against MRSA and is the preferred quinolone if treating skin infections suspected to be caused by MRSA. Other quinolones should be avoided due to high rates of MRSA resistance.

DRUG	DOSING	SAFETY/SIDE EFFECTS/MONITORING
Ciprofloxacin (_Cipro_, _Ciloxan_ eye drops, _Cetraxal_ ear drops) Tablet, suspension, injection, ointment, ophthalmic, otic Combination ear drops: + dexamethasone **(_Ciprodex_)** + fluocinolone (_Otovel_) + hydrocortisone (_Cipro HC_)	PO: 250-750 mg Q12H IV: 200-400 mg Q8-12H CrCl < 30 mL/min: Q18-24H	**BOXED WARNINGS** Tendon inflammation and/or rupture (often in the Achilles tendon) within hours/days of starting, or up to several months after completion of treatment; ↑ risk with concurrent use of systemic steroids, in organ transplant recipients or age > 60 years; discontinue immediately if symptoms occur Peripheral neuropathy; can last months to years after discontinuation of the drug and may become permanent; discontinue immediately if symptoms occur CNS effects (seizures, tremor, restlessness, confusion, hallucinations, depression, suicidal thoughts, paranoia, nightmares, insomnia,↑ intracranial pressure); use caution in patients with CNS disorders or with drugs that cause seizures or lower the seizure threshold (see the Seizures/Epilepsy chapter)
Levofloxacin Tablet, solution, injection, ophthalmic	PO/IV: 250-750 mg daily CrCl < 50 mL/min: Q48H and/ or ↓ dose	Avoid in patients with myasthenia gravis (may exacerbate muscle weakness) Use last-line for: acute bacterial sinusitis, acute exacerbation of chronic bronchitis and uncomplicated UTI **CONTRAINDICATIONS** Ciprofloxacin: concurrent administration of tizanidine
Moxifloxacin (_Avelox_, _Vigamox_ eye drops) Tablet, injection, ophthalmic	IV/PO: 400 mg Q24H No renal dose adjustments required	**WARNINGS** QT prolongation (highest risk with moxifloxacin > levofloxacin > ciprofloxacin); avoid in patients with known QT prolongation, or those with additive risks (hypokalemia, use of other drugs that prolong the QT interval – see the Arrhythmias chapter)
Delafloxacin (_Baxdela_) Tablet, injection	PO: 450 mg Q12H IV: 300 mg Q12H eGFR 15-29 mL/min/1.73 m²: dose adjustment required (IV only) eGFR < 15 mL/min/1.73 m²: not recommended (IV or PO)	Hypoglycemia and hyperglycemia Psychiatric disturbances (agitation, disorientation, lack of attention, nervousness, memory impairment, delirium) Avoid systemic quinolones in children and in pregnancy/breastfeeding due to the risk of musculoskeletal toxicity (exception: anthrax exposure) Aortic aneurysm and dissection (↑ risk with longer durations of therapy or history of peripheral vascular disease, atherosclerosis or prior aneurysms) Other: photosensitivity, hepatotoxicity, crystalluria (must stay hydrated)
Gatifloxacin (_Zymaxid_ eye drops)	No oral or injectable formulations	**SIDE EFFECTS** Nausea/diarrhea, headache, dizziness, serious skin reactions (SJS/TEN) **NOTES** Ciprofloxacin oral suspension: shake vigorously for 15 seconds before each dose; do not put through an NG or other feeding tube (the oil-based suspension adheres to tubing)
Ofloxacin **(_Ocuflox_** eye drops) Tablet, ophthalmic, otic	PO: 200-400 mg Q12H CrCl ≤ 50 mL/min: dose adjustment required	_Cipro_: can crush immediate-release tablets, mix with water and give via a feeding tube; hold tube feedings at least 1 hour before and 2 hours after the dose Moxifloxacin should not be used for UTIs (does not concentrate in the urine)

Quinolone Drug Interactions

- <u>Antacids</u> and other <u>polyvalent cations</u> (e.g., magnesium, aluminum, phosphate, calcium, iron, zinc), multivitamins, sucralfate, and bile acid resins <u>can chelate and inhibit quinolone absorption</u> and should not be taken at the same time (separate administration).

- The phosphate binders <u>lanthanum</u> carbonate and <u>sevelamer</u> can ↓ the serum concentration of oral quinolones; <u>separate administration</u>.

- Quinolones can ↑ the effects of warfarin.

- Quinolones can ↑ the effects of sulfonylureas, insulin and other hypoglycemic drugs.

- Caution with CVD, ↓ potassium and magnesium and with other <u>QT-prolonging drugs</u> (e.g., azole antifungals, antipsychotics, methadone, macrolides).

- Probenecid and NSAIDs can ↑ quinolone levels.

- Ciprofloxacin is a strong <u>CYP1A2 inhibitor</u> and a weak CYP3A4 inhibitor; ciprofloxacin can <u>↑ levels</u> of caffeine, <u>theophylline</u> and tizanidine by reducing metabolism.

KEY FEATURES OF QUINOLONES

Common Uses
- Varies by agent: pneumonia, UTIs, intra-abdominal infections, travelers' diarrhea

Respiratory Quinolones
- Levofloxacin, moxifloxacin
- Reliable *S. pneumoniae* activity (in pneumonia)

Antipseudomonal Quinolones
- Ciprofloxacin, levofloxacin

Moxifloxacin
- Only quinolone that is not renally adjusted (do not use for UTIs)

IV to PO Ratio 1:1
- Levofloxacin and moxifloxacin

Profile Review Tips
- Caution with CVD, ↓ K/Mg and with other QT-prolonging drugs (e.g., azole antifungals, antipsychotics, methadone, macrolides)
- Avoid in patients with a seizure history or if using antiseizure drugs
- Avoid in children

Counseling
- Avoid sun exposure, separate from polyvalent cations, monitor blood glucose (in diabetes)
- Watch for tendon rupture, neuropathy, CNS or psychiatric side effects

MACROLIDES

Macrolides bind to the <u>50S ribosomal subunit</u>, resulting in inhibition of protein synthesis. They have excellent coverage of <u>atypicals</u> (*Legionella, Chlamydia, Mycoplasma, Mycobacterium avium* complex) and also cover *S. pneumoniae, Haemophilus* and *Moraxella*, although these organisms have increasing rates of resistance to macrolides. Macrolides are treatment options for <u>community-acquired</u> upper and lower <u>respiratory tract infections</u> and certain sexually transmitted infections (e.g., <u>chlamydia</u>).

DRUG	DOSING	SAFETY/SIDE EFFECTS/MONITORING
Azithromycin (*Zithromax, Z-Pak,* Zithromax Tri-Pak, *AzaSite* eye drops) Tablet, suspension, injection, ophthalmic	Z-Pak: <u>500 mg on day 1, then 250 mg on days 2-5</u> Tri-Pak: <u>500 mg daily for 3 days</u> IV: 250-500 mg daily No renal dose adjustments required	**CONTRAINDICATIONS** History of cholestatic jaundice/hepatic dysfunction with prior use Clarithromycin and erythromycin: do not use with lovastatin or simvastatin, pimozide, ergotamine or dihydroergotamine Clarithromycin: concurrent use with colchicine in patients with renal or hepatic impairment **WARNINGS** <u>QT prolongation</u> (highest risk with erythromycin > azithromycin > clarithromycin); avoid in patients with known QT prolongation, or those with additive risks (hypokalemia, use of other drugs that prolong the QT interval – see the Arrhythmias chapter) <u>Hepatotoxicity</u>; use caution in patients with liver disease Exacerbation of myasthenia gravis Clarithromycin: caution in patients with <u>CAD</u> (↑ mortality has been documented ≥ 1 year after the end of a 2-week course of treatment) **SIDE EFFECTS** <u>GI upset</u> (diarrhea, abdominal pain, cramping), taste perversion, ototoxicity (rare, reversible), severe (but rare) skin reactions (SJS/TEN/DRESS)
Clarithromycin Tablet, suspension	PO: 250-500 mg Q12H or 1 gram (ER tablet) daily CrCl < 30 mL/min: dose adjustment required	
Erythromycin (*E.E.S., Ery-Tab, Erythrocin,* EryPed, Erygel topical) Capsule, tablet, suspension, injection, ophthalmic, topical E.E.S = erythromycin ethylsuccinate	Dosing varies by product E.E.S 400 mg = 250 mg erythromycin base or stearate No renal dose adjustments required	

Macrolide Drug Interactions

- <u>Erythromycin and clarithromycin</u> are major substrates of CYP3A4 and are <u>CYP3A4 inhibitors</u> (moderate for erythromycin, strong for clarithromycin). Some medications metabolized by CYP3A4 (e.g., <u>simvastatin</u>, <u>lovastatin</u>) are <u>contraindicated</u> in combination with these macrolides, and others may require close monitoring or should be used with caution. Some examples include apixaban, colchicine, dabigatran, rivaroxaban, theophylline and <u>warfarin</u>. Refer to the Drug Interactions chapter for more information.

- <u>Azithromycin</u> is a minor substrate of CYP3A4 and a weak inhibitor of CYP1A2 and P-gp; it has <u>fewer clinically significant drug interactions</u> than other macrolides.

- <u>All macrolides</u>: use caution with CVD, ↓ potassium and magnesium and with other <u>QT-prolonging drugs</u> (e.g., azole antifungals, antipsychotics, methadone, quinolones).

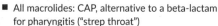

KEY FEATURES OF MACROLIDES

Common Uses

- All macrolides: CAP, alternative to a beta-lactam for pharyngitis ("strep throat")

- Azithromycin: COPD exacerbations, pertussis, chlamydia (in pregnant patients), prophylaxis for *Mycobacterium avium* complex, severe travelers' diarrhea (including dysentery)

- Clarithromycin: used in *H. pylori* treatment regimens (see the GERD & PUD chapter)

- Erythromycin ↑ gastric motility and is used for gastroparesis

Common Azithromycin Dosing (*Z-Pak*)

- Two 250 mg tablets PO x 1, then 250 mg PO daily x 4 days

QT Prolongation

- Caution with CVD, ↓ K/Mg and other QT-prolonging drugs (e.g., azole antifungals, antipsychotics, methadone, quinolones)

Drug Interactions

- Clarithromycin and erythromycin are CYP3A4 inhibitors; lovastatin and simvastatin are contraindicated (↑ risk of muscle toxicity)

TETRACYCLINES

Tetracyclines inhibit bacterial protein synthesis by reversibly binding to the <u>30S ribosomal subunit</u>. They cover many gram-positive bacteria (staphylococci, streptococci, enterococci, *Propionibacterium* spp.), gram-negative bacteria, including respiratory flora *(Haemophilus, Moraxella,* <u>atypicals</u>*)* and other unique pathogens (e.g., *Rickettsiae, Bacillus anthracis, Treponema pallidum,* other spirochetes).

<u>Doxycycline</u> has broader indications than the other tetracyclines, including respiratory tract infections (e.g., <u>CAP</u>), <u>tickborne/rickettsial diseases</u> and sexually transmitted infections (e.g., <u>chlamydia</u>). Doxycycline is an option for the treatment of mild <u>CA-MRSA</u> skin infections and <u>VRE</u> urinary tract infections.

DRUG	DOSING	SAFETY/SIDE EFFECTS/MONITORING
Doxycycline (*Vibramycin,* *Doryx,* *Oracea*) Capsule, tablet, suspension, syrup, injection	PO/IV: 100-200 mg daily in 1-2 divided doses Take with food to ↓ GI irritation (except take *Oracea* on an empty stomach) <u>No renal dose adjustments required</u>	**WARNINGS** <u>Children age < 8 years, pregnancy and breastfeeding</u> (suppresses bone growth and skeletal development, and permanently discolors teeth) <u>Photosensitivity</u>, tissue hyperpigmentation, severe skin reactions (DRESS/SJS/TEN), exfoliative dermatitis GI inflammation/ulceration (see Notes section) <u>Minocycline</u>: drug-induced lupus erythematosus (<u>DILE</u>)
Minocycline (*Minocin,* *Solodyn,* *Minolira*) Capsule, tablet, injection, topical	PO/IV: 200 mg x 1, then 50-100 mg Q12H No renal dose adjustments required	
Eravacycline (*Xerava*) Injection	1 mg/kg IV Q12H	**SIDE EFFECTS** N/V/D, rash
Omadacycline (*Nuzyra*) Tablet, injection	Dose varies by indication	**MONITORING** LFTs, renal function, CBC
Sarecycline (*Seysara*) Tablet	Dose based on body weight	**NOTES** <u>IV:PO ratio is 1:1</u> (doxycycline, minocycline)
Tetracycline Capsule	PO: 250-500 mg Q6H on an empty stomach CrCl ≤ 50 mL/min: dose adjustment required	Tablets and capsules should be taken with 8 oz of water; with <u>doxycycline, sit upright for at least 30 minutes</u> after dose to avoid esophageal irritation

Tetracycline Drug Interactions

- Antacids and other polyvalent cations (e.g., magnesium, aluminum, phosphate, calcium, lanthanum, iron, zinc), multivitamins, sucralfate, bismuth subsalicylate and bile acid resins can chelate and inhibit the absorption of tetracyclines. Separate administration. Dairy products should be avoided 1 hour before or 2 hours after tetracyclines.

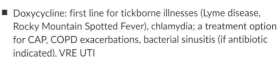

KEY FEATURES OF TETRACYCLINES

Common Uses

- Doxycycline and minocycline: CA-MRSA skin infections, acne

- Doxycycline: first line for tickborne illnesses (Lyme disease, Rocky Mountain Spotted Fever), chlamydia; a treatment option for CAP, COPD exacerbations, bacterial sinusitis (if antibiotic indicated), VRE UTI

- Tetracycline: used in *H. pylori* treatment regimens (see the GERD & PUD chapter)

Do not use in pregnancy, breastfeeding or children < 8 years old

SULFONAMIDES

Sulfamethoxazole (SMX) inhibits dihydrofolic acid formation, which interferes with bacterial folic acid synthesis. Trimethoprim (TMP) inhibits dihydrofolic acid reduction to tetrahydrofolate, resulting in inhibition of the folic acid pathway.

Sulfamethoxazole/trimethoprim has activity against staphylococci (including MRSA); *S. pneumoniae* and Group A *Streptococcus* activity is unreliable. Activity against gram-negative bacteria is broad and includes *Haemophilus, Proteus, E. coli, Klebsiella, Enterobacter, Shigella, Salmonella and Stenotrophomonas*. SMX/TMP is active against some opportunistic pathogens (*Nocardia, Pneumocystis, Toxoplasmosis*), but does not have activity against *Pseudomonas*, enterococci, atypicals or anaerobes.

DRUG	DOSING	SAFETY/SIDE EFFECTS/MONITORING
Sulfamethoxazole/ Trimethoprim (Bactrim, Bactrim DS, *Sulfatrim Pediatric)* Tablet, suspension, injection	Dose based on the TMP component **Severe Infections** PO/IV: 10-20 mg TMP/kg/day, divided Q6-12H (e.g., 2 DS tablets BID-TID)	**CONTRAINDICATIONS** Sulfa allergy, anemia due to folate deficiency, renal or hepatic disease, infants < 2 months **WARNINGS** Blood dyscrasias, including agranulocytosis and aplastic anemia
Single Strength (SS) 400 mg SMX/80 mg TMP	**Uncomplicated UTI** 1 DS tablet PO BID x 3 days	Skin reactions: SJS/TEN, thrombotic thrombocytopenic purpura (TTP) Hemolytic anemia: can be immune-mediated (identified with a positive Coombs test) or caused by G6PD deficiency (do not use with known deficiency); discontinue drug if hemolysis occurs
Double Strength (DS) 800 mg SMX/160 mg TMP	***Pneumocystis* Pneumonia (PCP) Prophylaxis** 1 DS or SS tablet daily	Hypoglycemia, thrombocytopenia Pregnancy (blocks folic acid metabolism, leading to congenital defects): use only if benefit outweighs risk (see ID II chapter for UTI treatment options)
All products are formulated with a SMX:TMP ratio = 5:1	**PCP Treatment** IV/PO: 15-20 mg TMP/kg/day divided Q6H CrCl 15-30 mL/min: dose adjustment required CrCl < 15 mL/min: not recommended	**SIDE EFFECTS** Photosensitivity, ↑ K, crystalluria (take with 8 oz of water), N/V/D, anorexia, skin rash, ↓ folate, false elevations in SCr (due to inhibition of creatinine tubular secretion), renal failure **MONITORING** Renal function, electrolytes, CBC, folate

Sulfonamide Drug Interactions

- SMX/TMP is a moderate-strong CYP2C8 and CYP2C9 inhibitor and can ↑ INR if used in combination with warfarin (see the Drug Interactions chapter for more information).

- SMX/TMP can enhance the toxic effects of methotrexate.

- The therapeutic effects of SMX/TMP can be diminished by the use of leucovorin or levoleucovorin.

- The risk for hyperkalemia will ↑ in patients with renal dysfunction or if used in combination with ACE inhibitors, ARBs, aliskiren, aldosterone receptor antagonists (ARAs), potassium-sparing diuretics, cyclosporine, tacrolimus, NSAIDs, drospirenone-containing oral contraceptives or canagliflozin.

KEY FEATURES OF SULFAMETHOXAZOLE/ TRIMETHOPRIM

Common Uses
- CA-MRSA skin infections, UTI, *Pneumocystis* pneumonia (PCP)

5:1 Ratio of SMX/TMP (Dose Based on TMP)
- Single strength (SS) tablet contains 80 mg TMP

- Double strength (DS) tablet contains 160 mg TMP – usual dose is one tablet BID

Sulfa Allergy
- Most sulfa allergies occur with SMX/TMP (rash/hives common)

- Rarely, severe skin reactions (e.g., SJS or TEN) can occur; if rash is accompanied by fever or systemic symptoms, seek emergency care

INR ↑ when used with warfarin. Use alternative antibiotic when possible.

ANTIBIOTICS FOR GRAM-POSITIVE INFECTIONS

VANCOMYCIN

Vancomycin is a glycopeptide that inhibits bacterial cell wall synthesis by binding to the D-alanyl-D-alanine cell wall precursor and blocking peptidoglycan polymerization. Vancomycin only covers gram-positive bacteria, including staphylococci (MRSA), streptococci, enterococci (not VRE) and *C. difficile* (using the PO route only).

DRUG	DOSING	SAFETY/SIDE EFFECTS/MONITORING
Vancomycin (*Vancocin*, Firvanq oral solution) Capsule, solution, injection First-line treatment for moderate-severe systemic MRSA infections Consider an alternative drug when MRSA MIC ≥ 2 mcg/mL	**Systemic Infections (IV Only)** IV: 15-20 mg/kg Q8-12H Dose based on total body weight CrCl 20-49 mL/min: Q24H CrCl < 20 mL/min: give one dose, then dose per levels Peripheral IV infusions should not exceed 5 mg/mL **C. difficile Infections (PO Only)** PO: 125 QID x 10 days 500 mg QID used for severe, complicated disease (in combination with IV metronidazole) No renal dose adjustments required	**WARNINGS** Ototoxicity and nephrotoxicity; caution with use of other nephrotoxic or ototoxic drugs or with prolonged high serum concentrations (dose adjustment required in renal impairment) PO formulation is used only for *C. difficile* colitis and enterocolitis, not for systemic infections; IV formulation is not effective for *C. difficile* (does not cross into the GI tract) Vancomycin infusion reaction (maculopapular rash, hypotension, flushing and chills) from too rapid of an infusion rate; do not infuse faster than 1 gram per hour **SIDE EFFECTS** Abdominal pain, nausea (oral route), phlebitis (irritation to vein), myelosuppression (neutropenia, thrombocytopenia), drug fever, severe skin reactions (SJS/TEN) **MONITORING** Renal function, drug levels (see below), WBC AUC/MIC ratio or steady state trough (drawn 30 minutes before the 4th or 5th dose) Serious MRSA infections (e.g., bacteremia, sepsis, endocarditis, pneumonia, osteomyelitis, meningitis): AUC/MIC ratio of 400-600 recommended or goal trough 15-20 mcg/mL Other infections (e.g., UTI, skin infections): goal trough 10-15 mcg/mL

Vancomycin Drug Interactions

- The risk of nephrotoxicity is ↑ when used with other nephrotoxic drugs (e.g., aminoglycosides, amphotericin B, cisplatin, polymyxins, cyclosporine, tacrolimus, loop diuretics, NSAIDs, radiographic contrast dye).

- Vancomycin can ↑ the risk of ototoxicity when used with other ototoxic drugs (e.g., aminoglycosides, cisplatin, loop diuretics).

LIPOGLYCOPEPTIDES

Lipoglycopeptides (with the generic name suffix "-vancin") inhibit bacterial cell wall synthesis by 1) binding to the D-alanyl-D-alanine portion of the cell wall, blocking polymerization and cross-linking of peptidoglycan, and 2) disrupting bacterial membrane potential and changing cell permeability (due to the presence of a lipophilic side chain). They have concentration-dependent activity against similar pathogens as vancomycin, but are only approved to treat skin and soft-tissue infections (SSTIs), except telavancin is also approved to treat hospital-acquired and ventilator-associated pneumonia.

DRUG	DOSING	SAFETY/SIDE EFFECTS/MONITORING
Telavancin (Vibativ)	IV: 10 mg/kg daily	**BOXED WARNINGS (TELAVANCIN)** Fetal risk – obtain pregnancy test prior to starting therapy; nephrotoxicity; ↑ mortality with pre-existing moderate to severe renal impairment (CrCl ≤ 50 mL/min) when compared to vancomycin in pneumonia trials **CONTRAINDICATIONS** Telavancin: concurrent use of IV unfractionated heparin (UFH)
Oritavancin (Orbactiv, Kimyrsa)	Single-dose IV regimen: 1,200 mg	Oritavancin: do not use IV UFH for 120 hours (5 days) after oritavancin administration due to interference (false elevations) with aPTT laboratory results **WARNINGS** Infusion reaction (similar to vancomycin) with rapid IV administration Oritavancin and telavancin: falsely ↑ aPTT/PT/INR but do not ↑ bleeding risk
Dalbavancin (Dalvance)	Single-dose IV regimen: 1,500 mg	Telavancin: QT prolongation Oritavancin: use a different antibiotic if osteomyelitis is confirmed or suspected Dalbavancin: ↑ ALT > 3x the upper limit of normal **NOTES** Telavancin, dalbavancin: renal dose adjustments required

Telavancin Drug Interactions

■ Avoid telavancin in patients with congenital long QT syndrome, known QT prolongation or decompensated heart failure. Use caution with other medications known to prolong the QT interval (see the Arrhythmias chapter).

DAPTOMYCIN

Daptomycin is a cyclic lipopeptide. It binds to cell membrane components, causing rapid depolarization; this inhibits all intracellular replication processes, including protein synthesis, and causes cell death. Daptomycin has concentration-dependent activity against most gram-positive bacteria, including staphylococci (MRSA) and enterococci (VRE). It has no activity against gram-negative pathogens.

DRUG	DOSING	SAFETY/SIDE EFFECTS/MONITORING
Daptomycin (Cubicin*) Do not use to treat pneumonia; drug is inactivated in the lungs by surfactant	SSTI: 4 mg/kg IV daily Bacteremia/right-sided endocarditis: 6 mg/kg IV daily (doses up to 10 mg/kg IV daily may be used in practice) CrCl < 30 mL/min: Q48H	**WARNINGS** Myopathy and rhabdomyolysis: discontinue in patients with s/sx and CPK > 1,000 units/L, or in asymptomatic patients with a CPK > 2,000 units/L; consider temporarily withholding other drugs that can cause muscle damage (e.g., statins) during treatment Can falsely ↑ PT/INR, but does not ↑ bleeding risk Peripheral neuropathy DRESS, eosinophilic pneumonia – generally develops 2-4 weeks after treatment initiation **SIDE EFFECTS** ↑ CPK, abdominal pain, pruritus, chest pain, edema, hypertension, acute kidney injury **MONITORING** CPK weekly (more frequent if on a statin or with renal impairment); muscle pain/weakness, s/sx of neuropathy, dyspnea **NOTES** Compatible with NS and LR (no dextrose)

Brand discontinued but name still used in practice.

OXAZOLIDINONES

Linezolid and tedizolid bind to the 50S subunit of the bacterial ribosome, inhibiting translation and protein synthesis. They have activity against similar pathogens as vancomycin (e.g., MRSA), but also cover VRE.

DRUG	DOSING	SAFETY/SIDE EFFECTS/MONITORING
Linezolid (Zyvox) Tablet, suspension, injection	PO/IV: 600 mg Q12H No renal dose adjustments required IV:PO ratio is 1:1	**CONTRAINDICATIONS** Do not use with or within 2 weeks of MAO inhibitors **WARNINGS** Duration-related myelosuppression (thrombocytopenia, anemia, leukopenia) when used > 14 days, peripheral and optic neuropathy when used > 28 days, serotonin syndrome, hypoglycemia (caution with insulin or other hypoglycemic drugs), hyponatremia, seizures, lactic acidosis, ↑ BP (caution and monitor BP in patients with uncontrolled hypertension and untreated hyperthyroidism) **SIDE EFFECTS** ↓ platelets, ↓ Hgb, ↓ WBC, headache, nausea, diarrhea, ↑ LFTs **MONITORING** Weekly CBC, HR, BP, BG (in diabetes), visual function **NOTES** Do not shake linezolid suspension
Tedizolid (Sivextro) Tablet, injection Approved for SSTI only	PO/IV: 200 mg daily No renal dose adjustments required IV:PO ratio is 1:1	**WARNINGS** Consider alternative treatment in patients with neutropenia **SIDE EFFECTS** Nausea, diarrhea, dizziness, infusion-related reactions

Linezolid/Tedizolid Drug Interactions

- Linezolid and tedizolid are reversible monoamine oxidase inhibitors. Avoid tyramine-containing foods and serotonergic drugs (see the Drug Interactions chapter).

- Linezolid can exacerbate hypoglycemic episodes; use caution in patients receiving insulin or oral hypoglycemic drugs (e.g., sulfonylureas).

ADDITIONAL BROAD-SPECTRUM DRUGS

TIGECYCLINE

Tigecycline (a glycylcycline) binds to the 30S ribosomal subunit and inhibits protein synthesis. It has broad-spectrum activity against gram-positive bacteria, including staphylococci (MRSA) and enterococci (VRE), gram-negative bacteria, anaerobes and atypical organisms. Among the gram-negatives, it has no activity against the "3 P's": *Pseudomonas*, *Proteus* and *Providencia*. Clinical use of tigecycline is limited (see Boxed Warning).

DRUG	DOSING	SAFETY/SIDE EFFECTS/MONITORING
Tigecycline (Tygacil) Injection	IV: 100 mg x 1 dose, then 50 mg Q12H Severe hepatic impairment: dose adjustment required No renal dose adjustments required	**BOXED WARNING** ↑ risk of death, use only when alternative treatments are not suitable **WARNINGS** Anaphylactic reactions (avoid in patients with a tetracycline-class allergy due to similar structure) Hepatotoxicity, pancreatitis, photosensitivity, bone growth suppression and teeth discoloration in children < 8 years old (avoid use) **SIDE EFFECTS** N/V (can be intractable), diarrhea, headache, dizziness, ↑ LFTs, rash/severe skin reactions (SJS) **NOTES** Do not use for bloodstream infections; it does not achieve adequate concentrations in the blood since it is lipophilic (drug distributes quickly out of the blood into tissues) Reconstituted solution should be yellow-orange; discard if not this color

POLYMYXINS

The polymyxin class consists of two drugs, colistimethate (sometimes referred to as colistin) and polymyxin B. Colistimethate is an inactive prodrug that is converted to colistin. Colistin and polymyxin B act as cationic detergents and damage the bacterial cytoplasmic membrane, causing leakage of intracellular substances and cell death. Polymyxins have activity against gram-negative bacteria, such as *Enterobacter* spp., *E. coli, Klebsiella pneumoniae* and *Pseudomonas aeruginosa* (but not *Proteus* spp.). Due to the risk of toxicities, they are used primarily for MDR gram-negative pathogens in combination with other antibiotics.

DRUG	DOSING	SAFETY/SIDE EFFECTS/MONITORING
Colistimethate (*Coly-Mycin M*) Injection can be used for inhalation administration	IV/IM: 2.5-5 mg/kg/day in 2-4 divided doses Solutions for inhalation must be mixed immediately prior to administration	**WARNINGS** Dose-dependent nephrotoxicity (monitor renal function), neurotoxicity (dizziness, headache, tingling, oral paresthesia, vertigo, respiratory paralysis from neuromuscular blockade) **NOTES** Assess dose carefully (can be units of colistimethate, mg of colistimethate or mg of colistin base activity)
Polymyxin B	IV: 15,000-25,000 units/kg/day divided every 12 hours 1 mg = 10,000 units polymyxin B	**BOXED WARNINGS** Dose-dependent nephrotoxicity (monitor renal function) Neurotoxicity (dizziness, tingling, numbness, paresthesia, vertigo, respiratory paralysis from neuromuscular blockade) Should only be administered to hospitalized patients Avoid concurrent or sequential use of other neurotoxic or nephrotoxic drugs

Polymyxin Drug Interactions

- Risk of nephrotoxicity is increased if used in combination with other nephrotoxic drugs, including aminoglycosides, amphotericin B, cisplatin, cyclosporine, loop diuretics, NSAIDs, radiocontrast dye, tacrolimus and vancomycin.

CHLORAMPHENICOL

Chloramphenicol reversibly binds to the 50S subunit of the bacterial ribosome, inhibiting protein synthesis. It has activity against gram-positive, gram-negative, anaerobic and atypical organisms; however, it is rarely used due to adverse effects, notably fatal blood dyscrasias (e.g., aplastic anemia, pancytopenia) and Gray syndrome (e.g., circulatory collapse, cyanosis, acidosis).

MISCELLANEOUS ANTIBIOTICS

CLINDAMYCIN

Clindamycin is a lincosamide that reversibly binds to the 50S subunit of the bacterial ribosome, inhibiting protein synthesis. It has activity against most gram-positive bacteria, including some CA-MRSA and anaerobes. It does not cover *Enterococcus* or gram-negative pathogens and has minimal gram-negative anaerobic activity.

DRUG	DOSING	SAFETY/SIDE EFFECTS/MONITORING
Clindamycin (*Cleocin*) Injection, capsule, solution Topical: **Cleocin-T, Clindagel,** *Clindacin Pac, Clindacin-P* Vaginal: *Clindesse, Cleocin*	PO: 150-450 mg Q6H IV: 600-900 mg Q8H No renal dose adjustments required	**BOXED WARNING** Colitis (*C. difficile*) **WARNING** Severe or fatal skin reactions (SJS/TEN/DRESS) **SIDE EFFECTS** N/V/D, rash, urticaria, ↑ LFTs (rare) **NOTES** An induction test (D-test) should be performed on *S. aureus* that is susceptible to clindamycin but resistant to erythromycin; a flattened zone between the disks (positive D-test) indicates inducible clindamycin resistance and clindamycin should not be used

METRONIDAZOLE AND RELATED DRUGS

These antibiotics cause a loss of helical DNA structure and strand breakage resulting in inhibition of protein synthesis. Metronidazole has activity against anaerobes and protozoal organisms. It is effective for bacterial vaginosis, trichomoniasis, giardiasis, amebiasis, C. difficile (though not preferred) and is used in combination regimens for intra-abdominal infections.

Tinidazole is structurally related to metronidazole, but its activity is limited to protozoa (giardiasis, amebiasis), trichomoniasis and bacterial vaginosis organisms. Secnidazole is only indicated for bacterial vaginosis and trichomoniasis.

DRUG	DOSING	SAFETY/SIDE EFFECTS/MONITORING
Metronidazole (Flagyl, Likmez) Tablet, capsule, injection, suspension Topical: MetroCream, Metrogel, MetroLotion, Noritate Vaginal: Nuvessa, Vandazole	PO/IV: 500-750 mg Q8-12H or 250-500 mg Q6-8H No renal dose adjustments required Take with food to ↓ GI upset IV:PO ratio is 1:1	**BOXED WARNING** Possibly carcinogenic based on animal data **CONTRAINDICATIONS** Pregnancy (1st trimester), use of alcohol or propylene glycol-containing products during treatment or within 3 days of treatment discontinuation (disulfiram reaction) Metronidazole: use of disulfiram within the past 2 weeks Tinidazole: breastfeeding **WARNINGS** CNS effects: seizures, peripheral neuropathy Metronidazole: aseptic meningitis, encephalopathy, optic neuropathy
Tinidazole Tablet	2 grams PO daily Take with food to minimize GI effects No renal dose adjustments required	**SIDE EFFECTS** Metallic taste, headache, nausea, furry tongue, dizziness, rash/severe skin reactions (SJS/TEN) **NOTES** See the ID II chapter for a discussion of use for STIs in pregnancy
Secnidazole (Solosec) Granule packet	PO: 2 gram single dose Sprinkle contents of 1 packet onto applesauce, yogurt, or pudding and consume within 30 minutes; do not chew the granules	**WARNINGS** Vulvovaginal candidiasis, possibly carcinogenic (based on animal data with structurally similar drugs) **SIDE EFFECTS** Headache, N/D

Metronidazole Drug Interactions

- Should not be used with alcohol (during and for 3 days after discontinuation of treatment) due to a potential disulfiram-like reaction (abdominal cramping, headaches, nausea/vomiting, flushing).
- Metronidazole is a weak inhibitor of CYP2C9 and can cause an ↑ INR in patients taking warfarin.

LEFAMULIN

Lefamulin is a first-in-class pleuromutilin. It inhibits bacterial protein synthesis by binding to the peptidyl transferase center of the 50S ribosomal subunit.

DRUG	DOSING	SAFETY/SIDE EFFECTS/MONITORING
Lefamulin (Xenleta) Tablet, injection	PO: 600 mg Q12H IV: 150 mg Q12H	**CONTRAINDICATIONS** Use with CYP3A4 substrates that prolong the QT interval **WARNINGS** Pregnancy (teratogenic), QT prolongation **SIDE EFFECTS** Diarrhea, nausea, injection site reactions

FIDAXOMICIN

Fidaxomicin inhibits RNA polymerase, resulting in inhibition of protein synthesis and cell death. It is used for _C. difficile_ infections.

DRUG	DOSING	SAFETY/SIDE EFFECTS/MONITORING
Fidaxomicin *(Dificid)* Tablet, suspension	PO: 200 mg BID x 10 days No renal dose adjustments required	**WARNINGS** Not effective for systemic infections – absorption is minimal **SIDE EFFECTS** N/V, abdominal pain, GI bleeding, anemia

RIFAXIMIN

Rifaximin inhibits bacterial RNA synthesis by binding to bacterial DNA-dependent RNA polymerase.

DRUG	DOSING	SAFETY/SIDE EFFECTS/MONITORING
Rifaximin *(Xifaxan)* Tablet	Travelers' diarrhea: 200 mg TID x 3 days Hepatic encephalopathy: 550 mg BID or 400 mg Q8H Irritable bowel syndrome w/diarrhea (IBS-D): 550 mg TID x 14 days No renal dose adjustments required	**SIDE EFFECTS** Peripheral edema, dizziness, headache, nausea, abdominal pain, rash/pruritus **NOTES** Not effective for systemic infections (< 1% absorption) Used off-label for _C. difficile_ infections (third or subsequent recurrence)

URINARY AGENTS

FOSFOMYCIN

Inactivates the enzyme pyruval transferase, which is critical in the synthesis of cell walls. It has activity against _E. coli_ (including ESBL-producing strains) and _E. faecalis_ (including VRE). A single-dose regimen is used for uncomplicated UTI (cystitis only).

DRUG	DOSING	SAFETY/SIDE EFFECTS/MONITORING
Fosfomycin *(Monurol)* Packet granules = 3 gram per packet	**Female, Uncomplicated UTI** 3 grams PO x 1, mixed in 3-4 oz of cold water	**SIDE EFFECTS** Headache, diarrhea, nausea **NOTES** Concentrates in the urine

NITROFURANTOIN

Nitrofurantoin is a bacterial cell wall, DNA, RNA and protein synthesis inhibitor. It is used for uncomplicated UTI (cystitis only). It covers *E. coli, Klebsiella, Enterobacter, S. aureus* and *Enterococcus* (including VRE).

DRUG	DOSING	SAFETY/SIDE EFFECTS/ MONITORING
Nitrofurantoin (Macrobid, Macrodantin) Capsule, suspension	*Macrodantin:* 50-100 mg PO QID x 3-7 days; 50-100 mg PO QHS for prophylaxis *Macrobid:* 100 mg PO BID x 5 days	**CONTRAINDICATIONS** Renal impairment (CrCl < 60 mL/min*): inadequate urine concentration and risk for accumulation of neurotoxins; history of cholestatic jaundice/hepatic dysfunction with previous use; pregnancy (at term) **WARNINGS** Optic neuritis, hepatotoxicity, peripheral neuropathy, pulmonary toxicity, G6PD deficiency (can cause hemolytic anemia; do not use if known deficiency) **SIDE EFFECTS** GI upset (take with food), headache, rash, brown urine discoloration (harmless) **NOTES** Concentrates in the urine

KEY FEATURES OF NITROFURANTOIN

Common Use
- Uncomplicated UTI (see ID II chapter for a discussion of use in pregnancy)

Do Not Use
- CrCl < 60 mL/min
- G6PD deficiency

Dosing
- Macro**bid** is BID
- Macrodantin is QID

Counseling
- Take with food to prevent nausea, cramping
- Can discolor the urine (brown)

*Per package labeling. Some sources (e.g., Beers Criteria) recommend use if CrCl > 30 mL/min.

TOPICAL DECOLONIZATION

MUPIROCIN NASAL OINTMENT

Mupirocin is a topical ointment used to eliminate staphylococci (MRSA) colonization of the nares. See the Common Skin Conditions chapter for a discussion of topical mupirocin use for infected skin lesions.

DRUG	DOSING	SAFETY/SIDE EFFECTS/MONITORING
Mupirocin	**Decolonization** ~500 mg in each nostril BID x 5 days	**SIDE EFFECTS** Headache, burning, localized irritation, rhinitis, pharyngitis

SUMMARY TABLES

COMMONLY USED DRUGS FOR SPECIFIC PATHOGENS

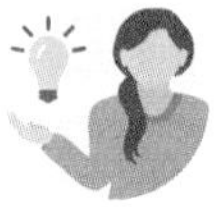

Methicillin-susceptible *Staphylococcus aureus* (MSSA)

Dicloxacillin, nafcillin, oxacillin

Cefazolin, cephalexin (and other 1st and 2nd generation cephalosporins)

Amoxicillin/clavulanate, ampicillin/sulbactam

Methicillin-resistant *Staphylococcus aureus* (MRSA)

Vancomycin (consider using alternative if MIC ≥ 2)

Linezolid

Daptomycin (not for pneumonia)

Ceftaroline

CA-MRSA SSTIs: SMX/TMP, doxycycline, clindamycin*

Vancomycin-resistant *Enterococcus* (VRE)

Pen G or ampicillin (*E. faecalis* only)

Linezolid

Daptomycin

Cystitis only: nitrofurantoin, fosfomycin, doxycycline

Atypical organisms

Azithromycin, clarithromycin

Doxycycline, minocycline

Quinolones

HNPEK

Beta-lactam/beta-lactamase inhibitor

Cephalosporins (1st generation covers PEK)

Carbapenems

Aminoglycosides

Quinolones

SMX/TMP

Pseudomonas aeruginosa

Piperacillin/tazobactam

Cefepime

Ceftazidime

Ceftazidime/avibactam

Ceftolozane/tazobactam

Carbapenems (except ertapenem)

Ciprofloxacin, levofloxacin

Aztreonam

Tobramycin

CAPES

Piperacillin/tazobactam

Cefepime

Carbapenems

Aminoglycosides

Extended-spectrum beta-lactamase (ESBL) producing gram-negative rods (*E. coli, K. pneumoniae, P. mirabilis*)

Carbapenems

Ceftazidime/avibactam

Ceftolozane/tazobactam

Carbapenem-resistant gram-negative rods (CRE)

Ceftazidime/avibactam

Colistimethate, polymyxin B

Meropenem/vaborbactam

Imipenem/cilastatin/relebactam

Gram-negative anaerobes (*Bacteroides fragilis*)

Metronidazole

Beta-lactam/beta-lactamase inhibitor

Cefotetan, cefoxitin

Carbapenems

Moxifloxacin (reduced activity)

C. difficile

Vancomycin (oral)

Fidaxomicin

Metronidazole

*A D-test must be performed before using clindamycin.
CA-MRSA SSTIs = community-acquired methicillin-resistant *Staphylococcus aureus* skin and soft tissue infections.
CAPES = *Citrobacter, Acinetobacter, Providencia, Enterobacter, Serratia.*
HNPEK = *Haemophilus, Neisseria, Proteus, E. coli, Klebsiella.*

STORAGE REQUIREMENTS: LIQUID ORAL ANTIBIOTICS*

REFRIGERATION REQUIRED AFTER RECONSTITUTION

Penicillin VK	Cefpodoxime	Fidaxomicin
Amoxicillin/Clavulanate	Cefprozil	Vancomycin oral
Cephalexin	Cefuroxime	Valganciclovir**
Cefadroxil	Cefaclor	

REFRIGERATION RECOMMENDED

Amoxicillin – improves taste

Oseltamivir** – increases shelf life

DO NOT REFRIGERATE

Cefdinir	Ciprofloxacin	Acyclovir**
Azithromycin	Levofloxacin	Fluconazole**
Clarithromycin – bitter taste, thickens/gels	Linezolid	Itraconazole**
Clindamycin – thickens, may crystallize	Metronidazole	Posaconazole**
Doxycycline	Nitrofurantoin	Voriconazole**
Erythromycin (E.E.S)	Sulfamethoxazole/Trimethoprim	Nystatin**

*Most oral suspensions should be discarded 10-14 days after reconstitution.
**Discussed in the ID III chapter.

STORAGE REQUIREMENTS: IV ANTIBIOTICS

Most IV medications are refrigerated; the list below represents a few that are not. See the Intravenous Medication Principles chapter for a complete list of drugs (including antibiotics) that should not be refrigerated.

DO NOT REFRIGERATE

Metronidazole	Sulfamethoxazole/Trimethoprim
Moxifloxacin	Acyclovir* – refrigeration causes crystallization

*Discussed in the ID III chapter.

RENAL DOSE ADJUSTMENTS

Many antibiotics are cleared through the kidneys and require dose adjustments based on renal function. This includes most beta-lactams and quinolones. See Key Drugs Guy for antibiotics that do not require renal adjustment.

KEY DRUGS

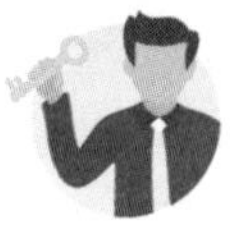

Antistaphylococcal penicillins
(e.g., dicloxacillin, nafcillin)

Azithromycin and erythromycin

Ceftriaxone

Clindamycin

Doxycycline

Metronidazole

Moxifloxacin

Linezolid

NO RENAL DOSE ADJUSTMENT REQUIRED

Others:

Fidaxomicin

Select tetracyclines (e.g., eravacycline, seracycline, omadacycline)

Rifaximin

Rifampin*

Tedizolid

Tigecycline

Tinidazole

Vancomycin (PO only)

*Discussed in the ID II chapter.

SPECIAL REQUIREMENTS

TAKE WITH/WITHOUT FOOD

Most antibiotics can be taken with food to decrease GI upset

Exceptions (take on an empty stomach):
Ampicillin oral capsules, levofloxacin oral solution, penicillin VK, tetracycline, doxycycline (*Oracea* brand only), rifampin*, isoniazid*, itraconazole oral solution*, voriconazole*

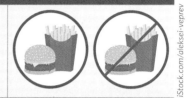

1:1 IV TO ORAL DOSING
For these drugs, the oral and IV doses are the same.

Azithromycin

Levofloxacin, moxifloxacin

Doxycycline, minocycline

Linezolid, tedizolid

Metronidazole

Sulfamethoxazole/Trimethoprim

Fluconazole*, isavuconazonium*, posaconazole* (oral tablets and IV), voriconazole*

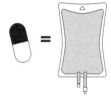

LIGHT PROTECTION DURING ADMINISTRATION
See the Intravenous Medication Principles chapter for a complete list of drugs (including antibiotics) that require specific light protection.

Doxycycline

Micafungin*

Pentamidine*

DILUENT COMPATIBILITY REQUIREMENTS
See the Intravenous Medication Principles chapter for a complete list of drugs (including antibiotics) that require specific diluents.

Compatible with dextrose only

Sulfamethoxazole/Trimethoprim

Amphotericin B* (conventional, *Abelcet, Ambisome*)

Pentamidine*

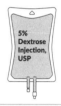

Compatible with saline only

Ampicillin

Ampicillin/Sulbactam

Ertapenem

Compatible with NS/LR only

Caspofungin*

Daptomycin

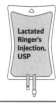

Discussed in the ID II-IV chapters.

KEY COUNSELING POINTS

See the Drug Formulations and Patient Counseling chapter for counseling language/layman's terminology.

ALL ANTIBIOTICS

- Proper storage (refrigeration or room temperature) and administration (with or without food) is essential.

- Shake suspensions (except linezolid) well.

- Antibiotics treat bacterial infections. They do not treat viral infections, such as the common cold.

- Complete the full course of therapy even if symptoms improve.

- Measure liquid doses carefully using the measuring device/syringe that comes with the medication. Do not use household spoons.

- Some oral liquid and chewable dosage forms contain phenylalanine. Do not use if you have phenylketonuria (PKU).

- Can cause:
  - ❏ Rash.
  - ❏ Nausea.
  - ❏ Diarrhea, including *C. difficile*-associated diarrhea (abdominal pain, cramps, watery or bloody stool).

QUINOLONES

- Can cause:
  - ❏ CNS effects, including seizures.
  - ❏ Hypo/hyperglycemia.
  - ❏ Peripheral neuropathy.
  - ❏ Photosensitivity.
  - ❏ QT prolongation.
  - ❏ Tendon inflammation (tendinitis) or tendon rupture. Can present with a "pop" or pain/swelling in the back of the ankle (Achilles), shoulder or hand.

- Avoid in pregnancy, breastfeeding and children.

- Drug interactions due to binding.

MACROLIDES

- Can cause:
  - ❏ GI upset.
  - ❏ QT prolongation.

Azithromycin

- *Z-Pak:* take two tablets on day 1, followed by one tablet daily on days 2 – 5.

TETRACYCLINES

- Avoid in pregnancy, breastfeeding and children < 8 years old.

- Drug interactions due to binding.

- Can cause photosensitivity.

Doxycycline (oral)

- Take with a full glass of water and remain upright for 30 minutes after the dose to avoid GI irritation.

SULFAMETHOXAZOLE/TRIMETHOPRIM

- Avoid in:
  - ❏ Pregnancy or breastfeeding.
  - ❏ Sulfa allergy.

- Can cause:
  - ❏ Photosensitivity.
  - ❏ Crystals in the urine. Take with a full glass of water.

METRONIDAZOLE

- Do not consume products containing alcohol while using this medication, and for at least three days afterward.

- Can cause:
  - ❏ Nausea.
  - ❏ Metallic taste in the mouth.

NITROFURANTOIN

- Take with food to ↓ nausea.

- Can cause:
  - ❏ Nausea.
  - ❏ Brown discoloration of urine (temporary and harmless).

MUPIROCIN NASAL OINTMENT

- Place an amount sufficient to cover the top of a cotton swab into each nostril. Press the nostrils at the same time and let go; do this many times (for about 1 minute) to spread the ointment into the nose.

- Wash hands after use.

- Can cause burning and itching in the nose.

Select Guidelines/References
Guidelines available at the Infectious Diseases Society of America website (www.idsociety.org)

CHAPTER 23

INFECTIOUS DISEASES II: BACTERIAL INFECTIONS

BACKGROUND

The Infectious Diseases I chapter should be reviewed first to gain a working knowledge of bacterial pathogens, microbiology reports, bacterial resistance and antimicrobial (antibiotic) drugs, including their spectrum of activity and pharmacokinetic/pharmacodynamic properties that play an important role in selecting the optimal treatment for infections.

PERIOPERATIVE ANTIBIOTIC PROPHYLAXIS

When a surgeon cuts into the skin during a surgical procedure, local bacterial flora at the incision site can cause contamination and subsequent infection. Skin flora (e.g., staphylococci and streptococci) are common causes of infection, with gram-negative and anaerobic organisms playing a role in select surgeries (e.g., intra-abdominal procedures). Intravenous (IV) antibiotics are given prior to surgery to reduce this risk. The preferred regimens and alternatives are shown in the Perioperative Antibiotic Selection table on the following page.

The recommended start time for antibiotics is based on drug half-life and infusion time to ensure adequate tissue concentrations are achieved by the time surgery begins. The Study Tip Gal flow diagram below provides details on the timing of antibiotics.

Timing of Perioperative Antibiotics

Prevent Infection — Hang before surgery

PRE-OPERATIVE (PRIOR TO SURGERY)

| Infuse antibiotic (e.g., cefazolin or cefuroxime)* within 60 min before first incision | If a quinolone or vancomycin is used,* start the infusion 120 min before first incision |

1g Cefazolin 50mL

INTRA-OPERATIVE (DURING SURGERY)

Additional doses may be administered for longer surgeries (e.g., > 4 hours) or if there is major blood loss

POST-OPERATIVE (AFTER SURGERY)

Antibiotics are not usually needed; if used, discontinue within 24 hours

See Perioperative Antibiotic Selection table on the next page.

CONTENT LEGEND

♦ = Study Tip Gal

PERIOPERATIVE ANTIBIOTIC SELECTION

- <u>Cefazolin</u>, a first-generation cephalosporin (or cefuroxime, a second-generation cephalosporin), is <u>preferred</u> for most surgeries to prevent methicillin-susceptible *S. aureus* (<u>MSSA</u>) and streptococcal infections.

- <u>Clindamycin</u> is an alternative if the patient has a <u>beta-lactam allergy</u>.

- In <u>gastrointestinal surgeries</u>, the prophylactic antibiotic regimen needs to cover skin flora plus broad <u>gram-negative</u> and <u>anaerobic</u> organisms.

- <u>Vancomycin</u> should be included in the regimen if <u>MRSA colonization or risk</u> is present. Vancomycin is also an alternative (instead of clindamycin) if the patient has a <u>beta-lactam allergy</u>.

SURGICAL PROCEDURE	RECOMMENDED ANTIBIOTICS*	BETA-LACTAM ALLERGY
Cardiac or vascular	Cefazolin or cefuroxime	Clindamycin or vancomycin
Orthopedic (e.g., joint replacement, hip fracture repair)	Cefazolin	
Gastrointestinal (e.g., appendectomy, colorectal surgery)	Cefazolin + metronidazole, cefotetan, cefoxitin, or ampicillin/sulbactam	Clindamycin or metronidazole + aminoglycoside or quinolone

For patients colonized with MRSA or procedures in hospitals with a high prevalence of post-operative MRSA infections, include vancomycin in the regimen.

MENINGITIS

Meningitis is an inflammation of the meninges (membranes) that cover the brain and spinal cord. The meninges swell, causing classic symptoms of <u>fever, headache</u>, nuchal rigidity (<u>stiff neck</u>) and <u>altered mental status</u>. Other symptoms include chills, vomiting, seizures, rash and photophobia. Meningitis symptoms must be quickly recognized and treated to avoid severe complications, including death.

<u>Diagnosis</u> is made via a <u>lumbar puncture (LP)</u>, during which a sample of <u>cerebrospinal fluid (CSF)</u> is collected for analysis (e.g., WBCs, protein, glucose); a <u>gram stain</u> and culture is also performed to help <u>guide</u> antibiotic treatment. A <u>high CSF pressure</u> (sometimes referred to as the "opening pressure") detected during the LP is another sign of possible infection. It is preferable to perform the LP prior to starting antibiotics; however, treatment should be initiated if the LP is delayed.

Meningitis is mostly caused by viruses but can be due to bacteria or fungi. The most common bacterial causes are *Neisseria meningitidis, Streptococcus pneumoniae* and *Haemophilus influenzae*; the risk of infection with these pathogens has decreased with routine vaccinations (see the Immunizations chapter). The risk of meningitis due to *Listeria monocytogenes* is higher in <u>neonates</u>, patients <u>age > 50 years</u> and <u>immunocompromised</u> patients.

ACUTE BACTERIAL MENINGITIS TREATMENT (COMMUNITY-ACQUIRED)

- The recommended empiric antibiotic regimens are based on the likely causative pathogens according to patient age and immune status (see <u>Study Tip Gal</u> on the following page). Aggressive (high) doses are used to adequately penetrate the CNS (e.g., ceftriaxone 2 grams Q12H).

- Antibiotic durations are pathogen-dependent:
  - ❑ 7 days for *N. meningitidis* and *H. influenzae*
  - ❑ 10 – 14 days for *S. pneumoniae*
  - ❑ At least 21 days for *Listeria monocytogenes*

- <u>Dexamethasone</u>, administered 15 – 20 minutes <u>prior to or with</u> the <u>first antibiotic dose</u>, can <u>prevent neurological complications</u> (e.g., hearing loss) and death from pneumococcal meningitis. Since the causative pathogen is not known at the time empiric treatment is initiated, it is appropriate to administer dexamethasone in all cases. The adult dose is 0.15 mg/kg (rounded to the nearest 10 mg) <u>IV</u> Q6H. Steroid treatment should be continued for 4 days. If *S. pneumoniae* is not identified as the cause of meningitis, dexamethasone should be discontinued.

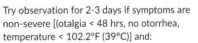

MENINGITIS: EMPIRIC TREATMENT*

COVER THE MOST COMMON BACTERIA
- *Streptococcus pneumoniae* and *Neisseria meningitidis* for most adult patients.
- Add coverage for *Listeria monocytogenes* in neonates, age > 50 years and immunocompromised patients.
- Add vancomycin in patients ≥ 1-month-old for double coverage of *Streptococcus pneumoniae*.

AGE < 1 MONTH (NEONATES)	AGE 1 MONTH TO 50 YEARS	AGE > 50 YEARS OR IMMUNOCOMPROMISED
Ampicillin (for *Listeria* coverage) + Cefotaxime, ceftazidime or cefepime ± Gentamicin	Ceftriaxone + Vancomycin	Ampicillin (for *Listeria* coverage) + Ceftriaxone + Vancomycin

Annasunny24/Shutterstock.com

DO NOT USE CEFTRIAXONE IN NEONATES
- Ceftriaxone can cause biliary sludging (solids that precipitate from bile) and kernicterus (brain damage from high bilirubin) in neonates.

If severe penicillin allergy (adults): treat with a quinolone (e.g., moxifloxacin) + vancomycin ± SMX/TMP (for Listeria coverage); obtain Infectious Diseases consult.

UPPER RESPIRATORY TRACT INFECTIONS

ACUTE OTITIS MEDIA (AOM)

Acute otitis media (AOM) is the most common childhood infection in the United States requiring antibiotic treatment. Signs and symptoms often have a rapid onset and can include bulging tympanic (eardrum) membranes, otorrhea (middle ear effusion/fluid), otalgia (ear pain), fever, crying and tugging or rubbing the ears.

- Most AOM is caused by viruses (antibiotics are ineffective).
- Bacterial infection is typically caused by *S. pneumoniae, H. influenzae* or *Moraxella catarrhalis*.
- Observation (without antibiotics) for 48 – 72 hours is an option for select patients age ≥ 6 months with non-severe AOM (see Study Tip Gal). Severe AOM is defined as having an ill appearance, otorrhea, otalgia > 48 hours or a temperature ≥ 102.2°F (39°C). Observation is not an option for children < 6 months old and antibiotics should be prescribed.

Antibiotic Treatment
- High-dose amoxicillin or amoxicillin/clavulanate are first-line (see the table on the following page). A high dose of amoxicillin is needed to cover most strains of *S. pneumoniae*.
- With amoxicillin/clavulanate, the formulation with the least amount of clavulanate should be used to decrease the risk of diarrhea. The target amoxicillin to clavulanate ratio is 14:1, making *Augmentin ES-600* (amoxicillin 600 mg and clavulanate 42.9 mg per 5 mL) a preferred formulation.
- In children with a non-severe penicillin allergy, the American Academy of Pediatrics (AAP) recommends a second- or third-generation cephalosporin as there is a

AOM TREATMENT IN KIDS: WHEN TO CONSIDER OBSERVATION

Try observation for 2-3 days if symptoms are non-severe [(otalgia < 48 hrs, no otorrhea, temperature < 102.2°F (39°C)] and:

- Age 6-23 months: symptoms in one ear only.
- Age ≥ 2 years: symptoms in one or both ears.

If symptoms do not improve, or worsen, use antibiotics.

Example
A physician gives a prescription for amoxicillin to a parent whose 18-month-old son has non-severe AOM on the right-side only, and advises the parent:

"Don't fill it right away; wait for a couple of days and see if he improves without medication. If he does not get any better, go ahead and get the medication filled."

low risk of cross-reactivity. Non-beta-lactam antibiotics that are suitable for use in children (e.g., azithromycin) have limited efficacy against typical AOM pathogens due to resistance.

- The treatment duration with oral medications is:
  - ❏ 10 days for children < 2 years
  - ❏ 7 days for ages 2 – 5 years
  - ❏ 5 – 7 days for ages ≥ 6 years

Acute Otitis Media: Antibiotic Treatment

FIRST-LINE TREATMENT	ALTERNATIVE TREATMENT (MILD PENICILLIN ALLERGY**)	TREATMENT FAILURE (NOT IMPROVED AFTER 2-3 DAYS)
Amoxicillin: 90 mg/kg/day in 2 divided doses or Amoxicillin/clavulanate*: 90 mg/kg/day of amoxicillin with 6.4 mg/kg/day of clavulanate, in 2 divided doses	Cefdinir 14 mg/kg/day in 1 or 2 doses	Amoxicillin/clavulanate (if amoxicillin was the initial therapy): 90 mg/kg/day of amoxicillin with 6.4 mg/kg/day of clavulanate, in 2 divided doses or Ceftriaxone 50 mg/kg IM daily for 3 days
	Cefuroxime 30 mg/kg/day in 2 divided doses	
	Cefpodoxime 10 mg/kg/day in 2 divided doses	
	Ceftriaxone 50 mg/kg IM daily for 1 or 3 days	

*Preferred in patients who have received amoxicillin in the past 30 days.
**Delayed-onset reaction (> 48 hours after the first antibiotic dose) appearing as a nonpruritic or mildly pruritic, maculopapular rash, but lacking systemic symptoms (e.g., hives, bronchospasm, anaphylaxis) or other serious reactions (e.g., Stevens-Johnson syndrome).

OVERVIEW OF NON-AOM UPPER RESPIRATORY TRACT INFECTIONS

The majority of upper respiratory tract infections are caused by viruses and antibiotics are not beneficial. With pharyngitis and sinusitis, antibiotics can be used if there is a suspicion for a bacterial cause, such as if symptoms are severe or chronic and/or if there is diagnostic evidence of a bacterial infection.

	COMMON COLD	INFLUENZA	PHARYNGITIS	ACUTE SINUSITIS
Typical Etiology	Respiratory viruses (rhinovirus, seasonal coronavirus)	Influenza virus	Respiratory viruses, Group A Streptococcus (*S. pyogenes*); commonly referred to as "strep throat"	Respiratory viruses, *S. pneumoniae*, *H. influenzae*, *M. catarrhalis*
Clinical Presentation	Sneezing, runny nose, mild sore throat and/or cough, congestion	Sudden onset fever, chills, fatigue, myalgia, dry cough, sore throat, headache Symptoms are more severe than the common cold	Sore throat, fever, swollen lymph nodes, white patches (exudates) on the tonsils There is an absence of cough, runny nose or congestion	Nasal congestion, purulent nasal discharge, facial/ear/dental pain or pressure, headache, fever
Criteria for Anti-Infective Treatment	None; generally resolves in a few days	Suspected or confirmed infection (e.g., positive rapid influenza antigen test) and: Symptoms < 48 hours, or Severe illness (e.g., hospitalized), or Symptoms plus risk factors for influenza complications	Rapid antigen test (tonsil swab) or throat culture positive for *S. pyogenes*	≥ 10 days of persistent symptoms or ≥ 3 days of severe symptoms (face pain, purulent nasal discharge, temperature > 102°F) or Worsening symptoms after initial improvement
Treatment Options	Symptomatic care: OTC analgesics, decongestants, cough suppressants, expectorants and/or antihistamines; see the Allergic Rhinitis, Cough & Cold chapter	Symptomatic care with or without antiviral therapy (see the Infectious Diseases III chapter)	Penicillin or amoxicillin Mild penicillin allergy: 1st or 2nd generation cephalosporin Severe reaction (e.g., anaphylaxis) to penicillin: macrolide (clarithromycin, azithromycin) or clindamycin	Amoxicillin/clavulanate or Symptomatic care for up to 7 days with OTC decongestants, antihistamines, expectorants and/or analgesics; antibiotics can be used if symptoms worsen or do not improve

LOWER RESPIRATORY TRACT INFECTIONS

ACUTE BRONCHITIS

Bronchitis is an inflammation of the mucous membranes of the bronchi. The key defining features include:

- Non-productive or productive cough lasting 1 – 3 weeks, chest wall tenderness, wheezing and/or rhonchi. Systemic symptoms (e.g., fever, chills, malaise) are rare.

- Usually preceded by an upper respiratory tract virus, such as rhinovirus, coronavirus or influenza virus.

- Bacterial causes are rare but can include *S. pneumoniae*, *H. influenzae* or atypical pathogens (e.g., *Mycoplasma pneumoniae*).

- Diagnosis is made by ruling out other causes of acute cough (e.g., pneumonia, COPD exacerbation). Chest X-ray findings are typically normal and cultures are not routinely performed.

- Antibiotics are not recommended. The symptoms are generally self-limiting and can be managed with supportive care (e.g., cough suppressants, expectorants, analgesics).

Pertussis

Acute bronchitis caused by *Bordetella pertussis* (and commonly known as whooping cough) can be distinguished from other causes of bronchitis by the characteristic series of forceful coughs followed by an inspiratory "whoop" sound. Diagnosis can be confirmed with a nasopharyngeal swab culture or PCR test for *B. pertussis*.

Pertussis is highly contagious and should be treated with macrolides (azithromycin, clarithromycin), which are highly effective at eradicating *B. pertussis* and preventing transmission to vulnerable populations (e.g., infants).

ACUTE BACTERIAL EXACERBATION OF COPD

- COPD is often diagnosed in older patients who smoke (or have a long history of smoking). The Global Initiative for Chronic Obstructive Lung Disease (GOLD) guideline defines a COPD exacerbation as an increase in symptoms that worsen over < 14 days.

- The three cardinal symptoms of a COPD exacerbation are: increased dyspnea, increased sputum volume and increased sputum purulence.

- Exacerbations can be triggered by viral infections, bacterial infections (e.g., *H. influenzae, M. catarrhalis, S. pneumoniae*), environmental pollution or an unknown cause.

- Supportive treatment (e.g., oxygen, systemic steroids, inhaled bronchodilators) is often adequate, but antibiotics should be administered to patients who meet select criteria (see diagram that follows).

MANAGEMENT OF ACUTE COPD EXACERBATION

Supportive treatment (e.g., oxygen, short-acting inhaled bronchodilators, IV or PO steroids)

↓

Antibiotics for 5-7 days if any one of the following are met:

- All three cardinal symptoms present: ↑ dyspnea, ↑ sputum volume and ↑ sputum purulence
- ↑ sputum purulence* + 1 additional symptom
- Mechanically ventilated

↓

Preferred antibiotics:

- Amoxicillin/clavulanate
- Azithromycin
- Doxycycline
- Respiratory quinolone

FGC/Shutterstock.com

Purulent sputum is thick and often yellow or green. If sputum purulence is increased, only 1 additional cardinal symptom (↑ dyspnea or ↑ sputum volume) is needed to justify antibiotic treatment.

COMMUNITY-ACQUIRED PNEUMONIA

Common pneumonia symptoms include shortness of breath, fever, cough with purulent sputum, pleuritic chest pain, rales (crackling noises in the lungs), tachypnea (increased respiratory rate) and decreased breath sounds. A chest X-ray is the gold standard diagnostic test and will have "infiltrates," "opacities" or "consolidations" to indicate pneumonia.

Community-acquired pneumonia (CAP) is a lung infection contracted outside of healthcare facilities and can be bacterial, viral or fungal (rare). When symptoms are mild (e.g., the patient is not hospitalized and is able to complete daily activities), it can be termed "walking pneumonia." Most bacterial cases are caused by *S. pneumoniae, H. influenzae, M. pneumoniae* and possibly *C. pneumoniae*.

Antibiotic regimens for CAP are designed to provide reliable activity against the likely causative pathogens, including resistant strains. The spectrum of activity of the specific antibiotic must be considered rather than using class trends (e.g., ciprofloxacin is not used for CAP; it is not a respiratory quinolone because it does not reliably cover *S. pneumoniae*). The usual duration of treatment for CAP is 5 – 7 days.

Outpatient CAP Treatment

Outpatient treatment of CAP requires an <u>assessment</u> for patient <u>comorbidities</u> that increase the risk of antibiotic resistance (e.g., <u>drug-resistant *S. pneumoniae*</u>) and therefore require <u>broader coverage</u>.

The <u>Study Tip Gal</u> and Case Scenario below describe a stepwise approach to selecting an empiric CAP regimen based on patient-specific criteria and known safety issues with select drugs/drug classes (as detailed in the Infectious Diseases I chapter). Lefamulin *(Xenleta)* and omadacycline *(Nuzyra)* are FDA-approved for CAP treatment but have not yet been incorporated into guidelines and are not included in the recommendations below.

OUTPATIENT CAP ASSESSMENT AND TREATMENT

Step 1: look for comorbidities (chronic heart, lung, liver or renal disease; diabetes mellitus; alcohol use disorder; malignancy; or asplenia)

Step 2: decide if the patient falls into the category of "Healthy" or "High Risk" (see below)

Step 3: choose one option within the assigned category; be sure to look for allergies, drug-disease interactions (e.g., quinolones and seizures), drug-drug interactions (e.g., QT prolongation) and culture results (if available)

PATIENT CHARACTERISTICS	RECOMMENDED EMPIRIC REGIMEN
Healthy (no comorbidities, see Step 1 above)	■ Amoxicillin high-dose (1 gram TID), or ■ Doxycycline, or ■ Macrolide (azithromycin or clarithromycin) if local pneumococcal resistance is < 25%

High Risk (with comorbidities, see Step 1 above)	■ Beta-lactam + macrolide or doxycycline
	
	  ❑ Amoxicillin/clavulanate or cephalosporin (e.g., cefpodoxime, cefuroxime) plus
	  ❑ Macrolide or doxycycline
	■ Respiratory quinolone monotherapy
	  ❑ Moxifloxacin or levofloxacin

CASE SCENARIO

RP is a 46-year-old female who presents to the urgent care clinic with shortness of breath, productive cough and a temperature of 100.8°F. A chest X-ray reveals a left lower lobe infiltrate. Her past medical history includes back pain and schizophrenia; she has a penicillin allergy (hives). Her scheduled medications include *Geodon* 40 mg PO BID and trazodone 50 mg PO QHS. Which empiric antibiotic regimen should RP receive for pneumonia?

Stepwise approach: RP's past medical history does not include any of the chronic comorbidities listed in Step 1. She is not at risk for drug-resistant *S. pneumoniae* and can be treated per the "Healthy" patient category. The choice is between high-dose amoxicillin, doxycycline or a macrolide. Amoxicillin should be avoided given her penicillin allergy. Macrolides can prolong the QT interval. Since *Geodon* and trazodone can also prolong the QT interval, causing additive risk, doxycycline would be the best choice in this patient with outpatient CAP.

Inpatient CAP Treatment

Selection of an empiric regimen is based on the severity of illness and often includes <u>IV antibiotics</u> initially.

Non-severe (admission to a general medicine unit):
■ <u>Beta-lactam + macrolide or doxycycline</u>

  ❑ Preferred beta-lactams: <u>ceftriaxone</u>, ceftaroline or <u>ampicillin/sulbactam</u>

■ <u>Respiratory quinolone monotherapy</u>

Severe (admission to the ICU):
■ Beta-lactam + macrolide

■ Beta-lactam + respiratory quinolone (<u>do not use quinolone monotherapy</u>)

Risk factors for *Pseudomonas* and/or MRSA:

■ <u>MRSA</u> (prior respiratory isolation or positive nasal swab): add coverage with <u>vancomycin or linezolid</u>.

■ *<u>Pseudomonas</u>* (prior respiratory isolation): use a beta-lactam antibiotic with activity against *Pseudomonas*, such as <u>piperacillin/tazobactam, cefepime</u>, ceftazidime, imipenem/cilastatin or <u>meropenem</u>.

■ <u>Hospitalization</u> and use of <u>parenteral antibiotics</u> in the <u>past 90 days</u>: use a regimen with antibiotics active against both MRSA and *Pseudomonas*.

HOSPITAL-ACQUIRED AND VENTILATOR-ASSOCIATED PNEUMONIA

Hospital-acquired pneumonia (HAP) has an onset > 48 hours after hospital admission. HAP is the leading infectious cause of death in ICU patients.

Ventilator-associated pneumonia (VAP) occurs > 48 hours after the start of mechanical ventilation and can lead to a prolonged duration of ventilation and hospitalization. The incidence of VAP can be reduced by proper hand-washing, elevating the head of the bed ≥ 30 degrees, weaning off the ventilator as soon as possible, removing nasogastric (NG) tubes when possible and discontinuing unnecessary stress ulcer prophylaxis (e.g., proton pump inhibitors).

Common pathogens in HAP and VAP

Nosocomial pathogens are common in HAP and VAP. The risk for MRSA and MDR gram-negative rods, including *P. aeruginosa*, *Acinetobacter* spp., *Enterobacter* spp., *E. coli* and *Klebsiella* spp., is increased.

Treatment of HAP and VAP

The degree of risk helps guide empiric treatment. The Study Tip Gal below lists the recommended antibiotics for coverage of MRSA and *Pseudomonas* in HAP and VAP and tips for selecting the correct regimen on the exam. Treat for 7 days; shorter or longer treatment durations may be indicated based on clinical, radiologic and laboratory parameters.

HAP/VAP: SELECTING AN EMPIRIC REGIMEN

All patients need an antibiotic for *Pseudomonas* and MSSA
- Example agents:
  - ❏ Cefepime
  - ❏ Piperacillin/tazobactam
  - ❏ Levofloxacin

Add vancomycin or linezolid if risk for MRSA
- Risk factors: IV antibiotic use in the past 90 days, MRSA prevalence in hospital unit is > 20% or uknown, prior MRSA infection or positive MRSA nasal swab
- Example regimens:
  - ❏ Cefepime + vancomycin
  - ❏ Meropenem + linezolid
  - ❏ Aztreonam + vancomycin

Use two antibiotics for *Pseudomonas* if risk for MDR gram-negative pathogens
- Risk factors: IV antibiotic use in the past 90 days, prevalence of gram-negative resistance in hospital unit is > 10%, hospitalized ≥ 5 days prior to the onset of VAP
- Example regimens (typically MRSA risk is also present):
  - ❏ Piperacillin/tazobactam + ciprofloxacin + vancomycin
  - ❏ Cefepime + gentamicin + linezolid

Antibiotics for *Pseudomonas* (do not use two beta-lactams together)
Beta-lactams: piperacillin/tazobactam, cefepime, ceftazidime, imipenem/cilastatin, meropenem

Levofloxacin or ciprofloxacin

Aztreonam

Aminoglycosides (typically tobramycin)*

---

*These agents are always used in combination with another antipseudomonal drug.

TUBERCULOSIS

Tuberculosis (TB) is caused by *Mycobacterium tuberculosis* (MTB), an aerobic, non-spore forming bacillus. It primarily infects the lungs but can disseminate (spread) to other organs. The disease has two phases: latent and active.

With latent disease, the immune system is able to contain the infection and the patient lacks symptoms. Active pulmonary TB is transmitted by aerosolized droplets (e.g., sneezing, coughing, talking) and is highly contagious. It most often presents with cough/hemoptysis (coughing up blood), purulent sputum, fever, night sweats and unintentional weight loss. Hospitalized patients require isolation in a single negative-pressure room and healthcare workers caring for them must wear a respirator mask (e.g., an N95 face mask).

Latent Tuberculosis Diagnosis

Latent disease can be diagnosed using the tuberculin skin test (TST), also called a purified protein derivative (PPD) test, or an interferon-gamma release assay (IGRA) blood test. With a TST, a solution is injected intradermally and the skin area must be inspected for induration (a raised area) 48 – 72 hours later (see criteria for a positive result in the box on the following page). The IGRA does not require a follow-up visit and is preferred in patients with a history of bacille Calmette-Guerin (BCG) vaccination (used in countries with high TB rates) because a false-positive TST can occur in these patients. Any patient with a positive TST or IGRA test should be screened for the presence of active TB (e.g., clinical symptoms, chest X-ray) before latent TB treatment is initiated.

DIAGNOSIS OF LATENT TB: CRITERIA FOR POSITIVE TB SKIN TEST (TST) RESULTS

≥ 5 mm induration
Close contacts of recent active TB cases
HIV infection
Immunosuppression (e.g., organ transplant recipients, chemotherapy)

≥ 10 mm induration
Immigrants from high burden countries
Clinical risk (e.g., IV drug use, diabetes)
Residents/employees of "high-risk" congregate settings (e.g., prisons, healthcare facilities, homeless shelters)

≥ 15 mm induration
Patients with no risk factors

Induration = raised area

Latent Tuberculosis Treatment

Treatment of latent TB with one of the following regimens greatly reduces the risk of developing active disease and the subsequent spread to others. In general, shorter regimens (e.g., 3 or 4 months) are preferred in most adults due to higher completion rates and less risk of hepatotoxicity compared to longer courses of isoniazid (INH). Drug interactions are the biggest barrier to rifampin- and rifapentine-based regimens (see the drug table on the following page).

Regimen options:

- INH and rifapentine once weekly for 12 weeks via directly observed therapy (DOT) or self-administered. Do not use this regimen in pregnant patients (fetal risk with rifapentine unknown).

- INH with rifampin daily for 3 months.

- Rifampin 600 mg daily for 4 months.

- INH 300 mg daily for 6 or 9 months.

  ❑ May be preferred in HIV-positive patients taking antiretroviral therapy (due to a lower risk of drug interactions). If used, a 9-month course of treatment is recommended.

Active Tuberculosis Diagnosis

The diagnosis of active TB is based on several findings. A positive TST or IGRA is likely, but the diagnosis must be confirmed. A chest X-ray showing a consolidation or cavitation (empty space) is suggestive of TB. Because MTB is an acid-fast bacilli (AFB), it can be detected with an AFB smear of a sputum sample; however, this test is not specific to MTB and a definitive diagnosis must be made via a sputum culture or polymerase chain reaction (PCR). MTB is a slow-growing organism; the final culture and susceptibility results can take up to 6 weeks.

Active Tuberculosis Treatment

Active TB treatment is divided into two phases (intensive and continuation). To avoid resistance, the preferred intensive phase regimen consists of four drugs: rifampin, isoniazid, pyrazinamide and ethambutol for two months (this regimen is known as "RIPE" therapy).

In the continuation phase (typically four months) treatment can be scaled back to two drugs (commonly rifampin and isoniazid) depending on the drug susceptibility of the isolate. The continuation phase is extended to seven months in select cases (e.g., the repeat sputum culture remains positive after two months of treatment, or if intensive phase treatment did not include pyrazinamide).

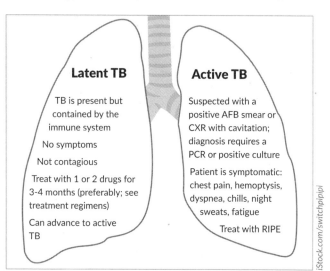

Latent TB

TB is present but contained by the immune system

No symptoms

Not contagious

Treat with 1 or 2 drugs for 3-4 months (preferably; see treatment regimens)

Can advance to active TB

Active TB

Suspected with a positive AFB smear or CXR with cavitation; diagnosis requires a PCR or positive culture

Patient is symptomatic: chest pain, hemoptysis, dyspnea, chills, night sweats, fatigue

Treat with RIPE

DOT is used to increase medication adherence and is preferred in select populations (homeless, drug-resistant disease, poor adherence, positive sputum smears and delayed culture positivity). Alternative dosing regimens (e.g., drugs administered 2 – 3 times per week) can be used in this setting. Daily dosing regimens are strongly encouraged if DOT is not possible.

TB can be resistant to INH or rifampin; if TB is resistant to both, it is called multidrug-resistant TB (MDR-TB). Resistant TB requires use of second-line agents and longer durations of treatment (up to 24 months). While many agents can be used, preferred drugs include quinolones (moxifloxacin or levofloxacin) or injectables (streptomycin, amikacin or kanamycin).

In extremely drug-resistant TB (XDR-TB), bedaquiline (*Sirturo*) can be used, but it has boxed warnings for QT prolongation and an increased risk of death compared to placebo. Pretomanid is approved for MDR-TB or XDR-TB of the lung, in combination with bedaquiline and linezolid. It has many side effects, including hepatotoxicity, peripheral neuropathy (can be severe), optic neuropathy, myelosuppression and QT prolongation.

PREFERRED ACTIVE TB REGIMEN (TOTAL TREATMENT DURATION: 6 MONTHS)

Intensive Phase	
4 drugs for 2 months (until cultures and susceptibilities are available)	RIPE: Rifampin (RIF) + Isoniazid (INH) + Pyrazinamide (PZA) + Ethambutol; daily or 5x per week
	Duration: 8 weeks
Continuation Phase	
2 drugs for 4 months (based on culture and susceptibility results)	INH and RIF; daily, 5x per week or 3x per week
	Duration: 18 weeks

RIPE Therapy for Active TB

DRUG	DOSING	SAFETY/SIDE EFFECTS/MONITORING
Rifampin *(Rifadin)*	10 mg/kg (max 600 mg) PO daily or 2-3x/week Doses differ for other indications Take on an empty stomach	**CONTRAINDICATIONS** Do not use with protease inhibitors **SIDE EFFECTS** ↑ LFTs, hemolytic anemia (detected with a positive Coombs test), flu-like syndrome, GI upset, rash/pruritus Orange-red discoloration of body secretions (saliva, urine, sweat, tears); can stain contact lenses, clothing and bedsheets **NOTES** Rifampin has many drug-drug interactions (see Rifampin Drug Interactions on the following page); rifabutin has fewer drug interactions and can replace rifampin in some cases (e.g., HIV patients taking protease inhibitors), though a drug-drug interaction screen is still needed
Isoniazid	5 mg/kg (max 300 mg) PO daily or 15 mg/kg (max 900 mg) 1-3x/week Take on an empty stomach Use pyridoxine (vitamin B6) 25-50 mg PO daily to ↓ the risk of INH-associated peripheral neuropathy	**BOXED WARNING** Severe (and fatal) hepatitis **CONTRAINDICATIONS** Active liver disease, previous severe adverse reaction to isoniazid **WARNINGS** Peripheral neuropathy, higher risk in patients predisposed to neuropathy (e.g., diabetes, HIV, renal failure, alcohol use disorder, elderly, malnourished); pyridoxine (vitamin B6) supplementation is recommended for these patients and patients who are pregnant or breastfeeding **SIDE EFFECTS** ↑ LFTs (usually asymptomatic), drug-induced lupus erythematosus (DILE), hemolytic anemia (detected with a positive Coombs test), agranulocytosis, aplastic anemia, hyperglycemia, headache, GI upset, pancreatitis, severe skin reactions (SJS/DRESS), optic neuritis
Pyrazinamide	20-25 mg/kg PO daily (max daily doses vary based on weight) CrCl < 30 mL/min: extend interval	**CONTRAINDICATIONS** Acute gout, severe hepatic damage **SIDE EFFECTS** ↑ LFTs, hyperuricemia/gout, GI upset, malaise, arthralgia, myalgia, rash
Ethambutol *(Myambutol)*	15-20 mg/kg (max 1.6 grams) PO daily or 25-30 mg/kg (max 2.4 grams) 3x/week or 50 mg/kg (max 4 grams) 2x/week CrCl < 50 mL/min: extend interval	**CONTRAINDICATIONS** Optic neuritis (risk vs. benefit decision); do not use in young children, unconscious patients or any patient who cannot discern and report visual changes **SIDE EFFECTS** ↑ LFTs, optic neuritis (dose-related), ↓ visual acuity, partial loss of vision/blind spot and/or color blindness (usually reversible), rash, headache, confusion, hallucinations, N/V

Rifampin Drug Interactions

- Rifampin is a potent inducer of CYP450 1A2, 2C8, 2C9, 2C19, 3A4 and P-glycoprotein. It can significantly ↓ the concentration and therapeutic effect of many other drugs, including:

  - Protease inhibitors (substitute rifabutin).

  - Warfarin (a very large ↓ in INR is common; requires increased doses of warfarin).

  - Oral contraceptives (↓ efficacy; requires additional backup contraceptive methods).

- Do not use rifampin with apixaban, rivaroxaban, edoxaban, or dabigatran.

- It is important to screen the medication profile for drug interactions with rifampin. See the Drug Interactions chapter for more information.

RIPE THERAPY FOR TB

MONITOR INFECTION
Sputum sample (for culture), symptoms and chest X-ray (are lungs clear or clearing up?)

DRUG-SPECIFIC KEY POINTS
All RIPE Drugs
↑ LFTs, including total bilirubin – monitor

Rifampin
Orange bodily secretions

Strong CYP450 inducer (can use rifabutin if unacceptable DDIs)

Flu-like symptoms

Isoniazid
Peripheral neuropathy: give with pyridoxine (vitamin B6) 25-50 mg PO daily

Monitor for symptoms of DILE

Rifampin and Isoniazid
Risk for hemolytic anemia (identified with a positive Coombs test)

Pyrazinamide
↑ uric acid – do not use with acute gout

Ethambutol
Visual damage (requires baseline and monthly vision exams)

Confusion/hallucinations

INFECTIVE ENDOCARDITIS

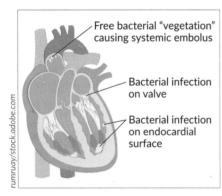

Free bacterial "vegetation" causing systemic embolus

Bacterial infection on valve

Bacterial infection on endocardial surface

rumruay/stock.adobe.com

An infection of the inner tissue of the heart, typically the heart valves, is called infective endocarditis (IE). Patients who have prosthetic heart valves, chronic IV access, IV drug use or frequent and chronic healthcare exposure are some of those who are most at risk. The majority of patients present with fever, with or without a heart murmur. IE is diagnosed using the Modified Duke Criteria, which includes an echocardiogram to visualize the vegetation and positive blood cultures. The three most common species of organisms that cause IE are staphylococci, streptococci and enterococci.

IE is generally fatal if left untreated. Empiric treatment often includes vancomycin and ceftriaxone. Definitive treatment, including antibiotic duration, is dependent on the pathogen, the type of infected valve (native or prosthetic) and the culture susceptibility results. Adding a second antibiotic (e.g.,

gentamicin) for synergy is recommended for infections that are more difficult to eradicate, such as with prosthetic valve infections or when treating more resistant organisms. In some cases, the risk of additive nephrotoxicity outweighs the benefit and it is left off the regimen (e.g., when vancomycin is used for streptococcal endocarditis in patients with a beta-lactam allergy).

In general, 4 – 6 weeks of IV antibiotic treatment is required; when prosthetic valves and/or more resistant organisms are involved, treatment durations are at the upper end of this range or longer. The duration of synergy (if used) varies from 2 – 6 weeks, depending on the organism being treated and the presence or absence of a prosthetic valve. When gentamicin is used for synergy, traditional dosing is typically used to target peak levels of 3 – 4 mcg/mL and trough levels < 1 mcg/mL. Extended interval dosing of aminoglycosides is less common when treating IE.

Some bacteria can form a biofilm (a surrounding protective layer), especially on prosthetic valves. This is difficult for some antibiotics to penetrate. Rifampin may be used in cases of staphylococcal prosthetic valve endocarditis due to its ability to treat organisms in a biofilm.

INFECTIVE ENDOCARDITIS TREATMENT

ORGANISM	PREFERRED ANTIBIOTIC REGIMEN
Viridans group streptococci	Penicillin or ceftriaxone (± gentamicin)
	If beta-lactam allergy, use vancomycin monotherapy
Staphylococci (MSSA)	Nafcillin or cefazolin (+ gentamicin and rifampin if prosthetic valve)
	If beta-lactam allergy, use vancomycin* (+ gentamicin and rifampin if prosthetic valve)
Staphylococci (MRSA)	Vancomycin* (+ gentamicin and rifampin if prosthetic valve)
Enterococci	For both native and prosthetic valve IE: penicillin or ampicillin + gentamicin, or ampicillin + high-dose ceftriaxone
	If beta-lactam allergy, use vancomycin + gentamicin
	If VRE, use daptomycin or linezolid

Daptomycin monotherapy is an alternative for MSSA and MRSA IE when the patient has a beta-lactam allergy and no prosthetic valve.

INFECTIVE ENDOCARDITIS DENTAL PROPHYLAXIS

The mouth contains bacteria that can enter the blood during dental procedures. The bacteria can travel to the heart, where they can settle on the myocardial lining, a heart valve or a blood vessel. IE after dental procedures is rare, but the risk is increased with certain cardiac conditions. In patients at high risk, antibiotics should be taken before all dental procedures that involve manipulation of gingival tissue (gums), the periapical region (near the root of the tooth) or perforation of the oral mucosa. Example procedures include root canals and tooth extractions (not routine cleanings). See the following table for the risk criteria and recommended prophylaxis regimens.

PATIENTS AT HIGH RISK FOR IE	ADULT PROPHYLAXIS REGIMENS*
Dental work needed, such as a root canal + **Select cardiac conditions, including:** ■ Artificial (prosthetic) heart valve or heart valve repaired with artificial material ■ History of endocarditis ■ Heart transplant with abnormal heart valve function ■ Certain congenital heart defects including heart/heart valve disease	All given as a single dose 30-60 minutes before the dental procedure **First line:** Amoxicillin 2 grams PO **If unable to take oral medication:** Ampicillin 2 grams IM/IV, or Cefazolin or ceftriaxone 1 gram IM/IV **If able to take oral medication but allergic to penicillin**:** Azithromycin or clarithromycin 500 mg, or Doxycycline 100 mg

In pediatric patients, use weight-based doses of the same antibiotics.
***In practice, cephalosporins may be considered if penicillin reaction is mild (no history of anaphylaxis, angioedema or urticaria); on the exam, look for a safer option.*

mariaaverburg/stock.adobe.com

INTRA-ABDOMINAL INFECTIONS

SPONTANEOUS BACTERIAL PERITONITIS

Spontaneous bacterial peritonitis (SBP), or primary peritonitis, is an infection of the peritoneal space that often occurs in patients with cirrhosis and ascites. Infection is suspected if an ascitic fluid sample (collected via a paracentesis) reveals ≥ 250 cells/mm³ PMNs (polymorphonuclear leukocytes).

Empiric treatment with ceftriaxone for 5 – 7 days is recommended to target the most likely pathogens (streptococci, *Proteus*, *E. coli*, *Klebsiella*). Alternatively, a carbapenem (e.g., meropenem) can be used in critically ill patients or those at risk for MDR pathogens. Patients who have received treatment for an initial SBP episode should be prescribed secondary prophylaxis with SMX/TMP or a quinolone (e.g., ciprofloxacin) to decrease the risk of subsequent infections.

OTHER INTRA-ABDOMINAL INFECTIONS

Common intra-abdominal infections encountered in clinical practice include appendicitis, cholecystitis (acute inflammation of the gallbladder due to an obstructive stone), cholangitis (infection of the common bile duct), secondary peritonitis (caused by ulceration, ischemia, obstruction, surgery) and diverticulitis.

If an abscess is present, it should be drained (referred to as source control) and sent for culture. Since intra-abdominal infections are usually polymicrobial, empiric antibiotic treatment should target multiple pathogens, including streptococci, enteric gram-negatives and anaerobes (e.g., *Bacteroides fragilis*).

If there is risk of MDR pathogens (e.g., critically ill, hospitalized > 48 hrs, antibiotics in past 90 days), coverage of *Pseudomonas* and other resistant organisms may be necessary.

Treatment can be accomplished with a single drug in some cases. If the antibiotic selected does not have anaerobic activity, an additional antibiotic (usually metronidazole) must be added (see the Infectious Diseases I chapter for a discussion of antibiotic spectrum of activity).

A treatment duration of 4 – 5 days is usually sufficient if source control is accomplished. Longer durations may be necessary in select patients (e.g., secondary bacteremia, lack of source control, immunosuppressed).

Treatment Options for Intra-Abdominal Infections

COMMUNITY-ACQUIRED (LOW RISK)	RISK FOR RESISTANT OR NOSOCOMIAL PATHOGENS*
Cover PEK, anaerobes, streptococci	Cover PEK, *Pseudomonas*, *Enterobacter*, anaerobes, streptococci ± enterococci
Possible regimens include:	Possible regimens include:
Ertapenem	Carbapenem (except ertapenem)
Moxifloxacin	Piperacillin/tazobactam
(Cefuroxime or ceftriaxone) + metronidazole	(Cefepime or ceftazidime) + metronidazole
(Ciprofloxacin or levofloxacin) + metronidazole	

*Ampicillin or vancomycin may be added to a cephalosporin-based regimen if Enterococcus coverage is needed; vancomycin may be included in the regimen if there is risk of MRSA.
PEK (enteric GNRs) = *Proteus, E. coli, Klebsiella*

SKIN AND SOFT-TISSUE INFECTIONS (SSTIs)

Skin and soft-tissue infections (SSTIs) can involve any or all layers of the skin (epidermis, dermis and subcutaneous fat), as well as underlying fascia and muscle. SSTIs usually result from the introduction of bacteria (e.g., staphylococci, streptococci) through breaks in the skin barrier, and less frequently from an infection that spreads from the bloodstream to the skin. Minor local skin trauma (e.g., cuts or abrasions, insect bites) can be the provoking event and can progress to a deeper infection.

SSTIs can be broadly divided into infections that are superficial (e.g., impetigo, furuncle, carbuncle) or infections that penetrate the subcutaneous tissues (e.g., cellulitis). They can be nonpurulent or purulent (contains pus), such as with an abscess. The severity of the infection (mild, moderate or severe) impacts the choice of antibiotics and the route (topical, PO or IV).

Antibiotics used for outpatient empiric treatment of common SSTIs are listed in the table on the following page. The list is not all-inclusive but represents commonly used oral antibiotics.

SSTI CLASSIFICATIONS

Mild infection
Systemic signs absent

Moderate infection
Systemic signs present

Severe infection
Systemic signs present, signs of a deeper infection (e.g., fluid-filled blisters, skin sloughing, hypotension or evidence of organ dysfunction), patient is immunocompromised or failed oral antibiotics + incision and drainage (for purulent infections).

Systemic signs:
Temperature > 100.4°F

Heart rate > 90 BPM

WBC > 12,000 or < 4000 cells/mm³

OUTPATIENT TREATMENT OF COMMON SKIN AND SOFT-TISSUE INFECTIONS

INFECTION	PRESENTATION	TREATMENT/COMMENTS
Superficial Infections		
Impetigo *S. pyogenes, S. aureus* (most often MSSA)  *FotoHelin/Shutterstock.com*	Common in children (contagious, spreads quickly). A blister-like rash (may be itchy or painful) found anywhere on the skin, usually around the nose, mouth, hands and arms. Pustules rupture and produce a thick, yellowish, clear fluid that dries and forms honey-colored crusts over the area.	Use warm, wet compresses to help remove dried crusts (but do not share personal towels and wash sheets/towels/clothing in hot water). **Limited, localized lesions:** Apply a topical antibiotic, typically mupirocin. Retapamulin (*Altabax*) and ozenoxacin (*Xepi*) are alternative treatments approved for impetigo. **Numerous, extensive lesions:** ■ Cephalexin 250-500 mg PO QID ■ Dicloxacillin 250-500 mg PO QID
Folliculitis/furuncle/ carbuncle *S. aureus*, including community-acquired MRSA (CA-MRSA)  *Alessandro Grandini/ stock.adobe.com*	Folliculitis: a superficial infection of hair follicles (looks like red pimples). Furuncle (boil): a purulent infection of the hair follicle. Carbuncle: a group of infected furuncles.	Folliculitis and small furuncles may require only warm compresses to ↓ inflammation and help with drainage. Incision & drainage (I&D) ± antibiotics is recommended for large furuncles and carbuncles. **Use an antibiotic that covers MSSA and MRSA:** ■ SMX/TMP DS 1-2 tablets PO BID ■ Doxycycline 100 mg PO BID Occasionally, folliculitis is due to a fungal infection and can be treated with ketoconazole cream.
Cellulitis (Non-Purulent Infections)		
Mild infection Streptococci, including *S. pyogenes* (Group A *Streptococcus*), *S. aureus*  *Blueee77/ Shutterstock.com*	Mild symptoms: localized pain, swelling, redness, warmth. Often occurs on the legs, generally unilateral, and can rapidly spread/expand.	**Antibiotic must be active against streptococci and MSSA:** ■ Cephalexin 500 mg PO QID ■ Dicloxacillin 500 mg PO QID ■ Beta-lactam allergy: clindamycin 300 mg PO QID Duration of treatment: 5 days (longer if no improvement within 5 days).
Abscess (Purulent Infections)		
Mild infection Commonly caused by *S. aureus*, including CA-MRSA  *Criniger kolio/ Shutterstock.com*	Initially appears as a localized fluid collection (abscess). Recurrent MRSA infections: consider nasal decolonization with nasal mupirocin, and skin decolonization with chlorhexidine or dilute bleach.	Source control with I&D of infected pus is recommended. **Use an antibiotic that covers MSSA and MRSA:** ■ SMX/TMP DS 1-2 tablets PO BID ■ Doxycycline 100 mg PO BID ■ Minocycline 200 mg PO x 1, then 100 mg PO BID ■ Clindamycin 300 mg PO QID ■ Linezolid 600 mg PO BID If cultures show MSSA, use cephalexin.

SEVERE SKIN AND SOFT TISSUE INFECTIONS

Severe infections or those in more complicated patients (e.g., failed initial treatment, immunocompromised) can lead to sepsis, requiring hospitalization and IV antibiotics. Once the patient is stable, it is often possible to transition to oral antibiotics to complete treatment.

INFECTION	NOTES	TREATMENT
Severe purulent	Duration of therapy: 7-14 days	Use antibiotics with MRSA activity: Vancomycin (goal trough 10-15 mcg/mL) Daptomycin Linezolid Others: ceftaroline, tedizolid, telavancin Once clinically stable, transition to PO antibiotics
Necrotizing fasciitis (i.e., severe nonpurulent) *S. pyogenes* (Group A *Streptococcus*), *S. aureus* (including MRSA), gram-negatives (e.g., *E. coli*), and anaerobes (e.g., *Clostridium* spp.)	A life-threatening, fast-moving type of skin infection that rapidly destroys tissue and can quickly penetrate down to the muscle. Presentation: intense pain/tenderness over affected skin and underlying muscle (often out of proportion with clinical findings), skin discoloration, edema, systemic signs. Requires emergency treatment in a hospital.	Urgent surgical debridement. Empiric therapy is broad: Vancomycin or daptomycin + beta-lactam (piperacillin/tazobactam, meropenem) + clindamycin (to suppress streptococcal toxin production)

DIABETIC FOOT INFECTIONS

Patients with diabetes are at high risk for foot ulcers because of neuropathic damage, compromised blood flow to the lower extremities (due to peripheral artery disease) and poor wound healing (due to hyperglycemia). It is imperative that patients follow proper foot care (see the Diabetes chapter) because ulcers can progress to foot infections (with erythema, edema, purulent discharge), which can lead to amputation.

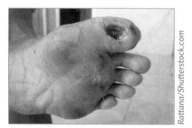

Rattana/Shutterstock.com

Most common cause of amputations. Starts in soft tissue, can spread into bone (osteomyelitis). Proper foot care is crucial to avoid infections.

Mild superficial infections without systemic symptoms can be treated with similar oral antibiotic regimens as mild SSTIs (see table on previous page). Patients with recent antibiotic exposure and/or those with moderate to severe presentations (e.g., requiring hospitalization) typically have polymicrobial infections and broad-spectrum empiric antibiotics targeting gram-positive and gram-negative organisms (see table below) are necessary. The ability to select a regimen that targets these pathogens, and possibly MDR organisms (e.g., MRSA, *Pseudomonas*) and/or anaerobes, is essential for the exam. Cultures should be performed in order to narrow therapy whenever possible.

ETIOLOGY	GRAM-POSITIVE	GRAM-NEGATIVE
Aerobic	*S. aureus* (including MRSA) Group A *Streptococcus* Viridans group streptococci *S. epidermidis*	*E. coli* *Klebsiella pneumoniae* *Proteus mirabilis* *Enterobacter cloacae* *Pseudomonas aeruginosa* (if significant water exposure)
Anaerobic (if limb ischemia or necrosis present)	*Peptostreptococcus* *Clostridium perfringens*	*Bacteroides fragilis* and others

SELECT TREATMENT REGIMENS FOR MODERATE TO SEVERE DIABETIC FOOT INFECTIONS

TYPE OF REGIMEN	TREATMENT OPTIONS	NOTES
No MRSA activity needed	Ampicillin/sulbactam	Start with IV then transition to PO
	Ertapenem	
	Ceftriaxone	**Treatment duration**
	Levofloxacin or moxifloxacin	■ 2-4 weeks (if no bone involvement)
Pseudomonas and/or MDR gram-negative activity needed	Piperacillin/tazobactam	■ 4-6 weeks for osteomyelitis (i.e., bone involvement), typically with IV antibiotics
	Cefepime	
	Meropenem, doripenem or imipenem/cilastatin	■ 2-5 days if amputation with no residual infection
MRSA activity needed	Add vancomycin, daptomycin or linezolid	
Anaerobic activity needed	Use a regimen with anaerobic activity (e.g., beta-lactam/beta-lactamase inhibitor combination, carbapenem) or add metronidazole	

URINARY TRACT INFECTIONS (UTIs)

Acute cystitis is an uncomplicated lower urinary tract infection (UTI) affecting the bladder and urethra. It is more common than upper UTIs, which occur in the kidneys (pyelonephritis) and are more severe. UTIs are more common in females than males, as the female urethra provides a shorter route for organisms to travel up into the bladder. Sexual intercourse can facilitate this movement; women who commonly develop UTIs after intercourse may be prescribed prophylactic antibiotics.

Infections in males are typically due to some type of abnormality or obstruction, such as an enlarged prostate. Other conditions that can increase the risk of infection include neurogenic bladder (e.g., spinal cord injury, stroke, multiple sclerosis), an obstruction (e.g., a kidney stone) or the presence of an indwelling catheter (see the Medication Safety & Quality Improvement chapter for a discussion of ways to reduce catheter-associated infections).

Cystitis can be diagnosed based on the typical symptoms (see box to the right). A urinalysis can aid in the diagnosis and is considered positive when there is evidence of pyuria (WBC > 10 cells/mm³), bacteria and positive leukocyte esterase and/or nitrites.

The presence of bacteria alone is not indicative of a UTI and does not require treatment (exception: asymptomatic bacteriuria in pregnancy). A positive urinalysis can be followed by a urine culture to identify a causative organism (see common pathogens in the table on the following page).

UTI SYMPTOMS

Cystitis (Lower UTI)
- Urgency and frequency (the feeling of needing to go often and quickly), including overnight (nocturia)
- Dysuria (painful urination, burning)
- Suprapubic tenderness
- Hematuria (blood in the urine)

Pyelonephritis (Upper UTI)
- Flank/costovertebral angle pain
- Abdominal pain, nausea and vomiting
- Fever, chills and malaise

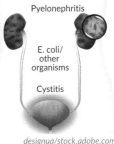

designua/stock.adobe.com
Artemida-psy/stock.adobe.com
rumruay/stock.adobe.com

UTI TREATMENT

DIAGNOSIS	DRUGS OF CHOICE		COMMENTS
Acute cystitis Common pathogens: *E. coli* (vast majority), *Proteus, Klebsiella, Staphylococcus saprophyticus*, enterococci	Nitrofurantoin *(Macrobid)* 100 mg PO BID x 5 days (contraindicated if CrCl < 60 mL/min) or SMX/TMP DS 1 tablet PO BID x 3 days (do not use if sulfa allergy or ≥ 20% *E. coli* resistance rate) or Fosfomycin 3 grams x 1 dose		Usually treated empirically as an outpatient. If no response with first-line treatment, check a urine culture and treat accordingly. Do not use moxifloxacin for UTIs (does not reach high levels in the urine). Prophylaxis: if ≥ 3 episodes in 1 year, can use SMX/TMP SS 1 tablet daily, nitrofurantoin 50 mg PO daily, or SMX/TMP DS 1 tablet after sexual intercourse. SMX/TMP and nitrofurantoin should be used in pregnant patients only if other options not available due to potential fetal risk.
	Alternative Options		
	Beta-lactam (amoxicillin/clavulanate or cephalosporin) x 5-7 days or Ciprofloxacin 250 mg PO BID x 3 days* or Levofloxacin 250 mg PO daily x 3 days* *Quinolones: do not use in children, pregnant patients, those with seizures, neuropathy or QT prolongation risk; watch for tendinitis/rupture and BG changes (especially in patients with diabetes)	Pregnancy: Amoxicillin Cephalexin Fosfomycin (if beta-lactam allergy) SMX/TMP Nitrofurantoin Pregnant women with acute cystitis (symptomatic) should be treated for 7 days See the following page for a discussion on asymptomatic bacteriuria during pregnancy	
Acute pyelonephritis Common pathogens: *E. coli, Proteus, Klebsiella* Less common pathogens: *Enterobacter, Serratia, Pseudomonas*, enterococci	**Moderately ill outpatient (PO)** If local quinolone resistance ≤ 10%: Ciprofloxacin 500 mg PO BID x 5-7 days Levofloxacin 750 mg PO daily x 5-7 days If local quinolone resistance > 10%: Ceftriaxone 1 gram IV/IM x 1, ertapenem 1 gram IV/IM x 1 or aminoglycoside extended-interval dose IV/IM x 1, then continue with a quinolone (as above) x 5-7 days Concern for quinolone adverse effects: SMX/TMP or beta-lactam (amoxicillin/clavulanate, cefdinir, cefadroxil or cefpodoxime) x 7-10 days **Severely ill hospitalized patient (IV)** Initial: ceftriaxone or a quinolone (ciprofloxacin or levofloxacin) Concern for resistance: piperacillin/tazobactam or a carbapenem (if ESBL-producing organism suspected) Step down to oral treatment options based on culture & susceptibility results Treatment duration: 5-10 days depending on regimen and clinical response		If risk for or documented *Pseudomonas* infection, consider piperacillin/tazobactam or an antipseudomonal carbapenem (meropenem, doripenem, imipenem/cilastatin). Last-line options (in adults with pyelonephritis or UTIs with systemic signs/symptoms and no other treatment options): Cefiderocol *(Fetroja)* Imipenem/cilastatin/relebactam *(Recarbrio)* Meropenem/vaborbactam *(Vabomere)* Plazomicin *(Zemdri)*

Urinary Analgesic

Phenazopyridine can help with dysuria (pain/burning with urination) but does not treat the infection.

DRUG	DOSING	SAFETY/SIDE EFFECTS/MONITORING	
Phenazopyridine *(Pyridium, Azo Urinary Pain Relief)* OTC and Rx	200 mg PO TID x 2 days (max) Take with 8 oz of water, with or immediately following food, to minimize stomach upset	**CONTRAINDICATIONS** Do not use in patients with renal impairment or liver disease **SIDE EFFECTS** Headache, dizziness, stomach cramps, body secretion discoloration **NOTES** Can cause red-orange coloring of the urine and other body fluids; contact lenses/clothes can be stained Hemolytic anemia with G6PD deficiency (discontinue if hemolysis occurs)	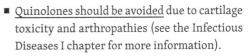 orange urine color

ASYMPTOMATIC BACTERIURIA IN PREGNANCY

Asymptomatic bacteriuria ($\geq 10^5$ bacteria/mL on a urinalysis) in pregnant women must be treated. If not treated, it can lead to pyelonephritis, premature birth and perinatal mortality.

- Beta-lactams are preferred (amoxicillin ± clavulanate or an oral cephalosporin).

- Nitrofurantoin, SMX/TMP or fosfomycin are alternatives in patients with a beta-lactam allergy. Nitrofurantoin and SMX/TMP may be reserved for when other options are not available; the American College of Obstetricians and Gynecologists (ACOG) suggests avoiding these agents in the 1st trimester, if possible, and there are safety risks when used later in pregnancy (SMX/TMP can cause hyperbilirubinemia and kernicterus in the newborn if used close to delivery, and nitrofurantoin should be avoided in the 3rd trimester due to the possibility of hemolytic anemia in the infant).

- Quinolones should be avoided due to cartilage toxicity and arthropathies (see the Infectious Diseases I chapter for more information).

CLOSTRIDIOIDES DIFFICILE INFECTION

The GI tract contains > 1,000 species of organisms as part of the normal flora. Antibiotics can eliminate much of the "healthy" bacteria, allowing an overgrowth of *Clostridioides difficile*, a gram-positive, obligate anaerobic, spore-forming rod. Some types of *C. difficile* release toxins (toxin A and B) that attack the intestinal lining, causing inflammation of the colon (colitis). Symptoms of *C. difficile* infection (CDI) include at least three, watery stools per day, abdominal cramps, fever and an elevated white blood cell count. Inflammation of the colon can lead to pseudomembranous colitis, which can progress to toxic megacolon and result in the need for colectomy or death. Other risk factors include recent healthcare exposure, use of proton pump inhibitors, advanced age, immunocompromised state, obesity and previous CDI.

CDI TREATMENT

Treatment recommendations vary based on whether it is the first infection or a recurrence, but in general, oral vancomycin or fidaxomicin are preferred (see Study Tip Gal on following page). Review the patient profile to determine the recommended treatment. Bezlotoxumab *(Zinplava)* is a monoclonal antibody that binds to toxin B and neutralizes its adverse effects. It has been shown to decrease the risk of CDI recurrence but does not treat the active infection and must be administered in conjunction with antibacterial therapy.

Fecal microbiota transplantation involves the introduction of healthy stool (not exposed to antibiotics) into the GI tract of a person with CDI to re-establish the intestinal microbiome and control the infection. It is typically recommended for later CDI recurrences and is performed as a medical procedure.

There are also microbiota products available for patients treated for recurrent CDI. These include *Rebyota* (a rectal suspension of live fecal microbiota) and *Vowst* (an oral capsule containing live fecal microbiota spores), which are taken after CDI treatment is completed to prevent future CDI episodes.

C. DIFFICILE GUIDELINE RECOMMENDATIONS

- When infection is suspected, discontinue unnecessary antibiotics and other possible causative agents (e.g., PPIs) if possible

- Isolate patients (in a single room with a dedicated bathroom; use contact precautions – gown and gloves)

- After patient care/visits: wash hands with soap and water (more effective than alcohol-containing hand sanitizers)

- Diagnosis: positive *C. difficile* stool toxin (enzyme immunoassay combined with a glutamate dehydrogenase test) or PCR

- Adjunct bezlotoxumab (i.e., in addition to antibacterial treatment) can be considered for high-risk patients: age ≥ 65 years, immunocompromised status, severe presentation and/or history of CDI within the past 6 months

1ST EPISODE	2nd EPISODE (1st Recurrence)	3rd OR SUBSEQUENT EPISODES
FDX 200 mg PO BID x 10 days, or VAN 125 mg PO QID x 10 days (standard regimen) MET 500 mg PO TID x 10 days (option only if non-severe* and treatments above are unavailable)	FDX 200 mg PO BID x 10 days, or VAN standard regimen followed by a prolonged pulse/tapered course** (the standard regimen without a prolonged taper is acceptable if MET was used for the initial episode)	FDX 200 mg PO BID x 10 days, or VAN standard regimen followed by a prolonged pulse/tapered course**, or VAN standard regimen followed by rifaximin 400 mg TID x 20 days, or Fecal microbiota transplantation

Fulminant/Complicated Disease

Diagnosed when significant systemic toxic effects are present, such as hypotension, shock, ileus or toxic megacolon; can occur with any episode/recurrence

VAN 500 mg PO/NG/PR QID + metronidazole 500 mg IV Q8H

FDX = fidaxomicin (Dificid); VAN = vancomycin; MET = metronidazole
*Non-severe = WBC < 15,000 cells/mm³ and SCr < 1.5 mg/dL.
**Example vancomycin tapered and pulsed regimen = 125 mg PO QID x 10 days, BID x 1 week, daily x 1 week, then 125 mg every 2-3 days for 2-8 weeks.

SEXUALLY TRANSMITTED INFECTIONS

Safe sex practices and education are important to prevent sexually transmitted infections (STIs). Condoms (male and female) can help decrease transmission. Oral sex has a much lower risk of HIV transmission than vaginal or anal sex, but still carries a risk for herpes, syphilis, hepatitis B, gonorrhea and human papillomavirus (HPV).

Screening should be performed for timely diagnosis of STIs and prevention of complications, including cervical cancer, infertility or transmission to partners. Sexual partners should be treated concurrently to prevent re-infection, except with bacterial vaginosis. See Study Tip Gal for usual symptoms of common STIs and the table on the next page for treatment recommendations (refer to the Infectious Diseases III chapter for a discussion of herpes simplex virus).

SYMPTOMS OF COMMON STIs

Chlamydia:	genital discharge or no symptoms
Gonorrhea:	genital discharge or no symptoms
Genital warts:	single or multiple pink/skin-toned lesions
Latent syphilis:	asymptomatic
Primary syphilis:	painless, smooth genital sores (chancre)

Females only

Bacterial vaginosis: vaginal discharge (clear, white or gray) that has a "fishy" odor and pH > 4.5; little or no pain

Trichomoniasis: yellow/green, frothy vaginal discharge with pH > 4.5; soreness, pain with intercourse

TREATMENT OF SEXUALLY TRANSMITTED INFECTIONS

INFECTION	DRUG OF CHOICE	DOSING/DURATION	ALTERNATIVES/NOTES
Syphilis (primary, secondary or early latent) *Treponema pallidum*, a spirochete Early latent: acquired within the past year, asymptomatic	Penicillin G benzathine (*Bicillin L-A*, do not substitute with *Bicillin C-R*)	2.4 million units IM x 1	Beta-lactam allergy ■ Doxycycline 100 mg PO BID x 14 days ■ If pregnant, nonadherent with treatment or unlikely to follow up, desensitize and treat with *Bicillin L-A* (see Study Tip Gal on next page) Diagnosis: positive non-treponemal test, such as a rapid plasma reagin (RPR) or Venereal Diseases Research Lab (VDRL) blood test, and treponemal assay
Syphilis (late latent or tertiary) Late latent: acquired > 1 year ago or unknown duration, asymptomatic	As above	2.4 million units IM weekly x 3 weeks (7.2 million units total)	Beta-lactam allergy ■ Doxycycline 100 mg PO BID x 28 days (see notes above for pregnant or nonadherent patients)
Neurosyphilis Can occur at any stage of disease	Penicillin G aqueous crystalline	3-4 million units IV Q4H x 10-14 days	Penicillin G procaine Beta-lactam allergy: desensitization followed by administration of penicillin G aqueous IV
Gonorrhea *Neisseria gonorrhoeae*, a gram-negative diplococcus Commonly diagnosed via urethral, vaginal, cervical, rectal and/or pharyngeal swabs	Ceftriaxone If chlamydia has not been excluded: add doxycycline (see below)	< 150 kg: 500 mg IM x 1 ≥ 150 kg: 1 gram IM x 1	Treatment is the same for pregnant patients If ceftriaxone is not available: cefixime 800 mg PO x 1 If cephalosporin allergy: gentamicin 240 mg IM x 1 + azithromycin 2 grams PO x 1 Ceftriaxone is most effective for pharyngeal infections (if severe cephalosporin allergy, consult an ID specialist)
Chlamydia *Chlamydia trachomatis*, an intracellular obligate gram-negative organism Testing as per gonorrhea	Non-pregnant: doxycycline Pregnant: azithromycin	100 mg PO BID x 7 days 1 gram PO x 1	Erythromycin base 500 mg PO QID x 7 days, or Levofloxacin 500 mg PO daily x 7 days Pregnancy: amoxicillin 500 mg PO TID x 7 days
Bacterial Vaginosis Many different organisms, including *Gardnerella vaginalis*	Metronidazole or Metronidazole 0.75% gel or Clindamycin 2% cream	500 mg PO BID x 7 days 1 applicator intravaginally daily x 5 days 1 applicator intravaginally at bedtime x 7 days	Clindamycin 300 mg PO BID x 7 days (or clindamycin ovules* 100 mg intravaginally at bedtime x 3 days), or Tinidazole 2 g PO daily x 2 days (or 1 g PO daily x 5 days), or Secnidazole 2 g PO x 1 dose Females with bacterial vaginosis should not douche
Trichomoniasis *Trichomonas vaginalis*, a flagellated protozoan	Metronidazole	Females: 500 mg PO BID x 7 days Males: 2 grams PO x 1	Pregnancy: metronidazole (per package labeling) is contraindicated in the 1st trimester, but based on additional safety data (and the adverse outcomes associated with infection), the CDC recommends metronidazole for trichomoniasis in all trimesters
Genital Warts Human papillomavirus (HPV) strains 6 & 11 *Gardasil* vaccine reduces the risk of genital warts as well as cervical and other cancers (see the Immunizations chapter)	Imiquimod cream (*Zyclara*)	Apply topically to clean, dry, warty tissue and wash off in 6-10 hours Apply 3x/week until cleared (or 16 weeks)	Treatment not required if asymptomatic (warts generally resolve spontaneously within one year) Local side effects of erythema, burning, scaling, ulcers and vesicles can occur with imiquimod treatment Imiquimod cream can weaken condoms and diaphragms and irritate anogenital mucosa; patients should abstain from sexual activity while the cream is on the skin

*Clindamycin ovules use a base that can weaken latex or rubber products (e.g., condoms); alternative contraception methods should be used within 72 hours of clindamycin ovules.

SYPHILIS: PENICILLIN DESENSITIZATION REQUIRED?

Syphilis must be treated with penicillin in select patients with a penicillin allergy because the alternative, doxycycline, is not suitable and poorly studied.

- A pregnant patient cannot take doxycycline due to the adverse effects on the fetus (suppressed bone growth and skeletal development).

- A patient with poor compliance/follow-up is at risk for treatment failure with a twice-daily regimen that must be taken for 14-28 days.

Per the CDC, follow these steps:

1. Confirm the allergic reaction with a skin test.

2. Temporarily desensitize the patient with an approved desensitization protocol.

3. Treat with IM penicillin G benzathine (*Bicillin L-A*).

COMMON TICKBORNE DISEASES

Tickborne infections are caused by a variety of bacteria that are carried by many ticks, fleas and lice. The diseases that commonly occur in humans are listed in the table below, along with the recommended treatments. Rocky Mountain spotted fever is the most common and most fatal of these illnesses in the U.S. Initial signs and symptoms include fever, headache, and muscle pain, followed 3 – 5 days later by an erythematous petechial rash (pinpoint or splotchy red spots caused by bleeding into the dermis).

DISEASE	ORGANISM	TREATMENT
Rocky Mountain Spotted Fever	*Rickettsia rickettsii* Gram-negative obligate intracellular bacteria	Doxycycline 100 mg PO/IV BID x 5-7 days (the drug of choice, including for pediatric patients)
Lyme Disease	*Borrelia burgdorferi, Borrelia mayonii* Spirochetes	Doxycycline 100 mg PO BID x 10 days, or Amoxicillin 500 mg PO TID x 14 days, or Cefuroxime 500 mg PO BID x 14 days
Ehrlichiosis	*Ehrlichia chaffeensis* Obligate intracellular bacteria	Doxycycline 100 mg PO/IV BID x 7-14 days

SELECT GUIDELINES/REFERENCES

Metlay JP, Waterer GW, Long AC, et al. Diagnosis and treatment of adults with community-acquired pneumonia. An official clinical practice guideline of the American Thoracic Society and Infectious Diseases Society of America. *Am J Respir Crit Care Med.* 2019;200:e45-e67.

Sterling TR, Njie G, Zenner D, et al. Guidelines for the treatment of latent tuberculosis infection: Recommendations from the National Tuberculosis Controllers Association and CDC, 2020. *MMWR Recomm Rep* 2020;69(No.RR-1):1-11.

Johnson S, Lavergne V, Skinner AM, et al. Clinical practice guideline by the Infectious Diseases Society of America (IDSA) and Society for Healthcare Epidemiology of America (SHEA): 2021 focused update guidelines on management of for *Clostridioides difficile* infection in adults. *Clinical Infectious Diseases.* 2021;73:e1029-e1044.

Workowski KA, Golan GA. Sexually transmitted infections treatment guidelines, 2021. *MMWR Recomm Rep* 2021;70(No. RR-4):1-187.

Other guidelines available from the Infectious Diseases Society of America (www.idsociety.org).

LYME DISEASE OR RINGWORM?

Lyme Disease

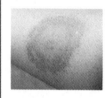

Bacterial (spirochete) infection *Borrelia burgdorferi* and *Borrelia mayonii*, spread by ticks

Erythema migrans: a "bull's-eye" rash (round, red with central clearing as it expands), achy joints, fever

Diagnosis: enzyme immunoassay (EIA) identifies antibodies
Treatment: doxycycline 100 mg BID PO/IV

Ringworm

Fungal infection *Tinea corporis*

1+ reddish, raised rings, can be itchy
Treatments: clotrimazole or another topical antifungal

AnastasiaKopa, Jane Rix/Shutterstock.com

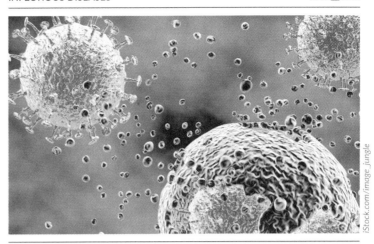

CHAPTER 24
INFECTIOUS DISEASES III: ANTIFUNGALS & ANTIVIRALS

SYSTEMIC FUNGAL INFECTIONS

Fungi are classified as either yeasts, molds or dimorphic species (see box). Certain types of fungi (including yeasts such as *Candida*) can colonize body surfaces and are considered to be normal flora in the intestine. They do not normally cause serious infections unless they contaminate a sterile space (e.g., the blood) or the immune system is weakened by drugs or diseases (e.g., chemotherapy, HIV), increasing the risk of opportunistic infections (see the Infectious Diseases IV: Opportunistic Infections chapter for more information).

Some fungi reproduce by spreading microscopic spores. The spores are often present in the air, where they can be inhaled or come into contact with the skin; they can cause a wide spectrum of diseases, from mild infections of the nail bed to severe infections such as meningitis or pneumonia. Invasive fungal infections are associated with high morbidity and mortality.

Dimorphic fungi exist as mold forms at lower temperatures and yeast forms at higher temperatures ("mold in the cold, yeast in the heat"). *Zygomycetes* refers to a class of fungi which includes *Mucor* and *Rhizopus* species; invasive disease caused by these species is commonly referred to as "mucormycosis."

Diagnosis of fungal infections can be made by culture, serologic studies or histologic features of a tissue specimen. *C. albicans* is the most susceptible of the *Candida* species to drug treatment. *C. glabrata* and *C. krusei* tend to be more difficult to treat due to resistance to certain azole antifungals. Of the molds, *Aspergillus* and *Zygomycetes* require the use of specific agents with an adequate spectrum of activity. Long-term, systemic antifungals are necessary for certain invasive fungal infections (e.g., *Cryptococcus, Coccidioides*) that occur in someone who is chronically immunosuppressed.

FUNGAL CLASSIFICATIONS

Yeasts	Molds
Candida species	*Aspergillus* species
C. albicans	
C. tropicalis	*Zygomycetes (Mucor*
C. parapsilosis	and *Rhizopus* species)
C. glabrata	
C. krusei	**Dimorphic fungi**
	Histoplasma
Cryptococcus	*capsulatum*
neoformans	
	Blastomyces
	dermatitidis
	Coccidioides immitis

CONTENT LEGEND

= Study
Tip Gal

AMPHOTERICIN B

Amphotericin B binds to ergosterol, altering cell membrane permeability and causing cell death. It is a broad-spectrum drug that can be used as initial treatment for many invasive fungal infections, including cryptococcal meningitis (in combination with flucytosine), histoplasmosis and mucormycosis. It is active against:

- Yeasts: most *Candida* species and *Cryptococcus neoformans*
- Molds: *Aspergillus* species and *Zygomycetes*
- Dimorphic fungi: *Histoplasma capsulatum*, *Blastomyces dermatitidis* and *Coccidioides immitis*

Amphotericin B deoxycholate (the conventional formulation) has many toxicities. The amphotericin B lipid formulations are a complex of the active medication and a lipid component; they are associated with fewer toxicities (e.g., decreased infusion reactions, decreased nephrotoxicity) compared to the conventional (deoxycholate) formulation.

FORMULATIONS	DOSING	SAFETY/SIDE EFFECTS/MONITORING
Conventional Formulation		**BOXED WARNINGS**
Amphotericin B Deoxycholate Injection	0.1-1.5 mg/kg/day	Medication errors confusing the lipid-based forms of amphotericin (*AmBisome* and *Abelcet*) and conventional amphotericin B (deoxycholate) have resulted in cardiopulmonary arrest and death; conventional amphotericin B doses should not exceed 1.5 mg/kg/day (verify product name and dosage if dose exceeds 1.5 mg/kg/day)
		SIDE EFFECTS Infusion-related: fever, chills, headache, malaise, rigors, ↓ or ↑ BP, thrombophlebitis, N/V Other: ↓ K, ↓ Mg, nephrotoxicity, anemia *AmBisome*: severe back/chest pain with the first dose
Lipid Formulations		**MONITORING**
Amphotericin B Lipid Complex (*Abelcet*) Injection	5 mg/kg/day	Renal function, LFTs, electrolytes (especially K and Mg), CBC **NOTES** Compatible with D5W only, lipid formulations must be filtered during preparation Amphotericin B deoxycholate (conventional formulation) requires premedication to reduce infusion-related reactions; give the following 30-60 minutes prior to the infusion:
Liposomal Amphotericin B (*AmBisome*) Injection	3-6 mg/kg/day	- Acetaminophen or NSAID - Diphenhydramine and/or hydrocortisone - NS boluses to ↓ the risk of nephrotoxicity - ± meperidine to ↓ the duration of severe rigors Both conventional and lipid formulations are yellow-orange in color

Amphotericin B Drug Interactions

- Additive risk of nephrotoxicity when used with other nephrotoxic agents, such as aminoglycosides, cisplatin, polymyxins, cyclosporine, loop diuretics, NSAIDs, radiocontrast dye, tacrolimus and vancomycin.
- Can ↑ the risk of digoxin toxicity due to hypokalemia. Use caution with any agent that ↓ potassium or magnesium since amphotericin decreases both. Scheduled replacement of potassium and/or magnesium should be considered.

FLUCYTOSINE

Flucytosine penetrates fungal cells and is converted to fluorouracil, which competes with uracil and interferes with fungal RNA and protein synthesis. Due to the development of resistance, flucytosine should not be used alone. It is recommended in combination with amphotericin B for the treatment of invasive cryptococcal (e.g., meningitis) or *Candida* infections.

DRUG	DOSING	SAFETY/SIDE EFFECTS/MONITORING
Flucytosine, 5-FC (*Ancobon*)	50-150 mg/kg/day PO divided Q6H CrCl ≤ 40 mL/min: adjustment required	**BOXED WARNING** Use with extreme caution in patients with renal dysfunction; monitor hematologic, renal and hepatic status **SIDE EFFECTS** Dose-related myelosuppression (anemia, neutropenia, thrombocytopenia), ↑ BUN/SCr, liver injury, ↑ bilirubin, many CNS effects, hypoglycemia, ↓ K, aplastic anemia

AZOLE ANTIFUNGALS

Azole antifungals decrease ergosterol synthesis and cell membrane formation. The coverage and indications of azoles vary widely, and their use is sometimes limited due to significant drug interactions caused by their CYP450 (mainly CYP3A4) inhibition. Ketoconazole was the first azole antifungal, but due to toxicities and many drug interactions, it is now most often used topically.

Fluconazole has activity against *C. albicans, C. parapsilosis* and *C. tropicalis.* It has limited efficacy against *C. glabrata* due to resistance, and *C. krusei* is considered fluconazole-resistant. Fluconazole can be used for many infections, including yeast infections (e.g., oral, esophageal, vaginal); a yeast infection in the mouth, called oral thrush or oral candidiasis, presents with white-colored, sore patches on the tongue and oral mucosa.

The primary uses for itraconazole are for the dimorphic fungi *(Blastomycoses* and *Histoplasma)* and nail bed infections (onychomycosis). Voriconazole is the treatment of choice for *Aspergillus.*

See the Common Skin Conditions chapter for treatment of non-invasive fungal infections (e.g., onychomycosis, vaginal candidiasis).

KEY ISSUES WITH AZOLE ANTIFUNGALS

Class Effects
- ↑ LFTs
- QT prolongation (except isavuconazonium)
- Many drug interactions

Drug-Specific Concerns
- Fluconazole: the only azole that requires renal dose adjustment
- Ketoconazole: hepatotoxicity has led to liver transplantation
- Itraconazole: can cause heart failure
- Voriconazole: can cause visual changes and phototoxicity
- Posaconazole:
  - Tablet dose ≠ suspension dose (due to different bioavailability)
  - Take with food

IV Administration
- IV to PO ratio is 1:1 for all azoles
- Drugs with sulfobutyl ether beta-cyclodextrin (SBECD) vehicle: voriconazole, posaconazole

---

DRUG	DOSING	SAFETY/SIDE EFFECTS/MONITORING
Fluconazole *(Diflucan)* Tablet, suspension, injection	50-800 mg PO/IV daily Vaginal candidiasis: 150 mg PO x 1 CrCl ≤ 50 mL/min: ↓ dose by 50%	**BOXED WARNINGS** **Itraconazole** Can worsen or cause heart failure; do not use to treat onychomycosis in patients with ventricular dysfunction or a history of heart failure Can cause ↑ plasma concentrations of certain drugs and can lead to QT prolongation and ventricular tachyarrhythmias, including Torsades de Pointes (TdP)
Itraconazole *(Sporanox, Tolsura)* Capsule, solution	200 mg PO daily or BID *Tolsura:* 130 mg PO daily or BID Formulations have different bioavailability and are not interchangeable; the oral solution is better absorbed Solution is taken on an empty stomach; capsules are taken with food Limited data on use in renal impairment (use with caution)	**Ketoconazole** Hepatotoxicity which has led to liver transplantation and/or death QT prolongation Use oral tablets only when other effective antifungal therapy is unavailable or not tolerated and the benefits outweigh the risks (hepatotoxicity, drug interactions) **WARNINGS** Hepatotoxicity Fluconazole: exfoliative skin reactions, not recommended in pregnancy
Ketoconazole Tablet, cream, foam, gel, shampoo *Nizoral A-D* shampoo is OTC	200-400 mg PO daily No adjustment in renal impairment	**SIDE EFFECTS** ↑ LFTs, QT prolongation, headache, N/V, abdominal pain, rash/pruritus, dizziness, hair loss (or possible hair growth) and altered hair texture with ketoconazole shampoo **NOTES** All azoles are cleared hepatically except fluconazole, which requires renal dose adjustment Fluconazole and voriconazole penetrate the CNS adequately to treat fungal meningitis (see voriconazole on the following page)

DRUG	DOSING	SAFETY/SIDE EFFECTS/MONITORING
Voriconazole (*Vfend, Vfend IV*) Tablet, suspension, injection	Loading dose: 6 mg/kg IV Q12H x 2 doses Maintenance dose: 4 mg/kg IV Q12H or 200 mg PO Q12H Mild-moderate hepatic impairment: reduce maintenance dose by 50% Severe hepatic impairment: only use if benefit outweighs risk, monitor closely CrCl < 50 mL/min: the intravenous vehicle SBECD accumulates; oral voriconazole is preferred Monitor SCr if IV voriconazole is used; change to oral when possible Therapeutic range (trough): 1-5 mcg/mL	**CONTRAINDICATIONS** Coadministration with barbiturates (long-acting), carbamazepine, efavirenz (≥ 400 mg/day), ergot alkaloids, pimozide, quinidine, rifabutin, rifampin, ritonavir (≥ 800 mg/day), sirolimus or St. John's wort **WARNINGS** Hepatotoxicity, visual disturbances (optic neuritis and papilledema), phototoxicity, QT prolongation (correct K, Ca and Mg prior to initiating treatment), nephrotoxicity, avoid in pregnancy, infusion-related reactions, serious skin reactions (SJS/TEN), skeletal adverse effects (fluorosis, periostitis), pancreatitis **SIDE EFFECTS** Visual changes (~20% - blurred vision, photophobia, altered color perception, altered visual acuity), ↑ LFTs, ↑ SCr, CNS toxicity (hallucinations, headache, dizziness), photosensitivity, ↑ or ↓ K **MONITORING** LFTs, renal function, electrolytes, visual function (when used > 28 days), trough concentrations (toxicity more likely with troughs > 5 mcg/mL) **NOTES** *Vfend*: take on an empty stomach, at least 1 hour before or after a meal; hold tube feedings for 1 hour before and after doses Use caution when driving at night due to vision changes Avoid direct sunlight Suspension: shake for 10 seconds before each use; do not refrigerate
Posaconazole (*Noxafil*) Delayed-release tablet, suspension, injection	Suspension: 200 mg TID or 400 mg BID Give with a full meal (during or within 20 minutes following a meal) Tablets: 300 mg PO BID on day 1, then 300 mg PO daily with food (can range from 100-400 mg/day, divided in 1-3 doses) IV: 300 mg BID on day 1, then 300 mg daily eGFR < 50 mL/min/1.73 m²: the intravenous vehicle SBECD can accumulate and worsen renal function; oral treatment is preferred	**CONTRAINDICATIONS** Coadministration with sirolimus, ergot alkaloids, pimozide, quinidine, atorvastatin, lovastatin and simvastatin **WARNINGS** QT prolongation (correct K, Ca and Mg prior to initiating treatment) Prescribing and dispensing errors: suspension and tablet are not interchangeable as dosing regimens differ (tablet is better absorbed) Neurotoxicity when used with vincristine, due to increased vincristine levels (seizures, peripheral neuropathy, SIADH, paralytic ileus) **SIDE EFFECTS** N/V/D, fever, headache, ↑ LFTs, rash, ↓ K, ↓ Mg, cough **MONITORING** LFTs, renal function, electrolytes, CBC
Isavuconazonium sulfate (*Cresemba*) Capsules, injection Prodrug of isavuconazole	IV/PO: 372 mg Q8H for 6 doses, then 372 mg daily No adjustment for renal dysfunction, use with caution in severe hepatic impairment Swallow capsules whole, do not crush or open	**CONTRAINDICATIONS** Use with strong CYP3A4 inhibitors or inducers, familial short QT syndrome (causes QT shortening, not prolongation) **WARNINGS** Hepatotoxicity, infusion-related reactions (hypotension, dyspnea, chills, dizziness, tingling and numbness), hypersensitivity reactions (anaphylaxis, SJS/TEN), teratogenic, drug interactions, particulates (undissolved intravenous drug) **SIDE EFFECTS** N/V/D, headache, injection site reactions, peripheral edema, ↓ K, ↑ LFTs **MONITORING** LFTs, electrolytes **NOTES** Requires a filter (0.2-1.2 micron) during administration due to possible particulates Capsules must be protected from moisture; original container has a desiccant

Azole Antifungal Drug Interactions

- <u>All</u> azoles are moderate-strong <u>CYP3A4 inhibitors</u>; monitor for drug interactions.

- Itraconazole and ketoconazole inhibit P-glycoprotein.

- <u>Fluconazole</u> and voriconazole <u>inhibit CYP2C9</u>, which can ↑ the effects of <u>warfarin</u>. <u>Monitor INR</u> and signs/symptoms of bleeding.

- Azoles can ↑ the concentrations of apixaban and rivaroxaban. Monitor for signs/symptoms of bleeding.

- Caution use in combination with other <u>QT-prolonging</u> drugs [e.g., antiarrhythmics, quinolones, macrolides, antidepressants (tricyclics, SSRIs, mirtazapine, trazodone, venlafaxine), antipsychotics, 5-HT3 receptor antagonists, others (see the Arrhythmias chapter)].

- <u>PPIs</u> and cimetidine can <u>decrease</u> the <u>absorption</u> of <u>posaconazole</u> suspension and should be stopped during therapy to avoid treatment failure.

- The absorption of <u>itraconazole (Sporanox brand capsules)</u> and <u>ketoconazole</u> requires an <u>acidic gut</u>; ↑ pH will ↓ absorption. Separate antacids two hours before and after doses.

  - ❑ If PPIs or H2RAs must be used while on ketoconazole, take with an acidic beverage (such as <u>non-diet cola</u>) to provide an <u>acidic environment for absorption</u>.

- Voriconazole:

  - ❑ Concentrations can ↑ dangerously when given with drugs that inhibit CYP2C19, 2C9 or 3A4, or with small dose increases. Exhibits first-order, followed by zero-order (non-linear), kinetics.

  - ❑ Do not use with barbiturates (long-acting), carbamazepine, efavirenz (≥ 400 mg/day), ergot alkaloids, pimozide, quinidine, rifabutin, rifampin, ritonavir (≥ 800 mg/day), sirolimus or St. John's wort.

ECHINOCANDINS

Echinocandins <u>inhibit</u> the <u>synthesis of beta (1,3)-D-glucan</u>, an essential component of the <u>fungal cell wall</u>. They are <u>effective against most</u> *Candida* species, including strains typically resistant to azole antifungals (e.g., *C. glabrata, C. krusei*). Though they have activity against *Aspergillus* species, they should only be used as part of a combination regimen, and other medications are generally preferred. Echinocandins are available <u>only as injections</u>. They are typically well-tolerated and are not associated with significant renal or hepatic toxicity.

DRUG	DOSING	SAFETY/SIDE EFFECTS/MONITORING
Caspofungin (Cancidas) Injection	70 mg IV on day 1, then 50 mg IV daily Moderate hepatic impairment: 70 mg IV on day 1, then 35 mg IV daily ↑ dose to 70 mg IV daily when used in combination with rifampin or other strong enzyme inducers	**WARNINGS** <u>Histamine-mediated symptoms</u> (rash, pruritus, facial swelling, flushing, hypotension) have occurred; anaphylaxis **SIDE EFFECTS** ↑ LFTs, headache, ↑ or ↓ K, ↓ Mg, fever, N/V/D, anemia, ↑ SCr, rash Caspofungin: severe skin reactions, including SJS/TEN
Micafungin (Mycamine) Injection	**Candidemia** 100 mg IV daily **Esophageal Candidiasis** 150 mg IV daily	**MONITORING** LFTs
Anidulafungin (Eraxis) Injection	**Candidemia** 200 mg IV on day 1, then 100 mg IV daily **Esophageal Candidiasis** 100 mg IV on day 1, then 50 mg daily	**NOTES** All except rezafungin are given <u>once daily</u> <u>Do not require dose adjustment in renal impairment</u> Very few drug interactions <u>Micafungin</u>: requires <u>light-protection during administration</u> (see the Intravenous Medication Principles Chapter)
Rezafungin (Rezzayo) Injection	**Candidemia and Invasive Candidiasis** 400 mg IV on day 1, then 200 mg IV weekly starting on day 8 for up to 4 doses	Rezafungin: reserve for patients with limited or no alternative options (due to limited clinical and safety data)

OTHER ANTIFUNGAL AGENTS

Superficial fungal infections are easier to treat than invasive fungal infections, and topical antifungal products are preferred in most cases (see the Common Skin Conditions chapter); systemic medications are considered second line. Griseofulvin has a narrow antifungal spectrum, is less effective than other systemic drugs (e.g., itraconazole, terbinafine) and requires prolonged courses. Nystatin suspension, clotrimazole troches/lozenges and buccal miconazole are useful for treating mild, localized *Candida* infections (e.g., thrush).

DRUG	DOSING	SAFETY/SIDE EFFECTS/MONITORING
Nystatin Suspension, tablet Topical forms: cream, ointment, powder	**Oral Candidiasis** Suspension: 400,000-600,000 units 4 times/day x 7-14 days **Intestinal Infections** Oral tablets: 500,000-1,000,000 units Q8H	**SIDE EFFECTS** N/V/D, stomach pain (otherwise low systemic risk due to minimal GI absorption) **NOTES** Suspension: swish in the mouth and retain for as long as possible (several minutes) before swallowing
Griseofulvin Tablet (microsize, ultramicrosize), suspension (microsize) Indicated for fungal infections of the skin, hair and nails	Microsize: 500-1,000 mg/day in 1-2 divided doses Ultramicrosize: 375-750 mg/day in 1-2 divided doses Duration of therapy depends on the site of infection: Tinea corporis: 2-4 weeks Tinea pedis: 4-8 weeks	**CONTRAINDICATIONS** Pregnancy, severe liver disease, porphyria **SIDE EFFECTS** Photosensitivity, ↑ LFTs, HA, rash, urticaria, dizziness, leukopenia, severe skin reactions **MONITORING** LFTs, renal function, CBC **NOTES** Cross reaction possible with penicillin allergy Take with a fatty meal to ↑ absorption or with food/milk to avoid GI upset
Terbinafine Tablet, topical Topical cream (OTC): *Lamisil AT*	250 mg/day in 1-2 divided doses without regard to meals	**CONTRAINDICATIONS** Chronic or active liver disease **WARNINGS** Hepatotoxicity, taste/smell disturbance (including permanent loss of taste or smell), depression, neutropenia, thrombotic thrombocytopenic purpura (TTP), hemolytic uremic syndrome (HUS), serious skin reactions (SJS/TEN/DRESS/ erythema multiforme), can cause/worsen systemic lupus erythematosus **SIDE EFFECTS** Headache, ↑ LFTs, skin rash, abdominal pain, pruritus, diarrhea, dyspepsia **MONITORING** CBC, LFTs
Clotrimazole 10 mg troche/lozenge Topical and vaginal forms (multiple brand names)	**Oropharyngeal Candidiasis** Prophylaxis: 10 mg 3 times/day Treatment: 10 mg 5 times/day x 7-14 days	**SIDE EFFECTS** ↑ LFTs, nausea, dysgeusia **NOTES** Allow troche to dissolve slowly over 15-30 minutes
Miconazole Buccal tablet (*Oravig*) Topical and vaginal forms (multiple brand names)	**Oropharyngeal Candidiasis** 50 mg (1 tablet) applied to the upper gum region daily for 7-14 days	**CONTRAINDICATIONS** Hypersensitivity to milk protein concentrate **SIDE EFFECTS** Local application site reactions (pain, burning, pruritus, edema, toothache)
Oteseconazole (*Vivjoa*) Only indicated for recurrent vulvovaginal candidiasis	600 mg x 1 on day 1, then 450 mg x 1 on day 2 Starting on day 14: 150 mg once weekly x 11 weeks	**CONTRAINDICATIONS** Pregnancy (or reproductive potential), breastfeeding, moderate-severe liver impairment (Child-Pugh class B or C) or eGFR < 30 mL/min/1.73 m² **SIDE EFFECTS** Nausea, headache, menstrual bleeding, vulvovaginal irritation or pain

Drug Interactions

- Griseofulvin: ↑ the metabolism of hormonal contraceptives (estrogen and progestin) which can lead to contraceptive failure. Use a nonhormonal form of contraception.

- Terbinafine is a strong CYP2D6 inhibitor and a weak/ moderate CYP3A4 inducer.

EMPIRIC TREATMENT FOR SELECT FUNGAL PATHOGENS/INFECTIONS*

PATHOGEN	PREFERRED REGIMEN	ALTERNATIVE REGIMEN
Candida albicans Oropharyngeal infection (thrush)	Mild disease: topical antifungals (clotrimazole, miconazole) Moderate-severe disease or HIV+: fluconazole	Nystatin
Candida albicans Esophageal infection	Fluconazole	Echinocandin
Candida krusei and glabrata** All Candida species bloodstream infections	Echinocandin	Amphotericin B, high-dose fluconazole (susceptible isolates only)
Aspergillus Invasive	Voriconazole	Amphotericin B, isavuconazonium
Cryptococcus neoformans Meningitis	Amphotericin B + flucytosine (5-FC)	High-dose fluconazole + flucytosine (5-FC)
Dermatophytes Nail bed infection	Terbinafine or itraconazole (confirm fungal infection prior to treatment); see the Common Skin Conditions chapter	Fluconazole

De-escalate and tailor therapy based on a culture and susceptibility report.
*See the Infectious Disease IV chapter for opportunistic fungal infections that affect immunocompromised patients.
**Candida krusei and glabrata are more resistant to azole antifungals.

ANTIFUNGAL KEY COUNSELING POINTS

See the Drug Formulations and Patient Counseling chapter for counseling language/layman's terminology.

AZOLE ANTIFUNGALS
- Can cause:
  - Liver damage.
  - QT prolongation (except isavuconazonium).
- Many drug interactions.

Ketoconazole and Itraconazole
- Itraconazole
  - Tablets and capsules: take with food.
  - Solution: take on an empty stomach.
  - Can cause heart failure.
- Possible drug interactions due to high gastric pH.

Posaconazole
- Posaconazole tablets: take with food.
- Posaconazole suspension: take with a full meal or oral liquid nutritional supplement.

Voriconazole
- Take on an empty stomach, at least one hour before or one hour after meals.
- Can cause:
  - Photosensitivity.
  - Vision changes.
- Store reconstituted oral suspension at room temperature.

NYSTATIN
- Oral suspension: shake well before using.

TERBINAFINE
- Oral terbinafine can cause liver damage.
- Can take several months after finishing treatment to see the full benefit of this drug (it takes time for new healthy nails to grow and replace the infected ones).

VIRAL INFECTIONS

Viruses depend on host cell metabolic processes for survival; for that reason, they are sometimes referred to as obligate intracellular parasites. Many viral infections have no effective drug treatment. Medications are available to treat influenza virus, COVID-19, herpes simplex virus [genital herpes, herpes labialis (cold sores) and systemic herpes virus infections], varicella zoster virus (VZV) and cytomegalovirus (CMV).

Treatments for viral infections work by directly inhibiting viruses (antiviral agents) or augmenting or modifying host defenses to the viral infection (immunomodulating agents). Antivirals target critical steps in the viral life cycle, such as entry into the cell or replication; since viruses depend on the host cell machinery for metabolism/replication, antivirals can also injure or destroy the host cell.

INFLUENZA

Influenza is a respiratory virus that affects 3 – 11% of the U.S. population annually, with peak activity typically occurring between late November and March. Influenza A and B are the strains that commonly infect humans. Many diagnostic tests are available to test for influenza (e.g., molecular assays, antigen detection tests). The rapid influenza diagnostic test is often done as a nasopharyngeal swab.

Both influenza A and B can cause severe illness leading to hospitalization and death, particularly in at-risk populations, including pregnant patients, immunocompromised patients, children < 5 years, adults ≥ 65 years, and those with comorbid conditions (e.g., diabetes, asthma, cardiovascular disease).

Influenza commonly presents with fever, chills, fatigue, myalgia, non-productive cough, sore throat and headache. It spreads via respiratory droplets (e.g., generated by coughing). A person with influenza can be contagious one day prior to developing symptoms and for up to 5 – 7 days after becoming ill.

The seasonal influenza vaccine is the most effective prevention for influenza infection and is recommended for all patients age ≥ 6 months who have no contraindications. See the Immunizations chapter for details.

Antivirals for Influenza

The Centers for Disease Control and Prevention (CDC) provides annual updates to the antiviral treatment recommendations based on the type of circulating virus each influenza season. Neuraminidase inhibitors (oseltamivir, zanamivir and peramivir) reduce the amount of virus in the body by inhibiting the enzyme which enables release of new viral particles from infected cells. They are active against influenza A and B, decreasing the duration of symptoms by about one day and reducing complications.

To be most effective, neuraminidase inhibitors should be started within 48 hours of illness onset. In hospitalized, severely ill patients and those at high risk of complications, neuraminidase inhibitors should still be started > 48 hours after symptom onset, though there is less benefit if started later, after the virus has already damaged respiratory epithelial cells.

Baloxavir marboxil is an endonuclease inhibitor approved for the treatment and post-exposure prevention of influenza. It has the advantage of being a single-dose regimen. Similar to neuraminidase inhibitors, it should be started within 48 hours of symptom onset.

The adamantanes (rimantadine and amantadine) were previously used to treat and prevent influenza A, but they are no longer recommended due to widespread resistance. Amantadine is used for Parkinson disease (see the Parkinson Disease chapter).

Neuraminidase Inhibitors

DRUG	DOSING	SAFETY/SIDE EFFECTS/MONITORING
Oseltamivir *(Tamiflu)* 30, 45, 75 mg capsules 6 mg/mL (60 mL) suspension *Stuart Monk/Shutterstock.com*	**Treatment, age > 12 years:** 75 mg BID x 5 days **Prophylaxis, age > 12 years:** 75 mg daily x 10 days CrCl ≤ 60 mL/min: adjustment required **Pediatric patients:** dose based on body weight	**WARNINGS** Neuropsychiatric events (sudden confusion, delirium, hallucinations, unusual behavior or self-injury), serious skin reactions (SJS/TEN), anaphylaxis **SIDE EFFECTS** Headache, nausea, vomiting, diarrhea, abdominal pain **NOTES** Preferred in pregnancy over other neuraminidase inhibitors Store reconstituted suspension at room temperature for 10 days or in the refrigerator for 17 days
Zanamivir *(Relenza Diskhaler)*	**Treatment, age ≥ 7 years:** 10 mg (two 5 mg inhalations) BID x 5 days **Prophylaxis, age ≥ 5 years:** 10 mg (two 5 mg inhalations) once daily x 10 days (household setting) or 28 days (community outbreak)	**WARNINGS** Neuropsychiatric events, bronchospasm (do not use in asthma/COPD or with any breathing problems); stop the drug if wheezing or breathing problems develop **SIDE EFFECTS** Headache, throat pain, cough
Peramivir *(Rapivab)* Injection	**Treatment (adult):** 600 mg IV as a single dose CrCl < 50 mL/min: adjustment required	**WARNINGS** Neuropsychiatric events, serious skin reactions (SJS/TEN), anaphylaxis, renal impairment **SIDE EFFECTS** Hypertension, insomnia, ↑ blood glucose, diarrhea, constipation, neutropenia, ↑ AST/ALT

Endonuclease Inhibitors

DRUG	DOSING	SAFETY/SIDE EFFECTS/MONITORING
Baloxavir marboxil *(Xofluza)* 20, 40 mg capsules 2 mg/mL (20 mL) suspension	**Treatment and prophylaxis, age ≥ 5 years:** ≥ 80 kg: 80 mg PO x 1 dose 20 to < 80 kg: 40 mg PO x 1 dose < 20 kg: 2 mg/kg PO x 1 dose Use with caution in renal or hepatic impairment (limited data)	**WARNINGS** Hypersensitivity, including skin reactions (erythema multiforme, urticaria) Monitor for secondary bacterial infections and treat accordingly **SIDE EFFECTS** Diarrhea **NOTES** Avoid administration with dairy products, antacids or other supplements containing polyvalent cations (e.g., calcium, magnesium, selenium, zinc) Store in original blister packaging Once reconstituted, administer the oral suspension within 10 hours (store at room temperature); dose may require more than 1 bottle

COVID-19

There are many different types of coronaviruses. Seasonal coronaviruses are a frequent cause of respiratory infections, including the common cold. Severe acute respiratory syndrome coronavirus 2 (SARS-CoV-2), a novel coronavirus that emerged in late 2019, causes coronavirus disease 2019 (COVID-19). It has a wide range of clinical presentations, from asymptomatic to severe illness requiring ICU admission and mechanical ventilation. Advanced age and comorbidities (e.g., cardiovascular or respiratory disease, diabetes, cancer) increase the risk of severe illness and death.

Like influenza, COVID-19 is spread through respiratory droplets released when coughing or sneezing. Spread can be reduced by isolating from others, wearing masks and frequent handwashing. Infected individuals may be contagious for up to 48 hours before symptom onset. Symptoms most often present within 4 – 5 days of exposure (up to 14 days) and can include fever, chills, cough, shortness of breath, fatigue, myalgia, loss of taste or smell, sore throat, runny nose and GI symptoms. Available vaccines to prevent COVID-19 are discussed in the Immunizations chapter.

COVID-19 Testing and Treatment

Generally, all symptomatic patients and select asymptomatic individuals (e.g., travelers, those with close contact with an infected person, people with repeated exposures, including healthcare workers) should be tested for COVID-19. Diagnosis usually involves a polymerase chain reaction (PCR) test using a nasopharyngeal swab specimen and/or a rapid antigen test, which is generally less sensitive than PCR. If testing is positive, the infected individual should isolate for at least 5 days after symptom onset and continue to wear a mask for 11 days. Consult the CDC, National Institutes of Health (NIH) and Infectious Diseases Society of America (IDSA) websites for the most current recommendations.

Symptomatic care (e.g., hydration, analgesics/antipyretics, antitussives) is appropriate in all patients. It is essential to counsel patients to seek medical care if symptoms worsen (e.g., new-onset dyspnea) or interfere with daily activities. The preferred outpatient treatment for patients at risk of progressing to severe COVID-19 (e.g., age > 50 years, not up-to-date with vaccinations, immunocompromised) is oral nirmatrelvir/ritonavir *(Paxlovid)*, which has a boxed warning for significant drug interactions due to the ritonavir component. Alternative therapies include IV remdesivir *(Veklury)* and oral molnupiravir *(Lagevrio)*.

Treatment of hospitalized patients can vary depending on disease severity (i.e., requirements for supplemental oxygen or mechanical ventilation), but can include systemic steroids (e.g., dexamethasone), antivirals (specifically remdesivir) and/or immunomodulator treatment (e.g., baricitinib, tocilizumab).

HERPES VIRUSES

There are hundreds of herpes viruses in existence, but not all are responsible for causing human disease. Clinically significant herpes viruses include herpes simplex viruses 1 and 2 (HSV-1, HSV-2), varicella zoster virus (VZV), cytomegalovirus (CMV), Epstein-Barr virus (EBV), human herpesviruses (HHV-6, HHV-7) and Kaposi sarcoma associated herpes virus (HHV-8).

Both HSV-1 and HSV-2 can cause various infections, including orofacial, esophageal, genital, ophthalmic, pulmonary and CNS (e.g., encephalitis) infections. HSV-1 is most commonly associated with oropharyngeal disease. HSV-2 is more closely associated with genital disease. Each virus is capable of causing infections clinically indistinguishable at both anatomic sites.

Antivirals for Herpes Simplex Virus and Varicella Zoster Virus

DRUG	SAFETY/SIDE EFFECTS/MONITORING
Acyclovir (Zovirax, Sitavig) Capsule, tablet, buccal tablet, suspension, injection, topical	**WARNINGS** Caution in patients with renal impairment, the elderly and/or those receiving nephrotoxic drugs; infuse acyclovir over at least 1 hour and maintain adequate hydration to reduce the risk of renal tubular damage Thrombotic thrombocytopenic purpura/hemolytic uremic syndrome (TTP/HUS) has been reported in immunocompromised patients
Valacyclovir (Valtrex) Tablet Prodrug of acyclovir	**SIDE EFFECTS** Malaise, headache, N/V/D, rash, pruritus, ↑ LFTs, neutropenia, transient burning or stinging with topical formulations (acyclovir) Anaphylaxis (famciclovir) ↑ BUN/SCr with crystal nephropathy (IV acyclovir)
Famciclovir Tablet Prodrug of penciclovir	**MONITORING** Renal function, LFTs, CBC **NOTES** Acyclovir dose is based on IBW, including in obese patients (see the Calculations IV chapter) ↓ dose and/or extend interval in renal impairment In general, 5 mg/kg IV acyclovir = 1,000 mg PO valacyclovir

Herpes Simplex Labialis (Cold Sores)

Cold sores are common and highly contagious. Children often contract the infection from family members; infection is usually due to HSV-1 in children but can be caused by HSV-2 due to adult oral/genital sex. The virus can shed when the patient is asymptomatic, but is more commonly spread when there are active lesions. Patients should avoid kissing and sharing drinks when the lesions are oozing.

Cold sores usually appear in the same location repeatedly. The most common site is the junction between the upper and lower lip. Triggers that cause sore outbreaks include stress/fatigue, stress to the skin (e.g., sun exposure, acid peels) and dental work. Patients should identify their triggers and attempt to avoid them.

Cold sore eruption is preceded by a prodrome (symptoms that occur before the lesions appear) of tingling, itching or soreness, which is the optimal time to take topical or oral medication to reduce blister duration. If recurrences are frequent (> 4 times/year), chronic suppression treatment may be warranted. OTC and prescription topicals shorten the duration of cold sores by up to one day; oral (systemic) antivirals shorten the duration by up to two days.

Topical Treatment for Herpes Labialis

DRUGS	DOSING	NOTES
Docosanol (Abreva) – OTC Cream	Apply 5x daily at first sign of outbreak, continue until healed.	Systemic antivirals are more effective. Marten_House/Shutterstock.com
Acyclovir (Zovirax) – Rx Cream	Apply 5x daily for 4 days (can be used on genital sores).	
Acyclovir (Sitavig) – Rx Buccal tablet	Apply 50 mg tablet as a single dose to the upper gum region.	
Penciclovir (Denavir) – Rx Cream	Apply every 2 hours during waking hours for 4 days.	

Systemic (Oral) Treatment of Herpes Labialis

EPISODE	ACYCLOVIR	VALACYCLOVIR	FAMCICLOVIR
Initial (treat for 7-10 days)	200 mg 5x daily or 400 mg TID	1 gram BID	250 mg 3x daily or 500 mg BID
Recurrence	400 mg TID x 5-10 days	2 grams BID x 1 day	1.5 grams x 1 dose
Chronic suppression	400 mg BID	500 mg or 1 gram daily	

Genital Herpes

Genital herpes, caused by HSV-2, is a chronic, life-long viral infection that affects 1 in 6 people in the U.S. The first episode of genital herpes usually begins within 2 – 14 days after exposure. Up to 50% of patients are asymptomatic, but others experience a prodrome of flu-like symptoms (fever, headache, malaise, myalgia) before the development of pustular or ulcerative lesions on external genitalia. Lesions usually begin as papules or vesicles that rapidly spread. Clusters of lesions form, crust and then re-epithelialize. Lesions are painful and associated with itching, dysuria and vaginal or urethral discharge.

Treatment must be initiated during the prodrome period or within one day of lesion onset. Acyclovir *(Zovirax)* is typically the least expensive regimen, but it must be dosed up to five times per day. Valacyclovir *(Valtrex)* is a prodrug of acyclovir; it can reach higher concentrations than oral acyclovir and the less frequent dosing can enhance adherence. If the virus is found to be resistant to acyclovir, it will be resistant to valacyclovir and (usually) famciclovir. Infections caused by acyclovir-resistant HSV are treated with foscarnet until the lesions heal.

Recurrent infections are not associated with systemic manifestations. Symptoms are localized to the genital area, are milder and of shorter duration. Patients typically experience a prodrome of mild tingling or shooting pain in the legs, hips, thighs or buttocks. Suppressive therapy (antivirals taken chronically) reduces the frequency of genital herpes recurrences by 70 – 80% and is recommended for patients who have frequent recurrences (e.g., > 6/year). With suppressive therapy, many report no symptomatic outbreaks and viral transmission is also reduced.

Oral Treatment of Genital Herpes in Non-HIV Patients

EPISODE	ACYCLOVIR	VALACYCLOVIR	FAMCICLOVIR
Initial (treat for 7-10 days)*	400 mg TID or 200 mg 5x daily	1 gram BID	250 mg TID
Recurrence	400 mg TID x 5 days or 800 mg BID x 5 days or 800 mg TID x 2 days	500 mg BID x 3 days or 1 gram daily x 5 days	125 mg BID x 5 days or 500 mg x 1, then 250 mg BID x 2 days or 1 gram BID x 1 day
Chronic suppression	400 mg BID	500 mg or 1 gram daily	250 mg BID

Treatment can be extended if healing is incomplete after 10 days of therapy.

Invasive HSV Infections

HSV is the most commonly identified cause of viral encephalitis in the U.S. HSV encephalitis occurs more frequently in young patients (ages 5 – 30 years) and older adults (age > 50 years). Hallmark symptoms include acute onset fever, focal neurologic symptoms and altered mental status. HSV encephalitis is treated with IV acyclovir 10 mg/kg/dose Q8H x 14 – 21 days. Other invasive infections (e.g., esophagitis and pneumonitis) occur infrequently, typically in the immunosuppressed population, and are treated with IV acyclovir 5 mg/kg/dose Q8H.

Varicella Zoster Virus and Herpes Zoster

Most adults in the U.S. had varicella zoster virus (chickenpox) infection during childhood. The virus can lie dormant in the nerve for decades without causing any symptoms. The recurrence of viral symptoms is called herpes zoster or shingles. An outbreak can occur as the patient ages and is often due to acute stress. Although herpes zoster can occur at any age, adults > 60 years old are most often affected. The shingles rash is distinctive; it can be itchy or tingly, is very painful and often manifests unilaterally (on one side of the body). Pharmacists should recognize the classic presentation of a shingles rash and inform patients to see a healthcare provider.

Antiviral therapy should be initiated at the earliest sign or symptom of shingles and is most effective when started within 72 hours of the onset of zoster rash. Pain can be treated with topical medications (*Lidoderm* patch, lidocaine gel), neuropathic pain medications (e.g., pregabalin, gabapentin, duloxetine, tricyclic antidepressants), NSAIDs or opioids. Most patients recover without long-term effects, but some will have chronic pain [called postherpetic neuralgia (PHN)], which can be debilitating. Older patients are more likely to experience PHN, non-pain complications, hospitalizations and interference with activities of daily living. The treatment of PHN is similar to the treatment of acute shingles pain.

The Advisory Committee on Immunization Practices (ACIP) recommends the shingles vaccines (*Shingrix*) in immunocompetent adults ≥ 50 years and adults ≥ 19 years who are or will be immunosuppressed. Patients previously vaccinated with *Zostavax* (no longer marketed) should be re-vaccinated with *Shingrix*. Patients who have had a previous shingles outbreak should be vaccinated to decrease the likelihood of recurrence and severity of PHN. See the Immunizations chapter.

Herpes Zoster (Shingles) Treatment

DRUG	DOSING	DESCRIPTION
Acyclovir (*Zovirax*)	800 mg PO 5x daily for <u>7 days</u> (or 10 days)	
Valacyclovir (*Valtrex*)	1 gram PO TID for <u>7 days</u>	
Famciclovir	500 mg PO TID for <u>7 days</u>	*Toey Toey/Shutterstock.com* <u>A cluster of fluid-filled blisters, often in a band</u> around one side of the waist, on one side of the forehead, around an eye or on the neck (less common on other areas of the body)

Cytomegalovirus

Cytomegalovirus (CMV) is a double-stranded DNA virus within the herpes family (HHV-5). CMV infection occurs in severely <u>immunocompromised</u> states (e.g., AIDS, transplant recipients) and most commonly causes <u>retinitis, colitis or esophagitis</u>. <u>Ganciclovir and valganciclovir</u> are the <u>treatments of choice for CMV</u> infection. <u>Foscarnet and cidofovir</u> should be <u>reserved</u> for <u>refractory cases</u>, as an alternative when treatment-limiting toxicities occur with ganciclovir and/or when the CMV strain is resistant to (val)ganciclovir. Maribavir *(Livtencity)* is an option for post-transplant CMV disease refractory to all other treatments.

Secondary prophylaxis (also called maintenance therapy) is necessary for some patients. <u>Letermovir *(Prevymis)*</u> is indicated for <u>CMV prophylaxis</u> in patients receiving a kidney transplant (if donor is CMV-positive/recipient CMV-negative) or bone marrow transplant (if recipient CMV-positive). Ganciclovir and <u>valganciclovir</u> are used for prophylaxis of CMV infection in solid organ transplant recipients at high risk (donor is CMV-positive/recipient is CMV-negative).

DRUG	DOSING	SAFETY/SIDE EFFECTS/MONITORING
Ganciclovir Injection *Zirgan* (ophthalmic gel)	Treatment: 5 mg/kg IV BID x 14-21 days Maintenance/prophylaxis: 5 mg/kg IV daily ↓ dose and extend interval when CrCl < 70 mL/min Injection: reconstitute with sterile water, <u>not</u> bacteriostatic water	**BOXED WARNINGS** <u>Myelosuppression</u>, carcinogenic, fetal toxicity, impaired fertility **SIDE EFFECTS** Fever, N/V/D, anorexia, ↑ SCr, seizures (rare), retinal detachment (in patients with CMV retinitis) **MONITORING** CBC with differential, SCr, retinal exam
Valganciclovir (*Valcyte*) Tablet, oral solution <u>Prodrug of ganciclovir</u> (with better bioavailability)	Treatment: 900 mg PO BID x 21 days Maintenance/prophylaxis: 900 mg PO daily ↓ dose and extend interval when CrCl < 60 mL/min	**NOTES** Females should use contraception during treatment and for 30 days after, males should use a barrier contraceptive for 90 days after Hazardous agent: special handling required Valganciclovir reconstituted <u>oral solution: refrigerate</u>; discard after 49 days
Cidofovir Injection CMV retinitis in HIV patients only	5 mg/kg/week IV x 2 weeks, then 5 mg/kg once every 2 weeks Renal impairment: ↓ dose or discontinue based on level of SCr increase (see Contraindications)	**BOXED WARNINGS** Nephrotoxicity, neutropenia, carcinogenic and teratogenic **CONTRAINDICATIONS** SCr > 1.5 mg/dL, CrCl ≤ 55 mL/min, urine protein ≥ 100 mg/dL (≥ 2+ proteinuria), sulfa allergy, use with or within 7 days of other nephrotoxic drugs, direct intraocular injection **SIDE EFFECTS** Myelosuppression (less than ganciclovir), metabolic acidosis **NOTES** Patient should receive hydration before each dose and probenecid before and after each dose to decrease nephrotoxicity Hazardous agent: special handling required

DRUG	DOSING	SAFETY/SIDE EFFECTS/MONITORING
Foscarnet (*Foscavir*) Injection CMV retinitis, resistant HSV	Induction: 90 mg/kg IV Q12H or 60 mg/kg Q8H x 2-3 weeks Maintenance: 90-120 mg/kg IV daily Renal impairment: ↓ dose and extend interval	**BOXED WARNINGS** Renal impairment (prehydration recommended); seizures due to electrolyte imbalances (can lead to status epilepticus or death) **SIDE EFFECTS** Electrolyte abnormalities (↓ K, ↓ Ca, ↓ Mg, ↓ Phos), ↑ BUN/SCr, QT prolongation **NOTES** Do not exceed maximum infusion rate (increases toxicity)
Letermovir (*Prevymis*) Tablet, injection CMV prophylaxis (select kidney and bone marrow transplant recipients)	480 mg PO/IV once daily Continue through day 100 post bone marrow transplantation Continue through day 200 post kidney transplantation Not recommended if severe hepatic impairment (Child-Pugh class C)	**CONTRAINDICATIONS** Concomitant administration with pimozide or ergot alkaloids, or pitavastatin and simvastatin (if also taking cyclosporine) **SIDE EFFECTS** Atrial fibrillation, tachycardia, peripheral edema, thrombocytopenia, N/V/D, fatigue, headache, cough **NOTES** IV vehicle (hydroxypropyl betadex) can accumulate if CrCl < 50 mL/min

Epstein-Barr Virus

Epstein-Barr virus (EBV) is a member of the herpes virus family. Infectious EBV is called mononucleosis or "mono." Most people get infected with EBV at some point in their lives; it is transmitted through bodily fluids, primarily saliva, and can spread by kissing, sharing drinks or food, or by contact with an object that has been in the mouth of an infected person (e.g., child's toys). Common symptoms include fatigue, fever, sore throat and swollen lymph nodes. Symptoms usually resolve in 2 – 4 weeks. No drug treatment or vaccine exists for mononucleosis.

Amoxicillin or ampicillin treatment in a child with EBV can cause a non-pruritic (i.e., non-itchy) rash that appears similar to an allergic reaction; it is not and should not be included as an "allergy" in the medical record.

ANTIVIRAL KEY COUNSELING POINTS

See the Drug Formulations and Patient Counseling chapter for counseling language/layman's terminology.

Oseltamivir
- Treatment should begin within two days of onset of influenza symptoms.
- Can cause delirium.

Acyclovir and Valacyclovir
- This medication does not cure herpes infections (cold sores, chickenpox, shingles or genital herpes). Use safe sex practices to lower transmission risk.
- Start treatment within 24 hours of the onset of symptoms.
- Acyclovir:
  - Drink plenty of fluids.
  - The topical cream can cause temporary burning or stinging.

Select Guidelines/References

Patterson TF, Thompson GR 3rd, Denning DW, et al. Practice Guidelines for the Diagnosis and Management of Aspergillosis: 2016 Update by IDSA. *Clin Infect Dis*. 2016;63:e1-e60.

Pappas PG, Kauffman CA, Andes DR, et al. Clinical Practice Guideline for Management of Candidiasis: 2016 Update by IDSA. *Clin Infect Dis*. 2016;62:409-17.

Uyeki TM, Bernstein HH, Bradley JS, et al. Clinical Practice Guidelines by the Infectious Diseases Society of America: 2018 Update on Diagnosis, Treatment, Chemoprophylaxis, and Institutional Outbreak Management of Seasonal Influenza. *Clin Infect Dis*. 2018;48:1003-1032.

COVID-19 Treatment Guidelines Panel. Coronavirus Disease 2019 (COVID-19) Treatment Guidelines. National Institutes of Health. Available at https://www.covid19treatmentguidelines.nih.gov/ (accessed 2023 Dec 20).

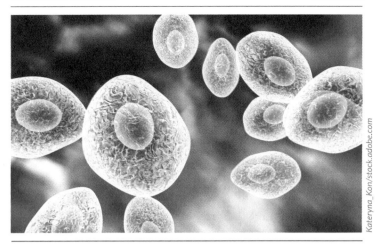

CHAPTER 25

INFECTIOUS DISEASES IV: OPPORTUNISTIC INFECTIONS

BACKGROUND

Immunocompromised patients are predisposed to opportunistic infections (OIs), which occur when the immune system is weak and unable to respond normally to invading bacteria, fungi, viruses and protozoa. The risk can be related to a disease or drug treatment that suppresses the immune system. Immunocompromised states include:

- Diseases that destroy key components of the immune response, primarily HIV with a CD4 T lymphocyte count < 200 cells/mm³ (which is a defining criteria for AIDS).

- Use of systemic steroids for 14 days or longer at a prednisone equivalent dose of ≥ 20 mg/day or ≥ 2 mg/kg/day.

- Asplenia (lack of a functioning spleen), due to sickle cell disease or splenectomy.

- Use of immunosuppressants for autoimmune conditions or post-transplant (e.g., TNF-alpha inhibitors).

- Use of cancer chemotherapy agents that destroy white blood cells, particularly if severe neutropenia (ANC < 500 cells/mm³) is present.

PRIMARY PROPHYLAXIS

Many OIs can be prevented with antimicrobials (e.g., antibiotics, antivirals); this is referred to as chemoprophylaxis, or simply prophylaxis. This is a key component of the management of patients with HIV, and the criteria for starting and stopping primary prophylaxis for the most common OIs is discussed in detail on the next page. Note that while *Candida* infections in the mouth/esophagus (e.g., thrush) are more likely in immunocompromised states, prophylaxis is not usually recommended.

Another important patient population at risk of infections (including OIs) are transplant recipients (including those receiving solid organ and bone marrow transplants). These patients have a greater risk of contracting infections in general; therefore, it is essential that they receive recommended vaccines before initiating immunosuppressive therapy (see the Immunizations and Transplant chapters). In addition, they have a high risk of:

- Viral infections, especially cytomegalovirus (CMV). CMV prophylaxis with letermovir (for kidney and bone marrow transplant recipients) or valganciclovir (for any solid organ transplant recipient) is common.

- *Pneumocystis jirovecii* pneumonia (PJP or PCP), which can be prevented with similar prophylaxis options as those used for patients with HIV (see table below).

PRIMARY PROPHYLAXIS REGIMENS IN HIV

The table below outlines select OIs, the CD4 count at which a patient with HIV becomes at risk for the infection, the primary prophylaxis regimens that can be used to prevent the infection and the criteria for discontinuing prophylactic therapy.

As with most infections, selection of an alternate (i.e., second-line) regimen is based on patient-specific factors (e.g., allergies, G6PD deficiency). For example, atovaquone, dapsone and pentamidine are options for PCP in the setting of a sulfa allergy, and atovaquone and pentamidine are options in the setting of a G6PD deficiency. Leucovorin is added to all pyrimethamine-containing regimens as rescue therapy to reduce the risk of pyrimethamine-induced myelosuppression.

OPPORTUNISTIC INFECTION	CRITERIA FOR STARTING	PRIMARY PROPHYLAXIS REGIMEN	CRITERIA FOR DISCONTINUING
Pneumocystis jirovecii pneumonia (PJP or PCP)	CD4 count < 200 cells/mm³ or AIDS-defining illness (see the Human Immunodeficiency Virus chapter)	**PREFERRED** SMX/TMP DS or SS daily **ALTERNATIVES** SMX/TMP DS 3x/week or Dapsone or Dapsone + pyrimethamine + leucovorin or Atovaquone or Atovaquone + pyrimethamine + leucovorin Inhaled pentamidine	CD4 count > 200 cells/mm³ for > 3 months and remains on ART
Toxoplasma gondii encephalitis	Toxoplasma IgG positive and CD4 count < 100 cells/mm³	**PREFERRED** SMX/TMP DS daily **ALTERNATIVES** SMX/TMP DS 3x/week or SS daily or Dapsone + pyrimethamine + leucovorin or Atovaquone or Atovaquone + pyrimethamine + leucovorin	CD4 count > 200 cells/mm³ for > 3 months and remains on ART
Mycobacterium avium complex (MAC)	Not recommended if ART is started immediately Initiate if not taking ART, CD4 count < 50 cells/mm³ and no active MAC infection	**PREFERRED** Azithromycin 1,200 mg weekly **ALTERNATIVES** Azithromycin 600 mg twice weekly or Clarithromycin 500 mg BID	Taking fully suppressive ART

ART = antiretroviral therapy

TREATMENT OF OPPORTUNISTIC INFECTIONS

The following table lists select OIs and the recommended medications for treatment, which is the same regardless of the cause of immunosuppression. After completing initial treatment, secondary prophylaxis is given to prevent recurrence of the infection in patients who continue to be at risk.

When treating thrush in patients with HIV, even with mild disease, systemic treatment is preferred (rather than localized treatment with agents such as clotrimazole, miconazole or nystatin).

OPPORTUNISTIC INFECTION	PREFERRED REGIMEN	ALTERNATIVE REGIMEN	SECONDARY PROPHYLAXIS
Candidiasis (oropharyngeal/ esophageal) Known as "thrush" Appears as a white film in the mouth/throat	Fluconazole	Oropharyngeal: itraconazole, posaconazole, topicals (e.g., clotrimazole troche, nystatin) Esophageal: voriconazole, isavuconazonium or an echinocandin (e.g., caspofungin)	Not usually recommended
Cryptococcal meningitis	Amphotericin B (liposomal preferred) + flucytosine	Fluconazole + flucytosine or Amphotericin B + fluconazole	Fluconazole (low dose)
Cytomegalovirus (CMV)	Valganciclovir or Ganciclovir	If toxicities to ganciclovir or resistant strains: foscarnet or cidofovir	None; for HIV, continue ART and maintain CD4 count > 100 cells/mm^3
Mycobacterium avium complex (MAC)	(Clarithromycin or azithromycin) + ethambutol	Add a 3rd or 4th agent using rifabutin, amikacin, streptomycin, moxifloxacin or levofloxacin	Same as treatment regimen
Pneumocystis jirovecii pneumonia (PJP or PCP)	SMX/TMP (high-dose, see the Infectious Diseases I chapter) ± prednisone or methylprednisolone Duration: 21 days	Pentamidine IV or Clindamycin + primaquine	Same as primary prophylaxis
Toxoplasmosis gondii encephalitis Risks: exposure to the parasite via ingestion of undercooked/raw meat or raw shellfish, or contact with cat feces/litter	Pyrimethamine + leucovorin + sulfadiazine	Clindamycin + pyrimethamine + leucovorin or SMX/TMP	Same as treatment (but with reduced doses)

Select Guidelines/References

Panel on Opportunistic Infections in HIV-Infected Adults and Adolescents. Guidelines for the Prevention and Treatment of Opportunistic Infections in HIV-Infected Adults and Adolescents: Recommendations from the Centers for Disease Control and Prevention, the National Institutes of Health, and the HIV Medicine Association of the Infectious Diseases Society of America. Available at https://clinicalinfo.hiv.gov/en/guidelines/hiv-clinical-guidelines-adult-and-adolescent-opportunistic-infections (accessed 2023 Nov 20).

National Comprehensive Cancer Network (NCCN) Clinical Practice Guidelines in Oncology. Prevention and Treatment of Cancer-Related Infections. Version 1.2023. Available at http://www.nccn.org/professionals/physician_gls/pdf/infections.pdf.

CONTENT LEGEND

💡 = Study
Tip Gal

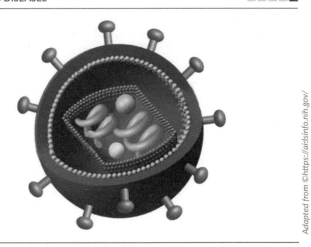

Adapted from ©https://aidsinfo.nih.gov/

CHAPTER 26

HUMAN IMMUNODEFICIENCY VIRUS

BACKGROUND

There are ~1.2 million people infected with human immunodeficiency virus (HIV) in the U.S., and ~13% of those are unaware that they are infected. Annually, ~35,000 people are newly diagnosed with HIV. If left untreated, HIV can progress to an advanced and severe stage of infection called acquired immunodeficiency syndrome (AIDS).

HIV CAUSES T-CELL DEATH

HIV is a single-stranded <u>RNA retrovirus</u> that uses the machinery in host <u>CD4 T-helper cells</u> (T cells) to replicate. Once replicated, the viral copies burst through the CD4 cell membrane, destroying the cell in the process. Billions of T cells are destroyed every day if HIV is not treated adequately with <u>antiretroviral therapy (ART)</u>.

- When HIV continues to replicate, the <u>viral load increases</u> and the <u>CD4 count decreases</u>.

- When the <u>CD4 count</u> falls <u>below 200 cells/mm³</u>, the immune system can no longer ward off <u>opportunistic infections (OIs)</u> (i.e., infections caused by normal environmental exposures that would not otherwise occur in a host with an intact immune system) and <u>specific malignancies</u> (e.g., Kaposi's sarcoma) related to AIDS.

TRANSMISSION

HIV infection is spread by direct contact between <u>infected body fluids</u> (blood, semen, vaginal or rectal secretions, or breast milk) and <u>mucus membranes</u> or <u>open wounds</u>. Most infections are caused by <u>unprotected (e.g., condomless) vaginal or rectal sex</u>, or <u>sharing injection</u> drug equipment, including needles. Infection can spread from a woman with HIV to her child during <u>pregnancy, childbirth</u> or <u>breastfeeding</u>. This is called <u>mother-to-child</u> or <u>vertical</u> transmission.

SCREENING AND DIAGNOSIS

SCREENING RECOMMENDATIONS

The CDC recommends routine HIV screening at least once for all patients who are 13 – 64 years old. Annual testing is recommended for patients with a history of other sexually transmitted infections (e.g., syphilis, gonorrhea), hepatitis or tuberculosis and for those that engage in the following high-risk activities:

- Sex with multiple partners and/or with someone whose sexual history is unknown
- Men who have sex with men
- Anal or vaginal sex with someone infected with HIV
- Sharing drug injection equipment (e.g., needles, syringes)

ACUTE HIV INFECTION

Acute HIV infection presents with non-specific flu-like symptoms that can last a few days to several weeks, including fever, myalgia, headache, lymphadenopathy (i.e., swollen lymph glands), pharyngitis and rash. An antibody response takes time to develop (weeks to months) and in most cases, is not fully able to fend off the virus. Patients become asymptomatic after this initial phase, but the virus continues to replicate and is capable of being transmitted.

PROGRESSION TO AIDS

AIDS is diagnosed when the CD4 count is < 200 cells/mm^3 or an AIDS-defining condition is present, which includes:

- Opportunistic infections (OIs) [e.g., *Mycobacterium avium* complex (MAC), *Pneumocystis jirovecii* pneumonia (PJP or PCP), *Cryptococcus neoformans, Histoplasmosis*, severe *Candida albicans* infections, including esophageal and bronchial thrush]. The prophylaxis and treatment of OIs is discussed in the Infectious Diseases IV: Opportunistic Infections chapter.
- Several cancers, including Kaposi's sarcoma.
- HIV wasting syndrome, a debilitating condition with loss of fat tissue (lipoatrophy), muscle mass and appetite (anorexia), and diarrhea. Treatment options to stimulate appetite include the cannabis-related drug dronabinol *(Marinol, Syndros)* and megestrol (a progestin).

DIAGNOSTIC TESTING

Diagnostic testing includes an initial screening for HIV antibodies and/or antigens, followed by a confirmatory test that distinguishes HIV-1 from HIV-2. If needed, a nucleic acid test detecting HIV RNA (i.e., viral load) may also be used (see algorithm on the next page). Antibodies can be detected in most people approximately 4 – 12 weeks after infection, but it can take up to 6 months in some cases and repeat testing may be needed.

DIAGNOSTIC TESTING ALGORITHM

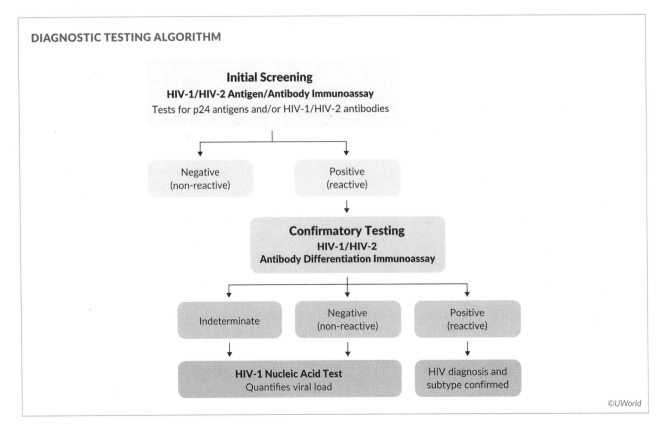

Initial Screening
HIV-1/HIV-2 Antigen/Antibody Immunoassay
Tests for p24 antigens and/or HIV-1/HIV-2 antibodies

Negative (non-reactive)

Positive (reactive)

Confirmatory Testing
HIV-1/HIV-2
Antibody Differentiation Immunoassay

Indeterminate

Negative (non-reactive)

Positive (reactive)

HIV-1 Nucleic Acid Test
Quantifies viral load

HIV diagnosis and subtype confirmed

©UWorld

Over-the-Counter HIV Testing

The _OraQuick In-Home HIV Test_ detects the presence of HIV antibodies and provides immediate results (other OTC test kits require that a sample be sent to a lab). Individuals with a positive _OraQuick_ result must follow up with a confirmatory laboratory test (see Diagnostic Testing Algorithm above).

To use the _OraQuick_ test, the upper and lower gums are swabbed with a test stick, which is then inserted into a test tube containing liquid. After 20 minutes, the result can be read (see image for interpretation). Testing sooner than 3 months after an exposure can lead to a false negative, due to the lag in antibody production.

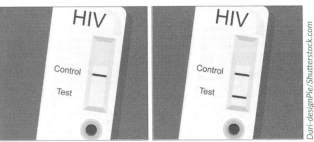

Dari-designPie/Shutterstock.com

1 line = negative result. The 1st line is the control line, which should always be present (indicates the test is valid).

2 lines = positive result. _OraQuick_ is like many other test kits (e.g., pregnancy): 2 lines indicates a positive result.

HIV REPLICATION STAGES AND ANTIRETROVIRAL SITES OF ACTION

It is <u>important to understand the stages</u> involved in <u>HIV viral replication</u> and know where <u>each drug class works</u>.

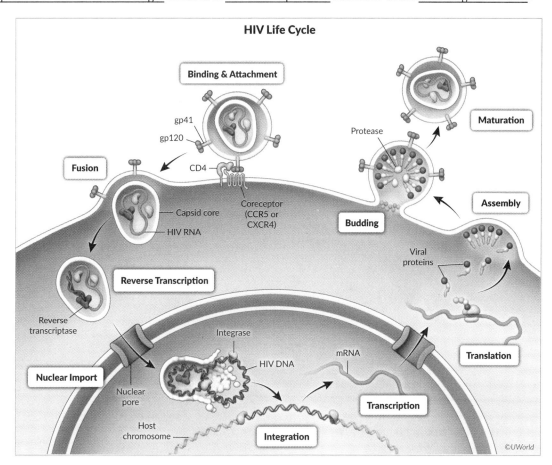

STAGE	DRUGS/DRUG CLASSES*
1. Binding and Attachment HIV attaches to a CD4 receptor and a co-receptor (CCR5 and/or CXCR4) on the surface of the host CD4 T cell.	CCR5 antagonist: maraviroc Attachment inhibitor: fostemsavir Post-attachment inhibitor: ibalizumab-uiyk
2. Fusion The HIV viral envelope fuses with the cell membrane. HIV enters the cell and releases its inner capsid, containing HIV RNA and viral enzymes.	Fusion inhibitor: enfuvirtide
3. Reverse Transcription HIV RNA is converted to HIV DNA by reverse transcriptase (an HIV enzyme).	NRTIs (e.g., emtricitabine) NNRTIs (e.g., rilpivirine)
4. Nuclear Import The HIV capsid is transported into the cell nucleus through a nuclear pore.	Capsid inhibitor: lenacapavir
5. Integration Inside the cell nucleus, integrase (an HIV enzyme) inserts HIV DNA into the host cell DNA.	INSTIs (e.g., bictegravir, dolutegravir)
6. Transcription and Translation Host cell machinery is used to transcribe and translate HIV DNA into HIV RNA and long-chain proteins (HIV building blocks).	None
7. Assembly New HIV RNA, proteins and enzymes (including protease) assemble at the cell surface.	Capsid inhibitor: lenacapavir
8. Budding and Maturation An immature virus pinches off the cell. Protease (an HIV enzyme) breaks up the long viral protein chains, forming the viral capsid and a mature virus that can infect other cells.	PIs (e.g., darunavir) Capsid inhibitor: lenacapavir

*See Drug Tables later in the chapter for more detail on mechanisms of action for each drug/drug class.
INSTI = integrase strand transfer inhibitor; NNRTI = non-nucleoside reverse transcriptase inhibitor; NRTI = nucleoside reverse transcriptase inhibitor; PI = protease inhibitor

ANTIRETROVIRAL THERAPY

The ART regimens currently available allow people with HIV to live long and healthy lives if <u>adherent to treatment</u>. Adherence is also important to <u>prevent resistance to ART</u>, which can develop quickly in patients who miss pills and/or are not taking recommended regimens.

INITIAL EVALUATION AND MONITORING

The initial evaluation and follow-up monitoring of patients with HIV is extensive. Vaccinations can be indicated (or contraindicated) based on the CD4 count (see the <u>Immunizations</u> chapter). Routine lab tests are listed below.

- <u>CD4 count</u>: the major <u>indicator of immune function</u>; determines the <u>need for OI prophylaxis</u> (see the Infectious Diseases IV chapter). The CD4 count <u>increases with ART</u>.

- <u>HIV viral load</u>: indicates how much HIV RNA is in the blood. It is the most important <u>indicator</u> of <u>ART response</u>. The viral load should decrease after starting ART. A high viral load after starting ART can be due to medication <u>non-adherence</u> or <u>drug resistance</u>.

- HIV genotypic testing: detects viral mutations that confer resistance to ART; assists in selecting therapy in treatment-naïve and/or treatment-experienced patients.

- Comprehensive metabolic panel (includes SCr and LFTs), CBC with differential, random or fasting lipid panel, random or fasting blood glucose level and a urinalysis.

- <u>Hepatitis B and C</u> screening.

- <u>Pregnancy</u> test (patients of child-bearing potential).

- <u>HLA-B*5701 allele</u> (if considering using <u>abacavir</u>) or a <u>tropism assay</u> (if considering using <u>maraviroc</u>).

TREATMENT INITIATION AND GOALS

<u>ART</u> should be started <u>as soon as possible</u> in <u>all HIV-infected individuals</u>. ART <u>treatment goals</u> include achieving and maintaining an <u>undetectable viral load</u>, restoring and preserving <u>immune function</u>, <u>reducing</u> HIV-associated morbidity (e.g., <u>OIs</u>) and mortality and <u>preventing transmission</u>.

The <u>Study Tip Gal</u> below shows the guideline-recommended <u>initial INSTI-based regimens</u> for <u>most patients</u> with newly diagnosed HIV. The table on the following page lists other <u>complete ART regimens</u> that are effective and tolerable if a preferred initial regimen is not suitable for a patient.

PREFERRED INITIAL ART REGIMENS IN MOST TREATMENT-NAÏVE ADULTS

BRAND	GENERIC COMPONENTS	COMMENTS
One-Pill, Once Daily (i.e., Single Tablet Regimens)*		**Most preferred regimens contain 2 NRTIs and 1 INSTI**
Biktarvy	Bictegravir / Emtricitabine / Tenofovir alafenamide	- Emtricitabine/tenofovir disoproxil fumarate *(Truvada)* or emtricitabine/tenofovir alafenamide *(Descovy)* make up the NRTI backbone in most regimens.
Triumeq	Dolutegravir / Abacavir / Lamivudine	
Dovato	Dolutegravir / Lamivudine	- Lamivudine and emtricitabine are interchangeable but should not be used together (both are cytosine analogs and would be antagonistic if taken concomitantly).
Two-Pills, Once Daily*		
Tivicay +	Dolutegravir +	**Dovato (1 NRTI + 1 INSTI) is an exception to the above**
Truvada	Emtricitabine / Tenofovir disoproxil fumarate	- Do not use in treatment-naïve patients if HIV RNA > 500,000 copies/mL, there is hepatitis B virus (HBV) coinfection (or status is unknown) or HIV genotypic testing is not performed (or resistance to either drug component is identified).
Tivicay +	Dolutegravir +	
Descovy	Emtricitabine / Tenofovir alafenamide	

Triumeq contains abacavir – extra testing is required!
- Test for the HLA-B*5701 allele before using. A positive result indicates a higher risk for a severe hypersensitivity reaction (HSR) and any abacavir-containing product is contraindicated.

Fixed-dose combinations have less flexibility with renal dosing
- *Biktarvy, Triumeq, Dovato, Truvada, Descovy*: do not use if CrCl < 30 mL/min.
  - ❑ Except for *Biktarvy*, the individual components of these drugs can be given separately to allow for renal dose adjustments.

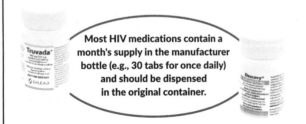

Most HIV medications contain a month's supply in the manufacturer bottle (e.g., 30 tabs for once daily) and should be dispensed in the original container.

Forance/Shutterstock.com

A "/" indicates that the generic components are available in the same pill.

ALTERNATIVE ART REGIMENS

There are multiple ways to "make" alternative ART regimens using single entity and/or combination products (see the Combination Antiretroviral Products tables later in the chapter). These regimens are less ideal because of lower barriers for resistance to develop (except PIs), lower patient tolerability, a higher potential for drug interactions and/or lower efficacy.

ALTERNATIVE ART REGIMENS

A complete HIV ART regimen has one "base" plus two NRTIs to serve as the "backbone." The "base" can be a PI, an NNRTI or an INSTI.

PI-based (boosted with cobicistat or ritonavir)
- Darunavir or atazanavir

NNRTI-based
- Efavirenz, rilpivirine or doravirine

INSTI-based
- Elvitegravir (only available in combination products)
- Raltegravir

NRTI backbone (2 drugs, 1 from each row)
- TDF or TAF or abacavir PLUS
- Emtricitabine or lamivudine

Complete regimen examples
- Rilpivirine + TDF + emtricitabine
- Raltegravir + TAF + emtricitabine

TDF = tenofovir disoproxil fumarate; TAF = tenofovir alafenamide

HIV TREATMENT DURING PREGNANCY

All pregnant patients with HIV should take ART during pregnancy for their own health and to prevent mother-to-child transmission. Most HIV medications are considered safe to use during pregnancy, without an increased risk of birth defects. Since breastfeeding can increase the risk of HIV transmission to the infant, replacement feeding with formula or banked pasteurized milk may be preferred.

Recommendations for Treatment-Naïve Pregnant Patients

In most cases, patients who are already taking an effective ART regimen should continue using the same regimen throughout their pregnancy. If not already taking ART, a regimen should be started as soon as possible.

Treatment should consist of three drugs: two NRTIs (e.g., abacavir/lamivudine, tenofovir alafenamide/emtricitabine) plus either an INSTI (dolutegravir preferred) or a boosted PI (darunavir preferred).

Perinatal Transmission Prophylaxis

Near the time of delivery, if a pregnant patient is newly diagnosed with HIV, the viral load is greater than 1,000 copies/mL or if the HIV status is unknown, IV zidovudine is administered to the mother and the newborn to prevent perinatal HIV transmission.

IMMUNE RECONSTITUTION INFLAMMATORY SYNDROME

Immune reconstitution inflammatory syndrome (IRIS) is a paradoxical (unexpected) worsening of a known underlying condition, or a previously unidentified condition, after ART is started or treatment is changed to a more effective regimen. As the immune system begins to recover, it becomes capable of mounting an inflammatory response, and symptoms of the underlying condition can become unmasked.

Key points about IRIS:

- It is more likely to occur when the CD4 count is low and begins to recover.
- Underlying conditions that can appear or worsen include common OIs, hepatitis B and C, herpes simplex virus (HSV), varicella zoster virus (VZV, shingles), autoimmune conditions and some cancers (e.g., Kaposi's sarcoma). In some cases, a known underlying condition will be treated for a short time prior to starting ART to help prevent IRIS.
- IRIS symptoms can range from mild (most common) to severe and are typically self-limiting. ART should be continued, and the unmasked condition should be treated.

DRUGS USED IN ART REGIMENS

DRUGS IN CLASS	MECHANISM OF ACTION	ADMINISTRATION
Nucleoside/Nucleotide Reverse Transcriptase Inhibitors (NRTIs)*		
Abacavir *(Ziagen)* **Emtricitabine** *(Emtriva)* **Lamivudine** *(Epivir)* **Tenofovir disoproxil fumarate,** TDF *(Viread)* **Tenofovir alafenamide,** TAF Only in combination products for HIV; ***Vemlidy*** is a single-entity product for HBV **Zidovudine** *(Retrovir)*	Competitively <u>inhibit</u> the <u>reverse transcriptase</u> enzyme, preventing the conversion of HIV RNA to HIV DNA NRTIs have a low barrier to resistance (i.e., resistance develops easily) **NAME TIP...** Remember the NRTIs with **Z ♥ LATTE**	Tenofovir (both formulations): <u>once daily</u> Abacavir and lamivudine: <u>once daily</u> and twice daily regimens Zidovudine: twice daily All NRTIs, except abacavir: <u>adjust dose</u> in <u>renal</u> impairment TDF oral powder: mix with 2-4 oz of soft food (applesauce, yogurt) to avoid a bitter taste; contains lactose Zidovudine: administered <u>IV</u> during <u>labor and delivery</u> to prevent perinatal HIV transmission (i.e., to the newborn)

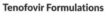

Many NRTI combination products are available; see the Combination Antiretroviral Products section later in the chapter.

NRTI KEY FEATURES AND SAFETY ISSUES

All NRTIs
- Warning: lactic acidosis and hepatomegaly with steatosis (fatty liver); boxed warning for zidovudine
- Common side effects: nausea, diarrhea

HBV and HIV Coinfection Boxed Warnings
- Severe acute HBV exacerbation can occur if emtricitabine, lamivudine or tenofovir-containing products are discontinued
- Do not use *Epivir-HBV* for the treatment of HIV (contains a lower dose of lamivudine than what is needed to treat HIV)

Abacavir
- Boxed warning: risk for hypersensitivity reaction (HSR)
  - ❏ Screen for HLA-B*5701 allele before starting; abacavir is contraindicated if positive (higher risk of HSR)
  - ❏ Patients must carry a medication card indicating that HSR (e.g., fever, rash, N/V/D, fatigue, dyspnea, cough) is an emergency
  - ❏ Never re-challenge patients with a history of HSR

Emtricitabine
- Hyperpigmentation of the palms of the hands or soles of the feet

Tenofovir Formulations
- Higher Risk with TDF vs. TAF
  - ❏ Renal impairment, including acute renal failure and Fanconi syndrome (renal tubular injury and electrolyte abnormalities)
  - ❏ Decreased bone mineral density: consider calcium/vitamin D supplementation and DEXA scan if at risk
- TAF is associated with lipid abnormalities
  - ❏ Monitor lipids if switching from TDF to TAF

Zidovudine
- Hematologic toxicity: neutropenia and anemia; macrocytosis (high MCV) is a sign of adherence

DRUGS IN CLASS	MECHANISM OF ACTION	ADMINISTRATION
Integrase Strand Transfer Inhibitors (INSTIs)		

Bictegravir Only in the combination drug ***Biktarvy*** **Cabotegravir** *(Vocabria, **Apretude**)* Also a component of ***Cabenuva*** **Dolutegravir** *(Tivicay)* Also a component of ***Triumeq, Dovato*** and *Juluca* **Elvitegravir** Only in the combination drugs ***Genvoya*** and ***Stribild*** **Raltegravir** *(Isentress, Isentress HD)*	Block the <u>integrase</u> enzyme, preventing HIV DNA from <u>inserting</u> into the host cell DNA Bictegravir and dolutegravir have a higher barrier to resistance than NRTIs, NNRTIs and other INSTIs ⸻ **NAME TIPS...** Generic names end in "-tegravir" Remember the INSTIs with **B CRED** ⸻	<u>Once daily</u>: *Biktarvy, Stribild, Genvoya, Isentress HD, Tivicay, Triumeq* and *Dovato (Tivicay* can be twice daily for treatment-experienced patients, those with INSTI resistance or those taking UGT1A1 or CYP3A4 inducers) <u>Twice daily</u>: *Isentress* CrCl < 70 mL/min: do not start *Stribild* CrCl < 50 mL/min: discontinue *Stribild* CrCl < 30 mL/min: do not start *Biktarvy* or *Genvoya* Cabotegravir PO *(Vocabria)*: indicated for optional lead-in treatment to assess tolerability prior to initiation of cabotegravir/rilpivirine *(Cabenuva)* injection, or as bridge therapy in patients who will miss a scheduled cabotegravir/rilpivirine injection for > 7 days Cabotegravir extended-release intramuscular injection *(Apretude)*: indicated only for <u>pre-exposure prophylaxis (PrEP)</u>; see HIV Prevention Strategies later in the chapter

---

INSTI KEY FEATURES AND SAFETY ISSUES

Side Effects and Warnings
- All INSTIs: weight gain, insomnia, rare risk of depression and suicidal ideation in patients with pre-existing psychiatric conditions

- Bictegravir, dolutegravir: ↑ SCr (by inhibiting tubular secretion) with no effect on GFR

- Raltegravir, dolutegravir:

   - ↑ CPK, myopathy and rhabdomyolysis

   - Hypersensitivity reaction (HSR): syndrome of rash, fever and symptoms of an allergic reaction

- Dolutegravir: hepatotoxicity (especially if coinfection with hepatitis B or C)

- Cabotegravir intramuscular: injection site reactions

Drug Interactions with Polyvalent Cations (↓ INSTI Absorption)
- In general, separate oral INSTIs from polyvalent cations (e.g., antacids, supplements) as taking them together can cause chelation, which can decrease efficacy*; exact timing (i.e., separation) may vary depending on the product

> **Cations and oral INSTIs**
> **do not go together!**
>
> Take INSTI **2 hours before** or
> **6 hours after** products containing
> Al, Ca, Mg or Fe
>
>

iStock.com/Ievgenii Volyk

Dolutegravir and bictegravir can be taken with calcium- or iron-containing supplements if also taken with food.

DRUGS IN CLASS	MECHANISM OF ACTION	ADMINISTRATION
Non-Nucleoside Reverse Transcriptase Inhibitors (NNRTIs)		

Efavirenz
 Component of *Symfi* and *Symfi Lo*

Rilpivirine *(Edurant)*
 Component of **Complera, Odefsey, Cabenuva** and *Juluca*

Doravirine *(Pifeltro)*
 Component of *Delstrigo*

Etravirine *(Intelence)*

Nevirapine

Non-competitively <u>inhibit</u> the <u>reverse transcriptase</u> enzyme, preventing the conversion of HIV RNA to HIV DNA

NNRTIs have a lower barrier to resistance than INSTIs or PIs

NAME TIPS...
Generic names contain "-vir-"

Remember the NNRTIs with **REDEN**

Rilpivirine
- Oral formulation
   - Take with a <u>meal</u> and water (do <u>not</u> substitute with a <u>protein</u> drink)
   - Requires an <u>acidic</u> environment for <u>absorption</u>; do <u>not use</u> with PPIs and <u>separate from H2RAs and antacids</u> (see <u>Study Tip Gal</u> below)
- Intramuscular formulation (part of the combination product *Cabenuva*)

Efavirenz
- Food increases the bioavailability and risk for CNS effects; take on an <u>empty stomach QHS</u> to ↓ (and sleep through) CNS effects

NNRTI KEY FEATURES AND SAFETY ISSUES

Used in alternative ART regimens (not first line in most patients): 1 NNRTI plus 2 NRTIs

All NNRTIs
- Hepatotoxicity and rash/severe rash, including SJS/TEN: highest risk with nevirapine

Efavirenz
- Psychiatric symptoms (depression, suicidal thoughts)
- CNS effects (impaired concentration, abnormal dreams, confusion), generally resolve in 2-4 weeks in most patients
- ↑ total cholesterol and triglycerides

Drug Interactions
- All NNRTIs are major CYP3A4 substrates (and some are substrates of other CYP enzymes)
   - Rilpivirine and doravirine: do not use with strong CYP3A4 inducers (phenytoin, rifampin, rifapentine, carbamazepine, oxcarbazepine, phenobarbital, St. John's wort)
- Efavirenz and etravirine are moderate CYP3A4 inducers (many drug interactions)
- Rilpivirine and acid suppressants (see image to the right)

Rilpivirine
- Depression
- ↑ SCr with no effect on GFR
- Do not use if initial viral load > 100,000 copies/mL and/or CD4 count < 200 cells/mm³ (higher failure rate)
- *Cabenuva* IM: injection site reacions

Rilpivirine needs an acidic gut for absorption.

 DO NOT USE WITH PPIs

 Separate H2RAs
Take H2RAs at least 12 hours before or 4 hours after rilpivirine

 Separate Antacids
Take antacids at least 2 hours before or 4 hours after rilpivirine*

Approximate; separation times vary between products.

DRUGS IN CLASS	MECHANISM OF ACTION	ADMINISTRATION

Protease Inhibitors (PIs)

Atazanavir (Reyataz)
  Component of *Evotaz*

Darunavir (Prezista)
  Component of **Symtuza** and *Prezcobix*

Fosamprenavir

Lopinavir / ritonavir* (*Kaletra*)

Tipranavir (*Aptivus*)

Inhibit the HIV protease enzyme, preventing long viral protein chains from being broken down into the smaller chains needed to produce mature (infectious) virus during the budding and maturation stage of the HIV life cycle

PIs (especially darunavir) have a high barrier to resistance

> **NAME TIP...**
> Generic names end in "-navir"

All PIs
- Recommended to take with a booster (ritonavir or cobicistat)
- No renal dose adjustments

Darunavir and atazanavir
- Take with food to ↓ GI upset

Atazanavir
- Needs an acidic gut for absorption (see Study Tip Gal below)

Ritonavir
- A protease inhibitor, but only used at low doses for pharmacokinetic boosting (see Boosters table on the next page)

*Co-formulated

PI KEY FEATURES AND SAFETY ISSUES

Used in alternative ART regimens (not first line in most patients): 1 PI (boosted with ritonavir or cobicistat) plus 2 NRTIs

All PIs
- Metabolic abnormalities: hyperglycemia/insulin resistance, dyslipidemia (↑ LDL, ↑ TGs), ↑ body fat and lipodystrophy
  - ❏ PIs ↑ CVD risk
- Hepatic dysfunction: ↑ LFTs, hepatitis, and/or exacerbation of preexisting hepatic disease
- Hypersensitivity reactions: rash (including SJS/TEN), angioedema, bronchospasm, anaphylaxis
- Common side effects: diarrhea, nausea
- All PIs are major CYP3A4 substrates and most are strong CYP inhibitors (see Drug Interactions Study Tip Gal on the next page)
  - ❏ Strong CYP3A4 inducers decrease PI concentrations

Darunavir, Fosamprenavir, Tipranavir
- Caution with sulfa allergy

Lopinavir/Ritonavir (Kaletra)
- Oral solution contains 42% alcohol: can cause a disulfiram reaction if taken with metronidazole

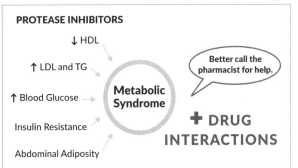

Atazanavir
- Hyperbilirubinemia (jaundice or scleral icterus, remember with "bananavir"): reversible, does not require discontinuation
- Requires acidic gut for absorption:
  - ❏ Separate from antacids and H2RAs
  - ❏ Avoid PPIs with unboosted atazanavir; take boosted atazanavir at least 12 hours after the PPI (dose should not exceed omeprazole 20 mg or equivalent)

DRUGS	ADMINISTRATION	KEY FEATURES
Pharmacokinetic Boosters (Enhancers)		
Ritonavir (Norvir) Oral powder and tablet Component of *Kaletra* and *Paxlovid* **Cobicistat (Tybost)** Component of **Genvoya**, **Stribild**, **Symtuza**, *Prezcobix* and *Evotaz*	**Ritonavir** 100 to 200 mg PO once or twice daily with the boosted drug (e.g., darunavir, atazanavir) and with food **Cobicistat** 150 mg PO daily with the boosted drug and with food ↑ SCr with no effect on GFR	■ Ritonavir and cobicistat are inhibitors of CYP3A4. They inhibit ART metabolism (e.g., PIs, elvitegravir), which increases (boosts) the ART level and therapeutic effect. ■ Ritonavir is a PI that is only used as a booster because it is not well tolerated at the higher doses needed for antiretroviral activity. Booster dosing is lower than treatment dosing (metabolic side effects less concerning). ■ Ritonavir and cobicistat are not interchangeable. Do not use both together. ■ Both have many drug interactions (see Study Tip Gal below).

PI AND PK BOOSTER DRUG INTERACTIONS

Knowing which ART combinations contain PIs and/or PK boosters can help to identify interactions with other CYP substrates, inhibitors and inducers.

Drug interactions for boosted PIs are likely greater than ritonavir or cobicistat alone, but a similar interaction is expected; it is always important to perform an interaction check.

Drugs that are contraindicated or should generally be avoided with boosted PIs due to a significant interaction*:

■ Alpha-1A blockers (alfuzosin, silodosin, tamsulosin)

■ Amiodarone, dronedarone

■ Anticoagulants/antiplatelets: apixaban, rivaroxaban, ticagrelor

■ Azole antifungals (voriconazole, posaconazole, itraconazole, isavuconazole)

■ Hepatitis C protease inhibitors (e.g., grazoprevir, glecaprevir)

■ Lovastatin and simvastatin

■ PDE-5 inhibitors used for pulmonary hypertension (sildenafil, tadalafil)

■ Strong CYP3A4 inducers (e.g., carbamazepine, phenytoin, rifampin, St. John's wort)

■ Systemic, inhaled and intranasal steroids (except beclomethasone)

*List not all inclusive, includes common drugs that could be tested.

DRUGS	MECHANISM OF ACTION	SAFETY ISSUES AND NOTES
Entry and Attachment Inhibitors		
CCR5 Antagonist Maraviroc (*Selzentry*) Tablet, solution	Blocks HIV from binding (and subsequently entering) the CD4 cell in virus strains that use the CCR5 co-receptor	**SAFETY ISSUES** Hepatotoxicity (boxed warning), hypersensitivity reactions (including SJS/TEN), orthostatic hypotension in patients with renal impairment Do not use if severe renal impairment (CrCl < 30 mL/min) and taking potent CYP3A4 inhibitors/inducers **BASELINE TEST REQUIRED** Must have tropism assay results before starting (determines if the HIV strain infecting the patient can only bind to the CCR5 co-receptor) If the HIV strain can bind to CXCR4 or mixed (CXCR4/CCR5) co-receptors, maraviroc will not work and HIV will still be able to enter the CD4 cell
Attachment Inhibitor Fostemsavir (*Rukobia*) Tablet	Converted to temsavir (active form), which binds to the gp120 subunit of HIV envelope proteins, inhibiting the interaction between the virus and the CD4 host cell	**SAFETY ISSUES** Do not use with strong CYP3A4 inducers Must maintain effective HBV treatment in patients coinfected with HBV Can ↑ SCr (higher risk if underlying renal disease) **NOTES** Indicated in combination with other ARTs in heavily treatment-experienced patients who are failing current therapy

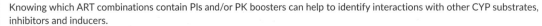

DRUGS	MECHANISM OF ACTION	SAFETY ISSUES AND NOTES
Entry and Attachment Inhibitors (Cont.)		
Post-Attachment Inhibitor Ibalizumab-uiyk (*Trogarzo*) IV injection administered by a healthcare professional	Monoclonal antibody that binds to a select domain of CD4 cell receptors, blocking entry of the virus into the cell	**SAFETY ISSUES** Infusion-related reactions (observe for 1 hour after the first infusion), diarrhea, dizziness, nausea, rash **NOTES** Indicated in combination with other ARTs in heavily treatment-experienced patients who are failing current therapy
Fusion Inhibitor Enfuvirtide (*Fuzeon*) Powder for injection (self-administered SC into the abdomen, the front of the thigh or the back of the arm)	Prevents HIV from fusing to the CD4 cell membrane, which prevents virus entry into the cell	**SAFETY ISSUES** Risk of bacterial pneumonia, hypersensitivity reactions Local injection site reactions (occur in nearly all patients): pain, erythema, nodules and cysts, ecchymosis, nausea, diarrhea and fatigue **NOTES** Reserved for use as salvage therapy in patients with extensive HIV resistance
Capsid Inhibitor		
Lenacapavir (*Sunlenca*) Tablet, SC injection Administered as an oral loading dose, followed by SC injection into the abdomen every 6 months	Inhibits multiple stages of the HIV life cycle, including capsid transport into the nucleus, virus assembly and capsid formation, resulting in a malformed capsid	**SAFETY ISSUES** Contraindicated with strong CYP3A4 inducers Local injection site reactions: erythema, induration, nodule, pain, swelling **NOTES** Indicated in combination with other ARTs in heavily treatment-experienced patients who are failing current therapy

COMBINATION ANTIRETROVIRAL PRODUCTS

Combination products lower the pill burden and improve adherence. The table below lists commonly used combination drugs and relevant notes. Additional notes on "first-line" (i.e., preferred initial) ART regimens are presented earlier in the chapter.

SINGLE TABLET REGIMENS

GENERIC NAME	BRAND	NOTES
Complete regimens (1 tablet once daily unless noted).		
INSTI-based		
Bictegravir / emtricitabine / tenofovir alafenamide	**Biktarvy**	*Biktarvy, Triumeq, Dovato:* first line.
Cabotegravir / rilpivirine	**Cabenuva**	*Cabenuva:* administered IM once monthly by a healthcare professional (may be preceded by lead-in treatment with oral cabotegravir to assess tolerability).
Dolutegravir / abacavir / lamivudine	**Triumeq**	*Cabenuva* and *Juluca:* only indicated to replace a stable ART regimen in patients with virologic suppression and no history of treatment failure or known resistance.
Dolutegravir / lamivudine	**Dovato**	
Dolutegravir / rilpivirine	Juluca	CrCl < 50 mL/min: do not start tenofovir disoproxil fumarate-containing products (< 70 mL/min for *Stribild*).
Elvitegravir / cobicistat / emtricitabine / tenofovir disoproxil fumarate	**Stribild**	CrCl < 30 mL/min: do not start tenofovir alafenamide-containing products.
Elvitegravir / cobicistat / emtricitabine / tenofovir alafenamide	**Genvoya**	*Stribild, Genvoya:* take with food (due to cobicistat component).

GENERIC NAME	BRAND	NOTES
NNRTI-based		
Doravirine / lamivudine / tenofovir disoproxil fumarate	*Delstrigo*	Same renal dosing criteria from previous page for tenofovir-containing products.
Efavirenz / emtricitabine / tenofovir disoproxil fumarate		Efavirenz-containing products: take on an empty stomach.
Efavirenz / lamivudine / tenofovir disoproxil fumarate	*Symfi, Symfi Lo*	Rilpivirine-containing products: take with food.
Rilpivirine / emtricitabine / tenofovir disoproxil fumarate	**Complera**	
Rilpivirine / emtricitabine / tenofovir alafenamide	**Odefsey**	
PI-based		
Darunavir / cobicistat / emtricitabine / tenofovir alafenamide	**Symtuza**	Take with food. Do not start if CrCl < 30 mL/min (contains tenofovir alafenamide).

OTHER COMBINATION PRODUCTS

GENERIC NAME	BRAND	NOTES

Must be used with additional ARTs to make a complete regimen.

GENERIC NAME	BRAND	NOTES
NRTI Combination Products (1 tablet daily unless noted)		
Abacavir / lamivudine	**Epzicom***	Epzicom: require baseline testing for HLA-B*5701 (contains abacavir).
Emtricitabine / tenofovir alafenamide	**Descovy**	Descovy, Truvada: part of first-line regimens. Do not use if CrCl < 30 mL/min [< 60 mL/min for Truvada if using for PrEP (see HIV Prevention Strategies section)].
Emtricitabine / tenofovir disoproxil fumarate	**Truvada**	
Lamivudine / zidovudine	Combivir	Combivir: twice daily.
Lamivudine / tenofovir disoproxil fumarate	Cimduo	Cimduo: do not use if CrCl < 50 mL/min.
PI Combination Products (1 tablet daily)		
Atazanavir / cobicistat	Evotaz	Take cobicistat-containing products with food.
Darunavir / cobicistat	Prezcobix	

*Brand discontinued but name still used in practice.

HIV PREVENTION STRATEGIES

TREATMENT AS PREVENTION

Treatment of HIV with current ART regimens is so effective that patients can achieve a viral load low enough to prevent infecting other people. When appropriate, PrEP and PEP are two other ways to reduce HIV infection risk before or after exposure (see the Study Tip Gal on the following page).

PRE-EXPOSURE PROPHYLAXIS (PrEP)

Pre-exposure prophylaxis (PrEP) is a strategy of prescribing ART to prevent HIV infection in patients who engage in high-risk activities.

PrEP Treatment Options
- An oral regimen of either *Truvada* or *Descovy*, taken daily, with no more than a 90-day supply provided at a time.
- A long-acting intramuscular injection of cabotegravir (*Apretude*) administered by a healthcare provider monthly for 2 doses, then every 2 months.

Before Starting PrEP
- Confirm that the patient is HIV-negative with an HIV antigen/antibody blood test (PrEP regimens are not appropriate to treat a person with HIV as resistance to commonly used treatments can develop).
- Ask about recent symptoms that could indicate HIV infection, due to the lag time in detectable antibody.
- Confirm CrCl ≥ 60 mL/min (if using *Truvada*) or ≥ 30 mL/min (if using *Descovy*). [Note: the CrCl cutoff for *Truvada* is higher for PrEP than when used for HIV treatment.]
- Screen for hepatitis B (if using oral PrEP) and sexually transmitted infections (STIs).

PrEP Follow-Up Visits

At each visit, <u>test for HIV</u> and <u>confirm a negative result</u> before refilling or administering PrEP treatment:

- *Truvada* and *Descovy*: <u>every 3 months</u>.
- Cabotegravir: 1 month after the first injection, then every 2 months.

Screening for STIs and monitoring of renal function and other drug adverse effects (e.g., lipid abnormalities with *Descovy*) is recommended during follow-up visits, but the suggested frequency varies between treatment strategies.

POST-EXPOSURE PROPHYLAXIS (PEP)

Post-exposure prophylaxis (<u>PEP</u>) is for <u>emergency</u> situations when a non-infected person is exposed to body fluids that are known to be or could be infected with HIV. The two types of PEP are: <u>nonoccupational (nPEP)</u> and <u>occupational (oPEP)</u>.

- <u>nPEP</u> can be used <u>after sex without a condom</u> (e.g., condom broke, unplanned sex, sexual assault), <u>injection drug use</u> or some other type of nonoccupational exposure.
- <u>oPEP</u> is typically used for healthcare personnel who are exposed to body fluids that could be infectious, such as from a <u>needlestick</u> injury (i.e., prick from a needle).
- For both types, treatment should be <u>started</u> as soon as possible <u>within 72 hours</u> (3 days) of the exposure and continued for <u>28 days</u>.
- The exposed individual should receive a baseline HIV antibody test and a follow-up test at 4 – 6 weeks, 3 months and 6 months after the exposure.

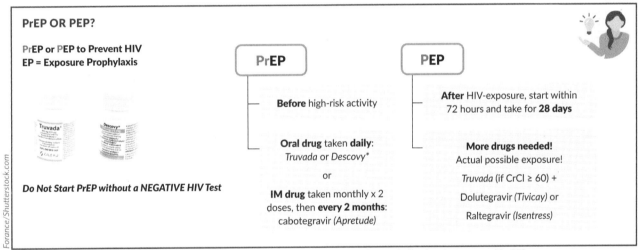

PrEP OR PEP?

PrEP or PEP to Prevent HIV
EP = Exposure Prophylaxis

Do Not Start PrEP without a NEGATIVE HIV Test

PrEP

Before high-risk activity

Oral drug taken **daily**:
Truvada or *Descovy**

or

IM drug taken monthly x 2 doses, then **every 2 months**: cabotegravir (*Apretude*)

PEP

After HIV-exposure, start within 72 hours and take for **28 days**

More drugs needed!
Actual possible exposure!

Truvada (if CrCl ≥ 60) +

Dolutegravir (*Tivicay*) or

Raltegravir (*Isentress*)

Forance/Shutterstock.com

*Descovy: not approved for PrEP in patients assigned female at birth (i.e., at risk of getting HIV from vaginal sex), and not approved for PEP.

KEY COUNSELING POINTS

See the Drug Formulations and Patient Counseling chapter for counseling language/layman's terminology.

All HIV Medications

- <u>Do not skip doses or stop taking HIV medications</u> unless instructed to do so by your healthcare provider (see strategies to improve adherence to the right); get refills before running out.

- <u>This medication is not a cure for HIV</u>. Do not share needles or other drug mixing equipment. Use safe sex practices.

- IRIS: do not stop taking ART; notify your healthcare provider of a new or worsening condition.

All NRTIs

- If you have hepatitis B, do not stop taking this medication without discussing with your healthcare provider, as a severe worsening of liver disease can occur.

- Can cause lactic acidosis.

Abacavir

- Before using this medication, your blood should be tested to see if you are at high risk for a severe reaction.

Emtricitabine

- This medication can cause darkened spots on the palms of the hands and on the soles of the feet.

Tenofovir Disoproxil Fumarate and Tenofovir Alafenamide

- Can cause (less with alafenamide):
  - ❑ Kidney impairment.
  - ❑ Low bone density/fracture risk.

All INSTIs

- This medication can interact with antacids. Take 2 hours before or 6 hours after this medication.

All NNRTIs

- Can cause:
  - ❑ Rash/severe rash.
  - ❑ Hepatotoxicity.

Efavirenz

- Take at bedtime on an empty stomach to reduce side effects.

- Can cause (at the start, improves in 2 – 4 weeks):
  - ❑ Depression/psychosis.
  - ❑ Confusion and abnormal dreams.

STRATEGIES TO IMPROVE ADHERENCE TO ANTIRETROVIRAL THERAPY

Multidisciplinary team approach (e.g., nurses, social workers, pharmacists, psychologists, physicians).

Accessible, non-judgmental healthcare team; establish a trusting relationship with the patient.

Evaluate the patient's knowledge of HIV disease, prevention and treatment, and provide information as needed; establish patient readiness to start ART and involve them in ART regimen selection.

Identify potential barriers to adherence (e.g., psychosocial or cognitive issues, substance abuse, low literacy, busy daily schedule, lack of prescription coverage and/or social support).

Assess adherence at every clinic visit, and simplify ART regimen when possible; provide positive reinforcement to foster adherence success.

Identify non-adherence and reasons for non-adherence (e.g., adverse effects from medications, complex regimen, difficulty swallowing large pills, forgetfulness, pill fatigue, food requirements, stigma, change or lapse of insurance coverage).

Provide resources (e.g., referrals for mental health and/or substance abuse treatment, prescription drug assistance programs, pillboxes, reminder tools, medication lists or calendars).

Rilpivirine

- Take with a full meal (not a protein drink) and water.

- Do not use proton pump inhibitors; take H2RAs 12 hours before or 4 hours after, and antacids 2 hours before or 4 hours after rilpivirine.

- Can cause depression.

All PIs

- Can cause high blood glucose, high triglycerides or body fat redistribution.

Atazanavir or Darunavir

- If taking ritonavir or cobicistat, make sure to take both at the same time.

- Take with food to decrease GI upset.

Atazanavir

- Do not take acid-suppressing medications with atazanavir.

- Can cause hyperbilirubinemia.

Darunavir, Fosamprenavir, Tipranavir

- Caution with sulfa allergy.

Select Guidelines/References

Guidelines for the Use of Antiretroviral Agents in Adults and Adolescents with HIV. Department of Health and Human Services. Available at: https://clinicalinfo.hiv.gov/en/guidelines/hiv-clinical-guidelines-adult-and-adolescent-arv/whats-new (accessed 2023 Nov 15).

Centers for Disease Control and Prevention: US Public Health Service: Preexposure Prophylaxis for the Prevention of HIV Infection in the United States – 2021 Update. Available at: https://www.cdc.gov/hiv/pdf/risk/prep/cdc-hiv-prep-guidelines-2021.pdf (accessed 2023 Nov 15).

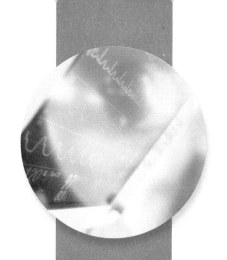
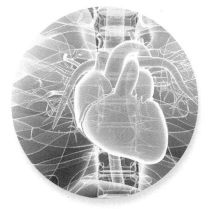
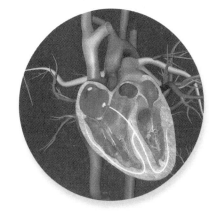

CARDIOVASCULAR CONDITIONS

CONTENTS

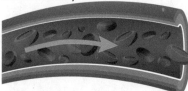

Normal Artery

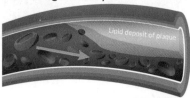

Narrowing of Artery

iStock.com/newannyart

CHAPTER 27
DYSLIPIDEMIA

BACKGROUND

Cholesterol is an important structural component of cell walls, a precursor in hormone synthesis and is used to produce bile acids.

Bile acids are needed to absorb lipids and fat-soluble vitamins. They are produced in the liver, then travel through the bile ducts (with free cholesterol and waste products) into the small intestine. They are then converted from bile acids to bile salts, which are returned back to the liver. This process of enterohepatic recycling can also affect drugs (see the Drug Interactions and Pharmacokinetics chapters for details).

Cholesterol is eliminated from the body either as free cholesterol or as bile acid.

ATHEROSCLEROSIS AND ASCVD

Although cholesterol is an essential substance in the body, elevated cholesterol increases the risk of atherosclerosis, which is the formation of plaque on the inner walls of the arteries from a buildup of fats, cholesterol and other substances.

Atherosclerosis is asymptomatic, but leads to atherosclerotic cardiovascular disease (ASCVD), which includes myocardial infarction, stroke/transient ischemic attack, stable angina and peripheral arterial disease (see image on following page).

Cholesterol in the body can be decreased by reducing the formation (as with statins), blocking the absorption (as with ezetimibe) or blocking enterohepatic recirculation of bile salts (as with bile acid sequestrants such as colesevelam).

CONTENT LEGEND

 = Study Tip Gal   = Key Drug Guy   = Required Formula

Atherosclerosis and ASCVD

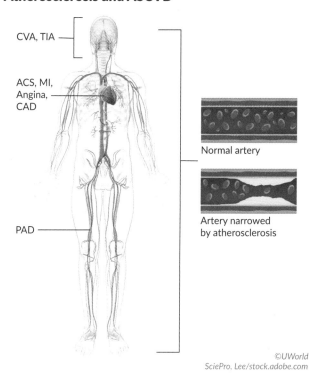

CVA, TIA

ACS, MI,
Angina,
CAD

PAD

Normal artery

Artery narrowed
by atherosclerosis

©UWorld
SciePro. Lee/stock.adobe.com

CHOLESTEROL (LIPOPROTEIN) TYPES AND NORMAL VALUES

Total cholesterol (TC) includes the three major types of lipoproteins: low-density lipoprotein (LDL), high-density lipoprotein (HDL) and very-low density lipoprotein (VLDL). These different types of cholesterol protect from or contribute to ASCVD risk.

- HDL ("good" cholesterol) takes cholesterol from the blood and delivers it to the liver for removal from the body. High HDL lowers ASCVD risk.

- Non-HDL includes the lipoproteins that contribute to ASCVD risk, such as LDL, VLDL and lipoprotein(a).

  ❑ Non-HDL is a strong predictor of ASCVD.

  ❑ Non-HDL calculation: non-HDL = TC – HDL

- High triglycerides (TGs), or hypertriglyceridemia, is associated with high ASCVD risk. TGs ≥ 500 mg/dL can cause acute pancreatitis.

Determining LDL Cholesterol

Lipid panels (i.e., TC, HDL, LDL, TG) are best taken after a 9 – 12 hour fast. Fasting is primarily needed for TG; they can be falsely elevated after eating. LDL is often reported with the panel. If LDL is not reported, it can be calculated using the Friedewald equation:

$$LDL = TC - HDL - \frac{TG}{5}$$

This formula is not used when the TGs are > 400 mg/dL; a falsely elevated TG level (i.e., the patient has not fasted) can result in a falsely low LDL calculation.

CASE SCENARIO

JS is a 47-year-old male with dyslipidemia and type 2 diabetes. He stopped taking his simvastatin about 5 months ago due to muscle aches. His cholesterol panel results are:
TC 202 mg/dL, HDL 36 mg/dL, TG 280 mg/dL.

Calculate the patient's LDL cholesterol:
Use the Friedewald equation: LDL = TC – HDL – (TG/5)

$$202 - 36 - \frac{280}{5} = 110 \text{ mg/dL}$$

CLASSIFICATION OF CHOLESTEROL AND TG LEVELS (MG/DL)	
NON-HDL	
< 130	Desirable
LDL	
< 100	Desirable
≥ 190	Very high
HDL	
≥ 40 (men)	Desirable
≥ 50 (women)	Desirable
Triglycerides	
< 150	Desirable
≥ 500	Very high*

HDL = high-density lipoprotein, LDL = low-density lipoprotein
*Severe hypertriglyceridemia is another term used for very high triglycerides.

CLASSIFICATION OF DYSLIPIDEMIA

Abnormal lipoprotein levels, called dyslipidemia, can be familial (genetic cause) or secondary (due to lifestyle and/or medical conditions).

FAMILIAL

Familial hypercholesterolemia (FH) is caused by genetic defects that result in severe cholesterol elevations. It includes heterozygous and homozygous familial hypercholesterolemia (HeFH and HoFH).

SECONDARY (OR ACQUIRED)

Dyslipidemia is most often caused by diet and a lack of physical activity. Medical conditions and select drugs can also cause or contribute to dyslipidemia (see Key Drugs Guy).

TREATMENT PRINCIPLES

Treatment of dyslipidemia is important, as lowering LDL by 1% reduces ASCVD risk by 1%. The American College of Cardiology and American Heart Association (ACC/AHA) provide guideline recommendations for cholesterol management. Recommendations for managing cholesterol in certain populations are also addressed in disease-specific guidelines (e.g., the ADA guidelines discuss cholesterol management in patients with diabetes).

CALCULATING ASCVD RISK

An online ASCVD risk calculator can be used to provide an estimate of an individual's risk of having a first cardiovascular event (e.g., MI, stroke) during the next 10 years. Healthcare providers use the estimated risk to determine whether they should prescribe risk-reducing treatments, including statins and antihypertensives. The clinician inputs the patient's:

- Sex, age (20 – 79 years), race and smoking status.
- TC, HDL and LDL, and whether a statin is used.
- Blood pressure, and whether antihypertensive treatment is used.
- Diabetes history and aspirin use.

KEY DRUGS

↑ LDL and TG
Diuretics
Efavirenz
Immunosuppressants (e.g., cyclosporine, tacrolimus)
Atypical antipsychotics
Protease inhibitors
↑ LDL Only
Fibrates
Fish oils (except *Vascepa*)
↑ TG Only
IV lipid emulsions
Propofol
Clevidipine
Bile acid sequestrants (~5%)
Conditions
Obesity, poor diet, alcohol use disorder, hypothyroidism, smoking, diabetes, renal/liver disease, nephrotic syndrome

SELECT DRUGS/CONDITIONS THAT CAN RAISE LDL AND/OR TRIGLYCERIDES

Others:
↑ LDL and TG
Retinoids
Systemic steroids
↑ LDL Only
Anabolic steroids
Progestins
SGLT2 inhibitors
↑ TG Only
Estrogen
Tamoxifen
Beta-blockers
Conditions
Pregnancy, polycystic ovarian syndrome, anorexia

Note that a risk score is not needed for patients with clinical ASCVD, diabetes or LDL ≥ 190 mg/dL, as all patients in these groups should be started on a statin.

If a risk-based treatment decision is still uncertain after a quantitative risk assessment, additional risk-enhancing factors should be considered. These factors include family history of premature ASCVD, metabolic syndrome, chronic kidney disease, history of preeclampsia or premature menopause, chronic inflammatory disorders, high CRP, high coronary artery calcium score (CAC) and abnormal ankle brachial index. The CAC measurement is helpful in deciding if statins should be initiated in those with a 10-year ASCVD risk of 7.5 – 19.9%. If the CAC score is ≥ 100 Agatston units, a statin is indicated.

NON-DRUG TREATMENT

Lifestyle modifications are an important part of management and include:

- Consuming a diet to maintain a healthy weight (BMI 18.5 – 24.9 kg/m^2). The diet should:

  ❏ Be rich in vegetables, fruits, whole grains and high-fiber foods, such as with plant-based and Mediterranean diets.

  ❏ Include healthy protein sources, such as low-fat dairy, poultry, fish and nuts.

  ❏ Limit intake of saturated fat, trans fat (partially hydrogenated), sweets, sugar-sweetened beverages and red meat.

  ❏ Be adjusted to appropriate calorie requirements.

- Engaging in aerobic physical activity 3 – 4 times per week, lasting 40 minutes/session (decreases LDL 3 – 6 mg/dL).

- Avoiding tobacco products and limiting alcohol use.

NATURAL PRODUCTS

Products that can be effective at lowering LDL include red yeast rice, which contains naturally occurring HMG-CoA reductase inhibitors in varying amounts, plant stanols, sterols and fibrous foods (found in psyllium, barley and oat bran).

OTC fish oils can be used to lower TG, but some products can increase LDL. Garlic is not considered effective for dyslipidemia.

DRUG TREATMENT

Statins are the drugs of choice for treating high LDL. If a patient needs additional LDL lowering or experiences statin-associated adverse effects, other cholesterol-lowering drugs may be used. Guidelines focus on adding ezetimibe and/or a proprotein convertase subtilisin/kexin type 9 monoclonal antibody (PCSK9 mAb) because of their effective LDL lowering and demonstrated cardiovascular benefits. The use of bempedoic acid and inclisiran is increasing due to growing evidence regarding their efficacy and beneficial outcomes.

LIVER DAMAGE

Many cholesterol-lowering drugs cause liver damage (niacin, fibrates, potentially statins and ezetimibe). These drugs should not be used if the AST or ALT is > 3 times the upper limit of normal, and LFTs should be monitored during treatment.

STATINS

Statins inhibit the enzyme 3-hydroxy-3-methylglutaryl coenzyme A (HMG-CoA) reductase, which prevents the conversion of HMG-CoA to mevalonate. This is the rate-limiting step in cholesterol synthesis.

Statins are grouped by intensity based on their LDL-lowering ability (see table on following page) and patients are categorized into statin benefit groups to determine the appropriate statin intensity at treatment initiation (see Study Tip Gal below). Amongst the available statins, only atorvastatin and rosuvastatin can provide high-intensity LDL lowering (i.e., ≥ 50% reduction from baseline).

DETERMINING STATIN TREATMENT INTENSITY BASED ON PATIENT RISK

STATIN BENEFIT GROUPS	PATIENT CRITERIA	STATIN TREATMENT
Secondary Prevention		
Clinical ASCVD	Includes CHD*, stroke/TIA or peripheral arterial disease thought to be of atherosclerotic origin	High-intensity**
Primary Prevention		
Primary severe dyslipidemia	Baseline LDL ≥ 190 mg/dL	High-intensity**
Diabetes and age 40-75 years	Multiple ASCVD risk factors	High-intensity**
	Regardless of 10-year ASCVD risk	Moderate-intensity
Age 40-75 years with LDL between 70-189 mg/dL	10-year ASCVD risk ≥ 20%	High-intensity**
	10-year ASCVD risk 7.5-19.9% + risk-enhancing factors	Moderate-intensity

*CHD = coronary heart disease, which includes a history of acute coronary syndrome (e.g., MI), stable angina, coronary or other arterial revascularization.
**Consider moderate-intensity statin if not a candidate for high-intensity or patient > 75 years with LDL 70-189 mg/dL.

Statin Treatment Intensity Definitions and Selection Options

	ATORVASTATIN	ROSUVASTATIN	SIMVASTATIN	PRAVASTATIN	LOVASTATIN	FLUVASTATIN	PITAVASTATIN
HIGH	40-80	20-40					
MODERATE	10-20	5-10	20-40	40-80	40	40 BID/80 XL	1-4
LOW			10	10-20	20	20-40	

High-intensity: ↓ LDL ≥ 50%; Moderate-intensity: ↓ LDL 30-49%; Low-intensity: ↓ LDL < 30%
Doses are in milligrams.

Statin Equivalent Doses

Equivalent doses (see Study Tip Gal) are used to change one statin to another. This might be needed in the case of drug escalation (to high-intensity dosing), drug interactions, intolerance or cost (see Case Scenario).

STATIN EQUIVALENT DOSES

Pitavastatin 2 mg

Rosuvastatin 5 mg

Atorvastatin 10 mg

Simvastatin 20 mg

Lovastatin 40 mg

Pravastatin 40 mg

Fluvastatin 80 mg

Remember: Pharmacists **R**ock **At S**aving **L**ives and **Pr**eventing **F**atty deposits

---

CASE SCENARIO

TM is a 57-year-old male with dyslipidemia. He is currently taking simvastatin 40 mg and his provider would like to switch to an equivalent atorvastatin dose.

Calculate the equivalent dose of atorvastatin:

$$\frac{Atorvastatin\ 10\ mg}{Simvastatin\ 20\ mg} = \frac{Atorvastatin\ X\ mg}{Simvastatin\ 40\ mg} \quad X = 20\ mg$$

A cholesterol panel is drawn before TM leaves the provider's office. The LDL is 195 mg/dL. The provider calls the pharmacy to change to a high-intensity regimen.

To change from moderate-intensity to high-intensity:
Increase the atorvastatin dose to 40 mg or 80 mg daily. Alternatively, change to rosuvastatin 20 mg or 40 mg daily.

Muscle Damage from Statins

Muscle damage is the most common adverse effect of statins. This generally presents as muscle soreness, tiredness or weakness that is symmetrical (on both sides of the body) in large muscle groups in the legs, back or arms. Symptoms usually occur within six weeks of starting treatment, but can develop at any time. These muscle effects can present with varying severity, such as:

- Myalgia: muscle soreness and tenderness
- Myopathy: muscle weakness ± CPK elevations
- Myositis: muscle inflammation
- Rhabdomyolysis: muscle symptoms with a very high CPK (> 10,000 IU/L) plus muscle protein in the urine (myoglobinuria), which can lead to acute renal failure

Coenzyme Q10 may provide benefit for mild muscle symptoms; however, the primary management includes holding the statin and rechallenging once symptoms resolve (see Study Tip Gal).

MANAGING MYALGIA

REDUCE THE RISK
Avoid drug interactions, including OTC products.

Do not use simvastatin 80 mg/day.

Do not use gemfibrozil + statin.

IF MYALGIA OCCURS
Hold statin, check CPK, investigate other possible causes.

After 2-4 weeks: re-challenge with the same statin at the same or a ↓ dose. Most patients will tolerate a re-challenge.

If myalgia returns, discontinue the statin. Once muscle symptoms resolve, use a low dose of a different statin; gradually ↑ dose.

If patient unable to tolerate a statin after at least two attempts, non-statin treatment may be considered.

Statins

DRUG	DOSING	SAFETY/SIDE EFFECTS/MONITORING
Atorvastatin (*Lipitor*, *Atorvaliq*) Tablet, suspension + amlodipine (*Caduet*)	10-80 mg daily	**CONTRAINDICATIONS** Breastfeeding, liver disease (including unexplained ↑ LFTs), concurrent use of strong CYP3A4 inhibitors (with simvastatin and lovastatin), concurrent use of cyclosporine (with pitavastatin) **WARNINGS** Muscle damage: myopathy/rhabdomyolysis with ↑ CPK ± acute renal failure; higher risk with higher doses (e.g., simvastatin 80 mg), advanced age, concurrent use of niacin, fibrates (e.g., gemfibrozil), hypothyroidism (uncontrolled), renal impairment
Fluvastatin (*Lescol XL*)	20-80 mg Immediate release: take daily in the evening *Lescol XL*: take daily	Do not use during pregnancy for most patients; can consider continuing statin for individuals at high risk for cardiovascular events Diabetes: ↑ A1C/fasting blood glucose; benefit of statin outweighs risk
Lovastatin (*Altoprev*)	20-80 mg Immediate release: take with the evening meal *Altoprev* (extended release): take at bedtime	Hepatotoxicity, with ↑ LFTs (rare) Rosuvastatin: proteinuria, hematuria – usually transient Atorvastatin: hemorrhagic stroke (if recent stroke or TIA); benefit of statin outweighs risk
Pitavastatin (*Livalo*, *Zypitamag*)	1-4 mg daily	**SIDE EFFECTS** Myalgia/myopathy **MONITORING** Lipid panel (TC, LDL, HDL, TG) at baseline, 4-12 weeks after starting or adjusting treatment, then every 3-12 months (usually annually)
Pravastatin (*Pravachol**)	10-80 mg daily	LFTs at baseline and if symptoms of hepatotoxicity (abdominal pain, jaundice) Myalgia/myopathy/rhabdomyolysis: check CPK if symptoms of muscle damage and SCr/BUN if decreased urine output
Rosuvastatin (*Crestor*, *Ezallor Sprinkle*)	5-40 mg daily May need to use lower doses in Asian patients – exposures are 2 times higher	**NOTES** Can take rosuvastatin, atorvastatin, pitavastatin, *Lescol XL* and pravastatin at any time of day *FloLipid* is taken on an empty stomach For CrCl < 30 mL/min, use lower starting doses of lovastatin, simvastatin and rosuvastatin
Simvastatin (*Zocor*, *FloLipid*) Tablet, suspension + ezetimibe (*Vytorin*)	10-40 mg daily in the evening Do not use 80 mg dose (↑ risk of myopathy)	For eGFR < 60 mL/min/1.73 m², use lower starting dose of pitavastatin **Lipid Effects** ↓ LDL ~20-55%, ↑ HDL ~5-15%, ↓ TG ~10-30%

Brand discontinued but name still used in practice.

Statin Drug Interactions

Drug interactions with statins <u>increase</u> the risk of <u>adverse effects</u> (e.g., muscle damage). Significant interactions are listed in the box to the right. Most interactions are CYP enzyme mediated, with <u>CYP3A4</u> being most common. Atorvastatin, lovastatin and simvastatin are CYP3A4 substrates. In general, <u>rosuvastatin</u> and <u>pravastatin</u> have <u>less drug interactions</u>.

Fibrates (especially gemfibrozil) and <u>niacin</u> can ↑ the risk of <u>myopathy</u> and rhabdomyolysis. Do not use statins with <u>gemfibrozil</u>.

Amlodipine can ↑ the concentration of atorvastatin, lovastatin and <u>simvastatin</u> (<u>max daily dose 20 mg/day</u>).

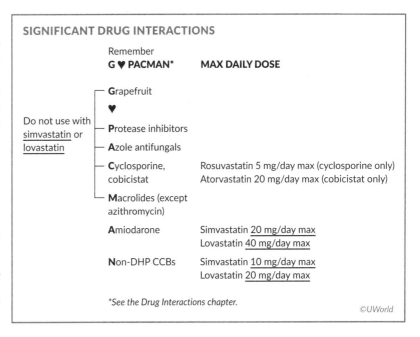

SIGNIFICANT DRUG INTERACTIONS

Remember
G ♥ PACMAN*   **MAX DAILY DOSE**

Do not use with simvastatin or lovastatin

- **G**rapefruit
- **♥**
- **P**rotease inhibitors
- **A**zole antifungals
- **C**yclosporine, cobicistat — Rosuvastatin 5 mg/day max (cyclosporine only) / Atorvastatin 20 mg/day max (cobicistat only)
- **M**acrolides (except azithromycin)

Amiodarone — Simvastatin 20 mg/day max / Lovastatin 40 mg/day max

Non-DHP CCBs — Simvastatin 10 mg/day max / Lovastatin 20 mg/day max

See the Drug Interactions chapter.

©UWorld

NON-STATIN TREATMENTS

Non-statin treatment may be warranted in patients who experience statin-associated adverse effects after multiple trials of a statin or when additional LDL-lowering is required (i.e., add-on treatment to a maximized dose of a statin).

Ezetimibe and/or PCSK9 mAbs are generally recommended as initial non-statin therapies in most clinical guidelines. Ezetimibe may be preferred, if LDL goals can be achieved (e.g., < 25% additional LDL lowering needed), because of cost and oral administration. PCSK9 mAbs are injectable and more expensive; the primary reason to choose a PCSK9 mAb over ezetimibe initially is if significant (e.g., > 25%) LDL lowering is needed.

Other treatment options include bempedoic acid (a cholesterol synthesis inhibitor) and inclisiran (an intracellular inhibitor of PCSK9 production). Of note, there is no benefit to using inclisiran and a PCSK9 mAb together because they have related mechanisms.

In select populations, fish oils and fibrates are used to target high triglycerides. Icosapent ethyl (a fish oil) is also recommended for ASCVD reduction in select patients. Bile acid sequestrants are rarely used, except when statins cannot be tolerated.

Determining Need for Add-On Treatment

PATIENT CRITERIA	LDL THRESHOLD TO ADD NON-STATIN THERAPY	PREFERRED TREATMENT
Clinical ASCVD and very high risk*	≥ 55 mg/dL	Ezetimibe and/or PCSK9 mAb
Clinical ASCVD not at very high risk* Clinical ASCVD and baseline LDL ≥ 190 mg/dL	≥ 70 mg/dL	
No clinical ASCVD with diabetes and/or 10-year ASCVD risk ≥ 20%	≥ 70 mg/dL	
No clinical ASCVD with baseline LDL ≥ 190 mg/dL	≥ 100 mg/dL	

History of multiple ASCVD events or one ASCVD event and multiple high-risk conditions (e.g., diabetes, hypertension, age ≥ 65 years, chronic kidney disease, smoking).

EZETIMIBE

Ezetimibe inhibits absorption of cholesterol in the small intestine.

DRUG	DOSING	SAFETY/SIDE EFFECTS/MONITORING
Ezetimibe (Zetia) + simvastatin (Vytorin) + bempedoic acid (Nexlizet)	10 mg daily eGFR < 60 mL/min/1.73 m²: do not exceed simvastatin 20 mg/day when using combination product (Vytorin)	**WARNINGS** Avoid use in moderate or severe hepatic impairment Skeletal muscle effects (e.g., myopathy, rhabdomyolysis), risk ↑ when combined with a statin Pregnancy: risks to fetus unknown (individualize therapy based on potential risk vs. benefit) Breastfeeding: generally not recommended **SIDE EFFECTS** Myalgia, arthralgia, pain in extremities, diarrhea, URTIs, sinusitis **MONITORING** LFTs at baseline and as clinically indicated thereafter **Lipid Effects (Ezetimibe Monotherapy)** ↓ LDL 18-23%, ↑ HDL 1-3%, ↓ TG 5-10%

Ezetimibe Drug Interactions

- When ezetimibe and cyclosporine are used together, the concentration of both can ↑; monitor levels of cyclosporine.
- Concurrent bile acid sequestrants ↓ ezetimibe; give ezetimibe two hours before or four hours after bile acid sequestrants.
- Can ↑ risk of cholelithiasis when used with fenofibrate and gemfibrozil. Do not use with gemfibrozil.

PROPROTEIN CONVERTASE SUBTILISIN/KEXIN TYPE 9 MONOCLONAL ANTIBODIES

The LDL receptor clears circulating LDL. Proprotein convertase subtilisin/kexin type 9 (PCSK9) is an enzyme that increases LDL receptor degradation. PCSK9 monoclonal antibodies (previously known as PCSK9 inhibitors) block the ability of PCSK9 to bind to the LDL receptor. They dramatically ↓ LDL cholesterol and reduce the risk of cardiovascular events. PCSK9 mAbs are indicated in patients with established ASCVD or familial hypercholesterolemia.

DRUG	DOSING	SAFETY/SIDE EFFECTS/MONITORING
Alirocumab (Praluent) 75 mg/mL, 150 mg/mL prefilled syringes or prefilled pen	75-150 mg SC once every 2 weeks or 300 mg (150 mg x 2 sites) SC monthly	**WARNINGS** Allergic reactions **SIDE EFFECTS** Injection site reactions, nasopharyngitis, influenza, URTIs, UTI, back pain (evolocumab), ↑ LFTs (alirocumab)
Evolocumab (Repatha, *Repatha SureClick, Pushtronex)* 140 mg/mL prefilled syringe or autoinjector 420 mg/3.5 mL prefilled cartridge	140 mg SC once every 2 weeks or 420 mg monthly The 420 mg dose is given as three consecutive 140 mg injections within 30 minutes or as a 420 mg single injection	**MONITORING** LDL at baseline and at 4-8 weeks to assess response **NOTES** Store in the refrigerator in the original carton to protect from light; can be kept at room temperature for up to 30 days, but then must be discarded Prior to administration, allow prefilled pen to warm to room temperature (~30 minutes, 45 minutes for *Pushtronex*) and inspect for particulate matter and discoloration **Lipid Effects** ↓ LDL ~60%, ↓ non-HDL ~35%, ↓ apoB ~50%, ↓ TC ~36%

BILE ACID SEQUESTRANTS/BILE ACID BINDING RESINS

These drugs bind bile acids in the intestine, forming a complex that is excreted in the feces. This non-systemic action results in partial removal of bile acids from enterohepatic circulation, preventing their reabsorption.

DRUG	DOSING	SAFETY/SIDE EFFECTS/MONITORING
Colesevelam (Welchol) 625 mg tablet, 3.75 gram granule packet Also approved for glycemic control in type 2 diabetes (↓ A1C ~0.5%)	3.75 grams daily or in divided doses with a meal and liquid	**CONTRAINDICATIONS** Cholestyramine: complete biliary obstruction Colesevelam: bowel obstruction, TG > 500 mg/dL, history of hypertriglyceridemia-induced pancreatitis **WARNINGS** Some formulations contain phenylalanine and should not be used in patients with PKU ↑ bleeding tendency due to vitamin K deficiency
Cholestyramine (*Prevalite*) Also approved for pruritus due to increased levels of bile acids 4 gram powder packet	Initial: 4 grams daily or BID Maintenance: 8-16 grams/day divided BID with meals (max 24 grams/day)	**SIDE EFFECTS** Constipation (may need dose reduction or laxative), abdominal pain, cramping, bloating, gas, ↑ TG, dyspepsia, nausea, esophageal obstruction **NOTES** Not recommended when TG are ≥ 300 mg/dL Cholestyramine packet: mix powder with 2-6 oz. water or non-carbonated liquid; sipping or holding the resin suspension in the mouth for prolonged periods may lead to changes in the surface of the teeth resulting in discoloration, erosion of enamel or decay; use good oral hygiene
Colestipol (*Colestid*) 1 gram tablet, 5 gram packet and granules	Tablets: 2 grams daily or BID (max 16 grams/day) Packet and granules: 5 grams daily or BID (max 30 grams/day)	Colesevelam is a treatment option for pregnant patients Colesevelam packet: empty 1 packet into a glass; add 8 oz. of water, fruit juice or diet soft drink and mix well Colestipol packet: empty 1 packet into at least 3 oz. of liquid and stir until mixed **Lipid Effects** ↓ LDL ~10-30%, ↑ HDL ~3-5%, no change or ↑ TG ~5%

Bile Acid Sequestrants Drug Interactions

- Colesevelam has fewer drug interactions than the other two bile acid sequestrants and is more commonly used. For cholestyramine or colestipol, take all other drugs at least 1 – 4 hours before or 4 – 6 hours after the bile acid sequestrant.

- Monitor INR more frequently in patients taking concurrent warfarin.

- Colesevelam can ↑ levels of metformin ER.

- The following medications should be taken four hours prior to colesevelam: cyclosporine, sulfonylureas, levothyroxine, olmesartan, phenytoin and oral contraceptives containing ethinyl estradiol and norethindrone.

- Bile acid sequestrants can ↓ absorption of fat-soluble vitamins (A, D, E, K), folate and iron. A multivitamin may be needed, but separate administration from the bile acid sequestrant.

FIBRATES

Fibrates are peroxisome proliferator-activated receptor alpha (PPARα) agonists, which upregulate the expression of apolipoprotein C2 (apoC-II) and apolipoprotein A1 (apoA-I). ApoC-II increases lipoprotein lipase activity leading to increased catabolism of VLDL particles. This will decrease TG significantly, but can lead to increased LDL in the setting of very high TG. The decreased TG can lead to an increase in HDL cholesterol.

DRUG	DOSING	SAFETY/SIDE EFFECTS/MONITORING
Fenofibrate, Fenofibric Acid **(Tricor, Trilipix,** *Fenoglide, Fibricor, Lipofen)*	Fenofibrate (micronized): 43-130 mg daily *Fenoglide:* 40-120 mg daily with meals *Fibricor:* 35-105 mg daily *Lipofen:* 50-150 mg daily with meals *Tricor:* 48-145 mg daily *Trilipix:* 45-135 mg daily	**CONTRAINDICATIONS** Severe liver disease, including primary biliary cirrhosis, severe renal disease (CrCl ≤ 30 mL/min), gallbladder disease, breastfeeding, concurrent use with repaglinide or simvastatin (gemfibrozil only) **WARNINGS** Myopathy, ↑ risk when coadministered with a statin (particularly in older adults, diabetes, renal failure, hypothyroidism), cholelithiasis, reversible ↑ SCr (> 2 mg/dL) **SIDE EFFECTS** Dyspepsia (gemfibrozil), ↑ LFTs (dose-related), abdominal pain, ↑ CPK, URTIs **MONITORING** LFTs, renal function
Gemfibrozil (Lopid)	600 mg BID, 30 minutes before breakfast and dinner	**NOTES** Reduce dose if CrCl 31-80 mL/min (fenofibrates) **Lipid Effects** ↓ TG ~20-50%, ↑ HDL ~15%, ↓ LDL ~5-20% (can ↑ LDL when TG are high)

Fibrate Drug Interactions

- Fibrates (especially gemfibrozil) can ↑ the risk of myopathy and rhabdomyolysis. Gemfibrozil should not be used with ezetimibe or statins.

- Colchicine can ↑ the risk of myopathy when coadministered with fenofibrate.

- Gemfibrozil is contraindicated with repaglinide as it can ↑ hypoglycemic effects.

- Fibrates can ↑ the effects of sulfonylureas and warfarin.

NIACIN

Niacin decreases the rate of hepatic synthesis of VLDL (decreases TG) and LDL and can also increase the rate of chylomicron TG removal from plasma. It alters the binding of HDL particles to scavenger receptor B-1 in the liver, which removes the cholesterol inside, but does not take up the HDL particle (i.e., HDL increases and is free to return to circulation for reverse cholesterol transport). Niacin is also known as nicotinic acid or vitamin B3, although doses for cholesterol reduction are much higher than doses found in multivitamin products.

DRUG	DOSING	SAFETY/SIDE EFFECTS/MONITORING
Niacin Immediate-release (IR) (crystalline): *Niacor* Extended-release (ER) Controlled-release (CR)/sustained-release (SR): *Slo-Niacin*, OTC	Titrate slowly IR: 250-3,000 mg in 3 divided doses with food ER: 500-2,000 mg at bedtime after a low-fat snack CR/SR: 250-750 mg daily with food	**CONTRAINDICATIONS** Active liver disease, active peptic ulcer disease or arterial bleeding **WARNINGS** Rhabdomyolysis with niacin doses ≥ 1 gram/day when combined with statins Hepatotoxicity ↑ BG, ↑ uric acid, ↓ phosphate Use with caution in patients with unstable angina or during the acute phase of an MI **SIDE EFFECTS** Flushing, pruritus (itching), vomiting, diarrhea, ↑ BG, hyperuricemia (or gout), nausea, cough, orthostatic hypotension, hypophosphatemia, ↓ platelets **MONITORING** LFTs at baseline, every 6-12 weeks for the first year and then every 6 months Blood glucose (if diabetic), uric acid (if gout history), INR (if on warfarin), lipid profile **NOTES** ER formulation is preferred due to less flushing and hepatotoxicity, but it is the most expensive To reduce flushing: take aspirin 325 mg (or ibuprofen 200 mg) 30-60 minutes before the dose; take with food, but avoid spicy food, alcohol and hot beverages (which can worsen flushing) Formulations of niacin are not interchangeable Flush-free niacins (inositol hexaniacinate or hexanicotinate), niacinamide or nicotinamide are not effective **Lipid Effects** ↓ LDL 5-25%, ↑ HDL 15-35%, ↓ TG 20-50%

Niacin Drug Interactions

- Take niacin 4 – 6 hours after bile acid sequestrants.

FISH OILS

Fish oils are also known as omega-3 fatty acids. Their mechanism is not completely understood; they may reduce hepatic synthesis of TG. Fish oils are indicated as an adjunct to diet when TG ≥ 500 mg/dL. Icosapent ethyl (*Vascepa*) is recommended for ASCVD risk reduction in select patients (clinical ASCVD or type 2 diabetes with additional risk factors) when triglycerides are 135 – 499 mg/dL despite use of a maximally tolerated statin.

DRUG	DOSING	SAFETY/SIDE EFFECTS/MONITORING
Omega-3 Acid Ethyl Esters (*Lovaza*) 1 gram capsule contains 465 mg eicosapentaenoic acid (EPA) and 375 mg docosahexaenoic acid (DHA)	4 capsules daily or 2 capsules BID	**WARNINGS** Use with caution in patients with known hypersensitivity to fish and/or shellfish Monitor LFTs in patients with hepatic impairment and LDL periodically *Lovaza:* can ↑ LDL levels; possible association with more frequent recurrences of symptomatic atrial fibrillation (AF) or flutter in patients with AF, particularly within the first months of initiation **SIDE EFFECTS** Eructation (burping), dyspepsia, taste perversions (*Lovaza*), arthralgia (*Vascepa*)
Icosapent ethyl (*Vascepa*) Contains 0.5 or 1 gram of icosapent ethyl, an ethyl ester of EPA	2 grams BID with food	**NOTES** Many OTC omega-3 fatty acid products are marketed as dietary supplements; only the prescription medications *Lovaza* and *Vascepa* are FDA-approved for TG lowering Stop prior to elective surgeries due to increased risk of bleeding **Lipid Effects** ↓ TG up to 45%, ↑ HDL ~9%, can ↑ LDL (up to 44% with *Lovaza*, no ↑ seen with *Vascepa*)

Fish Oil Drug Interactions

- Omega-3-fatty acids can prolong bleeding time; use caution when combined with other medications that can ↑ bleeding risk (e.g., antiplatelets, anticoagulants). Monitor INR in patients taking warfarin.

OTHER DRUGS

The drugs in the table below have more niche uses or are newer treatments whose place in therapy is still evolving.

DRUG CLASS	COMMENTS
Bempedoic Acid (*Nexletol*) + ezetimibe (*Nexlizet*) Tablet	MOA: inhibits cholesterol synthesis in the liver by inhibiting adenosine triphosphate-citrate lyase (ACL), an enzyme upstream of HMG-CoA reductase in the cholesterol synthesis pathway. Approved for HeFH or ASCVD in combination with a statin (i.e., add-on treatment) in patients who require additional LDL lowering. Significant adverse effects: hyperuricemia (and gout), tendon rupture.
Inclisiran (*Leqvio*) SC injection	MOA: inhibits intracellular production of PCSK9 via ribonucleic acid (RNA) interference, which results in increased activity of the LDL receptor. Approved for HeFH or primary hyperlipidemia in combination with a statin (i.e., add-on treatment) in patients who require additional LDL lowering. Do not use with PCSK9 mAb due to overlapping mechanism of action. Adverse effects: injection site reactions, arthralgia.
Lomitapide (*Juxtapid*) Capsule	MOA: prevents assembly of apoB-containing lipoproteins (LDL and VLDL) by inhibiting microsomal triglyceride transfer protein. Approved as an adjunct treatment for HoFH. Due to the risk of hepatotoxicity (a boxed warning), it is only available through the *Juxtapid* Risk Evaluation and Mitigation Strategy (REMS) program. Contraindications: active liver disease, pregnancy, concomitant use with moderate-strong CYP3A4 inhibitors.
Evinacumab (*Evkeeza*) IV infusion	MOA: monoclonal antibody that inhibits angiopoietin-like 3 (ANGPLT3), resulting in increased lipid metabolism; decreases LDL, HDL and TGs. Approved as an adjunct treatment for HoFH. Significant adverse effects: severe hypersensitivity reactions, including anaphylaxis.

KEY COUNSELING POINTS

See the Drug Formulations and Patient Counseling chapter for counseling language/layman's terminology.

See Drug Interactions section for each drug class.

ALL CHOLESTEROL MEDICATIONS

- Follow lifestyle recommendations, including heart-healthy eating habits and exercise.

Statins

- Take simvastatin and fluvastatin IR in the evening (if taken once daily), lovastatin IR with the evening meal and lovastatin ER at bedtime. Other statins can be taken at any time of the day.
- Can cause:
  - ❏ Muscle damage.
  - ❏ Liver damage.
- Avoid grapefruit.
- Avoid in pregnancy (teratogenic) in most cases.

Ezetimibe

- Can cause:
  - ❏ Muscle damage.
  - ❏ Liver damage.

PCSK9 Monoclonal Antibodies

- Inject subcutaneously into the thigh, abdomen or upper arm.
- Can cause:
  - ❏ Allergy/anaphylaxis.
  - ❏ Injection site reaction.
- Store in the refrigerator. Allow to warm to room temperature before injecting. Can be kept at room temperature for 30 days.

Bile Acid Sequestrants

- Take at mealtimes with plenty of water or other liquid.
- Can cause constipation.
- Reduces vitamin A, D, E and K absorption.

Fibrates

- *Lopid:* take twice daily, 30 minutes before breakfast and dinner.
- Can cause:
  - ❏ Muscle damage.
  - ❏ Liver damage.
  - ❏ Cholelithiasis (i.e., gallstones); contact prescriber for severe abdominal pain, nausea or vomiting.
  - ❏ Pancreatitis.

Niacin

- Extended release: take at bedtime after a low-fat snack.
- Other niacins: take with food.
- Can cause:
  - ❏ Hyperglycemia.
  - ❏ Liver damage.
  - ❏ Flushing (warmth, redness, itching and/or tingling of the skin). With extended-release formulation, flushing will occur mostly at night; use caution if awakened due to dizziness.
- To reduce flushing, take aspirin 325 mg (or ibuprofen 200 mg) 30 – 60 minutes before the dose. Taking with food and avoiding alcohol, hot beverages or spicy foods can also reduce flushing.

Fish Oil

- *Vascepa:* take with food.
- Can cause dyspepsia (all fish oils), burping, abnormal sense of taste (*Lovaza*) or joint pain (*Vascepa*).

Select Guidelines/References

Grundy SM, Stone NJ, Bailey AL, et al. 2018 AHA/ACC/AACVPR/ AAPA/ABC/ACPM/ADA/AGS/APhA/ASPC/NLA/PCNA guideline on the management of blood cholesterol: a report of the American College of Cardiology/American Heart Association Task Force on Clinical Practice Guidelines. *Circulation.* 2018;000:e000–e000. DOI: 10.1161/CIR.0000000000000625.

Lloyd-Jones DM, Morris PB, Ballantyne CM, et al. 2022 ACC expert consensus decision pathway on the role of nonstatin therapies for LDL-cholesterol lowering in the management of atherosclerotic cardiovascular disease risk. J Am Coll Cardiol. 2022;80:1366-1418.

CONTENT LEGEND

 = Study Tip Gal    = Key Drug Guy

CHAPTER 28

HYPERTENSION

BACKGROUND

Hypertension, or high blood pressure (BP), affects nearly half of all American adults and is a common disease managed in primary care. Hypertension is mostly asymptomatic, which can delay diagnosis and can contribute to medication non-adherence. Medication side effects, cost and pill burden can also lead to discontinuation of treatment. Uncontrolled hypertension places the patient at greater risk for heart disease, stroke and kidney disease. Pharmacists play a vital role in screening and monitoring patients and providing counseling about the importance of lifestyle management (e.g., healthy diet, sodium restriction, physical activity, smoking cessation) and medication adherence. Patient self-monitoring of blood pressure at home can improve motivation and treatment success.

ETIOLOGY AND PATHOPHYSIOLOGY

Most patients (~90%) have primary (essential) hypertension. The cause is unknown, but a combination of risk factors (e.g., obesity, sedentary lifestyle, excessive salt intake, smoking, family history, diabetes, dyslipidemia) is usually present. Secondary hypertension has an identifiable underlying cause, such as renal disease, adrenal disease (e.g., excess aldosterone secretion), obstructive sleep apnea or drugs (see Key Drugs Guy later in the chapter).

The pathophysiology of hypertension includes activation of the sympathetic nervous system (SNS) and renin-angiotensin-aldosterone system (RAAS). The resulting increase in neurohormone levels (e.g., norepinephrine, angiotensin II, aldosterone) can increase blood pressure. Most medications used to treat hypertension target one or both of these neurohormonal pathways (see the Neurohormonal Pathways Involved in Hypertension flow diagram on the next page).

NEUROHORMONAL PATHWAYS INVOLVED IN HYPERTENSION

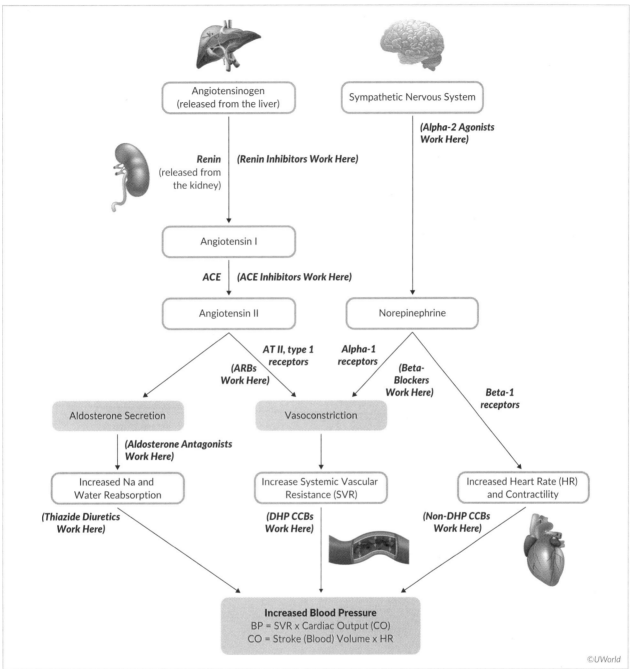

©UWorld

iStock.com/MariaAverburg, newannyart

DRUGS THAT CAN INCREASE BLOOD PRESSURE

Increased sympathomimetic activity
ADHD drugs (e.g., amphetamine)

Decongestants (e.g., pseudoephedrine, phenylephrine)

Recreational substances (e.g., cocaine, caffeine)

Antidepressants (e.g., TCAs, SNRIs, MAO inhibitors)

Increased sodium and water retention
NSAIDs

Immunosuppressants (e.g., cyclosporine)

Systemic steroids

Increased blood viscosity
Erythropoiesis-stimulating agents (e.g., epoetin alfa)

Other
Oral contraceptives (with higher estrogen content)

VEGF inhibitors (e.g., bevacizumab, sunitinib)

BLOOD PRESSURE MONITORING
Correct use of a blood pressure monitoring device

DO	DON'T
Go to the restroom and empty the bladder	Talk
Sit in a chair (both feet on the floor with back supported) and relax for at least 5 minutes	Lie down or sit without the back supported (e.g., on an examination table)
Use the correct cuff size	Drink caffeine, exercise or smoke for 30 minutes prior
Support the arm at heart level (e.g., resting on a desk)	Use a finger monitor or wrist monitor*
Wait 1-2 minutes in between measurements	

Self-monitoring (bring device and BP reading log to clinic visits)
Ambulatory BP monitoring device: typically worn continuously (i.e., for 24 hours) during daily activities and sleep; obtains readings every 15-60 minutes.

Home BP monitoring device: patient measures and records the average of at least 2 readings in the morning and evening before eating or taking any medications.

A wrist monitor is not ideal but may be necessary in select cases (e.g., if the appropriate cuff size is unavailable for an obese patient).

SCREENING AND DIAGNOSIS

Accurate measurement of BP (see Study Tip Gal) is essential for diagnosing hypertension and assessing if medication titration is needed. BP readings in the same individual can vary during the day due to stress, exercise, medications, eating and other activities of daily living. BP usually decreases during the night and increases again in the early morning.

A hypertension diagnosis should be based on an average of at least two readings obtained on at least two separate occasions. BP readings in a clinical office setting may be falsely elevated (e.g., white coat hypertension) and lead to inaccurate clinical decisions related to patient risk and treatment. Therefore, out-of-office BP monitoring with an ambulatory BP monitor or an automated home device is preferred.

The American College of Cardiology and American Heart Association (ACC/AHA) has defined four categories of BP in adults, based on systolic BP (SBP) and/or diastolic BP (DBP) readings:

- Normal: SBP < 120 mmHg and DBP < 80 mmHg
- Elevated: SBP 120 – 129 mmHg and DBP < 80 mmHg
- Hypertension:
  - Stage 1: SBP 130 – 139 mmHg or DBP 80 – 89 mmHg
  - Stage 2: SBP ≥ 140 mmHg or DBP ≥ 90 mmHg

LIFESTYLE MANAGEMENT

Lifestyle interventions are essential to prevent hypertension (in patients with normal or elevated BP) and to treat hypertension, alone or in conjunction with medications. Interventions proven to be effective in lowering BP include:

- Weight loss (1 kg of weight loss decreases BP by ~1 mmHg)
- A heart-healthy diet [e.g., DASH (Dietary Approaches to Stop Hypertension)] that is high in fruits, vegetables, fiber and low-fat dairy products, and low in saturated fats and sugar
- Adequate dietary potassium intake or supplementation, unless contraindicated (e.g., chronic kidney disease)
- Reduced sodium intake (< 1,500 mg daily)
- Routine physical activity
- Limited alcohol consumption (≤ 1 drink daily for women and ≤ 2 drinks daily for men)

Additional modifications to improve overall cardiovascular health, including tobacco cessation and adequate control of blood glucose and cholesterol, are also recommended.

NATURAL PRODUCTS

Although not recommended by the guidelines due to limited evidence for reducing BP, some patients may supplement drug treatment with natural medicines, such as garlic and fish oil. Patients should be advised that both of these natural products can increase bleeding risk.

TREATMENT PRINCIPLES (ACC/AHA)

- Emphasize lifestyle modifications throughout treatment.

- Drug treatment initiation is based on hypertension stage. An atherosclerotic cardiovascular disease (ASCVD) risk score may also be needed and can be assessed using an online tool (http://tools.acc.org/ASCVD-Risk-Estimator/).

  - ❏ See Study Tip Gal for details, including initial drug selection, BP goal and monitoring.

- Once-daily regimens and/or combination products (see table on next page) are preferred for medication adherence.

  - ❏ Most patients will require two or more drugs.

  - ❏ Agents from the four preferred drug classes should be selected first before considering alternative classes.

  - ❏ Do not use ACE inhibitors and ARBs in combination.

- When titrating medications, adding a second drug before reaching the maximum dose of the first medication can be more effective and cause fewer side effects.

- Patients with hypertension and select comorbid conditions (e.g., heart failure) should be treated according to the specific disease-state guideline recommendations. Refer to individual course book chapters as appropriate.

HYPERTENSION GUIDELINE RECOMMENDATIONS

WHEN TO START TREATMENT
- Stage 1 HTN (SBP 130-139 mmHg or DBP 80-89 mmHg) and any of the following:

  - ❏ Clinical CVD (stroke, heart failure or coronary heart disease)

  - ❏ 10-year ASCVD risk ≥ 10%

  - ❏ Does not meet BP goal after 6 months of lifestyle modifications

- Stage 2 HTN (SBP ≥ 140 mmHg or DBP ≥ 90 mmHg)

BP GOAL
- < 130/80 mmHg*

INITIAL DRUG SELECTION
- Use an agent from one of the preferred classes:

  - ❏ Thiazide diuretic**

  - ❏ Dihydropyridine calcium channel blocker (DHP CCB)**

  - ❏ Angiotensin-converting enzyme (ACE) inhibitor or angiotensin receptor blocker (ARB)

- CKD***: ACE inhibitor or ARB

- Start 2 drugs from the preferred classes when baseline average BP is > 20/10 mmHg above goal (e.g., > 150/90 mmHg)

MONITORING
- Check BP every month and titrate medication if not at goal

The KDIGO 2021 Blood Pressure in CKD Guideline recommends a goal SBP < 120 mmHg (if tolerated) for patients with hypertension and CKD (see Renal Disease chapter).
**May be preferred in self-identified black patients without CKD.*
***Stage 3 CKD (eGFR < 60 mL/min/1.73 m²) or albuminuria (for exam purposes, defined as urine albumin ≥ 30 mg/day or albumin:creatinine ratio ≥ 30 mg/g).*

PREGNANCY AND HYPERTENSION

Teratogenic drugs can cause fetal harm and should be discontinued if planning a pregnancy. ACE inhibitors, ARBs and the direct renin inhibitor (aliskiren) have a boxed warning for fetal toxicity in pregnancy and should be stopped immediately.

Other oral antihypertensive drugs can be used to treat non-severe chronic hypertension (hypertension occurring before pregnancy or 20 weeks gestation); drug treatment should be initiated if SBP ≥ 140 mmHg or DBP ≥ 90 mmHg.

Labetalol, nifedipine extended-release and methyldopa are recommended first-line treatments, although methyldopa may be less effective at lowering BP. The SBP should be maintained between 120 – 139 mmHg and the DBP between 80 – 89 mmHg.

Other hypertensive disorders of pregnancy include gestational hypertension and preeclampsia, which are both defined as new-onset hypertension after 20 weeks gestation. Preeclampsia is further characterized by the presence of proteinuria or significant end-organ dysfunction.

These conditions can be treated with the aforementioned oral agents, however the use of intravenous antihypertensives (e.g., labetalol, hydralazine) may be required for severe presentations. Additionally, in patients at high risk for preeclampsia (e.g., pre-existing hypertension, renal disease, diabetes, previous preeclampsia), daily low-dose aspirin is recommended after the first trimester.

COMBINATION BLOOD PRESSURE DRUGS

Tip: the brand names of many diuretic combinations end in HCT or -etic

ACE INHIBITOR OR ARB + DIURETIC
Lisinopril/Hydrochlorothiazide (Zestoretic)

Losartan/Hydrochlorothiazide (Hyzaar)

Olmesartan/Hydrochlorothiazide (Benicar HCT)

Valsartan/Hydrochlorothiazide (Diovan HCT)

Azilsartan/Chlorthalidone (Edarbyclor)

Benazepril/Hydrochlorothiazide (Lotensin HCT)

Candesartan/Hydrochlorothiazide (Atacand HCT)

Enalapril/Hydrochlorothiazide (Vaseretic)

Fosinopril/Hydrochlorothiazide

Irbesartan/Hydrochlorothiazide (Avalide)

Moexipril/Hydrochlorothiazide

Quinapril/Hydrochlorothiazide

Telmisartan/Hydrochlorothiazide (Micardis HCT)

ACE INHIBITOR OR ARB + CCB
Benazepril/Amlodipine (Lotrel)

Valsartan/Amlodipine (Exforge)

Olmesartan/Amlodipine (Azor)

Perindopril/Amlodipine (Prestalia)

Telmisartan/Amlodipine

Trandolapril/Verapamil

BETA BLOCKER + DIURETIC
Atenolol/Chlorthalidone (Tenoretic)

Bisoprolol/Hydrochlorothiazide (Ziac)

Metoprolol Tartrate/Hydrochlorothiazide

K-SPARING + THIAZIDE-TYPE DIURETIC
Triamterene/Hydrochlorothiazide (Maxzide, Maxzide-25)

Amiloride/Hydrochlorothiazide

Spironolactone/Hydrochlorothiazide (Aldactazide)

TRIPLE COMBINATIONS
Olmesartan/Amlodipine/Hydrochlorothiazide (Tribenzor)

Valsartan/Amlodipine/Hydrochlorothiazide (Exforge HCT)

THIAZIDE DIURETICS

Thiazide diuretics are inexpensive, effective and have mild side effects in most patients. They are one of four preferred drug classes that can be considered for initial hypertension treatment. Loop diuretics are used primarily in heart failure (see Chronic Heart Failure chapter).

Thiazides, including thiazide-type (e.g., hydrochlorothiazide) and thiazide-like (e.g., chlorthalidone) diuretics inhibit sodium reabsorption in the distal convoluted tubule (see Nephron diagram), causing increased excretion of sodium, chloride, water and potassium.

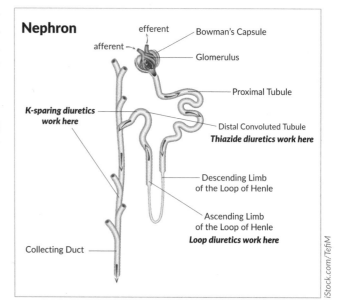

DRUG	DOSING	SAFETY/SIDE EFFECTS/MONITORING
Chlorthalidone Tablet	12.5-25 mg daily (daily doses > 25 mg/day have limited clinical benefit and ↑ risk of adverse effects)	**CONTRAINDICATIONS** Hypersensitivity to sulfonamide-derived drugs (not likely to cross-react – see Drug Allergies & Adverse Drug Reactions chapter); anuria **WARNINGS** Severe renal disease (can precipitate azotemia), progressive liver disease (fluid and electrolyte changes can precipitate hepatic coma), transient myopia or acute angle-closure glaucoma, can precipitate or exacerbate conditions such as systemic lupus erythematosus (SLE), gout, dyslipidemia and diabetes
Hydrochlorothiazide Tablet, capsule	12.5-50 mg daily (daily doses > 50 mg/day have limited clinical benefit and ↑ risk of adverse effects)	**SIDE EFFECTS** ↓ electrolytes: K, Mg, Na ↑ electrolytes/labs: Ca, UA, LDL, TG, BG
Chlorothiazide (*Diuril*) Oral suspension, injection	500-2,000 mg daily in 1-2 divided doses	Photosensitivity (including a small ↑ risk of non-melanoma skin cancer), impotence, dizziness, rash **MONITORING** Electrolytes, renal function, BP, fluid status (input and output, weight), BG (in diabetes)
Indapamide Tablet	1.25-2.5 mg daily	**NOTES** Thiazide diuretic effect is diminished when CrCl < 30 mL/min (except metolazone, which is indicated for volume overload in combination with a loop diuretic) Take early in the day to avoid nocturia
Metolazone Tablet	2.5-5 mg daily	Chlorothiazide is the only thiazide diuretic available IV Chlorthalidone is considered more effective at lowering BP due to a longer duration of action and increased potency Hypokalemia can be avoided with regular intake of potassium-rich foods, potassium supplements or concurrent use of a potassium-sparing diuretic

Thiazide Diuretic Drug Interactions

- All antihypertensives, including thiazide diuretics, can enhance the BP-lowering effects of other drugs; carefully monitor BP when using combinations of medications.

- Drugs that can cause sodium and water retention (e.g., NSAIDs) can decrease thiazide diuretic effectiveness; monitor BP closely if used in combination. If possible, avoid NSAIDs in patients with cardiovascular disease.

- Thiazide diuretics can ↓ lithium renal clearance and ↑ the risk of lithium toxicity. Consider decreasing the lithium dose if a thiazide diuretic is initiated and monitor lithium levels closely during concurrent treatment.

- Thiazide diuretics can ↑ dofetilide serum concentrations, leading to an ↑ risk of QT prolongation; do not use in combination.

CALCIUM CHANNEL BLOCKERS

There are two types of calcium channel blockers (CCBs), dihydropyridine (DHP) and non-dihydropyridine (non-DHP). They inhibit Ca ions from entering vascular smooth muscle and myocardial cells.

- DHP CCBs are more selective for vascular smooth muscle; this causes peripheral arterial vasodilation (which ↓ SVR and BP) and coronary artery vasodilation. Common side effects related to peripheral vasodilation include reflex tachycardia/palpitations, headache, flushing and peripheral edema.

- Non-DHP CCBs are more selective for the myocardium, making them less potent vasodilators. The decrease in BP produced by non-DHP CCBs is due to negative inotropic (↓ force of ventricular contraction) and negative chronotropic (↓ HR) effects.

Select agents (e.g., nifedipine, diltiazem, verapamil) have multiple long-acting formulations and not all generic products are therapeutically equivalent to the brand-name products (the *Orange Book* should be consulted to identify an AB-rated generic).

DIHYDROPYRIDINE CCBs

DHP CCBs have generic names that end in "-pine"; they are used for hypertension, chronic stable and vasospastic angina (see Stable Angina chapter), and Raynaud's phenomenon (cold/blue fingers secondary to peripheral vasoconstriction).

DRUG	DOSING	SAFETY/SIDE EFFECTS/MONITORING
Amlodipine (Norvasc, *Katerzia, Norliqva)* Tablet, suspension, solution	2.5-10 mg daily	**CONTRAINDICATIONS** Nicardipine should not be used in advanced aortic stenosis **WARNINGS** Hypotension (especially with severe aortic stenosis), worsening angina and/or MI, severe hepatic impairment, use caution in heart failure (see Notes)
Nicardipine (Cardene IV) Injection, IR capsule	IV: 5 mg/hr, ↑ by 2.5 mg/hr every 5-15 min to max dose of 15 mg/hr IR: 20-40 mg TID	Nifedipine IR: do not use for chronic hypertension or acute BP reduction in non-pregnant adults (significant hypotension, MI and/or death has occurred)
Nifedipine (Procardia XL, *Adalat CC*)* ER tablet, IR capsule	ER: 30-90 mg daily	**SIDE EFFECTS** Generally well-tolerated, can cause peripheral edema/headache/flushing/palpitations/reflex tachycardia/fatigue, nausea, gingival hyperplasia (or overgrowth) **MONITORING** Peripheral edema, BP, HR
Felodipine	2.5-10 mg daily	**NOTES** Amlodipine is considered safe if a DHP CCB must be used to lower BP in a patient with heart failure with reduced ejection fraction
Isradipine	2.5-5 mg BID	
Nisoldipine ER *(Sular)*	17-34 mg daily	Nifedipine ER is a drug of choice in pregnancy
Nisoldipine ER (original formulation)	20-40 mg daily	*Procardia XL*: OROS/gel matrix formulation (see Drug Formulations and Patient Counseling chapter) can leave a ghost tablet (empty shell) in the stool
Clevidipine *(Cleviprex)* Injection	1-21 mg/hr	**CONTRAINDICATIONS** Allergy to soybeans, soy products or eggs; defective lipid metabolism (e.g., lipoid nephrosis, hyperlipidemia with acute pancreatitis); severe aortic stenosis **WARNINGS** Hypotension, reflex tachycardia, infections (see Notes) **SIDE EFFECTS** Hypertriglyceridemia, headache, atrial fibrillation, nausea **MONITORING** BP, HR **NOTES** A lipid emulsion (provides 2 kcal/mL); milky-white in color Use strict aseptic technique due to infection risk; maximum time of use after vial puncture is 12 hrs

Brand discontinued but name still used in practice.

CASE SCENARIO

TW is a 54-year-old female admitted to the medical ICU with a hypertensive emergency. She is receiving clevidipine 50 mg/100 mL at a rate of 3 mg/hr. The bottle has 52 mL remaining at 1400.

- **How many calories per day is TW receiving from clevidipine?**
Calculate using the flow rate, product concentration and known kcal/mL provided.

$$\frac{3 \text{ mg}}{\text{hr}} \times \frac{24 \text{ hrs}}{\text{day}} \times \frac{100 \text{ mL}}{50 \text{ mg}} \times \frac{2 \text{ kcal}}{\text{mL}} = 288 \text{ kcal/day}$$

- **At what time should the bottle of clevidipine be removed and replaced?**
48 mL of clevidipine have been used. First, calculate how long the bottle has been hanging.

$$48 \text{ mL} \times \frac{50 \text{ mg}}{100 \text{ mL}} \times \frac{1 \text{ hr}}{3 \text{ mg}} = 8 \text{ hrs}$$

The bottle needs to be replaced every 12 hours (or in 4 more hours). It is currently 1400. A new bottle should be hung at 1800.

- **What other drugs may require similar calculations?**
Propofol (*Diprivan*) is another lipid emulsion that provides calories (1.1 kcal/mL) and requires tubing/vial changes every 12 hours (see Acute & Critical Care Medicine chapter for more information).

NON-DIHYDROPYRIDINE CCBs

The non-DHP CCBs, verapamil and diltiazem, are primarily used to control HR in certain arrhythmias (e.g., atrial fibrillation) and are sometimes used for hypertension and chronic stable and vasospastic angina.

DRUG	DOSING	SAFETY/SIDE EFFECTS/MONITORING
Diltiazem (*Cardizem, Tiazac,* Cardizem CD, Cardizem LA, Cartia XT, others) IR tablet, ER tablet (24-HR), ER capsule (12-HR), ER capsule (24-HR), injection	120-360 mg daily; max dose varies with product IR tablet: daily dose given in 4 divided doses ER capsule (12-HR): daily dose given in 2 divided doses	**CONTRAINDICATIONS** Hypotension (SBP < 90 mmHg) or cardiogenic shock; 2nd or 3rd degree AV block or sick sinus syndrome (unless patient has a functioning artificial ventricular pacemaker), atrial flutter or atrial fibrillation and an accessory bypass tract, concurrent use with an IV beta-blocker (IV CCBs only) Diltiazem: acute MI and pulmonary congestion Verapamil: severe left ventricular dysfunction **WARNINGS** Heart failure (may worsen symptoms), bradycardia, hypotension, acute liver injury/↑ LFTs, cardiac conduction abnormalities (diltiazem), hypertrophic cardiomyopathy (verapamil)
Verapamil (*Calan SR*,* Verelan, Verelan PM) IR tablet, ER tablet, ER capsule (24-HR), injection	120-480 mg daily IR: daily dose given in 3 divided doses ER: daily dose can be given in 1-2 divided doses *Verelan PM*: daily dose given QHS	**SIDE EFFECTS** Constipation (more with verapamil), gingival hyperplasia, edema (more with diltiazem), headache, dizziness, cutaneous hypersensitivity reactions (diltiazem) **MONITORING** BP, HR, ECG, LFTs **NOTES** IV:PO dose conversions are not 1:1

*Brand discontinued but name still used in practice.

Calcium Channel Blocker Drug Interactions

- Non-DHP CCBs: use caution with other drugs that ↓ HR, including beta-blockers, digoxin, clonidine, amiodarone and dexmedetomidine (*Precedex*).

- All CCBs (except clevidipine) are major substrates of CYP450 3A4. Check for drug interactions; it may be recommended to use caution or avoid concurrent use with strong CYP3A4 inducers or inhibitors. Do not use with grapefruit juice.

- Diltiazem and verapamil are substrates and inhibitors of P-gp and moderate inhibitors of CYP3A4; they can increase the concentration of many other drugs, such as select statins. Patients taking simvastatin or lovastatin should use lower doses (see Dyslipidemia chapter) or use a statin that is not metabolized by CYP3A4 (e.g., pitavastatin, pravastatin, rosuvastatin).

RENIN-ANGIOTENSIN-ALDOSTERONE SYSTEM INHIBITORS

Angiotensin II (Ang II) causes vasoconstriction and increased release of aldosterone, which results in sodium and water retention. RAAS inhibitors decrease BP by inhibiting the effects of Ang II. In addition to lowering BP, ACE inhibitors and ARBs have shown benefit for other disease states. For chronic kidney disease (e.g., eGFR < 60 mL/min/1.73 m^2 and/or albuminuria), they slow the progression of kidney damage by blocking the vasoconstricting effects of Ang II on the efferent arteriole in the nephron. This results in decreased filtration pressure and workload in the glomerulus. For heart failure, ACE inhibitors and ARBs protect the myocardium from the remodeling effects of Ang II and improve survival.

RAAS inhibitors should not be used in combination (e.g., ACE inhibitor + ARB) due to an increased risk for adverse effects (see RAAS Inhibitor Drug Interactions). Angioedema is a potentially fatal adverse effect that can occur with any RAAS inhibitor, although it is more common with ACE inhibitors than ARBs or aliskiren, and Black patients have a higher risk. For testing purposes, if a patient has a history of angioedema with any RAAS inhibitor, other RAAS inhibitors should be avoided.

ANGIOTENSIN-CONVERTING ENZYME INHIBITORS

ACE inhibitors end in "-pril." They block the conversion of angiotensin I (Ang I) to Ang II, resulting in ↓ vasoconstriction and ↓ aldosterone secretion. They also block the degradation of bradykinin, which is thought to contribute to the vasodilatory effects and characteristic side effects, such as a dry, hacking cough and angioedema.

DRUG	DOSING	SAFETY/SIDE EFFECTS/MONITORING
Benazepril (*Lotensin*)	10-40 mg daily in 1-2 divided doses	**BOXED WARNINGS** Can cause injury and death to the developing fetus when used in the 2nd and 3rd trimesters; discontinue as soon as pregnancy is detected
Enalapril (*Vasotec*, *Epaned* oral solution)	PO: 5-40 mg daily in 1-2 divided doses	
Enalaprilat (*Vasotec IV*)	IV (enalaprilat): 0.625-5 mg Q6H	**CONTRAINDICATIONS** Do not use with history of angioedema
Lisinopril (*Zestril*, *Prinivil, *Qbrelis* oral solution)**	5-40 mg daily	Do not use within 36 hrs of sacubitril/valsartan (*Entresto*) Do not use with aliskiren in patients with diabetes
Quinapril (*Accupril*)	10-80 mg daily in 1-2 divided doses	**WARNINGS** Angioedema
Ramipril (*Altace*)	2.5-20 mg daily in 1-2 divided doses	Hyperkalemia Renal impairment [(↑ risk with bilateral renal artery stenosis (avoid use)]
Captopril	12.5-150 mg daily in 2-3 divided doses	Hypotension/dizziness [(↑ risk if volume-depleted (e.g., concurrent diuretic use)]
Fosinopril	10-40 mg daily	
Moexipril	3.75-30 mg daily in 1-2 divided doses	**SIDE EFFECTS** See warnings; can also cause cough, headache
Perindopril	4-16 mg daily	**MONITORING** BP, K, renal function (↑ SCr), s/sx of angioedema
Trandolapril	1-4 mg daily	

*Brand discontinued but name still used in practice.

ANGIOTENSIN RECEPTOR BLOCKERS

ARBs end in "-sartan." They block Ang II from binding to the angiotensin II type-1 (underline{AT1}) receptor on vascular smooth muscle, preventing vasoconstriction, and on the adrenal gland, preventing aldosterone secretion and subsequent sodium and water retention.

DRUG	DOSING	SAFETY/SIDE EFFECTS/MONITORING
Irbesartan (*Avapro*)	150-300 mg daily	Same as ACE inhibitors except:
Losartan (*Cozaar*)	25-100 mg daily in 1-2 divided doses	Less cough Less angioedema No washout period required with sacubitril/valsartan (*Entresto*)
Olmesartan (*Benicar*)	20-40 mg daily	
Valsartan (*Diovan*)	80-320 mg daily	Additional safety issues unique to ARBs include:
Azilsartan (*Edarbi*)	40-80 mg daily	**WARNINGS** Olmesartan: sprue-like enteropathy – severe, chronic diarrhea with substantial
Candesartan (*Atacand*)	8-32 mg daily	weight loss; can occur months to years after drug initiation
Telmisartan (*Micardis*)	20-80 mg daily	**NOTES** Azilsartan: keep in original container to protect from light and moisture

DIRECT RENIN INHIBITOR

Aliskiren directly inhibits renin, which is responsible for the conversion of angiotensinogen to Ang I. A decrease in the formation of Ang I results in a decrease in the formation of Ang II.

DRUG	DOSING	SAFETY/SIDE EFFECTS/MONITORING
Aliskiren (*Tekturna*)	150-300 mg daily	Same as ACE inhibitors and ARBs except:
	Take with or without food but be consistent in administration with regard to meals	**CONTRAINDICATIONS** Do not use with ACE inhibitors or ARBs in patients with diabetes
	Avoid high fat foods (reduces absorption)	**NOTES** *Tekturna*: tablets must be protected from moisture

RAAS INHIBITOR DRUG INTERACTIONS

- All RAAS inhibitors ↑ the risk of hyperkalemia. Other medications that increase potassium (e.g., potassium-sparing diuretics) should be used cautiously. Patients should avoid salt substitutes that contain potassium chloride (instead of sodium chloride).

- Do not use more than one RAAS inhibitor together (e.g., ACE inhibitor + ARB) due to an ↑ risk of renal impairment, hypotension and hyperkalemia. Aliskiren in combination with an ACE inhibitor or ARB is specifically contraindicated in patients with diabetes.

- NSAIDs should be used cautiously in combination with ACE inhibitors or ARBs due to ↑ risk of renal impairment and diminished antihypertensive efficacy.

- ACE inhibitors and ARBs should not be used in combination with sacubitril/valsartan (*Entresto*). If switching from an ACE inhibitor to *Entresto*, or vice versa, a 36-hour washout period is required. See Chronic Heart Failure chapter for additional information.

- ACE inhibitors and ARBs can ↓ lithium renal clearance and ↑ the risk of lithium toxicity.

ADDITIONAL DRUGS FOR TREATING HYPERTENSION

POTASSIUM-SPARING DIURETICS

Triamterene and amiloride are potassium-sparing diuretics that exert their effects by directly blocking sodium channels in the late distal convoluted tubule and collecting duct of the nephron (see Nephron diagram earlier in the chapter). This increases sodium and water excretion but conserves potassium. Because sodium reabsorption is limited in this section of the nephron, these agents have minimal BP-lowering effects; they are primarily used in combination with thiazide diuretics (e.g., *Maxzide*) to counteract the mild potassium losses seen with thiazide diuretics.

The other potassium-sparing diuretics, spironolactone and eplerenone, are aldosterone receptor antagonists; they indirectly inhibit sodium channels by blocking the aldosterone receptor site and are the preferred add-on drugs for resistant hypertension (uncontrolled BP despite maximum tolerated doses of a DHP CCB + thiazide diuretic + ACE inhibitor or ARB). They are also used first line for heart failure. Spironolactone is a non-selective receptor antagonist (also blocks androgen), while eplerenone is a selective aldosterone receptor antagonist that does not exhibit endocrine side effects.

DRUG	DOSING	SAFETY/SIDE EFFECTS/MONITORING
Spironolactone (Aldactone, *CaroSpir* oral suspension)	25-100 mg daily in 1-2 divided doses	**BOXED WARNINGS** Amiloride and triamterene: hyperkalemia (K > 5.5 mEq/L) – more likely in patients with diabetes, renal impairment, or elderly patients **CONTRAINDICATIONS** Do not use with hyperkalemia, severe renal impairment, Addison's disease (spironolactone) or if taking strong CYP3A4 inhibitors (eplerenone)
Triamterene (*Dyrenium*) **+ HCTZ (Maxzide,** **Maxzide-25)**	50-300 mg daily in 1-2 divided doses + HCTZ: 37.5 mg/25 mg daily + HCTZ: 75 mg/50 mg daily	**SIDE EFFECTS** Hyperkalemia, ↑ SCr, dizziness, hyperchloremic metabolic acidosis (rare) Spironolactone: gynecomastia, breast tenderness, impotence, irregular menses, amenorrhea
Amiloride	5-10 mg daily in 1-2 divided doses	**MONITORING** BP, K, renal function, fluid status **NOTES**
Eplerenone (*Inspra*)	50-100 mg daily in 1-2 divided doses	*CaroSpir* suspension (also approved for use in heart failure and edema due to cirrhosis) is not therapeutically equivalent to *Aldactone* and dosing recommendations differ; doses > 100 mg can cause unexpectedly high concentrations; use a different formulation in this case

Potassium-Sparing Diuretic Drug Interactions

- Potassium-sparing diuretics ↑ the risk of hyperkalemia. There is an additive risk when these medications are used with other drugs that cause hyperkalemia (see Drug Interactions chapter) and/or potassium supplements.

- Eplerenone is a major substrate of CYP3A4; do not use with strong CYP3A4 inhibitors (e.g., ketoconazole, itraconazole, clarithromycin, ritonavir).

BETA-BLOCKERS

Beta-blockers mostly end in "-olol." They competitively block beta-1 and/or beta-2 adrenergic receptors; their actions at beta-1 receptors (located primarily in heart muscle) result in decreased HR and myocardial contractility, which decreases BP. Because beta-2 receptor blockade causes bronchoconstriction, a beta-1 selective agent is preferred in patients with bronchospastic disease (e.g., asthma, COPD) who require a beta-blocker. Carvedilol and labetalol also block alpha-1 receptors (located primarily in peripheral vasculature); this results in decreased peripheral vasoconstriction and provides additional BP lowering.

Beta-blockers with intrinsic sympathomimetic activity (ISA) (e.g., acebutolol, pindolol) partially stimulate beta receptors at rest while still blocking the effects of catecholamines (e.g., norepinephrine). While this may be useful in patients with bradycardia at rest who require beta-blockade, they are not recommended post-MI or in heart failure patients because they do not adequately decrease HR (and myocardial oxygen demand) compared to beta-blockers without ISA.

Beta-blockers are not recommended first-line for hypertension unless the patient has a comorbid condition for which beta-blockers are indicated (e.g., post-MI, stable angina, heart failure). Selection of a specific beta-blocker will depend on the condition being treated. For example, bisoprolol, carvedilol or metoprolol succinate should be used if treating heart failure with reduced ejection fraction.

DRUG	DOSING	SAFETY/SIDE EFFECTS/MONITORING
Beta-1 Selective Blockers		
Atenolol (Tenormin)	25-100 mg daily in 1-2 divided doses	**BOXED WARNINGS** Do not discontinue abruptly (particularly in patients with CAD/IHD); gradually taper dose over 1-2 weeks to avoid acute tachycardia, hypertension, and/or ischemia
Esmolol (Brevibloc) Injection	500 mg/kg IV bolus followed by 50 mcg/kg/min continuous IV infusion; titrate as needed to a maximum of 300 mcg/kg/min	**CONTRAINDICATIONS** Severe bradycardia; 2nd or 3rd degree AV block or sick sinus syndrome (unless a permanent pacemaker is in place); overt cardiac failure or cardiogenic shock Esmolol: pulmonary hypertension; use of IV non-DHP CCBs **WARNINGS** Use caution in patients with diabetes: can worsen hypoglycemia and mask hypoglycemic symptoms (see Diabetes chapter)
Metoprolol tartrate (Lopressor) Tablet, injection **Metoprolol succinate (Toprol XL, Kapspargo Sprinkle)** ER tablet, ER capsule	IR: 50-200 mg BID XL: 25-400 mg daily	Use caution with bronchospastic diseases (e.g., asthma, COPD) Use caution with Raynaud's/other peripheral vascular diseases (requires slow dose titration) and pheochromocytoma (requires adequate alpha-blockade first) Can mask signs of hyperthyroidism (e.g., tachycardia)
Acebutolol	200-1,200 mg daily in 1-2 divided doses	**SIDE EFFECTS** Bradycardia, hypotension, CNS effects (e.g., fatigue, dizziness, depression), impotence (less than thiazides), cold extremities (can exacerbate Raynaud's) **MONITORING** HR (↓ dose if symptomatic bradycardia), BP **NOTES** Oral drugs: titrate dose every 1-2 weeks (as tolerated), take without regard to meals (except Lopressor and Toprol XL should be taken with or immediately following food)
Betaxolol Betoptic S – ophthalmic	5-20 mg daily	Metoprolol tartrate IV is not equivalent to PO (IV:PO ratio is 1:2.5) When switching from metoprolol tartrate to metoprolol succinate, the same total daily dose of metoprolol should be used
Bisoprolol	2.5-20 mg daily	Kapspargo Sprinkle should be swallowed whole; for patients with difficulty swallowing, the capsule can be opened and the contents sprinkled on 1 teaspoonful of soft food (e.g., applesauce, yogurt or pudding) – the mixture must be swallowed within 60 min Toprol XL can be cut in half but should not be crushed or chewed For beta-1 selective drugs, remember: "AMEBBA" – Atenolol, Metoprolol, Esmolol, Bisoprolol, Betaxolol, Acebutolol

DRUG	DOSING	SAFETY/SIDE EFFECTS/MONITORING
Beta-1 Selective Blocker with Nitric Oxide-Dependent Vasodilation		
Nebivolol (Bystolic)	5-40 mg daily CrCl < 30 mL/min or moderate liver impairment, start at 2.5 mg daily	Same as above plus: **CONTRAINDICATIONS** Severe liver impairment (Child-Pugh class B or C) **SIDE EFFECTS** Fatigue, headache, nausea, diarrhea, ↑ TGs, ↓ HDL
Beta-1 and Beta-2 Blockers (Non-Selective)		
Propranolol (Inderal LA, Inderal XL, InnoPran XL, Hemangeol)** Tablet, ER capsule, oral solution, injection	IR: 80-640 mg in 2-4 divided doses LA: 80-640 mg daily XL: 80-120 mg daily	Same as for beta-1 selective blockers plus: **CONTRAINDICATIONS** Bronchial asthma **NOTES** Propranolol has high lipid solubility (lipophilic) and crosses the blood-brain barrier; this makes it useful for select non-cardiac conditions (e.g., migraine prophylaxis, essential tremor), but it is associated with more CNS side effects Non-selective beta-blockers are used to prevent variceal hemorrhage in patients with portal hypertension (see Hepatitis & Liver Disease chapter)
Nadolol (Corgard)	40-320 mg daily	
Pindolol	5-30 mg BID	
Timolol *Timoptic* – ophthalmic	10-30 mg BID	
Non-Selective Beta-Blockers and Alpha-1 Blockers		
Carvedilol (Coreg, Coreg CR) Tablet, ER capsule	IR: 6.25-25 mg BID CR: 20-80 mg daily	Same as for beta-1 selective and non-selective blockers plus: **CONTRAINDICATIONS** Severe hepatic impairment **WARNINGS** Intraoperative floppy iris syndrome (IFIS) has occurred in cataract surgery patients who were on or were previously treated with an alpha-1 blocker **SIDE EFFECTS** Weight gain, edema **NOTES** Take all forms of carvedilol with food to ↓ the rate of absorption and the risk of orthostatic hypotension Carvedilol CR has lower bioavailability than carvedilol IR; dosing conversions are not 1:1 (e.g., *Coreg* 3.125 mg BID = *Coreg CR* 10 mg daily)
Labetalol Tablet, injection	PO: 100-1,200 mg BID IV: 10-20 mg bolus, followed by 20-80 mg every 10 min or 0.5-2 mg/min continuous infusion titrated to a max of 10 mg/min	Same as above for carvedilol plus: **SIDE EFFECTS** Nausea **NOTES** Drug of choice in pregnancy Injection is commonly used in the hospital setting and can be administered by repeated IV push or slow continuous infusion

Beta-Blocker Drug Interactions

- Use caution when administering other drugs that ↓ HR, including diltiazem, verapamil, digoxin, clonidine, amiodarone and dexmedetomidine *(Precedex)*.

- Beta-blockers can enhance the hypoglycemic effects of insulin and sulfonylureas and mask some of the symptoms of hypoglycemia (e.g., shakiness, palpitations, anxiety); sweating, and possibly hunger, will still be present.

- Some beta-blockers can ↓ insulin secretion, causing hyperglycemia. Monitor blood glucose in diabetes.

- Carvedilol, propranolol, metoprolol and nebivolol are major substrates of CYP2D6. Monitor for drug interactions.

- Carvedilol and propranolol are inhibitors of P-gp and can increase the serum concentration of P-gp substrates (e.g., cyclosporine, dabigatran, digoxin, ranolazine).

CENTRALLY-ACTING ALPHA-2 ADRENERGIC AGONISTS

These drugs decrease BP by stimulating presynaptic alpha-2 adrenergic receptors in the brain; this decreases sympathetic outflow of norepinephrine, which leads to a reduction in SVR (and BP) and HR. Clonidine can be used for resistant hypertension and in patients who can not swallow (e.g., due to dysphagia, dementia) since it is available in a patch formulation. Since the patch is changed weekly, it can also help with adherence.

DRUG	DOSING	SAFETY/SIDE EFFECTS/MONITORING
Clonidine Tablet ER tablet: *Nexiclon XR* Patch: ***Catapres-TTS*** Injection: *Duraclon* – for epidural use only ***Kapvay*** – for ADHD	IR: 0.1-0.2 mg PO BID, max dose 2.4 mg daily ER: 0.17 mg QHS, max dose 0.52 mg QHS Patch: 0.1 mg/24 hr every 7 days; can titrate every 1-2 weeks up to 0.3 mg/24 hr strength patch	**WARNINGS** Do not discontinue abruptly (can cause rebound hypertension, sweating, anxiety, tremors); must taper gradually over 2-4 days **SIDE EFFECTS** Dry mouth, somnolence, fatigue, dizziness, constipation, ↓ HR, hypotension, impotence, headache, behavioral changes (irritability, confusion, anxiety, nightmares) Clonidine patch: skin rash, pruritus, erythema **MONITORING** BP, HR, mental status
Guanfacine IR **Guanfacine ER** **(Intuniv)** – for ADHD	0.5-2 mg QHS	**NOTES** Clonidine patch: apply weekly to a clean, dry and hairless area of skin on the upper outer arm or upper chest; remove before MRI; can apply the adhesive cover over the patch if it loosens; do not cut patch; takes 2-3 days to reach therapeutic effect; overlap is needed when transitioning from oral clonidine (consult package labeling)
Methyldopa	250 mg BID-TID; max dose is 3 grams daily	**CONTRAINDICATIONS** Concurrent use with MAO inhibitors and active liver disease **WARNINGS** Risk for hemolytic anemia (detected by a positive Coombs test), hepatic necrosis **SIDE EFFECTS** Drug-induced lupus erythematosus (DILE), edema or weight gain (control with diuretics), ↑ prolactin levels, transient sedation, headache **NOTES** Methyldopa can be used in pregnancy

DIRECT VASODILATORS

These drugs cause direct vasodilation of arterioles (little effect on veins), resulting in decreased SVR and BP.

DRUG	DOSING	SAFETY/SIDE EFFECTS/MONITORING
Hydralazine Tablet, injection	PO: 10-50 mg QID, max dose is 300 mg daily IM, IV: 10-20 mg Q4-6H PRN	**CONTRAINDICATIONS** Mitral valvular rheumatic heart disease, CAD **WARNINGS** Drug-induced lupus erythematosus (DILE – dose and duration related) **SIDE EFFECTS** Peripheral edema/headache/flushing/palpitations/reflex tachycardia, nausea/vomiting, peripheral neuritis, blood dyscrasias, hypotension **MONITORING** HR, BP, ANA titer
Minoxidil *Rogaine Mens,* *Rogaine Womens* – OTC topical for hair growth	5-40 mg daily in 1-3 divided doses, max dose is 100 mg daily	**BOXED WARNING** Potent vasodilator – can cause pericardial effusion (due to fluid retention) and angina exacerbations (due to reflex tachycardia); administer with a beta-blocker and loop diuretic **CONTRAINDICATION** Pheochromocytoma **SIDE EFFECTS** Hair growth, tachycardia, fluid retention (use caution in patients with heart failure or recent MI)

ALPHA-BLOCKERS

Alpha-blockers (e.g., doxazosin, prazosin, terazosin) inhibit alpha-1 adrenergic receptors, which results in peripheral vasodilation of arterioles and veins and a decrease in SVR. They are <u>not recommended</u> for hypertension but may be used in men who have hypertension and benign prostatic hyperplasia (see Benign Prostatic Hyperplasia chapter).

HYPERTENSIVE CRISES: URGENCIES AND EMERGENCIES

A hypertensive crisis is defined as an acute and <u>severe BP elevation</u> (generally ≥ 180/120 mmHg). The two types of crises are:

KEY IV MEDICATIONS FOR HYPERTENSIVE EMERGENCIES	
Clevidipine	Labetalol
Enalaprilat	Nicardipine
Esmolol	Nitroglycerin*
Hydralazine	Nitroprusside*

Vasodilators discussed in the Acute & Critical Care Medicine chapter

- Hypertensive <u>emergency</u>: patient has <u>acute target organ damage</u> that may be life-threatening (e.g., <u>encephalopathy, stroke, acute kidney injury, acute coronary syndrome</u>, aortic dissection, acute pulmonary edema).
  - ❏ Treat with <u>IV medications</u> (see <u>Key Drugs Guy</u>).
  - ❏ <u>Decrease BP by no more than 25% (within the first hour)</u>, then if stable, decrease to ~160/100 mmHg in the next 2 – 6 hours.
- Hypertensive <u>urgency</u> (severe asymptomatic hypertension): <u>no</u> evidence of <u>acute target organ damage</u>.
  - ❏ Treat with short-acting <u>oral medication</u> (e.g., captopril, clonidine) or restart chronic hypertension treatment.
  - ❏ Decrease BP <u>gradually over 24 – 48 hours</u>.

KEY COUNSELING POINTS

See the Drug Formulations and Patient Counseling chapter for counseling language/layman's terminology.

ALL HYPERTENSION PRODUCTS

- Can cause orthostasis.
- Check your blood pressure regularly.
- Take this medication as directed, even if you feel well.
  - ❏ Lowering blood pressure ↓ the risk of complications such as heart disease, kidney disease and stroke.

Thiazide Diuretics

- Take this medication early in the day (no later than 4 PM) to avoid getting up at night to go to the bathroom.
- Can cause:
  - ❏ Hyperglycemia.
  - ❏ Photosensitivity.
  - ❏ Sexual dysfunction.

Calcium Channel Blockers

- Can cause:
  - ❏ Peripheral edema.
  - ❏ Gingival hyperplasia.
- Ghost tablet in stool (*Procardia XL*).

ACE Inhibitors, ARBs and Aliskiren

- Avoid in pregnancy (teratogenic).
- Can cause:
  - ❏ Angioedema.
  - ❏ Dry, hacking cough.

Beta-Blockers

- Do not abruptly discontinue without consulting your healthcare provider.
- This medication can mask symptoms of low blood sugar. If you have diabetes, check blood sugar if you notice symptoms of sweating or hunger.
- Can cause sexual dysfunction.
- Take *Coreg/Coreg CR* with food.
- Take *Lopressor/Toprol XL* with or immediately after meals.

Clonidine

- Do not abruptly discontinue without consulting your healthcare provider.
- Patch: apply weekly to upper outer arm or chest. The white adhesive cover can be applied over the patch to keep it in place. Remove before an MRI. Do not cut the patch.
- Can cause sexual dysfunction.

Select Guidelines/References
2017 ACC/AHA/AAPA/ABC/ACPM/AGS/APhA/ASH/ASPC/NMA/PCNA guideline for the prevention, detection, evaluation, and management of high blood pressure: a report of the American College of Cardiology/American Heart Association Task Force on Clinical Practice Guidelines. *Hypertension* 2018;71:e13-e115.

CONTENT LEGEND

 = Study Tip Gal

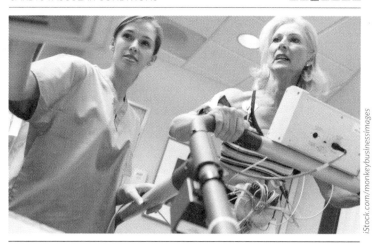

iStock.com/monkeybusinessimages

CHAPTER 29
STABLE ANGINA

BACKGROUND

Angina is chest pain, pressure, tightness or discomfort, usually caused by ischemia of the heart muscle or spasm of the coronary arteries. The chest pain is often described as "squeezing," "grip-like," "heavy" or "suffocating," and typically does not vary with position or respiration. In some patients (e.g., females, older adults, comorbid diabetes), angina may present as dyspnea, back pain or pain that mimics indigestion or GERD (e.g., burning, stabbing).

Stable angina, a type of chronic coronary disease (CCD), is associated with predictable chest pain, often brought on by exertion or emotional stress and relieved within minutes by rest or short-acting nitroglycerin. Unstable angina (UA) is a type of acute coronary syndrome (ACS); this is a medical emergency where the chest pain increases (in frequency, intensity or duration) and is not relieved with nitroglycerin or rest (see the Acute Coronary Syndromes chapter).

PATHOPHYSIOLOGY

Chest pain occurs when there is an imbalance between myocardial oxygen demand (workload) and supply (blood flow). Myocardial oxygen demand increases when the heart is working harder due to an increased heart rate, contractility or left ventricular wall tension [caused by increased preload (volume of blood returning to the heart) and/or afterload (systemic vascular resistance, or SVR)]. With stable angina, myocardial oxygen supply is often decreased due to atherosclerosis (plaque build up) within the inner walls of the coronary arteries. This is known as coronary artery disease (CAD); it causes narrowing of the arteries and reduced blood flow to the heart.

When chest pain is caused by coronary artery vasospasm, it is called vasospastic angina (or variant or Prinzmetal angina). This type of angina can occur at rest and can be caused by illicit drug use, particularly cocaine.

DIAGNOSIS

The risk factors for stable angina are similar to other types of heart disease, vascular disease and stroke, and include hypertension, smoking, dyslipidemia, diabetes, obesity and physical inactivity. To assess the likelihood of CAD and diagnose stable angina, a cardiac stress test or cardiac imaging is performed.

The cardiac stress test increases myocardial oxygen demand with either exercise (e.g., walking on a treadmill or pedaling a stationary exercise bicycle) or intravenous medications [adenosine, dipyridamole, dobutamine or regadenoson (Lexiscan)]. As myocardial oxygen demand increases, the patient is monitored for the development of symptoms (e.g., chest pain, dyspnea, lightheadedness), changes in heart rate and blood pressure or abnormalities (e.g., ST segment changes) on an ECG.

When the diagnosis of stable angina is certain, coronary angiography can be performed to assess the extent of atherosclerosis and need for revascularization.

EVALUATION OF STABLE ANGINA

History and physical

CBC, CK-MB, troponins (I or T), aPTT, PT/INR, lipid panel, glucose

ECG (at rest and during chest pain)

Cardiac stress test/stress imaging

Cardiac catheterization/angiography

NON-DRUG TREATMENT

Patients should be encouraged to follow a heart healthy diet (e.g., emphasizing fruits, vegetables, legumes, nuts, whole grains, lean proteins, < 2,300 mg/day of sodium, no trans fat), maintain a BMI of 18.5 – 24.9 kg/m², and maintain a waist circumference < 35 inches in females and < 40 inches in males.

Patients should engage in ≥ 150 minutes of moderate-intensity (or ≥ 75 minutes of high-intensity) aerobic activity per week, supplemented by an increase in daily lifestyle activities (e.g., walking breaks at work, gardening). Medically supervised programs, such as cardiac rehabilitation, are encouraged for at-risk patients.

Patients who smoke should quit, and secondhand smoke should be avoided. Alcohol intake should be limited to 1 drink/day (4 oz wine, 12 oz beer or 1 oz of spirits) for women and 1 – 2 drinks/day for men. Chronic NSAIDs should not be used.

DRUG TREATMENT

Stable angina is a type of atherosclerotic cardiovascular disease (ASCVD). Comorbid conditions (e.g., dyslipidemia, hypertension, diabetes) should be aggressively managed, and include the use of an ACE inhibitor or ARB (for hypertension and CAD) and a high-intensity statin (see the Dyslipidemia chapter). Vaccines (e.g., influenza, pneumococcal, COVID-19) should be administered per the Advisory Committee on Immunization Practices (ACIP) recommendations for patients with heart disease (see the Immunizations chapter).

The treatment goals for stable angina are to improve quality of life (by reducing chest pain episodes) and to prevent future cardiovascular events (e.g., MI, heart failure, death). This can be accomplished with an antiplatelet agent (for secondary prevention) and antianginal drug (to reduce chest pain).

Antiplatelet treatment prevents platelets from sticking together and forming a clot that can block an artery and reduce blood flow to the heart. Aspirin is the recommended antiplatelet; clopidogrel is used when there is an allergy or other contraindication to aspirin.

Dual antiplatelet therapy (DAPT) (e.g., concomitant aspirin and clopidogrel) is not useful for secondary prevention in patients with stable angina and is recommended only after recent ACS or percutaneous coronary intervention (PCI) (see the Acute Coronary Syndromes chapter). Low-dose rivaroxaban in combination with aspirin is indicated to reduce the risk of cardiovascular events in select patients with CAD or peripheral artery disease (PAD).

Antianginal treatment decreases myocardial oxygen demand or increases myocardial oxygen supply (see the Antianginal Treatment table later in the chapter). Beta-blockers, dihydropyridine (DHP) or non-dihydropyridine (non-DHP) calcium channel blockers (CCBs), or long-acting nitrates can be used to prevent symptoms. If the patient remains symptomatic with initial monotherapy, adding a second antianginal drug from a different therapeutic class is recommended. Ranolazine can be can be considered after these therapies, if needed. Short-acting nitroglycerin, as a sublingual (SL) tablet or translingual (TL) spray, is recommended for immediate relief of angina in all patients.

TREATMENT APPROACH FOR STABLE ANGINA

A – Antiplatelet and antianginal drugs

B – Blood pressure

C – Cholesterol (statins) and cigarettes (cessation)

D – Diet and diabetes

E – Exercise and education

ANTIPLATELET DRUGS

Aspirin irreversibly inhibits cyclooxygenase-1 and 2 (COX-1 and COX-2) enzymes, which results in decreased prostaglandin (PG) and thromboxane A2 (TXA2) production; TXA2 is a potent vasoconstrictor and inducer of platelet aggregation. Clopidogrel is a prodrug that irreversibly inhibits P2Y12 ADP-mediated platelet activation and aggregation. Refer to the Acute Coronary Syndromes chapter for an image depicting antiplatelet drug mechanisms of action.

DRUG	DOSING	SAFETY/SIDE EFFECTS/MONITORING
Aspirin (Bayer, Bufferin, Ecotrin, Ascriptin, Durlaza, Vazalore, others) OTC: tablet, chewable tablet, enteric-coated tablet, liquid-filled capsule, suppository Rx: ER capsule (Durlaza) + omeprazole (Yosprala) See the Pain chapter for more information on aspirin products	75-100 mg daily	**CONTRAINDICATIONS** NSAID or salicylate allergy; children and teenagers with a viral infection (due to the risk of Reye's syndrome, which has symptoms that include somnolence, N/V and confusion); rhinitis, nasal polyps or asthma (due to the risk of urticaria, angioedema or bronchospasm) **WARNINGS** Bleeding, including GI bleed/ulceration [↑ risk with heavy alcohol use or when used with other drugs that have bleeding risk (e.g., NSAIDs, anticoagulants, other antiplatelets)]; tinnitus (a sign of salicylate overdose) **SIDE EFFECTS** Dyspepsia, heartburn, bleeding, nausea **MONITORING** Symptoms of bleeding, bruising **NOTES** Used indefinitely in stable angina; ↓ incidence of CV events and death Non-enteric coated, chewable aspirin is preferred in ACS; if only enteric-coated (EC) aspirin is available, it should be chewed (325 mg) ER products (e.g., Durlaza) should not be used when rapid onset is needed (e.g., ACS, pre-PCI) To ↓ nausea, use EC or buffered product or take with food PPIs may be used to protect the GI tract from chronic aspirin use; consider the risks from chronic PPI use (↓ bone density, ↑ infection risk)
Clopidogrel (Plavix) Tablet	75 mg daily	**BOXED WARNING** Clopidogrel is a prodrug. Effectiveness depends on the conversion to an active metabolite, mainly by CYP450 2C19. Poor metabolizers of CYP2C19 exhibit higher cardiovascular events than patients with normal CYP2C19 function. Tests to check CYP2C19 genotype can be used as an aid in determining a therapeutic strategy. Consider alternative treatments in patients identified as CYP2C19 poor metabolizers. See the Pharmacogenomics chapter. **CONTRAINDICATIONS** Active serious bleeding (e.g., GI bleed, intracranial hemorrhage) **WARNINGS** Bleeding risk (stop 5 days prior to elective surgery); do not use with omeprazole or esomeprazole (see the Drug Interactions section); premature discontinuation (↑ risk of thrombosis); thrombotic thrombocytopenic purpura (TTP) **SIDE EFFECTS** Generally well tolerated, unless bleeding occurs **MONITORING** Symptoms of bleeding, Hgb/Hct as necessary **NOTES** Used in stable angina when there is a contraindication to aspirin

Antiplatelet Drug Interactions

- Most drug interactions are due to additive effects when antiplatelet drugs are used with other drugs that ↑ bleeding risk (e.g., anticoagulants, NSAIDs, SSRIs, SNRIs, some dietary supplements). See the Drug Interactions chapter.
- Aspirin: use caution in combination with other ototoxic drugs (see the Drug Interactions chapter).
- Clopidogrel: avoid moderate or strong CYP2C19 inhibitors (e.g., omeprazole, esomeprazole).

ANTIANGINAL TREATMENT

DRUG	MECHANISM OF CLINICAL BENEFIT	CLINICAL NOTES
Beta-Blockers See the Hypertension chapter for a complete review of beta-blockers	Reduce myocardial oxygen demand: ↓ HR, ↓ contractility and ↓ left ventricular wall tension	More effective than nitrates and CCBs for silent ischemia; avoid in vasospastic angina
Calcium Channel Blockers See the Hypertension chapter for a complete review of calcium channel blockers	Reduce myocardial oxygen demand: non-DHPs ↓ HR and contractility; DHPs ↓ SVR (afterload) Increase myocardial oxygen supply: all CCBs ↑ blood flow through coronary arteries	Slow-release or long-acting CCBs are effective; avoid nifedipine IR (short-acting DHP) DHPs are preferred when CCBs are used in combination with beta-blockers (due to the risk of excessive bradycardia when non-DHPs are used with beta-blockers) Preferred for vasospastic angina
Nitrates	Reduce myocardial oxygen demand: ↓ preload (free radical nitric oxide produces vasodilation of veins more than arteries) Increases myocardial oxygen supply: ↑ blood flow through collateral (non-atherosclerotic) arteries	**SL tablets or TL spray** Recommended for all patients for fast relief of anginal episodes **Long-acting nitrates** A nitrate-free interval is required to prevent tolerance (see the Nitrates table on next page)
Ranolazine (*Aspruzyo Sprinkle, Ranexa**)	Selectively inhibits the late phase Na current and ↓ intracellular Ca; can decrease myocardial oxygen demand by decreasing ventricular tension and oxygen consumption	**CONTRAINDICATIONS** Liver cirrhosis; do not use with strong CYP3A4 inhibitors or inducers **WARNINGS** QT prolongation Acute renal failure observed when CrCl < 30 mL/min **SIDE EFFECTS** Dizziness, headache, constipation, nausea **MONITORING** ECG, K, renal function **NOTES** Not for acute treatment of chest pain Can use as add-on treatment Has little to no clinical effects on HR or BP

Brand discontinued but name still used in practice.

Nitrates Used in Stable Angina*

FORMULATIONS	SAFETY/SIDE EFFECTS/MONITORING
Short-Acting Nitrates	**CONTRAINDICATIONS** Hypersensitivity to organic nitrates, do not use with PDE-5 inhibitors or soluble guanylate cyclase stimulators (e.g., riociguat) – see Nitrate Drug Interactions
Nitroglycerin SL tablet (Nitrostat) 0.3 mg, 0.4 mg, 0.6 mg	Short-acting nitrates: ↑ intracranial pressure, severe anemia, circulatory failure and shock
Nitroglycerin TL spray (NitroMist, Nitrolingual) 0.4 mg/spray	**WARNINGS** Hypotension, tachyphylaxis (tolerance/↓ effectiveness), can aggravate angina caused by hypertrophic cardiomyopathy
Long-Acting Nitrates	**SIDE EFFECTS** Headache, flushing, syncope, dizziness
Nitroglycerin ointment 2% (Nitro-Bid)	**MONITORING** BP, HR, chest pain
	NOTES **Short-acting nitrates** Used PRN for immediate relief of chest pain
Nitroglycerin transdermal patch (Nitro-Dur) 0.1, 0.2, 0.3, 0.4, 0.6, 0.8 mg/hr	Store nitroglycerin SL tablets in the original amber glass bottle and keep tightly capped after each use (to maintain potency)
Nitroglycerin ER capsule (Nitro-Time) 2.5 mg, 6 mg, 9 mg	**Long-acting nitrates** Require a 10-12 hour nitrate-free interval to ↓ tolerance (longer for some products)
Isosorbide mononitrate tablet IR: 10 mg, 20 mg ER: 30 mg, 60 mg, 120 mg	■ Patch: wear on for 12-14 hours, off for 10-12 hours; rotate sites; dispose of safely, away from children and pets ■ Ointment: dosed BID, 6 hours apart with a 10-12 hour nitrate-free interval
Isosorbide dinitrate IR (Isordil) IR: 5 mg, 10 mg, 20 mg, 30 mg, 40 mg	■ Isosorbide mononitrate: IR dosed BID, 7 hours apart (e.g., 8 AM and 3 PM); ER dosed once daily in the AM ■ Isosorbide dinitrate: IR dosed BID (same as above) or TID, take at 8 AM, 12 PM and 4 PM for a 14-hour nitrate-free interval (or similar) Isosorbide dinitrate in combination with hydralazine is the preferred combination for HFrEF

*IV nitroglycerin is discussed in the Acute & Critical Care Medicine chapter.

Nitrate Drug Interactions

■ Do not use long-acting nitrates in combination with PDE-5 inhibitors or soluble guanylate cyclase stimulators (e.g., riociguat); use caution with other antihypertensive medications and alcohol, as these combinations can cause a significant decrease in BP.

❏ Short-acting nitrates should not be used if a PDE-5 inhibitor was taken recently (avanafil in the past 12 hours, sildenafil or vardenafil in the past 24 hours or tadalafil in the past 48 hours). Occasionally, and with careful monitoring, nitrates can be used for an emergency (e.g., MI) in a patient who has recently taken a PDE-5 inhibitor.

Ranolazine Drug Interactions

■ Ranolazine is a major substrate of CYP3A4 and a minor substrate of CYP2D6 and P-gp. It is a weak inhibitor of CYP3A4, 2D6 and P-gp. Do not use with strong CYP3A4 inhibitors (e.g., protease inhibitors, cobicistat) or inducers.

KEY COUNSELING POINTS

See the Drug Formulations and Patient Counseling chapter for counseling language/layman's terminology.

ASPIRIN

- Can cause:
  - ❑ Bleeding/bruising.
  - ❑ Dyspepsia.
  - ❑ Allergic reaction.
  - ❑ Tinnitus or loss of hearing with overdose.

CLOPIDOGREL

- Can cause:
  - ❑ Bleeding/bruising.
  - ❑ Thrombotic thrombocytopenic purpura (TTP).

ALL NITRATE PRODUCTS

- Can cause:
  - ❑ Orthostasis.
  - ❑ Flushing and headache. Often a sign the medication is working. Usually goes away with time.
- Nitrate-free interval required with long-acting products.
- Drug interactions with phosphodiesterase-5 inhibitors.

SHORT-ACTING NITRATES

- Take one dose at first sign of chest pain.
- Call 911 immediately if chest pain persists after the first dose. Continue to take two additional doses at five minute intervals while waiting for the ambulance to arrive. Do not take more than three doses within 15 minutes.

Nitroglycerin SL Tablets

- Place the tablet under the tongue or between the inside of the cheek and the gums/teeth, and let it dissolve. Do not chew, crush or swallow.
- Slight burning or tingling sensation is not a sign of how well the medication is working.
- Keep tightly capped in the original amber glass bottle and store at room temperature. Remove one tablet only; do not let the other tablets get wet.

Nitroglycerin TL Spray

- Prime before first use and if not used within six weeks.
- Do not shake. Press the button firmly to release the spray onto or under the tongue. Close your mouth after the spray. Do not inhale the spray, and try not to swallow too quickly afterward. Do not spit or rinse the mouth for 5 – 10 minutes after the dose.

NITROGLYCERIN PATCH

- The chest is the preferred application site, though any area can be selected except the extremities below the knees or elbows.

NITROGLYCERIN OINTMENT

- Measure the dose of ointment with the dose-measuring applicator provided (see image below). Place the applicator on a flat surface, squeeze the ointment onto the applicator and place the applicator (ointment side down) on the chest or other desired area of the skin.
- Spread the ointment, using the dose-measuring applicator, lightly onto the skin. Do not rub into the skin. Tape the applicator into place.
- Can stain clothing. Cover the applicator completely.

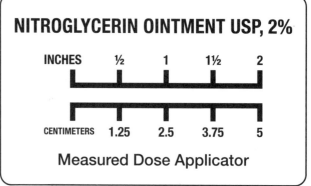

©UWorld

Select Guidelines/References
2023 AHA/ACC/ACCP/ASPC/NLA/PCNA guideline for the management of patients with chronic coronary disease. *Circulation.* 2023;148:e9-e119.

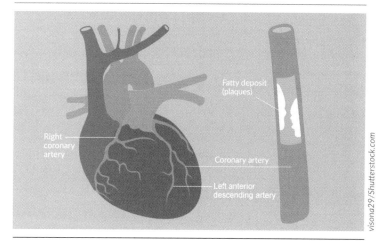

visona29/Shutterstock.com

CHAPTER 30
ACUTE CORONARY SYNDROMES

BACKGROUND

An acute coronary syndrome (ACS) results from plaque buildup (atherosclerosis) in the coronary arteries. The plaques are made up of fatty deposits that cause the arteries to narrow, making blood flow more difficult. The plaque can rupture, leading to clot (thrombus) formation and sudden, reduced blood flow (ischemia) to the heart. This causes an imbalance between myocardial oxygen supply and demand, resulting in symptoms (see section below) and/or cardiac muscle cell death (myocardial necrosis). Various risk factors (see box) can lead to plaque buildup, many of which are modifiable.

RISK FACTORS

Age: men > 45 years, women > 55 years (or early hysterectomy)	Known coronary artery disease
	Dyslipidemia
Family history: first-degree relative with a coronary event before 55 years (men) or 65 years (women)	Diabetes
	Chronic stable angina
Smoking	Lack of exercise
Hypertension	Excessive alcohol

SIGNS AND SYMPTOMS

The classic symptoms of an ACS include chest pain (often described as discomfort, pressure or squeezing) lasting ≥ 10 minutes, severe dyspnea, diaphoresis, syncope/presyncope and/or palpitations. The pain can radiate to the arms, back, neck, jaw or epigastric region. Females, the elderly and patients with diabetes are less likely to experience the classic symptoms. Symptoms can occur at rest, or may be precipitated by minimal exertion, exercise, cold weather, extreme emotions, stress or sexual intercourse. ACS is a medical emergency. Patients with a prescription for sublingual nitroglycerin (NTG) should use one dose every five minutes for up to three doses to relieve chest pain. If chest pain is not improved or is worse five minutes after the first dose, they should call 911 immediately.

DIAGNOSIS

ACS encompasses non-ST segment elevation acute coronary syndromes (NSTE-ACS) and ST-segment elevation myocardial infarction (STEMI). NSTE-ACS describes both unstable angina (UA) and non-ST segment elevation myocardial infarction (NSTEMI), which are indistinguishable upon presentation. The types of ACS are differentiated based on ECG findings, the detection of cardiac enzymes and the extent of blockage in the affected artery (see Study Tip Gal below).

A 12-lead ECG should be performed and evaluated within ten minutes at the site of first medical contact (which could be in an ambulance). Patients with an acute MI (STEMI or NSTEMI) should be urgently transported to a hospital with percutaneous coronary intervention (PCI) capability, if possible.

The measurement of biochemical markers (cardiac enzymes), released into the bloodstream when myocardial cells die, helps establish the diagnosis. Cardiac troponins I and T (TnI and TnT) are the most sensitive and specific biomarkers for ACS. Levels should be obtained at presentation and 3 – 6 hours after symptom onset in all patients with ACS symptoms. Creatine kinase myocardial isoenzyme (CK-MB) and myoglobin are less sensitive markers but may still be monitored in clinical practice.

COMPARING UA, NSTEMI AND STEMI

	UA	NSTEMI	STEMI
Symptoms	Chest pain (described in text)		
Cardiac Enzymes	Negative	Positive	Positive
ECG Changes	None or transient ischemic changes*		ST segment elevation**
Blockage	Partial blockage		Complete blockage

*ST segment depression or prominent T-wave inversion
**Meeting defined criteria in ≥ 2 contiguous leads (e.g., leads looking at the same area of the heart)

TREATMENT

Treatment is aimed at providing immediate relief of ischemia and preventing MI expansion and death.

PCI OR MEDICAL MANAGEMENT

PCI is a coronary revascularization procedure that involves inflating a small balloon inside a coronary artery to widen it and improve blood flow. Usually, a stent (metal mesh) is placed to keep the artery open.

- NSTE-ACS can be treated with medications alone (medical management) or with PCI (an early invasive strategy).

- A STEMI requires that the blocked arteries be opened as quickly as possible with PCI or fibrinolysis.

  ❑ PCI is preferred if it can be performed within 90 minutes of hospital arrival (optimal door-to-balloon time) or within 120 minutes of first medical contact (which could be in an ambulance).

  ❑ If PCI is not possible within 120 minutes of first medical contact, fibrinolytic therapy is recommended and should be given within 30 minutes of hospital arrival (door-to-needle time).

DRUG TREATMENT

A combination of antianginal, antiplatelet and anticoagulant medications are used in addition to PCI or fibrinolytics (see Study Tip Gal below and the summary table on the following page). These work by different mechanisms:

- Antianginals: decrease myocardial oxygen demand or increase supply (blood flow) to relieve ischemia.

- Antiplatelets: inhibit platelet aggregation to prevent clot formation/growth.

- Anticoagulants: inhibit clotting factors to prevent clot formation/growth.

DRUG TREATMENT OPTIONS FOR ACS

MONA-GAP-BA

Morphine	**G**PIIb/IIIa antagonists	Beta-blockers
Oxygen	**A**nticoagulants	ACE inhibitors
Nitrates	**P**2Y12 inhibitors	
Aspirin		

- NSTE-ACS: MONA-GAP-BA +/- PCI
- STEMI: MONA-GAP-BA + PCI or fibrinolytic (PCI preferred)

Colors correspond with the drug summary table on the following page

DRUGS FOR ACS (MONA-GAP-BA)

DRUG	CLINICAL BENEFIT	CLINICAL COMMENTS
Give these immediately (as needed)		
Morphine sulfate	Provides pain relief and helps anxiety	Not for routine use (has been shown to diminish antiplatelet effects); reserve for patients with unacceptable chest discomfort despite other treatments.
		Dose: 2-5 mg IV repeated at 5- to 30-minute intervals PRN. Monitor for hypotension, bradycardia, N/V, sedation and respiratory depression. See the Pain chapter for additional information.
Oxygen		Administer to patients with arterial oxygen saturation < 90% (SaO2 < 90%) or those with respiratory distress.
Nitrates	Antianginal: dilate coronary arteries and improve collateral blood flow; ↓ preload and afterload (modestly); reduces chest pain	Sublingual NTG (0.4 mg every 5 minutes x 3 doses) if not already administered and the patient has persistent chest pain, hypertension or heart failure. IV NTG can be considered if symptoms persist. Do not use IV NTG if SBP < 90 mmHg, HR < 50 bpm or the patient is experiencing a right ventricular infarction. PDE-5 inhibitors are contraindicated with NTG. See the Stable Angina and Sexual Dysfunction chapters for additional details.
Aspirin	See the Antiplatelet Drugs section and image on the following page	Non-enteric-coated, chewable aspirin (162-325 mg) should be given to all patients immediately if no contraindications are present (do not use extended-release aspirin products). A maintenance dose of aspirin 75 -100 mg daily should be continued indefinitely. If intolerant to aspirin, clopidogrel or ticagrelor (discussed later in this chapter) may be used.
Give these next [choice of drug/s relates to plan (PCI vs. CABG vs. medical management)]		
GPIIb/IIIa receptor antagonists	See the Antiplatelet Drugs section and image on the following page	Drugs include abciximab, eptifibatide and tirofiban.
Anticoagulants	Inhibit clotting factors and can reduce infarct size	Drugs include LMWHs (e.g., enoxaparin, dalteparin), UFH and bivalirudin (preferred for STEMI). See the Anticoagulation chapter.
P2Y12 Inhibitors	See the Antiplatelet Drugs section and image on the following page	Drugs include clopidogrel, prasugrel and ticagrelor.
Give within 24 hours (as needed); continue as an outpatient		
Beta-Blockers	Antianginal: ↓ BP, HR and contractility; ↓ ischemia, reinfarction and arrhythmias; prevent cardiac remodeling; ↑ long-term survival	An oral, low dose beta-blocker (beta-1 selective blocker without intrinsic sympathomimetic activity preferred) should be started within the first 24 hours unless contraindicated (e.g., decompensated heart failure, cardiogenic shock, HR < 45 bpm). If the patient has concomitant HFrEF that is stable, choose bisoprolol, metoprolol succinate or carvedilol (see the Chronic Heart Failure chapter). An IV beta-blocker or an oral long-acting non-dihydropyridine calcium channel blocker (verapamil or diltiazem) are alternative options used in some situations.
ACE Inhibitors	Inhibit angiotensin-converting enzyme (ACE) and block the production of angiotensin II; prevent cardiac remodeling; ↓ preload and afterload	An oral ACE inhibitor should be started within the first 24 hours and continued indefinitely in all patients with left ventricular ejection fraction (LVEF) < 40%), hypertension, diabetes or stable CKD, unless contraindicated (use an ARB if the patient is ACE inhibitor intolerant). Use of an ACE inhibitor in other patients may be reasonable. Do not use an IV ACE inhibitor within the first 24 hours due to the risk of hypotension. See the Hypertension chapter.

Medications to Avoid in the Acute Setting

- NSAIDs (except aspirin), whether nonselective or COX-2-selective, should not be administered during hospitalization due to ↑ risk of mortality, reinfarction, hypertension, cardiac rupture, renal insufficiency and heart failure.

- Immediate-release nifedipine should not be used due to ↑ risk of mortality.

ANTIPLATELET DRUGS

The antiplatelet drugs used in ACS <u>inhibit</u> <u>platelet aggregation</u> and clot formation by different mechanisms (see the platelet image to the right):

- Aspirin: <u>irreversibly inhibits COX-1</u> and <u>COX-2</u>, which <u>decreases</u> the production of <u>thromboxane A2 (TXA2)</u> (an inducer of platelet aggregation).

- P2Y12 inhibitors: <u>bind</u> to the platelet <u>adenosine diphosphate (ADP) P2Y12 receptor</u>, preventing ADP-mediated activation of the GPIIb/IIIa receptor complex.

- GPIIb/IIIa receptor antagonists: <u>block</u> the platelet glycoprotein IIb/IIIa receptor, which is the binding site for fibrinogen, von Willebrand factor and other ligands.

- Protease-activated receptor-1 antagonist: <u>binds</u> to the <u>PAR-1</u> receptor, preventing thrombin- and thrombin receptor agonist peptide-induced platelet aggregation.

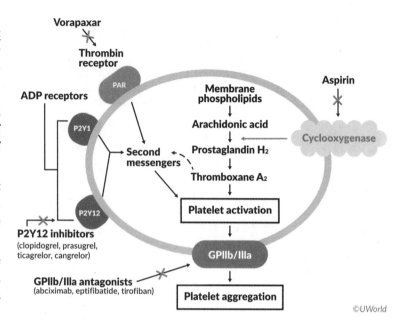

P2Y12 Inhibitors

<u>Clopidogrel and prasugrel</u> are structurally similar and are classified as <u>thienopyridines</u>. They are <u>prodrugs</u> that <u>irreversibly</u> <u>bind</u> to the <u>P2Y12 receptor</u>. Ticagrelor is not a prodrug and has reversible binding to the receptor. P2Y12 inhibitors are commonly <u>used with aspirin</u> after an ACS, which is called <u>dual antiplatelet therapy (DAPT)</u>. A higher one-time <u>loading dose</u> is required for P2Y12 inhibitors, either prior to PCI or at the time of diagnosis if PCI is not being performed, followed by a <u>maintenance dose</u>.

DRUG	DOSING	SAFETY/SIDE EFFECTS/MONITORING
Clopidogrel (*Plavix*) Tablet	LD: 300-600 mg PO (600 mg for PCI) MD: <u>75 mg PO daily</u> If age > 75 years and fibrinolytic therapy administered for STEMI, omit the loading dose and start 75 mg daily	**BOXED WARNINGS** Clopidogrel is a <u>prodrug</u>. Effectiveness depends on the <u>conversion</u> to an <u>active metabolite</u>, mainly by <u>CYP450 2C19</u>. Poor metabolizers of CYP2C19 exhibit higher cardiovascular events than patients with normal CYP2C19 function. <u>Tests to check CYP2C19 genotype</u> can be used as an aid in determining a therapeutic strategy. Consider alternative treatments in patients identified as CYP2C19 poor metabolizers. See the Pharmacogenomics chapter. **CONTRAINDICATIONS** Active <u>serious bleeding</u> (e.g., GI bleed, intracranial hemorrhage) **WARNINGS** <u>Bleeding risk (stop 5 days prior to elective surgery)</u>, do not use with <u>omeprazole or esomeprazole</u> (see P2Y12 Drug Interactions on the following page), premature discontinuation (↑ risk of thrombosis), thrombotic thrombocytopenic purpura (<u>TTP</u>) **SIDE EFFECTS** Generally well tolerated, unless <u>bleeding</u> occurs

DRUG	DOSING	SAFETY/SIDE EFFECTS/MONITORING
Prasugrel (*Effient*) Tablet Only indicated for ACS managed with PCI	LD: 60 mg PO (no later than 1 hour after PCI) MD: 10 mg PO daily with aspirin (5 mg daily if patient weighs < 60 kg) Once PCI is planned, give the dose promptly and no later than 1 hour after the PCI Protect from moisture; dispense in the original container	**BOXED WARNINGS** Significant, sometimes fatal, bleeding Not recommended in patients ≥ 75 years due to high bleeding risk, unless patient is considered high risk (diabetes or prior MI) Do not initiate if CABG likely, stop at least 7 days prior to elective surgery **CONTRAINDICATIONS** Active serious bleeding, history of TIA or stroke **WARNINGS** Bleeding risk, premature discontinuation (↑ risk of thrombosis), thrombotic thrombocytopenic purpura (TTP) **SIDE EFFECTS** Generally well-tolerated, unless bleeding occurs (higher risk than clopidogrel)
Ticagrelor (*Brilinta*) Tablet	LD: 180 mg MD: 90 mg PO BID for 1 year, then 60 mg BID Tablets can be crushed and mixed with water (to be swallowed or given via an NG tube)	**BOXED WARNINGS** Significant, sometimes fatal, bleeding After the initial aspirin dose of 162-325 mg, do not exceed a maintenance dose of 100 mg daily because higher daily doses reduce the effectiveness of ticagrelor Avoid use when CABG likely, stop 5 days before any surgery **CONTRAINDICATIONS** Active serious bleeding, history of intracranial hemorrhage **WARNINGS** Bleeding risk, severe hepatic impairment, bradyarrhythmias, premature discontinuation (↑ risk of thrombosis), thrombotic thrombocytopenic purpura (TTP) **SIDE EFFECTS** Bleeding, dyspnea (> 10%), ↑ SCr, ↑ uric acid
Cangrelor (*Kengreal*) Injection Only indicated as an adjunct to PCI in patients who are P2Y12 inhibitor naïve and are not receiving a GPIIb/IIIa inhibitor	30 mcg/kg IV bolus prior to PCI, then 4 mcg/kg/min IV infusion for 2 hours or for the duration of the procedure (whichever is longer)	**CONTRAINDICATIONS** Significant active bleeding **SIDE EFFECTS** Bleeding **NOTES** Effects are gone 1 hour after drug discontinuation Transition to one of the oral P2Y12 inhibitors after PCI

LD = loading dose, MD = maintenance dose

P2Y12 Inhibitor Drug Interactions

- Most drug interactions are due to additive effects when used with other drugs that ↑ bleeding risk. If an ACS patient experiences bleeding while on a P2Y12 inhibitor, it should be managed without discontinuing the P2Y12 inhibitor, if possible. Stopping the P2Y12 inhibitor (particularly within the first few months after ACS) ↑ the risk of subsequent cardiovascular events.

  ❏ NSAIDs, warfarin, SSRIs and SNRIs increase bleeding risk. See the Drug Interactions chapter.

- Clopidogrel: avoid in combination with the CYP2C19 inhibitors esomeprazole and omeprazole due to the risk of a decreased antiplatelet effect. Use caution with other CYP2C19 inhibitors.

- Ticagrelor is a major CYP3A4 substrate; avoid use with strong CYP3A4 inhibitors or inducers (see the Drug Interactions chapter). Avoid simvastatin and lovastatin doses greater than 40 mg/day.

- Monitor digoxin levels with initiation of or any change in ticagrelor dose.

- Clopidogrel increases the effects of repaglinide, which can cause hypoglycemia. Avoid using this combination.

Glycoprotein IIb/IIIa Receptor Antagonists

Eptifibatide and tirofiban have reversible blockade of the GPIIb/IIIa receptor. They are an option for medical management of ACS or patients receiving a PCI ± stent. Abciximab (which is not currently available) has irreversible blockade of the receptor and is only indicated for PCI ± stent. If used in PCI, the GPIIb/IIIa receptor antagonist is given with heparin.

DRUG	DOSING	SAFETY/SIDE EFFECTS/MONITORING
Eptifibatide (*Integrilin***) Injection	LD: 180 mcg/kg IV bolus (max 22.6 mg), repeat bolus in 10 min if undergoing PCI MD: 2 mcg/kg/min (max 15 mg/hr) IV infusion started after the first bolus; continue for 18-24 hrs after PCI or for 12-72 hrs if PCI was not performed CrCl < 50 mL/min: same LD, reduce MD to 1 mcg/kg/min (max 7.5 mg/hr)	**CONTRAINDICATIONS** Thrombocytopenia (platelets < 100,000 cells/mm^3) History of bleeding diathesis (i.e., a bleeding predisposition) Active internal bleeding Severe uncontrolled hypertension Recent major surgery or trauma (within the past 4 weeks for tirofiban and past 6 weeks for eptifibatide) History of stroke within 30 days or any history of hemorrhagic stroke (eptifibatide)
Tirofiban (*Aggrastat*) Injection	LD: 25 mcg/kg IV bolus over 5 min or less MD: 0.15 mcg/kg/min IV infusion for up to 18 hrs CrCl ≤ 60 mL/min: same LD, reduce MD to 0.075 mcg/kg/min	**SIDE EFFECTS** Bleeding, thrombocytopenia **MONITORING** Hgb, Hct, platelets, s/sx of bleeding, renal function
Abciximab* Injection	Not recommended for medical management (NSTE-ACS without PCI)	**NOTES** Do not shake vials Platelet function returns in ~4-8 hours after stopping eptifibatide or tirofiban

Currently unavailable in the U.S.
**Brand discontinued but name still used in practice.
LD = loading dose, MD = maintenance dose

Protease-Activated Receptor-1 Antagonist

Vorapaxar is indicated in patients with a history of MI or peripheral arterial disease (PAD) to reduce thrombotic cardiovascular events (e.g., CV death, MI, stroke, urgent coronary revascularization). This drug was used in addition to aspirin and/or clopidogrel in clinical trials.

DRUG	DOSING	SAFETY/SIDE EFFECTS/MONITORING
Vorapaxar (*Zontivity*) Tablet	2.08 mg (one tablet) PO daily	**BOXED WARNING** Bleeding risk (including ICH and fatal bleeding); do not use in patients with a history of stroke, TIA, ICH or active serious bleeding **WARNING** Do not use in severe liver impairment **SIDE EFFECTS** Bleeding, anemia

Vorapaxar Drug Interactions

■ Vorapaxar is a substrate of CYP3A4 and an inhibitor of P-gp. Avoid use with strong CYP3A4 inhibitors or inducers.

FIBRINOLYTICS

These medications cause fibrinolysis (clot breakdown) by binding to fibrin and converting plasminogen to plasmin. Fibrinolytics are used only for STEMI. Once a STEMI is confirmed on a 12-lead ECG, timing is critical to open the blocked artery or arteries as quickly as possible with either PCI or fibrinolytic therapy (see PCI or Medical Management earlier in the chapter). When fibrinolytic therapy is used, it should be given within 30 minutes of hospital arrival (door-to-needle time); survival is improved when fibrinolytics are given promptly. In the absence of contraindications, and when PCI is not available, fibrinolytic therapy is reasonable in STEMI patients who are still symptomatic within 12 – 24 hours of symptom onset.

DRUG	DOSING	SAFETY/SIDE EFFECTS/MONITORING
Alteplase *(Activase)* Recombinant tissue plasminogen activator (tPA, rtPA)* **Cathflo Activase** (single-use 2 mg vial) used to restore function of potentially clotted central lines and devices	Accelerated Infusion > 67 kg: 100 mg IV over 1.5 hrs, given as a 15 mg bolus, 50 mg over 30 min, then 35 mg over 1 hr ≤ 67 kg: 15 mg bolus, 0.75 mg/kg (max 50 mg) over 30 min, then 0.5 mg/kg (max 35 mg) over 1 hr (max 100 mg total)	**CONTRAINDICATIONS** Active internal bleeding or bleeding diathesis History of recent stroke Any prior intracranial hemorrhage (ICH) Recent intracranial or intraspinal surgery or trauma (in the last 2-3 months) Intracranial neoplasm, arteriovenous malformation or aneurysm Severe uncontrolled hypertension (unresponsive to emergency therapy)
Tenecteplase *(TNKase)*	Single IV bolus dose: < 60 kg: 30 mg 60-69 kg: 35 mg 70-79 kg: 40 mg 80-89 kg: 45 mg ≥ 90 kg: 50 mg	**SIDE EFFECTS** Bleeding (including ICH) **MONITORING** Hgb, Hct, s/sx of bleeding
Reteplase *(Retavase)*	2 dose regimen: 10 units IV, followed by 10 units IV given 30 minutes later	**NOTES** Alteplase contraindications and dosing differ when used for ischemic stroke (refer to the Stroke chapter)

*The abbreviation "tPA" is prone to errors; though it is used commonly, it is not recommended by ISMP.

SECONDARY PREVENTION AFTER ACS

ACS is one of the conditions included in the definition of atherosclerotic cardiovascular disease (ASCVD), discussed in the Dyslipidemia chapter. Taking the right medications after an ACS can reduce the risk of complications (e.g., heart failure) or future events. Many of the recommended medications will be taken indefinitely (see Study Tip Gal).

DRUGS FOR SECONDARY PREVENTION AFTER ACS

Aspirin
- Indefinitely (typically 81 mg per day), unless contraindicated

P2Y12 Inhibitor
- Medical management patients: ticagrelor or clopidogrel* with aspirin 81 mg for at least 12 months
- PCI-treated patients (including any type of stent): clopidogrel, prasugrel or ticagrelor with aspirin 81 mg for at least 12 months
    - ❏ Continuation of DAPT beyond 12 months may be considered in patients who are tolerating DAPT and are not at high risk of bleeding following coronary stent placement

Nitroglycerin
- Indefinitely (SL tablets or spray PRN)

Beta-Blocker
- 3 years; continue indefinitely in patients with heart failure or if needed for management of hypertension

ACE Inhibitor
- Indefinitely in patients with EF < 40%, hypertension, CKD or diabetes; consider for all MI patients with no contraindications

Aldosterone Antagonist (see Chronic Heart Failure chapter)
- Indefinitely in patients with EF ≤ 40% and symptomatic heart failure or diabetes receiving target doses of an ACE inhibitor and beta-blocker
- Contraindications: significant renal impairment (SCr > 2.5 mg/dL in men, SCr > 2 mg/dL in women) or hyperkalemia (K > 5 mEq/L)

Statin (see Dyslipidemia chapter)
- Indefinitely; high-intensity statin for most patients
- Patients ≥ 75 years of age: consider moderate- or high-intensity statin

In a patient with a STEMI that received fibrinolytics, clopidogrel is the guideline-recommended P2Y12 inhibitor.

OTHER CONSIDERATIONS

- Pain relief: patients with chronic musculoskeletal pain should use acetaminophen, nonacetylated salicylates, tramadol or small doses of narcotics before considering the use of NSAIDs. If these options are insufficient, it is reasonable to use nonselective NSAIDs such as naproxen (lowest CV risk). COX-2 selective NSAIDs have high CV risk and should be avoided.

- ACS + atrial fibrillation (AF): dual or triple antithrombotic therapy can be used in patients who require anticoagulation for AF and DAPT after PCI with a stent. If using triple therapy, use it for the shortest time possible. Clopidogrel is the preferred P2Y12 inhibitor for triple therapy and a transition to dual therapy (anticoagulant + P2Y12 inhibitor) can be considered after 4 – 6 weeks. Proton pump inhibitors should be prescribed in any patient with a history of GI bleeding while taking triple antithrombotic therapy.

- Lifestyle counseling should include smoking cessation, managing chronic conditions (such as hypertension and diabetes), avoiding excessive alcohol intake, encouraging physical exercise and a healthy diet.

KEY COUNSELING POINTS

Refer to the Stable Angina chapter for patient counseling on aspirin, nitrates and clopidogrel.

Select Guidelines/References

2017 ESC Guidelines for the Management of Acute Myocardial Infarction in Patients Presenting with ST-Segment Elevation. European Heart Journal. 2018 Jan, 39(2) 119-177.

2016 ACC/AHA Guideline Focused Update on Duration of Dual Antiplatelet Therapy in Patients With Coronary Artery Disease. J Am Coll Cardiol. 2016 Sep, 68(10) 1082-1115.

2014 AHA/ACC Guideline for the Management of Patients with Non-ST-Elevation Acute Coronary Syndromes. J Am Coll Cardiol. 2014 Dec, 64(24) e139-e228.

2013 ACCF/AHA Guideline for Management of ST-Elevation Myocardial Infarction. J Am Coll Cardiol. 2013 Jan, 61(4) e78-e140.

CONTENT LEGEND

 = Study Tip Gal   = Key Drug Guy

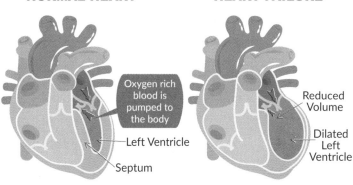

NORMAL HEART   **HEART FAILURE**

Oxygen rich blood is pumped to the body

Left Ventricle

Septum

Reduced Volume

Dilated Left Ventricle

iStock.com/Lin Shao-hua

CHAPTER 31
CHRONIC HEART FAILURE

BACKGROUND

Heart failure (HF) is a common condition in the U.S., especially in older adults. It is the primary diagnosis in over 1 million hospitalizations each year. Heart "failure" occurs when the heart is not able to supply sufficient oxygen-rich blood to the body, because of impaired ability of the left ventricle to either fill with or eject blood. This occurs due to a problem with systolic (contraction) or diastolic (relaxation) functions of the heart.

HF is commonly classified as either ischemic (due to decreased blood supply to the heart), such as from an MI, or non-ischemic, such as from long-standing uncontrolled hypertension. Less common causes include valvular disease, excessive alcohol intake, illicit drug use, congenital heart defects, viral infections, diabetes and cardiotoxic drugs/chest radiation.

DIAGNOSIS

Symptoms of HF are usually related to fluid overload, which commonly presents as shortness of breath (SOB) and edema (see Study Tip Gal on the next page). Patients can fluctuate between periods of stability and exacerbation (increased symptoms). Exacerbations frequently result in hospitalization and negatively impact quality of life.

An ultrasound of the heart (echocardiography or echo) is performed when HF is suspected. It provides an estimate of left ventricular ejection fraction (LVEF), or how much blood is pumped out of the left ventricle (the main pumping chamber of the heart) with each contraction. The term LVEF is used interchangeably with ejection fraction (EF). An EF < 40% indicates systolic dysfunction, or heart failure with reduced ejection fraction (HFrEF). HFrEF is the focus of this chapter, since it has well-defined treatment guidelines. Evidence-based treatments for other types of HF are also included as appropriate.

EJECTION FRACTION

EF	TERM	PRIMARY PROBLEM
55-70%	Normal	Normal
≥ 50%	Heart Failure with Preserved EF (HFpEF) Diastolic Dysfunction	Impaired ventricular relaxation and filling during diastole
41-49%	Heart Failure with Mildly Reduced EF (HFmrEF)	Likely mixed systolic and diastolic dysfunction
≤ 40%	Heart Failure with Reduced EF (HFrEF) Systolic Dysfunction	Impaired ability to eject blood during systole
≤ 40% at baseline but improves to > 40%	Heart Failure with Improved EF (HFimpEF)	EF improved with treatment; classified separately because treatments for HFrEF should be continued, despite higher EF

CLASSIFICATION SYSTEMS

The American College of Cardiology and the American Heart Association (ACC/AHA) recommend categorizing patients by HF stage (see table below). The staging system is used to guide treatment in order to slow progression of structural heart disease [e.g., left ventricular hypertrophy (LVH), low EF] in asymptomatic patients (stages A and B) or in symptomatic patients (stages C and D). "Biomarkers" in the definitions refer to BNP and NT-proBNP (discussed later). HF can also be classified by the level of limitation in physical functioning using the New York Heart Association (NYHA) classification system. Many drugs were studied based on the NYHA functional classification of patients, so this remains extremely relevant to drug therapy decisions.

ACC/AHA STAGING SYSTEM		NYHA FUNCTIONAL CLASS	
A	At risk for HF, but without symptoms, structural heart disease or elevated biomarkers. Examples: patients with hypertension, ASCVD or diabetes.		No corresponding category
B	Pre-HF; structural heart disease, abnormal cardiac function or elevated biomarkers, but without signs or symptoms of HF. Examples: patients with LVH, low EF, valvular disease.	I	No limitations of physical activity. Ordinary physical activity does not cause symptoms of HF (e.g., fatigue, palpitations, dyspnea).
Clinical Diagnosis of HF			
C	Structural and/or functional cardiac abnormalities with prior or current symptoms of HF. Example: a patient with known structural heart disease (e.g., LVH) plus shortness of breath, fatigue and reduced exercise tolerance.	I	No limitations of physical activity. Ordinary physical activity does not cause symptoms of HF.
		II	Slight limitation of physical activity. Comfortable at rest, but ordinary physical activity (e.g., walking up stairs) results in symptoms of HF.
		III	Marked limitation of physical activity. Comfortable at rest but minimal exertion (e.g., bathing, dressing) causes symptoms of HF.
		IV	Unable to carry on any physical activity without symptoms of HF, or symptoms of HF at rest (e.g., SOB while sitting in a chair).
D	Advanced (refractory) HF with severe symptoms or recurrent hospitalizations despite maximal treatment.	IV	Unable to carry on any physical activity without symptoms of HF, or symptoms of HF at rest (e.g., SOB while sitting in a chair).

SIGNS AND SYMPTOMS OF HEART FAILURE

Labs/Biomarkers

↑ BNP (B-type natriuretic peptide): normal is < 100 pg/mL

↑ NT-proBNP (N-terminal proBNP): normal is < 300 pg/mL

BNP and proBNP are used to distinguish between cardiac and non-cardiac causes of dyspnea

General Signs and Symptoms

Dyspnea (SOB at rest or upon exertion)

Cough

Fatigue, weakness

Reduced exercise capacity

Left-Sided Signs and Symptoms

Orthopnea: SOB when lying flat

Paroxysmal nocturnal dyspnea (PND): nocturnal cough and SOB

Bibasilar rales: crackling lung sounds heard on lung exam

S3 gallop: abnormal heart sound

Hypoperfusion (renal impairment, cool extremities)

Right-Sided Signs and Symptoms

Peripheral edema

Ascites: abdominal fluid accumulation

Jugular venous distention (JVD): neck vein distention

Hepatojugular reflux (HJR): neck vein distention from pressure placed on the abdomen

Hepatomegaly: enlarged liver due to fluid congestion

PATHOPHYSIOLOGY

TERMINOLOGY

Cardiac output (CO) is the volume of blood that is pumped by the heart in one minute. CO is determined by heart rate (HR) and stroke volume (SV), or the volume of blood ejected from the left ventricle during one complete heartbeat (cardiac cycle). SV depends on preload, afterload and contractility. The cardiac index (CI) relates the CO to the size of the patient, using the body surface area (BSA).

CO = HR x SV	CI = CO / BSA

COMPENSATORY MECHANISMS

HFrEF is a low cardiac output state. The body compensates by activating neurohormonal pathways to increase blood volume or the force or speed of contractions. This can temporarily increase CO, but chronically leads to myocyte damage and cardiac remodeling. This causes changes in the size, composition and shape of the heart (e.g., hypertrophy, dilatation).

The main pathways that are activated in HF are the renin-angiotensin-aldosterone system (RAAS), the sympathetic nervous system (SNS) and vasopressin (see diagram in Drug Treatment section). The neurohormones that normally balance these systems (e.g., natriuretic peptides) become insufficient.

RAAS and Vasopressin Activation

- Renin converts angiotensinogen to angiotensin I.
- Angiotensin I is converted to angiotensin II (Ang II) by angiotensin-converting enzyme (ACE).
- Ang II causes vasoconstriction and stimulates release of aldosterone from the adrenal gland and vasopressin from the pituitary gland.
- Aldosterone causes sodium and water retention and increases potassium excretion.
- Vasopressin causes vasoconstriction and water retention.

SNS Activation

- Norepinephrine (NE) and epinephrine (Epi) release cause an increase in HR, contractility (positive inotropy) and vasoconstriction.

LIFESTYLE MANAGEMENT

Patients with HF should be instructed to:

- Monitor and document body weight daily, in the morning after voiding and before eating.
- Notify the provider if weight ↑ by 2 – 4 pounds in one day or ≥ 5 pounds in one week, or if symptoms worsen (e.g., SOB with activity, or others listed in the Study Tip Gal on the previous page). A HF action plan should be provided and explained to the patient (see example at end of chapter).
- Avoid excessive sodium intake in all patients. Consider restricting to < 1,500 mg/day in those with hypertension.
- Restrict fluid (1.5 – 2 L/day) in stage D HF.
- Stop smoking. Limit alcohol intake. Do not use illicit drugs.
- Obtain recommended vaccines: influenza (annually) and pneumococcal vaccines per ACIP guidelines (see Immunizations chapter).
- Reduce weight to BMI < 30 kg/m^2 to decrease the heart's workload and preserve function.
- Exercise (or perform regular physical activity, if able).

Natural Products

- Omega-3 fatty acid (fish oil) supplementation is reasonable to ↓ mortality and cardiovascular hospitalizations.
- Hawthorn and coenzyme Q10 may improve HF symptoms.
- Avoid the use of products containing ephedra (ma huang) or ephedrine.

DRUGS THAT CAUSE OR WORSEN HEART FAILURE

Most drugs that cause or worsen HF cause fluid retention/ edema, increase blood pressure or have negative inotropic effects (see Key Drugs Guy below).

SELECT DRUGS THAT CAUSE OR WORSEN HEART FAILURE

KEY DRUGS

Remember: It's the
Drug **I**nformation **NATION**

Dipeptidyl peptidase 4 inhibitors
  ❑ Alogliptin, saxagliptin

Immunosuppressants
  ❑ TNF inhibitors (e.g., adalimumab, etanercept) and interferons

Non-dihydropyridine CCBs
  ❑ Diltiazem and verapamil (if LVEF < 50%)

Antiarrhythmics
  ❑ Class I agents (e.g., quinidine, flecainide) and dronedarone
  ❑ Amiodarone and dofetilide are preferred in patients with HF

Thiazolidinediones

Itraconazole

Oncology drugs
  ❑ Anthracyclines (doxorubicin, daunorubicin)

NSAIDs

Cilostazol

Systemic steroids

Sympathomimetics (stimulants), illicit drugs (e.g., cocaine)

Triptans

Oncology drugs: Some tyrosine kinase inhibitors (e.g., imatinib, lapatinib, sunitinib), trastuzumab, docetaxel

Excessive alcohol

DRUG TREATMENT

The diagram below reviews the pathophysiology and neurohormonal targets for select drugs used to treat HF. Guideline-directed medical therapy (GDMT) for HFrEF ↓ morbidity and mortality and consists of four main drug classes: a RAAS inhibitor [angiotensin receptor and neprilysin inhibitor (ARNI), ACE inhibitor or angiotensin receptor blocker (ARB)], an evidence-based beta-blocker, an aldosterone receptor antagonist (ARA) and a sodium-glucose cotransporter 2 (SGLT2) inhibitor (see Study Tip Gal). Medications may be started simultaneously (at low doses) or sequentially (without achieving target doses before initiating the next medication). The goal is for all medications to be titrated to target doses as tolerated.

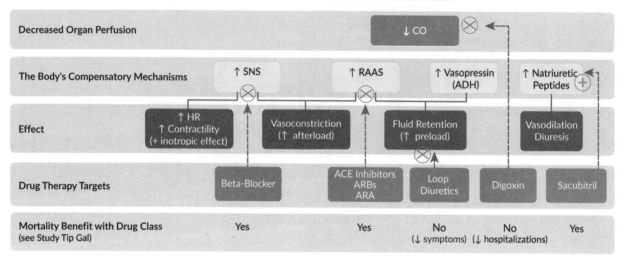

©UWorld

HFrEF TREATMENT

Guideline-Directed Medical Therapy (GDMT), recommended for all patients without contraindications

- **Angiotensin receptor and neprilysin inhibitor (ARNI), ACE inhibitor or angiotensin receptor blocker (ARB)**
  - ❑ ↓ morbidity and mortality
  - ❑ ARNI is preferred over an ACE inhibitor/ARB to further reduce morbidity and mortality
- **Beta-blocker (BB)**
  - ❑ Select agents provide benefit in ↓ mortality and hospitalizations
- **Aldosterone receptor antagonist (ARA)**
  - ❑ ↓ morbidity and mortality in NYHA Class II-IV HF
  - ❑ Must meet eGFR, SCr and potassium criteria for use
- **Sodium-glucose cotransporter 2 (SGLT2) inhibitor**
  - ❑ ↓ hospitalizations and mortality in patients with or without diabetes
  - ❑ Must meet eGFR criteria for use

Additional medications, add on in select patients

- **Loop diuretics**
  - ❑ Reduce blood volume, which ↓ edema and congestion; most HF patients need a loop diuretic for symptom relief
- **Hydralazine and nitrate (*BiDil*)**
  - ❑ ↓ morbidity and mortality in self-identified Black patients with NYHA Class III-IV HF when added to optimized (i.e., titrated to target doses) initial medications; can be considered for patients who cannot receive a RAAS inhibitor (e.g., ARNI, ACE inhibitor or ARB) due to intolerance or renal insufficiency.
- **Ivabradine**
  - ❑ ↓ risk of hospitalization and cardiovascular death in stable NYHA Class II-III HF with a resting heart rate ≥ 70 BPM in normal sinus rhythm on maximally tolerated dose of BB
- **Digoxin**
  - ❑ Provides a small ↑ in cardiac output, improves symptoms and ↓ cardiac hospitalizations (does not ↓ mortality); can be considered in patients who remain symptomatic with (or cannot tolerate) first-line therapies
- **Vericiguat**
  - ❑ ↓ risk of hospitalization and CV death after recent HF hospitalization or need for IV diuretics; can be used in select patients with worsening HF despite first-line therapies

OTHER TYPES OF HEART FAILURE

Patients with HFimpEF (i.e., baseline LVEF ≤ 40% but improves to > 40% with treatment) should continue recommended treatments to prevent relapse, even if they become asymptomatic.

In patients with HFmrEF (LVEF 41 – 49%) or HFpEF (LVEF ≥ 50%), SGLT2 inhibitors are recommended as they have demonstrated benefit in decreasing HF hospitalizations and cardiovascular mortality. Other treatments (e.g., ARNI/ACE inhibitor/ARB, BB, ARA, PRN diuretics) can also be considered, especially if LVEF is on the lower end of the spectrum (for each category) or they are needed to control comorbid conditions that can exacerbate HF (e.g., hypertension, heart rate control in atrial fibrillation).

RENIN-ANGIOTENSIN-ALDOSTERONE SYSTEM INHIBITORS

An ARNI, ACE inhibitor or ARB is recommended in all HF patients regardless of symptom severity. They ↓ RAAS activation (see specific mechanisms in the sections that follow), resulting in ↓ preload and afterload. They also ↓ cardiac remodeling, improve left ventricular function and ↓ morbidity and mortality. The clinical benefits are a class effect (i.e., any drug in the class can be used). Other important points include:

- Clinical trials established target doses that improve symptoms and increase survival. The goal is to titrate to the target dose, as tolerated, not to a goal BP.

- Combining an ACE inhibitor, ARB or ARNI with an ARA has added survival benefits; however, more than one RAAS inhibitor should not be combined with an ARA due to ↑ risk of hyperkalemia and renal insufficiency.

- Angioedema occurs more frequently with an ACE inhibitor or neprilysin inhibitor (than with an ARB). For testing purposes, do not use an ACE inhibitor, ARB or ARNI in patients with a history of angioedema due to any of these medications.

ANGIOTENSIN RECEPTOR AND NEPRILYSIN INHIBITOR

Entresto is a neprilysin inhibitor (sacubitril) combined with an ARB (valsartan). Neprilysin is the enzyme responsible for degradation of several beneficial vasodilatory peptides, including natriuretic peptides, adrenomedullin, substance P and bradykinin. These peptides counteract the effects of RAAS activation by causing vasodilation and diuresis.

An ARNI is indicated in NYHA Class II – IV patients to ↓ HF hospitalizations and cardiovascular death. It is a preferred first-line treatment in all patients with HFrEF, in place of an ACE inhibitor or ARB alone (should not be used in combination with an ACE inhibitor or ARB). Of note, *Entresto* is also FDA-approved for the treatment of HFpEF.

DRUG	DOSING	SAFETY/SIDE EFFECTS/MONITORING
Sacubitril/Valsartan **(Entresto)** Tablet	Start: 24/26 mg BID If previously taking a moderate-high dose ACE inhibitor or ARB: start 49/51 mg BID Target dose: 97/103 mg BID	**BOXED WARNING** Can cause injury and death to the developing fetus when used in the 2nd and 3rd trimesters; discontinue as soon as pregnancy is detected **CONTRAINDICATIONS** Do not use with or within 36 hours of an ACE inhibitor Do not use if history of angioedema Do not use with aliskiren in diabetes **WARNINGS** Angioedema, hyperkalemia, renal impairment [↑ risk with bilateral renal artery stenosis (avoid use)], hypotension/dizziness [↑ risk if volume-depleted (e.g., concurrent diuretic use)] **SIDE EFFECTS** See warnings; can also cause cough **MONITORING** BP, K, renal function (↑ SCr), s/sx of HF and angioedema **NOTES** Do not use with an ACE inhibitor or ARB No washout period required when switching from an ARB; take the first dose of sacubitril/valsartan when the next ARB dose was due

ACE INHIBITORS AND ANGIOTENSIN RECEPTOR BLOCKERS

ACE inhibitors block the conversion of angiotensin I to Ang II while ARBs block angiotensin II from binding to the angiotensin II type-1 (AT1) receptor. Both result in ↓ vasoconstriction and ↓ aldosterone secretion (refer to the Hypertension chapter). ACE inhibitors also block the degradation of bradykinin, which may contribute to the vasodilatory effects and the side effects of cough and angioedema.

DRUG	DOSING	SAFETY/SIDE EFFECTS/MONITORING
ACE Inhibitors – only those mentioned in the guidelines (see complete list in Hypertension chapter)		
Captopril	Start 6.25 mg TID, 1 hr before meals	**BOXED WARNING** Can cause injury and death to the developing fetus when used in the 2nd and 3rd trimesters; discontinue as soon as pregnancy is detected
	Target dose: 50 mg TID	
Enalapril (Vasotec, Epaned for oral solution)	Start 2.5 mg PO BID	**CONTRAINDICATIONS** Do not use with history of angioedema
	Target dose: 10-20 mg PO BID	Do not use within 36 hours of sacubitril/valsartan (Entresto)
Fosinopril	Start 5-10 mg daily	Do not use with aliskiren in diabetes
	Target dose: 40 mg daily	
Lisinopril (Zestril, Prinivil*, Qbrelis oral solution)	Start 2.5-5 mg daily	**WARNINGS** Angioedema, hyperkalemia, renal impairment [↑ risk with bilateral renal artery stenosis (avoid use)], hypotension/dizziness [↑ risk if volume-depleted (e.g., concurrent diuretic use)]
	Target dose: 20-40 mg daily	
Perindopril	Start 2 mg daily	
	Target dose: 8-16 mg daily	**SIDE EFFECTS** See warnings; can also cause cough, headache
Quinapril (Accupril)	Start 5 mg BID	
	Target dose: 20 mg BID	**MONITORING** BP, K, renal function (↑ SCr), s/sx of HF and angioedema
Ramipril (Altace)	Start 1.25-2.5 mg daily	
	Target dose: 10 mg daily	
Trandolapril	Start 1 mg daily	
	Target dose: 4 mg daily	
ARBs – only those mentioned in the guidelines (see complete list in Hypertension chapter)		
Candesartan (Atacand)	Start 4-8 mg daily	Same as ACE inhibitors except:
	Target dose: 32 mg daily	Less cough
Losartan (Cozaar)	Start 25-50 mg daily	Less angioedema
	Target dose: 50-150 mg daily	No washout period required with sacubitril/valsartan (Entresto)
Valsartan (Diovan)	Start 40 mg BID	
	Target dose: 160 mg BID	

*Brand discontinued but name still used in practice.

ARNI, ACE Inhibitor and ARB Drug Interactions

- Risk of hyperkalemia; use caution with other drugs that ↑ potassium (e.g., potassium-sparing diuretics). Avoid salt substitutes that contain potassium.

- Do not use more than one RAAS inhibitor together (e.g., ACE inhibitor + ARB/ARNI) due to ↑ risk of renal impairment, hypotension and hyperkalemia.

- Must have a 36-hour washout period when switching between an ACE inhibitor and Entresto. No washout needed if switching between an ARB and Entresto.

- Use caution with other drugs that ↓ blood pressure.

- Use with NSAIDs can ↑ risk of renal impairment (especially if elderly, volume depleted or compromised baseline renal function).

- Can ↓ lithium renal clearance and ↑ risk of lithium toxicity.

BETA-BLOCKERS

Beta-adrenergic receptor antagonists (beta-blockers) antagonize the effects of catecholamines (especially NE) at beta-1, beta-2 and/or alpha-1 adrenergic receptors. They ↓ vasoconstriction, improve cardiac function and ↓ morbidity and mortality. They are recommended for all HF patients. Unlike ACE inhibitors (or ARBs), the clinical benefits of beta-blockers are not considered a class effect. Only bisoprolol, carvedilol (IR and CR) and metoprolol succinate ER are recommended in the HF guidelines. The target doses demonstrated a survival benefit in clinical trials. Do not use beta-blockers with intrinsic sympathomimetic activity (ISA). Only discontinue beta-blockers during acute decompensated HF if hypotension or hypoperfusion is present.

DRUG	DOSING	SAFETY/SIDE EFFECTS/MONITORING
Beta-1 Selective Blockers		
Metoprolol succinate extended release *(Toprol XL, Kapspargo Sprinkle)* Metoprolol tartrate *(Lopressor)* is not recommended	Start 12.5-25 mg daily Target dose: 200 mg daily	**BOXED WARNING** Do not discontinue abruptly (particularly in patients with CHD/IHD); gradually taper over 1-2 weeks to avoid acute tachycardia, hypertension and/or ischemia **CONTRAINDICATIONS** Severe bradycardia; 2nd or 3rd degree AV block or sick sinus syndrome (unless a permanent pacemaker is in place); overt cardiac failure or cardiogenic shock **WARNINGS** Use caution in diabetes; can worsen hypoglycemia and mask hypoglycemic symptoms (see Diabetes chapter)
Bisoprolol	Start 1.25 mg daily Target dose: 10 mg daily	Use caution with bronchospastic diseases (e.g., asthma, COPD); beta-1 selective agent may be preferred Use caution with Raynaud's/other peripheral vascular diseases and pheochromocytoma Can mask signs of hyperthyroidism (e.g., tachycardia) **SIDE EFFECTS** Bradycardia, hypotension, CNS effects (e.g., fatigue, dizziness, depression), impotence, cold extremities (can exacerbate Raynaud's) **MONITORING** HR (↓ dose if symptomatic bradycardia), BP, s/sx of HF **NOTES** Metoprolol IV is not equivalent to PO (IV:PO ratio 1:2.5) *Toprol XL* can be cut in half (do no crush or chew); take with or immediately after meals *Kapspargo Sprinkle*: swallow whole; if needed, the capsule can be opened and the contents sprinkled on a teaspoonful of soft food (e.g., applesauce, yogurt or pudding)
Non-Selective Beta-Blocker and Alpha-1 Blocker		
Carvedilol *(Coreg, Coreg CR)*	**Immediate release** Start 3.125 mg BID Target dose: ≤ 85 kg: 25 mg BID > 85 kg: 50 mg BID **Controlled release** Start 10 mg daily Target dose: 80 mg daily	Same as above plus: **CONTRAINDICATION** Severe hepatic impairment, bronchial asthma **WARNING** Intraoperative floppy iris syndrome has occurred in cataract surgery patients who were on or were previously treated with an alpha-1 blocker **SIDE EFFECTS** Edema, weight gain **NOTES** Take with food (all forms) to ↓ the rate of absorption and the risk of orthostatic hypotension *Coreg CR*: swallow whole; if needed, the capsule can be opened and the contents sprinkled on a spoonful of applesauce Carvedilol CR has lower bioavailability than carvedilol IR; dose conversions are not 1:1 (e.g., *Coreg* 3.125 mg BID = *Coreg CR* 10 mg daily)

Beta-Blocker Drug Interactions

- Can enhance the hypoglycemic effects of insulin and sulfonylureas and can mask some symptoms of hypoglycemia (e.g., shakiness, palpitations, anxiety).
- Use caution with other drugs that ↓ HR (e.g., digoxin, verapamil, diltiazem, amiodarone).

- Carvedilol and metoprolol are CYP450 2D6 substrates; may interact with CYP2D6 inhibitors or inducers.
- Carvedilol inhibits P-gp and can ↑ concentrations of P-gp substrates (e.g., digoxin, cyclosporine, dabigatran, ranolazine).

ALDOSTERONE RECEPTOR ANTAGONISTS

Aldosterone receptor antagonists (ARAs) compete with aldosterone at receptor sites in the distal convoluted tubule and collecting ducts of the nephron. They ↓ sodium and water retention, cardiac remodeling (especially myocardial fibrosis) and the risk of sudden cardiac death. ARAs are a component of GDMT for HF. They ↓ morbidity and mortality and should be used first line in patients with NYHA Class II – IV HF. Spironolactone is non-selective; it also blocks androgen and exhibits endocrine side effects. Eplerenone is selective and does not exhibit endocrine side effects.

DRUG	DOSING	SAFETY/SIDE EFFECTS/MONITORING
Spironolactone (**Aldactone**, *CaroSpir* oral suspension) Tablet, oral suspension	Start 12.5-25 mg daily Target dose: 25-50 mg daily *CaroSpir*: start 10-20 mg daily; may ↑ to 37.5 mg daily	**CONTRAINDICATIONS** Do not use in hyperkalemia, severe renal impairment, Addison's disease (spironolactone) or if taking strong CYP3A4 inhibitors (eplerenone) **WARNINGS** Do not initiate for HF if K > 5 mEq/L, CrCl (eGFR) ≤ 30 or SCr > 2.0 mg/dL (females) or SCr > 2.5 mg/dL (males) **SIDE EFFECTS** Hyperkalemia, ↑ SCr, dizziness, hyperchloremic metabolic acidosis (rare) Spironolactone: gynecomastia, breast tenderness, impotence, irregular menses, amenorrhea
Eplerenone (*Inspra*) Tablet	Start 25 mg daily Target dose: 50 mg daily	Eplerenone: ↑ TGs **MONITORING** BP, K, renal function, fluid status, s/sx of HF **NOTES** *CaroSpir* suspension is not therapeutically equivalent to the tablets; *CaroSpir* doses > 100 mg can cause higher than expected concentrations; only use tablets when doses > 100 mg are needed

ARA Drug Interactions

- Risk of hyperkalemia; use caution with other drugs that ↑ potassium (e.g., RAAS inhibitor).
- Do not use triple combination of ACE inhibitor + ARB/ARNI + ARA due to ↑ risk of hyperkalemia and renal insufficiency.
- Use caution with other drugs that ↓ blood pressure.
- Eplerenone is a major substrate of CYP3A4. Do not use with strong CYP3A4 inhibitors (e.g., ketoconazole, itraconazole, clarithromycin, ritonavir).

SODIUM-GLUCOSE COTRANSPORTER 2 INHIBITORS

Sodium-glucose cotransporter 2 (SGLT2) inhibitors, many of which were originally approved for type 2 diabetes (see Diabetes chapter), have now shown benefit in treating HF. Though the mechanism responsible for benefit in HF is not well defined, it is likely related to reduced sodium reabsorption, diuresis and a decrease in preload and/or afterload. SGLT2 inhibitors are recommended first line for HF as a component of GDMT.

Select SGLT2 inhibitors and doses approved for HF (in patients with and without diabetes) to ↓ mortality and hospitalizations include:

- **Dapagliflozin (*Farxiga*)** 10 mg PO daily
- **Empagliflozin (*Jardiance*)** 10 mg PO daily

A dual SGLT1/2 inhibitor is approved to ↓ CV death, hospitalization and urgent visits for HF:

- **Sotagliflozin (*Inpefa*)** 200 – 400 mg PO daily

Warnings and side effects for SGLT2 inhibitors are the same as those seen when they are used to treat type 2 diabetes (see Diabetes chapter), and they should generally not be initiated for HF if eGFR < 20 – 25 mL/min/1.73 m² (cutoffs are medication-specific).

LOOP DIURETICS

Loop diuretics block sodium and chloride reabsorption in the thick ascending limb of the loop of Henle. They ↑ excretion of sodium, potassium, chloride, magnesium, calcium and water. The ↓ in fluid volume reduces congestive symptoms (↓ preload), making it easier for the heart to pump, and restores euvolemia ("dry" weight). They do not improve survival, but are often required for symptom control. The lowest effective dose should be used to prevent over-diuresis, which can cause hypotension and renal impairment. If response to loop diuretics is poor, adding a thiazide diuretic, such as metolazone, can be useful.

DRUG	DOSING	SAFETY/SIDE EFFECTS/MONITORING
Furosemide (**Lasix**, Furoscix) Tablet, injection, oral solution	Oral: 20-40 mg daily or BID Max 600 mg/day	**BOXED WARNING** Can cause profound diuresis resulting in fluid and electrolyte depletion **CONTRAINDICATIONS** Anuria, hepatic coma (bumetanide and torsemide only) **WARNINGS** Sulfa allergy (not likely to cross-react – see cautionary statement in Drug Allergies & Adverse Drug Reactions chapter); warning does not apply to ethacrynic acid
Bumetanide (**Bumex**) Tablet, injection	Oral: 0.5-1 mg daily or BID Max 10 mg/day	Ototoxicity including hearing loss, tinnitus and vertigo (more with ethacrynic acid or rapid IV administration) Acute kidney injury (due to excessive fluid loss) **SIDE EFFECTS** ↓ electrolytes: K, Mg, Na, Cl, Ca (different than thiazides which ↑ Ca) ↑ electrolytes/labs: HCO3 (metabolic alkalosis), UA, BG, TGs, total cholesterol Orthostatic hypotension, photosensitivity, myalgias
Torsemide (Soaanz) Tablet	Oral: 10-20 mg daily Max 200 mg/day	**MONITORING** Renal function, fluid status (input/output, weight), BP, electrolytes, s/sx of HF **NOTES** Take early in the day to avoid nocturia Furosemide injection: store at room temperature (refrigeration causes crystals to form, which may dissolve upon warming); solution must be clear, do not use if yellow in color
Ethacrynic Acid (Edecrin) Tablet, injection	Oral: 50-200 mg daily or divided Max 400 mg/day	*Furoscix* is a single-dose prefilled cartridge for use with an on-body infusor (administers drug as a SC infusion) Bumetanide and furosemide injections are light-sensitive (store in amber bottles); IV admixtures do not require light protection **Dose Conversions** Oral equivalent dosing: furosemide 40 mg = torsemide 20 mg = bumetanide 1 mg = ethacrynic acid 50 mg Furosemide IV:PO ratio 1:2 (furosemide 20 mg IV = furosemide 40 mg PO) Bumetanide and ethacrynic acid IV:PO ratio 1:1

Loop Diuretic Drug Interactions

- Avoid NSAIDs; the ↑ sodium and water retention can ↓ the effect of loop diuretics and may also cause renal impairment.
- Use caution with other drugs that ↓ blood pressure.
- Watch for additive diuresis and electrolyte abnormalities when used in combination with thiazide diuretics.
- Additive risk for ototoxicity when used with other ototoxic drugs (see the Drug Interactions chapter), especially in patients with impaired renal function.
- Can alter lithium levels leading to lithium toxicity or inadequate treatment.

CASE SCENARIO

A patient is being treated with furosemide 40 mg IV BID for an acute HF exacerbation. She is now ready for discharge and the team wants to send her home on bumetanide. What would be an equivalent oral dose of bumetanide?

First, determine the equivalent furosemide daily oral dose based on the current total daily dose of IV furosemide.

$$\frac{80 \text{ mg IV}}{X \text{ mg PO}} = \frac{1 \text{ mg IV}}{2 \text{ mg PO}}$$

X = 160 mg PO furosemide

Then, determine the equivalent daily oral dose of bumetanide.

$$\frac{160 \text{ mg PO furosemide}}{X \text{ mg PO bumetanide}} = \frac{40 \text{ mg PO furosemide}}{1 \text{ mg PO bumetanide}}$$

X = 4 mg PO bumetanide

HYDRALAZINE/NITRATE

Hydralazine is a direct arterial vasodilator which ↓ afterload. Nitrates ↑ the availability of nitric oxide, causing venous vasodilation and ↓ preload. The combination improves survival in HF (but to a lesser degree than ACE inhibitors) and can be used as an alternative in patients who cannot tolerate an ARNI, ACE inhibitor or ARB due to poor renal function, angioedema or hyperkalemia. The combination product *BiDil* is indicated in self-identified Black patients with NYHA Class III or IV HF who are symptomatic despite optimal treatment (e.g., ACE inhibitor or ARB, beta-blocker, ARA). There is no role for monotherapy with either hydralazine or an oral nitrate in the treatment of HF.

DRUG	DOSING	SAFETY/SIDE EFFECTS/MONITORING
Isosorbide Dinitrate/ Hydralazine (*BiDil*) Tablet	Start 20/37.5 mg TID (1 tab TID) Target dose: 40/75 mg TID (2 tabs TID)	See individual components below **WARNING** Worsening of ischemic heart disease **NOTES** No nitrate tolerance
Hydralazine Tablet, injection	Start 25-50 mg TID-QID Target dose: 300 mg/day in divided doses	**CONTRAINDICATION** Mitral valve rheumatic heart disease, CAD **WARNING** Drug-induced lupus erythematosus (DILE – dose and duration related) **SIDE EFFECTS** Peripheral edema/headache/flushing/palpitations/reflex tachycardia, nausea/vomiting, peripheral neuritis, blood dyscrasias, hypotension **MONITORING** HR, BP, ANA titer, s/sx of HF
Isosorbide dinitrate IR/ ER (*Isordil Titradose*) Preferred formulation for systolic HF Isosorbide mononitrate not listed in HF guidelines	Start 20-30 mg TID-QID Target dose: 120 mg daily in divided doses	**CONTRAINDICATIONS** Do not use with PDE-5 inhibitors or riociguat **SIDE EFFECTS** Hypotension, headache, dizziness, tachyphylaxis (need 10-12 hour nitrate-free interval), syncope **MONITORING** HR, BP, s/sx of HF **NOTES** Refer to the Stable Angina and Acute & Critical Care Medicine chapters for a discussion of nitrates used for other indications

BiDil Drug Interactions

- Do not use with PDE-5 inhibitors (e.g., avanafil, sildenafil, tadalafil, vardenafil) or riociguat. The combination can cause severe hypotension. Refer to the Sexual Dysfunction chapter for further discussion.

IVABRADINE

Ivabradine belongs to a class of drugs known as hyperpolarization-activated cyclic nucleotide-gated channel blockers. It disrupts the "funny" current (I_f) in the sinoatrial (SA) node, resulting in decreased rate of firing and ultimately ↓ HR. Ivabradine ↓ hospitalizations for worsening HF and may also reduce CV death. It is recommended as adjunct treatment in symptomatic (NYHA Class II – III) stable chronic HF (EF ≤ 35%). Patients must already be receiving GDMT, including target or maximally-tolerated doses of beta-blockers (unless contraindicated), and be in sinus rhythm with a resting HR ≥ 70 BPM.

DRUG	DOSING	SAFETY/SIDE EFFECTS/MONITORING
Ivabradine (Corlanor)	Starting dose: 5 mg PO twice daily; after two weeks, adjust dose based on HR Maintenance dose: 2.5-7.5 mg PO twice daily Target: resting HR between 50-60 BPM	**CONTRAINDICATIONS** ADHF; sick sinus syndrome, SA block or 3rd degree AV block (unless a permanent pacemaker is in place); clinically significant hypotension or bradycardia; HR maintained exclusively by a pacemaker; severe hepatic impairment; use with strong CYP3A4 inhibitors **WARNINGS** Can cause bradycardia which can ↑ risk of QT prolongation and ventricular arrhythmias; not recommended in 2nd degree AV block ↑ risk of atrial fibrillation Fetal toxicity (females should use effective contraception) **SIDE EFFECTS** Bradycardia, hypertension, luminous phenomena (phosphenes - seeing flashes of light) **MONITORING** HR, ECG, BP

Ivabradine Drug Interactions

- Do not use with moderate or strong CYP3A4 inhibitors or strong CYP3A4 inducers.
- Use caution with other drugs that ↓ HR (e.g., digoxin, beta-blockers, clonidine, non-DHP CCBs, amiodarone and dexmedetomidine).

DIGOXIN

Digoxin inhibits the Na-K-ATPase pump in myocardial cells, causing a positive inotropic effect (↑ CO), and exerts a parasympathetic effect, which slows AV nodal conduction, causing a negative chronotropic effect (↓ HR). It does not improve survival, but can ↓ HF related hospitalizations. It can be added to GDMT to improve symptoms, exercise tolerance and quality of life. It is usually added for ventricular rate control in patients with atrial fibrillation (AF), HFrEF and low blood pressure. The starting dose is based on renal function, body mass and age (lower dose if renal insufficiency, smaller or older). The dose is adjusted to maintain a serum concentration 0.5 – 0.9 ng/mL in HF. Since hypokalemia and hypomagnesemia ↑ the risk for digoxin toxicity, maintain potassium between 4 – 5 mEq/L and magnesium > 2 mEq/L.

DRUG	DOSING	SAFETY/SIDE EFFECTS/MONITORING
Digoxin (Digitek*, Lanoxin) Tablet, solution, injection	Typical dose: <u>0.125-0.25 mg</u> PO daily Loading dose not used in HF <u>CrCl < 60 mL/min: ↓ dose or frequency</u>; hold in acute renal failure ↓ dose by <u>20-25%</u> when switching from <u>PO to IV</u> **Therapeutic range (HF)** <u>0.5-0.9 ng/mL</u> (higher range used for atrial fibrillation)	**CONTRAINDICATIONS** Ventricular fibrillation **WARNINGS** 2nd/3rd degree heart block without a pacemaker, Wolff-Parkinson-White syndrome with AF, vesicant (avoid extravasation) **SIDE EFFECTS** Dizziness, visual/mental disturbances, headache, N/V, diarrhea **MONITORING** <u>Electrolytes, renal function, HR</u>, ECG, BP, and digoxin level (draw 12-24 hrs after dose) **TOXICITY** Symptoms: <u>N/V, loss of appetite</u>, abdominal pain, <u>blurred/double vision, greenish-yellow halos</u> (or altered color perception), confusion, delirium, <u>bradycardia, life-threatening arrhythmias</u> ↑ risk with <u>hypokalemia, hypomagnesemia and hypercalcemia</u> Hypothyroidism can ↑ digoxin levels **NOTES** Antidote: *DigiFab*

*Brand discontinued but name still used in practice.

Digoxin Drug Interactions

- Digoxin is a <u>substrate</u> of <u>P-gp</u> and CYP3A4 (minor). P-gp inhibitors will increase digoxin levels.

  - ❑ <u>Reduce digoxin dose by 50%</u> when starting <u>amiodarone</u> or dronedarone.

  - ❑ Use caution with concurrent administration of verapamil, cyclosporine, itraconazole, erythromycin, clarithromycin, quinidine, propafenone and others.

- Use caution with other drugs that <u>↓ HR</u> (e.g., <u>beta-blockers, clonidine, non-DHP CCBs, amiodarone</u> and dexmedetomidine).

VERICIGUAT

Vericiguat is a <u>soluble guanylate cyclase stimulator</u>, which increases cyclic GMP and leads to smooth muscle relaxation and vasodilation. It has been shown to reduce the risk of cardiovascular death and HF hospitalizations following a hospitalization for HF or need for IV diuretics in patients with chronic symptomatic heart failure (EF < 45%) on GDMT. Vericiguat can be used in select patients with HFrEF who are persistently symptomatic despite optimized first-line therapies.

DRUG	DOSING	SAFETY/SIDE EFFECTS/MONITORING
Vericiguat (Verquvo)	Initial: 2.5 mg PO daily with food; after two weeks, titrate dose as tolerated Target dose: 10 mg once daily with food	**BOXED WARNING** Do not use if pregnant; contraception required during use and for one month after stopping treatment **CONTRAINDICATIONS** Do not use with <u>riociguat</u> (another soluble guanylate cyclase stimulator) **SIDE EFFECTS** <u>Hypotension</u>, anemia, dyspepsia

Vericiguat Drug Interactions

- Vericiguat may enhance the hypotensive effects of phosphodiesterase-5 (PDE-5) inhibitors; this combination should be avoided.

- Patients taking long-acting nitrates (e.g., isosorbide mononitrate, isosorbide dinitrate) were excluded from studies because of the potential for increased hypotension.

POTASSIUM ORAL SUPPLEMENTATION

Potassium fluctuations are common in HF due to drugs that ↓ (loop diuretics) or ↑ (RAAS inhibitors, ARAs) potassium levels. Maintenance of normal potassium levels (3.5 – 5 mEq/L) is essential to reduce the already elevated arrhythmia risk. Potassium levels should be <u>checked</u> with <u>changes in renal function</u> and after any change in <u>diuretic, ARNI, ACE inhibitor, ARB or ARA dose</u>. Magnesium deficiency can aggravate hypokalemia. <u>Magnesium</u> should be checked and corrected (as needed) <u>prior to correcting the potassium level</u>.

<u>Potassium chloride (KCl)</u> is used <u>most commonly</u> when supplementation is needed (e.g., dietary sources alone are not sufficient), but some of the tablets and capsules are large and difficult to swallow (see <u>Study Tip Gal</u> and Case Scenario below for alternative options). Potassium chloride <u>injection</u> is a <u>concentrated electrolyte</u> and <u>high-alert medication</u> (see Acute & Critical Care Medicine chapter).

DRUG	DOSING	SAFETY/SIDE EFFECTS/MONITORING
Potassium chloride Extended-release capsules: *Klor-Con Sprinkle*, Micro-K** Extended-release tablets: **K-Tab, Klor-Con, Klor-Con 10, Klor-Con M10/M15/M20** Oral packet: **Klor-Con** Oral solution: <u>10% (20 mEq/15 mL)</u>, 20% (40 mEq/15 mL) Injection	**Prevention of hypokalemia:** 20-40 mEq/day in 1-2 divided doses **Treatment of mild hypokalemia:** 40-100 mEq/day in 2-4 divided doses; adjust dose according to laboratory values No more than 40 mEq should be given as a single dose to avoid GI discomfort	**CONTRAINDICATIONS** Hyperkalemia Solid oral formulations: delayed or obstructed passage through the GI tract **WARNINGS** Risk of <u>hyperkalemia</u>; use caution in renal impairment, with disorders that alter K (e.g., untreated Addison's disease) and with medications that ↑ K **SIDE EFFECTS** Abdominal pain/cramping, diarrhea, nausea, flatulence **MONITORING** K, Mg, Cl, pH, urine output **NOTES** Take with meals and a full glass of water to minimize the risk of GI irritation

*Brand discontinued but name still used in practice.

POTASSIUM CHLORIDE: A HARD PILL TO SWALLOW

Extended-release capsules
- Capsule contents can be sprinkled on a small amount of applesauce or pudding

Extended-release tablets
- *K-Tab, Klor-Con:* swallow whole; do not chew, crush, cut or suck on the tablet
- *Klor-Con M:* if difficult to swallow whole, it can be cut in half or dissolved in water (stir for 2 minutes and drink immediately); do not chew, crush, or suck on the tablet

Oral packet
- Dissolve contents in water and drink immediately

Oral solution
- KCl 10% = 20 mEq/15 mL (see Case Scenario)
- Mix each 15 mL with 6 oz of water

CASE SCENARIO

A 76-year-old woman who takes furosemide is started on *Klor-Con* 20 mEq TID. She has difficulty swallowing the large tablets and would like to switch to something that is easier to take. How many milliliters of KCl 10% oral solution would provide the same amount of daily potassium that she is receiving from *Klor-Con*?

First, determine the total daily dose of potassium from *Klor-Con*.

20 mEq x 3 doses/day = 60 mEq/day

Then, using the dose conversion for KCl 10% oral solution, calculate how many milliliters will provide the same total daily dose.

$$\frac{60 \text{ mEq}}{X \text{ mL}} = \frac{20 \text{ mEq}}{15 \text{ mL}}$$

X = 45 mL of KCl 10% oral solution

See the Calculations II: Compounding chapter for additional examples

IRON REPLACEMENT THERAPY

All patients with HF should be assessed for anemia, because anemia is associated with HF disease severity and mortality. Specifically, it is recommended that patients with HFrEF and iron deficiency receive intravenous iron treatment to improve exercise capacity and quality of life (see the Anemia chapter for further discussion of iron deficiency anemia and parenteral iron treatment).

CHRONIC HEART FAILURE MANAGEMENT/ACTION PLAN

EXCELLENT JOB!

- No new or worsening shortness of breath
- Usual amount of swelling in legs
- No weight gain
- No chest pain
- No change in usual activity

Weigh yourself every day

Eat a low salt diet

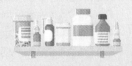

Take all your medications

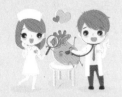

Go to your doctor appointments

BE CAREFUL!

Weight gain of:
- 2-4 pounds in 1 day
- More than 5 pounds in 1 week

Increased swelling (in abdomen and/or extremities) or coughing

Increased number of pillows to sleep

Shortness of breath with activity

You may need to change your medications (e.g., double the dose of your loop diuretic)

Call your doctor for instructions

WARNING!

Weight gain of more than 5 pounds in 1 week

Unable to sleep or lay flat due to shortness of breath

Dizziness, confusion, sadness or depression

Shortness of breath at rest, chest tightness or wheezing

Call your doctor <u>today</u> to report symptoms and request an appointment

<u>Call 911 if having severe chest pain</u>

©UWorld
iStock.com/Lin Shao-hua, drogatnev, Jane_Kelly, MedejaJa, pe-art

HEART FAILURE EXACERBATIONS AND QUALITY IMPROVEMENT

HF is the most common condition causing hospitalization in patients greater than 65 years old. HF admissions are caused by either new-onset HF (known as acute HF) or worsening HF (known as acute decompensated HF, or ADHF). ADHF presents with either worsening congestion and/or hypoperfusion. Treatment consists of IV loop diuretics, vasodilators and/or inotropes, which are discussed in the Acute & Critical Care Medicine chapter. Many HF hospitalizations are due to nonadherence with medications and/or lifestyle recommendations.

Lifestyle adherence is essential (discussed at the beginning of the chapter), including healthy eating and sodium restriction. Patients need to know what steps to take if symptoms worsen. The steps are outlined in the sample HF action plan on the previous page.

Avoidable HF admissions are a major cause of increased healthcare costs. Pharmacists are actively involved in quality improvement initiatives directed at decreasing hospital readmissions, such as medication optimization (ensuring the right medications are being used/appropriately titrated and harmful medications are not being used) and medication adherence strategies (25 – 50% of patients with HF report medication nonadherence).

KEY COUNSELING POINTS

See the Drug Formulations and Patient Counseling chapter for counseling language/layman's terminology.

ALL PATIENTS WITH HEART FAILURE

- Monitor and record body weight daily, in the morning after using the restroom and before eating.
- Limit salt intake. Choose foods with "no sodium added" or "low sodium." Avoid foods high in sodium, such as:
  - ❏ Prepared sauces and condiments (e.g., soy sauce, BBQ sauce, Worcestershire sauce, salsa)
  - ❏ Canned vegetables and soups
  - ❏ Frozen meals
  - ❏ Deli meat (e.g., sandwich meat, bacon, ham, hot dogs, sausage, salami)
  - ❏ Pickles, olives, cheese, nuts, chips
- Do not use NSAIDs (e.g., ibuprofen); they can worsen sodium and water retention and reduce the effectiveness of HF medications.

ARNI, ACE INHIBITORS AND ARBs

- Avoid in pregnancy (teratogenic).
- Can cause angioedema.
- ACE inhibitors and ARNI: tell your healthcare provider if you develop a dry, hacking cough.

BETA-BLOCKERS

- Do not suddenly stop taking this medication without consulting your healthcare provider.
- This medication can mask symptoms of low blood sugar. If you have diabetes, check your blood sugar if you notice symptoms of sweating or hunger.
- Can cause sexual dysfunction.
- Take *Coreg/Coreg CR* with food.

- Take *Toprol XL* with or immediately after meals.
- The *Coreg CR* capsule can be opened and the contents sprinkled on a small amount applesauce.
- The *Kapspargo Sprinkle* capsule can be opened and the contents sprinkled on a teaspoonful of applesauce, yogurt or pudding.

LOOP DIURETICS

- Take this medication early in the day (no later than 4 PM) to avoid getting up at night to use the bathroom.
- Can cause orthostasis.

DIGOXIN

- Digoxin levels and kidney function will be monitored regularly.
- Avoid dehydration; an overdose can occur more easily if you are dehydrated.
- Symptoms of overdose include nausea, vomiting, decreased appetite, vision changes (e.g., blurred or yellow/green vision), confusion and delirium.
- Many drug interactions.

Select Guidelines/References

2022 ACC/AHA/HFSA Guideline for the Management of Heart Failure. *J Am Coll Cardiol.* 2022;79:e263-e421.

2021 Update to the 2017 ACC Expert Consensus Decision Pathway for Optimization of Heart Failure Treatment: Answers to 10 Pivotal Issues About Heart Failure with Reduced Ejection Fraction. *J Am Coll Cardiol.* 2021;77(6):772-810.

2021 Universal Definition and Classification of Heart Failure Consensus Statement. https://www.onlinejcf.com/article/S1071-9164(21)00050-6/fulltext (accessed 2024 Jan 22).

CHAPTER CONTENT

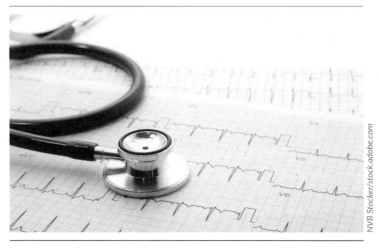

NVB Stocker/stock.adobe.com

CHAPTER 32
ARRHYTHMIAS

BACKGROUND

The cardiac conduction system is the electrical signaling system that coordinates the heartbeat and causes the atria and ventricles to contract, which pushes the blood forward. Blood flows in one direction in the body, through the heart chambers (from the atria to the ventricles), then to the lungs (to pick up oxygen) or to the body (to provide oxygen and nutrients), then back to the heart.

The "lub-dub" sounds (called S1 and S2) heard through auscultation (listening to the heart with a stethoscope) are made by the closing of heart valves that occur in sequence with each heartbeat and signal the beginning and end of ventricular systole (i.e., contraction). Sounds other than S1 and S2 are typically abnormal (e.g., S3, a murmur which is common in heart failure). Murmurs are caused by turbulent blood flow or regurgitation (i.e., blood flowing in the wrong direction).

A normal heartbeat has a relatively steady rate and a regular, coordinated rhythm. An arrhythmia is an abnormal heart rhythm, which can cause the heart to beat too slow (bradycardia) or too fast (tachycardia). Any change from the normal sequence of electrical impulses can cause an arrhythmia. When the electrical impulses are too fast, too slow, or erratic, the heart cannot pump blood efficiently, and symptoms can develop.

SYMPTOMS AND DIAGNOSIS

Some arrhythmias are silent (asymptomatic) and might only be detected during a medical exam. With other arrhythmias, patients can feel that the heart is beating very fast ("fluttering" in the chest) or abnormally ("skipping a beat"). Symptoms can include dizziness, shortness of breath, fatigue, lightheadedness and chest pain. In severe cases, arrhythmias can lead to syncope (loss of consciousness due to decreased cardiac output), heart failure or death.

CONTENT LEGEND

 = Study Tip Gal   = Key Drug Guy

An electrocardiogram (ECG) is used to diagnose arrhythmias. An ECG machine records the electrical activity of the heart using electrodes placed on the skin. An ECG can be obtained quickly in a clinic or ambulance, but it will only detect an arrhythmia present during the test.

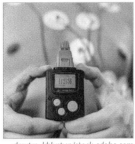

dmytro_khlystun/stock.adobe.com

A Holter monitor (see image to the left) is an ambulatory ECG device that records the electrical activity of the heart continuously for 24 – 48 hours. A Holter monitor or continuous ECG monitoring (in the hospital) can detect arrhythmias that are intermittent (i.e., the heart goes in and out of normal sinus rhythm). Other monitoring devices are available, such as event monitors (which record activity around the time of an arrhythmia), select smart watches and the Zio patch heart monitor. Zio is a wireless adhesive patch placed directly on the chest and worn for up to 14 days.

THE CARDIAC CONDUCTION PATHWAY

The cardiac conduction pathway consists of a group of specialized cardiac cells (myocytes) that send electrical impulses (signals) to the heart muscle, causing it to contract. The main components include the sinoatrial (SA) node, atrioventricular (AV) node, bundle of His, bundle branches and Purkinje fibers. The conduction pathway can be traced by following the numbers in the image below.

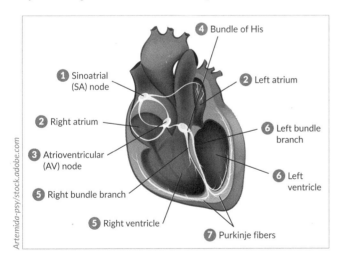

Artemida-psy/stock.adobe.com

1. The electrical impulse begins in the SA node, which is a cluster of cells located at the junction of the superior vena cava and the right atrium. The SA node is the heart's natural pacemaker; the frequency of its signals determines the pace, or heart rate. A normal heart rate is 60 to 100 BPM.

2. The impulse then travels from the SA node to the right and left atria, which causes the atria to contract.

3. When the signal reaches the AV node, electrical conduction slows down.

4. The impulse continues through the bundle of His and into the ventricles.

5. The bundle of His divides into the right bundle branch for the right ventricle, and

6. The left bundle branch for the left ventricle.

7. The signal continues to spread through the ventricles via the Purkinje fibers, which causes the ventricles to contract.

Normal sinus rhythm (NSR) has the characteristic appearance shown on the ECG printout and image below, with a distinct pattern for each heartbeat that represents the various waves (e.g., P and T waves) and segments (e.g., the QRS complex). Any disruption in the normal sequence of impulse conduction can result in an arrhythmia. For example, the SA node may fire at an abnormal rate or rhythm or damaged myocardial tissue can block or disrupt the electrical signal.

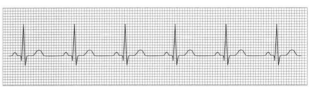

JYFotoStock/stock.adobe.com

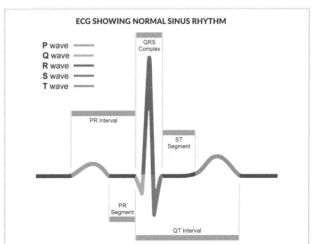

udaix/stock.adobe.com

ELECTRICAL SIGNALING: THE CARDIAC ACTION POTENTIAL

The cardiac action potential refers to the movement of ions through channels in the myocytes that cause the electrical impulses in the cardiac conduction pathway. In essence, the action potentials provide the electricity needed to power the cardiac conduction pathway. The cells in the SA node (pacemaker) have automaticity, which means that, unlike other myocytes, they initiate their own action potential (the cells spontaneously depolarize). The action potential of a ventricular myocyte is triggered when a threshold voltage is reached. This occurs in phases (see image below labeled with Phases 0, 1, 2, 3 and 4).

- Phase 0: a heartbeat is initiated when rapid ventricular depolarization occurs in response to an influx of sodium (Na); this causes ventricular contraction (represented by the QRS complex on the ECG).

- Phase 1: early rapid repolarization (Na channels close).

- Phase 2: a plateau in response to an influx of calcium (Ca) and efflux of potassium (K).

- Phase 3: rapid ventricular repolarization occurs in response to an efflux of K; this causes ventricular relaxation (represented by the T wave on the ECG).

- Phase 4: resting membrane potential is established; atrial depolarization occurs (represented by the P wave on the ECG).

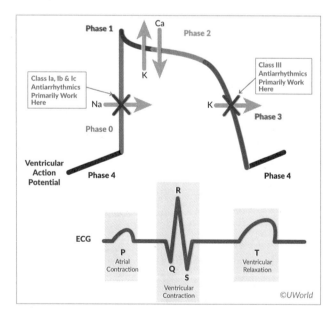

ARRHYTHMIAS

Abnormalities of the heart or its conduction system can alter the cardiac action potential and lead to arrhythmias. The most common cause of arrhythmias is myocardial ischemia or infarction. Other conditions resulting in damage to cardiac tissue can cause arrhythmias, including heart valve disorders, hypertension and heart failure.

Non-cardiac conditions that can trigger or predispose a patient to an arrhythmia include electrolyte imbalances (especially potassium, magnesium, sodium and calcium), elevated sympathetic states (e.g., hyperthyroidism, infection) and drugs (e.g., illicit drugs and drugs that prolong the QT interval).

Arrhythmias are generally classified into two broad categories based on their point of origin: supraventricular (originating above the AV node) and ventricular (originating below the AV node). Arrhythmias originating in or just below the AV node are called junctional rhythms, which are less common.

SUPRAVENTRICULAR ARRHYTHMIAS

These include sinus tachycardia, atrial fibrillation, atrial flutter, atrial tachycardia and supraventricular re-entrant tachycardias (formerly known as paroxysmal supraventricular tachycardias or PSVTs). Many patients have ongoing supraventricular arrhythmias (especially atrial fibrillation) without realizing it.

Atrial fibrillation (AF) is the most common type of arrhythmia and is discussed later in the chapter.

VENTRICULAR ARRHYTHMIAS

Common ventricular arrhythmias include premature ventricular contractions (PVCs), ventricular tachycardia and ventricular fibrillation. PVCs (also called skipped heartbeats) are relatively common and can occur in people with or without heart disease. PVCs can be related to stress or too much caffeine, nicotine or exercise.

A series of PVCs that result in a heart rate > 100 BPM is known as ventricular tachycardia (VT). Pulseless VT is a medical emergency and advanced cardiac life support (ACLS) should be initiated, whereas VT with a pulse can often be treated with antiarrhythmic drugs. All untreated VT can degenerate into ventricular fibrillation (completely disorganized electrical activation of the ventricles), which is also a medical emergency.

QT PROLONGATION & TORSADE DE POINTES

The QT interval is measured from the beginning of the QRS complex to the end of the T wave on an ECG. It reflects ventricular depolarization and repolarization and varies with heart rate (the QT interval is longer when the heart rate is slower). A QT interval can be used if the heart rate is ≤ 60 BPM; when the heart rate is > 60 BPM, a QT interval corrected for heart rate (QTc) is used. A QTc interval is considered prolonged when it is <u>> 440 – 460 milliseconds</u> (msec), but is more worrisome when markedly prolonged (> 500 msec).

<u>Prolongation of the QT interval</u> is a risk factor for <u>Torsade de Pointes (TdP)</u>, a particularly lethal ventricular tachyarrhythmia that can cause <u>sudden cardiac death</u>.

QT Prolongation Risk Factors

See the <u>Key Drugs Guy</u> for drugs that can prolong the QT interval. The risk of drug-induced QT prolongation increases with:

- <u>Higher doses</u> (risk is concentration-dependent).
- <u>Multiple</u> QT-prolonging <u>drugs</u> taken at the same time (additive effects).
- Reduced drug <u>clearance</u> due to renal disease, liver disease or drug <u>interactions</u> (e.g., enzyme inhibitors).
- Electrolyte abnormalities, including low potassium (<u>hypokalemia</u>), magnesium (<u>hypomagnesemia</u>) and calcium (hypocalcemia).
- Other <u>cardiac conditions</u> (e.g., heart failure, bradycardia).
- Female gender.

Some medications have specific recommendations to minimize the risk of QT prolongation (e.g., <u>maximum doses</u> for citalopram/escitalopram, avoidance of single IV doses > 16 mg for ondansetron, restricted use of droperidol).

QT Risk Requires Assessment

In addition to recognizing the drugs that prolong the QT interval, assessing a patient's risk for TdP is important. For example, if low-dose amitriptyline is being used for neuropathic pain, it is not particularly risky; but if the same patient is admitted to the hospital with hypokalemia and started on fluconazole and ondansetron, the level of concern would be heightened.

> **SELECT DRUGS THAT CAN INCREASE OR PROLONG THE QT INTERVAL**
>
> **Antiarrhythmics**
> Class Ia, Ic and III
>
> **Anti-infectives**
> Antimalarials (e.g., hydroxychloroquine)
>
> Azole antifungals (all except isavuconazonium)
>
> Macrolides
>
> Quinolones
>
> Lefamulin
>
> **Antidepressants**
> SSRIs (highest risk with citalopram and escitalopram)
>
> Tricyclic antidepressants
>
> Mirtazapine, trazodone, venlafaxine
>
> **Antiemetics**
> 5-HT3 receptor antagonists (e.g., ondansetron)
>
> Droperidol, metoclopramide, promethazine
>
> **Antipsychotics**
> First generation (e.g., haloperidol, chlorpromazine, thioridazine)
>
> Second generation (highest risk with ziprasidone)
>
> **Oncology medications**
> Androgen deprivation therapy (e.g., leuprolide)
>
> Tyrosine kinase inhibitors (e.g., nilotinib)
>
> Arsenic trioxide
>
> **Other**
> Cilostazol, donepezil, fingolimod, hydroxyzine, loperamide, methadone, ranolazine, solifenacin

ANTIARRHYTHMIC DRUGS

Antiarrhythmic drugs work by blocking the movement of ions in different phases of the action potentials that drive the cardiac conduction pathway. Select drugs can reduce conduction velocity and/or automaticity, or prolong the refractory period, which can slow or terminate the abnormal electrical activity causing the arrhythmia. However, antiarrhythmic drugs are not without risk. <u>Prior</u> to <u>starting</u> any drug for a non-life-threatening arrhythmia, <u>electrolytes</u> and a <u>toxicology screen</u> should be checked to identify any potentially reversible causes. <u>All antiarrhythmic drugs</u> have the potential to induce <u>proarrhythmia (causing a new arrhythmia or worsening the existing one)</u>. Risk of additive proarrhythmia can be minimized by <u>correcting electrolyte abnormalities</u> prior to antiarrhythmic use and throughout treatment.

MECHANISM OF ACTION

The Vaughan Williams classification system splits the antiarrhythmic drugs into categories based on their dominant electrophysiological effect or mechanism of action (see the Study Tip Gal); however, some drugs (e.g., amiodarone, sotalol) act via multiple mechanisms.

AMIODARONE

Amiodarone is a class III antiarrhythmic (K channel blocker) that also blocks Na and Ca channels and alpha and beta adrenergic receptors, making it useful for treating many different arrhythmias. Amiodarone is notable for a very long half-life (40 – 60 days) and a chemical structure containing iodine (see Basic Science Concepts chapter), which can impact thyroid function. Despite numerous toxicities, amiodarone is commonly prescribed and is a preferred antiarrhythmic in patients with heart failure.

DRUG	DOSING	SAFETY/SIDE EFFECTS/MONITORING
Amiodarone (*Nexterone, Pacerone*) Tablet, injection	**Pulseless VT/VF:** 300 mg IV push x 1, may repeat 150 mg IV push x 1 if needed **VT with pulse:** 150 mg IV bolus, then 1 mg/min x 6 hours, then 0.5 mg/min x 18 hours or longer **Secondary prevention of ventricular arrhythmias:** 800-1,600 mg/day x 1-3 weeks, then 600-800 mg/day x 4 weeks, then 400 mg/day **AF/atrial flutter – cardioversion (off-label):** 600-800 mg/day PO until a 10 gram loading dose is reached, then 200 mg daily **AF/atrial flutter – maintenance of NSR (off-label):** 400-600 mg/day for 2-4 weeks, then 100-200 mg daily	**BOXED WARNINGS** Pulmonary toxicity: check baseline chest X-ray, PFTs Hepatotoxicity: check baseline LFTs For life-threatening arrhythmias only; proarrhythmic, continuous ECG monitoring and cardiac resuscitation should be available for initiation **CONTRAINDICATIONS** Iodine hypersensitivity; sick sinus syndrome, 2nd/3rd-degree heart block, or bradycardia causing syncope (unless using artificial pacemaker); cardiogenic shock **WARNINGS** Hyper- and hypothyroidism (hypo is more common as amiodarone partially inhibits peripheral conversion of T4 to T3), visual impairment (optic neuropathy, corneal microdeposits), photosensitivity (blue-gray skin discoloration), neurotoxicity (peripheral neuropathy) Correct hypokalemia, hypomagnesemia, hypocalcemia prior to use Avoid in pregnancy (teratogenic) and when breastfeeding if possible **SIDE EFFECTS** Hypotension, bradycardia (may require ↓ infusion rate), photosensitivity (sun protection required), dizziness, tremor/ataxia, malaise/fatigue, nausea, drug-induced lupus erythematosus (DILE), severe skin reactions (SJS/TEN) **MONITORING** ECG, BP, HR, electrolytes LFTs every 6 months, thyroid function (TSH and free T4) and chest X-ray every 3-6 months, regular eye exams **NOTES** Oral/IV can provide rate control for AF (due to beta-blocking properties) when other measures are unsuccessful or contraindicated. **Intravenous** Infusions > 2 hours require a non-PVC container (e.g., polyolefin or glass); PVC tubing is okay Premixed IV bags: longer stability, non-PVC, available in common concentrations (e.g., *Nexterone* comes in non-PVC, non-DEHP GALAXY plastic container) Use 0.22 micron filter; central line preferable Incompatible with heparin (flush line with saline); many Y-site, additive incompatibilities

Amiodarone Drug Interactions

- Amiodarone can increase the level of many other drugs; it is a weak inhibitor of CYP450 2C9, 2D6, 3A4 and P-gp.

- Amiodarone is often given with drugs that it interacts with (common cardiovascular drug interactions are reviewed in the Drug Interactions chapter). When starting amiodarone:

  - ↓ digoxin by 50%, ↓ warfarin by 30 – 50% and do not exceed 20 mg/day of simvastatin or 40 mg/day of lovastatin (consider use of alternative statin).

- Additive effects can occur when used with other drugs that decrease HR, including non-dihydropyridine calcium channel blockers (non-DHP CCBs), digoxin, beta-blockers, clonidine and dexmedetomidine (Precedex).

- Sofosbuvir can enhance the bradycardic effect of amiodarone; do not use together.

OTHER ANTIARRHYTHMICS

Other antiarrhythmics work primarily by blocking sodium or potassium channels. Many of the drugs listed here have toxicities that limit their use, but lidocaine and adenosine are recommended in the ACLS algorithms for cardiac arrest (ventricular tachycardia/fibrillation) and tachycardia with a palpable pulse, respectively.

DRUG	DOSING	SAFETY/SIDE EFFECTS/MONITORING
Class Ia Drugs Block sodium channels		
Disopyramide (Norpace, Norpace CR) Capsule	400-600 mg/day	**BOXED WARNING** Reserve use for patients with life-threatening ventricular arrhythmias **CONTRAINDICATIONS** 2nd/3rd-degree heart block (unless patient has a functional artificial pacemaker), cardiogenic shock, congenital QT syndrome, sick sinus syndrome **WARNINGS** Proarrhythmic, hypotension, may exacerbate HF, can worsen BPH/urinary retention, narrow-angle glaucoma, myasthenia gravis (due to anticholinergic effects) **SIDE EFFECTS** Anticholinergic effects (e.g., dry mouth, constipation, urinary retention)
Quinidine Tablet	IR: 400 mg PO Q6H ER: 324-648 mg PO Q8-12H Take with food or milk to ↓ GI upset Different salt forms (IR vs ER) are not interchangeable (267 mg of gluconate = 200 mg of sulfate form)	**BOXED WARNING** May ↑ mortality in treatment of AF or atrial flutter and non-life-threatening ventricular arrhythmias **CONTRAINDICATIONS** Concurrent use of quinolones that prolong the QT interval or ritonavir; 2nd/3rd-degree heart block or idioventricular conduction delays (unless patient has a functional artificial pacemaker), thrombocytopenia, thrombotic thrombocytopenic purpura (TTP), myasthenia gravis **WARNINGS** Proarrhythmic, hepatotoxicity, hemolysis risk (avoid in G6PD deficiency), can cause positive Coombs test **SIDE EFFECTS** Drug-induced lupus erythematosus (DILE), diarrhea (35%), stomach cramping (22%), rash, lightheadedness Cinchonism (e.g., quinidine toxicity): symptoms include tinnitus, hearing loss, blurred vision, headache, delirium) **NOTES** Avoid changes in Na intake; ↓ Na intake can ↑ quinidine levels Alkaline foods/alkaline urine ↑ quinidine levels and can lead to toxicity

DRUG	DOSING	SAFETY/SIDE EFFECTS/MONITORING
Procainamide Injection	Active metabolite, N-acetyl procainamide (NAPA), is renally cleared; ↓ dose when CrCl < 50 mL/min **Therapeutic levels:** Procainamide: 4-10 mcg/mL NAPA: 15-25 mcg/mL Combined: 10-30 mcg/mL Draw level 6-12 hrs after IV infusion has started	**BOXED WARNINGS** Potentially fatal blood dyscrasias (e.g., agranulocytosis); monitor patient closely in the first 3 months and periodically thereafter Long-term use leads to positive antinuclear antibody (ANA) in 50% of patients, which can result in drug-induced lupus erythematosus (DILE) in 20-30% of patients Reserve use for patients with life-threatening ventricular arrhythmias **CONTRAINDICATIONS** Heart block, systemic lupus erythematosus, TdP **WARNINGS** Proarrhythmic **SIDE EFFECTS** Hypotension, rash **NOTES** Metabolism of procainamide to NAPA occurs by acetylation: slow acetylators are at risk for drug accumulation and toxicity; fast acetylators can have subtherapeutic drug concentrations and reduced efficacy Drug of choice for Wolff-Parkinson-White syndrome

Class Ib Drugs
Block sodium channels; useful for ventricular arrhythmias only (no efficacy in AF)

Lidocaine *(Xylocaine)* Injection	Bolus dosing: 1-1.5 mg/kg x 1, then 0.5-0.75 mg/kg every 5-10 minutes (max total dose 3 mg/kg) Continuous infusion: 1-4 mg/minute	**BOXED WARNINGS** Mexiletine: reserve use for patients with life-threatening ventricular arrhythmias, abnormal liver function seen in patients with CHF or ischemia **CONTRAINDICATIONS** 2nd/3rd-degree heart block (unless patient has a functional artificial pacemaker) Lidocaine: Wolff-Parkinson-White syndrome, Adam-Stokes syndrome, allergy to corn or corn-related products or amide-type anesthetics Mexiletine: cardiogenic shock
Mexiletine Capsule	150-300 mg PO Q8-12H; max 1.2 grams/day Take with food	**WARNINGS** Caution in the elderly, hepatic impairment and HF Mexiletine: blood dyscrasias, severe skin reactions (DRESS), proarrhythmic **NOTES** IV lidocaine is used for refractory VT/cardiac arrest; topical/local is primarily used for numbing; see the Acute & Critical Care Medicine and Pain chapters

Class Ic Drugs
Block sodium channels

Flecainide Tablet	50-100 mg PO Q12H; max 400 mg/day Store in tight, light-resistant container	**BOXED WARNINGS** When treating atrial flutter, 1:1 atrioventricular conduction may occur (i.e., rapid ventricular rate); pre-emptive negative chronotropic therapy (e.g., digoxin, beta-blockers) can ↓ the risk Proarrhythmic effects, especially in AF (do not use in chronic AF) Reserve use for patients with life-threatening ventricular arrhythmias **CONTRAINDICATIONS** 2nd/3rd-degree heart block (unless patient has a functional artificial pacemaker), cardiogenic shock, structural heart disease (e.g., heart failure, myocardial infarction), concurrent use of ritonavir **WARNINGS** Avoid use in severe hepatic and renal impairment **SIDE EFFECTS** Dizziness, visual disturbances, dyspnea

DRUG	DOSING	SAFETY/SIDE EFFECTS/MONITORING
Propafenone (Rythmol SR) IR tablet, ER capsule	IR: 150-300 PO Q8H ER: 225-425 mg PO Q12H	**BOXED WARNINGS** Reserve use for patients with life-threatening ventricular arrhythmias **CONTRAINDICATIONS** Sinoatrial and atrioventricular disorders (unless patient has a functional artificial pacemaker), sinus bradycardia, cardiogenic shock, hypotension, structural heart disease (e.g., heart failure, myocardial infarction), bronchospastic disorders, marked electrolyte imbalances **WARNINGS** Proarrhythmic **SIDE EFFECTS** Taste disturbance (metallic), dizziness, visual disturbances, N/V **NOTES** Propafenone has significant beta-blocking effects, negative inotropic and proarrhythmic properties (contraindicated in HF)

Class III Drugs
Primarily block potassium channels; see amiodarone discussed previously

DRUG	DOSING	SAFETY/SIDE EFFECTS/MONITORING
Dronedarone (Multaq) Tablet	400 mg PO Q12H Take with meals	**BOXED WARNINGS** Contraindicated in patients with decompensated HF (NYHA Class IV, or any NYHA class with a recent hospitalization due to HF) or permanent AF due to ↑ risk of death, stroke and HF **CONTRAINDICATIONS** Concurrent use of erythromycin, strong CYP3A4 inhibitors and QT-prolonging drugs, 2nd/3rd-degree heart block (unless patient has a functional artificial pacemaker), HR < 50 BPM, QTc ≥ 500 msec, PR interval > 280 msec, lung or liver toxicity from previous amiodarone use, hepatic impairment **WARNINGS** Hepatic failure, pulmonary toxicity (including fibrosis and pneumonitis), marked ↑ SCr, prerenal azotemia and acute renal failure (usually in the setting of heart failure or hypovolemia), avoid in pregnancy and nursing mothers **SIDE EFFECTS** Proarrhythmic, diarrhea, bradycardia, asthenia **NOTES** Unlike amiodarone, dronedarone does not contain iodine and has little effect on thyroid function Dronedarone is an inhibitor of CYP2D6, 3A4 and P-gp and a major substrate of CYP3A4; avoid use with strong inhibitors and inducers of CYP3A4 and with drugs that prolong the QT interval; ↓ digoxin dose by 50% and use lower doses of statins metabolized by CYP3A4, or use alternate statin; monitor INR if on warfarin
Dofetilide (Tikosyn) Capsule	500 mcg PO BID CrCl < 60 mL/min: ↓ dose CrCl < 20 mL/min: contraindicated	**BOXED WARNING** Must be initiated (or reinitiated) in a setting with continuous ECG monitoring, experienced staff and ability to assess CrCl for a minimum of 3 days; proarrhythmic (QT prolongation) **CONTRAINDICATIONS** Congenital or acquired long QT syndromes, prolonged QTc > 440 msec at baseline; do not use with cimetidine, dolutegravir, hydrochlorothiazide, itraconazole, ketoconazole, megestrol, prochlorperazine, trimethoprim, verapamil, bictegravir/emtricitabine/tenofovir (Biktarvy) (these drugs can inhibit renal tubular secretion of dofetilide) **SIDE EFFECTS** Ventricular tachycardias (e.g., TdP) **NOTES** A preferred antiarrhythmic in heart failure

DRUG	DOSING	SAFETY/SIDE EFFECTS/MONITORING
Sotalol (*Betapace AF, Betapace, Sotylize, Sorine*) Tablet, solution, injection	PO: 80-160 mg BID IV: 75-150 mg BID CrCl < 60 mL/min: ↓ frequency	**BOXED WARNINGS** Initiation (or reinitiation) and dosage increases should be done in a hospital with continuous ECG monitoring and experienced staff due to risk of VT and QT prolongation Adjust dosing interval based on CrCl to ↓ risk of proarrhythmia; QT prolongation is directly related to sotalol concentration **CONTRAINDICATIONS** 2nd/3rd-degree heart block (unless patient has a functional artificial pacemaker), congenital or acquired long QT syndrome, sinus bradycardia, uncontrolled HF, cardiogenic shock, asthma For *Betapace AF*, *Sotylize*, sotalol injection: QTc > 450 msec, bronchospastic conditions, CrCl < 40 mL/min, K < 4 mEq/L, sick sinus syndrome **WARNINGS** Proarrhythmic (↑ risk of TdP with QT prolongation), can worsen HF and cause bronchoconstriction **SIDE EFFECTS** Bradycardia, palpitations, chest pain, dizziness, fatigue, dyspnea, N/V **NOTES** Sotalol is a non-selective beta-blocker and K channel blocker *Betapace* should not be substituted with *Betapace AF*; *Betapace AF* is distributed with educational information specifically for patients with AF/atrial flutter
Ibutilide (*Corvert*) Injection	1 mg over 10 minutes (0.01 mg/kg < if 60 kg)	**BOXED WARNING** Proarrhythmic (administer with continuous ECG monitoring and experienced staff); confirm that benefits of maintaining NSR outweigh the risks **SIDE EFFECTS** Ventricular tachycardias (e.g., TdP), hypotension, QT prolongation **NOTES** Indicated only for pharmacologic cardioversion
Adenosine Activates adenosine receptors to ↓ AV node conduction		
Adenosine (*Adenocard**) Injection	6 mg IV push (may increase to 12 mg if not responding)	**CONTRAINDICATIONS** 2nd/3rd-degree heart block, sick sinus syndrome or symptomatic bradycardia (except in patients with a functional pacemaker), bronchospastic lung disease **SIDE EFFECTS** Transient new arrhythmia, facial flushing, chest pain/pressure, GI distress, transient ↓ in blood pressure, dyspnea **NOTES** Half-life < 10 seconds Used for supraventricular re-entrant tachycardias; do not use for ventricular tachycardia or for converting AF/atrial flutter

Brand discontinued but name still used in practice.

TREATMENT OF ATRIAL FIBRILLATION

AF occurs when multiple waves of electrical impulses in the atria result in an irregular (and usually rapid) ventricular response. The rapid ventricular rate can ↓ cardiac output (because the ventricles do not have time to fill), which can lead to hypotension and worsen ischemia and heart failure. Atrial flutter is more organized and regular than AF, but is still characterized by rapid atrial contraction and can progress to AF.

There are different stages of AF (see table below). Patients at risk for AF should make lifestyle modifications (e.g., weight loss, tobacco cessation, minimization of alcohol consumption and optimization of blood pressure and blood glucose control).

STAGES OF AF*			DEFINITION
1	At risk for AF		Presence of modifiable (e.g., obesity) and non-modifiable (e.g., male sex) risk factors associated with AF
2	Pre-AF		Evidence of structural or electrical findings that predispose a patient to AF (e.g., atrial flutter)
3	AF	Paroxysmal	Intermittent AF that terminates within 7 days of onset
		Persistent	Continuous AF sustained for > 7 days
		Long-standing persistent	Continuous AF sustained for > 12 months
		Successful ablation	Freedom from AF after percutaneous or surgical intervention
4	Permanent AF		No further attempts at rhythm control after discussion between patient and provider; a treatment choice rather than a characteristic of the arrhythmia itself

*The terms valvular and non-valvular AF have fallen out of favor, but may still be used in practice. Valvular AF refers to AF with moderate to severe mitral stenosis or with a mechanical heart valve.

Because of the disorganized depolarization of the atria in AF, the atria cannot adequately contract. Blood becomes stagnant in the atria, which ↑ risk of clot formation. A clot can embolize (break off and travel) to an artery in the brain, which can block blood flow and cause a stroke. To reduce clotting risk, patients with AF may require anticoagulation (see the Anticoagulation chapter).

Guideline-recommended treatment for most types of AF involves using one of two main strategies: rate control or rhythm control (see the Study Tip Gal below).

RATE CONTROL

The goal resting HR is < 80 BPM in patients with symptomatic AF; however, a more lenient goal of < 110 BPM may be reasonable in patients who are asymptomatic and have preserved left ventricular function.

Beta-blockers or non-DHP CCBs are recommended for controlling ventricular rate in patients with AF (see complete drug tables in the Hypertension chapter). Of note, patients with heart failure with reduced ejection fraction (HFrEF) should not receive a non-DHP CCB. Digoxin is not first line for ventricular rate control, but can be added for refractory patients or used in those who cannot tolerate the blood pressure lowering effect of beta-blockers or non-DHP CCBs.

AF: RATE VS. RHYTHM CONTROL & STROKE PROPHYLAXIS

Rate Control
- Patient remains in AF and takes medications to control the ventricular rate (or HR).
  - ❏ Beta-blockers or non-DHP CCBs are used (and sometimes digoxin).

Rhythm Control
- The goal is to restore and maintain NSR.
  - ❏ Class Ia, Ic or III antiarrhythmic drugs or electrical cardioversion.
- For permanent AF, avoid a rhythm-control strategy with antiarrhythmic drugs (risk outweighs the benefit).

Stroke Prophylaxis (see Anticoagulation chapter)
- Clots can form when a patient is in AF, which can embolize (causing a stroke).
- For many patients, it is safer to remain in AF with rate control than to try to restore NSR. A rate control strategy may require anticoagulation for stroke prevention, depending on the CHA_2DS_2-VASc score.
  - ❏ DOACs (e.g., apixaban, rivaroxaban) are preferred over warfarin for stroke prevention in non-valvular AF.
  - ❏ Warfarin is indicated for stroke prevention in patients with AF and a mechanical heart valve.
- When a rhythm control strategy is chosen, restoration and maintenance of NSR are not guaranteed. The decision about long-term anticoagulation will depend on the patient's clot risk.

Digoxin

Digoxin inhibits the Na-K-ATPase pump, causing a positive inotropic effect, and exerts a parasympathetic effect, which enhances vagal tone to slow conduction through the AV node, resulting in reduced HR (negative chronotropy).

DRUG	DOSING	SAFETY/SIDE EFFECTS/MONITORING
Digoxin (Digitek*, Lanoxin) Tablet, solution, injection	Typical dose: 0.125-0.25 mg PO daily Loading dose [called total digitalizing dose (TDD)]: 8-12 mcg/kg IBW Give ½ of the TDD as the initial dose, followed by ¼ of the TDD in 2 subsequent doses at 4-8 hour intervals (alternatively, give 0.25-0.5 mg once then can repeat 0.25 mg Q6H to a max of 1.5 mg over 24 hours) CrCl < 60 mL/min: ↓ dose or ↓ frequency; hold in acute renal failure ↓ dose by 20-25% when converting from oral to IV **Therapeutic range (AF)** 0.8-2 ng/mL (lower range used for HF)	**CONTRAINDICATIONS** Ventricular fibrillation **WARNINGS** 2nd/3rd-degree heart block without a pacemaker, Wolff-Parkinson-White syndrome with AF, vesicant (avoid extravasation) **SIDE EFFECTS** Dizziness, visual/mental disturbances, N/V, diarrhea **MONITORING** Electrolytes, renal function, HR, ECG, BP, and digoxin level (drawn 12-24 hrs after dose) **Toxicity** Symptoms: N/V, loss of appetite, abdominal pain, blurred/double vision, greenish-yellow halos (or altered color perception), confusion, delirium, bradycardia, life-threatening arrhythmias ↑ risk with hypokalemia, hypomagnesemia and hypercalcemia Hypothyroidism can ↑ digoxin levels **NOTES** Used in combination with a beta-blocker or non-DHP CCB for rate control (not usually given alone) Antidote: *DigiFab*

*Brand discontinued but name still used in practice.

Digoxin Drug Interactions

- Digoxin is a substrate of P-gp and CYP 3A4 (minor). Levels ↑ with P-gp inhibitors, including amiodarone, dronedarone, diltiazem, verapamil, clarithromycin, itraconazole and many other drugs. With amiodarone or dronedarone, ↓ digoxin dose by 50%.

- Additive effects can occur when used with other drugs that decrease HR, including amiodarone, non-DHP CCBs, beta-blockers, clonidine and dexmedetomidine (*Precedex*).

RHYTHM CONTROL

Rhythm control includes methods for conversion to and maintenance of NSR. There are two types of cardioversion:

- Electrical (or direct current) cardioversion is most effective. A high-energy shock is delivered through the chest wall, stopping the arrhythmia and allowing the sinus node to begin firing again in NSR (see image on the next page).

- Pharmacologic cardioversion may also be attempted with amiodarone (oral and IV), dofetilide, flecainide, ibutilide and propafenone.

Cardioversion carries a risk of thromboembolism. Anticoagulation is usually required before and after successful cardioversion, regardless of the patient's CHA$_2$DS$_2$-VASc score or method of cardioversion (see Anticoagulation chapter).

If NSR is restored, many antiarrhythmic options are available for maintenance of NSR. Recommended options include dofetilide, dronedarone, flecainide, propafenone or sotalol. Due to its toxicities, amiodarone is only recommended when other drugs have failed or are contraindicated.

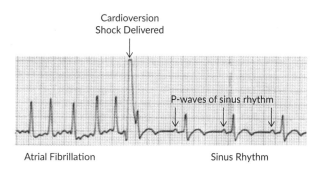

© Blausen.com staff (2014)

KEY COUNSELING POINTS

See the Drug Formulations and Patient Counseling chapter for counseling language/layman's terminology. See the Drug Interactions section for each class.

Amiodarone

- Can cause:
  - ❏ Lung damage.
  - ❏ Liver damage.
  - ❏ Eye damage (nerve damage and corneal deposits).
  - ❏ Hypothyroidism or hyperthyroidism.
  - ❏ Photosensitivity.
  - ❏ Skin discoloration to a blue-gray color. Not a harmful effect; usually goes away months after the medication is stopped.
- Avoid grapefruit.
- Many drug interactions (enzyme inhibitor).

Digoxin

- Early symptoms of overdose include loss of appetite and nausea. If this occurs, check heart rate. If bradycardic, a digoxin level should be checked.
- Symptoms of severe overdose include vision changes (e.g., blurred or yellow/green vision), confusion, hallucinations and feeling like you might pass out.
- Avoid dehydration; an overdose can occur more easily if you are dehydrated.
- Many drug interactions.

Select Guidelines/References

2023 ACC/AHA/ACCP/HRS Guideline for the Diagnosis and Management of Atrial Fibrillation: A Report of the American College of Cardiology/American Heart Association Joint Committee on Clinical Practice Guidelines. *J Am Coll Cardiol.* 2023; doi.org/10.1016/j.jacc.2023.08.017.

2017 AHA/ACC/HRS Guideline for Management of Patients with Ventricular Arrhythmias and the Prevention of Sudden Cardiac Death. *Circulation.* 2018;138:e272-e391.

Hemorrhagic Stroke	Ischemic Stroke
Hemorrhagic/blood leaks into brain tissue	Clot stops blood supply to an area of the brain

GraphicsRF/stock.adobe.com

CHAPTER 33
STROKE

BACKGROUND

A stroke, or cerebrovascular accident (CVA), occurs when blood flow to an area of the brain is interrupted. There are a few different types of stroke.

- Acute ischemic stroke can be caused by:
  - A thrombus (i.e., localized clot) that forms during a cerebral atherosclerotic infarction (similar to a myocardial infarction but in the brain). This is referred to as a non-cardioembolic stroke to indicate the origin is in the brain, not the heart.
  - An embolus (i.e., a clot) that forms in the heart and travels to the brain. This is referred to as a cardioembolic stroke. A common cause of cardioembolic stroke is atrial fibrillation (see the Arrhythmias and Anticoagulation chapters).
- Hemorrhagic stroke (bleeding in the brain), most often an intracerebral hemorrhage (ICH) or subarachnoid hemorrhage (SAH).

Approximately 87% of all strokes are ischemic, and 13% are hemorrhagic. When a stroke occurs, ischemia kills brain cells in the immediate area of injury. When brain cells die, they release chemicals that set off a chain reaction. Cells in the larger, surrounding area of ischemic brain tissue (i.e., penumbra) can die, resulting in permanent neurologic deficits or death.

A transient ischemic attack (TIA) is sometimes called a "mini-stroke; it is caused by a temporary clot (and blockage of blood flow) in the brain. Symptoms resemble acute ischemic stroke but resolve within minutes to a few hours with no permanent damage. TIAs are often a warning sign for acute ischemic stroke and should be medically managed with the same risk reduction strategies (see the Ischemic Stroke: Secondary Prevention section later in the chapter).

STROKE RISK FACTORS

The box below describes the modifiable and non-modifiable risk factors for stroke, many of which contribute to the development of atherosclerosis in cranial vasculature.

Modifiable risk factors	Non-modifiable risk factors
Hypertension – most important	Prior stroke or TIA
Atrial fibrillation	Advanced age (e.g., ≥ 80 years)
Dyslipidemia	Race (higher risk in African American patients)
Diabetes	
Physical inactivity	Genetic diseases (e.g., sickle cell disease)
Smoking	

PRESENTATION AND DIAGNOSIS

The American Stroke Association (ASA) and the American Heart Association (AHA) have public education campaigns to increase early recognition of stroke symptoms (see the Study Tip Gal below). Promptly calling 911 is essential, as brain tissue is rapidly lost as the stroke progresses (commonly stated as "time is brain").

SIGNS AND SYMPTOMS OF STROKE

ACT F.A.S.T.

Face drooping
Ask the person to smile. Does one side of the face droop or is it numb? Is the smile uneven?

Arm weakness
Ask the person to raise both arms. Does one arm drift downward?

Speech difficulty
Ask the person to repeat a simple sentence. Are the words slurred? Is the sentence repeated correctly?

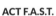

Time to call 911
If the person shows any of the symptoms above, even if they go away, call 911 immediately!

Once in the care of healthcare professionals, clinical assessment (e.g., history, physical exam, laboratory tests) and neurological assessment [e.g., use of the National Institutes of Health Stroke Scale (NIHSS)] help determine the severity of the stroke and guide treatment.

Brain imaging using computed tomography (CT) is ideally performed within 20 minutes of arrival to the emergency department to quickly identify whether the stroke symptoms are due to a hemorrhage. Drugs used to treat ischemic stroke can increase the risk of bleeding and can be harmful, or even fatal, in hemorrhagic stroke cases. Less commonly, magnetic resonance imaging (MRI) is performed.

ISCHEMIC STROKE: ACUTE MANAGEMENT

In addition to cardiac and respiratory support, the immediate goal of treatment is to restore blood flow to the ischemic area of the brain to obtain complete neurologic recovery. Intracranial pressure (ICP), cerebral perfusion pressure (CPP) and blood pressure (BP) should be monitored and controlled. Restoring blood flow may require mechanical removal of a clot (e.g., with stent retrievers), or the clot can be dissolved with intravenous fibrinolytic therapy if the patient arrives at the hospital in a timely manner after symptom onset.

ALTEPLASE

Alteplase is recombinant tissue plasminogen activator (tPA or rtPA). It binds to fibrin in a thrombus (clot) and converts plasminogen to plasmin, resulting in fibrinolysis. Alteplase is the only fibrinolytic drug FDA-approved to treat acute ischemic stroke. Tenecteplase, another fibrinolytic, is occasionally used off-label.

Patients are candidates for alteplase administration if there is no bleeding seen on brain imaging (i.e., CT scan has no acute abnormalities) and the following criteria for timing are met:

- Stroke symptom onset is ≤ 4.5 hours (guideline recommendation for most patients; FDA-approved timeline is symptom onset ≤ 3 hours).

- Alteplase can be administered within 60 minutes of hospital arrival (door-to-needle time).

Before administering alteplase, it should be established that the patient has no contraindications to use (see Study Tip Gal below and the Drug Table on the next page).

BLEEDING RISKS WITH ALTEPLASE

Alteplase breaks up existing clots → breaking up a clot increases the risk of bleeding

Before treatment, check that the patient isn't already at high bleeding risk. Select conditions and drugs that increase bleeding risk are contraindications to alteplase. They fit into these categories:

- Active internal bleed (e.g., ICH)

- Risk of internal bleed, due to:

  ❏ Severe hypertension (BP > 185/110 mmHg): if this is the only contraindication to treatment, BP should be lowered to < 185/110 mmHg with IV medications (e.g., labetalol, nicardipine) before proceeding with alteplase administration

  ❏ Other conditions (e.g., head trauma)

  ❏ Labs (e.g., elevated INR, low platelet count)

  ❏ Drug interactions (e.g., anticoagulant use)

DRUG	DOSING	SAFETY/SIDE EFFECTS/MONITORING
Alteplase *(Activase)* Injection ***Cathflo Activase*** (single-use 2 mg vial) used to restore function of potentially clotted central lines and devices	0.9 mg/kg (maximum dose 90 mg) Administer 10% of the calculated dose as a bolus over 1 minute then infuse the remainder over 60 minutes Must rule out hemorrhagic stroke before use (e.g., ICH, SAH)	**CONTRAINDICATIONS** Active internal bleeding or known bleeding diathesis History of recent stroke (within the past 3 months) Severe uncontrolled hypertension (BP > 185/110 mmHg – see Study Tip Gal on prior page and Monitoring below) Any prior intracranial hemorrhage (ICH) Other conditions that increase bleeding risk: recent (within 3 months) intracranial or intraspinal surgery or head trauma; presence of an intracranial neoplasm, arteriovenous malformation or aneurysm Labs that increase bleeding risk: INR > 1.7, aPTT > 40 seconds, platelet count < 100,000/mm³ Treatment-dose LMWH (within the previous 24 hours), use of a direct thrombin inhibitor or direct factor Xa inhibitor (within the previous 48 hours) or taking warfarin with an INR > 1.7 Blood glucose < 50 mg/dL **SIDE EFFECTS** Major bleeding (e.g., ICH) **MONITORING** Hgb, Hct, s/sx of bleeding Neurological assessments and BP (must be < 185/110 mmHg before alteplase is started and maintained at < 180/105 mmHg for at least 24 hours after the infusion) Head CT 24 hrs after treatment, before starting anticoagulants or antiplatelet drugs **NOTES** Contraindications and dosing differ when used for ACS (refer to the Acute Coronary Syndromes chapter) and pulmonary embolism, due to a higher risk of hemorrhagic conversion (i.e., brain bleed) in stroke If severe headache, acute hypertension, nausea, vomiting or worsening neurological function occurs, discontinue the infusion and obtain an emergent head CT The abbreviation "tPA" (or "TPA") is prone to errors; it is not recommended by ISMP

Contraindications are summarized from the package labeling and the AHA/ASA guidelines.

Alteplase Drug Interactions

- There is a risk for additive effects when used in combination with other drugs that can ↑ bleeding (see the Drug Interactions chapter for further discussion).

OTHER TREATMENTS

Aspirin

Initiation of aspirin 81 – 325 mg PO daily is recommended as soon as possible (within 48 hours) after stroke onset to prevent early recurrent stroke. Aspirin should not be given within 24 hours of fibrinolytic therapy.

Deep Vein Thrombosis (DVT) Prevention

DVT prophylaxis with intermittent pneumatic compression (IPC) devices is recommended. IPC devices are cuffs placed over the legs that periodically fill with air and squeeze the legs to increase blood flow.

If subcutaneous anticoagulants (unfractionated heparin or LMWH) are used, they should not be started within 24 hours of receiving alteplase.

Hypertension Management

See the Study Tip Gal on the previous page and the Drug Table above for BP criteria and management in patients who are eligible to receive alteplase.

If alteplase is not administered, IV antihypertensives (e.g., labetalol, nicardipine) may not be required unless BP is severely elevated (≥ 220/120 mmHg). In this case, a 15% reduction in BP during the first 24 hours after stroke onset is considered safe. Once neurologically stable, oral antihypertensive medications may be initiated (see the Ischemic Stroke: Secondary Prevention section).

Hyperglycemia Management

Maintain blood glucose levels in the range of 140 – 180 mg/dL and closely monitor to prevent hypoglycemia (which can mimic stroke symptoms).

ISCHEMIC STROKE: SECONDARY PREVENTION

The recommendations below reflect secondary prevention measures after the first occurrence of an ischemic stroke or TIA. Many of the same recommendations also apply to primary prevention of stroke.

TREATMENT OF MODIFIABLE RISK FACTORS

- Hypertension – blood pressure lowering treatment is often initiated after the first several days following a stroke. Thiazide diuretics, ACE inhibitors and ARBs have the best evidence for stroke risk reduction. A goal BP < 130/80 mmHg is recommended for most patients (see the Hypertension chapter). Lifestyle modifications are an important part of hypertension management (see below).

- Dyslipidemia – use a high-intensity statin (guidelines recommend atorvastatin 80 mg/day). In patients unable to achieve LDL goals, ezetimibe or a PCSK9 monoclonal antibody may be added to statin therapy (see the Dyslipidemia chapter).

- Diabetes – patients with no established history should be screened for diabetes in the post-stroke period; an A1C is the preferred test. Treat diabetes according to the most recent ADA guidelines (see the Diabetes chapter).

- Atrial fibrillation – cardioembolic stroke due to atrial fibrillation requires anticoagulation to prevent future strokes (see the Anticoagulation chapter).

- Lifestyle modifications – patients should be screened for obesity and counseled on lifestyle modifications for hypertension and cardiovascular risk reduction (e.g., smoking cessation, diet, exercise, weight loss).

  - Nutrition – a heart-healthy diet (e.g., a Mediterranean diet) emphasizing vegetables, fruits, fish, poultry, whole grains, legumes, nuts and olive oil is recommended. In addition, sodium restriction (e.g., < 1.5 grams/day) aids with blood pressure reduction.

  - Physical activity – if capable, patients should engage in at least 10 minutes of moderate-intensity exercise four days per week or 20 minutes of vigorous activity two days per week.

  - Weight reduction – maintain a BMI 18.5 – 24.9 kg/m^2 and a waist circumference < 35 inches for women and < 40 inches for men.

  - Alcohol intake – limit to ≤ 2 drinks/day for males and ≤ 1 drink/day for females.

ANTIPLATELET TREATMENT

For patients with non-cardioembolic ischemic stroke or TIA, antiplatelet therapy with aspirin, aspirin/extended-release dipyridamole or clopidogrel is recommended to reduce the risk of recurrent stroke, MI or death. Prasugrel is contraindicated in anyone with a history of TIA or stroke due to an increased risk of intracranial bleed.

The combination of clopidogrel and low-dose aspirin can be initiated within 24 hours of a minor ischemic stroke (i.e., NIHSS score ≤ 3, did not receive alteplase) and continued for 21 - 90 days. The combination should not be used long-term for secondary prevention of stroke or TIA as it increases the risk of hemorrhage. Rather, short-term dual antiplatelet therapy should be followed by antiplatelet monotherapy, continued indefinitely. This is different than the recommendations for dual antiplatelet therapy in heart disease (see the Stable Angina and Acute Coronary Syndromes chapters). Ticagrelor with aspirin can also be considered following a minor to moderate stroke (i.e., NIHSS score ≤ 5); this combination should not be continued beyond 30 days.

There is no added benefit to increasing the aspirin dose in patients already taking aspirin who have an ischemic stroke or TIA. Alternative antiplatelet are often considered, though no single drug or combination has been adequately studied in patients who have had an event while receiving aspirin.

Antiplatelet Drugs

Aspirin irreversibly inhibits cyclooxygenase-1 and 2 (COX-1 and 2) enzymes, resulting in decreased prostaglandin (PG) and thromboxane A2 (TXA2) production. TXA2 is a potent vasoconstrictor and inducer of platelet aggregation.

Dipyridamole (given with aspirin) inhibits the uptake of adenosine into platelets and increases cAMP levels, which inhibits platelet aggregation.

Clopidogrel is a prodrug that irreversibly inhibits P2Y12 ADP-mediated platelet activation and aggregation.

DRUG	DOSING	SAFETY/SIDE EFFECTS/MONITORING
Aspirin (*Bayer, Bufferin, Ecotrin,* Ascriptin, *Durlaza,* others) + omeprazole (*Yosprala*) <u>OTC</u>: tablet, chewable tablet, enteric coated tablet, suppository Rx: <u>ER</u> capsule (*Durlaza*), <u>delayed-release</u> tablet (*Yosprala*) See Pain chapter for more information on aspirin products	<u>50-325 mg daily</u> *Yosprala:* 81 mg/ 40 mg or 325 mg/ 40 mg daily Do not crush enteric-coated, delayed-release or ER products	**CONTRAINDICATIONS** NSAID or <u>salicylate allergy; children and teenagers</u> with viral infection due to risk of <u>Reye's syndrome</u> (symptoms include somnolence, N/V, confusion); rhinitis, nasal polyps or asthma (due to risk of urticaria, angioedema or bronchospasm) **WARNINGS** <u>Bleeding</u> [including GI bleed/ulceration, ↑ risk with heavy alcohol use or other drugs with bleeding risk (e.g., NSAIDs, anticoagulants, other antiplatelets)], <u>tinnitus</u> (salicylate <u>overdose</u>) **SIDE EFFECTS** <u>Dyspepsia, heartburn, bleeding,</u> nausea **MONITORING** Symptoms of bleeding, bruising **NOTES** To ↓ nausea, use EC or buffered product or take with food <u>PPIs</u> may be <u>used to protect the gut</u> with chronic NSAID use (e.g., *Yosprala* is indicated for those at risk of developing aspirin-associated gastric ulcers); <u>consider the risks</u> from chronic PPI use (↓ bone density, ↑ infection risk)
Extended-release dipyridamole/aspirin (*Aggrenox**) Capsule	200 mg/25 mg BID If intolerable headache: 200 mg/ 25 mg QHS (+ low-dose aspirin daily in the morning), then resume BID dosing within 1 week	As above for aspirin component plus: **WARNINGS** <u>Hypotension</u> and chest pain (in patients with coronary artery disease) can occur due to the <u>vasodilatory effects</u> of dipyridamole **SIDE EFFECTS** <u>Headache</u> (from the vasodilatory effects of dipyridamole) **NOTES** <u>Not interchangeable</u> with the individual components of aspirin and dipyridamole Amount of aspirin provided is not adequate for prevention of cardiac events (e.g., MI)
Clopidogrel (*Plavix*) Tablet	<u>75 mg daily</u>	**BOXED WARNINGS** Clopidogrel is a <u>prodrug</u>. Effectiveness depends on the <u>conversion</u> to an <u>active metabolite</u>, mainly by <u>CYP450 2C19</u>. Poor metabolizers of CYP2C19 exhibit higher cardiovascular events than patients with normal CYP2C19 function. <u>Tests to check CYP2C19 genotype</u> can be used as an aid in determining a therapeutic strategy. Consider alternative treatments in patients identified as CYP2C19 poor metabolizers. See the Pharmacogenomics chapter. **CONTRAINDICATIONS** Active <u>serious bleeding</u> (e.g., GI bleed, intracranial hemorrhage) **WARNINGS** <u>Bleeding risk: stop</u> 5 days <u>prior to elective surgery,</u> do not use with omeprazole or <u>esomeprazole</u> (see the Drug Interactions section), premature discontinuation (↑ risk of thrombosis), thrombotic thrombocytopenic purpura (<u>TTP</u>) **SIDE EFFECTS** Generally well tolerated, unless <u>bleeding</u> occurs **MONITORING** Symptoms of bleeding, Hgb/Hct as necessary **NOTES** Drug of choice in stroke/TIA if a <u>contraindication or allergy to aspirin</u>; do not use in combination with aspirin long-term for stroke prevention

Brand discontinued but brand name still used in practice.

Antiplatelet Drug Interactions

- Most drug interactions are due to <u>additive effects</u> with other drugs that can ↑ <u>bleeding risk</u> (e.g., <u>anticoagulants</u>, <u>NSAIDs, SSRIs, SNRIs, some herbals</u>). See the Drug Interactions chapter.

- Clopidogrel: <u>avoid</u> in combination with <u>omeprazole</u> and <u>esomeprazole</u> (other PPIs interact less) and use caution with other CYP2C19 inhibitors.

HEMORRHAGIC STROKE

Hemorrhagic strokes result in a significant amount of morbidity and mortality. Treatment is largely supportive and includes airway management, establishing hemostasis, monitoring (and lowering if needed) intracranial pressure, prevention or management of seizures, assessment for dysphagia, and control of blood pressure and blood glucose. Hospitalized patients with hemorrhagic stroke should use IPC devices on the legs to prevent DVT. Anticoagulants should not be used while a patient is bleeding.

INTRACEREBRAL HEMORRHAGE (ICH)

In addition to traditional stroke risk factors (e.g., hypertension), other common causes of ICH include trauma (e.g., a motor vehicle collision) or use of antithrombotic medications (e.g., anticoagulants). There is a high risk for rapid neurologic deterioration in the early hours of an ICH due to ongoing bleeding and enlargement of the brain hematoma.

Patients with a severe coagulation factor deficiency or thrombocytopenia should receive appropriate therapies (e.g., factor replacement, platelet infusions). As appropriate, anticoagulants should be discontinued and reversal agents should be administered (see the Anticoagulation chapter for information on reversal drugs). If there is clinical evidence of seizures, they should be treated, but prophylactic antiseizure medications (ASMs) should not be used.

Treating Elevated Intracranial Pressure

Increased intracranial pressure (ICP), caused by increased blood volume and edema in a relatively fixed intracranial space, is the primary complication of an ICH; it is a medical emergency that can lead to brain death. Interventions to lower ICP include elevating the head of the bed by at least 30 degrees and administering IV osmotic therapy with either hypertonic saline (e.g., NaCl 3%, NaCl 23.4%) or mannitol. These drugs increase plasma osmolarity, creating an osmotic gradient that draws water out of the brain parenchyma and into the intravascular space where it can then be renally excreted.

Mannitol

DRUG	DOSING	SAFETY/SIDE EFFECTS/MONITORING
Mannitol (Osmitrol) Injection	5%, 10%, 15%, 20%, 25% Mannitol 20%: 0.25-1 g/kg/dose IV Q6-8H PRN	**CONTRAINDICATIONS** Severe renal disease (anuria), severe hypovolemia, pulmonary edema or congestion, active intracranial bleed (except during craniotomy) **WARNINGS** CNS toxicity (can accumulate in the brain, causing rebound increases in ICP, if used for long periods of time as a continuous infusion; intermittent boluses preferred), extravasation (vesicant), nephrotoxicity, fluid and electrolyte imbalances (e.g., dehydration, hyperosmolar-induced hyperkalemia, acidosis, ↑ osmolar gap) **SIDE EFFECTS** Dehydration, headache, lethargy, ↑ or ↓ BP **MONITORING** Renal function, daily fluid intake and output, serum electrolytes, serum and urine osmolality, ICP, CPP **NOTES** Maintain serum osmolality < 300-320 mOsm/kg Inspect for crystals before administering; if crystals are present, warm the solution to redissolve Use a filter for administration with mannitol concentrations ≥ 20%

ACUTE SUBARACHNOID HEMORRHAGE (SAH)

SAH is bleeding in the space between the brain and the surrounding membrane (subarachnoid space). SAH usually results from a cerebral aneurysm rupture and results in a severe headache, often described as the "worst headache ever experienced." Surgical clipping or endovascular coiling to completely remove the aneurysm is performed when feasible to prevent rebleeding. Cerebral artery vasospasm can occur 3 – 21 days after the bleed, causing delayed cerebral ischemia; oral nimodipine has been shown to improve outcomes associated with vasospasm-induced ischemia and should be initiated in patients with SAH.

The use of prophylactic ASMs may be considered in the immediate post-hemorrhagic period to prevent seizures. The routine use of long-term ASMs is not recommended but may be considered for patients with known risk factors for delayed seizure disorder (e.g., prior seizure, intracerebral hematoma).

Nimodipine

Nimodipine is a dihydropyridine calcium channel blocker that is more selective for cerebral arteries due to increased lipophilicity. It is only indicated for SAH and is not used as an antihypertensive treatment.

DRUG	DOSING	SAFETY/SIDE EFFECTS/MONITORING
Nimodipine (*Nymalize*) Capsule, oral solution	60 mg PO Q4H x 21 days Swallow capsules whole; administer on an empty stomach, at least 1 hour before or 2 hours after meals Cirrhosis: 30 mg PO Q4H for 21 days (closely monitor)	**BOXED WARNINGS** Do not administer nimodipine IV or by other parenteral routes; death and serious life-threatening adverse events have occurred (including cardiac arrest, cardiovascular collapse, hypotension and bradycardia) when the contents of nimodipine capsules have been inadvertently injected parenterally (see Notes) **CONTRAINDICATIONS** ↑ risk of significant hypotension when used in combination with strong inhibitors of CYP3A4 (see the Drug Interactions section) **SIDE EFFECTS** Hypotension **MONITORING** CPP, ICP, BP, HR, neurological checks **NOTES** If capsules cannot be swallowed and the oral solution is unavailable, the capsule contents may be withdrawn with a parenteral syringe, then transferred to an oral syringe that cannot accept a needle and that can only administer medication orally or via nasogastric tube; the medication should be drawn up in the pharmacy to reduce medication errors Label oral syringes "For Oral Use Only" or "Not for IV Use" (including the oral syringe supplied with the commercially available solution)

Nimodipine Drug Interactions

- Nimodipine is a major substrate of CYP3A4; strong CYP3A4 inhibitors (e.g., clarithromycin, protease inhibitors, azole antifungals) are contraindicated. Avoid grapefruit juice. Strong CYP3A4 inducers (e.g., rifampin, carbamazepine, phenytoin, St. John's wort) can decrease the levels of nimodipine and should be avoided.

KEY COUNSELING POINTS

Refer to the Stable Angina chapter for patient counseling on aspirin and clopidogrel.

Select Guidelines/References
Guidelines for the early management of patients with acute ischemic stroke: 2019 update to the 2018 guidelines for the early management of acute ischemic stroke: A guideline for healthcare professionals from the American Heart Association/American Stroke Association. *Stroke.* 2019;50:e344-e418.

2018 Guidelines for the early management of patients with acute ischemic stroke. AHA/ASA. *Stroke.* 2018;49:e46-e99.

2021 Guideline for the prevention of stroke in patients with stroke and transient ischemic attack. AHA/ASA. *Stroke.* 2021;52(7):e364-e467.

Guidelines for the management of spontaneous intracerebral hemorrhage. AHA/ASA. *Stroke.* 2015;41:2108-2129.

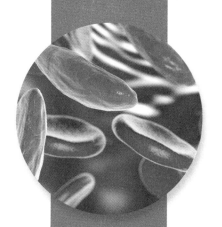
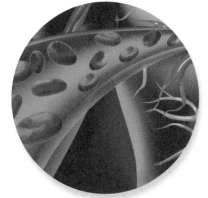
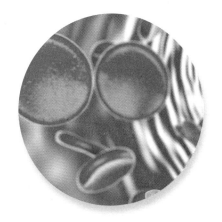

ANTICOAGULATION & BLOOD DISORDERS

CONTENTS

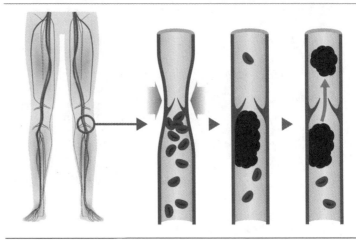

iStock.com/metamorworks

CHAPTER 34
ANTICOAGULATION

BACKGROUND

Anticoagulants are used to prevent blood clots from forming and to keep existing clots from becoming larger. They do not break down clots (like fibrinolytics). Anticoagulants are used in the prevention and treatment of venous thromboembolism (VTE), which refers to deep vein thrombosis (DVT) and/or pulmonary embolism (PE). Anticoagulants are also used in the immediate treatment of acute coronary syndromes (ACS) and for the prevention of cardioembolic stroke. The most common side effect of anticoagulants is bleeding, which can be fatal. Anticoagulants are high-alert medications for this reason.

CLOT FORMATION

Coagulation is the process by which blood clots form. A number of factors can lead to activation of the coagulation process, such as blood vessel injury, blood stasis (stopping or slowing of blood flow) and pro-thrombotic conditions.

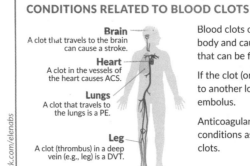

CONDITIONS RELATED TO BLOOD CLOTS

Brain
A clot that travels to the brain can cause a stroke.

Heart
A clot in the vessels of the heart causes ACS.

Lungs
A clot that travels to the lungs is a PE.

Leg
A clot (thrombus) in a deep vein (e.g., leg) is a DVT.

Blood clots can form anywhere in the body and cause serious conditions that can be fatal.

If the clot (or a piece of it) travels to another location, it is called an embolus.

Anticoagulants are used for conditions associated with blood clots.

iStock.com/elenabs

CONTENT LEGEND

☀ = Study Tip Gal

COAGULATION CASCADE

An important part of coagulation is the coagulation cascade which is a process that occurs through activation of a series of clotting factors.

Clotting factors are proteins made primarily by the liver. All of the clotting factors have an inactive and active form; the "a" next to a factor means "active/activated" (e.g., factor X is inactive and factor Xa is active). Once activated, a clotting factor will activate the next clotting factor in the sequence until fibrin is formed. The coagulation cascade has two pathways that lead to fibrin formation: the contact activation pathway (or the intrinsic pathway) and the tissue factor pathway (or the extrinsic pathway). Anticoagulants inhibit the coagulation cascade and prevent (or stop further) clot formation (See Study Tip Gal below).

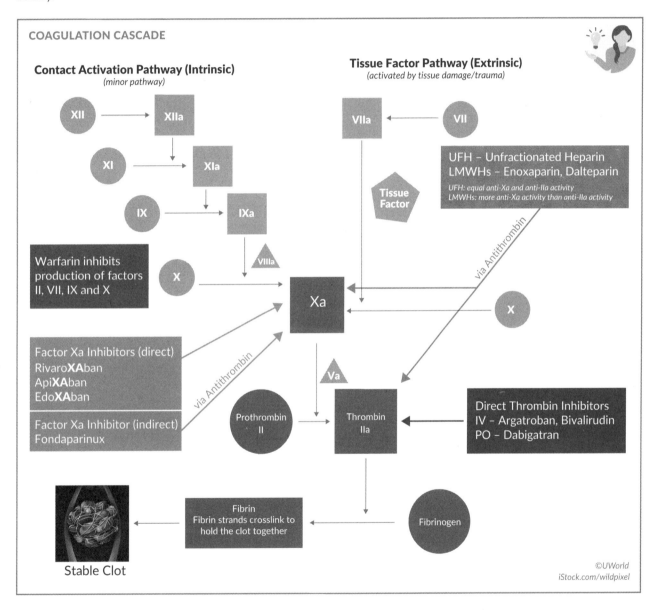

DRUG TREATMENT

Anticoagulants work by various mechanisms and routes of administration to prevent and treat a variety of conditions. An overview of some of these clinical conditions is included at the end of the chapter.

Parenteral anticoagulants are used for ACS treatment and prevention/treatment of VTE. Oral anticoagulants are used for prevention/treatment of VTE, as well as for cardioembolic stroke prevention in patients with atrial fibrillation (AF). These anticoagulants include warfarin (a vitamin K antagonist), factor Xa inhibitors and thrombin inhibitors. The oral factor Xa inhibitors and thrombin inhibitors are further classified as <u>direct-acting oral anticoagulants</u> (<u>DOACs</u>). For most conditions, DOACs are preferred over warfarin (see <u>Study Tip Gal</u> on right).

DOACs VERSUS WARFARIN

DOACs have fewer drug-drug interactions, less or comparable bleeding and a shorter onset and duration of action compared to warfarin

DOAC dosing is based on the indication and kidney/liver function – there is no need to adjust the dose based on the INR (as with warfarin)

DOACs are preferred for stroke prevention in AF

- BUT – if there is moderate-to-severe mitral stenosis or a mechanical heart valve, use warfarin

DOACs are preferred for VTE treatment

- BUT – if the patient has triple-positive antiphospholipid syndrome or a mechanical heart valve, use warfarin

Several organizations publish anticoagulation guidelines, including the <u>American College of Chest Physicians (CHEST)</u> and the American College of Cardiology/American Heart Association (ACC/AHA).

VITAMIN K ANTAGONISM

<u>Warfarin</u> is a <u>vitamin K antagonist</u>. Vitamin K is required for the carboxylation (activation) of clotting <u>factors II, VII, IX and X</u>. Without adequate vitamin K, the liver still produces the clotting factors, but they have reduced coagulant activity. Warfarin has a <u>narrow therapeutic range</u> and requires careful <u>monitoring</u> of the international normalized ratio (<u>INR</u>), which is <u>affected by</u> many <u>drugs</u> and <u>changes in dietary vitamin K</u>.

FACTOR Xa INHIBITION

<u>Antithrombin (AT)</u> is an endogenous (naturally occurring in the body) <u>anticoagulant</u>; it <u>inactivates thrombin</u> (factor IIa) and other proteases (e.g., <u>factor Xa</u>) involved in blood clotting. <u>Unfractionated heparin (UFH), low molecular weight heparins</u> (<u>LMWHs</u>) and <u>fondaparinux</u> work by <u>binding to AT</u> to cause a conformational change which <u>increases AT activity</u> 1,000-fold. UFH inhibits factor IIa (thrombin) and factor Xa equally while <u>LMWHs inhibit factor Xa to a greater degree</u> than UFH. <u>Fondaparinux</u> (*Arixtra*) has <u>selective</u> inhibition of factor Xa.

<u>Apixaban</u> (*Eliquis*), <u>edoxaban</u> (*Savaysa*) and <u>rivaroxaban</u> (*Xarelto*) work by <u>inhibiting factor Xa directly</u>. These oral medications are taken once or twice daily and require no laboratory monitoring for efficacy.

THROMBIN INHIBITION

<u>UFH and LMWH</u> indirectly inhibit thrombin and factor Xa through AT binding. <u>Direct thrombin inhibitors (DTIs) block thrombin directly</u>, decreasing the amount of fibrin available for clot formation. The <u>intravenous DTIs</u> (e.g., argatroban) are important clinically since they <u>do not cross-react with heparin-induced thrombocytopenia (HIT)</u> antibodies. <u>Dabigatran</u> (*Pradaxa*) is an <u>oral DTI</u>.

KEY POINTS

When studying the Anticoagulation, Acute Coronary Syndromes, Stable Angina and Stroke chapters, it can be difficult to determine when a fibrinolytic, antiplatelet or anticoagulant would be appropriate.

- Oral anticoagulants are used mainly in AF (for stroke prevention) and for DVT/PE (treatment and prevention). Oral medications like *Xarelto* or *Eliquis* are not indicated for the acute management of an ACS since platelet aggregation is the main target of drug therapy.

- Fibrinolytics break down existing clots but are associated with a very high risk of bleeding. They are used to immediately treat an acute ischemic stroke or STEMI when the patient could die without rapid restoration of blood flow.

- Antiplatelet drugs (e.g., aspirin, clopidogrel, ticagrelor) are used mainly for coronary artery disease (including ACS) and to prevent recurrent ischemic stroke/TIA. Dual antiplatelet therapy (DAPT) refers to using both aspirin and a P2Y12 inhibitor (e.g., clopidogrel) together, which is very common in patients who have had an ACS. Antiplatelet drugs are not sufficient for treating DVT/PE.

HIGH-ALERT MEDICATIONS

All anticoagulants can cause <u>significant bleeding</u> and are classified as "<u>high-alert</u>" medications by the Institute for Safe Medication Practices (ISMP). Bleeding events with anticoagulants put patients at increased risk for death. The <u>Joint Commission's National Patient Safety Goals</u> require policies and <u>protocols</u> to properly <u>initiate and manage anticoagulant therapy</u>. Patients receiving therapeutic anticoagulation should receive individualized care through a defined process that <u>includes standardized ordering, dispensing, administration, monitoring and patient/caregiver education</u>. Refer to the Medication Safety & Quality Improvement chapter for additional information. When pharmacists are involved in managing anticoagulants, patient care and outcomes are improved and costs are decreased.

The common types of visible bleeding and select causes are reviewed in the box below. In some cases, bleeding will not be visible, but can be identified from symptoms and/or labs. An <u>acute drop in hemoglobin</u> (e.g., ≥ 2 g/dL) could signify that bleeding is occurring (visible or not). Internal bleeding can occur anywhere, such as a retroperitoneal (behind the peritoneal space) bleed, a dissection (tear) within a blood vessel wall (e.g., aortic dissection) or an intracranial bleed (e.g., hemorrhagic stroke).

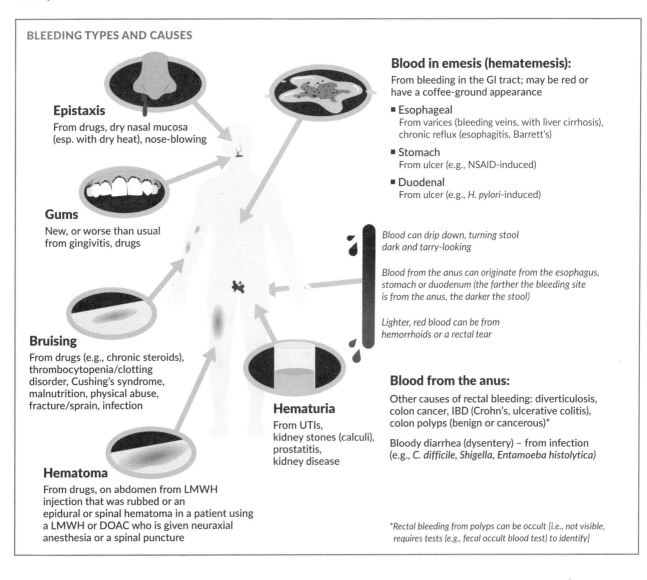

BLEEDING TYPES AND CAUSES

Epistaxis
From drugs, dry nasal mucosa (esp. with dry heat), nose-blowing

Gums
New, or worse than usual from gingivitis, drugs

Bruising
From drugs (e.g., chronic steroids), thrombocytopenia/clotting disorder, Cushing's syndrome, malnutrition, physical abuse, fracture/sprain, infection

Hematoma
From drugs, on abdomen from LMWH injection that was rubbed or an epidural or spinal hematoma in a patient using a LMWH or DOAC who is given neuraxial anesthesia or a spinal puncture

Blood in emesis (hematemesis):
From bleeding in the GI tract; may be red or have a coffee-ground appearance

- **Esophageal**
  From varices (bleeding veins, with liver cirrhosis), chronic reflux (esophagitis, Barrett's)

- **Stomach**
  From ulcer (e.g., NSAID-induced)

- **Duodenal**
  From ulcer (e.g., *H. pylori*-induced)

Blood can drip down, turning stool dark and tarry-looking

Blood from the anus can originate from the esophagus, stomach or duodenum (the farther the bleeding site is from the anus, the darker the stool)

Lighter, red blood can be from hemorrhoids or a rectal tear

Hematuria
From UTIs, kidney stones (calculi), prostatitis, kidney disease

Blood from the anus:
Other causes of rectal bleeding: diverticulosis, colon cancer, IBD (Crohn's, ulcerative colitis), colon polyps (benign or cancerous)*

Bloody diarrhea (dysentery) – from infection (e.g., *C. difficile, Shigella, Entamoeba histolytica*)

*Rectal bleeding from polyps can be occult [i.e., not visible, requires tests (e.g., fecal occult blood test) to identify]

UNFRACTIONATED HEPARIN

UFH binds to antithrombin (AT) and potentiates its ability to inactivate thrombin (factor IIa) and factor Xa (as well as factors IXa, XIa, XIIa and plasmin), thus preventing the conversion of fibrinogen to fibrin.

DRUG	DOSING	SAFETY/SIDE EFFECTS/MONITORING
Unfractionated Heparin Injection Premixed solution in D5W, NS or ½NS (25,000 units in 250 mL) Syringes, vials and flushes are available in many strengths (ranging from 1 unit/mL to 20,000 units/mL) and volumes (ranging from 1 to 30 mL)	**Prophylaxis of VTE** 5,000 units SC Q8-12H **Treatment of VTE** 80 units/kg IV bolus; 18 units/kg/hr infusion **Treatment of ACS/STEMI** 60 units/kg IV bolus; 12 units/kg/hr infusion Use total body weight for dosing Do not administer IM due to hematoma risk	**CONTRAINDICATIONS** Uncontrolled active bleed (e.g., intracranial hemorrhage), severe thrombocytopenia, history of HIT Some products contain benzyl alcohol as a preservative (do not use in neonates, infants, pregnancy and breastfeeding) and/or may be derived from animal tissue (do not use with pork allergy) **WARNING** Fatal medication errors: verify the correct concentration is chosen **SIDE EFFECTS** Bleeding (e.g., epistaxis, bruising, gingival, GI), thrombocytopenia, HIT, hyperkalemia, osteoporosis (with long-term use), alopecia **MONITORING** aPTT or anti-Xa level – check 6 hours after initiation and every 6 hrs until therapeutic, then every 24 hrs and with every dosage change aPTT therapeutic range is 1.5-2.5x control (per specific institutional protocol); anti-Xa therapeutic range typically 0.3-0.7 units/mL aPTT and anti-Xa monitoring are not required for SC (prophylactic) dosing Platelets, Hgb, Hct at baseline and daily (↓ in platelets > 50% from baseline suggests possible HIT) **NOTES** Antidote: protamine (see Antidotes and Reversal section) Unpredictable anticoagulant response (has variable and extensive binding to plasma proteins and cells) Continuous IV infusions are common for treating VTE and ACS because heparin has a rapid onset and short half-life (1.5 hrs); onset of SC is longer (20-30 mins) Heparin lock-flushes (*HepFlush*) are only used to keep IV lines open. Fatal errors, especially in neonates, have occurred when the incorrect heparin strength (higher concentration) was chosen. Heparin injection 10,000 units/mL and flushes 10 or 100 units/mL look and sound alike.

LOW MOLECULAR WEIGHT HEPARINS

LMWHs bind to AT and potentiate its ability to inactivate factor Xa and factor IIa which prevents conversion of fibrinogen to fibrin. The anti-factor Xa activity is much greater than the anti-factor IIa activity.

DRUG	DOSING	SAFETY/SIDE EFFECTS/MONITORING
Enoxaparin (Lovenox) Multidose vial (300 mg/3 mL) and prefilled syringes: 30 mg/0.3 mL 40 mg/0.4 mL 60 mg/0.6 mL 80 mg/0.8 mL 100 mg/mL 120 mg/0.8 mL 150 mg/mL 1 mg = 100 units anti-Xa activity	**Prophylaxis of VTE** 30 mg SC Q12H or 40 mg SC daily CrCl < 30 mL/min: 30 mg SC daily **Treatment of VTE and UA/NSTEMI** 1 mg/kg SC Q12H or 1.5 mg/kg SC daily (only for inpatient VTE treatment) CrCl < 30 mL/min: 1 mg/kg SC daily **Treatment of STEMI in patients < 75 years of age** 30 mg IV bolus plus a 1 mg/kg SC dose followed by 1 mg/kg SC Q12H (max 100 mg for the first two SC doses only) CrCl < 30 mL/min: 30 mg IV bolus plus a 1 mg/kg SC dose, followed by 1 mg/kg SC daily **Treatment of STEMI in patients ≥ 75 years of age** 0.75 mg/kg SC Q12H (no bolus - max 75 mg for the first two SC doses only) CrCl < 30 mL/min: 1 mg/kg SC daily (no bolus) Use total body weight for dosing	**BOXED WARNINGS** Patients receiving neuraxial anesthesia (epidural, spinal) or undergoing spinal puncture are at risk of hematomas and subsequent paralysis **CONTRAINDICATIONS** History of HIT, active major bleed, hypersensitivity to pork **SIDE EFFECTS** Bleeding, anemia, injection site reactions (e.g., pain, bruising, hematomas), ↓ platelets (thrombocytopenia, including HIT) **MONITORING** Platelets, Hgb, Hct, SCr Routine monitoring for efficacy is not required due to more predictable anticoagulant response than UFH If monitoring is needed, anti-Xa levels are used, not aPTT. Anti-Xa level monitoring is recommended in pregnancy and may be useful in renal insufficiency, obesity, low body weight, pediatrics, elderly Obtain peak anti-Xa levels 4 hours post SC dose; target range varies based on dosing frequency (once vs. twice daily) and indication (VTE treatment vs. prophylaxis) **NOTES** Antidote: protamine (see Antidotes and Reversal section) HIT antibodies have cross-sensitivity with LMWHs Do not expel air bubble from syringe prior to injection (can cause loss of drug)
Dalteparin (Fragmin)	**Prophylaxis of VTE** 2,500-5,000 units SC daily **Treatment of UA/NSTEMI** 120 units/kg (max 10,000 units) SC Q12H	Do not administer IM Store at room temperature

UFH/LMWH Drug Interactions

- Most drug interactions are due to additive effects with other drugs that can ↑ bleeding risk (other anticoagulants, antiplatelet drugs, some herbal supplements, NSAIDs, SSRIs, SNRIs, fibrinolytics). See the Drug Interactions chapter.

HEPARIN-INDUCED THROMBOCYTOPENIA

Heparin-induced thrombocytopenia (HIT) is an immune-mediated IgG drug reaction that has a high risk of venous and arterial thrombosis. The immune system forms antibodies against heparin bound to platelet factor 4 (PF4); the antibodies then join with heparin and PF4 to create a complex, and this complex binds to the Fc receptors on platelets. This causes platelet activation and a release of pro-coagulant microparticles.

HIT is a prothrombotic state and, if left untreated, can cause many complications, including heparin-induced thrombocytopenia and thrombosis (HITT). HITT leads to amputations, post-thrombotic syndrome and/or death. The estimated incidence of HIT is ~5% of patients exposed to heparin for more than four days. It is lower with a shorter duration of treatment. The probability of HIT can be assessed by calculating a 4 Ts score, which includes an evaluation of the following:

- **T**hrombocytopenia: an unexplained > 50% drop in platelet count from baseline is highly suspicious of HIT.
- **T**iming of platelet count drop: the typical onset of HIT occurs 5 – 10 days after the start of heparin or within hours if a patient has been exposed to heparin within the past three months.
- **T**hrombosis: can be a new suspected or confirmed thrombosis or skin lesions that are necrotizing or non-necrotizing.
- O**t**her causes: in addition to the criteria above, a ruling out (or inability to identify) other probable causes of HIT increases the likelihood of a diagnosis.

If there is a compatible clinical picture of HIT, a heparin-PF4 antibody enzyme-linked immunosorbent assay (ELISA) test, an immunoassay, is completed; results may be confirmed with a functional assay (e.g., serotonin release assay, heparin-induced platelet aggregation assay).

MANAGEMENT OF HIT COMPLICATED BY THROMBOSIS (HITT)

- If HIT is suspected or confirmed, stop all forms of heparin and LMWH, including heparin flushes and heparin-coated catheters. If the patient is on warfarin and diagnosed with HIT, the warfarin should be discontinued and vitamin K should be administered. Although the patient is at a high risk of thrombosis, warfarin use with a low platelet count has a high correlation with warfarin-induced limb gangrene and necrosis.
- For the immediate treatment of HIT, rapid-acting non-heparin anticoagulants (e.g., argatroban) are to be used.
- Do not start warfarin therapy until the platelets have recovered to ≥ 150,000 cells/mm³. Warfarin should be initiated at lower doses (5 mg maximum). Overlap warfarin with a non-heparin anticoagulant for a minimum of five days and until the INR is within the target range for at least 24 hours (i.e., as measured on two consecutive days). Argatroban can increase the INR; the value must be interpreted cautiously if argatroban is given with warfarin.
- If urgent cardiac surgery or PCI is required, bivalirudin is the preferred anticoagulant.

FACTOR Xa INHIBITORS

Apixaban *(Eliquis)*, edoxaban *(Savaysa)* and rivaroxaban *(Xarelto)* are direct factor Xa inhibitors that are administered orally. Fondaparinux *(Arixtra)* is an injectable synthetic pentasaccharide that selectively inhibits factor Xa via binding to antithrombin (AT), making it an indirect inhibitor of factor Xa. Fondaparinux is used off-label for HIT.

DRUG	DOSING	SAFETY/SIDE EFFECTS/ MONITORING
Oral Direct Factor Xa Inhibitors		
Apixaban *(Eliquis)* Tablet *Eliquis DVT/PE Starter Pack:* 30-day blister pack (for ease of prescribing for DVT/PE treatment) Missed Dose: Take immediately on the same day, then resume twice daily dosing; the dose should not be doubled to make up for a missed dose	**Nonvalvular AF (stroke prophylaxis)** 5 mg PO BID If patient has at least 2 of the following: age ≥ 80 years, body weight ≤ 60 kg or SCr ≥ 1.5 mg/dL, then give 2.5 mg BID **Treatment of DVT/PE** Initial: 10 mg PO BID x 7 days, then 5 mg PO BID Extended phase (after ≥ 6 months of initial treatment): 2.5 mg PO BID **Prophylaxis for DVT (after knee/hip replacement)** 2.5 mg PO BID (for 12 days after knee or 35 days after hip replacement surgery); give first dose 12-24 hours after surgery	**BOXED WARNINGS** All: patients receiving neuraxial anesthesia (epidural, spinal) or undergoing spinal puncture are at risk of hematomas and subsequent paralysis Premature discontinuation ↑ risk of thrombotic events Edoxaban only: reduced efficacy in nonvalvular AF patients with CrCl > 95 mL/min; do not use **CONTRAINDICATIONS** Active pathological bleeding **WARNINGS** Not recommended with prosthetic heart valves or triple-positive antiphospholipid syndrome (i.e., all 3 antiphospholipid antibodies are positive), avoid in patients with moderate to severe hepatic impairment
Rivaroxaban *(Xarelto)* Tablet, oral suspension *Xarelto Starter Pack:* 30-day blister pack containing 15 mg and 20 mg tablets (for ease of prescribing for DVT/PE treatment) Missed Dose: Administer the dose as soon as possible on the same day as follows: If taking 15 mg twice daily: take immediately to ensure intake of 30 mg/day (in this instance, two 15 mg tablets may be taken at once); then resume regular schedule on the following day If taking 10, 15 or 20 mg once daily: take immediately on the same day; otherwise skip	Doses ≥ 15 mg must be taken with food; 10 mg dose can be taken without regard to meals **Nonvalvular AF (stroke prophylaxis)** CrCl > 50 mL/min: 20 mg PO daily with evening meal CrCl 15-50 mL/min: 15 mg PO daily with evening meal CrCl < 15 mL/min: 15 mg PO daily (per manufacturer); limited data **Treatment of DVT/PE** Initial: 15 mg PO BID x 21 days, then 20 mg PO daily with food Extended phase (after ≥ 6 months of initial treatment): 10 mg PO daily CrCl 15-30 mL/min: use cautiously due to limited data CrCl < 15 mL/min: avoid use **Prophylaxis for DVT (after knee/hip replacement) and VTE (in acutely ill medical patients)** 10 mg PO daily for 12 days (knee replacement), 35 days (hip replacement) or 31 to 39 days (acutely ill medical patients) Give first dose 6-10 hours after knee/hip replacement surgery CrCl 15-30 mL/min: use cautiously due to limited data CrCl < 15 mL/min: avoid use **Reduction in the risk of major CVD events in CAD/PAD** 2.5 mg PO BID in combination with low-dose aspirin CrCl < 15 mL/min: 15 mg PO daily (per manufacturer); limited data	**SIDE EFFECTS** Generally well-tolerated, unless bleeding occurs Edoxaban: rash, ↑ LFTs **MONITORING** Hgb, Hct, SCr, LFTs; no monitoring of efficacy required **NOTES** Antidote for apixaban and rivaroxaban: andexanet alfa *(Andexxa)* All: can be crushed and put on applesauce or suspended in water to administer by NG tube Apixaban only: can be crushed and mixed in water, D5W or apple juice **Elective Surgery** Rivaroxaban, edoxaban: discontinue 24 hours prior Apixaban: discontinue 48 hours prior if moderate-high bleeding risk or 24 hours prior if low bleeding risk
Edoxaban *(Savaysa)* Tablet Missed Dose: Take immediately on the same day; the dose should not be doubled to make up for a missed dose	**Nonvalvular AF (stroke prophylaxis)** CrCl > 95 mL/min: do not use CrCl 51-95 mL/min: 60 mg daily CrCl 15-50 mL/min: 30 mg daily CrCl < 15 mL/min: not recommended **Treatment of DVT/PE** 60 mg daily, start after 5-10 days of parenteral anticoagulation CrCl 15-50 mL/min, body weight ≤ 60 kg or on certain P-gp inhibitors: 30 mg daily CrCl < 15 mL/min: not recommended	

DRUG	DOSING	SAFETY/SIDE EFFECTS/MONITORING
Injectable Indirect Factor Xa Inhibitor (SC)		

Fondaparinux *(Arixtra)* Prefilled syringes: 2.5 mg/0.5 mL 5 mg/0.4 mL 7.5 mg/0.6 mL 10 mg/0.8 mL Store at room temperature	**Prophylaxis of VTE** ≥ 50 kg: 2.5 mg SC daily < 50 kg: contraindicated **Treatment of VTE** < 50 kg: 5 mg SC daily 50-100 kg: 7.5 mg SC daily > 100 kg: 10 mg SC daily **Both Indications** CrCl 30-50 mL/min: use caution CrCl < 30 mL/min: contraindicated	**BOXED WARNING** Patients receiving neuraxial anesthesia (epidural, spinal) or undergoing spinal puncture are at risk of hematomas and subsequent paralysis **CONTRAINDICATIONS** Severe renal impairment (CrCl < 30 mL/min), active major bleed, bacterial endocarditis, thrombocytopenia with positive test for anti-platelet antibodies in presence of fondaparinux **SIDE EFFECTS** Bleeding (e.g., epistaxis, bruising, gingival, GI), anemia, local injection site reactions (rash, pruritus, bruising), thrombocytopenia **MONITORING** Platelets, Hgb, Hct, SCr, anti-Xa levels (3 hrs post-dose; routine monitoring not required) **NOTES** Do not expel air bubble from syringe prior to injection No antidote Do not administer IM

Factor Xa Inhibitor Drug Interactions

- Monitor for additive effects with other drugs that can ↑ bleeding risk (antiplatelet drugs, some herbals, NSAIDs, SSRIs, SNRIs, fibrinolytics). See the Drug Interactions chapter.

- Apixaban is a substrate of CYP450 3A4 (major) and P-gp. Avoid use with strong dual inducers of CYP3A4 and P-gp (e.g., carbamazepine, phenytoin, rifampin, St. John's wort). For patients receiving doses > 2.5 mg BID, the dose of apixaban should be decreased by 50% when coadministered with drugs that are strong dual inhibitors of CYP3A4 and P-gp (e.g., itraconazole, ketoconazole, ritonavir). For patients taking 2.5 mg BID, avoid these strong dual inhibitors.

- Rivaroxaban is a substrate of CYP3A4 (major) and P-gp. Avoid use with drugs that are combined P-gp and strong CYP3A4 inducers (e.g., carbamazepine, phenytoin, rifampin, St. John's wort) or combined P-gp and strong CYP3A4 inhibitors (e.g., ketoconazole, itraconazole, lopinavir/ritonavir, ritonavir, conivaptan). The benefit must outweigh the potential risks in patients who have a CrCl 15 – 80 mL/min and are receiving combined P-gp and moderate CYP3A4 inhibitors (e.g., diltiazem, verapamil, dronedarone, erythromycin).

- Edoxaban is a substrate of P-gp; avoid use with rifampin. When treating DVT/PE, reduce dose to 30 mg daily with verapamil, macrolides (azithromycin, clarithromycin, erythromycin) and oral itraconazole or ketoconazole.

- Cobicistat *(Tybost)*, *Stribild* and *Genvoya* (each containing cobicistat) can increase exposure to the factor Xa inhibitors. Rivaroxaban should not be used with any of these medications. Recommendations are product-specific for the other anticoagulants.

CONVERSION BETWEEN ANTICOAGULANTS

- From warfarin to another oral anticoagulant, stop warfarin and convert to:

  - ❑ **R**ivaroxaban when INR is < 3

  - ❑ **E**doxaban when INR is ≤ 2.5

  - ❑ **A**pixaban when INR is < 2

  - ❑ **D**abigatran when INR is < 2

  Remember: **READ**

- From oral Xa inhibitors (apixaban, edoxaban and rivaroxaban) to warfarin:

  - ❑ Stop Xa inhibitor. Start parenteral anticoagulant and warfarin at next scheduled dose.

  - ❑ Edoxaban only: refer to package labeling for conversion recommendations.

- From dabigatran to warfarin:

  - ❑ Start warfarin 1-3 days before stopping dabigatran (determined by renal function – refer to dabigatran labeling).

DIRECT THROMBIN INHIBITORS

These agents directly inhibit thrombin (factor IIa); they bind to the active site of free and clot-associated thrombin.

DRUG	DOSING	SAFETY/SIDE EFFECTS/MONITORING
Oral Direct Thrombin Inhibitor		
Dabigatran (Pradaxa) Capsule, oral packet (pellets) Missed Dose: Take immediately unless it is within 6 hours of next scheduled dose; the dose should not be doubled to make up for a missed dose	**Nonvalvular AF (stroke prophylaxis)** 150 mg BID CrCl 15-30 mL/min: 75 mg BID CrCl < 15 mL/min: avoid use **Treatment of DVT/PE and reduction in risk of recurrent DVT/PE** 150 mg BID, start after 5-10 days of parenteral anticoagulation CrCl ≤ 30 mL/min: avoid use **Prophylaxis of DVT/PE following hip replacement surgery** 110 mg on day 1, then 220 mg daily CrCl ≤ 30 mL/min: avoid use	**BOXED WARNINGS** Patients receiving neuraxial anesthesia (epidural, spinal) or undergoing spinal puncture are at risk of hematomas and subsequent paralysis Premature discontinuation ↑ risk of thrombotic events **CONTRAINDICATIONS** Active pathological bleeding, treatment of patients with mechanical prosthetic heart valves **WARNINGS** Not recommended for triple-positive antiphospholipid syndrome **SIDE EFFECTS** Dyspepsia, gastritis-like symptoms, bleeding (including GI bleeding) **MONITORING** Hgb, Hct, SCr; no monitoring of efficacy required **NOTES** Antidote: idarucizumab (Praxbind) Protect from moisture; dispense in original container and discard 4 months after opening Blister packs are good until the date on the pack Swallow capsules whole (do not break, chew, crush or open); do not administer by NG tube Can ↑ aPTT, PT/INR Discontinue if undergoing invasive surgery (1-2 days before if CrCl ≥ 50 mL/min, 3-5 days before if CrCl < 50 mL/min)
Injectable Direct Thrombin Inhibitors (IV)		
Argatroban Injection Indicated for HIT and in patients undergoing PCI who are at risk for HIT **Bivalirudin (Angiomax)** Injection Indicated for patients undergoing PCI, including those with HIT	**HIT** Argatroban: start at 2 mcg/kg/min, then titrate to target aPTT Max: 10 mcg/kg/min **PCI** IV bolus followed by an infusion; all are weight-based Used in patients with or at risk for HIT Argatroban: ↓ dose in hepatic impairment Bivalirudin: ↓ dose when CrCl < 30 mL/min .	**CONTRAINDICATIONS** Active major bleeding **SIDE EFFECTS** Bleeding (mild to severe), anemia **MONITORING** aPTT and/or activated clotting time, platelets, Hgb, Hct, renal function **NOTES** Safe with active HIT or history of HIT; no cross-reaction with HIT antibodies No antidote Argatroban can ↑ INR; if starting on warfarin concurrently, dose cautiously and do not use a loading dose of warfarin

Dabigatran Drug Interactions

- Dabigatran is a substrate of P-gp:

  - Avoid concurrent use with rifampin, or any P-gp inhibitor, if CrCl < 50 mL/min (or < 30 mL/min when taking dabigatran for nonvalvular AF).

  - Reduce dose to 75 mg BID if CrCl is 30 – 50 mL/min (when taking dabigatran for nonvalvular AF) and there is concurrent use of dronedarone or systemic ketoconazole.

  - Cobicistat (Tybost) and cobicistat-containing Stribild and Genvoya can increase exposure to dabigatran. Recommendations depend on renal function and indication for dabigatran.

- Monitor for additive effects with other drugs that can ↑ bleeding risk (antiplatelet drugs, some herbals, NSAIDs, SSRIs, SNRIs, fibrinolytics).

WARFARIN

Warfarin competitively inhibits the C1 subunit of the multi-unit vitamin K epoxide reductase (VKORC1) enzyme complex. This reduces the regeneration of vitamin K epoxide which decreases production of active clotting factors II, VII, IX and X and the anticoagulants protein C and S.

DRUG	DOSING	SAFETY/SIDE EFFECTS/MONITORING
Warfarin (Jantoven, *Coumadin*)* Tablet Missed Dose: Take immediately on the same day; do not double the dose the next day to make up for a missed dose	Healthy outpatients: ≤ 10 mg daily for first 2 days, then adjust dose per INR Lower doses (≤ 5 mg) for elderly, malnourished, taking drugs which can ↑ warfarin levels, liver disease, heart failure, or high risk of bleeding Take at the same time each day Highly protein bound (99%) See Study Tip Gal on the next page for tablet colors	**BOXED WARNINGS** Major or fatal bleeding **CONTRAINDICATIONS** Pregnancy (except with mechanical heart valves at high risk for thromboembolism), hemorrhagic tendencies, blood dyscrasias, malignant hypertension, noncompliance, recent or potential surgery of the eye or CNS, major regional lumbar block anesthesia or traumatic surgery resulting in large open surfaces, pericarditis or pericardial effusion, bacterial endocarditis, preeclampsia/eclampsia, possible miscarriage **WARNINGS** Tissue necrosis/gangrene, HIT (contraindicated as monotherapy in the initial treatment of active HIT), systemic atheroemboli and cholesterol microemboli (purple toe syndrome), presence of CYP2C9*2 or *3 alleles and/or polymorphism of VKORC1 gene may increase bleeding risk (routine genetic testing is not currently recommended; see Pharmacogenomics chapter) **SIDE EFFECTS** Bleeding/bruising (mild to severe), skin necrosis **MONITORING** Goal INR 2-3 (target 2.5): most indications (VTE, AF, bioprosthetic mitral valve, mechanical aortic valve, antiphospholipid syndrome) Goal INR 2.5-3.5 (target 3): high-risk indications such as a mechanical mitral valve, 2 mechanical heart valves or mechanical aortic valve with 1 additional risk factor (e.g., previous DVT, AF, hypercoagulable state) Begin INR monitoring after the initial 2 or 3 doses, or if on a chronic, stable dose of warfarin, monitor every 4-12 weeks Hct, Hgb, signs of bleeding **NOTES** Antidote: vitamin K (see Antidotes and Reversal section for details) Dental cleanings and single tooth extraction do not generally require a change in warfarin dosing if the INR is within the therapeutic range

*Brand discontinued but name still used in practice.

WARFARIN DRUG INTERACTIONS

Warfarin is a racemic mixture of two active enantiomers (R-warfarin and S-warfarin) that are metabolized by several CYP enzymes. S-warfarin is primarily metabolized via CYP2C9; R-warfarin is primarily metabolized via CYP3A4. S-warfarin is 3 – 5 times more potent than R-warfarin; this is why drugs that interact via CYP2C9 have a greater impact on the anticoagulant effect of warfarin.

Pharmacokinetic Interactions

- Warfarin is a substrate of CYP2C9 (major), 1A2 (minor), 2C19 (minor) and 3A4 (minor), and an inhibitor of CYP2C9 (weak) and 2C19 (weak). See Drug Interactions chapter.

- CYP2C9 inducers that can ↓ INR include carbamazepine, phenobarbital, phenytoin, rifampin (large ↓ in INR) and St. John's wort.

- CYP2C9 inhibitors that can ↑ INR include amiodarone, azole antifungals (e.g., fluconazole, ketoconazole, voriconazole), capecitabine, cimetidine, fluvastatin, fluvoxamine, metronidazole, tamoxifen, tigecycline, SMX/TMP and zafirlukast.

  - When starting amiodarone, ↓ the dose of warfarin by 30 – 50%.

  - Avoid use with tamoxifen.

- Other antibiotics: penicillins, including amoxicillin, some cephalosporins, quinolones and tetracyclines can ↑ the anticoagulant effect of warfarin – monitor INR.

- Check for CYP1A2, 2C19 and 3A4 interactions; these occur, but usually have less of an effect on INR.

Pharmacodynamic Drug Interactions

- The most common pharmacodynamic interactions are with NSAIDs, antiplatelet agents, other anticoagulants, SSRIs and SNRIs. These interactions ↑ bleeding risk, but the INR may not be increased.

- Drugs that ↑ clotting risk (e.g., estrogen and SERMs) should be discontinued if possible.

Dietary Supplements/Food Interactions

- Monitor the INR closely if patients are taking natural products with warfarin, but understand that some natural products can increase the risk of bleeding with or without increasing the INR.

  - ❏ ↑ bleeding risk when used with warfarin: chondroitin, dong quai, high doses of fish oils, the "5 Gs" (garlic, ginger, ginkgo, ginseng, glucosamine), vitamin E and willow bark (a plant salicylate).

  - ❏ ↓ effectiveness of warfarin: green tea, coenzyme Q10 and St. John's wort. American ginseng may decrease the effects of warfarin, but there is evidence that both American and Panax ginseng inhibit platelet aggregation, which potentially has the opposite effect (see increased bleeding risk above).

- Any additions of vitamin K will ↓ the INR. Check any nutritional products (including enteral nutrition) for vitamin K content. Stay consistent with the amount of vitamin K in the diet (see Foods High in Vitamin K box). Tube feeds should be held one hour before and after warfarin.

WARFARIN TABLET COLORS	
Pink (1 mg)	**P**each (5 mg)
Lavender (2 mg)	**T**eal (6 mg)
Green (2.5 mg)	**Y**ellow (7.5 mg)
Brown/Tan (3 mg)	**W**hite (10 mg)
Blue (4 mg)	
Remember:	
Please **L**et **G**reg **B**rown **B**ring **P**eaches **T**o **Y**our **W**edding	

FOODS HIGH IN VITAMIN K	
Spinach (cooked)	Turnip greens
Broccoli	Green onion
Brussel sprouts	Swiss chard
Collard greens	Endive
Kale	Parsley

Others: asparagus, cabbage, canola oil, cauliflower, coleslaw, lettuce (red leaf or butterhead), watercress, some teas

---

WARFARIN USE – KEY POINTS

- In healthy outpatients, the suggested initial starting dose of warfarin is ≤ 10 mg daily for the first two days, then adjust per INR values.

- In patients with acute DVT/PE, start warfarin while the patient is still receiving a parenteral anticoagulant (often on the first day) and continue both anticoagulants for a minimum of 5 days and until the INR is ≥ 2 for at least 24 hours (i.e., as measured on two consecutive days). Both criteria must be met.

- Routine pharmacogenomic testing is not recommended.

- Routine use of vitamin K supplementation is not recommended in patients taking warfarin.

- For patients with stable therapeutic INRs presenting with a single subtherapeutic (low) INR value, routinely bridging with UFH or LMWH is not recommended.

- For patients with previously stable therapeutic INRs who present with a single out-of-range INR of ≤ 0.5 below or above the therapeutic range, continue current dose and obtain another INR within 1 – 2 weeks.

- For patients with consistently stable INRs on warfarin therapy, INR testing can be done up to every 12 weeks rather than every 4 weeks.

- Warfarin is highly protein bound. Caution is advised with other highly protein bound drugs that may displace warfarin (e.g., phenytoin, valproic acid).

ANTIDOTES FOR REVERSAL

Bleeding is the major adverse effect of anticoagulants. Bleeding can be serious and fatal. Anticoagulation needs to be reversed if a patient experiences life-threatening bleeding or requires surgery.

Protamine combines with strongly acidic heparin to form a stable salt complex, neutralizing the anticoagulant activity of UFH and LMWH. Other drug-specific antidotes include: phytonadione (vitamin K), *Andexxa* and *Praxbind*. *Kcentra* and *Balfaxar* are indicated for the urgent reversal of warfarin. Prothrombin complex concentrates (PCCs) are sometimes used (off-label) for reversal of factor Xa inhibitors. If PCCs are used in this manner, monitoring of coagulation tests (PT, PTT, INR, anti-Xa) to assess reversal is not useful and is not recommended.

ANTIDOTE	DOSING	SAFETY/SIDE EFFECTS/MONITORING
For UFH/LMWH reversal		
Protamine sulfate Injection 10 mg/mL (5 mL, 25 mL)	**For IV UFH reversal** 1 mg protamine will reverse ~100 units of heparin Since UFH has a very short half-life, reverse the amount of heparin given in the last 2-2.5 hours Max dose: 50 mg **For LMWH reversal** Enoxaparin given within the last 8 hours: 1 mg protamine per 1 mg of enoxaparin (can neutralize ~60% of the anti-Xa activity of LMWH) Enoxaparin given > 8 hours ago: 0.5 mg protamine per 1 mg of enoxaparin Dalteparin: 1 mg protamine for each 100 anti-Xa units of dalteparin	**BOXED WARNINGS** Hypersensitivity: hypotension, cardiovascular collapse, non-cardiogenic pulmonary edema, pulmonary vasoconstriction **SIDE EFFECTS** Hypotension, bradycardia, flushing, anaphylaxis **MONITORING** aPTT or anti-Xa levels, cardiac monitoring (ECG, BP, HR) **NOTES** Rapid IV infusion causes hypotension Administer slow IV push (max rate of 50 mg over 10 minutes)
For reversal of the factor Xa inhibitors apixaban and rivaroxaban		
Andexanet alfa (*Andexxa*) Injection	Bolus, followed by infusion Dosing is specific to the Xa inhibitor, including the dose and when last taken	**BOXED WARNINGS** Thromboembolic risks, ischemic events, cardiac arrest, sudden death **SIDE EFFECTS** Injection site reaction, UTI, pneumonia, antibody development **NOTES** Not indicated for reversal of factor Xa inhibitors other than apixaban and rivaroxaban (though may be used off-label)
For dabigatran reversal		
Idarucizumab (*Praxbind*) Injection 2.5 g/50 mL single-use vial	5 grams IV (given as 2 separate 2.5 gram doses no more than 15 minutes apart)	**WARNINGS** Thromboembolic risks, risk of serious adverse reactions due to sorbitol excipient **SIDE EFFECTS** Headache, constipation, hypersensitivity reaction **NOTES** Do not confuse with idarubicin

ANTIDOTE	DOSING	SAFETY/SIDE EFFECTS/MONITORING
For <u>warfarin reversal</u>		
Vitamin K or phytonadione *(Mephyton)* 5 mg tablets 1 mg/0.5 mL, 10 mg/mL injection	1-10 mg <u>PO/IV</u> If given IV, infuse slowly; rate of infusion should not exceed 1 mg/min To ↓ risk of anaphylaxis, dilute dose in a minimum of 50 mL of compatible solution and administer using an infusion pump over at least 20 minutes	**BOXED WARNINGS** Severe reactions resembling <u>hypersensitivity reactions</u> (e.g., anaphylaxis) have occurred rarely during or immediately after IV (even with proper dilution and rate of administration) and IM administration; some patients had no previous exposure to phytonadione **SIDE EFFECTS** <u>Anaphylaxis</u>, flushing, rash, dizziness **NOTES** Requires <u>light protection</u> during administration <u>SC route not recommended due to variable absorption; IM route not recommended due to risk of hematoma</u> Orlistat and mineral oil ↓ absorption of oral vitamin K See specific dosing recommendations in Warfarin Reversal section
Four Factor Prothrombin Complex Concentrate (Human) *(Kcentra, Balfaxar)* Injection <u>Factors II, VII, IX, X, Protein C, Protein S</u>	IV dose is based on units of Factor IX per kg of body weight and patient's INR Do not repeat dose	**BOXED WARNINGS** Arterial and venous thromboembolic complications have been reported **CONTRAINDICATIONS** Known HIT (contains heparin); disseminated intravascular coagulation (DIC) (*Kcentra* only); IgA deficiency with antibodies to IgA (*Balfaxar* only) **WARNINGS** Made from human blood and may carry risk of transmitting infectious agents **SIDE EFFECTS** Headache, N/V/D, asthenia, hypotension, ↓ K, thrombotic events **NOTES** <u>Administer with vitamin K</u> Do not let drug back-up into line as it will clot Allow to reach room temperature prior to administration if refrigerated Each vial can have a different potency of multiple coagulation factors; actual potency is stated on the vial
Three Factor Prothrombin Complex Concentrate (Human) *(Profilnine)* Off-label	Dose based on weight and INR; give IV slowly Given with fresh frozen plasma (FFP) or factor VIIa	**WARNINGS** Contains <u>factors II, IX and X</u> but low or nontherapeutic levels of factor VII and should not be confused with *Kcentra*, which contains therapeutic levels of factor VII Made from human blood and may carry risk of transmitting infectious agents (e.g., viruses) **SIDE EFFECTS** Chills, fever, flushing, nausea, headache, risk of thrombosis **NOTES** Administer via slow infusion and give antihistamine to minimize side effects Administer with vitamin K
Factor VIIa Recombinant *(NovoSeven RT, Sevenfact)* Off-label	10-20 mcg/kg IV bolus over 5 minutes	**BOXED WARNINGS** Serious thrombotic events are associated with the use of factor VIIa

WARFARIN REVERSAL

Variable INRs are common in clinical practice. Elevated INRs are concerning due to an increased risk of bleeding. Vitamin K is used to reverse warfarin (to ↓ the INR more quickly); it can be used by itself or with other medications (e.g., *Kcentra*) for life-threatening bleeding. Bleeding (regardless of the INR) will warrant more serious intervention.

Oral formulations of vitamin K (generally at doses of 2.5 – 5 mg) are preferred for reversal in patients without significant or major bleeding. Vitamin K given subcutaneously (SC) has a slow onset and a variable response; avoid SC injections. Avoid the intramuscular (IM) route due to the risk of hematoma formation. Intravenous vitamin K should be used only when the patient is experiencing serious bleeding. IV injection is reported to cause anaphylaxis in 3 out of 100,000 patients; the risk can be reduced with proper dilution and slow infusion.

Use of Vitamin K for Overanticoagulation

SYMPTOMS/INR VALUE	WHAT TO DO
INR above therapeutic range but < 4.5 without bleeding	Reduce or skip warfarin dose. Monitor INR. Resume warfarin when INR therapeutic. Dose reduction may not be needed if INR elevation is due to transient or reversible factors.
Supratherapeutic INR of 4.5-10 without bleeding	Routine use of vitamin K is not recommended if no evidence of bleeding. Hold 1-2 doses of warfarin. Monitor INR. Resume warfarin at lower dose when INR therapeutic. Oral vitamin K can be used if urgent surgery is needed (≤ 5 mg, with additional 1-2 mg in 24 hours if needed) or bleeding risk is high (1-2.5 mg).
INR > 10 without bleeding	Hold warfarin. Give oral vitamin K 2.5-5 mg even if not bleeding. Monitor INR. Resume warfarin at a lower dose when INR is therapeutic.
Major bleeding	Hold warfarin. Give vitamin K 5-10 mg by slow IV injection and four-factor prothrombin complex concentrate (PCC). PCC suggested over fresh frozen plasma (FFP) due to risks of allergic reactions, infection transmission, longer preparation time, slower onset and higher volume.

PERIOPERATIVE MANAGEMENT OF PATIENTS ON WARFARIN

- Stop warfarin therapy approximately five days before major surgery. In patients with a mechanical heart valve, AF or VTE at high risk for thromboembolism, bridging therapy with LMWH or UFH is recommended (bridging means using therapeutic doses of the LMWH or UFH for a short period to prevent clotting). Discontinue therapeutic-dose SC LMWH 24 hours before surgery (stop the UFH IV therapy 4 – 6 hours before surgery). Patients at low risk for thromboembolism do not require bridging; stop the warfarin and restart after surgery when hemostasis is achieved.

- If INR is still elevated 1 – 2 days before surgery, give low-dose vitamin K (1 – 2 mg).

- If reversal of warfarin is needed in a patient requiring an urgent surgical procedure, give low-dose (2.5 – 5 mg) IV or oral vitamin K.

- Resume warfarin therapy 12 – 24 hours after the surgery, when there is adequate hemostasis.

VENOUS THROMBOEMBOLISM (VTE)

DIAGNOSIS

Symptoms of a DVT include <u>pain</u> in the affected limb and <u>unilateral lower extremity swelling</u>, while symptoms of a PE include <u>shortness of breath and chest pain</u>. DVTs can be diagnosed with an <u>ultrasound</u> (or MRI or venography, in some cases). A D-dimer (lab test) can aid in the diagnosis. If a PE is suspected, it is diagnosed with a pulmonary CT angiogram.

VTE PROPHYLAXIS

Risk factors for the development of VTE are shown below.

RISK FACTORS FOR VENOUS THROMBOEMBOLISM	
Modifiable:	**Non-modifiable:**
Acute medical illness	Increasing age
Immobility	Cancer or chemotherapy
Medications (e.g., SERMs, drugs containing estrogen, erythropoiesis-stimulating agents)	Previous VTE
	Inherited or acquired thrombophilia (e.g., antithrombin deficiency, factor V Leiden, antiphospholipid syndrome, protein C or S deficiency)
Obesity (BMI ≥ 30 kg/m²)	
Pregnancy and postpartum period	
Recent surgery or major trauma	Certain disease states (e.g., heart failure, nephrotic syndrome, respiratory failure)

Various guidelines provide specific recommendations for the prevention of VTE depending on the patient's level of risk. UFH, LMWHs, fondaparinux, rivaroxaban, apixaban and dabigatran are all approved for VTE prophylaxis (refer to the recommended doses in the drug tables). If patients have a contraindication to anticoagulants (such as an active bleed) or have a high risk for bleeding, they will need non-drug alternatives to prevent VTE. These options include intermittent pneumatic compression (IPC) devices or graduated compression stockings.

For <u>long-distance travelers</u> at risk for VTE (see <u>Study Tip Gal</u>), the following recommendations will ↓ VTE risk: <u>frequent ambulation, calf muscle exercises</u>, sitting in an aisle seat and <u>using graduated compression stockings</u> with 15 – 30 mmHg of pressure at the ankle during travel. Aspirin or anticoagulants should <u>not</u> be used.

VTE TREATMENT

Any VTE that is caused by surgery or a reversible risk factor should be <u>treated for three months</u>. Extending the duration of therapy is recommended if the VTE is unprovoked (unknown cause), as long as the patient's bleeding risk is low-to-moderate; this <u>extended phase</u> of therapy should utilize <u>reduced doses</u> of apixaban or rivaroxaban that are approved for this purpose (see drug table); full-dose anticoagulants are also acceptable if unable to utilize the medications approved at reduced doses. If the risk of bleeding is high, limit the treatment to three months. If a patient has two unprovoked VTE episodes, long-term treatment can be considered. <u>Estrogen-containing medications</u> and <u>selective estrogen receptor modulators</u> (SERMs) are <u>contraindicated</u> in patients with <u>history of, or current, VTE and should be discontinued</u>.

- For patients <u>without cancer, dabigatran and the oral factor Xa inhibitors</u> (rivaroxaban, apixaban and edoxaban) <u>are preferred over warfarin for the first three months</u> of treatment for a DVT in the leg or a PE.

- For patients <u>with cancer, the oral factor Xa inhibitors are preferred over other oral anticoagulants and LMWH.</u>

- In patients with an unprovoked DVT or PE who are stopping anticoagulation, aspirin is recommended to prevent recurrence (if there are no contraindications).

ATRIAL FIBRILLATION/FLUTTER

Patients with atrial fibrillation (AF) or atrial flutter can form clots in the heart (e.g., left atrial thrombus) that can travel to the brain and cause a cardioembolic stroke or transient ischemic attack (TIA). Stroke prevention is an important goal in patients with AF/atrial flutter (see Arrhythmias chapter).

Some patients with AF will undergo cardioversion (electrical or pharmacologic) to attempt to regain normal sinus rhythm. The recommended anticoagulation treatments to prevent atrial thrombus and subsequent stroke due to this procedure are shown in the box to the right.

> **ANTICOAGULATION FOR PATIENTS WITH AF WHO WILL UNDERGO CARDIOVERSION**
>
> - AF > 48 hours or unknown duration: anticoagulation for at least 3 weeks prior to and 4 weeks after cardioversion (when normal sinus rhythm is restored). If using warfarin, target an INR of 2–3.
>
> - AF ≤ 48 hours duration undergoing elective cardioversion: start full therapeutic anticoagulation at presentation, perform cardioversion, and continue full anticoagulation for at least 4 weeks while patient is in normal sinus rhythm.

For patients who remain in AF, the need for chronic anticoagulation therapy is based on stroke risk. Patients with AF and a mechanical heart valve have the highest risk for clotting/stroke. Patients with AF and a mechanical heart valve or mitral stenosis should only receive warfarin, as factor Xa inhibitors and DTIs are not approved for this population. The majority of patients with AF do not have heart valve involvement (previously referred to as nonvalvular AF), but they still require an evaluation of their stroke risk. The CHA_2DS_2-VASc scoring system is used to estimate stroke risk and guide therapy (see Study Tip Gal and table below).

CHA_2DS_2-VASc Scoring System

Count the number of risk factors the patient has, then select the recommended therapy. The higher the score, the greater the stroke risk and the more intensive the anticoagulant recommendations.

CHA_2DS_2-VASc SCORING SYSTEM
Add up the total number of risk factors (see table for treatment based on score).
C – CHF...1
H – HTN...1
A_2 – Age ≥ 75 Years 2
D – Diabetes...1
S_2 – Prior Stroke/TIA...2
V – Vascular Disease 1   (prior MI, PAD, aortic plaque)
A – Age 65-74 Years...1
Sc – Sex Category, Female.................................1

CHA_2DS_2-VASC SCORE	RISK OF STROKE	RECOMMENDED THERAPY
0 (males) 1 (females)	Low	No anticoagulation recommended.
1 (males) 2 (females)	Moderate	Oral anticoagulation may be considered.*
≥ 2 (males) ≥ 3 (females)	High	Oral anticoagulation is recommended. Non-vitamin K oral anticoagulant (DOAC**) is recommended over warfarin.

*Additional factors (e.g., AF burden, obesity, poorly controlled HTN) should be considered.
**DOAC: apixaban, rivaroxaban, edoxaban, dabigatran

HAS-BLED Scoring System

The HAS-BLED scoring system assesses bleeding risk in patients requiring anticoagulation for stroke prevention in AF. The decision to anticoagulate is individualized based on the risk of stroke (CHA_2DS_2-VASc) when compared to the risk of bleeding (HAS-BLED). The number of risk factors determines the score; the higher the score, the greater the risk of bleeding.

HAS-BLED SCORING SYSTEM
Add up the total number of risk factors.
H – HTN (SBP > 160 mmHg) 1
A – Abnormal Liver or Kidney Function.....................1-2
S – Prior Stroke...1
B – Bleeding Tendency or Predisposition.......................1
L – Labile INR (if on warfarin).............................1
E – Elderly (age > 65 years)................................1
D – Drugs (aspirin, NSAIDs), excess alcohol use 1-2

ANTICOAGULATION IN PREGNANCY

For prevention and treatment of VTE in pregnant women, LMWH is preferred. Pneumatic compression devices can be used alone or with LMWH in select patients. Since warfarin is teratogenic, women who require chronic warfarin therapy for mechanical heart valves or inherited thrombophilias are generally converted to LMWH during pregnancy. If necessary, they may be switched back to warfarin after the 13th week of pregnancy (i.e., after the first trimester), then back to LMWH closer to delivery. When LMWH is used in pregnancy, anti-Xa levels are recommended to monitor therapy. The oral factor Xa inhibitors and direct thrombin inhibitors have not been adequately studied in pregnancy and are not recommended.

KEY COUNSELING POINTS

See the Drug Formulations and Patient Counseling chapter for counseling language/layman's terminology.

FOR ALL ANTICOAGULANTS

- Can cause serious and life-threatening bleeding/bruising.
- Tell physicians and dentists that you are using this medication before any surgery is performed.
- Call your healthcare provider right away if you fall or injure yourself, especially if you hit your head.
- Avoid alcohol.
- Many drug interactions.
- Missed dose: take as soon as possible on the same day. Do not double the dose the next day to make up for a missed dose; see below for exceptions for dabigatran and rivaroxaban.

Dabigatran

- Take with a full glass of water; swallow capsules whole.
- Can cause dyspepsia.
- Only open one bottle of dabigatran at a time. After opening a bottle of dabigatran, use within four months.
- Keep dabigatran in the original bottle or blister package. Do not put dabigatran in pill boxes or pill organizers.
- Missed dose: if your next dose is less than six hours away, skip the missed dose.

Rivaroxaban

- Atrial fibrillation: take once daily with the evening meal.
- Blood clots in the veins of your legs or in the lungs: take once or twice daily, as prescribed, with food at the same time each day.
- Missed dose: if taken twice daily, can take two doses at the same time to make up for the missed dose.

Enoxaparin

- Subcutaneous injection; choose an area on the right or left side of your abdomen, at least two inches from the belly button (see image). Wash your hands and clean the site.

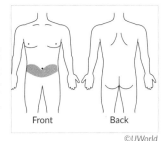

Front   Back

©UWorld

- Remove the needle cap by pulling it straight off the syringe. Do not twist the cap off as this can bend the needle.
- Do not expel the air bubble in the syringe prior to injection unless your healthcare provider has advised you to do so.
- Hold the syringe like a pencil. Pinch an inch of skin to make a fold. Insert the full length of the needle straight down at a 90-degree angle into the fold of the skin.
- Press the plunger with your thumb until the syringe is empty.
- Pull the needle straight out at the same angle that it was inserted, and release the skin fold.
- Point the needle down and away from yourself and others, and push down on the plunger to activate the safety shield.
- Do not rub the site of injection as this can lead to bruising. Place the used syringe in the sharps collector.

Warfarin

- Take at the same time every day.
- Ask your pharmacist if your tablet looks different.
- Can rarely cause:
  - ❏ Purple toe syndrome (painful toes and purple discoloration).
  - ❏ Death of skin tissue (with pain).
- Frequent blood monitoring required (INR).
- Consistent intake of vitamin K required (mainly found in green leafy vegetables).

Select Guidelines/References

Antithrombotic Therapy for VTE Disease: Second Update of the CHEST Guideline and Expert Panel Report. CHEST 2021;160(6):2247-2259.

Antithrombotic Therapy for VTE Disease: CHEST Guideline Expert Panel Report. CHEST 2016;149(2):315-352.

2023 ACC/AHA/ACCP/HRS Guidelines for Diagnosis and Management of Atrial Fibrillation. Circulation 2024;149:e1-e156.

CONTENT LEGEND

 = Study Tip Gal

 = Key Drug Guy

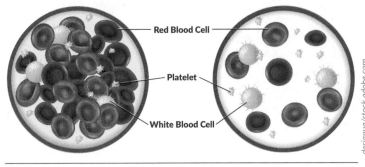

Normal Levels of Red Blood Cells   Anemic Levels of Red Blood Cells

Red Blood Cell

Platelet

White Blood Cell

designua/stock.adobe.com

CHAPTER 35
ANEMIA

BACKGROUND

Anemia is the most common blood disorder worldwide and it affects more than 3 million Americans. Anemia is a decrease in red blood cells (RBCs), hemoglobin (Hgb) and/or hematocrit (Hct) below the normal range for age and sex.

- Hgb is an iron-rich protein found in RBCs that carries oxygen from the lungs to the tissues.

- Hct is the percent of RBC volume compared to total blood volume.

- Reticulocytes (immature RBCs) are formed in the bone marrow where they take up Hgb and iron before being released into circulation. After 1 – 2 days, reticulocytes develop into erythrocytes (mature RBCs), which have a lifespan of about 120 days. Erythrocytes are removed from circulation by macrophages, mainly in the spleen.

Diagnosis of the underlying cause is essential. Anemia can occur due to impaired RBC or Hgb production, increased RBC destruction (hemolysis) or blood loss. Impaired RBC or Hgb production can result from nutritional deficiencies (e.g., iron, folate, vitamin B12) or it can be a complication of another medical disorder, such as chronic kidney disease (CKD) or a malignancy. Certain genetic conditions can cause anemia due to dysfunctional RBCs (see the Sickle Cell Disease chapter).

SYMPTOMS OF ANEMIA

A decrease in Hgb or RBC count results in decreased oxygen-carrying capacity of the blood. Most patients with mild anemia are asymptomatic, but if anemia becomes severe or prolonged, the reduced oxygen delivery to tissues can lead to symptoms of fatigue, weakness, shortness of breath, exercise intolerance, headache, dizziness and/or pallor. In chronic anemia, the heart compensates for reduced oxygen delivery by pumping faster (tachycardia). This can increase ventricular wall mass (i.e., cause hypertrophy) and lead to heart failure.

Glossitis (an inflamed, sore tongue), koilonychia (thin, concave, spoon-shaped nails) or pica (craving and eating non-foods, such as ice or clay) can develop with <u>iron deficiency anemia</u>. Patients with <u>vitamin B12 deficiency</u> can also develop glossitis as well as neurologic symptoms, including <u>peripheral neuropathy</u>, visual disturbances and psychiatric symptoms.

If sudden blood loss occurs, resulting in hypovolemia and hypotension, the patient can experience acute symptoms, such as chest pain, fainting, palpitations and tachycardia.

TYPES OF ANEMIA

Signs and symptoms alone are not sufficient to distinguish the type and cause of anemia, therefore laboratory tests are used.

- <u>Mean corpuscular volume (MCV)</u> reflects the size or average volume of RBCs, which classifies anemia as microcytic (<u>low MCV</u>), normocytic (normal MCV) or <u>macrocytic (high MCV)</u>. Likely causes of anemia can be determined from this classification (see flow diagram below).

Identifying the Cause of Anemia

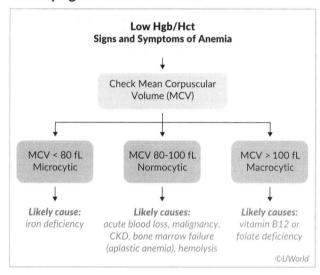

- <u>Iron studies</u> further evaluate <u>microcytic anemia</u>; they include serum iron (bound to transferrin), serum ferritin (iron stores), transferrin saturation (TSAT) (percent of transferrin binding sites occupied by iron) and total iron binding capacity (TIBC) (amount of transferrin binding sites available to bind iron, or unbound sites).

- <u>Vitamin B12 and folate levels</u> further evaluate <u>macrocytic anemia</u>. In addition, levels of methylmalonic acid and homocysteine (which require vitamin B12 and/or folate for metabolism) may be useful in confirming a diagnosis.

- The <u>reticulocyte count</u> is a measure of RBC production. The count is <u>low</u> in untreated <u>iron, folate or B12 deficiency</u> anemia and with <u>bone marrow suppression</u>. The reticulocyte count is high with acute blood loss or hemolysis.

LABORATORY TESTS IN ANEMIA*

CBC Components	Iron Studies
Hemoglobin (Hgb)	Serum iron
Hematocrit (Hct)	Serum ferritin
Red blood cell (RBC) count	Total iron binding capacity (TIBC)
Reticulocyte count	Transferrin saturation (TSAT)

RBC Indices	Additional Tests
Mean corpuscular volume (MCV)	Serum folate
Mean corpuscular hemoglobin (MCH)	Serum vitamin B12
Mean corpuscular hemoglobin concentration (MCHC)	Methylmalonic acid
	Homocysteine
Red blood cell distribution width (RDW)	

Refer to the Lab Values & Drug Monitoring chapter for normal laboratory ranges in adults.

IRON DEFICIENCY ANEMIA

<u>Iron deficiency</u> is the <u>most common</u> nutritional deficiency in the United States. Common causes are shown in the box below. Dietary iron is available in two forms: heme iron (found in meat and seafood) and non-heme iron (found in nuts, beans, vegetables and fortified grains, such as cereals). Heme iron is more readily absorbed than non-heme iron. Patients who follow a vegan or vegetarian diet may be more likely to consume foods with non-heme iron (the less absorbable form), which can make them more susceptible to iron deficiency.

Preventative measures can be used for some at-risk patient populations. For example, pregnant women are at risk of developing iron deficiency due to increased iron requirements for fetal and placental development. The CDC recommends low-dose iron supplementation (~30 mg/day) for all pregnant women, beginning at the first prenatal visit; this is usually included in a prenatal vitamin.

CAUSES OF IRON DEFICIENCY

Low Iron Intake
- Vegetarian or vegan <u>diet</u>, malnutrition

Blood Loss
- Acute (e.g., hemorrhage), chronic (e.g., <u>heavy menses</u>, blood donations, <u>peptic ulcer disease</u>, inflammatory bowel disease), drug-induced (e.g., NSAIDs, antiplatelets, anticoagulants)

Decreased Iron Absorption
- <u>High gastric pH</u> (e.g., use of PPIs), <u>GI disorders</u> (e.g., celiac disease, inflammatory bowel disease), gastrectomy, <u>gastric bypass</u>

Increased Iron Requirements
- <u>Pregnancy, lactation, infants</u>*, rapid growth (e.g., adolescence)

See the Dietary Supplements, Natural & Complementary Medicine chapter for infant iron requirements.

DIAGNOSIS AND TREATMENT OF IRON DEFICIENCY ANEMIA

The Study Tip Gal to the right summarizes the laboratory findings that are consistent with a diagnosis of iron deficiency anemia (IDA) and important treatment information.

Oral Iron

Most cases of IDA can be adequately treated with OTC oral iron supplements (many contain "fe," "fer" or "ferr" in the drug name). Higher doses of elemental iron do not result in a higher amount absorbed and can cause more adverse effects, therefore a single dose of an iron supplement taken daily or every other day is usually sufficient.

ASSESSING AND TREATING IRON DEFICIENCY ANEMIA

LABORATORY FINDINGS
- ↓ Hgb, MCV (< 80 fL), reticulocyte count, serum iron, ferritin and TSAT
- ↑ TIBC

TREATMENT: ORAL IRON THERAPY
- Common dosing: 1 tablet once daily or every other day
  - ❏ There is no difference in efficacy or adverse effects between products
- Take on an empty stomach (1 hr before or 2 hrs after meals) for best absorption
- Avoid H2RAs and PPIs; separate from antacids
- Sustained-release or enteric-coated formulations cause less GI irritation but are not recommended due to poor absorption

GOALS
- ↑ in Hgb after 1-2 weeks; continue treatment for 3-6 months or until iron stores return to normal

APPROXIMATE ELEMENTAL IRON IN ORAL PRODUCTS

Ferrous gluconate	12%
Ferrous sulfate	20%
Ferrous sulfate, dried	30%
Ferrous fumarate	33%
Carbonyl iron, polysaccharide iron complex, ferric maltol	100%

DRUG	DOSING	SAFETY/SIDE EFFECTS/MONITORING
Ferrous sulfate Tablet, elixir, oral solution, syrup	325 mg (65 mg elemental iron)	**BOXED WARNING** Accidental overdose of iron-containing products is a leading cause of fatal poisoning in children under age 6 years; keep iron out of reach of children; in the case of an accidental overdose, go to the emergency department or call a poison control center immediately (even if asymptomatic)
Ferrous sulfate, dried ER tablet	160 mg (50 mg elemental iron)	
Ferrous fumarate	324 mg (106 mg elemental iron)	**CONTRAINDICATIONS** Hemochromatosis, hemolytic anemia, hemosiderosis, patients receiving frequent blood transfusions
Ferrous gluconate	324 mg (38 mg elemental iron)	**SIDE EFFECTS** Gastrointestinal effects (in up to 70% of patients): constipation (dose related), dark and tarry stools, nausea, stomach upset
Carbonyl iron	90 mg (90 mg elemental iron)	**MONITORING** Hgb, Hct, iron studies, reticulocyte count
Polysaccharide iron complex Capsule, liquid	150 mg (150 mg elemental iron)	**NOTES** Treat constipation with a stool softener or laxative (see the Constipation & Diarrhea chapter for drugs used to treat constipation)
Ferric maltol (*ACCRUFeR*) Prescription only	30 mg (30 mg elemental iron)	May take with food if GI upset occurs (avoid milk products) Liquid preparations of ferrous sulfate may stain teeth The antidote for iron overdose is deferoxamine (*Desferal*)

Oral Iron Drug Interactions

- Antacids, H2RAs and PPIs ↓ iron absorption by ↑ gastric pH. Patients should take iron 2 hours before or 4 hours after taking antacids. H2RAs and PPIs raise gastric pH for up to 24 hours; separating the administration of these drugs from iron supplements does not improve absorption.

- Vitamin C (ascorbic acid) may minimally ↑ iron absorption by providing an acidic environment.

- Iron is a polyvalent cation that can ↓ absorption of other drugs by binding (i.e., chelating) with them in the GI tract to form nonabsorbable complexes. Separate administration from the following:

  - ❏ Quinolone and tetracycline antibiotics: take iron 2 hours before or 4 – 8 hours after the antibiotic.

  - ❏ Bisphosphonates: take iron ≥ 60 minutes after oral ibandronate or ≥ 30 minutes after alendronate or risedronate.

  - ❏ Levothyroxine: separate from iron by 4 hours.

  - ❏ Integrase strand transfer inhibitors (INSTIs): see the Human Immunodeficiency Virus chapter for details.

Intravenous (Parenteral) Iron

Parenteral iron increases Hgb faster than oral iron. As with oral iron, IV iron formulations demonstrate equal efficacy; choice is based on cost, formulary or insurance coverage. The total dose needed to replenish iron stores (e.g., 1,000 mg) can be provided in a single infusion, if desired. Due to the risk of more severe adverse reactions, as well as the cost of therapy, IV iron administration is typically restricted to the following patients:

- CKD on hemodialysis (most common use of IV iron) and/or receiving erythropoiesis-stimulating agents (ESAs).

- Unable to tolerate oral iron due to gastrointestinal side effects or failure of oral therapy (e.g., inflammatory bowel disease, celiac disease, certain gastric bypass procedures, *H. pylori*).

- Severe anemia (e.g., Hgb < 7 g/dL) or losing iron too fast for oral replacement (e.g., chronic blood loss).

- Patients who will not accept (e.g., for religious reasons) an RBC transfusion, which is the first-line treatment for acute blood loss or life-threatening anemia (of any cause) to achieve hemodynamic stability and prevent end-organ ischemia.

DRUG	SAFETY/SIDE EFFECTS/MONITORING
Iron sucrose *(Venofer)*	**BOXED WARNING** Iron dextran and ferumoxytol: serious and sometimes fatal anaphylactic reactions have occurred; a history of drug allergy or multiple drug allergies may ↑ this risk
Ferumoxytol *(Feraheme)*	Iron dextran: all patients should be given a test dose prior to the first full therapeutic dose; fatal reactions have occurred even in patients who tolerated the test dose
Iron dextran complex *(INFeD)*	**WARNING** All parenteral iron products carry a risk for hypersensitivity reactions (including anaphylaxis); premedication (e.g., diphenhydramine, methylprednisolone) is sometimes administered to high-risk patients
Ferric gluconate *(Ferrlecit)*	**SIDE EFFECTS** Nausea, vomiting, diarrhea, hypotension, dizziness, dyspnea, chest pain, muscle aches, peripheral edema, injection site reactions
Ferric carboxymaltose *(Injectafer)*	**MONITORING** Hgb, Hct, iron studies, reticulocyte count, vital signs, signs and symptoms of anaphylaxis
Ferric derisomaltose *(Monoferric)*	**NOTES** Give by slow IV injection or infusion to ↓ the risk of hypotension All agents are stable in NS; *Feraheme* is stable in NS or D5W

MACROCYTIC ANEMIA

Macrocytic anemia can be caused by <u>vitamin B12 or folate deficiency</u>, or both. <u>Pernicious anemia</u>, the most common cause of vitamin B12 deficiency, is an autoimmune condition caused by the development of <u>antibodies to intrinsic factor</u>, which is required for adequate vitamin B12 absorption in the small intestine. Pernicious anemia requires <u>lifelong parenteral vitamin B12 replacement</u>.

Other causes of macrocytic anemia include <u>alcohol use disorder, low intake</u> of vitamin B12 and/or folate (e.g., vegetarian or vegan diet), <u>decreased gastrointestinal absorption</u> (e.g., Crohn's disease, celiac disease, gastric bypass surgery, medications) and pregnancy. The <u>long-term</u> use (≥ 2 years) of <u>metformin, H2RAs or PPIs</u> can decrease the absorption of vitamin B12.

DIAGNOSIS AND TREATMENT OF MACROCYTIC ANEMIA

Patients with macrocytic anemia caused by vitamin B12 and/or folate deficiency will have <u>low Hgb and reticulocyte count</u> and <u>high MCV</u>; serum levels of vitamin B12 and/or folate will also be low. Since vitamin B12 is required for enzymatic reactions involving methylmalonic acid and homocysteine metabolism, they accumulate when vitamin B12 is deficient. Homocysteine metabolism also requires folate, therefore homocysteine levels can be elevated in folate deficiency, but methylmalonic acid levels may be normal if there is no deficiency of vitamin B12.

<u>Vitamin B12 deficiency</u> can result in <u>serious neurologic dysfunction</u>, including <u>cognitive impairment</u> and <u>peripheral neuropathy</u>. If vitamin B12 deficiency goes undiagnosed for more than three months, neurologic symptoms can become <u>irreversible</u>. The initial treatment of vitamin B12 deficiency typically involves vitamin B12 injections to bypass absorption barriers, followed by oral supplements, if appropriate. <u>Vitamin B12 injections</u> are <u>recommended first-line</u> for anyone with a severe deficiency or neurological symptoms.

<u>Folic acid deficiency</u> causes <u>ulcerations</u> of the tongue and <u>oral mucosa</u> and changes to skin, hair and fingernail pigmentation. <u>Oral folic acid</u> is usually sufficient to treat folic acid deficiency because typical doses are high enough to overcome any malabsorption and meet the recommended daily allowance.

Vitamin B12 and Folic Acid

DRUG	DOSING	SAFETY/SIDE EFFECTS/MONITORING
Cyanocobalamin, vitamin B12 (*Nascobal, Physicians EZ Use B-12*) Injection, lozenge, tablet (including ER and SL forms), SL liquid, <u>nasal spray</u>	IM or deep SC: 100-1,000 mcg daily/weekly/monthly depending on severity of the deficiency Oral/sublingual: 1,000-2,000 mcg daily *Nascobal*: 500 mcg in <u>one nostril once weekly</u>	**CONTRAINDICATIONS** Allergy to cobalt or vitamin B12 (an intradermal test dose is recommended for any patient suspected of vitamin B12 sensitivity prior to intranasal or injectable administration) **WARNINGS** Parenteral products may contain aluminum (which can accumulate and cause CNS and bone toxicity if renal function is impaired) or benzyl alcohol (which can cause fatal toxicity and "gasping syndrome" in neonates) **SIDE EFFECTS** Pain with injection Rash, polycythemia vera, pulmonary edema (all rare) **MONITORING** Hgb, Hct, vitamin B12, reticulocyte count
Folic acid, folate, vitamin B9 (*FA-8*) Tablet, capsule, injection	0.4-5 mg daily	**WARNINGS** As above for cyanocobalamin **SIDE EFFECTS** Bronchospasm, flushing, rash, pruritus, malaise (all rare) **MONITORING** Hgb, Hct, folate, reticulocyte count **NOTES** Folic acid can ↓ the serum concentration of fosphenytoin, phenytoin, primidone and phenobarbital

NORMOCYTIC ANEMIA

ANEMIA OF CHRONIC DISEASE

Erythropoietin (EPO) is a hormone produced by the kidneys that stimulates the bone marrow to produce RBCs. A deficiency of EPO contributes to anemia of chronic disease (e.g., CKD, malignancy). Iron therapy and erythropoiesis-stimulating agents (ESAs) are the primary treatments for anemia of chronic disease.

The KDIGO (Kidney Disease Improving Global Outcomes) guidelines recommend iron therapy in all patients with anemia of CKD if TSAT is ≤ 30% and ferritin is ≤ 500 ng/mL. IV iron is preferred, but a trial of oral iron may be used in patients not on hemodialysis (HD). If all correctable causes of anemia have been addressed and the Hgb remains < 10 g/dL, an ESA may be used.

ESAs are most commonly used in patients with CKD or malignancy. They may be initiated when the Hgb is < 10 g/dL and titrated up or down based on Hgb levels. Due to the risk of death and thrombosis, the dose should be decreased or interrupted when the Hgb approaches or exceeds 11 g/dL. Adequate iron stores are required for ESAs to be effective, therefore concurrent iron replacement therapy is often needed. Daprodustat (*Jesduvroq*) is an oral ESA indicated for CKD patients who have been receiving dialysis for at least four months. It increases erythropoietin levels and has a similar boxed warning and target Hgb levels as the parenteral ESAs.

Erythropoiesis-Stimulating Agents (ESAs)

DRUG	DOSING	SAFETY/SIDE EFFECTS/MONITORING
Epoetin alfa **(Epogen, Procrit,** *Retacrit*-biosimilar) IV, SC	**Chronic Kidney Disease** 50-100 units/kg IV or SC 3x/week **Cancer (on chemotherapy)** 150 units/kg SC 3x/week or 40,000 units SC weekly	**BOXED WARNINGS** ↑ risk of death, MI, stroke, VTE, thrombosis of vascular access Use the lowest effective dose required to reduce the need for blood transfusions Chronic kidney disease: ↑ risk of death, serious cardiovascular events and stroke when Hgb level > 11 g/dL Select cancers: shortened overall survival and/or ↑ risk of tumor progression or recurrence; not indicated when the anticipated outcome is cure; discontinue when chemotherapy completed Perisurgery (epoetin alfa): DVT prophylaxis is recommended due to ↑ risk of DVT **CONTRAINDICATIONS** Uncontrolled hypertension, pure red cell aplasia (PRCA) that begins after treatment Epoetin alfa: neonates, infants, pregnancy and lactation (multidose vials contain benzyl alcohol)
Darbepoetin alfa **(Aranesp)** IV, SC Available as a single-dose prefilled syringe (needle included)	**Chronic Kidney Disease** HD: 0.45 mcg/kg IV or SC weekly or 0.75 mcg/kg IV or SC every 2 weeks Non-HD: 0.45 mcg/kg IV or SC every 4 weeks **Cancer (on chemotherapy)** 2.25 mcg/kg SC weekly or 500 mcg SC every 3 weeks	**WARNINGS** Hypertension, seizures, serious allergic reactions, serious skin reactions (SJS/TEN) Epoetin alfa: contains albumin from human blood (remote risk for transmission of viral diseases) **SIDE EFFECTS** Arthralgia/bone pain, fever, headache, pruritus/rash, N/V, cough, dyspnea, edema, injection site pain, dizziness **MONITORING** Hgb, Hct, TSAT, serum ferritin, BP **NOTES** IV route is recommended for patients on hemodialysis Store in the refrigerator; protect from light; discard multidose vials 21 days after initial entry Do not shake The darbepoetin half-life is 3-times longer than epoetin alfa (allows weekly administration)

DRUG-INDUCED HEMOLYTIC ANEMIA

Hemolytic anemia develops when RBCs are destroyed prematurely (i.e., before their normal 120-day lifespan). There are many possible causes; this discussion will focus on drug-induced etiologies, which can have an acute onset of severe symptoms, including typical anemia findings (e.g., fatigue, dyspnea) plus those associated with RBC destruction (e.g., jaundice, dark urine, splenomegaly).

The two most common mechanisms by which drug-induced hemolytic anemia occurs are:

- Immune-mediated hemolysis, where the medication binds to the RBC surface and triggers the development of antibodies that lead to RBC destruction. This type can be identified with a positive direct Coombs test, which detects antibodies that are stuck to the surface of RBCs.

- Hemolysis in the setting of glucose-6-phosphate dehydrogenase (G6PD) deficiency (an inherited disorder). The G6PD enzyme protects RBCs from oxidant injury; without sufficient levels of G6PD, RBCs hemolyze after exposure to oxidative stress. Most individuals with known G6PD deficiency do not need treatment but must avoid certain high-risk medications, foods (e.g., fava beans), severe stress and other known triggers. Drug-induced hemolytic anemia caused by G6PD deficiency will typically result in a negative direct Coombs test.

The Key Drugs Guy below lists medications that can cause hemolytic anemia via these mechanisms. If hemolysis develops and the patient has a positive direct Coombs test or is identified as G6PD deficient, the offending agent should be discontinued.

SELECT DRUGS THAT CAN CAUSE HEMOLYTIC ANEMIA

Immune-Mediated (+Coombs Test)	G6PD Deficiency
Penicillins	Dapsone
Cephalosporins	Methylene blue
Isoniazid	Nitrofurantoin
Levodopa	Pegloticase
Methyldopa	Rasburicase
Rifampin	Primaquine
Quinidine	Quinidine
Quinine	Quinine
Sulfonamides	Sulfonamides

KEY COUNSELING POINTS

See the Drug Formulations and Patient Counseling chapter for counseling language/layman's terminology.

Oral Iron
- Take on an empty stomach.
- Can cause:
  - Constipation.
  - Dark stools.
- Drug interactions due to:
  - High gastric pH.
  - Binding.

ESAs
- Can cause:
  - Blood clots.
  - Hypertension.
- Do not shake the vial or syringe; this will ruin the medication and it will not work.
- ESA injection sites:

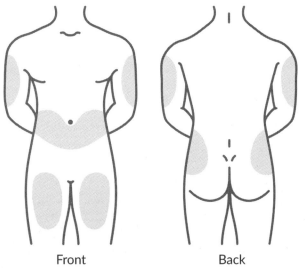

Front   Back

iStock.com/Barbulat

Select Guidelines/References
Camaschella C. Iron deficiency. *Blood.* 2019:133:30-39.

Ning S, Zeller MP. Management of iron deficiency. *Hematology Am Soc Hematol Educ Program.* 2019:2019:315-322.

Kidney Disease: Improving Global Outcomes (KDIGO) Anemia Work Group. KDIGO Clinical Practice Guideline for Anemia in Chronic Kidney Disease. Kidney Int Suppl. 2012;2:279-335.

CONTENT LEGEND

🔑 = Key Drug Guy

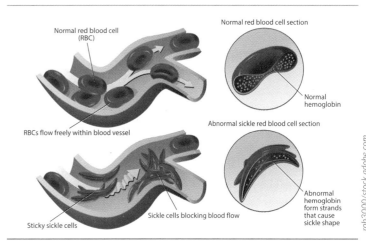

Normal red blood cell (RBC)

RBCs flow freely within blood vessel

Normal red blood cell section

Normal hemoglobin

Abnormal sickle red blood cell section

Abnormal hemoglobin form strands that cause sickle shape

Sticky sickle cells

Sickle cells blocking blood flow

rob3000/stock.adobe.com

CHAPTER 36
SICKLE CELL DISEASE

BACKGROUND

Red blood cells (RBCs) contain adult hemoglobin (HgbA) and are shaped like a donut without the hole. They have the flexibility to move through large and small blood vessels to deliver oxygen to the tissues. RBCs have a lifespan of ~120 days.

Sickle cell disease (SCD) is a group of inherited RBC disorders that most commonly affects the African American population. It results from a genetic mutation in the genes that encode hemoglobin (see the Pharmacogenomics chapter for a discussion on genetic inheritance). Patients with homozygous inheritance of the sickle cell gene (i.e., they have two copies of the mutated gene) have RBCs that contain abnormal hemoglobin, called hemoglobin S (i.e., HgbS or sickle hemoglobin). This causes RBCs to be rigid with a concave "sickle" shape. Sickled RBCs hemolyze after 10 – 20 days, which causes anemia.

The irregularly shaped RBCs cannot transport oxygen effectively and they stick together, blocking smaller blood vessels (known as vascular occlusion) and causing a wide array of complications. Symptoms of SCD develop approximately 2 – 3 months after birth. This is because a fetus and young infants have RBCs with fetal hemoglobin (HgbF), which blocks the sickling of RBCs. A hemoglobin electrophoresis test or high-performance liquid chromatography (HPLC) can be used to measure the amount of each Hgb (A, F and S) in the blood.

ACUTE AND CHRONIC COMPLICATIONS

Vascular occlusion prevents oxygen from reaching the tissues, causing them to become ischemic. This can lead to different types of sickle cell crises (see the box on the following page), the most common of which is vaso-occlusive crisis (VOC), or acute pain crisis. VOC most commonly occurs in the lower back, legs, hips, abdomen and chest, and can last for days or weeks. If the pain is in the chest and there is evidence of a pulmonary infection, it is called acute chest syndrome. Acute chest syndrome is life-threatening and is the leading cause of death in SCD.

Due to the risk of stroke, females with SCD should not use estrogen; progestin-only contraceptives, levonorgestrel intrauterine devices (IUDs) and barrier methods are preferred for contraception.

The most common chronic complications of SCD are chronic pain, avascular necrosis (bone death), pulmonary hypertension and renal impairment.

SICKLE CELL DISEASE COMPLICATIONS

Acute	Chronic
Acute chest syndrome	Avascular necrosis (bone death)
Anemia	Depression and stress
Cholecystitis (gallbladder infection)	Gallstones
	Leg ulcers
Infection	Pain
Multiorgan failure (kidneys, liver, lung)	Pregnancy complications (including fetal death)
Priapism (painful and prolonged erection)	Pulmonary hypertension
	Recurrent priapism
Splenic sequestration	Renal impairment
Stroke	Retinopathy
Vaso-occlusive crisis (acute pain crisis)	

INFECTION RISK

A healthy spleen has several physiologic roles, including the removal of old or damaged RBCs. It aids in immune function, making and storing white blood cells and clearing some types of bacterial pathogens from the body, particularly the encapsulated organisms *Streptococcus pneumoniae*, *Haemophilus influenzae* and *Neisseria meningitidis*. In SCD, the spleen becomes fibrotic and shrinks in size due to repetitive sickling and infarctions. This causes functional asplenia (decreased or absent spleen function), typically within the first year of life. Patients with functional asplenia are at an increased risk for serious infections; they require immunizations and prophylactic antibiotics and should seek immediate medical attention for a temperature > 101.3°F.

NON-DRUG TREATMENT

Blood transfusions protect against many of the life-threatening complications of SCD by providing RBCs with HgbA. Stroke, acute chest syndrome and severe anemia are acute complications that warrant treatment with blood transfusions. When administering chronic monthly blood transfusions, the goal Hgb level should be no higher than 10 g/dL post-infusion. One of the risks of blood transfusions is iron overload, which can lead to hemosiderosis (excess iron that impairs organ function). Chelation therapy to remove excess iron is discussed on the following page.

The only cure for SCD is bone marrow transplantation, but due to the high risks involved as well as the substantial cost, it is not a widely used approach.

DRUG TREATMENT

Drug classes used in SCD are immunizations and antibiotics to reduce infection risk, chelation therapy to manage iron overload from blood transfusions, and analgesics to control pain.

Hydroxyurea is the primary disease-modifying therapy for SCD. Other treatments include L-glutamine, voxelotor and crizanlizumab, which can all be used alone or in combination with hydroxyurea.

IMMUNIZATIONS AND ANTIBIOTICS

Infections are a major cause of death, especially in children < 5 years of age. Sepsis and meningitis, due to *S. pneumoniae*, *H. influenzae, N. meningitidis* and *Salmonella* spp., can occur. The risk of infections caused by atypical organisms (*Chlamydophila* and *Mycoplasma pneumoniae*) is increased. Vaccinations are essential to prevent infection (see the Key Drugs Guy).

Prophylactic oral penicillin reduces the risk of death from invasive pneumococcal infections in young children. Infants who screen positive for SCD at birth should be initiated on twice daily penicillin and treated until age five years. If a patient undergoes surgical removal of the spleen, or if invasive pneumococcal infection develops despite penicillin prophylaxis, it should be continued indefinitely.

KEY VACCINES IN SICKLE CELL DISEASE

Routine Childhood Series
- *Haemophilus influenzae* type B (Hib)
- Pneumococcal conjugate vaccine [PCV15 *(Vaxneuvance)* or PCV20 *(Prevnar 20)*]

Additional Vaccines For Functional Asplenia
- Meningococcal conjugate vaccine (MenACWY) series plus routine boosters *(Menveo, MenQuadfi)*
- Meningococcal serogroup B *(Bexsero, Trumenba)**
- Pneumococcal vaccines – if never received as a child, give one of the following regimens**:
  - ❏ PCV20 *(Prevnar 20)* x 1, or
  - ❏ PCV15 *(Vaxneuvance)* x 1 followed by PPSV23 *(Pneumovax 23)* ≥ 8 weeks later

*At age ≥ 10 years
**At age ≥ 19 years

IRON CHELATION TREATMENT

Iron overload from chronic blood transfusions damages the liver, heart and other organs. Chelation therapy is used to remove excess iron stores from the body. Oral chelating drugs, such as deferasirox *(Exjade, Jadenu)* and deferiprone *(Ferriprox)*, are commonly used. Due to the side effect profile of both drugs, treatment is typically prescribed, dispensed and monitored by specialty clinics and pharmacies.

ANALGESICS

Mild to moderate pain can often be managed at home with rest, fluids, application of warm compresses to affected areas and the use of NSAIDs or acetaminophen. For severe pain and VOC, acute management must be guided by the patient's self-reported pain severity; outpatient analgesic use should be reviewed and an analgesic administered within 30 minutes of triage. Patients with severe pain and VOC will require IV administration of opioids or patient-controlled analgesia (PCA). Refer to the Pain chapter for a detailed discussion of analgesics.

HYDROXYUREA

Hydroxyurea is a disease-modifying drug that stimulates production of HgbF. Long-term use of hydroxyurea reduces the frequency of acute pain crises, episodes of acute chest syndrome and the need for blood transfusions. It is indicated for all adults with ≥ 1 moderate-severe pain crisis or acute chest syndrome in one year, or chronic pain affecting their quality of life. It is also recommended in all pediatric patients age 9 months – 18 years regardless of disease severity.

DRUG	DOSE	SAFETY/SIDE EFFECTS/MONITORING
Hydroxyurea *(Droxia, Hydrea, Siklos)* Capsule, tablet	Start: *Droxia:* 15 mg/kg once daily *Siklos:* 20 mg/kg once daily ↑ by 5 mg/kg/day every 8-12 weeks to a goal absolute neutrophil count (ANC) of 2,000-4,000 cells/mm^3 Max: 35 mg/kg/day Use IBW or TBW, whichever is less, when calculating daily dose Round doses to the nearest capsule size CrCl < 60 mL/min: dose adjustment required	**BOXED WARNINGS** Myelosuppression (↓ WBCs and platelets), malignancy (leukemia, skin cancer) **WARNINGS** Fetal toxicity, avoid live vaccinations, skin ulcers, macrocytosis, pulmonary toxicity ↑ risk of pancreatitis, hepatotoxicity and peripheral neuropathy when used with antiretroviral drugs **SIDE EFFECTS** ↑ LFTs, uric acid, BUN and SCr; N/V/D, alopecia, hyperpigmentation or atrophy of skin and nails, low sperm counts (males) **MONITORING** CBC with differential every 2-4 weeks during treatment initiation and titration, then every 2-3 months once a stable dose is achieved; if toxicity (ANC < 2,000 cells/mm^3, platelets < 80,000 cells/mm^3) occurs, hold hydroxyurea until the bone marrow recovers, then restart at a dose 2.5-5 mg/kg/day lower HgbF, LFTs, uric acid, renal function, baseline pregnancy test **NOTES** Contraception required for males and females during treatment and for 6-12 months after discontinuation; do not breastfeed during treatment Hazardous drug – wear gloves when dispensing and wash hands before and after contact (see the Compounding chapters) Folic acid supplementation is recommended to prevent macrocytosis Clinical response can take 3-6 months

Hydroxyurea Drug Interactions

- Additive risk of myelosuppression if used in combination with other immunosuppressants (e.g., topical or systemic tacrolimus, clozapine, deferiprone, leflunomide, natalizumab, tofacitinib).

L-GLUTAMINE

L-glutamine is an amino acid shown to reduce acute complications of SCD (e.g., number of pain crises requiring parenteral analgesics, number and duration of hospitalizations, occurrence of acute chest syndrome). The mechanism of action is not fully known, but it is thought to decrease oxidative stress, which can damage sickled RBCs.

DRUG	DOSE	SAFETY/SIDE EFFECTS/MONITORING
L-glutamine (Endari) Oral powder (5 grams per packet)	TBW < 30 kg: 5 grams twice daily TBW 30-65 kg: 10 grams twice daily TBW > 65 kg: 15 grams twice daily	**SIDE EFFECTS** Constipation, flatulence, nausea, headache, pain (abdominal, extremities, back, chest), cough **NOTES** Mix each dose in 8 oz. of a cold or room temperature beverage (e.g., water, milk, apple juice), or 4-6 oz. of food (e.g., applesauce, yogurt); drug does not need to completely dissolve before administration

VOXELOTOR

Voxelotor inhibits hemoglobin S (HgbS) polymerization, which prevents red blood cell sickling.

DRUG	DOSE	SAFETY/SIDE EFFECTS/MONITORING
Voxelotor (Oxbryta) Tablet	1.5 grams once daily ↓ dose if taking with strong CYP450 3A4 inhibitors, ↑ dose if taking CYP3A4 inducers	**WARNINGS** Hypersensitivity reactions, lab test interference with measurement of Hgb subtypes (A, F, S) **SIDE EFFECTS** Headache, fatigue, abdominal pain, diarrhea, nausea **NOTES** Swallow tablets whole – do not crush, chew or cut

CRIZANLIZUMAB

Crizanlizumab is a monoclonal antibody that reduces the frequency of VOC. It binds and inhibits P-selectin, which is involved in adhesion of sickled erythrocytes to vessels (causing vaso-occlusion).

DRUG	DOSE	SAFETY/SIDE EFFECTS/MONITORING
Crizanlizumab (Adakveo) Injection	5 mg/kg IV every 2 weeks x 2 doses, then 5 mg/kg every 4 weeks	**WARNINGS** Infusion-related reactions, lab test interference with platelet counts **SIDE EFFECTS** Nausea, arthralgias, fever

KEY COUNSELING POINTS

See the Drug Formulations and Patient Counseling chapter for counseling language/layman's terminology.

HYDROXYUREA

- Anyone handling the medication (patient or caregiver) should wear disposable gloves to reduce the risk of exposure. Wash hands before and after handling. The capsules should not be opened.

- Can cause infections.

- Avoid in pregnancy (teratogenic). Effective contraception required for sexually active males and females of reproductive potential, both during and after treatment.

- Live vaccines must be avoided. Check with your provider before getting any vaccines.

Select Guidelines/References
National Heart, Lung, and Blood Institute. Evidence-based management of sickle cell disease. Expert panel report, 2014. https://www.nhlbi.nih.gov/sites/default/files/media/docs/sickle-cell-disease-report%20020816_0.pdf.

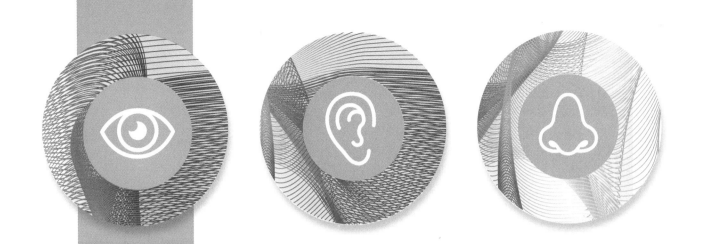

EYES, EARS, NOSE & SKIN CONDITIONS

CONTENTS

CONTENT LEGEND

 ✱ = Study Tip Gal

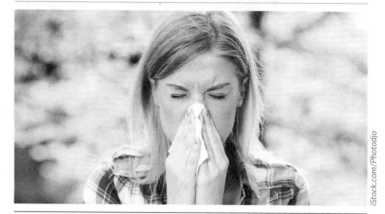

iStock.com/Photodjo

CHAPTER 37

ALLERGIC RHINITIS, COUGH & COLD

ALLERGIC RHINITIS

BACKGROUND

Allergic rhinitis, commonly called hay fever or simply "allergies," causes cold-like symptoms [congestion, rhinorrhea (runny nose), sneezing, sinus pressure and itchy eyes]. Colds are caused by a virus; allergic rhinitis is caused by exposure to an allergen (e.g., pollen, dust, pet dander). Refer to the figure below that distinguishes between colds and allergic rhinitis. Allergic rhinitis can be easily spotted when a person has a few quick sneezes in succession (due to an exposure to an allergen) with watery, itchy red eyes and an itchy nose and throat.

Allergic rhinitis symptoms can be intermittent (e.g., exposure to animal dander when visiting a friend's home) or chronic (e.g., symptoms that last for months whenever the pollen count is elevated).

Allergic rhinitis can cause discomfort, missed days at school and work and lost productivity. Untreated symptoms can lead to chronic sinusitis, otitis media (in children) and asthma exacerbations.

Many patients with asthma have allergic rhinitis; both are inflammatory reactions to some type of trigger.

COLDS VS. ALLERGIES

The symptoms of the common cold and allergies are very similar, which can make it difficult to tell the difference between the two.

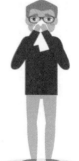

COLD	ALLERGY
Sneezing	Sneezing
Runny nose	Runny nose
Thick, dark mucus	Thin, clear mucus
Sore throat	Wheezing
Body aches	Red, watery eyes
Symptoms take about three days to appear and usually last for about a week	Symptoms can last for days or months after contact with allergens

iStock.com/AnnaViolet

NON-DRUG TREATMENT

Avoiding exposure to known or suspected allergens, if possible, will reduce symptoms (e.g., it might be possible to avoid triggers from dust mites, but it may not be possible to avoid chronic exposure to air pollution). An IgE-mediated skin prick test (see picture) or blood test can determine patient-specific allergens.

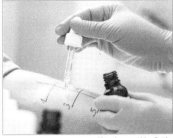

iStock.com/AlexRaths

Common allergens include:

- Pollens from trees, grasses and weeds
- Molds, both indoor and outdoor
- Dust mites that live in bedding, carpeting and other items that hold moisture
- Animal dander from furred animals such as cats, dogs, horses and rabbits

Ventilation systems with high-efficiency particulate air (HEPA) filters reduce some allergens (pollen, mold), but these systems can be expensive and are not effective for everyone.

Vacuuming carpets, drapes and upholstery with a HEPA vacuum cleaner often (at least weekly) reduces allergens. Dust mites can be reduced by removing carpets and upholstered furniture, encasing pillows, mattresses and box springs in allergen-impermeable covers and washing bedding and soft toys in hot water weekly.

When air pollutants are triggers, outdoor activities may need to be limited when air is unhealthy. The air quality index (AQI) rates the local air as good to hazardous. The AQI is useful for other conditions in which the air quality can affect breathing, including asthma, other types of lung disease and heart disease.

Pollen counts can be monitored when pollen is a trigger. When the pollen count is high, it is best to have patients stay indoors, with the windows closed and with the air conditioner on.

Nasal Irrigation and Wetting Agents

Nasal irrigations and wetting agents provide symptom relief by reducing nasal stuffiness, runny nose and sneezing. Nasal gels with petrolatum (Allergen Block) can be applied around the nostrils to physically block pollens and allergens from entering the nose. These products are considered safe for most populations, including children and pregnant women.

Wetting agents are commercially available (e.g., Ocean, Little Remedies, Simply Saline) and contain saline, propylene or polyethylene glycol, which provide moisture and reduce irritation to the nasal passages. Nasal irrigation (e.g., NeilMed Sinus Rinse) uses an isotonic (0.9%) or hypertonic (2 – 3.5%) saline solution, made with salt and water, to rinse out allergens and mucus, improve ciliary function and reduce swelling. Premixed saline packets are commercially available or a salt solution can be prepared at home. A homemade or store-bought saline mixture must be combined with distilled, sterile or previously boiled and cooled water. Tap water (known as drinking, or potable, water) should not be used; it contains organisms that are safe to ingest orally (killed by stomach acid) but can cause infections when used for nasal irrigation.

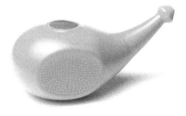

iStock.com/rob_lan

Nasal irrigations can be administered using a syringe or neti pot. A neti pot is a popular product that looks like a small teapot (see above). The prepared saline solution is placed in the neti pot, then poured into one nostril and drained out of the other nostril while breathing through the mouth. The most common side effects are mild nasal stinging or burning which are increased at higher concentrations of saline. After each use, the neti pot should be rinsed out with distilled, sterile or previously boiled water and allowed to air dry. Pots should never be shared with others.

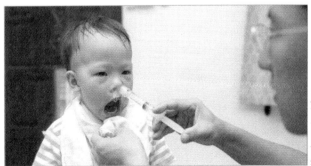

iStock.com/yaoinlove

DRUG TREATMENT

Selecting appropriate medication treatment depends on the severity of illness and symptoms. Intranasal steroids are first line for chronic, moderate-to-severe symptoms. Milder, intermittent symptoms can be treated with oral antihistamines. Decongestants can be used if congestion is present. Antihistamines and decongestants are available in both oral and nasal formulations. Ophthalmic medications for red, itchy eyes (e.g., allergic conjunctivitis) can be found in the Common Conditions of the Eyes & Ears chapter.

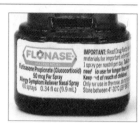

Eric Glenn/Shutterstock.com

Intranasal Steroids

Intranasal steroids work by decreasing inflammation. They are considered first-line treatment for moderate-severe symptoms. They are especially effective in reducing the nasal symptoms of allergic rhinitis (e.g., sneezing, itching, rhinorrhea, congestion). Several intranasal steroids come OTC for use in adults and pediatric patients. Note that the same steroids used to treat allergic rhinitis and asthma have different brand names and delivery systems. For example, fluticasone for allergic rhinitis comes in a nasal inhaler as *Flonase* ("-nase" for nasal), and for asthma it comes in an oral inhaler as *Flovent*.

DRUG	DOSING	SAFETY/SIDE EFFECTS/MONITORING
Budesonide **(Rhinocort Allergy)** OTC	Adult: 1 spray per nostril daily (max 4 sprays per nostril daily) Age ≥ 6 yrs: 1 spray per nostril daily (max 2 sprays per nostril daily)	**WARNINGS** Avoid use if recent nasal septal ulcers, nasal surgery, or recent nasal trauma due to delayed wound healing High doses for prolonged periods can cause: adrenal suppression, ↓ growth velocity (pediatrics) and immunosuppression
Fluticasone **(Flonase Allergy Relief, Flonase Sensimist, Children's Flonase, Xhance)** Rx and OTC + azelastine (Dymista)	Adult and children ≥ 12 yrs: 1-2 sprays per nostril daily Age 2-11 yrs: 1 spray per nostril daily	Use caution in patients with cataracts and/or glaucoma; ↑ intraocular pressure (IOP), open-angle glaucoma and cataracts have occurred with prolonged use **SIDE EFFECTS** Epistaxis (nose bleeds), headache, dry nose, unpleasant taste, localized infection
Triamcinolone **(Nasacort Allergy 24HR, Nasacort Allergy 24HR Children*)** OTC	Adult and children age ≥ 6 yrs: 1-2 sprays per nostril daily Age 2-5 yrs: 1 spray per nostril daily	**MONITORING** Growth (pediatrics), vision changes, eye exams in long-term use, signs/symptoms of oral thrush and/or adrenal suppression
Beclomethasone (Beconase AQ, Qnasl, Qnasl Children's)	Adult: 1-2 sprays per nostril BID (Beconase AQ); 2 sprays per nostril daily (Qnasl)	If using regularly for several months, recommend periodic nasal exams to evaluate for nasal septal perforation or ulcers
Ciclesonide (Omnaris, Zetonna)	Adult: 2 sprays per nostril daily (Omnaris); 1 spray per nostril daily (Zetonna)	**NOTES** Can take up to one week to get full relief Budesonide and beclomethasone are the preferred nasal steroids in pregnancy
Flunisolide	Adult: 2 sprays per nostril BID or TID	Shake bottle well before each use
Mometasone (Nasonex 24HR Allergy) Rx and OTC Nasal implant: Sinuva + olopatadine (Ryaltris)	Adult: 2 sprays per nostril daily	Discard device after total number of labeled doses, even if the bottle does not feel completely empty

*Brand discontinued but name still used in practice.

Antihistamines

Oral antihistamines are commonly used for <u>mild-moderate disease</u>. They are effective in reducing symptoms of itching, sneezing, rhinorrhea and other types of immediate hypersensitivity reactions, but have <u>little effect on nasal congestion</u>. Antihistamines work by blocking histamine at the <u>histamine-1 (H1) receptor site</u>. <u>First-generation</u> antihistamines, including hydroxyzine and meclizine, cause <u>more sedation</u> than second-generation antihistamines. The <u>second-generation</u> agents are generally <u>preferred</u> since they cause less sedation and cognitive impairment. Promethazine is a first-generation antihistamine that can be seen in cough and cold combination products (see later in chapter). Antihistamines can help if symptoms of allergic conjunctivitis (e.g., itchy, red eyes) are present (see the Common Conditions of the Eyes & Ears chapter for more information).

DIPHENHYDRAMINE IN PHARMACY; IT'S EVERYWHERE

Diphenhydramine is a first-generation antihistamine, but it is used for many indications, such as:

- Treatment of acute allergic reactions (+/- epinephrine, depending on severity)
- Prevention of allergic reactions (included in most premedication regimens for high-risk drugs)
- Allergic rhinitis
- Cough (has antitussive properties)
- Sleep (sedating)
- Dystonic reactions (anticholinergic properties)
- Motion sickness

Because of its wide range of effects, it can worsen some disease states (e.g., BPH, constipation, dementia, glaucoma)

Keith Homan/Shutterstock.com

DRUG	DOSING	SAFETY/SIDE EFFECTS/MONITORING
Select First-Generation Oral Antihistamines		
Diphenhydramine **(Benadryl**, many others) Capsule, tablet, chewable, elixir, strip, syrup, injection, cream, gel, solution, spray Rx and OTC	Adult: <u>25 mg PO Q4-6H or 50 mg PO Q6-8H</u> (max 300 mg/day) Age 6-11 yrs: 12.5-25 mg PO Q4-6H (max 150 mg/day) Age < 6 yrs: <u>do not use OTC</u> unless directed by a healthcare provider	**CONTRAINDICATIONS** Neonates or premature infants, breastfeeding **WARNINGS** <u>Avoid in the elderly</u> (due to strong anticholinergic effects; Beers criteria) and in children < 2 years Can cause CNS depression/sedation
Chlorpheniramine (Aller-Chlor, others) Tablet, syrup OTC	IR (adult): 4 mg PO Q4-6H (max 24 mg/day) ER (adult): 12 mg PO Q12H (max 24 mg/day)	Use with caution in patients with cardiovascular disease, <u>prostate enlargement, glaucoma</u>, asthma, pyloroduodenal obstruction and thyroid disease Do not use with MAO inhibitors (especially clemastine or carbinoxamine)
Doxylamine Unisom SleepTabs - for sleep Tablet OTC	Adult: 12.5-25 mg PO Q4-6H (max 75 mg/day)	Age restrictions vary for OTC use, check the product labeling (e.g., do not use diphenhydramine in children < 6 years or doxylamine in children < 12 years) **SIDE EFFECTS** <u>Somnolence, cognitive impairment</u>, strong <u>anticholinergic effects</u> (dry mouth, blurred vision, urinary retention, constipation) and seizures/arrhythmias at higher doses
Clemastine Tablet, syrup	Adult: 1.34-2.68 mg PO Q8-12H (max 8.04 mg/day)	**NOTES** First-generation antihistamines should not be taken by lactating women; second-generation agents preferred Should be discontinued ≥ 72 hours prior to allergy skin testing
Carbinoxamine (Karbinal ER, RyVent) Tablet, liquid	IR (adult): 4-8 mg PO Q6-8H ER (adult): 6-16 mg PO Q12H	Can cause photosensitivity; use sunscreens and wear protective clothing while taking FDA issued a Safety Alert regarding reports of abuse/misuse of diphenhydramine by teenagers leading to serious heart problems, seizures, coma or death

DRUG	DOSING	SAFETY/SIDE EFFECTS/MONITORING
Second-Generation Oral Antihistamines		
Cetirizine (Zyrtec Allergy, Zyrtec Childrens Allergy, others) Capsule, tablet, solution, syrup, chewable, ODT, injection Rx and OTC **+ pseudoephedrine (Zyrtec-D)** OTC	Adult and children ≥ 6 yrs: 5-10 mg PO daily (max 5 mg daily in elderly) Age 2-5 yrs: 2.5-5 mg PO daily	**CONTRAINDICATIONS** Levocetirizine: end-stage renal disease (CrCl < 10 mL/min), hemodialysis, infants and children 6 months to 11 years of age with renal impairment **WARNINGS** Can cause CNS depression/sedation, especially when used with other sedating drugs Use with caution in the elderly and in renal or hepatic impairment **SIDE EFFECTS** Somnolence can still be seen (more with cetirizine and levocetirizine), headache **NOTES** Fexofenadine: take with water (not fruit juice due to ↓ absorption); avoid administration with aluminum or magnesium-containing products Should be discontinued ≥ 72 hours prior to allergy skin testing If using in pregnancy, loratadine and cetirizine are preferred Cetirizine and levocetirizine have a fast onset and may work best for some patients More sedating: cetirizine and levocetirizine Less sedating: fexofenadine and loratadine Some formulations of fexofenadine, loratadine and desloratadine contain phenylalanine (avoid with PKU)
Levocetirizine (Xyzal Allergy 24HR, Xyzal Allergy 24HR Childrens) Tablet, solution Rx and OTC	Adult and children ≥ 12 yrs: 5 mg PO QHS Age 6-11 yrs: 2.5 mg PO QHS Age 6 mos-5 yrs: 1.25 mg PO QHS	
Fexofenadine (Allegra Allergy, Allegra Allergy Childrens) Tablet, suspension, ODT OTC **+ pseudoephedrine (Allegra-D)** OTC	Adult and children ≥ 12 yrs: 60 mg PO BID or 180 mg PO daily Age 2-11 yrs: 30 mg PO BID	
Loratadine (Claritin, Claritin Childrens, Alavert) Tablet, capsule, chewable, solution, syrup, ODT OTC **+ pseudoephedrine (Claritin-D)** OTC	Adult and children ≥ 6 yrs: 10 mg PO daily or 5 mg PO BID (RediTabs) Age 2-5 yrs: 5 mg PO daily	
Desloratadine (Clarinex) Tablet, ODT + pseudoephedrine (Clarinex-D 12 Hour)	Adult: 5 mg PO daily	
Intranasal Antihistamines		
Azelastine (Astepro Allergy) OTC and Rx + fluticasone (Dymista)	Adult: 1-2 sprays per nostril BID	**SIDE EFFECTS** Bitter taste, headache, somnolence, nasal irritation, epistaxis, sinus pain **NOTES** Helps with nasal congestion; can be combined with an intranasal steroid (increases cost and risk for side effects)
Olopatadine (Patanase)	Adult: 2 sprays per nostril BID	

Decongestants

Decongestants are <u>alpha-adrenergic agonists</u> (sympathomimetics). They cause <u>vasoconstriction</u>, which decreases sinus vessel engorgement and mucosal edema and makes them effective at reducing sinus and nasal congestion. If a product contains a <u>D after the name</u> (such as *Mucinex D)*, it usually <u>contains</u> a decongestant such as <u>phenylephrine or pseudoephedrine</u> (see <u>Study Tip Gal</u> on combination products later in chapter). <u>Phenylephrine</u> has <u>poor</u> oral absorption. It comes as a <u>nasal spray</u>, but lasts for a <u>shorter time</u> and causes more side effects than the popular <u>oxymetazoline spray</u>. <u>Pseudoephedrine</u> is an <u>effective systemic decongestant</u>; pseudoephedrine is a <u>precursor</u> to <u>methamphetamine</u>, and has restricted distribution (see box to the right).

COMBAT METHAMPHETAMINE EPIDEMIC ACT 2005

To combat the methamphetamine epidemic, there are restricted sales of <u>non-prescription</u> products containing <u>pseudoephedrine, phenylpropanolamine</u> and <u>ephedrine</u>, since these can all be <u>converted</u> easily to <u>methamphetamine</u>.

Products must be kept <u>behind the counter</u> or in a locked cabinet, usually located in the pharmacy.

A logbook of any sale more than a single-dose package (maximum of 60 mg) is kept. For any sale above this amount, the customer must show a government-issued photo ID (e.g., driver's license, ID card or US passport).

Customers record their name, date and time of sale and signature in the logbook. Staff must verify that the name matches the photo ID, the date and time are correct, record the customer address (can be done by swiping the driver's license electronically) and what the person received as well as the quantity purchased.

Under federal law <u>the maximum amount allowed for purchase is 3.6 grams per day, and 9 grams in a 30-day period</u>.

Logbook must be kept secured for a minimum of 2 years and be readily available upon request by board inspectors or law enforcement. It cannot be shared with the public.

Many states have their own restrictions in addition to the federal restrictions, such as age restrictions, prescription required or stricter quantity limits.

DRUG	DOSING	SAFETY/SIDE EFFECTS/MONITORING
Systemic (Oral)		
Phenylephrine *(Sudafed PE,* others) Tablet, liquid, solution OTC Injection: used as a vasopressor (see Acute & Critical Care Medicine chapter)	Adult: 10 mg PO Q4H PRN (max 60 mg/day) Age 6-11 yrs: 5 mg PO Q4H PRN (max 30 mg/day) Age 4-5 yrs: 2.5 mg PO Q4H PRN (max 15 mg/day)	**CONTRAINDICATIONS** <u>Do not use within 14 days of MAO inhibitors</u> **WARNINGS** <u>Avoid in children < 2 years (FDA), < 4 years (package labeling)</u> Use with <u>caution</u> in patients with <u>CV disease</u> and uncontrolled hypertension (can ↑ BP), hyperthyroidism (can worsen), diabetes (can ↑ BG), bowel obstruction, glaucoma (can ↑ IOP), <u>BPH</u> (can cause <u>urinary retention</u>), renal impairment, seizure disorder, the elderly
Pseudoephedrine *(Sudafed, Nexafed, Zephrex-D,* others) Tablet, liquid, syrup Rx and <u>non-prescription behind the counter</u> (see box above)	Adult: 60 mg PO Q4-6H PRN, or 120 mg ER PO Q12H, or 240 mg ER PO daily (max 240 mg/day) Age 6-11 yrs: 30 mg PO Q4-6H PRN (max 120 mg/day) Age 4-5 yrs: 15 mg PO Q4-6H PRN (max 60 mg/day)	**SIDE EFFECTS** Cardiovascular stimulation (<u>tachycardia, palpitations, ↑ BP</u>), CNS stimulation (anxiety, tremors, <u>insomnia</u>, nervousness, restlessness, fear, hallucinations), ↓ appetite, dizziness, headache **NOTES** <u>Oral decongestants should be avoided in the first trimester of pregnancy</u> Phenylephrine has low bioavailability (≤ 38%); pseudoephedrine is more effective Onset of 15-60 minutes
Topicals (Intranasal)		
Oxymetazoline 0.05% *(Afrin,* Vicks Sinex 12 Hour, Zicam Extreme Congestion Relief) OTC	Adult and Children ≥ 6 yrs: 2-3 sprays per nostril Q12H PRN	**CONTRAINDICATIONS** Oxymetazoline: do not use for more than 3 days **WARNINGS** Do not use with MAO inhibitors Use with caution in patients with CV disease and uncontrolled hypertension, thyroid disease, diabetes and <u>BPH</u>
Phenylephrine 0.25%, 0.5%, 1% *(Little Remedies Decongestant Drops, Neo-Synephrine,* others) OTC	Adult: 2-3 sprays of 0.25% to 1% per nostril Q4H PRN	**SIDE EFFECTS** <u>Rhinitis medicamentosa (rebound congestion if used longer than 3 days)</u>, nasal stinging, burning and dryness (vehicle-related), sneezing, trauma from the tip of the device **NOTES** Fast onset (5-10 minutes)

Additional Allergy Medications

Intranasal Cromolyn

Intranasal cromolyn (*NasalCrom*) is an OTC mast cell stabilizer used for treatment and prophylaxis of allergic rhinitis. It must be started at the onset of allergy season and used regularly (not PRN) to be effective. Symptoms will start to improve in 3 – 7 days, but maximal effect can take ≥ 2 – 4 weeks of continued use. Intranasal cromolyn is not as effective as other agents but it is safe to use in children ≥ 2 years old and in pregnancy.

Oral Leukotriene Receptor Antagonist

Montelukast (*Singulair*) is the only leukotriene modifying agent indicated for the treatment of both allergic rhinitis and asthma. It is commonly used in children. The FDA issued a boxed warning for montelukast, resulting from the risk of serious neuropsychiatric side effects. For allergic rhinitis, montelukast should be reserved for those who are unable to be treated effectively with other medications. See the Asthma chapter for more information.

Intranasal Ipratropium

This drug is effective for decreasing rhinorrhea by causing nasal dryness (it is not effective for other nasal symptoms).

Immunotherapy

Immunotherapy is a preventative treatment for allergies, either through subcutaneous (SC) injections or sublingual (SL) treatments. They work by slowly increasing exposure to the allergen, making the immune system less sensitive to the substance. Long-term immunotherapy can improve the underlying allergic disease and relieve symptoms even after stopping treatment. It is recommended to treat for a minimum of three years.

SC allergy shots are the traditional method of treatment, which must be given in a medical office. An alternative option is SL treatment. The four FDA-approved SL treatments for allergic rhinitis are tailored to specific allergens. The first dose must be given in a medical office where the patient can be monitored for at least 30 minutes afterward for signs of an allergic reaction (boxed warning). If tolerated, subsequent doses can be taken at home. The patient should have an epinephrine auto-injector while on SL immunotherapy.

- *Oralair* contains five different grass pollen extracts.
- *Grastek* contains Timothy grass pollen extract.
- *Ragwitek* contains ragweed pollen extract.
- *Odactra* contains house dust mite allergen extract.

COUGH AND COLD

BACKGROUND

The common cold, a viral infection of the upper respiratory tract, is caused by over 200 viruses, including rhinoviruses and coronaviruses. It is transmitted by mucus secretions (via patient's hands) or by the air (from coughing or sneezing). Coughing or sneezing into the elbow or into a tissue is preferable over coughing into a hand, which can then touch surfaces and spread illness. Transmission is best prevented by frequent hand washing with soap or soap substitutes (e.g., hand sanitizer). Refer to the Medication Safety & Quality Improvement chapter for correct hand washing technique, and to the Infectious Diseases II chapter for a table of common upper and lower respiratory infections. Colds are usually self-limiting, but are a leading cause of absenteeism in work and school due to bothersome symptoms.

DRUG TREATMENT

Treatment of cough and cold is based on the presenting symptoms; each patient will present differently and require different treatment. The goal of treatment is to reduce duration and frequency of symptoms to allow the patient to feel better and return to normal activities.

Natural Products Used for Colds

Zinc, in various formulations including lozenges, is used for cold prevention and treatment. Zinc lozenges or syrup might decrease cold duration if used correctly and at first signs of symptoms (taken every two hours while awake, starting 24 – 48 hours of symptom onset). For this purpose zinc supplements are rated as "possibly effective" by the *Natural Medicines Database*. Zinc lozenges can cause mouth irritation, a metallic taste and nausea. They should not be used for more than five to seven days, as long-term use can cause copper deficiency. Zinc nasal formulations were removed from the market due to causing loss of smell.

Vitamin C (ascorbic acid) supplements are commonly used, but they have little to no efficacy for cold prevention. Some data has shown a decrease in the duration of the cold by 1 – 1.5 days at doses of 1 – 3 grams/day. There might also be a dose-dependent response; doses of at least 2 grams/day appear to work better than 1 gram/day. Vitamin C is rated as "possibly effective" for cold treatment by the *Natural Medicines Database*. High doses of vitamin C (4 g/day or greater) can cause diarrhea and possibly kidney stones. Echinacea is rated as "possibly effective" for cold treatment.

With any of these products, it is important to use the correct dose from a reputable manufacturer. *Airborne* and *Emergen-C Immune+* are popular products that contain a variety of ingredients, including vitamin C, vitamin E, zinc and echinacea.

Expectorants

Cough associated with colds is usually nonproductive (i.e., a dry cough). If productive cough is present, expectorants can be used to thin mucus and move secretions up and out of the respiratory tract.

DRUG	DOSING	SAFETY/SIDE EFFECTS/MONITORING
Guaifenesin (Mucinex, Robitussin Mucus + Chest Congestion,* Robafen*) Tablet, liquid, syrup, packet **+ dextromethorphan (Robafen DM, Robitussin DM*)** OTC	Adult: 200-400 mg PO Q4H PRN, or 600-1,200 mg ER PO Q12H (max 2.4 g/day) Age 6-11 yrs: 1,200 mg/day (max) Age 4-5 yrs: 600 mg/day (max)	**SIDE EFFECTS** Nausea (dose-related), vomiting, dizziness, headache, rash, diarrhea, stomach pain **NOTES** OTC: do not use ER tablets in children < 12 years of age Some formulations contain phenylalanine (avoid with PKU)

Brand discontinued but name still used in practice.

Cough Suppressants

Cough suppressants are used for dry, nonproductive cough or to suppress productive cough at night to allow for restful sleep. Dextromethorphan and opioids, such as codeine and hydrocodone, have a high affinity for several regions of the brain, including the medullary cough center, suppressing the cough reflex. Benzonatate suppresses cough by a topical anesthetic action on the respiratory stretch receptors.

Opioids and dextromethorphan have abuse potential (see the Pain chapter for opioid boxed warnings). Dextromethorphan acts as a serotonin reuptake inhibitor. At usual antitussive doses, it does not have addictive properties, but at high doses it acts as an NMDA-receptor blocker leading to euphoria and hallucinations similar to the illicit substance PCP. Due to its abuse potential, many states ban the sale of dextromethorphan to minors < 18 years of age. Codeine products containing one or more non-codeine active ingredient (e.g., guaifenesin) and no more than 200 mg of codeine/100 mL are scheduled as C-V drugs. Codeine is a known drug of abuse, particularly in combination with promethazine.

DRUG	DOSING	SAFETY/SIDE EFFECTS/MONITORING
Dextromethorphan (Delsym, Robafen Cough, Robitussin Cough*) Capsule, liquid, lozenge, suspension, strips OTC **+ guaifenesin (Robafen DM, Robitussin DM*)** OTC	Adult: 10-20 mg PO Q4H PRN, or 30 mg PO Q6-8H PRN, or 60 mg ER PO Q12H PRN (max 120 mg/day) Age 6-12 yrs: max 60 mg/day Age 4-6 yrs: max 30 mg/day	**CONTRAINDICATIONS** Do not use within 14 days of an MAO inhibitor **WARNINGS** Serotonin syndrome (if co-administered with other serotonergic drugs), use with caution in patients who are CYP450 2D6 poor metabolizers or with CYP2D6 inhibitors, debilitated (e.g., sedated, confined to a supine position) **SIDE EFFECTS** N/V, drowsiness, CNS depression (especially when used with other sedating drugs) **NOTES** If the product name has DM at the end, such as *Robitussin DM*, it contains dextromethorphan OTC: do not use in children < 4 years
Codeine C-II (single entity used for pain) C-V (combination products used for cough and cold: see table on following page)	Adult: 7.5-120 mg PO as single dose or divided doses	**BOXED WARNING** Respiratory depression and death have occurred in children who received codeine following tonsillectomy and/or adenoidectomy and had evidence of being ultra-rapid metabolizers of codeine due to a CYP450 2D6 polymorphism; deaths have also occurred in nursing infants after being exposed to high concentrations of morphine from mothers who were ultra-rapid metabolizers **CONTRAINDICATIONS** Do not use in children < 12 years of age (any indication) or in children < 18 years of age after tonsillectomy and/or adenoidectomy **NOTES** The FDA recommends to avoid codeine-containing cough and cold products for patients < 18 years of age (see the Pain and Pediatric Conditions chapters)
Benzonatate (Tessalon Perles)	Adult: 100-200 mg PO TID PRN (max 600 mg/day)	**WARNINGS** Do not use in children < 10 years of age; accidental ingestion and fatal overdose has been reported **SIDE EFFECTS** Somnolence, confusion, hallucinations
Diphenhydramine (Benadryl) Rx and OTC	Adult: 25 mg PO Q4H PRN (max 150 mg/day)	See First-Generation Oral Antihistamines table

Brand discontinued but name still used in practice.

Decongestants

Systemic and nasal decongestants, discussed previously, are used to relieve congestion and rhinorrhea.

Analgesics/Antipyretics

Analgesics and antipyretics such as acetaminophen and ibuprofen are used to relieve sore throat, body malaise and fever. They are often added to combination products for cough/cold. Use caution <u>not</u> to <u>exceed the maximum</u> daily dosing for acetaminophen or ibuprofen if multiple medications are being used. See the Pain chapter for more information.

Select Cough and Cold Combination Products

See the <u>Study Tip Gal</u> below for methods to help recognize the ingredients in combination products.

DRUG	ADULT DOSING
Dextromethorphan/promethazine	15 mg/6.25 mg per 5 mL; 5 mL PO Q4-6H PRN (max 30 mL/day)
Brompheniramine/pseudoephedrine/dextromethorphan **(Bromfed DM)** Rx and OTC	2 mg/30 mg/10 mg per 5 mL; 10 mL PO Q4H PRN (max 60 mL/day)
Promethazine/codeine <u>C-V</u>	6.25 mg/10 mg per 5 mL; 5 mL PO Q4-6H PRN (max 30 mL/day)
Promethazine/phenylephrine/codeine (Promethazine VC/Codeine) <u>C-V</u>	6.25 mg/5 mg/10 mg per 5 mL; 5 mL PO Q4-6H PRN (max 30 mL/day)
Guaifenesin/codeine (G Tussin AC) <u>C-V</u>	100 mg/10 mg per 5 mL; 10 mL PO Q4H PRN (max 60 mL/day)
Guaifenesin/codeine/pseudoephedrine (Coditussin DAC, Virtussin DAC) <u>C-V</u>	100 mg/10 mg/30 mg per 5 mL; 10 mL PO Q4H PRN (max 40 mL/day)
Chlorpheniramine/hydrocodone **(TussiCaps, Tussionex*)** <u>C-II</u>	Capsule: 8 mg/10 mg per capsule; 1 capsule PO Q12H PRN (max 2 caps/day) Suspension: 8 mg/10 mg ER per 5 mL; 5 mL PO Q12H PRN (max 10 mL/day)
Chlorpheniramine/codeine (Tuzistra XR) C-III	4 mg/20 mg ER per 5 mL; 10 mL PO Q12H PRN (max 20 mL/day)

Brand discontinued but name still used in practice.

COUGH AND COLD COMBINATION PRODUCTS: WHAT'S IN A NAME?

The name of a combination cough/cold product can tell you what it contains. This is based on either the symptom it treats or the abbreviation included in the name (e.g., *Robitussin Cough + Chest Congestion DM* contains dextromethorphan, a cough suppressant identified with the abbreviation DM and guaifenesin, an expectorant for chest congestion). Some commonly used abbreviations are:

D = decongestant (e.g., phenylephrine or pseudoephedrine); example: *Mucinex D* = guaifenesin + pseudoephedrine

PE = **p**henyl**e**phrine; example: *Sudafed PE* = phenylephrine

DM = **d**extro**m**ethorphan; example: *Robafen DM* = guaifenesin + dextromethorphan

AC = contains codeine; example: *G Tussin AC* = guaifenesin + codeine

Guaifenesin is a mucolytic (thins out mucus); example: *Mucinex*

Analgesic in combination cough and cold products is usually acetaminophen

Antihistamines (e.g., diphenhydramine, chlorpheniramine, brompheniramine) are common and cause sedation; the night-time products, and some anytime products, contain an antihistamine

Cough and Cold Products in Children

If a young child has a cold, it is safe and useful to recommend proper hydration, nasal bulbs for gentle suctioning, saline drops/sprays (*Ocean* and generics) and vaporizers/humidifiers. Ibuprofen and acetaminophen can be used, if needed, for fever or pain (see the Pain and Pediatric Conditions chapters for more information).

PEDIATRIC COUGH AND COLD TREATMENT - CAUTION NEEDED

CHILDREN < 18 YEARS
- Avoid codeine and hydrocodone-containing cough and cold products (FDA)

CHILDREN < 4 YEARS
- Avoid OTC cough and cold products (package labeling)

CHILDREN < 2 YEARS
- Avoid OTC cough and cold products (FDA)
- Avoid promethazine (FDA)
- Avoid topical menthol and camphor (package labeling)

Cough and cold products generally do not offer much symptom relief to young children, while having potentially serious side effects. Many of the products contain multiple ingredients, which increases the risk of accidental overdose if combined with other medications. Symptoms due to cough and cold are self-limiting and drug treatment is often not necessary. The FDA does not recommend OTC drug treatment for cough and cold symptoms in children ≤ 2 years old, but most manufacturers include product labeling to avoid in children ≤ 4 years old. Some combination products have additional labeling restrictions for use only in children ≥ 6 years of age.

Do not use promethazine in any form in children < 2 years old because of the risk of fatal respiratory depression. Due to the risk of adverse events (e.g., slowed breathing, overdose,

misuse), the FDA recommends against using prescription cough and cold products containing codeine or hydrocodone in patients ≤ 18 years old. When used to treat pain, codeine and hydrocodone do not have the same restrictions (see the Pain and Pediatric Conditions chapters for more complete information).

Topical products containing menthol (e.g., *Vicks VapoRub*) can be applied to the chest and neck (never directly to the nose) to help open the airways and suppress cough. Such products should not be used in children < 2 years of age, as camphor and menthol can cause serious side effects (e.g., CNS toxicity) if ingested. *Vicks BabyRub* contains petrolatum, eucalyptus oil, lavender oil, rosemary oil and aloe extract and is considered relatively safe, but lacks sufficient efficacy data.

KEY COUNSELING POINTS

See the Drug Formulations and Patient Counseling chapter for nasal spray administration instructions.

ANTIHISTAMINES

- Some formulations contain phenylalanine. Do not use if you have phenylketonuria (PKU).

Select Guidelines/References

Dykewicz MS, Wallace DV, Amrol DJ, et al. Rhinitis 2020: A practice parameter update. J Allergy Clin Immunol. 2020;146(4):721-767.

Handbook of Nonprescription Drugs: An Interactive Approach to Self-Care, 20th Edition. December 2020.

Seidman MD, Gurgel RK, Lin SY et al. Clinical Practice Guideline: Allergic Rhinitis. Otolaryngology-Head and Neck Surgery. 2015;152(IS):S1-S43.

GLAUCOMA

damage to optic nerve

abnormal pressure inside eye

iStock.com/TefiM

CHAPTER 38

COMMON CONDITIONS OF THE EYES & EARS

BACKGROUND

Many eye and ear conditions can be treated with topical medications that are applied directly to the eye or ear. By applying the medication directly to the specific location, instead of systemically, adverse effects are minimized.

The various formulations of topical eye and ear medications are shown in the box below. The eyes are more sensitive than the ears. Eye drops can be used in the ear, but never use ear drops in the eyes. The ear drops may not have an appropriate pH, may not be isotonic and may not be sterile. Correct administration technique is key for each medication to work.

EYE & EAR PRESCRIPTION INTERPRETATION

ABBREV.	MEANING	CAUTION
AD AS AU	Right Ear Left Ear Each Ear	These abbreviations can be mistaken (interchanged) for each other and can mean other things; know how to interpret them, but it is safer to write them out (e.g., use right eye instead of OD)
OD OS OU	Right Eye Left Eye Each Eye	

Memory tip: A is from the Latin for ear (auris), O is for eye (oculus), D is for right (dextra) and S is for left (sinistra)

iStock.com/Sudowoodo

EYE AND EAR FORMULATIONS

- Solutions: 1 drop = 0.05 mL.

- Suspensions: shake well.

- Ointments: apply to the conjunctival sac or over lid margins (for blepharitis). Ointments can make vision blurry. Do not use with contact lenses.

- Gels: with cap on, invert and shake once to get the medication into the tip before instilling into the eye.

GLAUCOMA

Glaucoma is a disease of the eye that results in damage to the optic nerve and loss of the visual field (i.e., the vision straight ahead and the peripheral vision, measured by the visual field test). In most cases, the intraocular pressure (IOP) is above the normal range of 12 – 22 mmHg. IOP can be increased from genetics, age and medications (see Key Drugs Guy). The goal of treatment is to reduce IOP.

There are two main forms of glaucoma. Open-angle glaucoma is the most common type. It often presents without symptoms and is treated with eye drops or surgery. Angle-closure, or closed-angle glaucoma, is a sharp, sudden increase in IOP due to a blockage. This type of glaucoma usually presents with eye pain, headaches and decreased vision and is a medical emergency that is treated surgically.

DRUGS THAT CAN INCREASE IOP

Anticholinergics (e.g., antihistamines, oxybutynin, tolterodine, benztropine, scopolamine, trihexyphenidyl, tricyclic antidepressants)

Decongestants (e.g., pseudoephedrine)

Chronic steroids, especially eye drops such as prednisolone (Pred Forte)

Topiramate (Topamax)

DRUG TREATMENT

Glaucoma treatments decrease IOP by targeting the aqueous humor (fluid in the eye) in two main ways (see Study Tip Gal). Prostaglandin (PG) analogs are used commonly as initial treatment. PG analogs are the most effective drugs at decreasing IOP (~30%); they are safe and are used once daily. Ophthalmic beta-blockers (e.g., timolol), another common class of drugs, decrease IOP by ~22%. A beta-blocker is preferable if the pressure is high in one eye only because the darkening of the iris and eyelash thickening seen with PG analogs is not desirable in only one eye (see drug table below). If monotherapy does not sufficiently decrease IOP, consider switching to a different medication or using combination therapy.

GLAUCOMA TREATMENT GOAL: DECREASE IOP

Strategies:
- Reduce aqueous humor production (make less fluid)
  - ❏ Beta-blockers, like timolol
  - ❏ Carbonic anhydrase inhibitors, like dorzolamide
- Increase aqueous humor outflow (move fluid out)
  - ❏ Prostaglandin analogs, like latanoprost
- Or, do both: often achieved with add-on treatment
  - ❏ Alpha-2 agonists, like brimonidine

Adequate treatment requires good eye drop technique and a high level of adherence. The correct way to administer eye drops is described in the Drug Formulations and Patient Counseling chapter. Because glaucoma often presents with no symptoms, adherence can be a major issue. Counseling on proper administration technique and the importance of adherence is critical.

DRUG	DOSING	SIDE EFFECTS/CLINICAL CONCERNS
Prostaglandin Analogs: increase aqueous humor outflow		
Bimatoprost (Lumigan) **Latanoprost (Xalatan, Xelpros)** + netarsudil (Rocklatan) **Travoprost (Travatan Z)** Latanoprostene bunod (Vyzulta) Tafluprost (Zioptan) **Bimatoprost (Latisse)** is indicated for eyelash hypotrichosis (inadequate growth of eyelashes) to ↑ eyelash growth; do not use with prostaglandin analogs indicated for glaucoma	1 drop QHS Do not exceed once daily dosing; can decrease efficacy Select products contain the preservative benzalkonium chloride (BAK); remove contact lenses before use	**WARNINGS** Ocular effects: darkening of the iris, eyelid skin and eyelashes; eyelash length and number can increase; contamination of multiple-dose ophthalmic solutions can cause bacterial keratitis **SIDE EFFECTS** Blurred vision, stinging, increased pigmentation of the iris/eyelashes, eyelash growth/thickening, foreign body sensation **NOTES** Travatan Z and Xelpros do not contain BAK (a different preservative is used); can be used in patients with a past reaction to BAK or dry eye Zioptan comes as 10 single-use, preservative-free containers in a foil pouch; discard each container after use Latanoprost, latanoprostene bunod and tafluprost should be stored in the refrigerator before opening; once opened, store at room temperature Naming tip: –prost = prostaglandin analog

DRUG	DOSING	SIDE EFFECTS/CLINICAL CONCERNS
Beta-Blockers: reduce aqueous humor production		
Timolol 0.25% and 0.5% (Timoptic, Timoptic-XE, Istalol, Timolol GFS, Betimol, Timoptic Ocudose) **+ dorzolamide (Cosopt, Cosopt PF)** + brimonidine (Combigan) Betaxolol (Betoptic S) Carteolol Levobunolol (Betagan)	*Timolol*: 1 drop daily or BID *Timoptic-XE, Timolol GFS* (gels): daily Gels: shake once before use; wait 10 minutes after administering other eye drops before inserting gel Select products contain the preservative BAK; remove contact lenses before use	**CONTRAINDICATIONS** Sinus bradycardia; heart block > 1ˢᵗ degree (except in patients with a pacemaker); cardiogenic shock; uncompensated cardiac failure; bronchospastic disease **SIDE EFFECTS** Burning, stinging, bradycardia/fatigue, bronchospasm with non-selective agents, itching of the eyes or eyelids, changes in vision, increased light sensitivity **NOTES** All are non-selective beta-blockers except betaxolol; betaxolol is less likely to cause pulmonary adverse effects in patients with chronic lung disease (e.g., asthma/COPD) *Cosopt PF* (the PF stands for "preservative-free") is packaged in single-use containers Some products contain sulfites, which can cause allergic reactions
Cholinergics (Miotics): increase aqueous humor outflow		
Carbachol (Miostat) Pilocarpine (Isopto Carpine)	1-2 drops up to TID Solution: 1-2 drops up to 4 times per day Select products contain the preservative BAK; remove contact lenses before use	**SIDE EFFECTS** Poor vision at night (due to pupil constriction), corneal clouding, burning (transient), hypotension, bronchospasm, abdominal cramps/GI distress **NOTES** Use with caution in patients with a history of retinal detachment or corneal abrasion
Carbonic Anhydrase Inhibitors: reduce aqueous humor production		
Dorzolamide (Trusopt) **+ timolol (Cosopt, Cosopt PF)** Brinzolamide (Azopt) + brimonidine (Simbrinza) Acetazolamide – oral, injection Methazolamide – oral	*Trusopt*: 1 drop TID *Cosopt*: 1 drop BID *Azopt*: 1 drop TID Acetazolamide 250 mg PO 1-4 times per day, or 500 mg ER PO BID Select ophthalmic products contain the preservative BAK; remove contact lenses before use	**WARNINGS** Sulfonamide allergy: caution due to the risk of systemic exposure and cross reactivity (especially with oral formulations) **SIDE EFFECTS** Eye drops: burning, blurred vision, blepharitis, dry eye Oral (acetazolamide): CNS effects (ataxia, confusion), photosensitivity/skin rash (including risk of SJS and TEN), anorexia, nausea, risk of hematological toxicities **NOTES** Acetazolamide is used infrequently for glaucoma; it is used for the prevention and treatment of acute mountain (altitude) sickness Naming Tip: –zolamide = caution with sulfonamide allergy
Adrenergic Alpha-2 Agonists: increase aqueous humor outflow, reduce aqueous humor production		
Brimonidine (Alphagan P) + timolol (Combigan) + brinzolamide (Simbrinza) Apraclonidine (Iopidine) Brimonidine (Lumify) (OTC) is indicated for ocular redness	*Alphagan P* and *Iopidine* are dosed TID Select products contain the preservative BAK; remove contact lenses before use	**WARNINGS** CNS depression: caution with heavy machinery, driving **SIDE EFFECTS** Sedation, dry mouth, dry nose
Rho Kinase Inhibitors: increase aqueous humor outflow		
Netarsudil (Rhopressa) + latanoprost (Rocklatan)	1 drop daily in the evening Contains the preservative BAK; remove contact lenses before use	**SIDE EFFECTS** Burning/eye pain, corneal disease, conjunctival hemorrhage and conjunctival hyperemia (excess blood vessels) **NOTES** Store in the refrigerator before opening; once opened, store at room temperature for ≤ 6 weeks

CONJUNCTIVITIS

Conjunctivitis, also known as "pink eye," occurs in one or both eyes. Symptoms include swelling, itching, burning and redness of the conjunctiva, the protective membrane that lines the eyelids and covers the white part of the eye (the sclera). Conjunctivitis can be due to a virus, bacteria, an allergen or some type of ocular irritant, such as a chemical or contact lenses. In most cases, conjunctivitis causes only mild discomfort, does not harm vision and will clear without medical treatment. In some cases, treatment is required.

Viral and bacterial conjunctivitis occur mostly in young children and are highly contagious. Infected children should stay at home and only return to school once treatment begins, unless there are systemic symptoms. To prevent the spread of the infection, any patient with viral or bacterial conjunctivitis should be instructed to:

- Avoid touching their eyes
- Use proper hand hygiene and wash their hands thoroughly and frequently
- Change towels and washcloths daily, and do not share towels with others
- Discard eye cosmetics, particularly mascara

Chemical conjunctivitis has no specific drug treatment and is not described in the following table. The irritant should be flushed out of the eyes with saline, and inflammation can be reduced with an NSAID or a steroid eye drop. If contact lenses caused the irritation, they should not be used until the condition clears. It might be helpful to change the type of contact lenses or the brand of disinfectant solution. If the condition is severe, such as a burn, or the chemical is dangerous or unknown, refer for emergency care.

TREATMENT OF CONJUNCTIVITIS BY TYPE

Conjunctivitis is usually viral and self-limiting. With bacterial or allergic conjunctivitis, treatments are helpful. Antibiotics are only indicated for bacterial conjunctivitis. If antibiotics are used, the full treatment course should be completed. These treatments can be combined with symptomatic treatment (see Symptom-Based Ophthalmic Treatments on the following page).

TYPE	CAUSES	TREATMENT
Viral	Adenovirus (most common), other viruses Most infections are mild, but some can be severe (e.g., caused by zoster virus or HIV)	No topical treatment for common viral conjunctivitis; the infection runs its course over several days to three weeks
Bacterial	*Staphylococcus aureus, Streptococcus pneumoniae, Haemophilus influenzae, Moraxella catarrhalis* More severe cases caused by *Neisseria gonorrhoeae* or *Chlamydia*, which requires systemic treatment	Select topical antibiotic eye drops or ointments: **Moxifloxacin (*Vigamox*)** **Neomycin/Polymyxin B/Dexamethasone (*Maxitrol*)** **Ofloxacin (*Ocuflox*)** **Trimethoprim/Polymyxin B (*Polytrim*)** Azithromycin (*AzaSite*) – store in the refrigerator, stable for 14 days at room temperature Besifloxacin (*Besivance*) Ciprofloxacin (*Ciloxan*) Erythromycin Gentamicin (*Gentak*) Neomycin/Bacitracin/Polymyxin B (*Neo-Polycin*) Tobramycin (*Tobrex*) Tobramycin/Dexamethasone (*TobraDex, TobraDex ST*) Sulfacetamide (*Bleph-10*)
Allergic	Common allergens include pollen, dust mites, animal dander, molds **USAGE NOTES:** Prednisolone/steroid eye drops are often used acutely for a severe reaction, but not long term due to risk of ↑ IOP Ophthalmic decongestants can be used to decrease redness caused by allergic conjunctivitis (see Symptom-Based Ophthalmic Treatments on the next page)	**MAST CELL STABILIZERS** Cromolyn Lodoxamide (*Alomide*) Nedocromil (*Alocril*) **ANTIHISTAMINES** **Azelastine** **Olopatadine (*Pataday*)** (OTC) Cetirizine (*Zerviate*) Epinastine **ANTIHISTAMINE/MAST CELL STABILIZER** **Ketotifen (*Alaway, Zaditor*)** (OTC) Alcaftadine (*Lastacaft*)

BLEPHARITIS

Blepharitis (eyelid inflammation) most commonly involves the eyelid margins (where the eyelashes come out of the skin). In many patients, the condition is chronic and difficult to treat, and in others, it is an acute, short-term condition. The primary symptoms are inflamed, irritated and itchy eyelids. The preferred treatment includes application of a warm compress over the eye for a few minutes to loosen the crusty deposits, then use of a warm, moist washcloth (water plus a few drops of baby shampoo) to wipe away the debris. In some cases, antibiotic ointments, steroid eye drops and/or artificial tears are helpful.

OTHER OCULAR CONDITIONS

SYMPTOM-BASED OPHTHALMIC TREATMENTS

Symptoms can accompany the diseases previously discussed (e.g., conjunctivitis) or they can occur independently. Common ophthalmic symptoms include inflammation, dry eye and eye redness. Inflammation can be reduced with a cold compress and either an NSAID eye drop (if mild) or a steroid eye drop (if severe). Artificial tears can help with a "gritty"

feeling and alleviate dryness. Chronic dry eye requires more aggressive treatment. Instruct patients to return for follow-up if they do not recover within a few days.

WHY DO MOST EYE DROPS BURN?

Most bottles of eye drops contain multiple doses. Since the drops are being put into the eyes, the bottle must remain free from contamination. A preservative is often added to prevent the growth of microorganisms. The most common preservative used in eye drops is benzalkonium chloride (BAK).

- Preservatives are toxic to bacteria and are irritating to the sensitive tissues in the eyes, which leads to burning/stinging after administration.
  - Some drugs found in eye drops can also cause irritation.
- Contact lenses trap the drug and preservatives against the surface of the eye, making irritation worse.
  - Lenses should be removed before using eye drops and wait 15 minutes after administration before reinserting.
  - This is especially important with drops containing BAK as these can damage the eyes when used with contacts.
- Some eye drops have preservative-free formulations for those unable to tolerate the side effects.
  - Example: *Cosopt PF* (the PF stands for preservative-free).

See the Drug Formulations and Patient Counseling chapter for eye drop administration instructions.

SYMPTOM	EXAMPLES OF TREATMENT	USAGE NOTES
Inflammation	**STEROIDS** **Prednisolone (Pred Forte, Pred Mild)** Dexamethasone (*Maxidex, Ozurdex*) Fluorometholone (*Flarex, FML Forte, FML Liquifilm* suspension, ointment) Loteprednol (*Alrex, Lotemax* suspension, ointment, gel) **NSAIDS** **Ketorolac (Acular,** *Acular LS, Acuvail*) Nepafenac (*Ilevro, Nevanac*) Bromfenac Diclofenac Flurbiprofen	Steroid eye drops should be used short-term due to risk of ↑ IOP
Dryness	*Refresh* (OTC) *Systane* (OTC) *Liquifilm Tears* (OTC) Others	Often referred to as Artificial Tears Contain common lubricants – mineral oil, glycerin, propylene glycol, dextran, hypromellose Administered multiple times daily, as needed
Chronic Dry Eye Disease	**Cyclosporine Emulsion Eye Drops (Restasis)** Lifitegrast (*Xiidra*) Loteprednol (*Eysuvis*) Varenicline nasal spray (*Tyrvaya*)	*Restasis* is indicated for keratoconjunctivitis sicca (severe, chronic dry eye syndrome)
Redness	**Naphazoline (Clear Eyes Redness Relief)** (OTC) **Naphazoline/Pheniramine (Naphcon A, Visine A)** (OTC) **Tetrahydrozoline (Visine)** (OTC) Brimonidine (*Lumify*) (OTC)	Can be used to treat allergic conjunctivitis

MEDICATION INDUCED OPHTHALMIC ISSUES

Medications can cause ocular adverse effects. Most disappear once the drug is discontinued (such as blurry vision from an anticholinergic). In other cases, the damage can be permanent (such as vision loss with a PDE-5 inhibitor). Patients must be instructed to report visual changes immediately; in most cases, the damage is reversible if the medication is stopped quickly. See the Key Drugs Guy on the next page for specific medications and their effects.

COMMON DRUGS KNOWN TO CAUSE VISION CHANGES OR DAMAGE

Retinal changes/retinopathy
Chloroquine

Hydroxychloroquine

Optic neuropathy
Amiodarone (plus corneal deposits)

Ethambutol

Linezolid

Intraoperative floppy iris syndrome (IFIS); causes difficulty in cataract surgery
Alpha-blockers (e.g., tamsulosin)

Color discrimination
Digoxin (with toxicity) – yellow/green vision

PDE-5 inhibitors (e.g., sildenafil) – greenish tinge around objects

Voriconazole – color vision changes

Vision loss/abnormal vision
Digoxin (with toxicity) – blurriness, halos

PDE-5 inhibitors – vision loss (one or both eyes; can be permanent)

Isotretinoin – ↓ night vision (can be permanent), dryness, irritation

Topiramate – visual field defects

Vigabatrin – permanent vision loss (high risk)

Voriconazole – abnormal vision, photophobia

COMMON EAR CONDITIONS

Common conditions treated in the ear include ear wax (cerumen) impaction and pain, such as from an outer ear infection (otitis externa). Tinnitus (ringing, roaring or buzzing sounds) is caused by drug toxicity (e.g., salicylates), noise exposure, or it can be idiopathic. There is no effective drug treatment for tinnitus.

EAR WAX (CERUMEN) BLOCKAGE

Ear blockage occurs when wax (cerumen) accumulates in the ear or becomes too hard to wash away naturally. For patients with symptoms (e.g., earache, hearing loss), it is removed in a medical office (manually or with irrigation) or with the use of cerumenolytics in a medical office or at home. Cerumenolytics soften ear wax, allowing it to be cleared from the ear more easily. Examples include water, saline solution, mineral oil, hydrogen peroxide and carbamide peroxide (Debrox). Use should be limited to 3 – 5 days, with follow-up after this time (see the Drug Formulations and Patient Counseling chapter for administration instructions).

OTITIS EXTERNA

Otitis externa (also known as swimmer's ear) is inflammation in the outer part of the ear, most commonly caused by an acute bacterial infection. Swimming is a risk factor because excess moisture remaining in the ear promotes microbial growth. Using earplugs while swimming and drying the ear after can prevent recurrent infections. Mild cases of otitis externa can be treated with ear drops containing acetic acid and a glucocorticoid (VoSol HC). Moderate to severe infections require topical otic antibiotics. Pain can be treated with systemic analgesics (e.g., ibuprofen, acetaminophen). During treatment, patients should stay out of the water, avoid flying due to the pressure changes and avoid the use of headphones and earplugs.

Common antibiotics include:

- Ciprofloxacin and dexamethasone (Ciprodex)

- Ciprofloxacin and hydrocortisone (Cipro HC)

- Neomycin, colistin, hydrocortisone and thonzonium (Cortisporin-TC)

KEY COUNSELING POINTS

See the Drug Formulations and Patient Counseling chapter for counseling language/layman's terminology and eye drop and ear drop administration instructions.

ALL EYE DROPS

- Can cause stinging/burning (except for preservative-free).

- Wait 5 minutes in between two drops of the same medication.

- Wait 5 – 10 minutes in between drops of two different medications.

- Apply gels last. Wait 10 minutes after the last eye drop before use.

- Remove contact lenses prior to using eye drops. Wait 15 minutes to reinsert.

Prostaglandin Analogs

- Darkening of the iris and an increase in eyelash growth can occur.

- Do not use with bimatoprost (Latisse). Latisse can reduce the effectiveness of other prostaglandins.

Select Guidelines/References
American Academy of Ophthalmology Glaucoma Committee. Preferred Practice Pattern Guidelines. Primary Open-Angle Glaucoma 2020. https://www.aao.org/preferred-practice-pattern/primary-open-angle-glaucoma-ppp (accessed 2023 Jan 17).

THE STRUCTURE OF THE SKIN

CHAPTER 39
COMMON SKIN CONDITIONS

BACKGROUND

Patients in the community setting often ask pharmacists for recommendations for skin conditions. A pharmacist should be able to recognize certain skin conditions, such as a blemish that could be skin cancer (see the Oncology chapter) or the discoloration of skin and secretions caused by certain medications (see Study Tip Gal below). If recommending OTC treatment, the patient should be counseled to seek further help if the condition does not improve or worsens.

SELECT DRUGS THAT CAN DISCOLOR SKIN AND SECRETIONS

BROWN
Entacapone
Levodopa
Methyldopa

BROWN/YELLOW
Nitrofurantoin

BLACK/GREEN
Iron (black stool)

ORANGE/YELLOW
Sulfasalazine

YELLOW-GREEN
Propofol

RED-ORANGE
Phenazopyridine
Rifampin

RED
Anthracyclines

BLUE
Methylene blue
Mitoxantrone

BLUE-GRAY
Amiodarone

NATURAL PRODUCTS

Several natural products are frequently used to treat or prevent skin conditions. Aloe is a natural product produced from the aloe vera plant that is used for many skin conditions, including sunburn and psoriasis; it may provide a soothing effect when used as a gel or lotion. Tea tree oil is used for a variety of skin conditions, such as acne. It may be helpful for onychomycosis (depending on the dose and application schedule) but will not eradicate the infection in most patients. Oral or topical lysine is used for cold sore (herpes simplex labialis) prevention and treatment. Biotin is a vitamin used for hair loss and brittle nails. Topical vitamin D is used in skin conditions, such as diaper rash and psoriasis.

ACNE VULGARIS

Most people develop acne vulgaris (commonly known as acne) at some point in their life, but it primarily develops in adolescents during puberty. Androgen (male sex hormone) activity is the primary determinant of acne; the presence of bacteria (e.g., *Cutibacterium acnes*) and sebum in oil (sebaceous) glands also contribute. Acne mainly appears on the face, chest, shoulders and back. Diets with a high glycemic index or dairy can worsen acne.

Acne lesions are classified as whiteheads (closed comedones), blackheads (open comedones), papules, pustules and nodules (sometimes called "cysts"). Treatment is determined by severity: mild (few, occasional pimples), moderate (inflammatory papules) or severe (nodules). Acne is primarily treated with OTC benzoyl peroxide and salicylic acid, retinoids, topical or systemic (oral) antibiotics and systemic isotretinoin (see Study Tip Gal on the following page).

- Benzoyl peroxide (BPO) is an effective OTC medication and is recommended for most patients with acne. It is also available by prescription, including in combinations with hydrocortisone, adapalene or antibiotics (e.g., erythromycin, clindamycin).

- Salicylic acid is available OTC in several different formulations, including washes, "medicated pads" and lotions.

- Retinoids (e.g., topical tretinoin) are vitamin A derivatives that primarily work by reducing cohesion (i.e., stickiness) of follicular epithelial cells, increasing epithelial cell turnover and unblocking pores to prevent acne. They are also used to reduce wrinkles. Most are available by prescription only for treating acne; adapalene (*Differin gel 0.1%*) is the only retinoid available OTC.

  - Retinoids are teratogenic. They must be avoided in pregnancy or breastfeeding (see Drug Use in Pregnancy and Lactation chapter).

  - They are well-tolerated when used topically; mild skin irritation (redness, drying) and photosensitivity can occur. Retinoids should be applied nightly, using a pea-sized amount. This can be decreased to every other night if irritation occurs. A moisturizer, followed by sunscreen, should be used each morning.

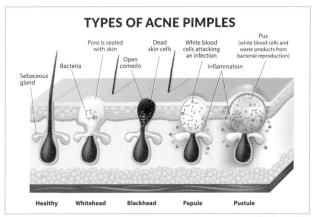

TYPES OF ACNE PIMPLES

Healthy Whitehead Blackhead Papule Pustule

iStock.com/ttsz

- Retinoids take 4 – 12 weeks to work, and acne can worsen initially. Minocycline can be used with topical retinoids to help reduce worsening. Tazarotene often works better than tretinoin; it is used for difficult cases.

- The oral retinoid isotretinoin has many safety considerations. Isotretinoin is FDA-approved for severe, recalcitrant nodular acne only, though it is also used off-label for moderate, treatment-resistant acne. Pregnancy, lipid and liver function tests are required (as part of its iPLEDGE REMS program).

- Some women find benefit with oral contraceptive pills, especially if the acne occurs around the menstrual cycle or if irregular menstruation or symptoms of excess androgen are present.

- Spironolactone is an aldosterone receptor antagonist with antiandrogen effects. It is not FDA-approved for acne but is recommended as a useful treatment for some females.

- Azelaic acid (*Azelex, Finacea*) is a topical dicarboxylic acid available OTC and by prescription as a cream, foam or gel for acne and rosacea.

- Clascoterone (*Winlevi*) is a topical androgen receptor inhibitor cream. It can be used as an alternative for the treatment of mild acne in patients age 12 and older.

ACNE TREATMENT SUMMARY

Acne treatment is determined by acne severity and success of past treatments.

	MILD	MODERATE	SEVERE
FIRST-LINE TREATMENT	Topicals: BPO or retinoid or Topicals: combination*	Topicals: combination* or PO antibiotic + BPO + topical retinoid (+/– topical antibiotic)	Topicals: combination* + PO antibiotic or PO isotretinoin
ALTERNATIVE TREATMENT	Add topical retinoid or BPO, switch to another retinoid or topical dapsone	Other combination*, switch PO antibiotic, add combined OCP or spironolactone (females) or PO isotretinoin	Switch PO antibiotic, add combined OCP or spironolactone (females) or PO isotretinoin (if not previously tried)

Topical combination therapy includes the following: BPO + topical antibiotic, BPO + retinoid or BPO + retinoid + topical antibiotic.

DRUGS	NOTES	SAFETY/COUNSELING
Topical Retinoids		
Tretinoin (Atralin, Renova, Retin-A, Retin-A Micro, Altreno, *Avita*) Rx: cream, gel, lotion Clindamycin/tretinoin gel (*Veltin, Ziana*) Tretinoin/BPO cream (*Twyneo*) **Adapalene (Differin)** OTC: gel (*Differin* gel 0.1%) Rx: adapalene/BPO gel (*Epiduo, Epiduo Forte*) Tazarotene Rx: cream (*Tazorac*), foam (*Fabior*), gel (*Tazorac*), lotion (*Arazlo*) Halobetasol/tazarotene lotion (*Duobrii*) Trifarotene Rx: cream (*Aklief*)	Topical retinoids should be avoided in pregnancy *Retin-A Micro* (microsphere gel) and *Avita* (polymerized cream or gel): slower release, less skin irritation Tazarotene: contraindicated in pregnancy, lotion (*Arazlo*) is approved in individuals aged 9 years and older *Altreno:* 0.05% lotion form of tretinoin, less irritating *Fabior:* stronger, more irritating	Limit sun exposure. Apply daily, usually at bedtime, about 20 minutes after washing face. If irritation occurs, use lower strength or decrease frequency to every other night. May need to reduce contact initially (wash off if skin is irritated). A pea-sized amount is sufficient (for facial application); it should be smoothed over the entire surface of the face, not just on acne. Avoid salicylic acid scrubs or astringents; will worsen irritation. Wash only with mild soap twice daily. Takes 4-12 weeks to see response; may worsen acne initially.
Other Topical Acne Products		
Benzoyl peroxide (BPO) OTC: many products including *Benzac, Clearasil, PanOxyl* Rx: BPO/hydrocortisone (*Vanoxide-HC*)	Start with 2.5-5% BPO, generally adequate and less irritating than the higher strengths	Can bleach clothing and hair. Limit sun exposure.
TOPICAL ANTIBIOTICS AND COMBINATIONS (All available as Rx only) Erythromycin/BPO (*Benzamycin*) Clindamycin/BPO (*BenzaClin, Acanya, Neuac, Onexton*) Minocycline foam (*Amzeeq*) **OTHERS** OTC: **Salicylic acid** (*Clearasil,* and others) OTC: **Azelaic acid** lower strengths (*Paula's Choice, The Ordinary,* and others) Rx: **Azelaic acid** cream, gel, foam (*Azelex* 15%, *Finacea* 20%) Rx: Dapsone gel (*Aczone*) Rx: Clascoterone cream (*Winlevi*)	*Benzamycin* and *BenzaClin:* Add indicated amount of purified water to the vial (70% ethyl alcohol for *Benzamycin*) and immediately shake to completely dissolve medication (use additional purified water to bring level up to the mark if needed) Add the solution in the vial to the gel; stir until homogenous (1 to 1.5 minutes) Place a 3-month expiration date on the label following mixing *Benzamycin* is kept refrigerated *BenzaClin* is kept at room temp *Winlevi:* Keep refrigerated before dispensing; store at room temperature after dispensing	Clindamycin topicals: Clean face, shake (if lotion), apply a thin layer once or twice daily. Avoid contact with eyes; if contact occurs, rinse with cold water. Takes 2-6 weeks for effect and up to 12 weeks for full benefit. Minocycline topical: See oral antibiotics section (next page) Dapsone gel: Avoid in G6PD deficiency. Clascoterone: HPA axis suppression may occur during or after treatment; more likely with use over a large surface area, prolonged use, and use with occlusive dressings. Apply a thin layer twice daily after washing and drying the skin.

DRUGS	NOTES	SAFETY/COUNSELING
Oral Retinoids		
Isotretinoin (*Absorica, Amnesteem,* *Claravis, Myorisan, Zenatane*) Rx: capsules 0.5-1 mg/kg/day, divided BID with food for 15-20 weeks.	Only FDA-approved for severe, refractory nodular acne. Patients who can get pregnant must sign patient information/informed consent form about birth defects if the fetus is exposed to isotretinoin. Must have had 2 negative pregnancy tests prior to starting treatment. Do not get pregnant for 1 month before, while taking the drug, or for 1 month after the drug is stopped. Do not breastfeed or donate blood until at least 1 month has passed after the drug is stopped. Do not use with vitamin A supplements, tetracyclines, progestin-only contraceptives, St. John's wort or steroids. Must swallow capsule whole, or puncture and sprinkle on applesauce or ice cream – this may irritate the esophagus.	**BOXED WARNING** Birth defects have been documented; must not be used by patients who are pregnant or may become pregnant. Can only be dispensed by a pharmacy registered and activated with the pregnancy REMS (iPLEDGE) program. 1-month Rx at a time, fill within 7 days with yellow sticker attached. **WARNINGS** Dry skin, chapped lips, dry eyes/eye irritation (may cause difficulty wearing contact lenses), ↓ night vision (may be permanent), arthralgias, skeletal hyperostosis (calcification of ligaments that attach to the spine), osteoporosis, psychiatric issues (depression, psychosis, risk of suicide), ↑ cholesterol (TG) and BG. **Counseling:** pregnancy testing must be repeated on a monthly basis. 2 forms of birth control are required (cannot use a progestin-only pill). Carry bottled water, eye drops and lip balm.
Oral Antibiotics Used for Acne		
Minocycline (*Minocin, Solodyn,* *Minolira,* *Ximino*) Rx: capsule, tablet IR formulations: 50-100 mg PO BID; may be used by patients ≥ 8 years XR formulations: 1 mg/kg PO daily; only approved for use in patients ≥ 12 years Sarecycline (*Seysara*) Rx: tablet	Doxycycline and minocycline are more effective than tetracycline in eradicating *C. acnes*. Sulfamethoxazole/trimethoprim is also used. Erythromycin is used less commonly due to resistance. Sarecycline is a tetracycline derivative for non-nodular moderate to severe acne.	Can cause photosensitivity, rash in susceptible patients, dizziness, diarrhea, somnolence. Like other tetracyclines, can cause fetal harm if administered during pregnancy. May cause permanent discoloration in teeth if used when teeth are forming (up to 8 years of age).

COLD SORES

- Cold sores (herpes simplex labialis) are common and highly contagious. Infection is typically caused by herpes simplex virus type 1 (HSV-1), but it can be caused by HSV-2 transmitted through oral/genital sex. The virus spreads mostly with active lesions; kissing and sharing drinks can transmit the infection.

- Sore eruption is preceded by prodromal symptoms (e.g., tingling, itching, soreness). In most patients, the sore reappears in the same location; the most common site is the junction between the upper and lower lip. Sore or lesion outbreaks can be triggered by fatigue, stress, dental work and skin irritation (e.g., sun exposure, acid peels).

- The prodromal period is the optimal time to start treatment (topical or oral) to reduce blister duration. If recurrences are frequent (> 4 times/year), daily medications for chronic suppression can be used. OTC and prescription topicals can shorten the outbreak duration by up to one day. Oral (systemic) antivirals shorten the duration by up to two days.

- The natural product lysine is used commonly for cold sore prevention and treatment.

DRUGS	NOTES	SAFETY/COUNSELING
OTC **Docosanol (*Abreva*)** **Rx** **Acyclovir topical cream/ointment (*Zovirax*)** Acyclovir buccal tablets (*Sitavig*) Penciclovir topical cream (*Denavir*)	Oral antivirals are more effective (see Infectious Diseases III chapter). 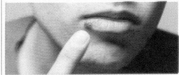 *Lolostock/Shutterstock.com*	*Abreva* cream: apply 5x daily at first sign of outbreak, continue until healed. *Zovirax* cream: apply 5x daily for 4 days (can be used on genital sores). *Sitavig* tablet: apply one 50 mg tablet as a single dose to the upper gum region. *Denavir* cream: apply every 2 hours during waking hours for 4 days.

DANDRUFF

- Seborrheic dermatitis is a common form of eczema that causes flaking, itchy skin on the face, back, chest or scalp. Dandruff is a mild form of seborrheic dermatitis that involves the scalp, causing white, itchy flakes of dead skin cells in the hair. These flakes can fall on the shoulders, back or clothing.

- Dandruff can be due to either eczema or fungal (yeast) overgrowth, and is worsened by hormones, the weather or shampoo.

- An inexpensive OTC dandruff shampoo can be tried first. If this is ineffective, ketoconazole antifungal shampoo can be used.

DRUGS	NOTES	SAFETY/COUNSELING
OTC **Ketoconazole 1% shampoo (Nizoral A-D), selenium sulfide (Selsun*, Dandrex), pyrithione zinc (Head & Shoulders), coal tar shampoos (T/Gel),** Suave or store brand "dandruff" shampoos **Rx** **Ketoconazole 2% shampoo (Nizoral*)** Ketoconazole topical comes in many formulations for dandruff or seborrheic dermatitis (see notes above): cream, foam, gel & shampoo	 *lovemydesigns/Shutterstock.com*	Rub shampoo in well, leave in for 5 minutes, then rinse out. Shampoo daily. If the shampoo stops working, switch products. **Nizoral A-D** Apply twice weekly, for up to 8 weeks. Do not use if open sores on scalp. Can cause skin irritation.

*Brand discontinued but name still used in practice.

ALOPECIA (HAIR LOSS)

Hair tends to gradually thin as part of the natural aging process. Other causes of hair loss include hormonal changes, medical conditions and medications.

- The most common cause of hair loss is hereditary male-pattern baldness, and less commonly, female-pattern baldness.

- Hormonal changes in women that can result in hair loss are usually associated with pregnancy, childbirth or menopause.

- Some medical conditions that can cause hair loss include hypothyroidism, scalp infections and some autoimmune conditions (e.g., lupus, alopecia areata).

- Chemotherapeutics frequently cause alopecia due to their cytotoxic effects on rapidly dividing cells, such as hair cells. Other drugs that can cause alopecia include valproate, lamotrigine, tacrolimus, heparin, interferons and some oral contraceptives.

- Biotin, zinc, selenium and vitamin D deficiency can contribute to hair loss.

- Medications work modestly for hair loss; many people will seek cosmetic solutions or surgical intervention (e.g., hair transplantation).

DRUGS	NOTES	SAFETY/COUNSELING
Finasteride (Propecia) Rx: tablet 1 mg daily; can take ≥ 3 months to begin to see effect **Finasteride (Proscar)** is a 5-alpha reductase type 2 inhibitor approved for BPH	Must be used indefinitely or condition reappears Do not dispense to patients taking finasteride (Proscar) for BPH	**CONTRAINDICATION** Pregnancy **WARNING** Hazardous drug for females of childbearing potential, can harm a male fetus **SIDE EFFECTS** Lower dose than Proscar; lower risk of sexual side effects; see the Benign Prostatic Hyperplasia (BPH) chapter for further details
Baricitinib (Olumiant) Rx: tablet	Janus kinase inhibitor approved for severe alopecia areata Treatment may need to be continued to maintain improvement	**BOXED WARNINGS** Serious infections (e.g., herpes zoster) and higher rates of malignancy, thrombosis, major cardiovascular events and mortality

DRUGS	NOTES	SAFETY/COUNSELING
Minoxidil topical (*Rogaine,* others) OTC: 5% foam, 2% and 5% solution Minoxidil tablets (Rx) <u>indicated for hypertension</u> (very rarely used)	5% strength is more effective but causes more facial hair growth Must be used indefinitely or condition reoccurs	Flammable; do not use near a heat source Can be used by males or females
Bimatoprost (*Latisse*) Rx: solution <u>For thinning eyelashes (hypotrichosis)</u> *iStock.com/Marina79*	<u>Do not use with prostaglandin analogs</u> used for <u>glaucoma (IOP may increase)</u>	May cause itchy eyes and/or eye redness. Eyelid skin darkening may occur, may be reversible. Hair growth may occur in other skin areas that the solution frequently touches. <u>Apply nightly</u>, with applicator brush, to the <u>skin at the base</u> of the <u>upper eyelashes</u> only (do not apply to the lower lid). Blot any excess. Repeat on other eye. Dispose of applicator after one use. If stopped, lashes will return to their previous appearance.

ECZEMA (ATOPIC DERMATITIS)

Eczema is a general term for many types of skin inflammation and is used interchangeably with the term atopic dermatitis.

- Eczema is most common in young children and infants but can occur at any age.
- Eczema appears as <u>itchy, red, dry skin rashes</u> and may turn into <u>crusty, scaly</u> sores.
- Common sites affected include the elbows, behind the knees/ears, face (often the cheeks), buttocks, hands and feet.
- Patients should avoid triggers such as environmental irritants, allergens (e.g., soaps, perfumes), stress or weather changes.

- <u>Hydration and moisturizers</u> reduce disease severity. Prescription or OTC <u>antihistamines</u> may help reduce itching.
- Treatment can include <u>topical steroids (occasional oral courses</u>, if needed) or topical <u>calcineurin inhibitors</u>.
- Topical phosphodiesterase-4 inhibitors [crisaborole (*Eucrisa*)] and topical Janus kinase inhibitors [ruxolitinib (*Opzelura*)] are options for mild to moderate cases.
- In severe, refractory cases, monoclonal antibodies such as dupilumab (*Dupixent*), oral immunosuppressants (e.g., cyclosporine, methotrexate) or oral Janus kinase inhibitors [e.g., abrocitinib (*Cibinqo*)] may be used. Other systemic immunosuppressants may be used off-label (see the Systemic Steroids & Autoimmune Conditions chapter).

DRUGS	NOTES	SAFETY/COUNSELING
OTC Moisturizers with petrolatum, lanolin (*Aquaphor*, *Eucerin*, *Keri* or store brands) **Rx** **Topical steroids** See "Inflammation and Rash" and "Potencies of Topical Steroids" sections in this chapter. **Topical calcineurin inhibitors** Tacrolimus (*Protopic*) – ointment Pimecrolimus (*Elidel*) – cream Other treatments: **Topical phosphodiesterase-4 inhibitor** Crisaborole (*Eucrisa*) – 2% ointment **Monoclonal antibodies (interleukin receptor antagonists)** Dupilumab (*Dupixent*) – SC injection Tralokinumab (*Adbry*) – SC injection **Janus kinase inhibitors** Abrocitinib (*Cibinqo*) – oral tablet Upadacitinib (*Rinvoq*) – oral tablet Ruxolitinib (*Opzelura*) – cream	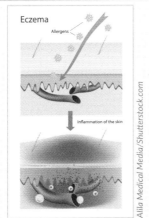 Eczema Allergens Inflammation of the skin *Alila Medical Media/Shutterstock.com*	**All topical products:** <u>Wash hands after application</u> Apply a thin layer only to the affected skin twice a day Use the smallest amount needed to control symptoms **Topical calcineurin inhibitors:** <u>Do not use in children < 2 years of age; associated with lymphoma and skin cancer</u> Avoid exposure to natural or artificial sunlight Side effects can include headache, skin burning, itching, cough and flu-like symptoms **Monoclonal antibodies:** Avoid use of live vaccines Injection site reactions and upper respiratory tract infections are common side effects **Janus kinase inhibitors:** Boxed warnings include serious <u>infections</u> (e.g., herpes zoster) and higher rates of <u>malignancy, thrombosis</u>, major cardiovascular events and mortality

HYPERHIDROSIS

Hyperhidrosis is excessive sweating; it is diagnosed based on a physical exam and history of symptoms. Treatment depends on where the excessive sweating occurs on the body (e.g., underarms, hands, feet).

DRUGS	NOTES	SAFETY/COUNSELING
Rx Glycopyrronium topical *(Qbrexza)* **OTC** Antiperspirants *(Secret Clinical Strength, Certain Dri and others)*	*Qbrexza* is a topical anticholinergic.	**Glycopyrronium topical *(Qbrexza)*:** Do not use in medical conditions that can be exacerbated by anticholinergics (e.g., glaucoma, ulcerative colitis, myasthenia gravis). Use on clean, dry skin; use one premoistened pad for both underarms. Wash hands with soap and water afterward.

FUNGAL INFECTIONS: SKIN

Tinea pedis, cruris, corporis and topical *Candida* infections are covered in this section. For vaginal infections, onychomycosis and diaper rash, see separate sections in this chapter.

ATHLETE'S FOOT *(TINEA PEDIS)*

- A fungal infection of the foot caused by various fungi (commonly *trichophyton rubrum*).

- Symptoms include feet itching, peeling, redness, mild burning and sometimes sores. This is a common infection, particularly among those using public pools, showers and locker rooms.

- Diagnosis is usually based on nonspecific symptoms, such as itching. If the diagnosis is unclear, skin cells can be scraped off and viewed under a microscope as confirmation.

- Treated topically with antifungals, except in severe cases.

JOCK ITCH *(TINEA CRURIS)*

- Affects the genitals, inner thighs and buttocks.

- The rash is red, itchy and can be ring-shaped.

- Jock itch is not very contagious but can be spread person-to-person with close contact.

- Keep the skin dry (use a clean towel after showering) and treat with a topical antifungal. Creams work best.

- Change underwear at least daily.

RINGWORM *(TINEA CORPORIS)*

- Not a worm, but a fungal skin infection.

- Ringworm can appear anywhere on the body and typically looks like circular, red, flat sores (one or more, may overlap), usually with dry, scaly skin. Occasionally the ring-like presentation is not present – just itchy, red skin. The outer part of the sore is raised while the skin in the middle appears normal.

- Can spread person-to-person or by contact with infected animals.

- Most cases are treated topically.

- *Tinea capitis* is "ringworm" on the scalp. This affects primarily young children, mostly in crowded, lower-income situations and requires systemic therapy, with the same drugs used for onychomycosis.

CUTANEOUS (SKIN) *CANDIDA* INFECTIONS

- Topical *Candida* infections cause red, itchy rashes, most commonly in the groin, armpits or anywhere the skin folds. The infection can be in unusual places, such as under the breasts, if the skin is moist.

- More likely in patients with obesity because they often have more skin folds. Diabetes is another risk factor.

- Fungal infections can occasionally appear on the skin next to a fingernail. For a suspected bacterial infection in this area, OTC antibiotic topicals or mupirocin can be used.

- *Candida* can cause diaper rash in infants (see Diaper Rash section).

FUNGAL TREATMENTS FOR THE SKIN

DRUGS	NOTES	SAFETY/COUNSELING
OTC **Terbinafine (Lamisil AT)** Cream, gel, spray **Butenafine (Lotrimin Ultra)** Cream **Clotrimazole (Lotrimin AF,** Pro-Ex Antifungal, Shopko Athletes Foot) Cream **Miconazole (Lotrimin AF,** Cruex, Desenex Jock Itch) Powder, spray Miconazole/petrolatum (Baza) – for moisture barrier, used in geriatrics **Tolnaftate (Tinactin)** Cream, powder, spray **Undecylenic acid** (Toelieva, others) **Rx** **Betamethasone/Clotrimazole (Lotrisone):** for tinea with inflammation/itching Cream, lotion **Ketoconazole** (Extina) Cream, foam Luliconazole (Luzu) 1% cream	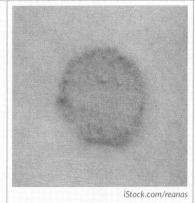 *iStock.com/reanas* *Tinea corporis* (ringworm) – the name "ringworm" is a misnomer; this is a fungal infection. The rings can be single or overlap. Topical antifungals come in creams, ointments, gels and solutions.	If infection is on the foot, do not walk barefoot (to avoid spreading it); wear sandals in public showers (to avoid catching it). Apply medication 1-2 inches beyond the rash. Use for at least 2-4 weeks, even if it appears healed. Reduce moisture to the infected area. Creams work best and are used in most cases. Solutions can be easier to apply in hairy areas. Powders do not work well for treatment but may be used for prevention, such as in shoes after a gym workout; use cotton socks. Note the same name in OTC products (Lotrimin AF) can refer to different active ingredients; be careful with recommendations to avoid mix-ups.

FUNGAL INFECTIONS: TOENAIL & FINGERNAIL

- Onychomycosis, a fungal infection of the nail often caused by *tinea unguium,* can cause pain, discomfort, nail disfigurement and physical limitations (e.g., difficulty standing, walking).

- Topical drugs are limited to mild cases and patients who cannot tolerate systemic therapies; they are not potent enough to cure most infections.

- Itraconazole and terbinafine are indicated and commonly used to treat fungal nail infections; fluconazole and posaconazole are used off-label. Griseofulvin is rarely used.

- It takes a long time for the nail bed appearance to improve – sometimes up to a year in toenails. Toenails take longer to treat than fingernails and are more commonly infected.

- Pulse therapy (intermittent) can be used to reduce costs and possibly toxicity but may not be as effective.

- A 20% potassium hydroxide (KOH) smear is essential for diagnosis as other conditions can produce a similar presentation.

DRUGS	NOTES	SAFETY/COUNSELING
Rx **Terbinafine** – oral (topical is *Lamisil AT*; used for fungal skin infections) 250 mg PO daily for 6 weeks (fingernail) or 12 weeks (toenail) Itraconazole (*Sporanox*) – oral 200 mg PO daily x 12 weeks or "pulse-dosing" (fingernails only): 200 mg BID x 1 week, 3 weeks off then repeat 1-week course Ciclopirox (*Loprox*) – topical, used QHS Tavaborole (*Kerydin*) – topical oxaborole antifungal Efinaconazole (*Jublia*) – topical azole antifungal	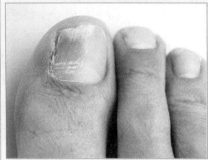 iStock.com/Manuel-F-O Ciclopirox is used in combination with orals; poor efficacy when used alone Tavaborole and efinaconazole are applied topically x 48 weeks	Systemic drugs used for nail fungal infections are hepatotoxic (monitor LFTs), QT-prolonging (avoid in QT risk) and CYP450 3A4 substrates and inhibitors (see Infectious Diseases III chapter for systemic azoles). Nausea and diarrhea are common. Itraconazole: boxed warning to avoid use in heart failure. Requires gastric acid for absorption; cannot use with strong acid-suppressing drugs. Terbinafine (oral): primary side effects include headache, rash, nausea and risk of hepatotoxicity. Recurrence is common. Practice proper foot care and keep the nails dry. Keep blood glucose controlled. Do not smoke.

FUNGAL INFECTIONS: VAGINAL

Vaginal fungal infections are common. Approximately 75% of women will have at least one episode, and half of these women will have recurrence; a small percentage of women have chronic infections. Hormones affect the pH of the vagina, making menstruating women more susceptible. Treatment decisions around menstruation are important, as infections occur most commonly during the week before menstruation. Women can begin treatment during or after menstruation. Tampons should not be used with vaginally inserted medications.

- Vaginal fungal infections are more common during pregnancy. Pregnant patients should consult their physician. Longer treatment courses (i.e., 7 – 10 days) are required.
- Symptoms primarily include itching with possible soreness and pain (burning) during urination or sex. Some women have a cottage-cheese like discharge (white, thick, clumpy).
- Diagnosis can be confirmed with a vaginal culture to check for fungal growth, while a pH test can be used to help rule out other conditions. A pH > 4.5 is consistent with bacterial vaginosis or trichomoniasis infection.
  - ❏ OTC test kits are available to test vaginal pH.
- Testing is not necessary if the woman has been seen by a physician for the initial infection and is able to recognize the symptoms. Self-treatment with OTC products is appropriate.
- If there are more than four infections in a year, or if symptoms recur within two months, refer to the physician to rule out any causative underlying conditions (e.g., diabetes, HIV, pregnancy, irritation from repeated douching or use of lubricants).

- Women taking high-dose estrogen, hormone replacement therapy, steroids, other immune-suppressing drugs or antibiotics are at elevated risk. Antibiotic use can kill the normal flora and lead to fungal overgrowth.
- Lactobacillus or yogurt with active cultures is thought to reduce infection occurrence; however, this is rated as "possibly ineffective" by the *Natural Medicines Database*.
- If self-treating, counsel that the creams and suppositories are oil-based medications that can weaken latex condoms and diaphragms and will not provide adequate pregnancy protection. Patients should avoid sexual intercourse during treatment.
- Patients can take the following steps to reduce their risk of future infections:
  - ❏ Keep the vaginal area clean
  - ❏ Wipe from front to back after using the restroom
  - ❏ Use cotton underwear and avoid tight-fitting clothing
  - ❏ Change pads/tampons often
  - ❏ Remove wet swimsuits or clothing promptly
  - ❏ Avoid using vaginal douches, sprays or other products that can alter vaginal pH

DRUGS	NOTES	SAFETY/COUNSELING
Mild-moderate, infrequent infection: 1, 3 or 7 day treatment with vaginal cream, ointment or vaginal suppository/tab **OTC, topical** **Clotrimazole** **Miconazole (_Monistat 3_, others)** **Rx, topical** **Butoconazole (_Gynazole-1_, others)** Terconazole **Rx, oral** **Fluconazole (_Diflucan_)** 150 mg PO x 1 Ibrexafungerp (_Brexafemme_) 300 mg PO BID x 1 day Complicated infections, pregnancy: 7–10 days treatment, or refer to healthcare provider **Recurrent vulvovaginal candidiasis:** Oteseconazole (_Vivjoa_) - indicated for prevention of infection in females (not of reproductive potential)	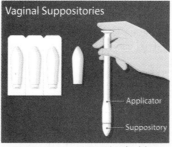 Vaginal Suppositories — Applicator — Suppository _rumruay/stock.adobe.com_ Always counsel on ways to avoid future infections (see previous text) A male sexual partner can be tested if female partner's infections are recurrent (not common)	**Counseling for OTC antifungals:** Prior to using the product, wash the external genital area with mild soap and water, and pat dry with a towel. Insert applicator, suppository or vaginal tab at night before bed. Lying down immediately after insertion helps retain the medicine inside the vagina; a protective pad can be used. The creams and suppositories are oil-based medications that can weaken latex condoms and diaphragms; avoid sexual intercourse. If you get your menstrual cycle during treatment, you may continue the treatment. Do not use tampons during treatment. Complete entire course of treatment. Medical care is warranted if symptoms persist/return within 2 months after using an OTC product, or if > 4/year.

DIAPER RASH

Diaper rash is very common in infants and toddlers. Their skin is sensitive, and when exposed to urine, stools and friction from a diaper moving back and forth, a rash appears. Once the skin is damaged, it is susceptible to bacteria and yeast overgrowth.

Prevention
- Change diapers often; do not cover diapers with plastic.
- Clean the area well with unscented wipes or plain water.
- Leave the diaper off, when possible, to let the skin air-dry.
- Use a skin protectant:
  - ❏ Petrolatum ointment (_A & D Ointment_, store brands) is a good preventative ointment containing vitamins A & D.
  - ❏ Petrolatum with zinc oxide (a desiccant, used to dry out the skin) may be preferable for babies prone to rash.

Treatment
- Clotrimazole, miconazole, nystatin: for stubborn rashes, if yeast is thought to be involved.
- Hydrocortisone 0.5 – 1% cream can be applied twice a day, but not for more than several days at a time. Hydrocortisone can be used in combination with topical antifungals.

DRUGS	SAFETY/COUNSELING
OTC **Petrolatum/zinc oxide (_Desitin_, _Boudreaux's Butt Paste_, _Triple Paste_)** Petrolatum (_A&D Ointment_, others) **Rx** Miconazole/zinc oxide/petrolatum (_Vusion_)	Infants should be referred to the physician (especially if under 6 months); refer toddlers if condition appears serious or worsens. Diaper rashes can have more than one contributing organism. Topical antibiotics can be needed if bacterial involvement is suspected. Topical antifungals can be needed if fungal involvement is suspected. Low-potency topical steroids may be used short-term.

HEMORRHOIDS

Hemorrhoids are swollen blood vessels in the lower rectum. They are often the result of constipation and straining during a bowel movement. Rectal tissue is sensitive and has a rich blood vessel supply, making it susceptible to swelling or engorgement. Common symptoms include pruritus, burning and rectal bleeding with <u>bright red blood</u>.

- If dietary fiber intake is low, <u>increasing fiber intake can help reduce straining</u>. Soluble fiber products such as <u>psyllium</u> absorb water in the intestine and promote peristalsis, making the stool easier to pass. A stool softener (such as docusate) can help reduce straining.

- Phenylephrine (*Preparation H*, others) is a <u>vasoconstrictor</u> that <u>shrinks the hemorrhoid</u> and <u>reduces burning and itching</u>.

- Hydrocortisone (*Anusol-HC, Preparation H*, others) comes in anal suppositories and various topicals, including creams and wipes. These reduce itching and inflammation.

- Witch hazel *(Tucks Medicated Cooling Pads)* is a mild astringent that can relieve mild itching.

- Barriers (skin protectants) to reduce irritation from stool/urine are helpful in some cases (petrolatum, others – see Diaper Rash section).

- There are many combination products. Some contain mineral oil (skin protectant), zinc oxide (desiccant) or pramoxine (anesthetic).

DRUGS	NOTES	SAFETY/COUNSELING
OTC **Phenylephrine topical** *(Preparation H*, others)	Recommend suppositories for internal hemorrhoids and topical creams/ointments/wipes for external symptoms.	Clean the skin first with mild soap and warm water. Gently pat dry. Apply ointment externally up to 5 times daily. For suppository: hold wrapped suppository container with rounded end up, separate the foil tabs and slowly peel apart, remove from the wrapper, insert into the rectum up to 4 times daily, especially at night and after bowel movements.

PINWORM (VERMICULARIS)

Pinworm infection most commonly occurs in <u>children</u> and <u>presents as anal itching</u>. Anthelmintics (i.e., drugs used to kill parasitic worms), such as mebendazole, <u>pyrantel pamoate</u> and albendazole, are active against *Enterobius vermicularis*. The "tape" test is used to <u>identify eggs: stick a piece of tape around the anus in the morning</u> prior to voiding/defecating. The tape is removed and brought to a healthcare provider, who examines it under a microscope to look for eggs. It <u>can take up to three tape tests to identify</u> the eggs. Pinworms are often resistant to treatment; reinfection is common. Wash hands frequently and treat the entire household.

DRUGS	NOTES	SAFETY/COUNSELING
OTC **Pyrantel pamoate** *(Reese's Pinworm Medicine)* Suspension **Rx** (systemic worm infections, many types) Albendazole Mebendazole *(Emverm)*		Pyrantel causes headaches and dizziness. It is given as a single dose and repeated in 2 weeks to eliminate reinfection. Mebendazole and albendazole cause <u>headache, nausea</u> and are <u>hepatotoxic</u>. Treatments for <u>systemic worm infections</u> are toxic. In some cases, such as treating CNS infections, <u>steroids and antiseizure medications</u> will be given with the anthelmintic. When treating systemic infections, albendazole must be taken with a <u>high-fat</u> meal (to increase absorption).

LICE AND SCABIES

Scabies (mites) and lice are spread mainly through close body contact and treated with some of the same medications. For example, permethrin can be used to treat either of these conditions, though the concentrations and formulations are different. Permethrin cream 5% is used to treat scabies, while permethrin lotion 1% (Nix) is available OTC and is used to treat lice. Nix can also be purchased in shampoo and spray formulations. Topical ivermectin (Sklice) is approved to treat head lice and is available without a prescription. Oral ivermectin (Stromectol) can be used in patients who weigh at least 15 kg, though use is off-label for both conditions, and it can be difficult to tolerate. Possible adverse effects of oral ivermectin include lymph node enlargement, arthralgias, skin tenderness, pruritus and fever.

- Lice, *Pediculus humanus capitis*, occurs most commonly in elementary school-age children.

- Topical OTC drugs are generally first-line, such as pyrethrins and permethrin, though the efficacy of pyrethrins has decreased due to resistance. Avoid these products with a chrysanthemum or ragweed allergy.

- Malathion lotion 0.5% (Ovide) is an organophosphate only for use on persons 6 years of age and older. It can cause skin irritation and is flammable; do not smoke or use electrical heat sources (e.g., hair dryers, heated curlers, flat irons) near hair that is saturated with malathion.

- Lindane shampoo 1% is no longer available; it was removed from the market due to neurotoxicity.

- If the same medication has been used several times, it may be ineffective, and a different medication should be used.

- Repeating the procedure and removing the nits (louse eggs) from hair, bedding and elsewhere is essential:

  - Wash clothes and bedding in hot water, followed by a hot dryer.

  - If something cannot be washed, seal it in an air-proof bag for two weeks or dry clean. Vacuum the carpet well. Soak combs and brushes in hot water for 10 minutes. Make sure to check other family members in the household.

  - Do not use conditioner (including combination shampoo + conditioner) before using lice medicine. Do not re-wash the hair for 1 – 2 days after treatment.

  - Most products must be left on the hair for 10 minutes before rinsing to be effective; malathion should be left on for 8 – 12 hours.

  - After treatment, use a nit comb to remove nits and lice every 2 – 3 days. Continue to check for 2 – 3 weeks to be sure all lice and nits are gone.

  - Most products, except for *Sklice*, require re-treatment on days 7 – 10 to kill any surviving hatched lice before they produce new eggs. Check the product package since timing of re-treatment can vary.

DRUGS	NOTES	SAFETY/COUNSELING
LICE **OTC** **Permethrin 1% lotion (Nix)**, ages 2 + months **Pyrethrin/Piperonyl butoxide (RID**, LiceMD), ages 2 + years Ivermectin lotion (Sklice), ages 6 + months **Rx** Spinosad (Natroba), ages 6 + months Malathion lotion (Ovide), ages 6 + years **SCABIES** **Rx** Permethrin 5% cream Ivermectin oral (Stromectol)	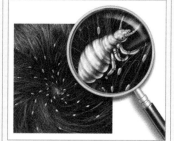 iStock.com/wildpixel	Drug of choice for lice: OTC topical treatment such as permethrin or pyrethrin/piperonyl butoxide. Repeat treatment on day 9. Malathion: flammable, do not use near heat source or open flame. Spinosad: works well, expensive. In addition to OTC treatment, remove the live lice and nits by inspecting the hair in 1-inch segments and using a lice comb. Nits are "cemented" to the hair shaft and do not fall off after treatment. Many OTC products require removal of live lice and nits for maximum efficacy. Nit removal requires multiple efforts, which should be continued for at least 2 weeks after treatment. See above.

MINOR WOUNDS

Minor wounds include cuts, abrasions, bites and burns. Some can be effectively treated with simple first aid, while others, depending on the severity, may need more medical attention than first aid can provide. Puncture wounds should be referred to a medical provider. Make sure tetanus vaccine is current (booster every 10 years, after series has been completed). If the wound is dirty, a repeat tetanus vaccine may be required if it is > 5 years since vaccination.

Some chronic wounds (e.g., pressure ulcers) require management by wound care providers. Debridement of chronic wounds is often needed to remove the damaged or contaminated tissue since it can prevent healing. There are several methods of debridement, but the most common method is enzymatic debridement, which is done with the application of collagenase ointment (Santyl). Other debridement methods, including surgical debridement, are used for more complicated wounds.

CUTS, LACERATIONS AND ABRASIONS

- Lacerations are irregular wounds with ragged edges, with the potential for deeper skin damage and bruising under the skin. A cut is different than a laceration because the edges will be more uniform or regular.

- After cleaning, if the bleeding does not stop, or the wound extends far below the surface layers of the skin, seek medical attention because it may require stitches to close the wound. If the wound is not deep, regular bandaging should allow it to close over time.

- Antibiotic ointment can be applied prior to bandaging.

- Tissue adhesives (e.g., *Band-Aid Liquid Bandage, Nexcare Skin Crack Care*, others) create a polymer layer, which binds to the skin; this keeps the wound clean and protected from moisture. Some contain topical analgesics.

- *Wound Seal* is a topical powder that can be used over a bleeding wound to quickly form a scab and reduce the risk of infection.

- Abrasions are minor injuries to the top layer of skin and are primarily treated with simple first aid.

- Abrasions (e.g., a skinned knee) should be cleaned thoroughly; apply antibiotic ointment and bandage if desired.

BITES

- Animal and human bites are associated with a high risk of infection; these should always be evaluated by a healthcare provider.

- Bites from certain spiders in the U.S. can be deadly, such as the brown recluse, black widow and hobo spiders. See the Toxicology & Antidotes chapter.

- Spiders tend to stay hidden and are not aggressive; bites can usually be avoided by inspecting and shaking out clothing or equipment prior to use and wearing protective clothing. If bitten, stay calm, identify the type of spider if possible, wash with soap and cold water, apply a cold compress with ice, elevate the extremity and get emergency medical care.

- Minor, harmless insect bites can be treated with a topical steroid or oral antihistamine (such as diphenhydramine) to reduce itching.

BURNS

- Burns can be characterized as:
  - ❑ First degree (red/painful, minor swelling)
  - ❑ Second degree (thicker, produces blisters, very painful)
  - ❑ Third degree (damage to all layers of skin, appears white or charred).

- Burns from chemical exposure or in immunosuppressed patients should be referred for emergency medical care.

- If the burn is first or second degree, OTC treatment is acceptable if the area is less than two inches in diameter and not located on the face, over a major joint or on the feet or genitals. In diabetes, even a mild foot burn could lead to amputation. Vigilance is required.

- Minor burns should be treated first by running the burn under cool water or soaking in cool water for 5 – 20 minutes.

- Do not apply ice as it can further damage injured skin. Bandages should be applied if the skin is broken, or if blisters pop.

- Burned skin itches as it heals. Skin that has been burned is more sensitive to the sun for up to a year.

- Ointments (e.g., *Aquaphor*) should be applied to minor burns to protect the skin, retain moisture and reduce scarring risk.

- Silver sulfadiazine (*Silvadene; SSD*) can be used topically to reduce infection risk and promote healing. If the skin is broken, systemic toxicity could occur. Do not use with sulfa allergy or G6PD deficiency (due to hemolysis risk).

DRUGS	NOTES	SAFETY/COUNSELING
OTC **Polymyxin/bacitracin/neomycin,** triple antibiotic ointment **(Neosporin Original,** store brands) For neomycin allergy, use *Polysporin* (bacitracin and polymyxin) or bacitracin alone; either is sufficient **Rx** **Mupirocin** *(Bactroban*)* is an <u>antibiotic</u> cream or ointment; <u>very good staph and strep coverage</u>, including MRSA **Bacitracin/neomycin/polymyxin B/ hydrocortisone (Cortisporin** ointment) is a popular Rx topical used for superficial skin infections Collagenase *(Santyl)* – topical debriding drug for chronic wounds	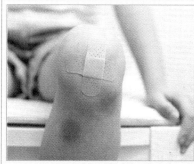 *iStock.com/DmitriMaruta* If the wound is not in an area that will get dirty or be rubbed by clothing, it does not need to be covered. Leaving a wound uncovered helps it stay dry and heal.	**Application of topical antibiotics** Clean the affected area and apply a small amount of medication (an amount equal to the surface area of the tip of a finger) to the affected area 1 to 3 times daily. If the area can get dirty (such as a hand) or be irritated by clothing, cover with an adhesive bandage (e.g., *Band-Aid*) or with sterile gauze and adhesive tape +/– antibiotic ointment. Change dressing/s daily. Burns require a moist (but not wet) environment for healing. Apply either an ointment or a bandage designed for burns.

*Brand discontinued but name still used in practice.

POISON IVY, OAK AND SUMAC

- <u>Poison ivy, oak or sumac poisoning</u> is an <u>allergic reaction</u> that results from <u>touching the sap</u> of these plants, which <u>contain the toxin urushiol</u>.
- See the image below for the appearance of each of the leaves. Poison oak and ivy are known for leaves in clusters of three.
- The sap may be on the plant, in the ashes of burned plants, on an animal or on other objects that came in contact with the plant (e.g., clothing, garden tools and sports equipment).
- Small amounts of urushiol can remain under a person's fingernails for days unless removed with good cleaning.

DRUGS	NOTES	SAFETY/COUNSELING
OTC Aluminum acetate solution *(Boro-Packs, Domeboro Soothing Soak)* Colloidal oatmeal *(Aveeno)* Calamine lotion/pramoxine (anesthetic): *(Caladryl, IvaRest)* *Zanfel* works by binding urushiol (the toxin) – low evidence for efficacy	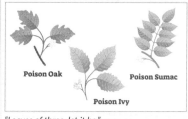 *"Leaves of three, let it be."*	Aluminum acetate is an <u>astringent</u> (drying agent). Wash the urushiol off with soap and water carefully, including under fingernails and on clothing. <u>Topical or oral steroids will help (oral needed in severe rash)</u>. Cold compresses can help.

VectorMine/stock.adobe.com

INFLAMMATION AND RASH

- The primary treatment for skin irritation is topical steroids. Two strengths of hydrocortisone (HC) are available OTC, 0.5% and 1%; all other topical steroids are prescription only.

- The steroid vehicle influences the strength of the medication. Usual potency, from highest to lowest: ointment > creams > lotions > solutions > gels > sprays.

- Thin skin on the face, eyelids and genitals is highly susceptible to topical steroid side effects; low potency steroids should be used on these areas and skin folds (e.g., armpits, groin, under the breasts) where the absorption is higher.

- Local (skin) steroid side effects, if used long-term, include skin thinning, pigment changes (lighter or darker), telangiectasia (i.e., spider veins or small blood vessels visible through the skin), rosacea, perioral dermatitis and acne, increased risk of skin infections, delayed wound healing, irritation/burning/peeling and possibly contact dermatitis.

- For urticaria (hives), second-generation antihistamines (e.g., cetirizine) are preferred over first-generation antihistamines (e.g., diphenhydramine) due to better tolerability. Higher doses are used, and the "non-sedating" antihistamines can still cause sedation at higher doses. First-generation antihistamines can be given at bedtime. See the Allergic Rhinitis, Cough & Cold chapter.

- Histamine-2 receptor antagonists (e.g., famotidine) are helpful in some patients with urticaria/hives. Hydroxyzine is often prescribed (see table).

DRUGS	NOTES	SAFETY/COUNSELING
OTC Lowest potency: **Hydrocortisone** 0.5% (infants) and 1% for mild conditions, thin skin (groin area, elderly) and for children HC 1% lotion (*Aquanil HC*) **Rx** Higher potency: see chart on the next page	Common topical steroids, ranked by potency, are included in the table on the following page. Use ointments for thick or dry skin. Ointments have low water content (reduced absorption) and form a skin barrier. See the Nonsterile Compounding chapter. Use lotions, gels and foams for hairy skin. No evidence for use of topical diphenhydramine, can use systemic but caution due to side effects. Skin should be lubricated (hydrated) with moisturizers for most conditions. Camphor, menthol, local anesthetics (often in combo creams with HC) can help relieve itching. Severe rash will likely require oral steroids for 1-2 weeks.	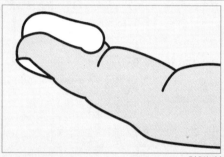 ©UWorld The "fingertip" unit is used to estimate amount: from the fingertip to the 1st joint provides enough medication to cover one adult hand (about ½ g). Encourage patient not to use more than directed as overuse has risks (see above). Do not apply for longer than 2 weeks. Apply the high-potency Rx steroids once daily. Apply OTC/lower potency steroids 1-2x daily. It is common to see a higher potency product, followed by a lower potency product, to treat acute inflammation.
Hydroxyzine (Vistaril)	Used for general urticaria (hives) with severe itching. Dose is 25 mg PO TID-QID.	Anticholinergic side effects, primarily sedation and dry mouth.

POTENCIES OF TOPICAL STEROIDS

Very High Potency

Clobetasol propionate 0.05% Lotion/Shampoo/Spray (Clobex), Cream/ Ointment (Temovate*), Foam (Olux), Gel

Fluocinonide 0.1% Cream (Vanos)

Betamethasone dipropionate 0.05% Ointment (Diprolene), Gel/Lotion

Halobetasol propionate 0.05% Lotion (Ultravate), Cream/Ointment

Diflorasone diacetate 0.05% Ointment

High Potency

Betamethasone dipropionate 0.05% Cream (Diprolene AF*)

Fluocinonide 0.05% Ointment

Mometasone furoate 0.1% Ointment

Desoximetasone 0.05% Gel (Topicort), 0.25% Cream (Topicort)

Diflorasone diacetate 0.05% Cream

Halcinonide 0.1% Cream (Halog)

High-Medium Potency

Fluocinonide 0.05% Cream

Betamethasone valerate 0.12% Foam (Luxiq)

Desoximetasone 0.05% Cream (Topicort)

Fluticasone propionate 0.005% Ointment

Medium Potency

Mometasone furoate 0.1% Lotion

Triamcinolone acetonide 0.1% Cream (Triderm), 0.147 mg/g **Spray (Kenalog)**

Fluocinolone acetonide 0.025% Cream/Ointment (Synalar)

Flurandrenolide 0.05% Ointment (Cordran)

Lower Potency

Desonide 0.05% Lotion (DesOwen)

Fluocinolone acetonide 0.01% Shampoo (Capex), 0.025% Cream (Synalar), 0.01% Cream

Flurandrenolide 0.05% Cream, Lotion/Tape (Cordran)

Fluticasone propionate 0.05% Cream/Lotion

Hydrocortisone butyrate 0.1% Cream/Lotion/Ointment/Solution (Locoid)

Hydrocortisone probutate 0.1% Cream (Pandel)

Prednicarbate 0.1% Cream

Mild Potency

Alclometasone dipropionate 0.05% Cream/Ointment

Desonide 0.05% Gel, Cream (Tridesilon), Foam (Verdeso)

Fluocinolone acetonide 0.01% Oil (Derma-Smoothe/FS), Solution (Synalar), Cream

Lowest Potency

Hydrocortisone Cream: 0.5%, **1% (Cortizone-10),** 2.5% (MiCort-HC); Lotion: 1%/2%; Ointment: 0.5%/1%/2.5%

*Brand discontinued but still used in practice.

SUNSCREENS AND SUN PROTECTION

- Applying sunscreen is important due to the risk of sun damage and skin cancer. Keep in mind that sunscreen blocks vitamin D production in the skin, and many Americans are vitamin D deficient.

- It is advisable to stay out of the sun when it is strongest (between 10AM – 4PM). The damaging ultraviolet (UV) rays penetrate clouds; this applies to overcast days as well. Another way to avoid sun exposure is to wear protective clothing.

- Sunscreen that provides UVA (A for aging – causes damage below the skin surface) and UVB (B for burning) protection should be applied to exposed skin. Both UVA and UVB contribute to skin cancer. A "broad-spectrum" sunscreen should be chosen that protects against both UVA and UVB.

- SPF stands for sun protection factor, which is a measure of how well the sunscreen deflects UVB rays.

- Some dermatologists and the American Academy of Pediatrics (AAP) recommend a minimum SPF 15 and others like the American Academy of Dermatology (AAD) recommend a minimum SPF 30. Sunscreen should be applied liberally at least every two hours and reapplied after swimming or sweating. The AAP recommends keeping babies less than 6 months old out of the sun.

TIME TO BURN (TTB)

> TTB (with sunscreen in min) = SPF x TTB (without sunscreen)

- How SPF works: if someone would normally burn in 10 minutes, an SPF of 5 would extend the time they would burn to 50 minutes (5 x 10 = 50). Regardless of the SPF and calculated TTB, sunscreens only provide skin protection for a couple of hours and need to be reapplied frequently.

- Sunscreen labeling is no longer permitted to use "waterproof" or "sweatproof" since they all wash off, at least partially, in the water. A sunscreen can claim to be "water-resistant," but only for 40 – 80 minutes. Always reapply after swimming or sweating.

- The AAD recommends chemical sunscreens with any of the following ingredients: oxybenzone, avobenzone, octisalate, octocrylene, homosalate or octinoxate.

  ❏ Oxybenzone can be irritating to the skin (uncommon).

- Physical sunscreens may be used as an alternative to chemical sunscreens. Zinc oxide and titanium dioxide are physical sunscreens recommended by the AAD.

- Products claiming to be oral sunscreens are not effective substitutes for topical sunscreen and should not be recommended.

Select Guidelines/References

Zaenglein AL, Pathy AL, Schlosser BJ, et al. Guidelines of care for the management of acne vulgaris. *J Am Acad Derm* 2016; 74:945-973.

Sidbury R, Alikhan A, Bercovitch L, et al. Guidelines of care for the management of atopic dermatitis in adults with topical therapies. *J Am Acad Derm* 2023; S0190-9622.

Nolt D, Moore S, Yan AC, et al. Committee on Infectious Diseases, Committee on Practice and Ambulatory Medicine, Section on Dermatology. Head Lice. *Pediatrics* 2022; 150(4):e2022059282.

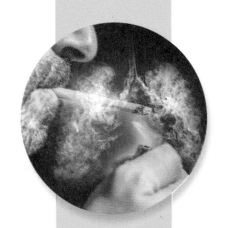
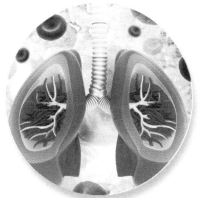
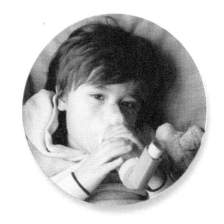

PULMONARY CONDITIONS & TOBACCO CESSATION

CONTENTS

WORLD HEALTH ORGANIZATION (WHO) CLINICAL CLASSIFICATION OF PULMONARY HYPERTENSION

Group 1: pulmonary arterial hypertension (PAH) – includes idiopathic, heritable, drug- and toxin-induced, disease-associated (e.g., connective tissue diseases, HIV infection, portal hypertension) and persistent pulmonary hypertension of a newborn

Group 2: pulmonary hypertension due to left heart disease

Group 3: pulmonary hypertension due to lung diseases and/or hypoxia

Group 4: chronic thromboembolic pulmonary hypertension (CTEPH)

Group 5: pulmonary hypertension with unclear or multifactorial mechanisms

CONTENT LEGEND

 — Key Drug Guy

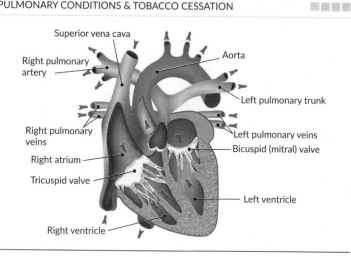

Superior vena cava · Aorta · Right pulmonary artery · Left pulmonary trunk · Right pulmonary veins · Left pulmonary veins · Right atrium · Bicuspid (mitral) valve · Tricuspid valve · Left ventricle · Right ventricle

iStock.com/ElenBushe

CHAPTER 40

PULMONARY ARTERIAL HYPERTENSION

BACKGROUND

Pulmonary hypertension (PH) is characterized by continuous high blood pressure in the pulmonary arteries. A normal pulmonary artery pressure (PAP) ranges from 8 – 20 mmHg when resting. PH is defined as a mean PAP (mPAP) ≥ 25 mmHg in the setting of normal fluid status. Other hemodynamic parameters are affected as well.

CLASSIFICATION

PH may occur secondary to various disease states. The World Health Organization (WHO) classifies PH into five groups (see the box to the left). The primary focus of this chapter is Group 1, pulmonary arterial hypertension (PAH). When there is no identifiable cause, it is called primary, or idiopathic, PAH. Secondary causes include genetic inheritance, connective tissue diseases, advanced liver disease and HIV infection. Less commonly, medications can be the causative factor (see the Key Drugs Guy on the following page).

Treatment of PH groups 2 – 5 is aimed at the underlying causes. Group 2 is pulmonary venous hypertension, which arises from left-sided heart disease (e.g., left ventricular systolic or diastolic dysfunction, valvular disease, congenital heart disease). Group 3 is PH due to hypoxia or chronic lung diseases, such as COPD, pulmonary fibrosis or emphysema. Group 4 is chronic thromboembolic PH (CTEPH), which occurs in a minority of pulmonary embolism (PE) survivors. Anticoagulation is recommended for CTEPH (i.e., warfarin, with an INR goal of 2 – 3). Group 5 is PH caused by conditions that do not fit in the above categories (e.g., sarcoidosis).

SELECT DRUGS THAT CAN CAUSE PAH

Cocaine

Fenfluramine

Methamphetamine/amphetamine

SSRI use during pregnancy [↑ risk of persistent pulmonary hypertension of a newborn (PPHN)]

Weight-loss drugs (diethylpropion, phendimetrazine, phentermine)

PATHOPHYSIOLOGY

PAH stems from an imbalance in vasoconstrictor and vasodilator substances. Vasoconstrictor substances [e.g., endothelin-1, thromboxane A2 (TXA2)] are increased, and vasodilating substances (e.g., prostacyclins) are decreased. Vasoconstriction results in reduced blood flow and high pressure within the pulmonary vasculature. In addition, there is an imbalance between cell proliferation and apoptosis (cell death) in the walls of the pulmonary arteries. The increasing amount of pulmonary artery smooth muscle cells causes pulmonary artery walls to thicken and form scar tissue (vasoproliferation).

As the walls thicken and scar, the arteries become increasingly narrower. These changes make it difficult for the right ventricle to pump blood through the pulmonary arteries and into the lungs due to the increased pressure. As a result of working harder, the right ventricle becomes enlarged, and right heart failure develops. Heart failure is the most common cause of death in people who have PAH.

Symptoms of PAH include fatigue, dyspnea, chest pain, syncope, edema, tachycardia and/or Raynaud's phenomenon. In Raynaud's, reduced blood supply causes discoloration and coldness in the fingers, toes and occasionally other areas.

There is no cure for PAH, but in the last decade, knowledge of the disease has increased significantly and many more treatment options have become available. Without treatment, life expectancy is three years. In some cases, a lung or heart-lung transplant may be an option for younger patients.

NON-DRUG TREATMENT

Patients with PAH should follow a sodium-restricted diet of ≤ 2.4 grams/day to help manage volume status, especially if they have right ventricular failure. Medications which increase sodium and water retention (e.g., NSAIDs) should

be avoided. Routine immunizations against influenza and pneumococcal pneumonia are advised. Exposure to high altitudes may contribute to hypoxic pulmonary vasoconstriction and may not be tolerated. Oxygen is used when needed to maintain oxygen saturation above 90%.

DRUG TREATMENT

A right heart catheterization is performed to confirm the diagnosis of PAH. During the right heart catheterization, short-acting vasodilators (e.g., inhaled nitric oxide, IV epoprostenol, IV adenosine) are administered for vasoreactivity testing. The response to acute vasoreactivity testing determines which vasodilator medications should be used (see the PAH Treatment Algorithm on the next page).

If testing results in the mPAP falling by at least 10 mmHg to an absolute value less than 40 mmHg, the patient is considered a responder and should be initially treated with an oral calcium channel blocker (CCB). Approximately 10% of patients are candidates for CCB therapy, though only half of these will have a sustained response. The CCBs used most frequently are long-acting nifedipine, diltiazem and amlodipine. The use of verapamil is not recommended due to its more pronounced negative inotropic effects relative to diltiazem.

Non-responders to vasoreactivity testing and positive responders who fail CCB therapy need to be treated with more potent vasodilating drugs. These include prostacyclin analogues and receptor agonists, endothelin receptor antagonists (ERAs), phosphodiesterase-5 (PDE-5) inhibitors and/or a soluble guanylate cyclase (sGC) stimulator. In most cases, drug therapy will reduce symptoms and improve exercise tolerance. Parenteral prostacyclin analogues, specifically IV epoprostenol, have been shown to decrease mortality. Some patients will require combination therapy.

Supportive therapies for PAH may include loop diuretics (for volume overload) and digoxin (to improve cardiac output or control heart rate in atrial fibrillation). Biochemical changes (↑ TXA2, ↓ prostacyclin), along with other altered pathways, lead to a pro-thrombotic state and increased risk of blood clots. The need for anticoagulation is assessed on a case-by-case basis; if used, warfarin is the preferred agent and it should be titrated to an individualized patient INR goal (e.g., 1.5 – 2.5, 2 – 3) based on thromboembolic risk and the presence of comorbid conditions (e.g., atrial fibrillation). Referral to a PAH specialty center is important to assess the feasibility of transplantation.

PAH TREATMENT ALGORITHM

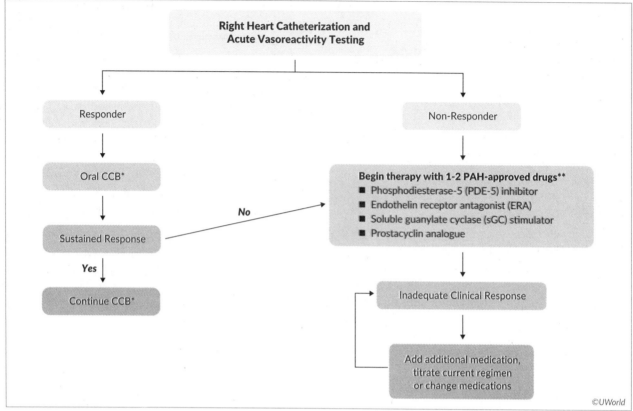

*Usually long-acting nifedipine, diltiazem or amlodipine.
**When selecting medications, consider disease severity and patient-specific factors (e.g., drug interactions, compliance, suitability for home IV therapy). For World Health Organization Functional Classification (WHO-FC) Class IV (i.e., unable to be physically active and with signs of right heart failure, which may be present at rest), first-line treatment is an IV prostacyclin analogue.*

PROSTACYCLIN ANALOGUES (OR PROSTANOIDS) AND RECEPTOR AGONISTS

Prostacyclin synthase is reduced in PAH, causing decreased production of prostacyclin I2 (a vasodilator with anti-proliferative effects) in pulmonary artery smooth muscle cells. Prostacyclin analogues (prostanoids) are potent vasodilators (of both pulmonary and systemic vascular beds) and inhibitors of platelet aggregation. The prostacyclin receptor agonist selexipag (*Uptravi*) is structurally different but works similarly. Epoprostenol and treprostinil can be administered by continuous IV infusion at home using an ambulatory infusion pump.

DRUG	DOSING	SAFETY/SIDE EFFECTS/MONITORING
Epoprostenol (Flolan, Veletri) AKA prostacyclin Continuous IV infusion via central venous catheter	Start at 2 ng/kg/min; ↑ by 1-2 ng/kg/min in 15 minute intervals based on clinical response; usual dose is 25-40 ng/kg/min (can be higher)	**CONTRAINDICATIONS** Epoprostenol: heart failure with ↓ left ventricular ejection fraction Treprostinil (oral): severe hepatic impairment (Child-Pugh Class C) **WARNINGS** Vasodilation reactions (hypotension, flushing, headache, dizziness) Rebound PH (with interruption or large decreases in dose), which can be fatal Increased risk of bleeding
Treprostinil *Remodulin:* continuous SC or IV (central venous catheter) infusion *Tyvaso:* inhalation solution and dry powder inhaler (DPI) *Orenitram:* oral, ER tablet	*Remodulin:* start at 1.25 ng/kg/min and ↑ at weekly intervals, up to 40-80 ng/kg/min (and possibly more) *Tyvaso:* start with 16 mcg (DPI) or 18 mcg (solution) 4 times/day while awake; ↑ every 1-2 weeks to target dose of 48-64 mcg per session (DPI) or 54 mcg per session (solution) *Orenitram:* start at 0.25 mg BID or 0.125 mg TID, ↑ every 3-4 days up to the maximum tolerated dose; take with food	Chronic IV infusions: sepsis and bloodstream infections (use sterile technique when preparing parenteral drug and educate patients about infusion site care) Treprostinil (*Orenitram*): oral tablet shell does not dissolve (ghost tablet) and can lodge in a diverticulum **SIDE EFFECTS** Hypotension, flushing, jaw pain, headache, dizziness, N/V/D, edema, musculoskeletal pain (e.g., myalgia), tachycardia, flu-like syndrome, anxiety, tremor, thrombocytopenia IV/SC infusions: infusion-site pain, especially with SC *Remodulin* (~85%) Treprostinil (inhaled) and iloprost: cough and mouth/throat irritation
Iloprost (*Ventavis*) Inhalation	2.5-5 mcg/inhalation given 6-9 times/day, no more than once every 2 hours	**NOTES** Parenteral agents (*Flolan, Veletri, Remodulin*) are very potent vasodilators; avoid interruptions and sudden, large dose reductions Due to the short half-lives of epoprostenol (~6 minutes) and parenteral treprostinil (~4 hours), immediate access to a backup pump, infusion sets and medication is essential
Selexipag (*Uptravi*) Tablet, IV infusion	Start with 200 mcg BID and ↑ at weekly intervals to maximum dose of 1600 mcg BID	Epoprostenol: must protect from light before reconstitution and during infusion Reconstituted solutions of *Flolan* require use of ice packs for stability; *Veletri* and *Remodulin* are thermostable (no need for ice packs)

Prostacyclin Analogue and Receptor Agonist Drug Interactions

- The effects of antihypertensive, antiplatelet and anticoagulant agents can be increased.

- Treprostinil levels are increased by CYP450 2C8 inhibitors (e.g., gemfibrozil) and decreased by CYP2C8 inducers (e.g., rifampin). Strong CYP2C8 inhibitors should be avoided with selexipag.

CASE SCENARIO

AM is a 42-year-old female (weight 85 kg) in the ICU with pulmonary arterial hypertension. At home she mixes 9.5 mL of 1 mg/mL treprostinil (*Remodulin*) with 40.5 mL of sterile water. She sets her pump to 0.06 mL/hr.

- **What is her dose in ng/kg/min? Round to the nearest tenth.**

Step 1: determine how many milligrams of treprostinil (*Remodulin*) are mixed with sterile water.

$$9.5 \text{ mL} \times \frac{1 \text{ mg}}{\text{mL}} = 9.5 \text{ mg}$$

Step 2: calculate the concentration by dividing the milligrams of treprostinil (*Remodulin*) by the total volume (drug plus diluent).

$$\frac{9.5 \text{ mg}}{(40.5 \text{ mL} + 9.5 \text{ mL})} = 0.19 \text{ mg/mL}$$

Step 3: calculate the dose in ng/kg/min using dimensional analysis.

$$\frac{\left[\dfrac{0.06 \text{ ml}}{\text{hr}} \times \dfrac{1 \text{ hr}}{60 \text{ min}} \times \dfrac{0.19 \text{ mg}}{\text{mL}} \times \dfrac{1{,}000{,}000 \text{ ng}}{1 \text{ mg}} \right]}{85 \text{ kg}} = 2.2 \text{ ng/kg/min}$$

- **The pharmacy has treprostinil (*Remodulin*) 2.5 mg/mL in stock. How many milliliters of the pharmacy stock supply should be used to prepare the same treprostinil (*Remodulin*) concentration AM uses at home?**

$$9.5 \text{ mg} \times \frac{\text{mL}}{2.5 \text{ mg}} = 3.8 \text{ mL treprostinil (Remodulin)}$$

ENDOTHELIN RECEPTOR ANTAGONISTS

Endothelin is a vasoconstrictor with cellular proliferative effects. ERAs block endothelin receptors on pulmonary artery smooth muscle cells.

DRUG	DOSING	SAFETY/SIDE EFFECTS/MONITORING
Bosentan (*Tracleer*) Tablet	< 40 kg: 62.5 mg BID ≥ 40 kg: 62.5 mg BID (for 4 weeks), then 125 mg BID	**BOXED WARNINGS** Teratogenic (women of childbearing potential must have a negative pregnancy test prior to initiation of therapy and monthly thereafter) Bosentan: hepatotoxicity (↑ ALT/AST and liver failure) Available only through individual REMS programs (Bosentan REMS Program, Ambrisentan REMS Program and *Opsumit* REMS Program); prescribers, pharmacies and patients must enroll (only female patients required to be enrolled in the Ambrisentan and *Opsumit* REMS programs)
Ambrisentan (*Letairis*) Tablet	5 mg daily, may ↑ to 10 mg daily after 4 weeks if tolerated	**CONTRAINDICATIONS** Pregnancy Bosentan: use with cyclosporine or glyburide Ambrisentan: idiopathic pulmonary fibrosis **WARNINGS** Hepatotoxicity, ↓ Hgb/Hct, fluid retention (e.g., pulmonary edema, peripheral edema), decreased sperm counts
Macitentan (*Opsumit*) Tablet	10 mg daily	Bosentan: hypersensitivity reactions (e.g., rash, angioedema, anaphylaxis, DRESS) **SIDE EFFECTS** Headache, upper respiratory tract infections (e.g., nasal congestion, cough, bronchitis), flushing, hypotension **MONITORING** LFTs, bilirubin, Hgb/Hct, pregnancy tests

Endothelin Receptor Antagonist Drug Interactions

- Bosentan is a substrate and inducer of CYP3A4 and 2C9; monitor for drug interactions. Levels of bosentan can increase with CYP2C9 (e.g., amiodarone, fluconazole) and CYP3A4 (e.g., ritonavir) inhibitors. Concurrent use of cyclosporine or glyburide is contraindicated. Bosentan can decrease the effectiveness of hormonal contraceptives (at least one barrier method of contraception, if not two, is recommended).

- Ambrisentan is a substrate of CYP3A4 (major), CYP2C19 (minor) and P-gp. Cyclosporine can increase the serum concentration of ambrisentan; limit the dose of ambrisentan to 5 mg daily when given with cyclosporine.

- Macitentan is a substrate of CYP3A4 (major) and CYP2C19 (minor). Strong CYP3A4 inhibitors and inducers should be avoided with macitentan.

PHOSPHODIESTERASE-5 INHIBITORS

PDE-5 is responsible for the degradation of cyclic guanosine monophosphate (cGMP). Increased cGMP concentrations lead to pulmonary vasculature relaxation and vasodilation.

DRUG	DOSING	SAFETY/SIDE EFFECTS/MONITORING
Sildenafil (*Revatio*, *Liqrev*) Tablet, oral suspension, injection ***Viagra*** – erectile dysfunction	IV: 10 mg TID Oral: 20 mg TID, taken 4-6 hours apart	**CONTRAINDICATIONS** Avoid use with nitrates or riociguat *Revatio*: avoid taking with protease inhibitors (e.g., atazanavir, ritonavir, others) **WARNINGS** Hearing loss (with or without tinnitus and dizziness), vision loss [rare but may be due to nonarteritic anterior ischemic optic neuropathy (NAION)], hypotension, priapism (seek emergency medical care if erection lasts > 4 hours), pulmonary edema
Tadalafil (*Adcirca*, *Alyq*, *Tadliq*) Tablet, oral suspension ***Cialis*** – erectile dysfunction, BPH	40 mg daily 20 mg daily if mild-moderate renal or hepatic impairment CrCl < 30 mL/min or severe hepatic impairment: avoid use	**SIDE EFFECTS** Headache, epistaxis, flushing, dyspepsia, extremity or back pain, N/D

PDE-5 Inhibitor Drug Interactions

- Do not give with other PDE-5 inhibitors used for erectile dysfunction.

- Do not use with nitrate medications (see Stable Angina chapter) or the sGC stimulator riociguat as the potential for excessively low blood pressure is increased. Taking nitrates is an absolute contraindication to the use of PDE-5 inhibitors.

- Use caution with concurrent use of alpha-1 blockers or other antihypertensives as PDE-5 inhibitors can increase the risk of hypotension. When tadalafil is used for PAH, alpha 1-blockers are not recommended for comorbid BPH. Alcohol can enhance hypotension with PDE-5 inhibitors.

- PDE-5 inhibitors are major substrates of CYP3A4; avoid use of strong CYP3A4 inhibitors and inducers.

SOLUBLE GUANYLATE CYCLASE STIMULATOR

Soluble guanylate cyclase (sGC) is a receptor for endogenous nitric oxide. Riociguat (*Adempas*) sensitizes sGC to endogenous nitric oxide and directly stimulates the receptor at a different binding site. This increases cGMP, leading to relaxation and antiproliferative effects in the pulmonary artery smooth muscle cells. Riociguat is approved for use in both PAH and CTEPH.

DRUG	DOSING	SAFETY/SIDE EFFECTS/MONITORING
Riociguat (*Adempas*) Tablet	Start with 0.5-1 mg TID, increasing by 0.5 mg TID every 2 weeks if SBP > 95 mmHg; max dose is 2.5 mg TID	**BOXED WARNINGS** Teratogenic (women of childbearing potential must have a negative pregnancy test prior to initiation of therapy and monthly thereafter) Available only through the *Adempas* REMS Program; prescribers, pharmacies and female patients must enroll **CONTRAINDICATIONS** Pregnancy, use of PDE-5 inhibitors or nitrates **WARNINGS** Hypotension, bleeding, pulmonary edema **SIDE EFFECTS** Headache, dyspepsia, dizziness, N/V/D

Riociguat Drug Interactions

- Do not use with nitrate medications (any formulation – see Stable Angina chapter) or PDE-5 inhibitors as the potential for excessively low blood pressure is increased. Specifically, riociguat should not be administered within 24 hours of sildenafil, or within 24 hours before or 48 hours after tadalafil.

- Smoking increases riociguat clearance; the dose may need to be decreased with smoking cessation.

- Separate from antacids by > 1 hour.

- Riociguat is a major substrate of CYP3A4, 2C8 and P-gp; monitor for drug interactions and dose adjustments.

PULMONARY FIBROSIS

Pulmonary fibrosis (PF) is <u>scarred</u> and <u>damaged lung tissue</u>. The common presentation is exertional <u>dyspnea</u> with a nonproductive cough. As the condition worsens, breathing becomes more labored. There are various causes of PF, including toxin exposure (e.g., asbestos, silica), medical conditions and drugs (see <u>Key Drugs Guy</u>). Often the contributing factor is not identified, and the PF is called idiopathic pulmonary fibrosis (IPF).

If the condition is drug-induced, the offending drug should be discontinued. Aside from treatment with chronic oxygen supplementation, two drugs are now available for IPF. Both pirfenidone (*Esbriet*) and nintedanib (*Ofev*) slow the rate of decline in lung function. In addition to these two drugs, several of the drugs approved for PAH (particularly sildenafil) may be used off-label for IPF. The prognosis of IPF is poor; five-year survival is approximately 20 – 30% once diagnosed.

Select Guidelines/References

Therapy for pulmonary arterial hypertension in adults. *Chest.* 2019;155:565-586.

2015 ESC/ERS guidelines for the diagnosis and treatment of pulmonary hypertension. *Eur Heart J.* 2016;37:67-119.

SELECT DRUGS THAT CAN CAUSE PULMONARY FIBROSIS

KEY DRUGS

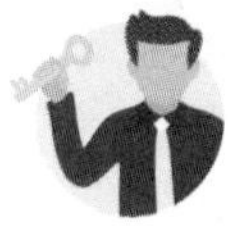

Amiodarone/dronedarone

Bleomycin

Busulfan

Carmustine

Others:

Nitrofurantoin

Sulfasalazine

CONTENT LEGEND

Study
Tip Gal

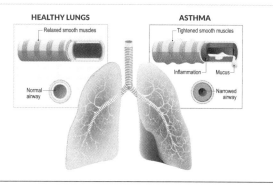

HEALTHY LUNGS — Relaxed smooth muscles — Normal airway

ASTHMA — Tightened smooth muscles — Inflammation — Mucus — Narrowed airway

iStock.com/ttsz

CHAPTER 41
ASTHMA

BACKGROUND

Asthma is a disease that affects the airways (bronchi) of the lungs. It is a common chronic disease among children. Asthma is characterized by chronic airway inflammation and bronchoconstriction (narrowed airways). The inflammation and bronchoconstriction cause airflow obstruction, which results in expiratory airflow limitation (difficulty with exhalation). This results in recurrent episodes of wheezing, breathlessness, chest tightness and coughing, which are the classic symptoms of asthma. The symptoms can vary over time and in intensity, often occurring more frequently at night or on awakening. They can also be worsened by exposure to triggers (see next section).

The inflammation and bronchoconstriction in asthma are reversible with medication (and sometimes spontaneously). Patients with asthma can live successful and active lives if they adhere to treatment and follow an asthma action plan. The most common complication is exacerbations, also called asthma attacks, which can range from mild to severe, and in some cases, can be fatal. There is no cure for asthma, but it can be controlled.

ENVIRONMENTAL TRIGGERS AND COMORBID CONDITIONS

The triggers that cause an asthma attack vary; some people will have bronchoconstriction from a pet, and others will not. Patients need to learn their personal triggers and avoid them when possible. If the trigger cannot be avoided, acute treatment may be needed. Some of the most common triggers are listed below, including comorbid conditions.

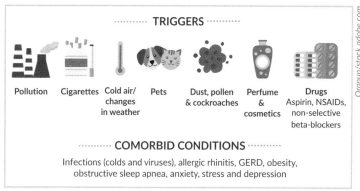

Orapun/stock.adobe.com

TRIGGERS

Pollution | Cigarettes | Cold air/ changes in weather | Pets | Dust, pollen & cockroaches | Perfume & cosmetics | Drugs Aspirin, NSAIDs, non-selective beta-blockers

COMORBID CONDITIONS

Infections (colds and viruses), allergic rhinitis, GERD, obesity, obstructive sleep apnea, anxiety, stress and depression

DIAGNOSIS AND ASSESSMENT

There are many types of asthma. When classic symptoms are present, a detailed history and physical examination can help define the type, along with triggers, environmental factors and comorbid conditions that can contribute to disease severity. Most types of asthma result from the activation of inflammatory mediators (e.g., histamine, leukotrienes, cytokines) and an increase in inflammatory cells (e.g., mast cells, eosinophils) that contribute to the disease process. Some patients have a genetic predisposition for severe allergic asthma, which is mediated by immunoglobulin E (IgE), or severe eosinophilic asthma. Both can require specialized treatments in addition to the use of routine inhaled medications.

An asthma diagnosis is confirmed with spirometry, which is performed in a medical facility (not at home). Spirometry assesses how well the lungs work with various pulmonary function tests, including:

- Forced expiratory volume in 1 second (FEV1): how much air can be forcefully exhaled in one second
- Forced vital capacity (FVC): the maximum volume of air exhaled after taking a deep breath
- FEV1/FVC: the percentage of total air capacity ("vital capacity") that can be forcefully exhaled in one second (the speed of the exhale)

To diagnose asthma, pulmonary function tests should be measured at baseline and after use of a short-acting bronchodilator (e.g., albuterol) to test for reversibility. The Study Tip Gal below describes the diagnostic criteria.

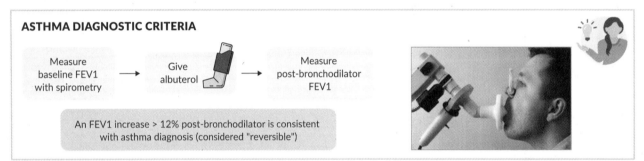

ASTHMA DIAGNOSTIC CRITERIA

Measure baseline FEV1 with spirometry → Give albuterol → Measure post-bronchodilator FEV1

An FEV1 increase > 12% post-bronchodilator is consistent with asthma diagnosis (considered "reversible")

Other tests that may be involved in diagnosing asthma include fractional exhaled nitric oxide (FeNO) and the peak expiratory flow rate (PEFR). FeNO measures nitric oxide in exhaled breath and can indicate the level of airway inflammation. PEFR is measured using a peak flow meter and is typically used for monitoring control as part of the asthma action plan, but it can be used at initial diagnosis. PEFR and peak flow meters are described in more detail later in the chapter.

TREATMENT PRINCIPLES

Long-term asthma management should focus on reducing impairment (e.g., symptoms, frequency of rescue inhaler use, limitations to normal activity) and risks (exacerbations, hospitalizations and medication adverse events). Initiating, monitoring and adjusting treatment follows a step-wise and continuous process.

There are two major guidelines used for treating asthma: the Global Initiative for Asthma (GINA) and the NHLBI's Expert Panel Report (EPR). The GINA guidelines are considered the gold standard, as they are published annually; they are "global" guidelines, so are not specific to the United States. The treatment recommendations in this chapter follow the GINA guidelines.

INITIAL ASTHMA ASSESSMENT

The intensity (or step) of initial treatment is primarily based on the frequency of daytime symptoms and nighttime awakenings. The table below describes the clinical assessment for each step. The Asthma Treatment Algorithm discussed later in the chapter provides the corresponding treatment. Asthma severity is then determined based on how well the treatment controlled the patient's symptoms.

Symptoms	Clinical Assessment and Treatment Intensity (or Step)			
	Step 1	Step 2	Step 3	Steps 4 and 5
Daytime symptoms	< 2x/month	≥ 2x/month but < 4-5 days/week	Most days	Daily
Nighttime awakenings	None	None	≥ 1x/week	≥ 1x/week

GENERAL TREATMENT APPROACH

- Select treatment according to the initial assessment of asthma symptoms (see the table on the previous page and the Asthma Treatment Algorithm later in the chapter).

- Follow up in 2 – 6 weeks. At <u>each visit</u>:

  - ❏ Assess adherence to medications.

  - ❏ Perform medication counseling (confirm <u>appropriate inhaler technique</u> and understanding of maintenance versus rescue treatment). See the detailed instructions on technique, <u>priming</u> and <u>cleaning</u> of select inhalers at the end of the chapter.

  - ❏ Assess control of risk factors, triggers and comorbid conditions.

  - ❏ Review the asthma action plan (see example later in the chapter).

  - ❏ Address patient concerns.

  - ❏ Assess asthma control/severity and <u>step up, maintain or step down treatment</u>. Do not step up therapy until the items above have been addressed; there might be other factors contributing to poor asthma control (e.g., incorrect inhaler technique, lack of adherence) and increasing doses of medications and/or adding other drugs can increase side effects without providing additional benefit.

- Follow up visits can decrease to 1 – 6 months once control is gained, and to every three months if a step down in treatment is planned.

CONTROLLING RISK FACTORS

Patients with asthma should avoid exposure to <u>tobacco smoke</u> and those who smoke should <u>quit</u>, or be strongly encouraged to quit at each healthcare visit. Physical activity should not be avoided, even in those with exercise-induced bronchospasm.

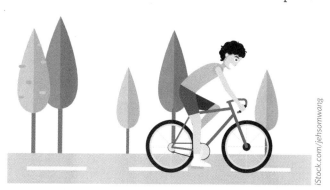

iStock.com/jehsomwang

Triggers should be identified and avoided, if possible. Some triggers should not be avoided (e.g., laughter) and others are difficult to avoid (e.g., stress, infections). Comorbid conditions should be treated to improve asthma control.

An <u>annual influenza vaccine</u> is recommended in all patients 6 months of age or older, including those with asthma. <u>Pneumococcal</u> and COVID-19 vaccines should be kept up to date; see Immunizations chapter for details.

Any patient with persistent asthma and a clear connection between symptoms and exposure to an <u>allergen</u> should have skin or in vitro testing performed to assess <u>sensitivity</u>. Treatment with subcutaneous allergen immunotherapy should be used, if indicated, based on the test results.

DRUG TREATMENT

Asthma drugs come in <u>oral, inhaled and injectable</u> formulations. <u>Inhaled forms</u> deliver drugs directly into the <u>lungs</u>, have <u>reduced toxicity</u> and are the <u>preferred</u> delivery vehicle. Drugs used to treat asthma are classified as relievers (rescue inhalers) or controllers (maintenance drugs). The table below describes the different classes of asthma medications and the primary role or place in treatment for each.

<u>Relievers, or rescue inhalers, rapidly open airways</u> within minutes of inhalation to treat <u>acute symptoms</u> (i.e., they make breathing easier). The preferred reliever regimen is the combination of a <u>low-dose inhaled corticosteroid (ICS) + formoterol</u>. Alternatively, a <u>short-acting beta-2 agonist</u> (SABA) can be used but should be administered at the <u>same time as an ICS</u>. In addition to treating acute asthma symptoms, relievers can be used to prevent <u>exercise-induced bronchospasm</u> (EIB).

<u>Controllers, or maintenance inhalers</u>, are taken on a <u>daily basis</u> to <u>reduce inflammation</u> and maintain asthma control. <u>ICS</u> are the <u>mainstay of treatment</u>. Doses are categorized as low, medium or high and can be escalated (by increasing the number of inhalations per dose or increasing to a higher strength inhaler), if indicated, based on asthma severity.

ASTHMA MEDICATION CLASS	NOTES
Relievers (Rescue Drugs)	
Low-dose <u>ICS + formoterol</u> (combination inhaler)	<u>Preferred</u> reliever regimen; may be referred to as an anti-inflammatory reliever (AIR)
	Used intermittently (<u>as needed</u>) for acute asthma <u>symptoms</u>
	Formoterol is a long-acting beta-2 agonist (LABA) with fast onset; this combination <u>reduces</u> the risk of <u>exacerbations</u> compared to SABA alone
Inhaled <u>short-acting beta-2 agonist</u> (SABA)	Used intermittently (<u>as needed</u>) for acute asthma <u>symptoms</u> (an alternative to the preferred therapy of ICS-formoterol)
	Quickly <u>reverses bronchoconstriction</u>
	SABAs do not treat underlying inflammation; they should be used <u>with an ICS</u> (taken as needed at the same time as the SABA, or taken daily as a controller medication). A combined ICS-SABA (another type of AIR) is an alternative option.
Systemic steroids	Injections: used during exacerbations
	Oral: used during <u>exacerbations</u> or for <u>severe asthma</u> that is difficult to control with other drug combinations
	Use should be limited as much as possible due to the risk of adverse effects (see the Systemic Steroids & Autoimmune Conditions chapter)
Inhaled epinephrine	Available OTC; can be used intermittently for acute treatment of mild asthma only
	Not included in asthma guidelines
Inhaled short-acting muscarinic antagonists (SAMAs); also called inhaled anticholinergics	Can be used in combination with a SABA during exacerbations
Controllers (Maintenance Drugs)	
<u>Inhaled corticosteroids (ICS)</u>	<u>First-line for all patients</u> with asthma; the most effective anti-inflammatory drugs
<u>Inhaled long-acting beta-2 agonists (LABAs)</u>	Used <u>in combination with ICS</u> (should <u>never</u> be used <u>alone</u> for asthma due to an increased risk of serious adverse outcomes)
	<u>Preferred add-on</u> agents to ICS
Oral leukotriene receptor antagonists (<u>LTRAs</u>)	Alternative option to LABA in combination with ICS; can also be added to ICS/LABA treatment
	Most commonly used in <u>children</u>
Theophylline (oral or IV)	Least desirable option for add-on treatment due to significant adverse effects, drug interactions and the need to <u>monitor serum drug concentrations</u>
Inhaled long-acting muscarinic antagonists (<u>LAMAs</u>); also called inhaled anticholinergics	Can be used as <u>add-on</u> treatment in patients with a history of exacerbations despite ICS/LABA treatment
Injectable <u>monoclonal antibodies</u> (SC or IV)	Add-on treatment in persistent severe asthma:
	Omalizumab: for <u>severe allergic asthma</u>
	Mepolizumab, reslizumab, benralizumab and dupilumab: for <u>severe eosinophilic asthma</u>
	Tezepelumab: for <u>severe asthma</u> (regardless of eosinophil counts or biomarkers)

ASTHMA TREATMENT ALGORITHM

The <u>algorithm</u> below shows the recommended treatment of asthma at each step of therapy per the GINA guidelines, with as-needed rescue inhalers shown in blue (left side) and maintenance inhalers show in green (right side). The <u>preferred regimens</u> are those that <u>use low-dose ICS-formoterol rescue therapy</u>. For steps 3 and higher, ICS-formoterol is used for rescue therapy if the same combination is also used for maintenance therapy; this is called maintenance and reliever therapy (MART).

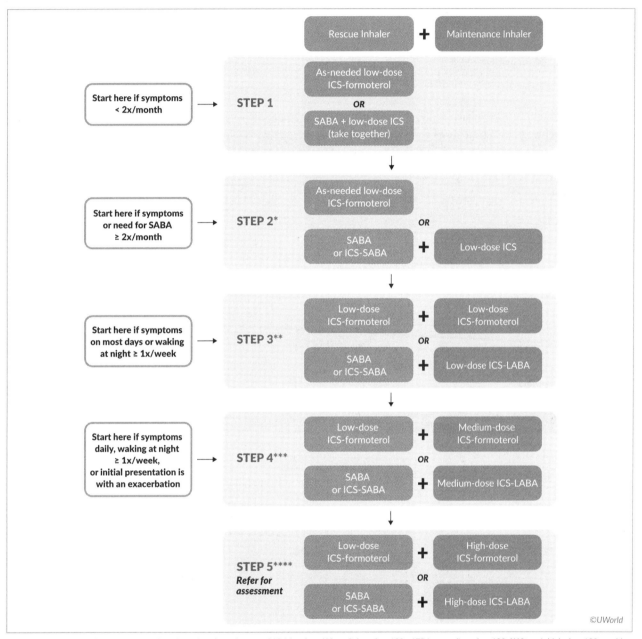

*Alternative treatments: *Step 2: LTRA, or low-dose ICS taken whenever SABA is taken. **Step 3: low-dose ICS + LTRA or medium-dose ICS. ***Step 4: high-dose ICS or add on tiotropium or LTRA. ****Step 5: consider adding tiotropium, oral steroid, or injectable treatments (e.g., omalizumab, mepolizumab, reslizumab, tezepelumab).*

Assessing Asthma Control

Asthma control should be assessed at each visit using the following four yes/no questions:

- Daytime asthma <u>symptoms > twice/week</u>?

- Any nighttime awakenings due to asthma?

- SABA reliever treatment used > twice/week? (Note: only for patients using SABA therapy.)

- Is activity limited due to asthma?

The number of questions answered "yes" determines the level of asthma control and how to adjust treatment:

Well-controlled: no questions answered "yes." Maintain current step (or step down if controlled for ≥ 3 months).

Partly controlled: 1 – 2 questions answered "yes." Step up 1 step.

Uncontrolled: 3 – 4 questions answered "yes." Step up 1 – 2 steps and consider a short course of oral steroids.

BETA-2 AGONISTS

Beta-2 agonists bind to beta-2 receptors, which causes relaxation of bronchial smooth muscle and leads to bronchodilation. SABAs are used as needed (rescue therapy) for acute asthma symptoms. They were previously used as monotherapy in Step 1 of the treatment algorithm, but due to an increased risk of exacerbations, they are no longer recommended this way. SABAs should only be used with an ICS (either taken as needed, at the same time as the SABA, or daily). They can also be used for other reversible airway diseases, such as colds, allergies and bronchitis.

LABAs are used as part of rescue therapy (e.g., ICS + formoterol) or as maintenance therapy beginning in Step 3 of treatment. LABAs should be used only in combination with an ICS. If not already part of the treatment regimen, a LABA should be added to medium-dose ICS before increasing to high-dose ICS, as this leads to more rapid improvement in symptoms and lung function, and a reduction in exacerbations.

DRUG	DOSING	SAFETY/SIDE EFFECTS/MONITORING
Short-Acting Beta-2 Agonists (SABAs)		
Albuterol (ProAir HFA, ProAir RespiClick, Proventil HFA, Ventolin HFA, ProAir Digihaler) 90 mcg/inh, 0.5% and 0.083% nebulizer solution, oral syrup + budesonide (Airsupra)	MDI/DPI: 1-2 inhalations Q4-6H PRN Nebulizer: 1.25-5 mg Q4-8H PRN PO forms are available but not recommended	**WARNINGS** Caution in CVD, glaucoma, hyperthyroidism, seizures, diabetes **SIDE EFFECTS** Nervousness, tremor, tachycardia, palpitations, cough, hyperglycemia, ↓ K **MONITORING** Number of days of SABA use, symptom frequency, peak flow, pulmonary function tests, BP, HR, blood glucose, K
Levalbuterol (Xopenex, Xopenex HFA) 45 mcg/inh, nebulizer solution	MDI: 1-2 inhalations Q4-6H PRN Nebulizer: 0.63-1.25 mg Q6-8H PRN (max = 1.25 mg three times daily)	**NOTES** MDIs (HFA products): shake well before use Levalbuterol contains the R-isomer of albuterol Epinephrine inhaler: FDA-approved for mild symptoms in intermittent asthma only
Epinephrine (Asthmanefrin Refill) OTC	Should not be used since it is non-selective	Most albuterol inhalers contain 200 inhalations/canister; the exception is Ventolin HFA, which is available as 200 inhalations/canister and 60 inhalations/canister EIB: use 2 inhalations 5 minutes prior to exercise
Long-Acting Beta-2 Agonists (LABAs)		
Salmeterol (Serevent Diskus) 50 mcg/inh	DPI: 1 inhalation BID	Side effects and monitoring are the same as SABAs plus: **BOXED WARNINGS** ↑ risk of asthma-related deaths; should only be used in asthma patients who are currently receiving but are not adequately controlled on an inhaled corticosteroid ↑ risk of asthma-related hospitalizations in pediatric and adolescent patients **NOTES** Maintenance inhaler only; not for acute bronchospasm

INHALED CORTICOSTEROIDS

Corticosteroids inhibit the inflammatory response. They block the late-phase reaction to allergens, reduce airway hyper-responsiveness and are potent and effective anti-inflammatory medications. ICSs reduce asthma symptoms, increase lung function, improve quality of life and reduce the risk of exacerbations. They are used as needed in combination with formoterol or a SABA for acute symptoms (rescue treatment), and as monotherapy or combination therapy (with a LABA) to control symptoms (maintenance treatment).

DRUG	DOSING	SAFETY/SIDE EFFECTS/MONITORING
Beclomethasone (QVAR RediHaler) 40, 80 mcg/inh	MDI: 1-4 inhalations BID	**CONTRAINDICATIONS** Primary treatment of status asthmaticus or acute episodes of asthma
Budesonide		
Pulmicort Flexhaler: 90, 180 mcg/inh	DPI: 1-4 inhalations BID	**WARNINGS** High doses for prolonged periods of time can cause adrenal suppression, ↑ risk of fractures, growth retardation (in children) and immunosuppression
Pulmicort Respules: nebulizer suspension	Nebulizer: 0.25-0.5 mg daily or BID in children age 1-8 years	
+ formoterol (Symbicort, Breyna) + albuterol (Airsupra)		**SIDE EFFECTS** Dysphonia (difficulty speaking), oral candidiasis (thrush), cough, headache, hoarseness, URTIs, hyperglycemia
Fluticasone		
Flovent HFA*: 44, 110, 220 mcg/inh	MDI: 2 inhalations BID	**MONITORING** Use of SABA/rescue inhaler, symptom frequency, peak flow; growth (children/adolescents), s/sx adrenal insufficiency; s/sx of thrush; bone mineral density
Flovent Diskus*: 50, 100, 250 mcg/inh	DPI: 1-2 inhalations BID	
Arnuity Ellipta: 100, 200 mcg/inh	DPI: 1-2 inhalations daily	
ArmonAir Digihaler: 55, 113, 232 mcg/inh	DPI: 1 inhalation BID	
+ salmeterol (Advair Diskus, Advair HFA, AirDuo RespiClick, AirDuo Digihaler, Wixela Inhub)		**NOTES** Rinse mouth with water and spit out after each use to prevent thrush; can use a spacer device with an MDI to decrease risk
+ vilanterol (Breo Ellipta)		Alvesco: MDI that does not need to be shaken before use
Mometasone		Budesonide: only ICS available as a nebulized solution; used commonly in young children
Asmanex HFA: 100, 200 mcg/inh	MDI: 1-2 inhalations BID	Pulmicort Respules: only use with a jet nebulizer connected to an air compressor; do not use an ultrasonic nebulizer
Asmanex: 110, 220 mcg/inh	DPI: 1-2 inhalations daily	QVAR RediHaler: breath-activated aerosol with characteristics of a DPI and MDI; do not shake or use with a spacer; does not need priming or activation
+ formoterol (Dulera)		
Ciclesonide (Alvesco): 80, 160 mcg/inh	MDI: 1-2 inhalations BID	ArmonAir and AirDuo Digihalers: contain a built-in electronic module that detects, records and stores data (detects when the inhaler is used and measures inspiratory flow)

*Brand discontinued but name still used in practice.

Categorization of Inhaled Corticosteroid Daily Doses

DRUG	LOW DAILY DOSE	MEDIUM DAILY DOSE	HIGH DAILY DOSE
Beclomethasone MDI 40 or 80 mcg/inh	100-200 mcg	> 200-400 mcg	> 400 mcg
Budesonide DPI 90 or 180 mcg/inh	200-400 mcg	> 400-800 mcg	> 800 mcg
Ciclesonide MDI 80, 160 mcg/inh	80-160 mcg	> 160-320 mcg	> 320 mcg
Fluticasone MDI: 44, 110 or 220 mcg/inh	100-250 mcg	> 250-500 mcg	> 500 mcg
DPI: 50, 100 or 250 mcg/inh	100-250 mcg	> 250-500 mcg	> 500 mcg
Mometasone MDI: 100 or 200 mcg/inh	200-400 mcg	200-400 mcg	> 400 mcg
DPI: 110 or 220 mcg/inh	110-220 mcg	> 220-440 mcg	> 440 mcg

CONTROLLER (MAINTENANCE) INHALERS

There are many inhaled products available to treat respiratory conditions. This can create confusion in terms of proper use for specific disease states. The table below categorizes the different classes of controller medications for asthma and chronic obstructive pulmonary disease (COPD). ICS and ICS/LABA combinations are preferred for asthma, whereas LABA, LAMA or LAMA/LABA combinations are preferred for COPD. Some ICS/LABA combinations are approved for COPD and can be used in select patients (see the COPD chapter for treatment recommendations).

Combination inhalers increase adherence to treatment which improves disease control. Combination ICS/LABA products are considered safer for asthma, as they reduce the risk of using a LABA alone. Because of this, combination ICS/LABA inhalers do not have the boxed warning for asthma-related deaths that single-entity LABAs have. Note that this table does not include short-acting (rescue) medications.

DRUG CLASS	ASTHMA	COPD
ICS	**Beclomethasone (QVAR RediHaler)** **Budesonide (Pulmicort Flexhaler)** **Fluticasone (Flovent HFA, Flovent Diskus, Arnuity Ellipta,** ArmonAir Digihaler) Ciclesonide (Alvesco) Mometasone (Asmanex HFA, Asmanex)	No single ICS product is FDA-approved for COPD
LABA	**Salmeterol (Serevent Diskus)**	**Salmeterol (Serevent Diskus)** Formoterol (Perforomist – nebulizer) Arformoterol (Brovana – nebulizer) Olodaterol (Striverdi Respimat)
LAMA	**Tiotropium (Spiriva Respimat** only)	**Tiotropium (Spiriva HandiHaler, Spiriva Respimat)** Aclidinium (Tudorza Pressair) Revefenacin (Yupelri – nebulizer) Umeclidinium (Incruse Ellipta)
ICS/LABA	**Budesonide/formoterol (Symbicort, Breyna)** **Fluticasone/salmeterol (Advair Diskus, Advair HFA,** AirDuo RespiClick, AirDuo Digihaler, Wixela Inhub) **Mometasone/formoterol (Dulera)** **Fluticasone/vilanterol (Breo Ellipta)**	**Budesonide/formoterol (Symbicort, Breyna)** **Fluticasone/salmeterol (Advair Diskus,** Wixela Inhub) **Fluticasone/vilanterol (Breo Ellipta)**
LAMA/LABA	No combination LAMA/LABA products are FDA-approved for asthma	Aclidinium/formoterol (Duaklir Pressair) Glycopyrrolate/formoterol (Bevespi Aerosphere) Tiotropium/olodaterol (Stiolto Respimat) Umeclidinium/vilanterol (Anoro Ellipta)
LAMA/LABA/ICS	**Umeclidinium/vilanterol/fluticasone (Trelegy Ellipta)**	**Umeclidinium/vilanterol/fluticasone (Trelegy Ellipta)** **Glycopyrrolate/formoterol/budesonide (Breztri Aerosphere)**

INHALED DELIVERY DEVICES

Inhaler devices come as metered-dose inhalers (MDIs) or dry powder inhalers (DPIs), including breath-actuated DPIs. Recognizing the type of inhaler is important as it impacts the technique the patient needs to use and the education required (see the Patient Self-Management and Education section later in the chapter).

KEY DIFFERENCES BETWEEN MDIs AND DPIs

FEATURES	MDIs	DPIs
Brand name identifiers	*HFA*, *Respimat* or no suffix (e.g., *Symbicort, Dulera*)	*Diskus, Ellipta, Pressair, HandiHaler, RespiClick, Flexhaler*
Dose delivery	Aerosolized liquid	Fine powder
Propellant	Some use a propellant (HFA)	No propellant
Administration	Slow, deep inhalation while pressing the canister (hand-breath coordination)	Quick, forceful inhalation (breath activated dose delivery; no need to press anything)
Spacer	Can be used for most (but not *QVAR RediHaler* or *Respimat* products) Helpful in patients incapable of hand-breath coordination and decreases risk of thrush (with ICS)	Cannot be used
Shaking prior to use	Required for all products except: *QVAR RediHaler, Alvesco* and *Respimat* products, and *Atrovent HFA* (discussed in the COPD chapter)	Do not shake
Priming	Before first use and if not used for a certain period of time (see the Key Counseling Points section later in the chapter)	Not needed except for *Flexhaler* (prior to first use)

Note: QVAR RediHaler is a breath-activated aerosol, which has characteristics of both a DPI and MDI (see the ICS table).

LEUKOTRIENE MODIFYING AGENTS

Leukotrienes are mediators of airway inflammation. Leukotriene receptor antagonists (LTRAs) reduce airway edema, constriction and inflammation. Montelukast inhibits leukotriene D4 (LTD4), while zafirlukast inhibits both LTD4 and LTE4. Zileuton, a 5-lipoxygenase inhibitor, inhibits leukotriene formation.

DRUG	DOSING	SAFETY/SIDE EFFECTS/MONITORING
Montelukast (Singulair) Tablet, chewable tablet, packet Also approved for allergic rhinitis and exercise-induced bronchoconstriction	10 mg daily in the evening Age 6-14 years: 5 mg daily in the evening Age 1-5 years: 4 mg daily in the evening EIB: 5 mg (6-14 years) or 10 mg (≥ 15 years) 2 hours before exercise	**BOXED WARNINGS** Montelukast: neuropsychiatric events (e.g., serious behavior and mood-related changes, including suicidal thoughts or actions) **CONTRAINDICATIONS** Zafirlukast and zileuton: hepatic impairment **WARNINGS** Neuropsychiatric events; monitor for signs of aggressive behavior, hostility, agitation, hallucinations, depression, suicidal thinking
Zafirlukast (*Accolate*) Tablet	20 mg BID Age 5-11 years: 10 mg BID Take 1 hour before or 2 hours after meals (empty stomach)	Systemic eosinophilia (montelukast and zafirlukast) **SIDE EFFECTS** Headache, dizziness, abdominal pain, ↑ LFTs, URTIs **MONITORING** LFTs (zafirlukast and zileuton), mood or behavior changes (montelukast)
Zileuton (*Zyflo*) Tablet, ER tablet	*Zyflo*: 600 mg QID ER tablet: 1,200 mg BID within 1 hour after morning and evening meals Age < 12 years: not recommended	**NOTES** Montelukast granules: can be administered directly in the mouth, dissolved in a small amount (5 mL) of breast milk or formula or mixed with a spoonful of applesauce, carrots, rice or ice cream (do not mix with anything else); use within 15 minutes of opening the packet Zafirlukast: protect from moisture and light; dispense in original container

Leukotriene Modifying Agents Drug Interactions

- Montelukast is a minor substrate of CYP450 3A4 and 2C8/9 and a weak inhibitor of CYP2C8/9.

  - Gemfibrozil can ↑ levels of montelukast; lumacaftor can ↓ levels of montelukast.

- Zafirlukast is a major substrate of CYP2C9. It inhibits CYP2C9 (moderate) and CYP2C8 (weak).

- Zafirlukast can ↑ levels of theophylline and CYP2C9 substrates (e.g., warfarin).

  - Erythromycin and theophylline ↓ zafirlukast levels.

- Zileuton is a minor substrate of CYP1A2, 2C9 and 3A4, and a weak inhibitor of CYP1A2. It can ↑ levels of theophylline, propranolol and warfarin.

THEOPHYLLINE

Theophylline blocks phosphodiesterase, causing an increase in cyclic adenosine monophosphate (cAMP) and release of epinephrine from adrenal medulla cells. This results in bronchodilation, but it also causes diuresis, CNS and cardiac stimulation and gastric acid secretion. Use of theophylline is limited by ↓ effectiveness, drug interactions and adverse effects.

DRUG	DOSING	SAFETY/SIDE EFFECTS/MONITORING
Theophylline (Elixophyllin, Theo-24) ER capsule, ER tablet, elixir, oral solution, injection Active metabolites are caffeine and 3-methylxanthine	Oral loading dose: 5 mg/kg IBW (or TBW if < IBW) Oral maintenance dose: 300-600 mg daily **Therapeutic range** 5-15 mcg/mL Measure peak level at steady state, after 3 days of oral dosing	**WARNINGS** Can exacerbate cardiovascular arrhythmias, peptic ulcer disease and seizure disorders **SIDE EFFECTS** Nausea, vomiting, headache, insomnia, ↑ HR, tremor, nervousness Toxicity: persistent vomiting, arrhythmias, seizures **MONITORING** Theophylline levels, HR, CNS effects (insomnia, irritability), use of rescue inhaler **NOTES** Aminophylline contains 2:1 theophylline and ethylenediamine To convert aminophylline to theophylline, multiply by 0.8*; to convert theophylline to aminophylline, divide by 0.8 *Remember: ATM (Aminophylline → Theophylline Multiply)

Theophylline Interactions

Theophylline has saturable kinetics (first-order kinetics, followed by zero-order kinetics). In the higher end of the therapeutic range, small dose increases can result in large increases in theophylline concentrations (see the Pharmacokinetics chapter).

- Theophylline is a substrate of CYP1A2 (major), 3A4 and 2E1 (minor).

- CYP1A2 inhibitors that ↑ theophylline levels: cimetidine, ciprofloxacin, fluvoxamine, propranolol and zileuton.

- CYP3A4 inhibitors that ↑ theophylline levels: clarithromycin and erythromycin.

- Other drugs that ↑ theophylline levels: zafirlukast, alcohol, allopurinol, disulfiram, estrogen-containing oral contraceptives, methotrexate, pentoxifylline, propafenone and verapamil.

- Drugs that ↓ theophylline levels: carbamazepine, fosphenytoin, phenobarbital, phenytoin, primidone, rifampin, ritonavir, levothyroxine, St. John's wort and tobacco/marijuana smoking.

- Theophylline can ↓ lithium (via ↑ renal excretion) and zafirlukast.

- Conditions/foods that ↑ theophylline levels (due to ↓ theophylline clearance): CHF, cirrhosis or liver disease, acute pulmonary edema, cor pulmonale, fever, hypothyroidism, shock and high carbohydrate/low protein diet.

- Conditions/foods that can ↓ theophylline levels (due to ↑ theophylline clearance): low carbohydrate/high-protein diet, daily consumption of charbroiled beef, cystic fibrosis and hyperthyroidism.

ANTICHOLINERGICS

Anticholinergics, also called muscarinic antagonists, inhibit muscarinic cholinergic receptors and reduce the intrinsic vagal tone of the airway, leading to bronchodilation. Short-acting anticholinergics (e.g., ipratropium) are sometimes used in combination with SABAs in hospitalized patients with acute exacerbations. A long-acting anticholinergic, tiotropium (Spiriva Respimat), is FDA-approved for asthma in patients ≥ 6 years of age with a history of exacerbations despite ICS/LABA therapy. Anticholinergics should not be used alone in asthma; they are add-on treatments to be used with an ICS. Refer to the COPD chapter for more information on anticholinergics.

MONOCLONAL ANTIBODIES FOR SEVERE ASTHMA

Treatment with a monoclonal antibody can be considered for patients with severe asthma that remains uncontrolled despite maximized treatment with inhaled medications. These monoclonal antibodies are biologic, injectable medications that each have unique indications based on their molecular targets. For example, the interleukin antagonists are only appropriate for patients with eosinophilic asthma (i.e., an elevated blood eosinophil count). The patient's specific asthma phenotype should be determined prior to starting treatment to ensure appropriate drug selection.

DRUG	ADMINISTRATION	NOTES
IgG Monoclonal Antibody: inhibits IgE binding to the IgE receptor on mast cells and basophils		
Omalizumab *(Xolair)*	Administer SC every 2 or 4 weeks; dose and frequency based on pretreatment IgE serum levels and body weight Initiate in a healthcare setting under medical supervision (≥ 3 doses) Self-administration can be considered (after 3 doses) if specific criteria are met	Indication: severe allergic asthma Allergic asthma should be documented before use with a positive skin test or in vitro reactivity to a perennial aeroallergen Boxed warning for anaphylaxis (can occur at any point in treatment); patients must be observed after administration
Interleukin Receptor Antagonists: block interleukins (cytokines responsible for the growth, differentiation, recruitment, activation and survival of eosinophils) to reduce inflammation; all block interleukin 5 with the exception of dupilumab, which blocks interleukins 4 and 13		
Mepolizumab *(Nucala)*	Administer SC every 4 weeks	Indication: severe eosinophilic asthma
Reslizumab *(Cinqair)*	Administer IV once every 4 weeks	Reslizumab: boxed warning for anaphylaxis; patients must be observed after administration
Benralizumab *(Fasenra, Fasenra Pen)*	Administer SC every 4 weeks x 3 doses, then every 8 weeks	Mepolizumab, dupilumab and *Fasenra Pen:* can be administered at home by a patient or caregiver
Dupilumab *(Dupixent)*	Administer SC every other week	
Human Thymic Stromal Lymphopoietin Blocker: reduces multiple biomarkers of inflammation		
Tezepelumab *(Tezspire)*	Administer SC every 4 weeks	Indication: severe asthma (of any type) Can be administered at home by a patient or caregiver

SPECIAL SITUATIONS

EXERCISE-INDUCED BRONCHOSPASM: *PREVENT IT*

A SABA or low-dose ICS plus formoterol, taken 5 – 15 minutes before exercise, is preferred to prevent most EIB. The effects of the SABA will last 2 – 3 hours, while the duration of the ICS plus formoterol can last up to 12 hours. Salmeterol (a LABA) can be used as an alternative to a SABA if a longer duration of symptom control is needed; it should be taken 30 minutes before exercise. If the patient is using a LABA for asthma maintenance, they should not use additional doses for EIB. LABAs should never be used alone for persistent asthma.

Montelukast can be taken two hours prior to exercise and lasts up to 24 hours. It is effective in only 50% of patients. Patients taking montelukast for asthma, or any other indication, should not take an additional dose to prevent EIB.

EIB is often a marker of inadequate asthma control. It might be necessary to start or increase a controller medication (e.g., an ICS) to control the EIB.

PREGNANCY: *KEEP CONTROL*

Asthma control can worsen during pregnancy. To ensure oxygen supply to the fetus, it is safer to treat asthma with medications than to have poorly controlled asthma. Down-titration of medications is not recommended, and exacerbations should be treated aggressively. An ICS should be continued during pregnancy and is still the preferred controller (either as needed or daily).

CASE SCENARIO

SG is a 35-year-old female with asthma. She brings a prescription for *Advair Diskus* to the pharmacy and requests a refill on her *ProAir RespiClick*. You review her medication refill history and see that she filled prescriptions for *Pulmicort Flexhaler* 3 weeks ago and *ProAir RespiClick* approximately 2 months ago.

SG tells you that she is stopping her *Pulmicort Flexhaler* and starting the *Advair Diskus* instead. She says she uses her *ProAir RespiClick* about 3 times a day, on at least 3 days of the week. She feels like she cannot have as active of a social life as she would like due to asthma attacks.

How would you assess SG's asthma control?
SG is not well controlled, as she uses her SABA inhaler *(ProAir RespiClick)* more than 2 days a week and has limitations to normal activity.

Is the change in treatment appropriate?
A step up in treatment is needed. The change from an ICS to an ICS/LABA combination product is appropriate.

What counseling points about her treatment are important for SG?

■ Follow the specific instructions for inhaler technique.

■ Use *Advair Diskus* twice daily to help control asthma symptoms. It is not a rescue medication.

■ Rinse the mouth and spit after each dose of *Advair Diskus* to prevent thrush (an infection in the mouth).

■ Use *ProAir RespiClick* as needed for shortness of breath. Using it more than twice weekly means asthma is not well controlled. If *ProAir RespiClick* is used too often, it can cause palpitations, nervousness or tremor.

■ Monitor the counter on the *ProAir RespiClick* to make sure it does not run out before the next refill.

■ Avoid triggers known to make asthma worse.

PATIENT SELF-MANAGEMENT AND EDUCATION

INHALERS

Most patients (up to 80%) cannot use their inhaler correctly, which results in little or no medication reaching the lungs. This contributes to poor symptom control and increased exacerbations. Patient counseling and assessing inhaler technique is essential. Up to 50% of adults and children do not take their controller medications as prescribed; this is often unintentional and due to a lack of education, cost or forgetfulness. Assessing adherence is important when evaluating asthma control.

Patients should be aware of how to monitor the doses remaining in an inhaler. Some inhalers have an internal dose counter. Most controller inhalers are designed to last one month when the patient is adherent to therapy. SABA rescue inhalers can last a varying amount of time depending on use, but for a patient with good asthma control, an albuterol inhaler should last about 12 months (or 3 – 4 months for the smaller *Ventolin HFA* inhaler with 60 inhalations/canister). It is useful for patients to know when the inhaler should run out. Refer to the table below for examples of the number of days that commonly used inhalers will last.

DRUG	INHALATIONS	EXAMPLE DOSAGE	SUPPLY
Maintenance Inhalers			
Advair Diskus	60	1 inhalation BID	30 days (60/2 inhalations daily)
QVAR RediHaler	120	1-2 inhalations BID	30 days (120/4 inhalations daily)
Mometasone *(Asmanex)*	60	2 inhalations daily	30 days (60/2 inhalations daily)
SABA Rescue Inhalers			
Albuterol MDI	200	2 inhalations per dose, used twice weekly (4 inhalations/week)	50 weeks (200/4 inhalations weekly)
Ventolin HFA	60		15 weeks (60/4 inhalations weekly)

Timing and Order of Use

If prescribed > 1 inhalation of medication at a time, the patient should wait 60 seconds between each one. If using more than one inhaler, the sequence of inhalers is important. Bronchodilators (beta-2 agonists and anticholinergics) work faster than ICS. Using bronchodilators first will open the airways quickly, allowing the ICS to travel deeper into the lungs.

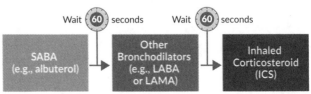

NEBULIZERS

A nebulizer is a device that <u>turns liquid medication into a fine mist</u>. The fine mist can be inhaled through a face mask or mouthpiece into the lungs. Nebulizers use natural breathing, making medication delivery easy for infants, children and the elderly. There are three types of nebulizers: jet, ultrasound and mesh. Check the medication information to see which nebulizer device is recommended.

Albuterol comes as a nebulizer solution in both unit dose packaging and a 20 mL vial. The two common concentrations are 0.083% solution (contains 2.5 mg/3 mL), and 0.5% solution (contains 2.5 mg/0.5 mL). The 0.083% solution is a ready-to-use preparation that can be placed directly into the nebulizer; no dilution is required. Concentrated solutions (i.e., ≥ 0.5%) must be diluted with normal saline prior to use.

SPACERS

"Spacer" is a generic term for different types of open tubes that are placed between the mouthpiece of an MDI and the mouth of the patient to help with medication delivery. Spacers are especially useful for <u>children</u> and anyone with <u>dexterity issues</u> (i.e., difficulty pressing down and breathing in at the same time with an MDI), and they reduce the risk of thrush (see the <u>Study Tip Gal</u>). They should <u>never</u> be used with a <u>DPI</u>. <u>Clean</u> spacers at least once a <u>week</u> (in warm, soapy water).

WITH A SPACER, MORE DRUG GETS INTO THE LUNGS

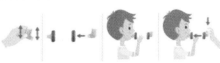

Spacers are helpful for children and anyone that has difficulty with hand-breath coordination (e.g., pressing down on the inhaler while breathing in at the same time) with an MDI. Plus, spacers reduce the risk of thrush from inhaled corticosteroids.

Common spacers: *AeroChamber, OptiHaler, OptiChamber*

PEAK FLOW METERS

Peak flow meters are handheld devices that measure the <u>peak expiratory flow rate (PEFR)</u>, which is the maximum flow rate from a forceful exhalation, starting from fully inflated lungs. The patient's best PEFR is called their <u>personal best</u> (PB), which can be measured by <u>spirometry</u>. The measurement takes into account the patient's <u>height, gender and age</u> because the PEFR depends on the muscular strength of the patient. Patients can measure their PB themselves by taking peak flow readings twice a day (morning and evening) for 2 – 3 weeks when asthma is in good control. The highest reading that occurs most frequently is the PB.

Peak flow meters are beneficial in patients with frequent asthma exacerbations, moderate to severe asthma (Steps 3 – 5), poor perception of airflow obstruction or unexplained response to environmental factors. When used correctly, peak flow meters can identify exacerbations early (even before the patient is symptomatic), allowing treatment to begin sooner.

An <u>asthma action plan</u> is developed by the healthcare provider so the patient knows how to manage symptoms <u>at home</u> and avoid hospitalizations due to an exacerbation. The action plan uses the patient's PB and outlines "zones" of control (based on the percentage of their PB). Each "zone" is then given a specific action to follow (see the example on the next page).

Peak Flow Meter Technique

- Use the peak flow meter <u>every morning</u> upon awakening and <u>before</u> the use of any asthma medications. <u>Proper technique</u> and <u>best effort</u> are essential. Less than the best effort can lead to taking unnecessary medication.

- Move the indicator to the bottom of the numbered scale. Stand up straight. Exhale comfortably.

- Inhale as deeply as possible. Place lips firmly around the mouthpiece, creating a tight seal.

- Blow out as <u>hard</u> and as <u>fast</u> as possible. <u>Write down</u> the PEFR.

- Repeat steps two more times, with enough rest in between. Record the <u>highest value</u>.

- Compare the peak flow value to your personal asthma action plan and follow the steps as instructed.

Peak Flow Meter Care

- Always use the same brand of peak flow meter.

- <u>Clean</u> at least <u>once a week</u> using warm water and mild soap; if you have an infection, clean the meter more frequently. Rinse gently; do not use brushes to clean the inside of the peak flow meter. Do not place peak flow meters in boiling water. Allow the meter to air dry before using again.

ZONES OF AN ASTHMA ACTION PLAN

<u>Green zone (> 80 – 100% of personal best)</u>
- Indicates "<u>all clear</u>" – good control
- Patients are instructed to follow <u>routine maintenance</u> plan

<u>Yellow zone (50 – 80% of personal best)</u>
- Indicates "<u>caution</u>" – worsening lung function
- Patient-specific intervention required (<u>action plan</u>) – usually an increase in rescue inhaler use and the addition or increase of other medications

<u>Red zone (< 50% of personal best)</u>
- Indicates "<u>medical alert</u>" – seek medical attention
- Action plan includes using a rescue inhaler, possibly steroids or going to the <u>emergency department</u>

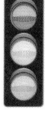

SAMPLE ASTHMA ACTION PLAN (ADULT)

Asthma Action Plan

For: _____ Doctor: _____ Date: _____

Doctor's Phone Number: _____ Hospital/Emergency Department Phone Number: _____

GREEN ZONE

Doing Well

- No cough, wheeze, chest tightness, or shortness of breath during the day or night
- Can do usual activities

And, if a peak flow meter is used,

Peak flow: more than _____
(80 percent or more of my best peak flow)

My best peak flow is: _____

Take these long-term control medicines each day (Include an anti-inflammatory).

Medicine	How much to take	When to take it
_____	_____	_____
_____	_____	_____
_____	_____	_____
_____	_____	_____
_____	_____	_____

| Before exercise | ❏ _____ | ❏ 2 or ❏ 4 puffs _____ | 5 minutes before exercise |

YELLOW ZONE

Asthma is Getting Worse

- Cough, wheeze, chest tightness, or shortness of breath, or
- Waking at night due to asthma, or
- Can do some, but not all, usual activities

-Or-

Peak flow: _____ to _____
(50 to 79 percent of my best peak flow)

My best peak flow is: _____

First Add: quick-relief medicine—and keep taking your GREEN ZONE medicine.

➡ _____ ❏ 2 or ❏ 4 puffs, every 20 minutes for up to 1 hour
(rescue inhaler) ❏ Nebulizer, once

Second **If your symptoms (and peak flow, if used) return to GREEN ZONE after 1 hour of above treatment:**
➡ ❏ Continue monitoring to be sure you stay in the green zone.
-Or-
If your symptoms (and peak flow, if used) do not return to GREEN ZONE after 1 hour of above treatment:
❏ Take: _____ ❏ 2 or ❏ 4 puffs or ❏ Nebulizer
(rescue inhaler)
❏ Add: _____ mg per day For _____ (3–10) days
(oral steroid)

❏ Call the doctor ❏ before/ ❏ within _____ hours after taking the oral steroid.

RED ZONE

Medical Alert!

- Very short of breath, or
- Quick-relief medicines have not helped, or
- Cannot do usual activities, or
- Symptoms are same or get worse after 24 hours in Yellow Zone

-Or-

Peak flow: less than _____
(50 percent of my best peak flow)

Take this medicine:

❏ _____ ❏ 4 or ❏ 6 puffs or ❏ Nebulizer
(rescue inhaler)

❏ _____ mg
(oral steroid)

Then call your doctor NOW. Go to the hospital or call an ambulance if:

- You are still in the red zone after 15 minutes AND
- You have not reached your doctor.

DANGER SIGNS
- Trouble walking and talking due to shortness of breath
- Lips or fingernails are blue

- **Take 4 or 6 puffs of your quick-relief medicine AND**
- **Go to the hospital or call for an ambulance _____ NOW!**
  (phone)

Adapted from ©www.nhlbi.nih.gov

CASE SCENARIO

ES is a 29-year-old male with asthma. He comes into the pharmacy asking for help interpreting his peak flow readings. He states that he feels fine, but is worried that his peak flow readings are declining. ES is able to demonstrate appropriate use of the peak flow meter, and reports that he has been checking at the appropriate time (first thing in the morning, before medications and taking the best of three readings). His personal best (PB) is 480 mL, and his readings from the last few days are as follows:

> Monday: 400 mL (83% PB)
> Tuesday: 388 mL (81% PB)
> Wednesday: 420 mL (88% PB)

What zone is ES in?
ES is in the green zone. All readings fall within 80–100% of his personal best.

What steps should ES take today?
ES should be advised to follow the instructions in his specific asthma action plan. Make sure this is filled out to include his medications (rescue and maintenance) and personal range of each zone:

- Green Zone (> 80%) = > 384 mL

- Yellow Zone (50–80%) = 240 mL–384 mL

- Red Zone (< 50%) = < 240 mL

Since he feels well and his peak flow readings are in the green zone, he should continue his maintenance medications. His action plan might include using a rescue inhaler prior to exercise. For anyone with asthma, it is important to avoid triggers and monitor for symptoms, regardless of peak flow readings.

KEY COUNSELING POINTS

SELECT METERED-DOSE INHALERS

Albuterol *(Ventolin HFA, ProAir HFA)*, budesonide/formoterol *(Symbicort, Breyna)*, fluticasone *(Flovent HFA)*, mometasone/formoterol *(Dulera)*, others

STEP 1	STEP 2	STEP 3
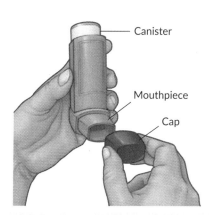	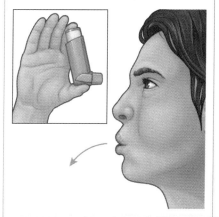	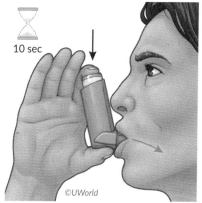

Canister

Mouthpiece

Cap

10 sec

©UWorld

Make sure the canister is fully inserted into the actuator (if it comes separately). Always use the actuator that came with the canister. Shake the inhaler well for 5 seconds immediately before each spray (except for *QVAR RediHaler, Atrovent HFA, Respimat* products or *Alvesco*, which do not need to be shaken). Remove cap from the mouthpiece and check mouthpiece for foreign objects prior to use.

Breathe out fully through your mouth, expelling as much air from your lungs as possible. Holding the inhaler upright (as shown in the picture), place the mouthpiece into your mouth and close your lips around it.

While breathing in slowly and deeply through your mouth, press the top of the canister all the way down with your index finger. Right after the spray comes out, take your finger off the canister. After you have inhaled all the way, take the inhaler out of your mouth and close your mouth. Hold your breath as long as possible, up to 10 seconds, then breathe normally. If another inhalation is needed, wait 1 minute and repeat Steps 1-3. Place cap back on the mouthpiece after use.

For any inhaler that contains an ICS (e.g., *Symbicort, Breyna, Dulera*): rinse your mouth with water and spit out the water to prevent thrush. Do not swallow the water.

TO PRIME

Ventolin HFA, ProAir HFA
Spray 4 times (3 for *ProAir*) away from the face, shaking between sprays. Prime again if > 14 days from last use or if you drop it.

Flovent HFA, Dulera
Spray 4 times away from the face, shaking between sprays. Prime again with just 1 spray if > 7 days from last use (> 5 days for *Dulera*).

Symbicort, Breyna
Spray 2 times away from the face, shaking between sprays. Prime again if > 7 days from last use or if you drop it.

TO CLEAN

Ventolin HFA, ProAir HFA
To prevent medication buildup and blockage, remove the metal canister (do not let this get wet) and rinse the mouthpiece only under warm running water for 30 seconds, then turn upside down and rinse under warm water for another 30 seconds. Shake to remove excess water and let air dry. Clean at least weekly.

Flovent HFA
Use a clean cotton swab dampened with water to clean the small circular opening where the medication sprays out. Gently twist the swab in a circular motion to remove any medication buildup. Do not take the canister out of the plastic actuator. Wipe the inside of the mouthpiece with a damp tissue. Let air dry overnight.

Symbicort, Breyna, Dulera
Wipe the inside and outside of the mouthpiece opening with a clean, dry cloth. Do not put into water. Clean every 7 days.

SELECT DRY POWDER INHALERS

Fluticasone/salmeterol (*Advair Diskus*)

STEP 1	STEP 2	STEP 3	STEP 4	STEP 5
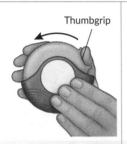	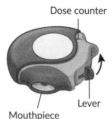	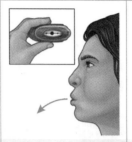	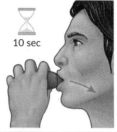	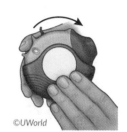
Hold the *Diskus* in your left hand and put the thumb of your right hand in the thumb grip. Push the thumb grip away from you as far as it will go until the mouthpiece appears and the *Diskus* snaps into position.	Hold the *Diskus* in a level, flat position with the mouthpiece towards you. Slide the lever away from the mouthpiece until it clicks.	Before using, breathe out fully while holding the *Diskus* <u>away from your mouth</u>. Do not tilt the *Diskus*.	Put the mouthpiece to your lips. Breathe in <u>quickly</u> and <u>deeply</u> through the inhaler. <u>Do not breathe in through your nose</u>. Remove the *Diskus* from your mouth and hold your breath as long as possible, up to 10 seconds. Then, breathe out slowly.	Close the *Diskus* by putting your thumb in the thumb grip and sliding it as far back towards you as it will go, until the *Diskus* clicks shut. <u>Rinse your mouth with water and spit out</u> the water to prevent thrush. Do not swallow the water.

TO CLEAN
<u>Do not wash</u> the *Diskus*. Store in a dry place.

Budesonide (*Pulmicort Flexhaler*)

STEP 1	STEP 2	STEP 3	STEP 4	STEP 5
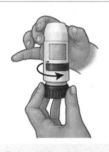	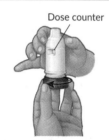	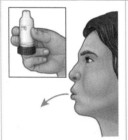	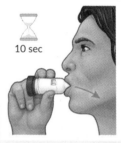	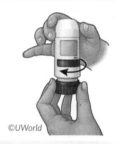
Twist off the white cover.	Holding the inhaler with one hand, <u>twist the brown base</u> fully in one direction as far as it will go with the other hand. Twist it back again in the other direction as far as it will go. You will hear a "click" during one of the twisting movements. The dose is now loaded (note: only one dose is loaded at a time, no matter how often you twist the brown base, but the dose counter will continue to advance).	Hold the inhaler upright in one hand. Turn your <u>head away</u> from the inhaler and breathe out fully.	Place the mouthpiece in your mouth and close your lips around the mouthpiece. Breathe in <u>deeply</u> and <u>forcefully</u> through the inhaler. Remove the inhaler from your mouth and breathe out.	Replace the white cover on the inhaler and twist shut. <u>Rinse your mouth with water and spit out the water</u> to prevent thrush.

TO PRIME
Twist off the white cover. Holding the inhaler upright, <u>twist the brown base</u> fully in one direction as far as it will go and then fully back. You will hear a "click" during one of the twisting motions. Repeat twisting motion again (back and forth). The inhaler is <u>now primed</u> and ready to load your first dose. This inhaler does <u>not</u> need to be <u>primed again</u> (even after long periods of no use).

TO CLEAN
<u>Wipe</u> the mouthpiece with a <u>dry tissue</u> weekly. Do not use water or immerse it in water.

Albuterol *(ProAir RespiClick)*, fluticasone/salmeterol *(AirDuo RespiClick)*

STEP 1	STEP 2	STEP 3

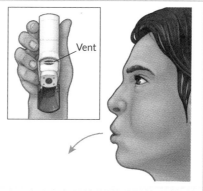

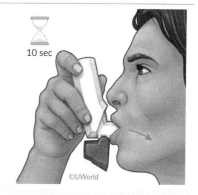

Make sure the cap is closed before each dose. Hold the inhaler upright as you open the cap fully. Open the cap all the way back until you hear a "click." Your inhaler is now ready to use. Do not open the cap unless you are taking a dose. Note: opening and closing the cap without inhaling a dose will waste medication and can damage your inhaler.	Turn your head away from the inhaler so you do not breathe into the mouthpiece. Breathe out through your mouth and push as much air from your lungs as you can.	Put the mouthpiece in your mouth and close your lips around it. Breathe in quickly and deeply through your mouth, until your lungs feel completely full of air. Do not let your lips or fingers block the vent above the mouthpiece. Hold your breath for as long as possible, up to 10 seconds. Remove the inhaler from your mouth. Check the dose counter on the back of the inhaler to make sure you received the dose. Close the cap over the mouthpiece after each use of the inhaler. Make sure the cap closes firmly into place. For *AirDuo RespiClick*: rinse your mouth with water and spit out the water to prevent thrush. Do not swallow the water.

TO PRIME
None needed.

TO CLEAN
Keep your inhaler dry and clean at all times. Do not wash or put any part of your inhaler in water. If the mouthpiece needs cleaning, gently wipe it with a dry cloth or tissue after using.

ALL PATIENTS WITH ASTHMA

See the Drug Formulations and Patient Counseling chapter for language/layman's terminology.

- Always have your rescue inhaler with you for asthma attacks.
- If asthma symptoms get worse, or if you increase the use of your rescue inhaler for asthma attacks, contact your healthcare provider right away.

MONTELUKAST *(SINGULAIR)*

- Take in the evening.
- Can cause suicidal ideation, behavior and mood changes.
- Do not use more than one dose within 24 hours. If using daily for another indication, do not take another dose to prevent exercise-induced asthma.
- Oral granules:
  - ❏ Administer within 15 minutes of opening the packet.
  - ❏ Can be mixed with a teaspoonful of baby formula, breast milk, applesauce, mashed carrots, rice or ice cream or given directly in the mouth.

BUDESONIDE *(PULMICORT RESPULES)*

- Store upright, protected from light, at room temperature.
- Ampules should be used within two weeks of opening the aluminum package.
- Gently swirl the ampule in a circular motion before use.
- Rinse mouth with water and spit it out after each dose. If a face mask was used, wash face after each treatment.

Select Guidelines/References

Global Initiative for Asthma (GINA). Global Strategy for Asthma Management and Prevention, 2023. http://www.ginasthma.org.

National Heart, Lung and Blood Institute. Expert Panel Report 3: Guidelines for the Diagnosis and Management of Asthma. August 2007.

National Heart, Lung and Blood Institute. 2020 Focused Updates to the Asthma Management Guidelines: A Report from the National Asthma Education and Prevention Program Coordinating Committee Expert Panel Working Group. December 2020.

CONTENT LEGEND

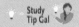
Study Tip Gal

Healthy   Emphysema

Alveolar membranes breakdown

Healthy   Chronic Bronchitis

Inflammation and excess mucus

tolgasez33/stock.adobe.com

CHAPTER 42

CHRONIC OBSTRUCTIVE PULMONARY DISEASE (COPD)

BACKGROUND

Chronic obstructive pulmonary disease (COPD) is a respiratory condition that causes obstructed airflow from the lungs. It is one of the leading causes of death worldwide. COPD is most commonly caused by tobacco smoke, but can be caused by other air pollutants (e.g., smoke from fires or coal burning, marijuana, occupational hazards). Long-term exposure to these gases or particles causes chronic inflammation in the lungs, eventually resulting in emphysema and/or bronchitis.

Emphysema is the destruction of the small passages in the lungs, called alveoli. Bronchitis (or bronchiolitis) is inflammation and narrowing of the bronchial tubes and results in mucus production. Individuals with alpha-1 antitrypsin (AAT) deficiency, a genetic condition, have a higher risk of developing COPD because AAT helps protect the lungs from damage caused by inflammation.

DIAGNOSIS

COPD should be suspected in any patient with chronic, progressive symptoms [e.g., dyspnea (shortness of breath), cough, sputum production, wheezing] and risk factors (e.g., tobacco smoke exposure). Other common reasons for shortness of breath and cough should be ruled out, such as asthma, chronic heart failure and pulmonary infections (e.g., tuberculosis).

Asthma is the most difficult to differentiate from COPD (see Study Tip Gal on the following page). The limitation of airflow in asthma is reversible with medication. In COPD, the limitation of airflow is not fully reversible and progresses over time, leading to a gradual loss of lung function.

Spirometry is required to assess lung function and make a diagnosis of COPD. It provides an objective measurement of airflow obstruction and is the most reproducible test available. Spirometry measures the total amount of air a person can breathe out (forced vital capacity, or FVC) and the amount of air exhaled in one second (forced expiratory volume, or FEV1). A post-bronchodilator FEV1/FVC < 0.70 confirms a diagnosis of COPD.

KEY DIFFERENCES BETWEEN COPD AND ASTHMA

FEATURE	COPD	ASTHMA
Age of onset	Usually > 40 years	Usually < 40 years
Smoking history	Usually > 20 years	Uncommon
Sputum production	Common	Infrequent
Allergies	Uncommon	Common
Symptoms	Persistent	Intermittent and variable
Disease process	Progressive, worsens over time	Stable, does not worsen over time
Exacerbations	A common complication	A common complication
First-line treatment	Bronchodilators	Inhaled corticosteroids

COPD ASSESSMENT

A COPD assessment includes the following four components:

- Degree of airflow limitation
- Symptom assessment
- Risk of exacerbations
- Presence of comorbidities

DEGREE OF AIRFLOW LIMITATION

The post-bronchodilator FEV1, assessed using spirometry, determines the severity of airflow limitation. The GOLD guidelines use a grading system of 1 – 4 to classify patients based on spirometry results. The grade assignment is used to assess prognosis and disease progression.

Severity of Post-Bronchodilator Airflow Limitation

GRADE	SEVERITY	AIRFLOW LIMITATION
In patients with FEV1/FVC < 0.70		
GOLD 1	Mild	FEV1 ≥ 80% predicted
GOLD 2	Moderate	FEV1 50-79% predicted
GOLD 3	Severe	FEV1 30-49% predicted
GOLD 4	Very severe	FEV1 < 30% predicted

SYMPTOM ASSESSMENT

Scoring systems are used for symptom assessment and are integral to selecting drug treatment. The two most commonly used scoring systems are described below; higher scores indicate worse symptoms.

- Modified British Medical Research Council (mMRC) dyspnea scale: assesses breathlessness, with scores ranging from 0 – 4.
- COPD Assessment Test (CAT): assesses a range of symptoms (e.g., cough, mucus production, chest tightness, energy level, breathlessness), with scores ranging from 0 – 40.

The application of these two scoring systems is shown in the Combined Assessment of COPD chart and case scenarios on the following page.

RISK OF EXACERBATIONS

A COPD exacerbation is an increase in respiratory symptoms that worsen over < 14 days. The risk of exacerbations increases as airflow limitation worsens. Hospitalization for an exacerbation is associated with an increased risk of death. Taking measures to prevent and quickly treat exacerbations is an important component of COPD management.

COMORBIDITIES

Comorbid conditions, such as cardiovascular diseases, osteoporosis, diabetes, depression, anxiety, skeletal muscle dysfunction, respiratory infections and lung cancer should be monitored and treated appropriately. Poor control of comorbid conditions can independently influence mortality and hospitalizations.

COMBINED ASSESSMENT OF COPD

The combined assessment of COPD focuses on symptom assessment and risk of exacerbations as the critical components that drive treatment. Symptoms should be assessed using the mMRC or CAT, and history of exacerbations in the past year should be documented. The patient is then assigned to a group (A, B or E), which determines the initial treatment warranted (see Initial Pharmacologic Therapy on the following page).

An exacerbation is classified as moderate if it required treatment with an oral steroid ± antibiotics.

CASE SCENARIOS

These examples illustrate how the combined assessment is used to direct treatment.

Patient 1: a 62-year-old male with FEV1/FVC < 0.7 and FEV1 40% predicted has a CAT score of 16 and no exacerbations in the past year. *Assessment:* confirmed diagnosis of COPD, GOLD grade 3, group B.

Patient 2: a 62-year-old female with FEV1/FVC < 0.7 and FEV1 40% predicted has a CAT score of 16 and 2 exacerbations in the past year, one of which required hospitalization. *Assessment:* confirmed diagnosis of COPD, GOLD grade 3, group E.

Both patients have the same disease severity (based on FEV1 and CAT scores). In both cases, better symptom control is needed, but patient 2 requires more intensive treatment due to her history of exacerbations. See the section on Initial Pharmacologic Therapy to review the differences in treatment recommendations.

NON-DRUG TREATMENT

Smoking cessation is an essential management strategy proven to slow the progression of COPD. Healthcare providers should encourage all tobacco users to quit using proven strategies (see Tobacco Cessation chapter). Vaccinations reduce the risk of hospitalizations and death due to serious respiratory illness. Patients with COPD should receive all age-appropriate vaccines per ACIP recommendations, including an annual influenza vaccine and pneumococcal vaccinations (see Immunizations chapter).

To improve outcomes, it is essential to routinely assess inhaler technique (see detailed instructions on inhaler use, priming and cleaning at the end of the chapter) and adherence. Pulmonary rehabilitation programs help improve quality of life and symptoms. Long-term oxygen treatment has been shown to increase survival in patients with severe resting hypoxemia.

DRUG TREATMENT

The medications used to treat COPD decrease symptoms and/or prevent complications, such as exacerbations and hospitalizations. A patient's treatment regimen should be individualized based on CAT and/or mMRC score and risk of exacerbations (see the ABE assessment chart to the left and initial treatment recommendations in the table below).

Bronchodilators are the first-line treatment for all patients. A short-acting beta-2 agonist (SABA) or short-acting muscarinic antagonist (SAMA) can be used as needed for patients with intermittent symptoms, or a long-acting beta-2 agonist (LABA) and/or long-acting muscarinic antagonist (LAMA) may be appropriate.

Inhaled corticosteroids (ICS) (see Asthma chapter) are recommended in select patients with a history of exacerbations and an eosinophil count (a marker of inflammation) ≥ 300 cells/μL. ICS have a risk of adverse effects (e.g., pneumonia, oral candidiasis, hoarse voice) that can limit their use (see the Escalation of Treatment algorithm on the following page). An ICS is not recommended in patients with lower eosinophil counts (< 100 cells/μL) because there is no demonstrated benefit.

Combination treatment is often required (e.g., LABA + LAMA ± ICS); in this case, use of a single inhaler containing 2 - 3 medications is preferred to improve adherence. All patients receiving long-acting bronchodilators should be prescribed a SABA and/or SAMA to relieve acute symptoms as needed.

Other, less commonly used treatments include azithromycin and the phosphodiesterase-4 (PDE-4) inhibitor roflumilast, which are used in only the most severe cases. Long-term monotherapy with oral steroids is not recommended.

INITIAL PHARMACOLOGIC THERAPY

PATIENT GROUP	RECOMMENDED TREATMENT*
A	A bronchodilator: SAMA PRN, SABA PRN, LAMA or LABA**
B	LAMA + LABA
E	LAMA + LABA If blood eosinophils ≥ 300 cells/μL, consider: LAMA + LABA + ICS

*All patients receiving LAMA and/or LABA treatment should receive rescue therapy with a SABA and/or SAMA.

**Long-acting bronchodilators (i.e., LAMA or LABA) are preferred over short-acting bronchodilators (i.e., SAMA or SABA), except for patients with only occasional dyspnea.

ESCALATION OF TREATMENT

An assessment of inhaler use and adherence, non-pharmacologic measures, symptoms and exacerbations is repeated at each follow-up visit. If there was an appropriate response to treatment, no medication changes are necessary. If the response was not appropriate, treatment should be escalated based on the primary concern (dyspnea or exacerbations).

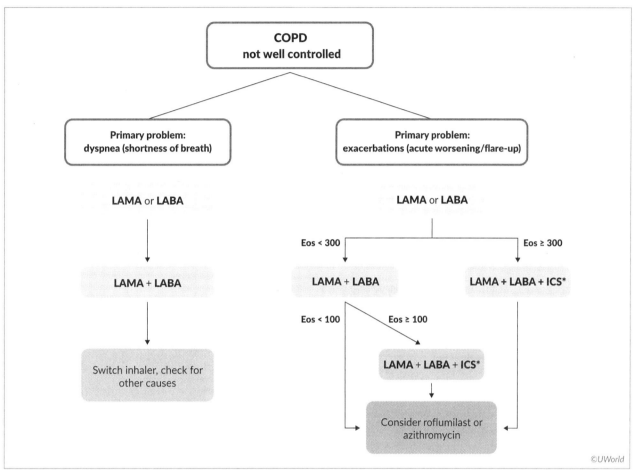

Eos = blood eosinophils (cells/μL)
*De-escalate (remove ICS) or decrease ICS dose if significant adverse effects occur (consider risk of increased exacerbations).

COPD EXACERBATIONS

COPD exacerbations can be caused by respiratory tract infections (viral or bacterial) or other factors, such as increased air pollution. Treatment includes a SABA with or without a SAMA. If the exacerbation is moderate or severe, injectable or oral systemic steroids are typically used. If there is sputum purulence with increased sputum volume or dyspnea, or if mechanical ventilation is required, antibiotics should be used (see Infectious Diseases II chapter).

INHALER PRODUCTS

Inhaled medications are preferred for COPD. There are two categories of inhalers: metered-dose inhalers (MDIs) and dry powder inhalers (DPIs). Consult the Asthma chapter for a review of the differences between these two inhaler types and for a list of maintenance inhalers that are indicated in asthma vs. COPD. A review of appropriate technique is provided for select inhalers at the end of this chapter and the Asthma chapter.

MUSCARINIC ANTAGONISTS/ANTICHOLINERGICS

Muscarinic antagonists (also called anticholinergics) cause bronchodilation by blocking the constricting action of acetylcholine at M3 muscarinic receptors in bronchial smooth muscle. Medications in this class are generally well tolerated.

DRUG	DOSING	SAFETY/SIDE EFFECTS/MONITORING
Short-acting muscarinic antagonist (SAMA)		**WARNINGS** Use with caution in patients with narrow-angle glaucoma, urinary retention, benign prostatic hyperplasia or bladder neck obstruction
Ipratropium bromide (Atrovent HFA) 17 mcg/inh	MDI: 2 inhalations Q4-6H PRN	
Nebulizer solution 0.02%	Nebulizer: 0.5 mg Q6-8H PRN	**SIDE EFFECTS** Dry mouth, upper respiratory tract infections (nasopharyngitis, sinusitis), cough, bitter taste
+ albuterol (Combivent Respimat) 20 mcg ipratropium + 100 mcg albuterol/inh	MDI: 1 inhalation Q4-6H PRN	
Nebulizer solution 0.5 mg ipratropium + 2.5 mg albuterol per 3 mL	Nebulizer: 3 mL Q4-6H PRN	**MONITORING** S/sx at each visit, smoking status, COPD questionnaires, annual spirometry
Long-acting muscarinic antagonists (LAMAs)		**NOTES** Avoid spraying in the eyes
Tiotropium		
Spiriva HandiHaler 18 mcg capsule	DPI: inhale contents of 1 capsule via HandiHaler device daily (requires 2 puffs)	HandiHaler devices are DPIs that come with a capsule that is placed into the device; do not swallow the capsules by mouth
Spiriva Respimat 2.5 mcg/inh	MDI: 2 inhalations daily	
+ olodaterol (Stiolto Respimat)		Pressair devices are DPIs that have an indicator window that turns from green to red if the dose was inhaled properly
Aclidinium (Tudorza Pressair) 400 mcg/inh	DPI: 1 inhalation BID	
+ formoterol (Duaklir Pressair)		ICS-containing products: rinse mouth with water and spit to prevent oral candidiasis (thrush)
Glycopyrrolate (only in combination products)	MDI: 2 inhalations BID	
+ formoterol (Bevespi Aerosphere)		
+ formoterol/budesonide (Breztri Aerosphere)		
Revefenacin (Yupelri) 175 mcg/inh nebulizer solution	Nebulizer: 175 mcg daily	
Umeclidinium (Incruse Ellipta) 62.5 mcg/inh	DPI: 1 inhalation daily	
+ vilanterol (Anoro Ellipta)		
+ vilanterol/fluticasone (Trelegy Ellipta)		

BETA-2 AGONISTS

Beta-2 agonists bind to beta-2 receptors in the lung, causing relaxation of bronchial smooth muscle and bronchodilation. LABAs can be used as monotherapy only for COPD, not asthma (see Boxed Warning below). SABAs are discussed in more detail in the Asthma chapter.

DRUG	DOSING	SAFETY/SIDE EFFECTS/MONITORING
Long-acting beta-2 agonists (LABAs)		**BOXED WARNINGS** LABAs increase the risk of asthma-related deaths when used alone; they should only be used in asthma patients who are currently receiving but are not adequately controlled on an inhaled corticosteroid
Salmeterol (Serevent Diskus) 50 mcg/inh **+ fluticasone (Advair Diskus, Wixela Inhub)**	DPI: 1 inhalation BID	
Formoterol (Perforomist) 20 mcg/2 mL nebulizer solution **+ budesonide (Symbicort, Breyna)** + glycopyrrolate (Bevespi Aerosphere) **+ glycopyrrolate/budesonide (Breztri Aerosphere)** + aclidinium (Duaklir Pressair)	Nebulizer: 20 mcg BID MDI: 2 inhalations BID DPI: 1 inhalation BID	**CONTRAINDICATIONS** Status asthmaticus, acute episodes of asthma or COPD, monotherapy in the treatment of asthma **SIDE EFFECTS** Nervousness, tremor, tachycardia, palpitations, hyperglycemia, ↓ K, cough
Arformoterol (Brovana) 15 mcg/2 mL nebulizer solution	Nebulizer: 15 mcg BID	**MONITORING** S/sx at each visit, smoking status, COPD questionnaires, annual spirometry
Olodaterol (Striverdi Respimat) 2.5 mcg/inh + tiotropium (Stiolto Respimat)	MDI: 2 inhalations daily	**NOTES** Arformoterol contains the R-isomer of formoterol ICS-containing products: rinse mouth with water and spit to prevent oral candidiasis (thrush)
Vilanterol (only in combination products) 25 mcg/inh **+ fluticasone (Breo Ellipta)** + umeclidinium (Anoro Ellipta) **+ umeclidinium/fluticasone (Trelegy Ellipta)**	 DPI: 1 inhalation daily	

PHOSPHODIESTERASE-4 INHIBITOR

Roflumilast is a PDE-4 inhibitor that ↑ cAMP levels, leading to a reduction in lung inflammation. This medication should be used in combination with at least one long-acting bronchodilator; its use is reserved for patients with very severe COPD, chronic bronchitis and a history of exacerbations.

DRUG	DOSING	SAFETY/SIDE EFFECTS/MONITORING
Roflumilast (Daliresp) Tablet	Start 250 mcg PO daily for 4 weeks (to improve tolerability), then 500 mcg PO daily	**CONTRAINDICATIONS** Moderate to severe liver impairment **WARNINGS** Weight loss, psychiatric events (depression, mood changes) including suicidality **SIDE EFFECTS** Diarrhea, nausea, ↓ appetite, insomnia, headache **MONITORING** S/sx at each visit, LFTs, smoking status, COPD questionnaires, annual spirometry

Roflumilast Drug Interactions

- Roflumilast is a substrate of CYP450 3A4 and 1A2. Use with strong enzyme inducers (e.g., carbamazepine, phenobarbital, phenytoin, rifampin) is not recommended. Use with CYP3A4 inhibitors or dual CYP3A4 and CYP1A2 inhibitors (e.g., erythromycin, ketoconazole, fluvoxamine, cimetidine) will ↑ roflumilast levels.

KEY COUNSELING POINTS

SELECT METERED-DOSE INHALERS

Ipratropium bromide (*Atrovent HFA*)

STEP 1	STEP 2	STEP 3
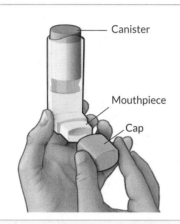	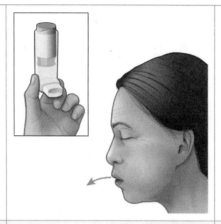	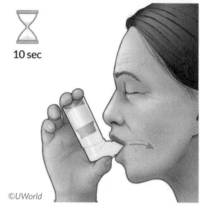
Make sure the canister is fully inserted into the actuator (if it comes separately). The *Atrovent HFA* plastic actuator should only be used with the *Atrovent HFA* canister. Remove the protective dust cap from the mouthpiece and check mouthpiece for foreign objects prior to use. You do not have to shake *Atrovent HFA* before using it.	Breathe out fully through your mouth. Holding the inhaler upright (as shown in the picture), place the mouthpiece into your mouth and close your lips around it. Keep your eyes closed so that no medication will be sprayed into your eyes.	While breathing in slowly and deeply through your mouth, press the top of the canister all the way down with your index finger. Hold your breath as long as possible, up to 10 seconds, then breathe out slowly. If another inhalation is needed, wait at least 15 seconds and repeat Steps 1-3. Place cap back on the mouthpiece after use.

TO PRIME

Spray 2 times away from the face. Prime again if > 3 days from last use.

TO CLEAN

Remove the dust cap and metal canister (do not let this get wet) and rinse the mouthpiece under warm running water for 30 seconds. Shake to remove excess water and let air dry. Clean at least weekly.

Respimat products:

- **Albuterol/ipratropium** *(Combivent Respimat)*
- **Olodaterol** *(Striverdi Respimat)*
- **Olodaterol/tiotropium** *(Stiolto Respimat)*
- **Tiotropium** *(Spiriva Respimat)*

STEP 1	STEP 2	STEP 3
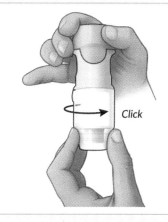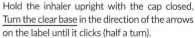	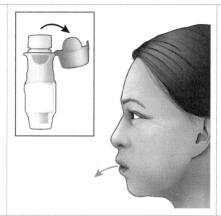	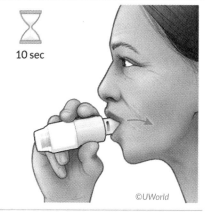
Hold the inhaler upright with the cap closed. <u>Turn the clear base</u> in the direction of the arrows on the label until it clicks (half a turn).	<u>Open the cap</u> until it snaps fully open. Turn head away from the inhaler and <u>breathe out</u> slowly and fully.	Close lips around the end of the mouthpiece without covering the air vents. While taking a slow, deep breath through your mouth, <u>press</u> the dose release button and continue to breathe in slowly. Hold <u>your breath as long as possible, up to 10 seconds</u>. Close the cap when finished.

©UWorld

To simplify these steps for patient counseling, think: **TOP**

 T   **O**   **P**

TURN	**OPEN**	**PRESS**
the clear base	the cap and close your lips around the mouthpiece	the dose-release button and inhale

TO ASSEMBLE DEVICE FOR FIRST USE	**TO PRIME**	**TO CLEAN**
With the cap closed, press the safety catch while pulling off the clear base. Do not touch the piercing element located inside the bottom of the clear base. Write the discard by date on the inhaler's label (which is 3 months from the date the cartridge is inserted). Push the narrow end of the cartridge into the inhaler and push down firmly until it clicks into place. Put the clear base back into place until it clicks. Do not remove the clear base or the cartridge once assembled.	Hold the inhaler upright with the cap closed. Turn the clear base in the direction of the arrows on the label until it clicks (half a turn). Flip the cap until it snaps fully open. Point the inhaler toward the ground away from your face. Press the dose release button. Close cap. Repeat these steps over again until a spray is visible. Once the spray is visible, repeat the steps 3 more times to make sure the inhaler is prepared for use. If inhaler is not used for > 3 days, release 1 spray toward the ground to prepare the inhaler. If inhaler has not been used for > 21 days, follow priming instructions above for initial use.	Clean the mouthpiece, including the metal part inside the mouthpiece, with a <u>damp cloth or tissue weekly</u>.

SELECT DRY POWDER INHALERS

Tiotropium (*Spiriva HandiHaler*)

STEP 1	STEP 2	STEP 3	STEP 4	STEP 5
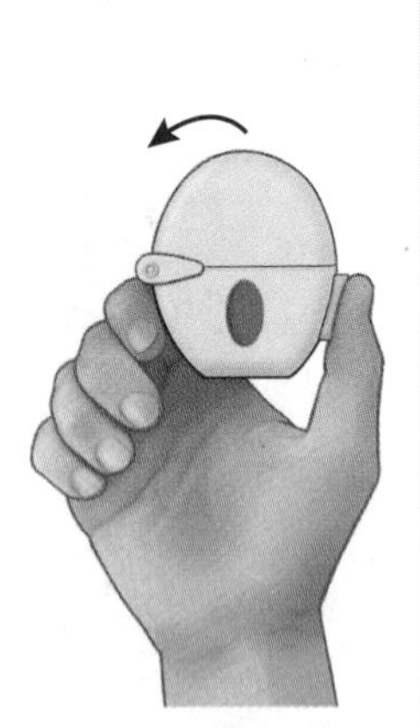	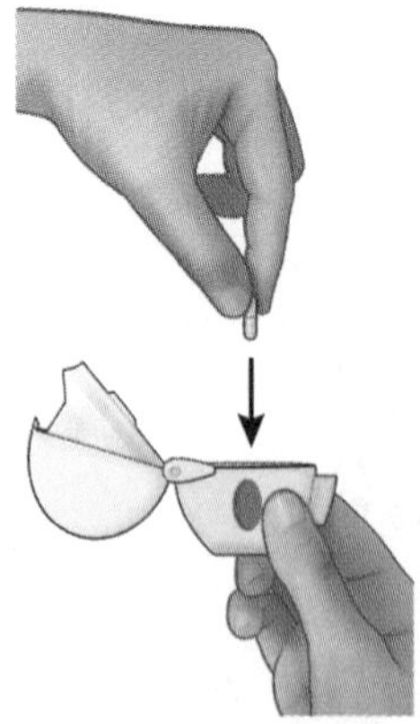	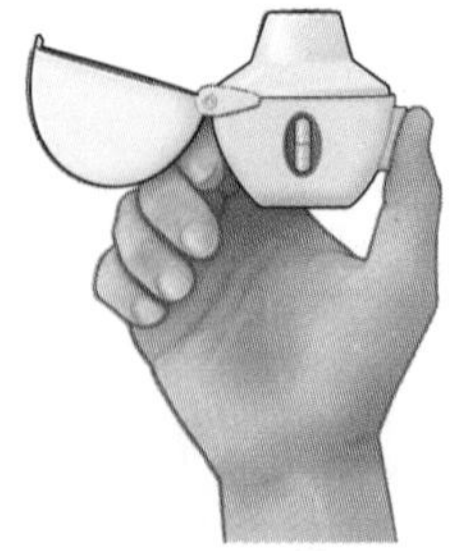	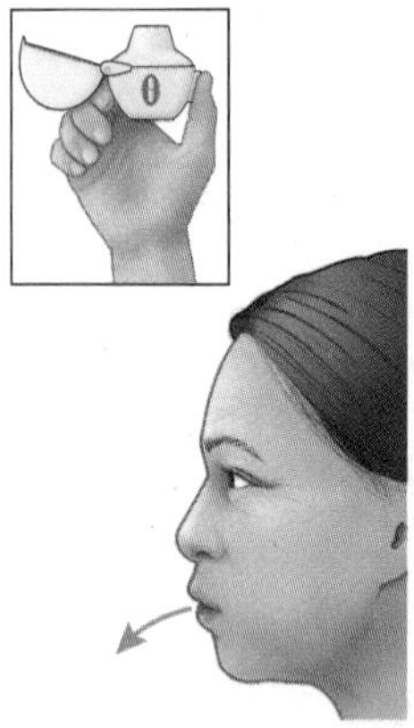	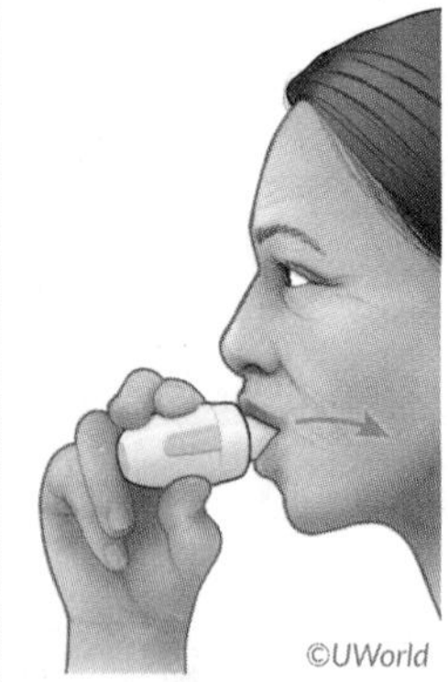
Open the *HandiHaler* device by pressing on the green button and lifting the cap upwards. Open the mouthpiece by pulling the mouthpiece ridge up and away from the base so the center chamber is showing.	Remove a *Spiriva* capsule from the blister pack and insert it into the chamber (do NOT swallow the capsule). Firmly close the mouthpiece against the gray base until you hear a click.	Press the green piercing button once until it is flat (flush) against the base, then release. Do not shake the device.	Turn head away from the inhaler and breathe out fully.	Raise the *HandiHaler* to your mouth in a horizontal position and close your lips around the mouthpiece. Breathe in deeply and fully. You should hear or feel the *Spiriva* capsule vibrate (rattle). Remove inhaler from your mouth and hold your breath for as long as is comfortable. Breathe normally. To get the full dose, you must inhale twice from each capsule. Repeat steps 4 and 5, breathing out fully, then breathing in deeply and fully through the inhaler. Tip out the used capsule into a trash can after 2 inhalations. Do not touch the capsule. Close the device lid.

©UWorld

TO CLEAN

Clean inhaler monthly, or as needed. Rinse inhaler under warm water. Make sure any powder build-up is removed. Let air dry. It takes 24 hours to air dry the *HandiHaler* device after it is cleaned.

Aclidinium *(Tudorza Pressair)*, aclidinium/formoterol *(Duaklir Pressair)*

STEP 1	STEP 2	STEP 3	STEP 4
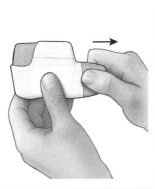	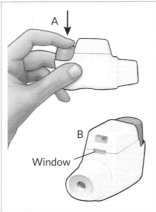	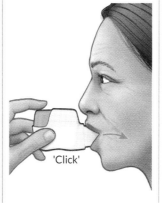	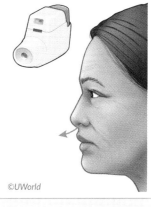
Remove the protective cap by lightly squeezing the arrows marked on each side of the cap and pulling outwards. Check the mouthpiece for foreign objects.	Hold the inhaler with the mouthpiece facing you and the green button straight above. Before putting into your mouth, press the green button all the way down and release. Check the control window; the dose is ready for inhalation if it changed from <u>red to green</u>. Breathe out completely, away from the inhaler.	Put your lips tightly around the mouthpiece. <u>Breathe in quickly</u> and <u>deeply</u> through your mouth. Breathe in until you hear a <u>"click"</u> sound and keep breathing in to get the full dose. Do not hold down the green button while breathing in.	Remove the inhaler from your mouth and hold your breath for as long as comfortable. Then breathe out slowly away from the inhaler. Place the protective cap on the inhaler. Check that the control <u>window has turned to red</u> which indicates the full dose has been inhaled correctly.

In Step 2 image: "A", "Window", "B" labels. In Step 3 image: "'Click'". ©UWorld

TO CLEAN

Routine cleaning is not required. If needed, wipe the outside of the mouthpiece with a dry tissue or paper towel.

Ellipta products:

- **Fluticasone (*Arnuity Ellipta*)**
- **Fluticasone/vilanterol (*Breo Ellipta*)**
- **Umeclidinium (*Incruse Ellipta*)**

- **Umeclidinium/vilanterol (*Anoro Ellipta*)**
- **Umeclidinium/vilanterol/fluticasone (*Trelegy Ellipta*)**

STEP 1	STEP 2	STEP 3
	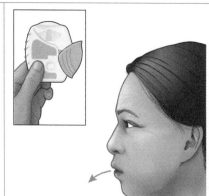	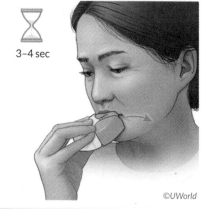
Open the cover of the inhaler by sliding the cover down to expose the mouthpiece. You should hear a "click." The counter will count down by 1 number, indicating that the inhaler is ready to use. If you open and close the cover without inhaling the medication, the dose will be lost. It is not possible to accidentally take a double dose or an extra dose in 1 inhalation.	While holding the inhaler away from your mouth, breathe out fully. Do not breathe out into the mouthpiece.	Put the mouthpiece between your lips and close your lips firmly around it. Take one long, steady, deep breath in through your mouth. Do not block the air vent with your fingers. Remove inhaler from mouth and hold your breath for 3-4 seconds or as long as comfortable. Breathe out slowly and gently. Close the inhaler. For ICS products: rinse your mouth with water and spit out the water to prevent thrush.

TO CLEAN
Routine cleaning is not required. If needed, you can clean the mouthpiece using a dry tissue before you close the cover.

Select Guidelines/References

Global Strategy for the Diagnosis, Management, and Prevention of COPD, 2024 Report. Global Initiative for Chronic Obstructive Lung Disease (GOLD). http://www.goldcopd.org (accessed 2023 Nov 15).

THE "5 A'S" MODEL FOR TREATING TOBACCO USE AND DEPENDENCE

<u>Ask</u> about tobacco use
Identify and document tobacco use status for every patient at every visit.

<u>Advise</u> to quit
In a clear, strong and personalized manner, urge every tobacco user to quit.

<u>Assess</u> readiness to quit
Is the tobacco user willing to quit at this time (e.g., in the next month)?

<u>Assist</u> in quit attempt
For the patient willing to make a quit attempt, offer medication (if appropriate) and provide, or refer for, behavioral counseling.

For patients unwilling to quit at this time, provide motivational interventions designed to encourage a future quit attempt.

For the recent quitter or any patient with remaining challenges, provide relapse prevention.

<u>Arrange</u> follow up
For the patient willing to make a quit attempt, arrange follow-up visits within the first week after the quit date.

For patients unwilling to make a quit attempt at this time, address tobacco dependence and willingness to quit at the next clinic visit.

CONTENT LEGEND

 Study Tip Gal    Required Formula

---

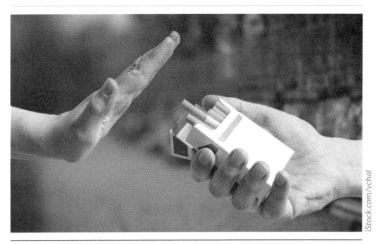

iStock.com/vchal

CHAPTER 43

TOBACCO CESSATION

BACKGROUND

Smoking is the leading cause of preventable death in the U.S. and a known risk factor for heart disease, stroke, pregnancy complications, COPD, multiple cancers and many other diseases. In some cases, disease risk (e.g., lung cancer) is related to an individual's <u>pack-year smoking history</u>, which can be calculated using the formula below.

$$\text{Pack-year smoking history} = \text{cigarette packs / day} \times \text{number of years smoked}$$

For example, a patient who has smoked 2 packs (i.e., 40 cigarettes) per day for 10 years has a 20 pack-year smoking history.

Tobacco use disorder is a chronic disease that often requires repeated interventions and multiple attempts to quit. Nicotine and other chemicals in cigarettes activate nicotinic receptors; this leads to an increase in dopamine release and activation of the dopamine reward system, making quitting difficult. However, effective treatments are available that can assist in quitting and significantly increase long-term abstinence rates. It is essential for healthcare providers to <u>ask patients about tobacco use</u>, document the response and provide treatment (see the "5 A's" Model). A national network of tobacco quit-lines is available by telephone for patients at 1-800-QUIT-NOW (1-800-784-8669).

TREATMENT PRINCIPLES

<u>Counseling</u> is an essential component of tobacco cessation treatment, and two especially effective methods are behavioral counseling (e.g., problem-solving skills training) and social support. A strong correlation exists between quitting success and counseling intensity (i.e., length and number of counseling sessions).

<u>Medications</u> should be <u>encouraged</u> for <u>all patients</u> attempting to quit, <u>except</u> when medically <u>contraindicated</u>. Medications reduce

withdrawal symptoms, including anxiety, irritability, depression, insomnia, poor concentration, restlessness, increased appetite and an urge to smoke (cravings). The combination of counseling and medication is more effective than using either strategy alone.

There are several effective, first-line options:

- Five nicotine replacement therapies (NRTs): patch, gum, lozenge, inhaler or nasal spray.
- Two non-nicotine drugs: bupropion and varenicline.

Combining two drugs, such as using a nicotine patch with short-acting NRT (e.g., gum) or a nicotine patch with varenicline, is effective and can be used first-line.

EXCEPTIONS TO DRUG TREATMENT

Behavioral counseling is preferred over drugs for several patient populations due to limited evidence of safety or effectiveness of smoking cessation medications. This includes pregnant women, adolescents, smokeless tobacco users (e.g., chewing tobacco) and "light" smokers (e.g., < 10 cigarettes a day).

ELECTRONIC CIGARETTES

Electronic nicotine delivery systems, such as electronic cigarettes or e-cigarettes, are not recommended for smoking cessation due to health concerns; they increase carcinogen exposure and can cause e-cigarette or vaping product use associated lung injury (EVALI) and nicotine addiction.

SMOKING AND DRUG INTERACTIONS

The non-nicotine chemicals in tobacco smoke induce CYP450 enzymes, primarily CYP450 1A2. Smokers who quit no longer have CYP1A2 induction and, as a result, can experience side effects from supratherapeutic levels of caffeine, theophylline, fluvoxamine, olanzapine, clozapine and the R-isomer (less potent isomer) of warfarin.

Women ≥ 35 years of age who smoke should not take estrogen-containing oral contraceptives due to an increased risk of cardiovascular events.

VACCINATIONS IN SMOKERS

Smokers age 19 – 64 years old should receive a pneumococcal vaccine, an annual influenza vaccine and all age-appropriate vaccines (see the Immunizations chapter).

DRUG TREATMENT

NICOTINE REPLACEMENT THERAPY (NRT)

Nicotine replacement therapy (NRT) provides nicotine without the use of tobacco; this helps to ease withdrawal symptoms and break the habit of smoking. Combination therapy with the long-acting patch and a short-acting NRT (e.g., gum or lozenge) is more effective than monotherapy and can be recommended first-line.

DRUG	DOSING	SAFETY/SIDE EFFECTS/MONITORING
Nicotine patch (**NicoDerm CQ,** others) OTC	Initial dose is based on the number of cigarettes smoked per day See Study Tip Gal on next page	**WARNINGS** Avoid in immediate post-MI period, life-threatening arrhythmias, severe or worsening angina and pregnancy* Inhaler/nasal spray: avoid in asthma, COPD and other chronic respiratory diseases
Nicotine gum (**Nicorette,** others) OTC **Nicotine lozenge** (**Nicorette Mini,** others) OTC	Initial dose is based on the timing of the first cigarette smoked upon waking up See Study Tip Gal on next page	**SIDE EFFECTS** Insomnia, headache, dizziness, nervousness, dyspepsia Patch: vivid dreams, skin irritation Inhaler: mouth and throat irritation, cough, rhinitis Nasal spray: nasal irritation, watery eyes, sneezing, transient changes in taste and smell
Nicotine inhaler (Nicotrol) Rx	6-16 cartridges daily for up to 12 wks, then taper frequency of use over 6-12 wks Use up to 6 months	**NOTES** The FDA prohibits sale of nicotine products to individuals < 21 years of age; identification required to purchase Patch: highest adherence rate; remove before an MRI
Nicotine nasal spray (Nicotrol NS) Rx	1 dose = 1 spray in each nostril; use 1-2 doses per hour, ↑ PRN for symptom relief Min: 8 doses/day Max: 5 doses/hr or 40 doses/day Use up to 3 months	Gum and lozenge (sugar-free): 4 mg strength can reduce or delay weight gain; acidic beverages/foods ↓ buccal absorption, do not eat/drink 15 minutes before or during use Inhaler: mimics the hand to mouth smoking action, providing a coping mechanism Nasal spray: fastest delivery (useful for rapid relief of withdrawal symptoms); has the highest risk of dependence

*Package labeling warns of NRT use in these situations, but in practice, the decision is based on comparing the risks of smoking to the potential risks of NRT.

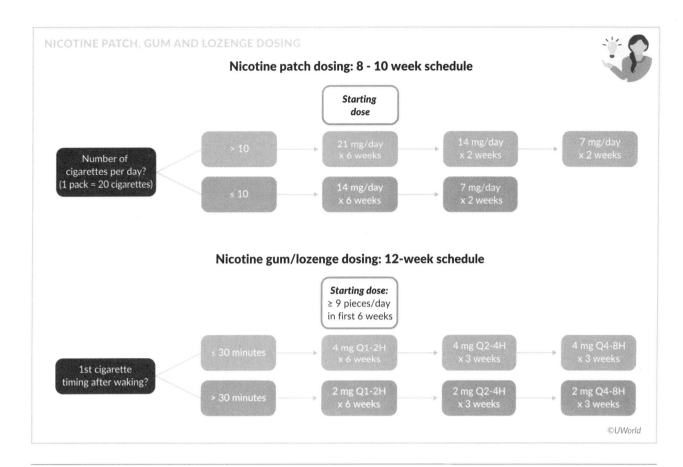

BUPROPION

Bupropion blocks neuronal reuptake of dopamine and/or norepinephrine, resulting in reduced cravings and other withdrawal symptoms. Since bupropion works by reducing cravings, it should be started before the quit date. It does not need to be tapered when it is discontinued.

DRUG	DOSING	SAFETY/SIDE EFFECTS/MONITORING
Bupropion SR (*Zyban**) Tablet For depression: ***Wellbutrin SR,*** ***Wellbutrin XL,*** *Aplenzin, Forfivo XL,* bupropion IR For seasonal affective disorder: ***Wellbutrin XL,*** *Aplenzin*	Start 1-2 weeks before quit date SR: 150 mg QAM for 3 days, then 150 mg BID Max dose: 300 mg/day Adjust dose for renal and hepatic impairment Use up to 6 months	**BOXED WARNING** Increased risk of suicidal thinking and behavior in children, adolescents and young adults taking antidepressants **CONTRAINDICATIONS** Seizure disorder; history of anorexia/bulimia; concurrent use with MAO inhibitors, linezolid or IV methylene blue; abrupt discontinuation of alcohol or sedatives **WARNINGS** Serious neuropsychiatric events (e.g., mood changes, hallucinations, paranoia, aggression, anxiety), activation of mania/hypomania, hypertension, angle-closure glaucoma, rash (including SJS) **SIDE EFFECTS** Dry mouth, insomnia, tremors, weight loss, agitation, anxiety, tachycardia, headache, sweating, nausea/vomiting, constipation **NOTES** Do not use with other forms of bupropion (see Depression chapter for more information) Delays weight gain To ↓ insomnia, take the 1st dose upon waking up and the 2nd dose 8 hours after the 1st dose If no significant progress by week 7, consider discontinuation

*Brand discontinued but name still used in practice.

VARENICLINE

Varenicline is a partial neuronal alpha-4 beta-2 nicotinic receptor agonist. It causes low-level stimulation of the receptor while blocking the ability of nicotine to bind. This relieves symptoms of nicotine withdrawal and inhibits the surges of dopamine responsible for the reinforcement and reward associated with smoking. Similar to bupropion, varenicline should be started before the quit date because it works by reducing cravings. It does not need to be tapered when it is discontinued. The American Thoracic Society recommends varenicline over bupropion, and varenicline plus NRT over varenicline monotherapy.

DRUG	DOSING	SAFETY/SIDE EFFECTS/MONITORING
Varenicline (*APO-Varenicline, Chantix**) Tablet Starter pack available with 0.5 mg tablets (11) and 1 mg tablets (42) *Tyrvaya* - nasal spray for dry eyes	Start 1 week before quit date Days 1-3: 0.5 mg daily Days 4-7: 0.5 mg BID Day 8 (quit date) and beyond: 1 mg BID CrCl < 30 mL/min: 0.5 mg daily titrated to max 0.5 mg BID Use for 12 weeks; can use another 12 weeks to maintain success	**WARNINGS** Serious neuropsychiatric events (e.g., agitation, depression, suicidal thoughts/behaviors), seizures, ↑ effects of alcohol, somnambulism (sleepwalking), accidental injury (e.g., traffic accidents), CVD risk, hypersensitivity reactions (e.g., angioedema, SJS) **SIDE EFFECTS** Nausea (~30%, dose-dependent), insomnia, vivid dreams, headache, constipation, vomiting **NOTES** To ↓ nausea, take after eating with a full glass of water; can reduce dose if needed To ↓ insomnia, take 2nd dose earlier than bedtime If unable to abruptly quit smoking on day 8, decrease smoking by 50% in the first 4 weeks, an additional 50% in weeks 5-8, with complete cessation by week 12 Efficacy has not been demonstrated in those ≤ 16 years old (not recommended)

Brand discontinued but name still used in practice.

TREATMENT CONSIDERATIONS FOR TOBACCO CESSATION

- All smokers should be offered medications unless it is contraindicated, they are pregnant or they are an adolescent.
- The combination of the nicotine patch + gum, lozenge or bupropion is more effective than the patch alone.
- Varenicline is more effective than bupropion, and varenicline + nicotine patch is more effective than varenicline alone.

WEIGHT GAIN	DEPRESSION	DENTURES	ASTHMA/COPD	SKIN CONDITIONS	SEIZURES
Use	**Use**	**Avoid**	**Avoid**	**Avoid**	**Avoid**
Gum, lozenge or bupropion SR (all delay weight gain)	Bupropion SR	Gum	Inhaler, nasal spray	Patch	Bupropion, varenicline

---

KEY COUNSELING POINTS

See the Drug Formulations and Patient Counseling chapter for counseling language/layman's terminology.

NICOTINE PATCH ADMINISTRATION

- At the start of each day, remove a new patch from the pouch; save the pouch to throw away used patches.
- Remove the backing and apply the sticky side of the patch to a clean, dry and relatively hairless area of the skin; press the patch firmly onto the skin for ~10 seconds.
- Wear for 24 hours (especially if cravings begin when you wake up). If vivid dreams or trouble sleeping occur, remove the patch prior to bedtime (after about 16 hours) and apply a new one in the morning.
- Discard the patch by folding the sticky ends together, place it back in the pouch and put it in a trash can with a lid to keep away from children and pets.
- Wash your hands after applying (and removing) the patch.
- Rotate the application site; do not apply to the same site for at least one week. Skin reactions can occur but generally go away in a few days. Topical hydrocortisone can help with minor skin irritation.
- Never cut the patch or wear more than one patch at a time.

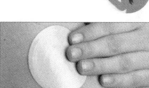

Use gum or lozenges to help with cravings while using the patch

NICOTINE GUM

HOW TO CHEW NICOTINE GUM

- Chew slowly until there is a tingle or peppery flavor in the mouth.
- Park it between the cheek and gum.
- When the tingle or flavor goes away, begin chewing slowly again until it returns, then park the gum again.
- Repeat until most of the flavor or tingle is gone (~30 minutes).
- Do not eat or drink 15 minutes before or during chewing.

NICOTINE LOZENGE

- Do not eat or drink for 15 minutes before or during use.
- Do not chew or swallow. Allow it to dissolve slowly. Move the lozenge from one side of the mouth to the other until it has completely dissolved (~20 – 30 minutes).
- May cause a warm or tingling sensation.
- Do not use more than one lozenge at a time or continuously use one lozenge after another.

NICOTINE INHALER

- Inhale deeply into the back of the throat or puff in short breaths.
- Each cartridge provides about 20 minutes of active puffing and is only good for one day after opening.
- Clean the mouthpiece with soap and water regularly.
- Keep at room temperature; cold temperatures reduce the amount of nicotine inhaled.

NICOTINE NASAL SPRAY

- Tilt head back slightly and spray once in each nostril while breathing through the mouth. Do not sniff, swallow or inhale through the nose.
- Can cause sneezing, coughing, watery eyes, runny nose and a hot peppery feeling in the back of the throat.

BUPROPION

- Start taking one week before desired quit date.
- Can cause:
  - Suicidal ideation.
  - Insomnia (avoid near bedtime).
- Do not use if you have a seizure disorder, anorexia or bulimia.

VARENICLINE

- Start taking one week before desired quit date.
- Can cause:
  - Suicidal ideation or depression.
  - Insomnia.
  - Nausea.
  - Impairment of ability to drive or properly operate heavy machinery.
- Can increase the effects of alcohol. Reduce the amount of alcohol consumed.

Select Guidelines/References

Barua RS, Rigotti NA, et al. 2018 ACC Expert Consensus Decision Pathway on Tobacco Cessation Treatment. J Am Coll of Cardiol. 2018;72:3332-65.

Treating Tobacco Use and Dependence: 2008 Update (last reviewed February 2020). Agency for Healthcare Research and Quality, Rockville, MD. http://www.ahrq.gov/prevention/guidelines/tobacco/index.html.

Leone FT, Zhang Y, Evers-Casey S, et al. Initiating pharmacologic treatment in tobacco-dependent adults. An official American Thoracic Society clinical practice guideline. American Journal of Respiratory and Critical Care Medicine. 2020;202(2):e5-e31.

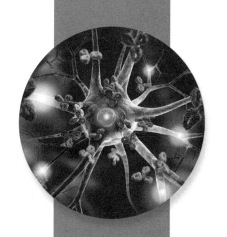
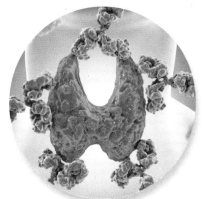
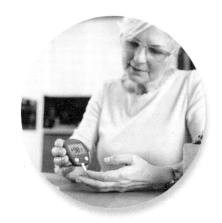

ENDOCRINE CONDITIONS

CONTENTS

CONTENT LEGEND

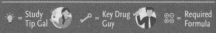

☼ = Study Tip Gal   🌐 = Key Drug Guy   ⚏ = Required Formula

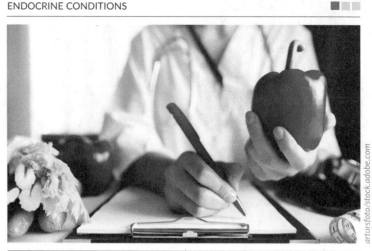

artursfoto/stock.adobe.com

CHAPTER 44
DIABETES

BACKGROUND

Diabetes is a common condition in the United States, affecting > 35 million Americans (just over 1 in 10). The central problem in all types of diabetes is that blood glucose (BG) remains high (hyperglycemia) due to decreased insulin secretion from the pancreas, decreased insulin sensitivity (i.e., how responsive cells are to insulin) or both. Chronic hyperglycemia can lead to damage throughout the body, including organ and nerve damage.

Insulin is a hormone produced by beta-cells (also called islet cells) in the pancreas. It is responsible for moving glucose out of the blood and into body cells to be used as energy. The glucose is either moved to muscle cells (primarily) for immediate use or stored for later use by liver cells (as glycogen, the quick glucose reserve) or adipose (fat) cells.

Insulin is counter-balanced by glucagon; they have opposite effects, as shown in the diagram below. Glucagon is produced by alpha-cells in the pancreas and works when BG is low. Glucagon pulls glucose back into the blood by releasing glucose from glycogen. If glycogen is depleted, glucagon will signal fat cells to make ketones as an alternative energy source.

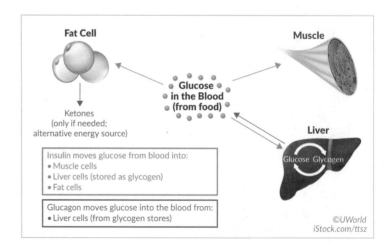

Insulin moves glucose from blood into:
• Muscle cells
• Liver cells (stored as glycogen)
• Fat cells

Glucagon moves glucose into the blood from:
• Liver cells (from glycogen stores)

©UWorld
iStock.com/ttsz

TYPES OF DIABETES

TYPE 1 DIABETES

Type 1 diabetes (T1D) accounts for ~5 – 10% of all cases. It is caused by an autoimmune destruction of beta-cells in the pancreas. Once the beta-cells are destroyed, insulin cannot be produced. Without insulin, glucose cannot enter muscle cells to be used for energy. The body then goes into starvation mode and starts to metabolize fat into ketones to use as an alternative energy source. Because ketones are acidic, high ketone levels can cause diabetic ketoacidosis (DKA), which is a medical emergency (discussed later in this chapter).

Most T1D is diagnosed in children, but it can develop at any age. Family history is the biggest risk factor. It can be difficult to distinguish between T1D and type 2 diabetes (T2D), especially early in the disease; testing for islet autoantibodies (an autoimmune marker) and C-peptide (a substance released by the pancreas only when insulin is released) can be done to differentiate between T1D and T2D. The C-peptide level is very low or absent (undetectable) in T1D.

Patients with T1D must be treated with insulin and should be screened for other autoimmune disorders (e.g., thyroid disorders, celiac disease). Teplizumab (Tzield) is a monoclonal antibody that is FDA-approved to delay the onset of symptomatic disease in T1D.

TYPE 2 DIABETES

T2D accounts for ~90 – 95% of all cases and is due to both insulin resistance (decreased insulin sensitivity) and relative insulin deficiency. The pancreatic beta-cells produce less insulin over time as they become damaged. Hyperglycemia develops gradually, which is why the onset of T2D often goes unnoticed. T2D is strongly associated with obesity, physical inactivity, family history and the presence of other comorbid conditions (see Risk Factors section). T2D is usually diagnosed in older patients and can be managed with lifestyle modifications alone (in a small number of patients) or in combination with oral and/or injectable medications.

PREDIABETES

Prediabetes means there is an increased risk of developing diabetes. In prediabetes, the BG is higher than normal, but not high enough for a diabetes diagnosis. Following dietary and exercise recommendations reduces the risk of progression from prediabetes to diabetes.

Metformin can be used to help improve BG levels, especially in patients with a BMI ≥ 35 kg/m², age 25 – 59 years and women with a history of gestational diabetes mellitus (GDM). Annual monitoring for development of diabetes and treatment of modifiable cardiovascular disease (CVD) risk factors are recommended.

DIABETES IN PREGNANCY

There are two types of diabetes in pregnancy:

- Diabetes that is present prior to becoming pregnant, or
- Diabetes that develops during pregnancy [gestational diabetes mellitus (GDM)]; typically diagnosed in the second or third trimester

In both types, BG goals are more stringent than in the non-pregnant population (see Study Tip Gal titled Glycemic Targets in Diabetes). Hyperglycemia during pregnancy can lead to an infant that is larger than normal (macrosomia) and an increased risk for developing obesity and diabetes later in life (for both the mother and the baby).

Most pregnant women are tested for GDM at 24 – 28 weeks gestation using the oral glucose tolerance test (OGTT) (see Diagnosis section). Hyperglycemia, if present, should be treated first with lifestyle modifications (diet and exercise). If medication is needed, insulin is preferred. Metformin and glyburide are sometimes used.

SCREENING & DIAGNOSIS

RISK FACTORS

The presence of multiple risk factors increases the likelihood of prediabetes and T2D. Major risk factors include:

- Age
- Physical inactivity
- Overweight (BMI ≥ 25 kg/m² or ≥ 23 in Asian-Americans)
- High-risk race or ethnicity: African-American, Asian-American, Latino/Hispanic-American, Native American or Pacific Islander
- History of gestational diabetes
- A1C ≥ 5.7% (i.e., prediabetes)
- First-degree relative with diabetes (sibling or parent)
- HDL < 35 mg/dL and/or TG > 250 mg/dL
- Hypertension (≥ 130/80 mmHg or taking BP medication)
- CVD history or smoking history
- Conditions that cause insulin resistance (e.g., acanthosis nigricans, polycystic ovary syndrome)

SYMPTOMS

The classic symptoms of hyperglycemia include:

- Polyuria (excessive urination)
- Polyphagia (excessive hunger or increased appetite)
- Polydipsia (excessive thirst)

Other symptoms include fatigue, blurry vision and weight loss. In T1D, the initial presentation is often DKA due to the total insulin deficiency.

SCREENING

Everyone, even those with no other risk factors, should be tested beginning at 35 years old. In addition, all asymptomatic adults who are overweight (BMI ≥ 25 or ≥ 23 in Asian-Americans) or obese with at least one other risk factor (e.g., physical inactivity) should be tested. If the result is normal, repeat testing every 3 years at a minimum. Screening should also be considered for patients taking drugs that increase blood glucose (see Drugs that Affect Blood Glucose later in the chapter) and those with HIV or pancreatitis.

DIAGNOSIS

There are three types of tests used to identify if prediabetes or diabetes is present:

1. Hemoglobin A1C (or simply A1C) indicates the average BG over approximately the past 3 months.

2. Plasma glucose gives the BG at that moment. Fasting plasma glucose (FPG) is taken after fasting for ≥ 8 hours.

3. The OGTT determines how well glucose is tolerated by measuring the BG level 2 hours after drinking a liquid that is high in sugar (glucose).

No single test is preferred. The criteria for diagnosing diabetes are shown in the Study Tip Gal below. A positive test should be confirmed with a second abnormal test result from either the same sample or a new sample, unless there is a clear clinical diagnosis (e.g., classic symptoms of hyperglycemia plus a random BG ≥ 200 mg/dL).

DIAGNOSTIC CRITERIA FOR DIABETES

	A1C (%)	FPG (mg/dL)	Random BG (mg/dL)	OGTT, 2-hr BG (mg/dL)
Diabetes	≥ 6.5	≥ 126	≥ 200*	≥ 200
Prediabetes	5.7-6.4	100-125		140-199

*In addition to classic symptoms of hyperglycemia.

TREATMENT GOALS

The treatment goals for A1C, preprandial glucose (before meals) and postprandial glucose (PPG, which is BG measured after eating) are shown in the Study Tip Gal below.

GLYCEMIC TARGETS IN DIABETES

	A1C (%)	Preprandial (mg/dL)	1-hr PPG (mg/dL)	2-hr PPG (mg/dL)
Not Pregnant	< 7*	80-130		< 180
Pregnant		< 95	< 140	< 120

*A lower A1C goal may be acceptable if it can be reached without significant hypoglycemia. A less-stringent goal of < 8% may be appropriate (e.g., if patient has severe hypoglycemia or a limited life-expectancy).

Typically, the A1C is measured with a blood sample sent to a lab. Point-of-care A1C test kits provide immediate results and can be used to assess blood glucose control (but are not typically recommended for diagnosis). Patients can measure their own BG using a glucose meter or with a continuous glucose monitoring (CGM) device (discussed later).

Testing Frequency

Glycemic control (e.g., A1C, time in range) should be assessed:

- Quarterly (every 3 months) if not meeting goals

- Biannually (every 6 months, or twice per year) if at goal

Interpreting the A1C with the eAG

It can be difficult to understand how an A1C value correlates with BG values measured on a glucose meter. The estimated average glucose (eAG) is an interpretation of the A1C value that makes it appear similar to a glucose meter value.

- An A1C of 6% is equivalent to an eAG of 126 mg/dL. Each additional 1% increases the eAG by ~28 mg/dL.

Example: an A1C of 7% is 126 + 28 ≅ 154 eAG.

LIFESTYLE MODIFICATIONS

Weight Loss

- Monitor measurements (e.g., BMI, waist circumference) annually.

- Goal weight loss is ≥ 5% of body weight if overweight or obese (for some, 10 – 15% is recommended). Medications and/or surgery may be needed (see Weight Loss chapter).

Individualized Medical Nutrition Therapy

- Consume natural forms of carbohydrates and sugars (i.e., from vegetables, fruits, whole grains, legumes, dairy).

- Limit alcohol consumption (≤ 1 drink/day for women, ≤ 2 drinks/day for men).

- Patients with T1D should use carbohydrate-counting, where the prandial (mealtime) insulin dose is adjusted to the carbohydrate intake. A carbohydrate serving is measured as 15 grams, which is approximately one small piece of fruit, 1 slice of bread or ⅓ cup of cooked rice/pasta.

Physical Activity

- Perform at least 150 minutes of moderate-intensity aerobic activity per week spread over at least 3 days.

- Reduce sedentary (long hours of sitting) habits by standing every 30 minutes, at a minimum.

Smoking Cessation

- Encourage all patients who smoke to quit; this includes tobacco, e-cigarettes and cannabis.

Natural Products

- Although evidence is limited, cinnamon, alpha lipoic acid, chromium, magnesium and ginseng are commonly used.

COMPREHENSIVE CARE

In addition to glycemic control, treatment is aimed at preventing the long-term complications of diabetes. Left untreated, diabetes damages nearly all parts of the body. Complications are categorized as microvascular (small vessel) or macrovascular (large vessel), as shown in the Study Tip Gal to the right.

Diabetes is the top cause of lower-extremity amputations, kidney disease and blindness. The primary cause of death is cardiovascular disease, which is twice as likely to occur in these patients compared to the general population.

The American Diabetes Association (ADA) provides recommendations for monitoring, preventing and treating complications of uncontrolled diabetes (see diagram below).

DIABETES COMPLICATIONS

Microvascular Disease
Retinopathy

Diabetic kidney disease (i.e., nephropathy)

Peripheral neuropathy (i.e., loss of sensation, often in the feet), ↑ risk of foot infections and amputations

Autonomic neuropathy (gastroparesis, loss of bladder control, erectile dysfunction)

Macrovascular Disease*
Coronary artery disease (CAD), including MI

Cerebrovascular disease, including stroke (CVA)

Peripheral artery disease (PAD)

Macrovascular disease is the same as atherosclerotic cardiovascular disease (ASCVD)

Antiplatelet Therapy (Aspirin)

- Aspirin 75-162 mg/day (usually given as 81 mg/day) is recommended for ASCVD secondary prevention (e.g., post-MI).
  - ❏ If allergy: use clopidogrel 75 mg/day.
- Not recommended for primary prevention (in most); the risk of bleeding is about equal to the benefit. Can consider if high risk.
- CAD/PAD: aspirin + low-dose rivaroxaban can be added.
- Used in pregnancy to ↓ risk of preeclampsia.

Diabetic Retinopathy

- T2D: eye exam with dilation at diagnosis.
  - ❏ If retinopathy, repeat annually. If not, repeat every 1-2 yrs.

Vaccinations

Recommended, in addition to all age-appropriate vaccines:
- Hepatitis B virus (HBV) series.
- Influenza, annually.
- Pneumococcal, COVID-19 and RSV vaccines per ACIP guidelines (see Immunizations chapter).

Neuropathy

- Annually: a 10-g monofilament test and 1 other test (e.g., pinprick, temperature, vibration) to assess sensation.
- Comprehensive foot exam at least annually. If high-risk, refer to podiatrist.

Treatment options: gabapentin, pregabalin, SNRIs (e.g., duloxetine), tricyclic antidepressants or sodium channel blockers.

Bone Health

- Monitor bone mineral density via DXA every 2-3 yrs for adults age > 65 (or earlier with risk factors).
- Consider treatment for T-score ≤ -2.0 or with fragility fracture.

See Osteoporosis, Menopause & Testosterone Use chapter for details on treatment options.

Cholesterol Control

Statin Treatment in Patients with Diabetes*
- High-intensity statin** for:
  - ❏ Comorbid ASCVD; LDL goal < 55 mg/dL.
  - ❏ Age 40-75 years with ≥ 1 ASCVD risk factor; LDL goal < 70 mg/dL.
- Moderate-intensity statin for:
  - ❏ Age 40-75 years (no ASCVD).
  - ❏ Age 20-39 years with ASCVD risk factors.

Add-On Treatment (to Maximally Tolerated Statin)
- Ezetimibe or a PCSK9 inhibitor if LDL remains above goal.
- Icosapent ethyl (*Vascepa*) if LDL is controlled but TGs are 135–499 mg/dL in patients with ASCVD or risk factors.

Monitoring: lipid panel at statin initiation, 4-12 weeks after initiation and dose changes, then annually.

Statin alternatives (if intolerant): bempedoic acid or PCSK9 inhibitor.
**Atorvastatin 40-80 mg or rosuvastatin 20-40 mg daily.*

Diabetic Kidney Disease

- Defined as $eGFR < 60$ mL/min/1.73 m^2 and/or albuminuria (urine albumin ≥ 30 mg/24 hrs or UACR ≥ 30 mg/g).
- Monitor urinary albumin and eGFR annually if normal kidney function.*

Treatment
- ACE inhibitor or ARB.
- SGLT2 inhibitor (if eGFR ≥ 20 mL/min/1.73 m^2).
- Finerenone (once on a maximally tolerated dose of ACE inhibitor or ARB).

UACR = urine albumin-to-creatinine ratio.
More frequent monitoring (e.g., 2-4 times a year) is recommended in patients with CKD (based on severity/stage of disease).

Blood Pressure Control

- BP goal: < 130/80 mmHg

Treatment
- No albuminuria or CAD: thiazide, DHP CCB, ACE inhibitor or ARB.
- Albuminuria or CAD: ACE inhibitor or ARB.

FOOT CARE COUNSELING

Counseling on proper foot care is essential for patients with diabetes, as they may not be able to feel damage or injury to the feet. Patients should be instructed to wash, dry and examine their feet daily, as well as moisturize the top and bottom of their feet (but not between the toes). They should wear socks and shoes, elevate the feet when sitting and trim their toenails with a nail file (to avoid sharp edges from a clipper). The patient's feet should also be examined at each office visit, and they should have an annual foot exam by a podiatrist.

TREATMENT FOR TYPE 2 DIABETES

The goals of treatment are to maintain BG levels in the target range (while avoiding hypoglycemia) and to reduce long-term complications of hyperglycemia. The ADA guidelines provide recommendations for initial treatment and add-on therapy (see Study Tip Gal below). Initial treatment depends on comorbidities and patient-specific factors.

- Start a GLP-1 agonist or SGLT2 inhibitor with proven benefit at baseline if the patient has ASCVD, heart failure or chronic kidney disease.

- Start two drugs at baseline if A1C is 8.5 – 10%.

- Insulin can be used initially for severe hyperglycemia (A1C > 10% or BG ≥ 300 mg/dL), evidence of catabolism (e.g., weight loss) or if symptoms of hyperglycemia are present (e.g., polyuria, polydipsia); see Insulin section. Outside of these scenarios, if injectable medications are needed for A1C lowering, GLP-1 agonists or GLP-1/GIP agonists are preferred over insulin.

- Add medications if the A1C remains above goal and continue until A1C goal is met. Treatment is driven by patient-specific factors (e.g., glycemic efficacy, effect on weight, cost, risk of hypoglycemia).

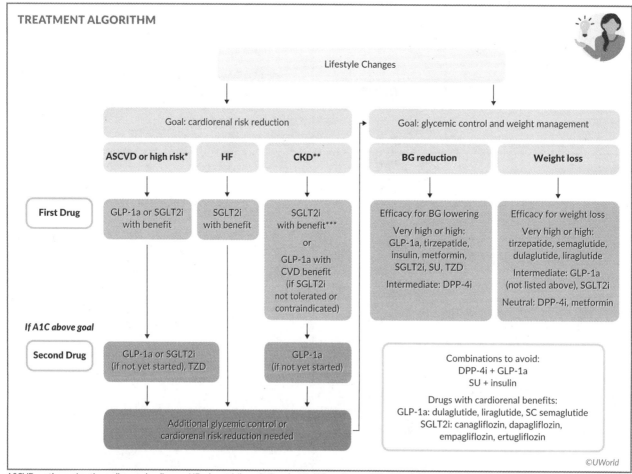

TREATMENT ALGORITHM

ASCVD = atherosclerotic cardiovascular disease, HF = heart failure, CKD = chronic kidney disease, BG = blood glucose, GLP-1a = glucagon-like peptide 1 receptor agonist, SGLT2i = sodium-glucose cotransporter 2 inhibitor, TZD = thiazolidinedione, SU = sulfonylurea, DPP-4i = dipeptidyl peptidase 4 inhibitor.
*High risk: age ≥ 55 with two or more additional risk factors (e.g., obesity, hypertension, smoking, dyslipidemia, albuminuria).
**Defined as eGFR < 60 mL/min/1.73 m² and/or urine albumin ≥ 30 mg/24 hr.
***SGLT2i recommended if eGFR ≥ 20 mL/min/1.73 m² at initiation; continue until dialysis or transplant. GLP-1a preferred for glycemic control if eGFR < 30 mL/min.

NON-INSULIN MEDICATIONS FOR TYPE 2 DIABETES

GLUCAGON-LIKE PEPTIDE 1 (GLP-1) AND GLUCOSE-DEPENDENT INSULINOTROPIC POLYPEPTIDE (GIP) AGONISTS

Glucagon-like peptide 1 (GLP-1) agonists are analogs of the incretin hormone GLP-1, which ↑ glucose-dependent insulin secretion, ↓ glucagon secretion, slows gastric emptying, improves satiety and can result in weight loss. Glucose-dependent insulinotropic polypeptide (GIP) agonists are analogs of GIP, which has similar effects to GLP-1.

Liraglutide, dulaglutide and SC semaglutide are recommended in patients with ASCVD (or high risk) and as an alternative in CKD because of their demonstrated cardiovascular benefits. GLP-1 and GLP-1/GIP agonists are all subcutaneous injections available in either single-dose or multidose pens, except semaglutide which also comes as an oral tablet. Some are available in combination with long-acting insulin. GLP-1 and GLP-1/GIP agonist names end in "-tide."

DRUG	DOSING	SAFETY/SIDE EFFECTS/MONITORING
GLP-1 Agonists		**BOXED WARNING**
Liraglutide *(Victoza)* *Saxenda* – for weight loss	0.6 mg SC daily x 1 week, then ↑ to 1.2 mg SC daily; can ↑ to 1.8 mg SC daily	All (except *Byetta*): risk of thyroid C-cell carcinomas; do not use if personal or family history of medullary thyroid carcinoma (MTC) or with Multiple Endocrine Neoplasia syndrome type 2 (MEN 2) **WARNINGS**
Dulaglutide *(Trulicity)*	0.75 mg SC once weekly; can ↑ to 4.5 mg SC once weekly	Pancreatitis (can be fatal, risk factors: gallstones, alcoholism or ↑ TGs), acute kidney injury, gallbladder disease Not recommended in patients with severe GI disease, including gastroparesis (drug-induced ileus has been reported)
Semaglutide *(Ozempic* – SC, *Rybelsus* – oral)* *Wegovy* – for weight loss	SC: 0.25 mg SC once weekly x 4 weeks, then ↑ to 0.5 mg SC weekly; can ↑ to 2 mg SC weekly PO: 3 mg PO daily x 30 days, then ↑ to 7 mg daily; can ↑ to 14 mg	*Byrdureon BCise*: serious injection-site reactions (e.g., abscess, cellulitis, necrosis) with or without SC nodules *Ozempic*, *Trulicity* and *Mounjaro*: ↑ complications with diabetic retinopathy
Exenatide *(Byetta)*	5 mcg SC BID for 1 month; can ↑ to 10 mcg SC BID CrCl < 30: not recommended	**SIDE EFFECTS** Weight loss, nausea/vomiting/diarrhea (reduced with dose titration), hypoglycemia, injection site reactions Tirzepatide: increased heart rate
Exenatide ER *(Bydureon BCise)*	2 mg SC once weekly eGFR < 45: not recommended	**NOTES** ↓ A1C 0.5-1.5%; ↓ postprandial BG, low hypoglycemia risk (unless used with insulin)
Dual GLP-1 and GIP Agonist (also called "twincretin")		Do not use with DPP-4 inhibitors (overlapping mechanism)
Tirzepatide *(Mounjaro)* *Zepbound* – for weight loss	2.5 mg SC weekly x 4 weeks, then ↑ to 5 mg SC weekly; can ↑ to 15 mg SC weekly	*Byetta*: give dose within 60 minutes before meals; *Rybelsus*: take dose ≥ 30 minutes before first food/drink/medications of the day with 4 oz of plain water Pen needles are not provided with *Byetta* or *Victoza*; provided with all others (which are the weekly injections) Glucose lowering may not be seen with initial doses (titrated to reduce GI side effects)

eGFR units: mL/min/1.73 m², CrCl units: mL/min

GLP-1 Agonist Drug Interactions

- These drugs slow gastric emptying and can reduce the absorption of orally administered drugs. Use caution with narrow therapeutic index drugs or drugs that require threshold concentrations for efficacy (e.g., antibiotics, oral contraceptives).

  - *Mounjaro, Zepbound:* patients using oral hormonal contraceptives are advised to switch to a non-oral or barrier method of contraception for 4 weeks after initiation and for 4 weeks after each dose escalation.

- Exenatide: can ↑ the INR in patients on warfarin, monitor INR.

GLP-1 Agonist Injection Counseling

Injection technique is similar to insulin administration (see Insulin Injection Counseling later in the chapter).

- Injectable GLP-1 agonists are administered subcutaneously in the abdomen (alternatively in the back of the upper arms, outer thighs or upper buttocks).

- Attach a new pen needle for each injection (if not already attached). Follow the manufacturer's instructions for priming the pen (e.g., once for each new pen).

- After cleaning the hands and injection site, pinch a portion of the injection area and insert the pen needle at 90 degrees.

- Press the injection button and count 5 – 10 seconds before removing the needle.

- Rotate injection sites with each injection.

- Properly dispose of needles in a sharps disposal container. Do not store pens with a needle attached to reduce the risk of contamination or drug leakage.

SODIUM-GLUCOSE COTRANSPORTER 2 INHIBITORS

The sodium-glucose cotransporter 2 (SGLT2) protein, expressed in the proximal renal tubules, is responsible for the reabsorption of filtered glucose. By inhibiting SGLT2, these drugs reduce reabsorption of glucose and ↑ urinary glucose excretion, which ↓ BG concentrations.

Canagliflozin, dapagliflozin, empagliflozin and ertugliflozin have shown benefits in patients with HF, CKD and/or ASCVD; they are recommended for diabetes treatment when these comorbid conditions are present, and select drugs are also approved for HF and CKD in patients without diabetes (see the Chronic Heart Failure and Renal Disease chapters for details).

Dosing and eGFR thresholds for use vary by drug and indication, but most guidelines now recommend use if eGFR ≥ 20 mL/min/1.73 m^2. SGLT2 inhibitor names end in "-gliflozin."

DRUG	DOSING	SAFETY/SIDE EFFECTS/MONITORING
Canagliflozin (*Invokana*)	100 mg daily prior to the first meal of the day; can ↑ to 300 mg daily eGFR 30-59: max dose 100 mg/day	**WARNINGS** Ketoacidosis (can occur with BG < 250 mg/dL) – risk ↑ with acute illness, dehydration and renal impairment, D/C prior to surgery to ↓ risk
Dapagliflozin (*Farxiga*)	5 mg daily in the morning; can ↑ to 10 mg daily	Genital mycotic infections, urinary tract infections (including urosepsis and pyelonephritis), necrotizing fasciitis (perineum) Hypotension, AKI and renal impairment (due to intravascular volume depletion)
Empagliflozin (*Jardiance*)	10 mg daily in the morning; can ↑ to 25 mg daily	Canagliflozin and bexagliflozin: ↑ risk of leg and foot amputations (higher risk with history of amputation, PAD, peripheral neuropathy and/or diabetic foot ulcers); risk of fractures
Bexagliflozin (*Brenzavvy*)	20 mg daily in the morning	**SIDE EFFECTS** ↑ urination, ↑ thirst, hypoglycemia, ↑ Mg/PO4
Ertugliflozin (*Steglatro*)	5 mg daily in the morning; can ↑ to 15 mg daily	Canagliflozin: hyperkalemia risk when used with other drugs that increase potassium **NOTES** ↓ A1C 0.7-1%, low hypoglycemia risk (unless used with insulin)
		Use not recommended in dialysis

eGFR units: mL/min/1.73 m^2

SGLT2 Inhibitor Drug Interactions

- ↑ risk of intravascular volume depletion (causing hypotension and acute kidney injury) if used in combination with diuretics, RAAS inhibitors or NSAIDs.

- Uridine diphosphate glucuronosyltransferase (UGT) inducers (e.g., rifampin, phenytoin, phenobarbital) can ↓ levels of canagliflozin; consider using higher dose (up to 300 mg) if used in combination and eGFR ≥ 60 mL/min/1.73 m^2.

BIGUANIDE

Metformin primarily works by ↓ hepatic glucose production, ↑ insulin sensitivity and ↓ intestinal absorption of glucose. Metformin is a first-line treatment option for T2D and can be used in prediabetes. Use of metformin is dependent on eGFR.

DRUG	DOSING	SAFETY/SIDE EFFECTS/MONITORING
Metformin **(Fortamet, Glumetza,** *Glucophage*,* *Glucophage XR*,* *Riomet)* IR: 500, 850, 1,000 mg ER: 500, 750, 1,000 mg *Riomet* liquid: 500 mg/5 mL	IR: 500 mg daily or BID ER: 500-1,000 mg daily (usually with dinner) Titrate weekly, usual maintenance dose: 1,000 mg BID Max dose: 2,000-2,550 mg/day (varies by product) Give with a meal to ↓ GI upset	**BOXED WARNING** Lactic acidosis – risk ↑ with renal impairment, contrast dye, excessive alcohol or drugs (e.g., topiramate) and hypoxia **CONTRAINDICATIONS** eGFR < 30, acute or chronic metabolic acidosis (includes DKA) **WARNINGS** Not recommended to start if eGFR 30-45; reassess if eGFR < 45 during treatment, may need dose reduction Vitamin B12 deficiency with long-term use: symptoms can include peripheral neuropathy and cognitive impairment; monitor B12 levels periodically (every 1-2 years) **SIDE EFFECTS** GI effects: diarrhea, nausea, flatulence, cramping; usually transient (resolve over time) **NOTES** ↓ A1C 1-2%, weight neutral, no hypoglycemia ER: swallow whole; can leave a ghost tablet (empty shell) in the stool Dose titration recommended to reduce GI effects; glucose-lowering effect may not be seen with initial doses

eGFR units: mL/min/1.73 m².
*Brand discontinued but name still used in practice.

Metformin Drug Interactions

- Intra-arterial iodinated contrast media (used for imaging studies) can cause renal dysfunction, leading to an ↑ risk of lactic acidosis. Discontinue metformin before the imaging procedure. Metformin can be restarted 48 hours after the procedure if eGFR is stable.

INSULIN SECRETAGOGUES

Sulfonylureas (SUs) and meglitinides are known as insulin secretagogues; they work by stimulating insulin secretion from the pancreatic beta-cells to decrease postprandial BG. Meglitinides have a faster onset (15 – 60 minutes) and a shorter duration of action compared to the SUs. Older, first generation SUs (chlorpropamide, tolazamide and tolbutamide) have a risk of prolonged hypoglycemia and should not be used. Meglitinide names end in "-glinide" and SU names start with "G" and end in "-ide."

Sulfonylureas

DRUG	DOSING	SAFETY/SIDE EFFECTS/MONITORING
Glipizide **(Glucotrol XL,** *Glucotrol*, Glipizide XL)*	IR: 5 mg daily, titrate to a max dose of 40 mg/day Doses > 15 mg should be divided BID XL: 5 mg daily, titrate to a max dose of 20 mg/day	**CONTRAINDICATIONS** Sulfa allergy (not likely to cross-react, see Drug Allergies & Adverse Drug Reactions chapter), T1D, DKA **WARNINGS** Hypoglycemia [(decreased risk with short-acting drugs (e.g., glipizide)]
Glimepiride **(Amaryl)**	1-2 mg daily, titrate to a max dose of 8 mg/day	**SIDE EFFECTS** Weight gain, nausea **NOTES** ↓ A1C 1-2%; ↓ efficacy after long-term use (as pancreatic beta-cell function declines)
Glyburide **Micronized glyburide** **(Glynase)**	Glyburide: 2.5-5 mg daily, titrate to a max dose of 20 mg/day *Glynase*: 1.5-3 mg daily, titrate to a max dose of 12 mg/day	Glipizide IR: take 30 minutes before a meal; all other products are taken with breakfast or the first meal of the day; may need to hold doses if NPO *Glucotrol XL* is an OROS formulation and can leave a ghost tablet (empty shell) in the stool Glimepiride, glyburide not preferred in elderly (on the Beers criteria) due to hypoglycemia risk Patients with G6PD deficiency can be at increased risk of hemolytic anemia with sulfonylureas

*Brand discontinued but name still used in practice.

Meglitinides

DRUG	DOSING	SAFETY/SIDE EFFECTS/MONITORING
Repaglinide	0.5-2 mg 2-4 times daily AC Max dose: 16 mg daily Take within 30 minutes before meals	**WARNINGS** Hypoglycemia, caution with severe liver/renal impairment **SIDE EFFECTS** Weight gain, headache, upper respiratory tract infections (URTIs)
Nateglinide	60-120 mg up to 3 times daily AC Take 1-30 minutes before meals	**NOTES** ↓ A1C 0.5-1.5% Skip dose if meal is skipped

Sulfonylurea and Meglitinide Drug Interactions

- Insulin in combination with either SUs or meglitinides ↑ risk of hypoglycemia and should be avoided. Use caution with other drugs that can decrease BG (see Hypoglycemia section).

- SUs are CYP2C9 substrates; use caution with 2C9 inducers or inhibitors.

- Gemfibrozil and clopidogrel can ↑ repaglinide, leading to ↓ BG. Repaglinide is contraindicated with gemfibrozil.

- Alcohol can ↑ the risk for delayed hypoglycemia when taking insulin or insulin secretagogues.

DIPEPTIDYL PEPTIDASE 4 INHIBITORS

Dipeptidyl peptidase 4 (DPP-4) inhibitors prevent the enzyme DPP-4 from breaking down incretin hormones, glucagon-like peptide 1 (GLP-1) and glucose-dependent insulinotropic polypeptide (GIP), which enhances the effects of these incretins. These hormones help to regulate BG levels by ↑ glucose-dependent insulin secretion from the pancreatic beta-cells and ↓ glucagon secretion (which ↓ hepatic glucose production) from pancreatic alpha-cells. DPP-4 inhibitor names end in "-gliptin."

DRUG	DOSING	SAFETY/SIDE EFFECTS/MONITORING
Sitagliptin **(Januvia)**	100 mg daily eGFR 30-45: 50 mg daily eGFR < 30: 25 mg daily	**WARNINGS** Pancreatitis, severe arthralgia (joint pain), acute renal failure, bullous pemphigoid (blisters/erosions requiring hospitalization)
Linagliptin **(Tradjenta)**	5 mg daily No renal dose adjustments	Risk of heart failure seen with saxagliptin and alogliptin, but warning added for class Alogliptin: hepatotoxicity
Saxagliptin (Onglyza)	2.5-5 mg daily eGFR < 45: 2.5 mg daily	**SIDE EFFECTS** Generally well tolerated, can cause nasopharyngitis, URTIs, headache, rash
Alogliptin (Nesina)	25 mg daily CrCl 30-59: 12.5 mg daily CrCl < 30: 6.25 mg daily	**NOTES** ↓ A1C 0.5-0.8%, weight neutral, low hypoglycemia risk Do not use with GLP-1 agonists (overlapping mechanism)

CrCl units: mL/min, eGFR units: mL/min/1.73 m²

DPP-4 Inhibitor Drug Interactions

- Saxagliptin is a major substrate of CYP450 3A4 and P-gp. Limit the dose to 2.5 mg with strong CYP3A4 inhibitors, including protease inhibitors (e.g., atazanavir, ritonavir), clarithromycin, itraconazole, ketoconazole.

- Linagliptin is a major substrate of CYP3A4 and P-gp. Linagliptin levels are ↓ by strong CYP3A4 and P-gp inducers (e.g., carbamazepine, phenytoin, rifampin, St. John's wort).

THIAZOLIDINEDIONES

Thiazolidinediones (TZDs) are peroxisome proliferator-activated receptor gamma (PPARγ) agonists that ↑ peripheral insulin sensitivity (↑ uptake and utilization of glucose by the peripheral tissues, also known as insulin sensitizers). TZD names end in "-glitazone." Pioglitazone is the only TZD currently available; rosiglitazone, another TZD, is no longer available in the U.S.

DRUG	DOSING	SAFETY/SIDE EFFECTS/MONITORING
Pioglitazone **(Actos)**	Initial: 15-30 mg daily Max dose: 45 mg daily	**BOXED WARNINGS** Can cause or exacerbate heart failure, do not use with NYHA Class III/IV heart failure **WARNINGS** Edema (including macular edema), risk of fractures, hepatic failure, can stimulate ovulation (which can lead to unintended pregnancy), ↑ risk of bladder cancer (do not use in patients with a history of bladder cancer) **SIDE EFFECTS** Peripheral edema, weight gain, URTIs, myalgia **NOTES** ↓ A1C 0.5-1.4%, low risk of hypoglycemia (unless used with insulin) Benefit seen in nonalcoholic steatohepatitis (NASH) and for stroke/myocardial infarction risk reduction in patients with history of stroke and insulin resistance/prediabetes

Thiazolidinedione Drug Interactions

- TZDs are major substrates of CYP2C8; use caution with CYP2C8 inducers (e.g., rifampin) or inhibitors (e.g., gemfibrozil).

OTHER MEDICATIONS

The following classes of drugs are not used routinely for the treatment of T2D, but can be used in specific situations.

DRUG CLASS	COMMENTS
Alpha-Glucosidase Inhibitors Acarbose Miglitol (Glyset)	MOA: inhibit the metabolism of complex carbohydrates and disaccharides (e.g., sucrose), which delays glucose absorption. Do not cause hypoglycemia alone, but if hypoglycemia occurs due to another drug, it cannot be treated with sucrose (present in fruit juices, table sugar or candy); glucose tablets or gel need to be purchased to treat hypoglycemia. Each dose should be taken with the first bite of each meal. GI side effects are common (flatulence, diarrhea, abdominal pain).
Bile Acid Binding Resins Colesevelam (Welchol)	Also indicated for dyslipidemia (see Dyslipidemia chapter). Constipation is the most common side effect. Can bind to and decrease absorption of other drugs and fat-soluble vitamins (A, D, E, K).
Dopamine Agonist Bromocriptine (Cycloset)	Contraindicated in patients with syncopal migraines (can cause hypotension and orthostasis) and those who are postpartum and/or breastfeeding (inhibits lactation). Should not be used with metoclopramide or other dopamine agonists.
Amylin Analog Pramlintide (Symlin) SC injection	MOA: helps control postprandial glucose by slowing gastric emptying, which suppresses glucagon secretion following a meal and ↑ satiety. Can be used in type 1 or type 2 diabetes, administered SC prior to each major meal. Skip dose if skipping meal. Significant hypoglycemia risk; must reduce mealtime insulin dose by 50% when starting. Contraindicated in gastroparesis. Side effects include nausea, vomiting, anorexia and weight loss.

COMBINATIONS

METFORMIN + SU
Metformin/glipizide
Metformin/glyburide

METFORMIN + TZD
Metformin/pioglitazone (Actoplus Met)

METFORMIN + DPP-4 INHIBITOR
Metformin/alogliptin (Kazano)
Metformin/linagliptin (Jentadueto, Jentadueto XR)
Metformin/sitagliptin (Janumet, Janumet XR)
Metformin/saxagliptin (Kombiglyze XR)

METFORMIN + SGLT2 INHIBITOR
Metformin/canagliflozin (Invokamet, Invokamet XR)
Metformin/dapagliflozin (Xigduo XR)
Metformin/empagliflozin (Synjardy, Synjardy XR)
Metformin/ertugliflozin (Segluromet)

METFORMIN + SGLT2 INHIBITOR + DPP-4 INHIBITOR
Metformin/empagliflozin/linagliptin (Trijardy XR)

SULFONYLUREA + TZD
Glimepiride/pioglitazone (Duetact)

DPP-4 INHIBITOR + TZD
Alogliptin/pioglitazone (Oseni)

DPP-4 INHIBITOR + SGLT2 INHIBITOR
Linagliptin/empagliflozin (Glyxambi)
Saxagliptin/dapagliflozin (Qtern)
Sitagliptin/ertugliflozin (Steglujan)

GLP-1 AGONIST + LONG-ACTING INSULIN
Liraglutide/insulin degludec (Xultophy)
Lixisenatide/insulin glargine (Soliqua)

Does not include premixed insulins - see Insulin section

INSULIN

In an individual without diabetes, the pancreas controls the release of insulin in the body. It provides a consistent level (or basal amount) of insulin at all times, then releases more insulin when the BG is elevated postprandially (after meals). In a patient with diabetes, <u>insulin</u> can be administered to <u>mimic</u> the <u>normal physiologic process</u>. Insulin cannot be given orally; it is given as a <u>subcutaneous injection</u> (most common), <u>intravenously</u> (less often, usually for acutely high BG) or inhaled (uncommon).

Insulin is a <u>high-alert medication</u>, which means it has a <u>high risk</u> of causing <u>patient harm</u> and requires extra care during handling and administration. Insulin is a high-alert medication primarily due to <u>human errors</u>, such as <u>misreading</u> measurements, using the <u>wrong</u> insulin <u>type, strength, dose or frequency</u> and <u>skipping meals</u>.

INSULIN PROPERTIES AND TYPES

The graph below shows the <u>onset, peak</u> and <u>duration of action</u> of the common insulin types, which must be understood in order to design an insulin regimen and to make <u>adjustments</u> when the BG trends too high or too low. The table that follows describes how the different types of insulins are used and their major safety issues. Basal and rapid-acting insulins are called <u>insulin analogs</u>; when basal insulin is used with mealtime rapid-acting insulin, the profile is <u>analogous</u> (similar) to the <u>natural pattern of insulin secretion</u> from the pancreas.

Basal Insulin

- <u>Basal insulin</u> includes <u>glargine</u> (red line), <u>detemir</u> (blue line) and ultra-long acting <u>degludec</u> (pink line). These insulins are "<u>peakless</u>" with an <u>onset of 3 – 4 hours</u> and duration ≥ 24 hours. They mainly impact <u>fasting glucose</u>.

Intermediate-Acting Insulin

- <u>Insulin NPH</u> (yellow line) is <u>intermediate</u>-acting but it can be used as a basal insulin. NPH has an <u>onset of 1 – 2 hours</u>, and it <u>peaks</u> at <u>4 – 12 hours</u>, which can cause <u>hypoglycemia</u>. BG control is further complicated by the <u>variable</u>, unpredictable <u>duration</u> of action (<u>14 – 24 hours</u>).

- The P in NPH is for <u>protamine</u>, which helps to delay absorption/extend the duration of effect. Lispro-protamine and aspart-protamine, have the same onset, peak and duration as NPH; they come in premixed solutions only, combined with standard rapid-acting insulins (aspart and lispro).

Rapid-Acting and Short-Acting Insulin

- <u>Rapid-acting</u> insulin (purple line) includes aspart, lispro and glulisine. These provide a <u>bolus</u> dose, similar to the pancreas releasing a burst of insulin in response to food. They have a fast <u>onset (~15 min)</u>, peak in <u>1 – 2 hours</u> and have a <u>duration of 3 – 5 hours</u> (gone by the next meal).

- <u>Regular</u> insulin U-100 (green line) is considered a <u>short-acting insulin</u>; it can be given as a bolus at mealtimes like rapid-acting insulin, but has a slower onset and lasts longer than needed for a meal. Regular insulin has an <u>onset of 30 minutes, peaks at ~2 hours and lasts 6 – 10 hours</u>.

Other Insulins (Not Included in Graph)

- <u>Regular U-500</u> is a very <u>concentrated</u> insulin. The onset is the same as regular insulin U-100, but the duration is closer to NPH; it can last up to 24 hours. It is often dosed twice daily or TID, before meals.

- <u>Inhaled insulin</u> is not used commonly. It is a <u>mealtime</u> insulin with fast absorption through the lungs.

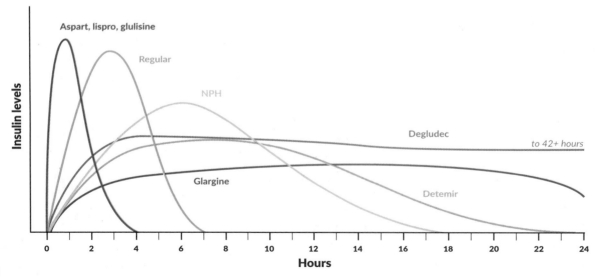

©UWorld

INSULIN SAFETY ISSUES AND NOTES; APPLIES TO ALL INJECTABLE INSULIN, EXCEPT WHERE NOTED

CONTRAINDICATIONS
- Do not administer during episodes of hypoglycemia.

WARNINGS
- Hypoglycemia, hypokalemia (insulin facilitates K+ entry into cells, and is used to treat hyperkalemia).

SIDE EFFECTS
- Weight gain: insulin causes excess glucose to move into adipose cells, and increases body fat and lean mass and stimulates appetite.

- Lipoatrophy: loss of SC fat at the injection site (which disfigures skin) and lipohypertrophy: accumulation of fat lumps under the injection site. Avoid both by rotating injection sites and using analog insulins (lower risk than with older insulins).

STORAGE AND ADMINISTRATION NOTES
- Most vials are 10 mL (a few products are also available in 3 mL, which helps decrease waste in an institutional setting) and most pens are 3 mL.

- Insulin concentrations are 100 units/mL, unless noted otherwise (discussed later in the chapter).

- Do not shake; turn suspensions (NPH, protamine mixes) up and down slowly or roll between hands. Do not freeze or expose to extreme heat.

- Unopened insulin vials and pens are stored in the refrigerator. Open vials and pens can be kept at room temperature (see Room Temperature Stability of Insulin chart later in the chapter). It is more painful/uncomfortable to inject cold insulin.

- Pen devices should never be shared (even if the needle is changed) due to the risk for transmission of blood-borne pathogens.

- Any percentage mixture of NPH and regular (or rapid-acting) insulins can be made by mixing the two insulins in the same syringe; regular insulin (and rapid-acting) is clear and is drawn up (into the syringe) first, before the NPH, which is cloudy.

Rapid-Acting (Bolus) Insulin	
Aspart (Novolog, Fiasp) **Lispro (Humalog**, Admelog, Lyumjev) Lispro U-200 (Humalog U-200) Insulin Glulisine (Apidra) Clear and colorless Apidra SoloStar pens contain glulisine Humalog KwikPens contain lispro Novolog FlexPens contain aspart	▪ Inject SC 5-15 minutes before meals to have insulin available when glucose from the meal is absorbed. ❑ Lispro can also be administered right after eating. ❑ Fiasp and Lyumjev can be injected with the first bite or within 20 minutes of starting a meal. ▪ Used as prandial insulin (to prevent high BG from a meal) and for correction doses (often using a sliding scale) when BG is high. ▪ Preferred insulin type for insulin pumps (discussed later in the chapter). ▪ Aspart and lispro insulins come in premixed insulins with intermediate-acting protamine insulin. ▪ Co-formulations with faster absorption: Fiasp is formulated with niacinamide (vitamin B3) and Lyumjev is formulated with treprostinil and citrate.
Inhaled insulin (Afrezza)	▪ Contraindicated in any lung disease, including asthma and COPD; do not use Afrezza in smokers. ▪ Can cause acute bronchospasm, cough and throat pain. ▪ Requires lung monitoring with pulmonary function tests (FEV1). Replace inhaler every 15 days.

Short-Acting (Bolus) Insulin	
Regular (Humulin R, Novolin R, Novolin R ReliOn) Clear and colorless Rx and OTC Myxredlin is a ready-to-use (RTU) regular insulin IV solution (100 mL bag)	▪ Inject SC 30 minutes before meals to have insulin available when the glucose from the next meal is absorbed. ▪ Used as prandial insulin and for correction doses (often using a sliding scale) when BG is high. ▪ Regular insulin is preferred for IV infusions, including in parenteral nutrition; it is less expensive than other insulins and when administered as a continuous IV infusion, the onset is immediate. IV regular insulin should be prepared in a non-PVC container. ▪ Often given with NPH twice daily, 30 min before breakfast and dinner. Lunch is covered by the NPH, and possibly some residual regular insulin. This regimen requires just 2 injections per day (since the insulins can be mixed).
Concentrated Regular U-500 (Humulin R U-500)	▪ Five times as concentrated as regular insulin; many safety risks. Recommended only when patients require > 200 units of insulin per day. ▪ The prescribed dose of Humulin R U-500 should always be expressed in units of insulin. ▪ All patients using the U-500 insulin vial must be prescribed U-500 insulin syringes to avoid dosing errors; see the Syringes and Needles section for details. ▪ Do not mix with any other insulin; only administer as SC injection (not IV, IM or in an insulin pump).

Intermediate-Acting (Basal) Insulin

NPH (*Humulin N, Novolin N, Novolin N ReliOn*) Cloudy Rx and OTC	■ Given as a basal insulin, typically dosed <u>twice daily</u> as an add-on to oral drugs. Can be a less expensive alternative, but causes more <u>hypoglycemia</u>. ■ If nocturnal hypoglycemia occurs with NPH dosed once daily QHS, the dose can be split (e.g., 2/3 QAM, 1/3 QHS).

Long-Acting (Basal) Insulin

Insulin detemir (*Levemir*) **Insulin glargine (*Lantus, Toujeo, Basaglar*)** Interchangeable biosimilars to *Lantus*: *Rezvoglar, Semglee* Clear and colorless	■ Usually injected <u>once daily</u>; detemir may need to be given twice daily. ■ Caution required: *Lantus* is <u>100 units/mL</u> and *Toujeo* is a <u>concentrated</u> insulin glargine with <u>300 units/mL</u> (an option when > 20 units/day of insulin glargine is needed). ■ *Toujeo* has max effect by the 5th day; the coverage may not be adequate initially. ■ *Lantus* and *Toujeo* [and the rapid-acting insulins *Admelog* (lispro) and *Apidra* (glulisine)] are made by the same manufacturer and all of them use the same *SoloStar* pen. ■ <u>Do not mix</u> with any other insulins. ■ Pending state law restrictions, interchangeable biosimilars to *Lantus* can be substituted without a separate prescription or provider intervention.

Ultra-Long-Acting (Basal) Insulin

Insulin degludec (*Tresiba*)	■ Insulin degludec comes in a vial and the *Tresiba FlexTouch* pen. The vial has 100 units/mL. *Tresiba FlexTouch* pens come in <u>100 units/mL and 200 units/mL</u>. ■ *Tresiba* can be useful when insulin detemir or glargine causes nocturnal hypoglycemia.

Premixed Insulin

70/30 MIXES **70% NPH/30% regular** **(*Humulin 70/30, Novolin 70/30*)** Rx and OTC 70% aspart protamine/30% aspart (*Novolog Mix 70/30*) **75/25 MIX** 75% lispro protamine/25% lispro (*Humalog Mix 75/25*) **50/50 MIX** 50% lispro protamine/50% lispro (*Humalog Mix 50/50*)	■ Given BID (before breakfast and dinner), or sometimes TID (mixes with rapid-acting insulin). ❑ If the mixture contains <u>rapid-acting</u> insulin: inject <u>15 minutes</u> before a meal. ❑ If the mixture contains <u>regular</u> insulin: inject <u>30 minutes</u> before a meal. ■ In premixed insulins, the percentage of NPH or protamine insulin is listed <u>first</u> and the percentage of short-acting or rapid-acting insulin is listed <u>second</u> (e.g., *Humulin 70/30* contains 70% NPH and 30% regular). ■ NPH or protamine (which are both cloudy) make the premixed insulins cloudy. **CASE SCENARIO** A 35-year-old female injects *Humulin 70/30* 60 units before breakfast and 20 units before dinner. **What is her TDD of regular insulin?** *Humulin 70/30* is 70% NPH and 30% regular. The regular insulin dose in the morning is 60 units x 0.3 = 18 units. The regular insulin dose in the evening is 20 units x 0.3 = 6 units. The TDD of regular insulin is 24 units.

Drug Interactions with Insulin

■ <u>Avoid</u> concurrent use of insulin with <u>sulfonylureas or meglitinides</u>. May need to ↓ insulin dose when used with drugs that can cause hypoglycemia, including SGLT2 inhibitors, GLP-1 agonists, TZDs and DPP-4 inhibitors.

■ Pramlintide: <u>must reduce mealtime insulin by 50%</u> when <u>starting</u> pramlintide to avoid <u>severe hypoglycemia</u>.

■ May need to ↓ insulin dose when used with direct acting antivirals (DAAs) for hepatitis C treatment due to the risk of hypoglycemia.

INSULIN AVAILABLE OTC

<u>Regular, NPH and premixed 70% NPH/30% regular insulins</u> can be sold <u>OTC</u> or can be dispensed with a prescription for insurance coverage. All basal and rapid-acting insulins are available by prescription only.

INSULIN DOSING AND CALCULATIONS

STARTING INSULIN IN TYPE 2 DIABETES

If an injectable medication is needed to reduce the A1C in T2D, a GLP-1 receptor agonist is preferred and should be considered first. If the patient is already on a GLP-1 agonist (or a GLP-1 agonist is not appropriate), insulin should be started. An exception is when using insulin initially to treat very high BG at diagnosis (A1C > 10% or BG ≥ 300 mg/dL) or if symptoms of catabolism are present (e.g., DKA). If insulin is required, combination with a GLP-1 agonist is recommended for greater efficacy. Starting insulin in T2D should follow a step-wise approach (see image below).

Starting Insulin in Type 2 Diabetes

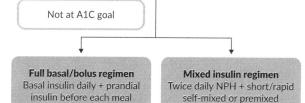

Add basal insulin
10 units SC daily or 0.1-0.2 units/kg/day SC
Titrate based on fasting plasma glucose (FPG)

If FPG not at goal or signs that prandial insulin is needed (e.g., FPG at goal or below goal, but A1C above goal)

Add prandial insulin
4 units or 10% of basal dose SC once daily prior to largest meal
Titrate based on prandial blood glucose; add on doses prior to other meals if needed

Not at A1C goal

Full basal/bolus regimen
Basal insulin daily + prandial insulin before each meal

Mixed insulin regimen
Twice daily NPH + short/rapid self-mixed or premixed

©UWorld

STARTING INSULIN IN TYPE 1 DIABETES

All people with T1D require insulin. Most are treated with an insulin pump or multiple daily injections of insulin designed to mimic the normal pattern of insulin secretion. Rapid-acting injectable insulins and long-acting basal insulins are preferred (over short- and intermediate-acting insulins) because they cause less hypoglycemia risk and better mimic the physiologic pattern of insulin made by the body.

STARTING A BASAL-BOLUS INSULIN REGIMEN IN TYPE 1 DIABETES

The typical starting dose for T1D is 0.5 units/kg/day.

Insulin is dosed using total body weight (TBW).

Commonly, 50% of the total daily dose (TDD) is administered as basal insulin and 50% as prandial (bolus) insulin. Steps:

1. Calculate the TDD (0.5 units/kg/day, using TBW).

2. Divide the TDD into 50% basal insulin and 50% bolus (rapid-acting) insulin.

3. Divide the bolus insulin evenly among 3 meals (or allocate more insulin for larger meals and less for smaller meals).

CASE SCENARIO

Start a basal-bolus regimen with *Lantus* and *Humalog* in a patient with type 1 diabetes that weighs 84 kg.

1. Calculate the TDD:
   0.5 units/kg/day x 84 kg = 42 units

2. Split the dose in half for basal and rapid-acting insulin:
   21 units Lantus and 21 units Humalog

3. Split rapid-acting insulin into 3 even doses:
   7 units Humalog TID AC

Regimen: 21 units *Lantus* daily and 7 units *Humalog* TID AC

Starting a Regimen with NPH and Regular Insulin

NPH and regular insulin regimens are not preferred; neither insulin has a profile that can mimic the natural insulin release from the pancreas as well as basal and rapid-acting insulin combinations. However, the lower cost and ability to use less injections (since these insulins can be mixed) make this type of regimen more feasible for some.

The starting TDD of insulin is the same as with basal-bolus regimens. However, NPH is given twice daily with 30% of the TDD in the morning and 20% of the TDD in the evening. The remaining 50% of the TDD is given as regular insulin.

TREATMENT WITH AN INSULIN PUMP

Pumps can provide excellent BG control and require less daily insulin injections. Users must be motivated, willing to test their BG frequently and be able to understand the pump's operation. Prior experience with multiple daily injections is a requirement for switching to a pump.

Pumps hold insulin in a reservoir (see image on the next page). The insulin runs out of the pump through tubing to a small infusion set placed on the skin, usually on the abdomen, through a small cannula (needle) that inserts under the skin. The cannula tip rests in subcutaneous fatty tissue, where the insulin is released. The insulin reservoir, tubing and infusion set need to be replaced regularly.

Insulin pumps deliver <u>rapid-acting</u> insulin (preferred) by two complementary methods, <u>continuous</u> and <u>bolus</u> dosing.

1. <u>Continuous</u> doses: <u>small amounts</u> of <u>insulin</u> are released every few minutes to provide a <u>basal</u> insulin level.

2. <u>Bolus</u> doses: pumps can be programmed to release a number of insulin units to <u>match</u> the <u>carbohydrates</u> in a meal. The bolus dose is calculated by the patient's <u>insulin to carbohydrate ratio</u> (ICR), see Mealtime Insulin Dosing Options section. The bolus dose is adjusted based on the current BG level (e.g., if low, use less insulin).

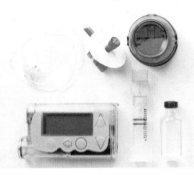

The insulin is held in a reservoir that is inserted into the pump.
The tubing connects the pump to the infusion set, which has a cannula that inserts under the skin.

iStock.com/Click_and_Photo

CASE SCENARIO

RC, a 47-year-old male with type 2 diabetes, takes *Toujeo* 18 units SC QHS and *Novolog* 5 units SC TID AC. He presents with two days of BG readings, taken before meals and at bedtime.

	BREAKFAST	LUNCH	DINNER	BED
Day 1 (mg/dL)	105	118	200	126
Day 2 (mg/dL)	97	115	197	122

What adjustment should be made to RC's insulin regimen?

The *Novolog* dose taken prior to lunch should be increased.

Explanation: the goal range for preprandial blood glucose is 80-130 mg/dL. The readings are all within the normal range except for the readings before dinner. The high readings before dinner indicate that RC is not taking enough insulin before lunch. The lunchtime dose should be increased.

Fasting BG is most affected by the basal insulin. If the pre-breakfast readings were high, the *Toujeo* dose should be increased.

If the readings at dinner were taken postprandially (instead of preprandially), the *Novolog* dose before dinner should be increased.

ADJUSTING INSULIN BASED ON BLOOD GLUCOSE TRENDS

BG readings from a meter can be written on a paper log or downloaded from a meter's memory (see later section on Blood Glucose Monitoring). Changes to an insulin dose are not based on single measurements; there needs to be a <u>trend</u> showing that the BG runs too high or too low. BG is ideally checked before breakfast (FPG), lunch and dinner and at bedtime. A high or low BG reading is reflective of the <u>insulin dose prior</u> to that reading; look backwards to see which insulin/s are active and could be contributing to the trend.

Adjusting Basal Insulin

<u>Fasting</u> BG <u>highs</u> or <u>lows</u>, and/or similar trends that last most of the day (except with BG spikes after eating), typically indicate that the <u>basal insulin</u> dose needs to be changed.

- Low fasting BG trend: ↓ the <u>basal</u> or <u>NPH</u> insulin dose.
- High fasting BG trend: ↑ the <u>basal</u> or <u>NPH</u> insulin dose.

Adjusting Mealtime Insulin

If the postprandial BG is high or low <u>following</u> the <u>same meal</u> on most days, the <u>regular</u> or <u>rapid-acting</u> insulin dose taken prior to that meal should be <u>increased</u> for <u>high BG</u>, or <u>decreased</u> for <u>low BG</u>.

If the <u>preprandial</u> BG is high or low <u>before</u> the <u>same meal</u> (e.g., lunch) on most days, the <u>regular</u> or <u>rapid-acting</u> insulin dose taken before the previous meal (e.g., breakfast) should be <u>increased</u> for <u>high BG</u>, or <u>decreased</u> for <u>low BG</u>.

MEALTIME INSULIN DOSING OPTIONS

Option 1: Use the Same Insulin Dose Every Time

The mealtime (rapid-acting or regular) insulin dose can the same everyday for a meal (e.g., 20 units of insulin lispro before dinner).

- This assumes that the grams of carbohydrates eaten at dinner every day is about the same.
- This method results in high or low BG when the carbohydrate intake is higher or lower, respectively.

Option 2: Calculate an Insulin Dose at Each Meal

When different amounts of carbohydrates are eaten at each meal (which is common), a simple calculation can provide the right amount of rapid-acting or regular insulin needed.

- The bolus dose is calculated with the <u>insulin-to-carbohydrate ratio (ICR)</u>.
- The ICR indicates the <u>grams</u> of <u>carbohydrates</u> covered by <u>1 unit of insulin</u>.
- There are two variations of the ICR formula, depending on the type of insulin being used. <u>Regular</u> insulin uses the <u>Rule of 450</u>, and <u>rapid-acting</u> insulin uses the <u>Rule of 500</u>. The <u>TDD of insulin</u> used in the formula should account for <u>both</u> long-acting and short- or rapid-acting insulins included in the regimen.

ICR: Rule of 450 *for REGULAR*

$$\frac{450}{\text{total daily dose of insulin (TDD)}} = \begin{array}{l}\text{grams of carbohydrates}\\ \text{covered by 1 unit of regular}\\ \text{insulin}\end{array}$$

ICR: Rule of 500 *for RAPID-ACTING*

$$\frac{500}{\text{total daily dose of insulin (TDD)}} = \begin{array}{l}\text{grams of carbohydrate}\\ \text{covered by 1 unit of rapid-}\\ \text{acting insulin}\end{array}$$

CASE SCENARIO

ST is a 70 kg female with T1D who uses an insulin lispro pump. The continuous (basal) dose delivered by the pump in a 24 hour period is 26 units of insulin lispro. The average daily amount of insulin lispro administered as bolus doses with meals is 24 units.

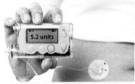

Click and Photo/Shutterstock.com

Calculate the ICR.

ST uses rapid-acting insulin. Use the Rule of 500.

$$\frac{500}{\text{total daily dose of insulin (TDD)}} = \begin{array}{l}\text{grams of carbohydrate}\\ \text{covered by 1 unit of}\\ \text{rapid-acting insulin}\end{array}$$

$$\frac{500}{50 \text{ units}} = 10$$

She has an ICR of 1:10, which means 1 unit of rapid-acting insulin covers 10 grams of carbohydrates.

ST will eat a hamburger (24 g carbohydrate) and fries (28 g carbohydrate) for lunch. She adds up the total carbohydrates and divides by 10 to calculate the bolus dose:

$$\frac{24 \text{ g (bun)} + 28 \text{ g (fries)}}{10 \text{ (her ICR)}} = 5.2 \text{ units}$$

ST enters 5.2 units on the pump. If she was using a syringe or pen to inject, she would round to the nearest whole number.

CORRECTION DOSES FOR ELEVATED BLOOD GLUCOSE

BG that is higher than the targeted range can be corrected with a bolus called a correction dose.

1. The first step is to calculate the correction factor, which indicates how much the BG will be lowered (in mg/dL) by 1 unit of insulin.

   ❏ To calculate the correction factor, use the 1,500 Rule for regular insulin and the 1,800 Rule for rapid-acting insulin. The TDD of insulin used in the formula should account for both long-acting and short- or rapid-acting insulins included in the regimen.

Correction Factor – 1,500 Rule *for REGULAR*

$$\frac{1,500}{\text{total daily dose of insulin (TDD)}} = \begin{array}{l}\text{correction factor for 1 unit}\\ \text{of regular insulin}\end{array}$$

Correction Factor – 1,800 Rule *for RAPID-ACTING*

$$\frac{1,800}{\text{total daily dose of insulin (TDD)}} = \begin{array}{l}\text{correction factor for 1 unit}\\ \text{of rapid-acting insulin}\end{array}$$

2. Next, calculate the correction dose, which is the total units of insulin needed to return the BG to the target range. The formula for the correction dose is the same for both regular and rapid-acting insulin.

Correction Dose *for BOTH TYPES*

$$\frac{(\text{blood glucose now}) - (\text{target blood glucose})}{\text{correction factor}} = \text{correction dose}$$

CASE SCENARIO

JJ is a 35-year-old male with T2D currently treated with *Lantus* 50 units SC QHS and *Novolog* 15 units SC TID AC.

1. What is JJ's correction factor?

Since *Novolog* is a rapid-acting insulin, use the Rule of 1,800 to calculate JJ's correction factor.

$$\frac{1,800}{\text{total daily dose of insulin (TDD)}} = \begin{array}{l}\text{correction factor for}\\ \text{1 unit of rapid-acting}\\ \text{insulin}\end{array}$$

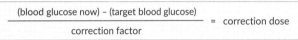

50 units Lantus + 45 units Novolog = 95 units ← TDD

$$\frac{1,800}{95 \text{ units}} = 18.947 = 19 \xleftarrow{} \begin{array}{l}\text{Round to the}\\ \text{nearest whole \#}\end{array}$$

A correction factor of 19 means 1 unit of rapid-acting insulin will lower the BG by 19 mg/dL.

2. JJ has a target premeal BG of 120 mg/dL. He checks his BG before dinner and it is 200 mg/dL. What dose of *Novolog* should JJ administer before dinner?

Determine the correction dose using the formula:

$$\frac{(\text{blood glucose now}) - (\text{target blood glucose})}{\text{correction factor}} = \begin{array}{l}\text{correction}\\ \text{dose}\end{array}$$

$$\frac{200 \text{ mg/dL} - 120 \text{ mg/dL}}{19} = 4 \text{ units}$$

Add the correction dose to the number of units JJ usually administers before meals to get the dose he needs before dinner: 4 units + 15 units = 19 units *Novolog*

INSULIN CONVERSIONS

Most insulin conversions are 1:1 (the same dose is used), but the regimen might need to be split up differently. The exceptions involve converting twice daily NPH and different forms of glargine; see the Study Tip Gal on the next page.

INSULIN ADMINISTRATION

INSULIN STRENGTHS AND CONTAINERS

Most insulin products contain 100 units/mL of insulin. Some insulins have > 100 units/mL; these are concentrated insulins (see below). Insulin is available in:

- Vials (usually 10 mL); insulin is drawn up with an insulin syringe. *Humulin R U-500* comes in a 20 mL vial. A few products come in a 3 mL vial (primarily for use in an institutional setting to decrease waste; 10 mL vials are more commonly dispensed for patient use).

- Pens; insulin is ready to inject once a needle is attached. Pens are dialed to the number of units needed. All pens contain 3 mL of insulin, except *Toujeo*, which is available in two sizes: 1.5 mL and 3 mL.

All insulin pens are multi-dose; needles must be dispensed with all insulin pens. Some pens are disposable, and others have replaceable cartridges.

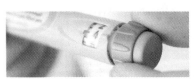

Insulin pens are easy to use; simply dial the units to inject.

Orawan Pattarawimonchai/Shutterstock.com

Example of providing a 20-unit dose of *Lantus* 100 units/mL with a pen or with a vial and syringe:

- The *Lantus Solostar* pen would be dialed to 20 units, which would provide 0.2 mL.

- The *Lantus* 10 mL vial provides the same dose by drawing up 0.2 mL with a U-100 syringe.

Concentrated Insulin

Injecting high doses of U-100 insulin requires a volume that can feel uncomfortable and, with very high doses (> 100 units), can require more than one syringe. Concentrated

insulin is useful to reduce the volume of the injection, but can be fatal when used incorrectly. Fortunately, most concentrated insulin comes in pens, which are simply dialed to the correct dose. The concentrated insulin that comes in both a pen and a vial is regular insulin U-500, which has higher risk.

INSULIN THAT COMES CONCENTRATED

Rapid-Acting Insulin
Humalog KwikPen, *Lyumjev KwikPen* (lispro): 200 units/mL

Short-Acting Insulin
Humulin R U-500 KwikPen and vial: 500 units/mL

Long-Acting Insulin
Tresiba FlexTouch pen (degludec): 200 units/mL
Toujeo SoloStar, *Toujeo Max SoloStar* pens (glargine): 300 units/mL

Example of providing an 80-unit dose with *Tresiba FlexTouch* U-100 and U-200:

Pens of either strength would be dialed to 80 units. The difference is the volume of the injection.

- An 80-unit dose with U-100 is 0.8 mL.

- An 80-unit dose with U-200 is 0.4 mL (half the volume).

Concentrated Regular Insulin U-500

Humulin R U-500 is five times as concentrated as regular insulin U-100. It is useful for patients taking > 200 units/day, but has a high risk for dosing errors.

Methods to avoid dosing errors with U-500 insulin:

- The prescribed dose of *Humulin R U-500* should always be expressed in units of insulin. Only dispense with U-500 syringes (see Selecting an Insulin Syringe section).

- *Humulin R U-500 KwikPen* provides up to 300 units with one injection and has a lower risk of dosing errors.

INSULIN STABILITY

Unused insulin vials, pens and cartridges are stored in the refrigerator. The expiration date of insulin that has been stored in the refrigerator is the manufacturer's expiration date on the label.

Once the insulin is in use it can be kept at room temperature, but the manufacturer's expiration date no longer applies. Insulin stored at room temperature must be used within a specific number of days based on the type of insulin (see Study Tip Gal below). This is an important counseling point for patients.

Notice in the table that most insulin is stable at room temperature for 28 days including all rapid-acting insulin. The insulins with shorter stability are typically pens.

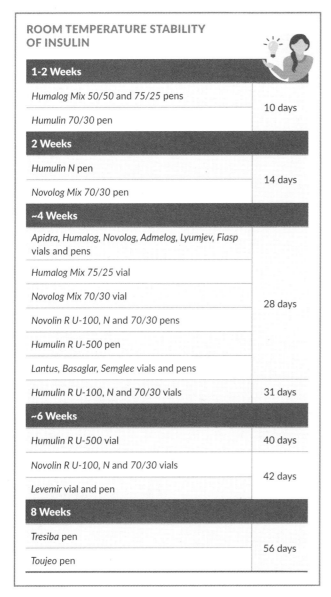

ROOM TEMPERATURE STABILITY OF INSULIN	
1-2 Weeks	
Humalog Mix 50/50 and 75/25 pens	10 days
Humulin 70/30 pen	
2 Weeks	
Humulin N pen	14 days
Novolog Mix 70/30 pen	
~4 Weeks	
Apidra, Humalog, Novolog, Admelog, Lyumjev, Fiasp vials and pens	28 days
Humalog Mix 75/25 vial	
Novolog Mix 70/30 vial	
Novolin R U-100, N and 70/30 pens	
Humulin R U-500 pen	
Lantus, Basaglar, Semglee vials and pens	
Humulin R U-100, N and 70/30 vials	31 days
~6 Weeks	
Humulin R U-500 vial	40 days
Novolin R U-100, N and 70/30 vials	42 days
Levemir vial and pen	
8 Weeks	
Tresiba pen	56 days
Toujeo pen	

SYRINGES AND NEEDLES

Selecting an Insulin Syringe

Use the smallest U-100 syringe that will hold the units of insulin. The unit markings are in smaller increments on smaller syringes, which increases the accuracy of insulin measurements.

- 0.3 mL syringe for less than 30 units
- 0.5 mL syringe for 30 – 50 units
- 1 mL syringe for 51 – 100 units

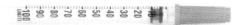

A 1 mL U-100 insulin syringe holds up to 100 units. Use smaller syringes to inject up to 50 units.

khuntapol/Shutterstock.com

Humulin R U-500 insulin vials can only be dispensed with U-500 syringes. The U-500 vials have a dark green cap and the U-500 syringes (Rx only) have dark green needle covers. In contrast, U-100 syringes have orange caps. A U-500 syringe holds up to 250 units; a U-100 1 mL syringe holds up to 100 units.

Selecting an Insulin Pen Needle

Needles are chosen by the length and the gauge (thickness). The higher the gauge, the thinner the needle [e.g., 28G (thickest) – 32G (thinnest)]. The 32G cannula has a width of ~2 human hairs. Shorter needles and higher-gauge needles cause less pain.

- The shortest needles are 4 mm and 5 mm in length and are preferred for most pens. They do not require the skin to be pinched during administration and are good for thinner patients and children.

- 8 mm needles are long enough for most patients; pinch up the skin before injecting.

- 12.7 mm (1/2 inch) needles may be needed for obese patients; pinch up the skin before injecting.

Common brands for needles and syringes include BD, Comfort EZ and Easy Touch. Needles require a prescription in some states.

INSULIN INJECTION COUNSELING

1. Get supplies. Wash hands.

2. Check insulin for discoloration and particles. Discard if present.

3. If insulin contains NPH or protamine, it is a suspension and needs to be resuspended (do not shake):

   ❏ Vials: roll the bottle gently between the hands.

   ❏ Pens: invert (turn upside-down) 4 – 5 times.

4. Clean the injection site (area of the skin) with an alcohol swab. If using a vial, wipe the top (after removing the plastic cover) with an alcohol swab.

5. Pens:

    ❏ Use a <u>new needle</u> for each injection. Prior to each injection, <u>prime the needle</u> by turning the knob to <u>2 units</u> (can vary based on the insulin), face the needle away from you and press the injection button.

    ❏ Turn the dosing knob to the correct number of units, then inject (see number 7, below).

6. Vials:

    ❏ Use a new syringe for each injection; syringes come with a needle already attached. Inject an equal volume of air into the vial before withdrawing the insulin. Limit bubbles in the syringe.

    ❏ If <u>mixing NPH</u> and <u>regular or rapid-acting</u> insulin in the same syringe, the <u>clear</u> insulin (regular or rapid-acting) should be drawn into the syringe <u>before</u> the <u>cloudy</u> (NPH) insulin. Tip: inject air into the cloudy insulin first, then inject air into the clear insulin before withdrawing it out.

7. Insulin is best absorbed in the <u>abdomen (preferred)</u>. Alternative sites for injection: posterior upper arm, superior buttocks and lateral thigh area (shaded areas of image).

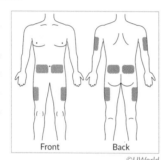

Front   Back
©UWorld

8. With needles > 5 mm, gently <u>pinch a 2-inch</u> portion of skin between your thumb and first finger (typically not required with shorter needles).

9. Insert the needle all the way in. Pens are injected <u>straight down</u> (at a 90-degree angle). Syringes are injected at <u>90 degrees for most</u> or <u>45 degrees</u> if the patient is <u>thin</u>.

10. Press the injection button (pen) or plunger (syringe) all the way down to inject the insulin. Count <u>5 – 10 seconds</u> before removing the needle.

11. <u>Rotate injection sites</u> around the abdomen regularly to prevent skin damage.

12. <u>Properly dispose</u> of needles or entire syringes (see below). Do not store pens with needle attached.

DEVICE DISPOSAL

Used needles, syringes, single-dose pens (with needles attached) and lancets should be placed in a <u>sharps disposal container</u> and taken to a disposal site. Locations are provided by the local public health agency. Alternatively, a heavy plastic milk bottle (not glass) or metal coffee can works well.

BLOOD GLUCOSE MONITORING

Blood glucose monitoring (<u>BGM</u>) refers to patients tracking their BG using a <u>glucose meter</u> or a <u>continuous glucose monitor (CGM)</u>. CGMs are taped to the skin and have a probe that passes through the skin and into the fatty tissue. The probe provides measurements of the <u>glucose level</u> in the <u>interstitial fluid</u> between the cells. CGM also provides a percent time in range, a useful metric of glycemic control.

PREPARING TO USE A GLUCOSE METER

- If the meter requires calibration, recalibrate each time a new canister of test strips is opened, if the meter was left in extreme cold or heat, if it was dropped or if the BG value does not match what the patient is feeling.

- <u>Keep</u> the <u>test strips</u> in the <u>original container</u>, with the <u>cap closed</u>. Light and air damage test strips. Check the <u>expiration date</u>; expired test strips can give false results.

- Wash hands vigorously, using warm water.

- Dry hands thoroughly; water can dilute the blood sample and give a false result.

- Allow arm to hang down for 30 seconds so blood can pool into the fingertips. Do not squeeze the finger.

TESTING WITH A GLUCOSE METER

- Insert test strip into meter.

- Prick <u>side of fingertip</u> (side is less painful) with a lancet.

- Apply a drop of blood to the test strip.

- Record the result in a logbook, or the meter might store the results.

- Dispose of the used lancet in a sharps container.

Alternative Site Testing

- Some meters are approved to test blood from both the fingertip and <u>alternative</u> sites (<u>forearm, palm or thigh</u>), which can hurt less than the side of a fingertip.

- Alternative testing sites are useful <u>only</u> when the <u>BG is steady</u>. The BG level can be ~20 minutes old. Do <u>not</u> use when the <u>BG is changing quickly</u> (e.g., after <u>eating</u>, after <u>exercise</u>, when <u>hypoglycemia</u> is suspected).

- The lancing device might need to have a special cap screwed onto the tip to use on an alternative site.

HYPOGLYCEMIA

Hypoglycemia is defined as a <u>BG < 70 mg/dL</u>. Low BG can have <u>severe consequences</u>, including <u>falls</u>, motor vehicle accidents and death. Each episode contributes to irreversible <u>cognitive impairment</u>.

HYPOGLYCEMIA SYMPTOMS

Symptoms include dizziness, anxiety/irritability, shakiness, headache, diaphoresis (sweating), hunger, confusion, nausea, ataxia, tremors, palpitations/tachycardia and blurred vision.

Severe hypoglycemia can cause seizures, coma and death. All episodes of hypoglycemia are dangerous and should be reported to the prescriber. Monitoring with a CGM can help by displaying the BG every few minutes and sounding an alert when the BG level falls too low. CGM should be considered for individuals at high risk for hypoglycemia (e.g., T1D, multiple insulin injections).

HYPOGLYCEMIA TREATMENT

Conscious and Able to Swallow

Pure glucose, in tablets or gel, is preferred, but any form of carbohydrate that contains glucose will work (see image). Added fat (e.g., a chocolate candy bar) is not recommended; it slows absorption and prolongs hypoglycemia. To treat, follow the "rule of 15":

1. Ingest 15 – 20 grams of glucose or simple carbohydrates.

2. Recheck BG after 15 minutes.

3. If hypoglycemia continues, repeat steps 1 & 2.

4. Once BG is normal, eat a small meal or snack.

Unconscious

When oral treatment is not possible, treat with dextrose (if there is IV access) or with glucagon. Caregivers of someone at high risk for hypoglycemia should know how to administer glucagon 1 mg SC injection (*GlucaGen, Gvoke*), dasiglucagon injection (*Zegalogue*) or glucagon nasal spray (*Baqsimi*). If using glucagon, place the patient in a lateral recumbent position (on side) to protect the airway and prevent choking when consciousness returns.

DRUG-INDUCED HIGH OR LOW BLOOD GLUCOSE

DRUGS THAT CAUSE HYPOGLYCEMIA

- Insulin is the primary cause of drug-induced hypoglycemia.

- Sulfonylureas and meglitinides ("insulin secretagogues") and pramlintide are high-risk.

  - Glyburide and glimepiride are not recommended in the elderly due to hypoglycemia risk.

- GLP-1 agonists, DPP-4 inhibitors, SGLT2 inhibitors and TZDs have a low risk for hypoglycemia when used alone. When used in combination with insulin or a sulfonylurea, the risk is higher, and the insulin or sulfonylurea dose may need to be lowered.

Raise Blood Sugar with 15 Grams of Simple Carbs

4 oz. (1/2 cup) of Juice   8 oz. (1 cup) Milk   4 oz. Regular Soda (not diet)

1 Tablespoon Sugar, Honey or Corn Syrup   3-4 Glucose Tablets or 1 Serving Glucose Gel (follow package instructions)

- Alcohol, especially if taken on an empty stomach, can cause hypoglycemia when used with insulin or sulfonylureas.

- Caution: beta-blockers can enhance the hypoglycemic effects of insulin and sulfonylureas and mask some of the symptoms of hypoglycemia (e.g., shakiness, palpitations, anxiety); sweating, and possibly hunger, will still be present. Counsel to recognize symptoms and test BG if unsure.

DRUGS THAT CAUSE HYPERGLYCEMIA

It is preferable, but not always possible, to avoid drugs that increase BG (see Key Drugs Guy). If not avoidable (e.g., using tacrolimus post-transplant), the increase in BG will need to be managed.

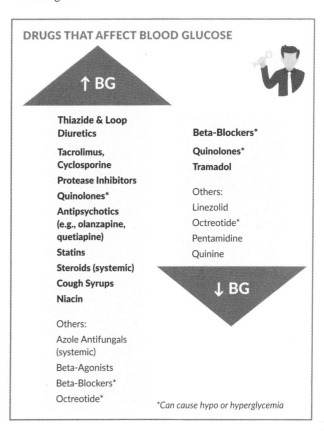

DRUGS THAT AFFECT BLOOD GLUCOSE

↑ BG

Thiazide & Loop Diuretics

Tacrolimus, Cyclosporine

Protease Inhibitors

Quinolones*

Antipsychotics (e.g., olanzapine, quetiapine)

Statins

Steroids (systemic)

Cough Syrups

Niacin

Beta-Blockers*

Quinolones*

Tramadol

Others:
Linezolid
Octreotide*
Pentamidine
Quinine

↓ BG

Others:
Azole Antifungals (systemic)

Beta-Agonists

Beta-Blockers*

Octreotide*

*Can cause hypo or hyperglycemia

INPATIENT GLUCOSE CONTROL

Treatment should be initiated for hospitalized patients with persistent hyperglycemia (defined as BG ≥ 180 mg/dL), and maintained within a target range of 100 – 180 mg/dL for noncritically ill (non-ICU) patients and 140 – 180 mg/dL for critically ill (ICU) patients, although more stringent goals might be appropriate for select ICU patients.

The use of sliding scale insulin (SSI) alone to control BG in the hospital setting is discouraged. This method of administering insulin in response to elevated BG levels is reactionary (treats BG after it becomes elevated, rather than preventing elevated BG) and leads to poor outcomes. In addition, most sliding scales used are not patient-specific. See the Sliding Scale Example below.

- Insulin is used for most hospitalized patients; the regimen depends primarily on oral intake.
- If oral intake is adequate, a regimen with basal, bolus (prandial) and correction doses (usually added to the mealtime bolus dose) is preferred.
- A basal and correction dose strategy is recommended if the patient is not eating well (poor intake).
- Correction dose insulin is given when BG is already high. Like sliding scale insulin, the insulin dose given will correlate with the BG, on a scale. The difference is that the correction dose scale is designed for a specific patient. It is based on the patient's insulin sensitivity factor (same as the correction factor), which indicates how much the BG will drop with each unit of insulin.

Sliding scales, like the one below, and correction dose insulin use rapid-acting or regular insulin. Rapid-acting insulin will lower the BG quicker, and is preferable.

SLIDING SCALE EXAMPLE	
BLOOD GLUCOSE READING (MG/DL)	**INSTRUCTION**
< 60	Hold insulin; contact MD
150-200	Give 2 units of insulin
201-250	Give 4 units of insulin
251-300	Give 6 units of insulin
301-350	Give 8 units of insulin
351-400	Give 10 units of insulin
401-450	Call MD

HYPERGLYCEMIC CRISES

DIABETIC KETOACIDOSIS

Diabetic ketoacidosis (DKA) is a life-threatening crisis with high BG, ketoacidosis and ketonuria (i.e., ketones in the urine). DKA occurs most often in patients with T1D, but can occur in T2D. DKA is commonly the initial presentation in T1D or is caused by insulin omission (e.g., unable to afford insulin) or subtherapeutic insulin dosing (e.g., increased insulin requirements due to a stressor, such as an infection).

In DKA, ketones are present because triglycerides and amino acids are used for energy, which produces free fatty acids (FFAs) that are converted to ketones by glucagon. Insulin normally prevents this conversion, but in DKA, insulin is absent or severely lacking. DKA can be recognized by:

- BG > 250 mg/dL
- Ketones (urine and serum, result in "fruity" breath), abdominal pain, nausea and vomiting, dehydration
- Anion gap acidosis (arterial pH < 7.35, anion gap > 12)

HYPEROSMOLAR HYPERGLYCEMIC STATE

Hyperosmolar hyperglycemic state (HHS) has a higher mortality rate than DKA, but is less common. HHS commonly occurs in patients with T2D. The primary cause is illness (e.g., infection, stroke) that leads to less fluid intake. This, along with fluid shifts and osmotic diuresis, leads to severe dehydration with altered consciousness. Ketones are not present because in T2D the patient still makes insulin. HHS is recognized by:

- Confusion, delirium
- BG > 600 mg/dL, with high (> 320 mOsm/L) serum osmolality
- Extreme dehydration
- pH > 7.3, bicarbonate > 15 mEq/L

Severe hyperglycemia can decrease sodium concentrations; sodium levels may require correction in HHS (or DKA).

DKA AND HHS TREATMENT

The primary treatment is aggressive fluids (first) and insulin to treat the hyperglycemia

FLUIDS first for all patients
Start with NS
When blood glucose reaches 200 mg/dL, change to D5W½NS

REGULAR insulin infusion (regular is preferable in IV solutions)
1) 0.1 units/kg bolus, then 0.1 units/kg/hr continuous infusion OR
2) 0.14 units/kg/hr continuous infusion

PREVENT hypokalemia
Insulin shifts K+ into cells; serum K+ will fall
Monitor K+ and keep serum level between 4-5 mEq/L

TREAT acidosis if pH < 6.9; acidosis may be corrected by fluids
Give sodium bicarbonate if needed

SELECTING DRUG TREATMENT

The Study Tip Gal below summarizes some of the key safety issues seen with diabetes medications, and the following Case Scenario highlights how these safety issues could appear in exam questions. More examples can be found in the QBank.

SUMMARY OF DRUG SAFETY ISSUES

IF PRESENT	AVOID
Thyroid cancer, including medullary thyroid carcinoma	GLP-1 agonists, GLP-1/GIP agonists
Gastroparesis, GI disorders	GLP-1 agonists, GLP-1/GIP agonists, pramlintide
Genital infection/UTI	SGLT2 inhibitors
Heart failure	TZDs, alogliptin, saxagliptin
Hypoglycemia	Insulin, sulfonylureas, meglitinides, pramlintide
Hypotension/dehydration	SGLT2 inhibitors
Hypokalemia	Insulin
Ketoacidosis	SGLT2 inhibitors (can occur when BG < 250 mg/dL)
Lactic acidosis	Metformin; ↑ risk with renal impairment, alcoholism
Osteopenia/osteoporosis	Canagliflozin and bexagliflozin (↓ BMD, fractures), TZDs (fractures)
Pancreatitis	DPP-4 inhibitors, GLP-1 agonists, GLP-1/GIP agonists
Peripheral neuropathy, PAD, foot ulcers	Canagliflozin, bexagliflozin
Sulfa allergy, severe	Sulfonylureas (or use cautiously)
Renal insufficiency (eGFR or CrCl < 30)	Metformin, exenatide, glyburide; may need to start insulin at a lower dose
Weight gain/obesity	Sulfonylureas, meglitinides, TZDs, insulin

CASE SCENARIO

CS is a 56-year-old female with hypertension, diabetes and a past MI. At her last clinic visit 3 months ago, her A1C was 8.6% despite treatment with metformin ER 2,000 mg PO daily and *Januvia* 100 mg PO daily. At that time, *Invokana* 100 mg PO daily was added to her regimen. CS also takes aspirin, rosuvastatin, lisinopril, *Coreg CR* and hydrochlorothiazide for her hypertension and ASCVD.

At the current visit, CS complains of dry mouth, weakness, dizziness and lightheadedness. On a couple of occasions she has nearly fainted. These symptoms began approximately 2 months ago.

What do CS's symptoms likely describe?
CS has symptoms of dehydration and hypotension.

Which medications could be associated with these symptoms?
The addition of *Invokana* (canagliflozin) to her medication regimen put CS at risk for these adverse effects. *Invokana* decreases blood glucose by excreting it in the urine; water is also excreted with glucose. The use of diuretics and antihypertensive medications could be contributing to the problem due to additive effects.

What laboratory abnormalities could occur with this combination of medications?
CS is at risk for acute kidney injury. Evaluate for elevated BUN, SCr and assess the eGFR. Check an anion gap and ketones; if they are elevated, this is a sign of ketoacidosis, which can occur with *Invokana*.

If asked to select an alternative diabetes medication, what should be selected?
There are a number of treatment options for diabetes management. CS's history of ASCVD will dictate the next treatment option. An SGLT2 inhibitor was appropriate, but due to side effects, she should be switched to a GLP-1 agonist with benefit (e.g., dulaglutide, liraglutide, SC semaglutide). Her DPP-4 inhibitor [sitagliptin (*Januvia*)] would need to be discontinued when this is started (should not be used in combination with a GLP-1 agonist).

KEY COUNSELING POINTS

See the Drug Formulations and Patient Counseling chapter for counseling language/layman's terminology.

GLP-1 Agonists and GLP-1/GIP Agonists

- Subcutaneous injection (except *Rybelsus*). Rotate injection sites. See GLP-1 Agonist Injection Counseling section for details.
- *Byetta*: give within 60 minutes before meals; *Rybelsus*: take 30 minutes before breakfast; others can be taken anytime.
- *Trulicity, Bydureon BCise, Ozempic, Mounjaro*: inject once a week. The needles are inside the box or built into the pen.
- *Byetta, Victoza*: needles need to be purchased.
- If injection has been in the refrigerator, leave at room temperature 15 minutes before using.
- *Bydureon BCise*: shake the injection vigorously to ensure medication is evenly mixed. Look in the window to check for drug particles; if present, shake again.
- Can cause:
  - ❑ Nausea, diarrhea, decrease in appetite, weight loss.
  - ❑ Pancreatitis and gallbladder disease.
  - ❑ Kidney damage, especially from dehydration due to severe vomiting or diarrhea.
  - ❑ *Bydureon BCise*: injection-site reactions (abscesses, nodules).
  - ❑ *Ozempic, Mounjaro, Trulicity*: diabetic retinopathy.

SGLT2 Inhibitors

- Can cause:
  - ❑ Hypotension.
  - ❑ Ketoacidosis. Stop prior to surgery to reduce risk.
  - ❑ Severe UTIs and genital fungal infections.
  - ❑ Canagliflozin and bexagliflozin: amputation risk (avoid if foot problems, neuropathy), fractures.

Metformin

- Can cause:
  - ❑ Lactic acidosis.
  - ❑ Diarrhea, nausea; usually goes away. Taking with food and using long-acting metformin will help.
- With long-term metformin, take a vitamin B12 supplement.
- Long-acting formulations of metformin can leave a ghost tablet in the stool.

Thiazolidinediones

- Can cause:
  - ❑ Heart failure (cause or worsen).
  - ❑ Weight gain.
  - ❑ Bone fractures.

DPP-4 Inhibitors

- Can cause:
  - ❑ Pancreatitis.
  - ❑ Renal impairment.
  - ❑ Severe arthralgia.
  - ❑ Saxagliptin and alogliptin: heart failure.

Sulfonylureas/Meglitinides

- Take sulfonylureas with breakfast, except glipizide IR (take 30 minutes before meals).
- Take meglitinides within 30 minutes before meals. Do not take if skipping the meal.
- Can cause:
  - ❑ Hypoglycemia.
  - ❑ Weight gain.

Insulins

- Subcutaneous injection (except *Afrezza*). Rotate injection sites. See Insulin Injection Counseling section for details.
- Can cause:
  - ❑ Hypoglycemia.
  - ❑ Hypokalemia.
  - ❑ Weight gain.
- Store unopened insulin pens/vials in the refrigerator. Once opened, store at room temperature and discard after the designated number of days (for that type of insulin).

Pramlintide

- When starting, reduce dose of mealtime insulin by 50%. Inject before meals. Do not mix with insulin.

Alpha Glucosidase Inhibitors

- Can cause flatulence and diarrhea.
- Do not cause hypoglycemia. If you get hypoglycemia (from another medication), treat with glucose tablets or gel.

Select Guidelines/References

American Diabetes Association (ADA). Standards of Medical Care in Diabetes–2024. Diabetes Care 2024;47 (suppl 1):S1-S321.

AACE Consensus Statement on the Comprehensive Type 2 Diabetes Management Algorithm - Executive Summary. *Endocr Pract.* 2020 Jan;26(1):107-139.

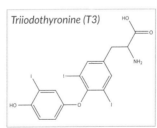

Thryoid Gland (front view)

Larynx

Right Lobe

Isthmus

Thryoid Gland

Left Lobe

Trachea

Parathyroid Glands

Back View

iStock.com/VectorMine

CHAPTER 45
THYROID DISORDERS

BACKGROUND

The thyroid gland is located in the neck, below the Adam's apple and in front of the trachea (windpipe). The gland is shaped like a butterfly, with two symmetrical lobes. The lobes sit on each side of the trachea, connected by a stretch of tissue called the isthmus. The thyroid gland produces thyroid hormones, which regulate metabolism, including the chemical processes needed to maintain life: cardiac and nervous system functions, body temperature, muscle strength, skin dryness, menstrual cycles, weight and cholesterol levels. Hyperthyroidism (overactive thyroid) and hypothyroidism (underactive thyroid) are the most common thyroid disorders.

PATHOPHYSIOLOGY

Triiodothyronine (T3)

iStock.com/chromatos

The two thyroid hormones produced by the thyroid gland are triiodothyronine, known as T3, and thyroxine, known as T4. The thyroid gland is the only organ that can absorb iodine, which is required for the production of both hormones (see T3 structure). T3 is primarily formed from the breakdown of T4. A small percentage (< 20%) is produced by the thyroid gland directly. T3 is more potent than T4 but has a shorter half-life.

Thyroid hormone production is regulated by thyroid-stimulating hormone (TSH), also referred to as thyrotropin. TSH is secreted by the pituitary gland, which is located in the brain and regulates growth and development.

CONTENT LEGEND

 = Study Tip Gal

 = Key Drug Guy

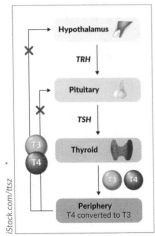

TRH = Thyrotropin Releasing Hormone
TSH = Thyroid-Stimulating Hormone

Negative Feedback Loop

Feedback loops are used to regulate the production of hormones secreted by the pituitary and thyroid glands, including T3 and T4. When the level of circulating (free) T4 increases, it inhibits the secretion of TSH. Less TSH will lead to a decrease in T4 production.

T3 and T4 are transported in the blood and are largely bound to proteins. Free T4 (FT4) is the unbound, active form that is monitored in patients with thyroid disorders.

SELECT DRUGS AND CONDITIONS THAT CAN CAUSE HYPOTHYROIDISM

KEY DRUGS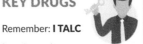

Remember: **I TALC**

Interferons*

Tyrosine kinase inhibitors (e.g., sunitinib)

Amiodarone*

Lithium

Carbamazepine

Conditions:
Hashimoto's Disease

Others:
Oxcarbazepine
Eslicarbazepine
Phenytoin

Conditions:
Iodine deficiency
Pituitary failure
Surgical removal of thyroid gland
Congenital hypothyroidism
Thyroid gland ablation with radioactive iodine
External irradiation

Can also cause hyperthyroidism (see Hyperthyroidism section)

HYPOTHYROIDISM

Hypothyroidism is a deficiency in T4, and consequently, an elevation in TSH. Hypothyroidism occurs more commonly in females (~80% of cases) and with increased age. When T4 decreases, the body slows down and the classic symptoms of low metabolism (e.g., fatigue and weight gain) appear. Hypothyroidism can cause depression, infertility, cardiovascular disease and other symptoms related to slow metabolism (see Study Tip Gal below).

The most common cause of hypothyroidism is Hashimoto's disease, an autoimmune condition in which a patient's own antibodies attack the thyroid gland. Drugs and conditions can cause hypothyroidism (see Key Drugs Guy).

Myxedema coma is an uncommon but potentially fatal complication of hypothyroidism that can occur when hypothyroidism is left untreated for a long time, or when hypothyroidism decompensates. It is a life-threatening emergency characterized by poor circulation, hypothermia and hypometabolism. The initial treatment for myxedema coma is IV levothyroxine.

S/SX OF HYPOTHYROIDISM

Cold intolerance/sensitivity	Myalgias
Dry skin	Weakness
Fatigue	Depression
Muscle cramps	Bradycardia
Voice changes	Coarse hair or loss of hair
Constipation	Menorrhagia (heavier than normal menstrual periods)
Weight gain	
Goiter (possible; can be due to low iodine intake)	Memory and mental impairment

DIAGNOSIS

A diagnosis of hypothyroidism is made using two laboratory test results:

- Low free T4: normal range 0.9 – 2.3 ng/dL
- High TSH: normal range 0.3 – 3 mIU/L

Screening should be considered in patients > 60 years old.

MONITORING

Thyroid function tests include TSH, FT4 and total T3. TSH is the primary test to monitor thyroid function in those receiving thyroid hormone replacement with drug treatment (occasionally FT4 is ordered with TSH). The TSH level and symptoms should be monitored every 4 – 6 weeks until levels are normal, then 4 – 6 months later, then yearly. It is important to monitor thyroid function as the patient ages because a reduction in thyroid hormone replacement dose can be required. Too high of a thyroid hormone replacement dose in elderly patients can cause atrial fibrillation and fractures. Serum FT4 is monitored in addition to TSH in central hypothyroidism (rare), which is a defect in pituitary production of TSH. FT4 is also monitored when treating hypothyroidism in pregnancy.

DRUG TREATMENT

The goals of treatment are to resolve symptoms, achieve euthyroid state (i.e., normal levels of thyroid hormones) and avoid over-treatment; excessive doses of thyroid hormone will cause hyperthyroidism. Patients should be counseled on symptoms of both hypo- and hyperthyroidism. Levothyroxine (T4) is the drug of choice for hypothyroidism. A consistent preparation (i.e., the same formulation and manufacturer) is preferred to minimize variability from refill to refill. Some patients state they feel better using other thyroid hormone formulations, including liothyronine (T3, such as *Cytomel)* or desiccated thyroid (T3 and T4, such as *Armour Thyroid)*, although these are generally not recommended. Desiccated thyroid is called "natural thyroid" and is dosed in grains. It is not recommended because it can contain variable amounts of T3 and T4.

Levothyroxine has many drug interactions and unique administration recommendations due to binding; see the table below and the Drug Interactions section for details.

Iodine supplementation with kelp or other iodine-containing functional foods is not required in the U.S. because most table salt has iodine added (iodized salt). This has eliminated almost all U.S. cases of iodine deficiency goiter. Individuals who are restricting salt intake can consume foods high in iodine (e.g., dairy, seafood, meat, some breads) and can take a multivitamin containing iodine.

Hypothyroidism Treatment

DRUG	DOSING	SAFETY/SIDE EFFECTS/MONITORING
Levothyroxine (T4) **(Synthroid, Levoxyl, Unithroid,** *Euthyrox, Tirosint, Tirosint-SOL)* Capsule, tablet, injection, oral solution Drug of choice Check the therapeutic equivalence of a generic to a brand in the *Orange Book*. Not all generic levothyroxine formulations are A-rated to various brands.	Full replacement dose = 1.6 mcg/kg/day (IBW) Start with full replacement dose in otherwise healthy, young (< 50 years of age) patients with markedly ↑ TSH Start with partial replacement dose in milder hypothyroidism and those with comorbidities If known CAD, start with 12.5-25 mcg daily Elderly patients often need 20-25% less per kg; may require < 1 mcg/kg/day	**BOXED WARNING** Ineffective and potentially toxic when used for obesity or weight reduction, especially in euthyroid patients; high doses can cause serious, life-threatening toxic effects, particularly when used with some anorectic drugs (e.g., sympathomimetic amines) **CONTRAINDICATIONS** Uncorrected adrenal insufficiency **WARNINGS** ↓ dose in cardiovascular disease (chronic hypothyroidism predisposes to coronary artery disease), ↓ bone mineral density which can lead to osteoporosis
Thyroid, Desiccated USP **(T3 and T4) (Armour Thyroid,** *Nature-Throid, NP Thyroid, Westhroid, WP Thyroid)* Tablet	Start 15-30 mg daily (15 mg in cardiac disease); titrate in 15 mg increments Usual dose is 60-120 mg daily	**SIDE EFFECTS** Hyperthyroid symptoms can occur when the dose is too high: ↑ HR, palpitations, sweating, weight loss, arrhythmias, irritability **MONITORING** TSH levels and clinical symptoms every 4-6 weeks until levels are normal, then 4-6 months later, then yearly; serum FT4 in select patients **NOTES** Highly protein bound (> 99%)
Liothyronine (T3) **(Cytomel,** *Triostat)* Tablet, injection	Start 25 mcg daily; titrate in 12.5-25 mcg increments Usual dose is 25-75 mcg daily	Dose reduction may be necessary as the patient ages **Levothyroxine PO** Should be taken with water at the same time each day for consistent absorption, at least 60 minutes before breakfast or at bedtime (at least three hours after the last meal) Levothyroxine tablet colors are standard; they do not change between manufacturers (see Study Tip Gal on tablet colors) **Levothyroxine IV** IV to PO ratio is 0.75:1; use immediately upon reconstitution
Liotrix (T3 and T4 in 1:4 ratio) *(Thyrolar)* Tablet	Start 25 mcg levothyroxine/6.25 mcg liothyronine daily Usual dose is 50-100 mcg levothyroxine/ 12.5-25 mcg liothyronine	**Levothyroxine oral solution** Can be given undiluted or diluted (in water only); store in original container **Thyroid, Desiccated USP** Natural porcine-derived thyroid that contains both T3 and T4; less predictable potency and stability **Liothyronine** Shorter half-life causes fluctuations in T3 levels

LEVOTHYROXINE TABLET COLORS

Remember: **O**rangutans **W**ill **V**omit **O**n **Y**ou **R**ight **B**efore **T**hey **B**ecome **L**arge, **P**roud **G**iants.

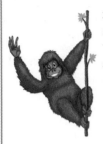

25 mcg – orange
50 mcg – white (no dye)
75 mcg – violet
88 mcg – olive
100 mcg – yellow
112 mcg – rose
125 mcg – brown
137 mcg – turquoise
150 mcg – blue
175 mcg – lilac
200 mcg – pink
300 mcg – green

iStock.com/colematt

DRUG INTERACTIONS

Drugs that ↓ the effect of thyroid replacement hormone treatment:

- Drugs that ↓ levothyroxine absorption:
  - ❑ Antacids and polyvalent cations containing iron, calcium, aluminum or magnesium, multivitamins (containing ADEK, folate, iron), cholestyramine, orlistat *(Xenical, Alli)*, sevelamer and sucralfate: separate doses by four hours from thyroid replacement therapy.
  - ❑ Sodium polystyrene sulfonate and patiromer *(Veltassa)*: separate doses by three hours from thyroid replacement therapy.
  - ❑ Lanthanum: separate doses by two hours from thyroid replacement therapy.
- Estrogen, SSRIs and hepatic inducers ↓ thyroid hormone levels.
- Beta-blockers, amiodarone, propylthiouracil (PTU) and systemic steroids can ↓ the effectiveness of levothyroxine by ↓ the conversion of T4 to T3.
- Thyroid hormone is highly protein bound (> 99%). Drugs can cause protein-binding site displacement (e.g., phenytoin).

Thyroid hormone replacement treatment can change the concentration or effect of these drugs:

- ↑ effect of warfarin (e.g., ↑ PT/INR)
- ↓ levels of theophylline

KEY COUNSELING POINTS

See the Drug Formulations and Patient Counseling chapter for counseling language/layman's terminology.

LEVOTHYROXINE

- Drug interactions due to binding.
- Take this medication with water, 60 minutes before breakfast or at bedtime (at least three hours after your last meal). Take this medication every day, even if you feel well.
- If you get a prescription refill and your new pills look different, speak to the pharmacist.
- Tell your prescriber if you become pregnant; it is likely that your dose will need to be increased during pregnancy or if you plan to breastfeed.
- Requires blood work on a regular basis (at least annually).

HYPERTHYROIDISM

Hyperthyroidism (overactive thyroid or thyrotoxicosis) occurs when there is over-production of thyroid hormones. FT4 is high, TSH is low, and symptoms are nearly opposite of those seen in hypothyroidism. Hyperthyroidism can significantly accelerate metabolism, causing weight loss, agitation, heat intolerance and other symptoms (see Study Tip Gal below).

Left untreated, hyperthyroidism can cause tachycardia, arrhythmias, heart failure and osteoporosis.

S/SX OF HYPERTHYROIDISM

Heat intolerance or increased sweating	Insomnia
Weight loss	Tremor
Agitation, nervousness, irritability, anxiety	Thinning hair
Palpitations and tachycardia	Goiter (possible)
Fatigue and muscle weakness	Exophthalmos (protrusion of the eyeballs), diplopia
Frequent bowel movements or diarrhea	Light or absent menstrual periods

Causes

The most common cause of hyperthyroidism is <u>Graves' disease</u>, which most commonly occurs in females aged 30 – 50 years. Graves' disease is an <u>autoimmune</u> disorder (like Hashimoto's), but instead of destroying the thyroid gland, the <u>antibodies stimulate the thyroid</u> to produce too much T4. Less common causes include thyroid nodules and thyroiditis (inflammation of the thyroid). <u>Drug-induced causes</u> of <u>hyperthyroidism</u> include <u>iodine, amiodarone and interferons</u>. Excess iodine increases the synthesis and release of thyroid hormone. Iodine-induced hyperthyroidism can be due to excess iodine in the diet or <u>exposure to radiographic contrast media</u>. Excessive doses of thyroid hormone can cause hyperthyroidism.

DRUG TREATMENT

Treatment involves antithyroid <u>medications</u>, destroying part of the gland via <u>radioactive iodine</u> (RAI-131) or <u>surgery</u>. RAI-131 has historically been considered the preferred treatment in Graves' disease, but all three treatment options are effective and relatively safe. With any option, the patient can be treated with <u>beta-blockers</u> first for <u>symptom control</u> (to reduce <u>palpitations, tremors and tachycardia</u>). Propylthiouracil (PTU) or methimazole can be used as a temporary measure until surgery is complete. It takes <u>1 – 3 months of treatment</u> with antithyroid medications at <u>high doses</u> to <u>control symptoms</u>. Once symptoms are controlled, <u>the dose</u> should be <u>reduced</u> to <u>prevent hypothyroidism</u> from occurring.

Hyperthyroidism Treatment

DRUG	DOSING	SAFETY/SIDE EFFECTS/MONITORING
Thionamides: <u>inhibit synthesis of thyroid</u> hormones by blocking the oxidation of iodine in the thyroid gland; PTU also inhibits <u>peripheral conversion</u> of T4 to T3		
Propylthiouracil (PTU) Tablet	50-150 mg Q8H initially until euthyroid (higher doses for more severe hyperthyroidism), followed by dose reduction	**BOXED WARNINGS (PTU)** <u>Severe liver injury and acute liver failure</u> <u>Pregnancy: PTU preferred in 1st trimester</u> (due to increased risk of fetal abnormalities from methimazole) **WARNINGS** <u>Hepatotoxicity</u>, bone marrow suppression (rare, includes <u>agranulocytosis</u>), drug-induced lupus erythematosus (<u>DILE</u>), vasculitis **SIDE EFFECTS** <u>GI upset</u>, headache, rash (exfoliative dermatitis, pruritus), fever, constipation, loss of taste/taste perversion, lymphadenopathy, bleeding
Methimazole *(Tapazole)* Tablet	Mild hyperthyroidism: 5 mg Q8H initially until euthyroid (↑ doses for more severe hyperthyroidism), then 5-15 mg daily	**MONITORING** FT4 and T3 every 4-6 weeks until euthyroid, TSH, CBC, LFTs and PT Patient must monitor for liver toxicity (abdominal pain, yellow skin/eyes, dark urine, nausea, weakness) and infection (high fever or severe sore throat) **NOTES** Take with food to reduce GI upset <u>Methimazole</u> is the <u>drug of choice</u> (due to a lower risk of liver damage) except in certain situations, noted below <u>PTU</u> is preferred in <u>thyroid storm</u> and if methimazole is not tolerated <u>Pregnancy: PTU</u> is preferred in the <u>1st trimester</u> (see Boxed Warning); <u>methimazole</u> can be used in the <u>2nd and 3rd trimesters</u> (to ↓ the risk of liver toxicity from PTU)

DRUG	DOSING	SAFETY/SIDE EFFECTS/MONITORING
Iodides: temporarily inhibit secretion of thyroid hormones; T4 and T3 levels will be reduced for several weeks but effect will not be maintained		
Potassium iodide and iodine solution (*Lugol's Solution*) Oral solution	Preparation for thyroidectomy: 5-7 drops Q8H for 10 days prior to surgery (off-label)	**CONTRAINDICATIONS** Hypersensitivity to iodide or iodine, dermatitis herpetiformis, hypocomplementemic vasculitis, nodular thyroid condition with heart disease **SIDE EFFECTS** Rash, metallic taste, sore throat/gums, GI upset, urticaria, hypo/hyperthyroidism with prolonged use
Saturated solution of potassium iodide (*SSKI, ThyroSafe*) Oral solution	Preparation for thyroidectomy: 1-2 drops Q8H for 10 days prior to surgery (off-label)	**MONITORING** Thyroid function tests, s/sx of hyperthyroidism **NOTES** Dilute in a glassful of water, juice, or milk; take with food or milk to ↓ GI upset *SSKI* is also used as an expectorant

POTASSIUM IODIDE USE AFTER EXPOSURE TO RADIATION

Potassium iodide (KI) blocks the accumulation of radioactive iodine in the thyroid gland, thus preventing thyroid cancer. Potassium iodide should be taken as soon as possible after radiation exposure on the advice of public health or emergency management personnel only. The correct dose must be used; higher doses do not offer greater protection. Refer to the CDC website for age-specific dosing based on the duration of radiation exposure (https://emergency.cdc.gov/radiation/ki.asp). Iodized salt and foods do not contain enough iodine to block radioactive iodine and are not recommended.

THYROID STORM

Thyroid storm is a life-threatening medical emergency characterized by decompensated hyperthyroidism that can be precipitated by infection, trauma, surgery, radioactive iodine treatment or non-adherence to antithyroid medication. It is important to recognize symptoms so that treatment can be implemented promptly (see Study Tip Gal).

S/SX OF THYROID STORM		
Fever (> 103°F)	Agitation	
Tachycardia	Delirium	
Tachypnea	Psychosis	
Dehydration	Coma	
Profuse sweating		

DRUG TREATMENT

- Antithyroid drug therapy (PTU is preferred; 500 – 1,000 mg loading dose, then 250 mg PO Q4H)

  PLUS

- Inorganic iodide therapy such as *SSKI* 5 drops (in water or juice) PO Q6H or *Lugol's Solution* 4 – 8 drops PO Q6 – 8H

  PLUS

- Beta-blocker (e.g., propranolol 40 – 80 mg PO Q6H)

  PLUS

- Systemic steroid (e.g., dexamethasone 2 – 4 mg PO Q6H)

  PLUS

- Aggressive cooling with acetaminophen and cooling blankets and other supportive treatments (e.g., antiarrhythmics, insulin, fluids, electrolytes)

The antithyroid drug should be given ≥ 1 hour before iodide to block synthesis of thyroid hormone. PTU tablets can be crushed and administered through an NG tube if needed.

THYROID DISEASE AND PREGNANCY

PREGNANCY AND HYPOTHYROIDISM

Untreated maternal hypothyroidism has been associated with loss of pregnancy, low birth weight, premature birth and lower IQ in children. Levothyroxine is safe in pregnancy and is the recommended treatment. Pregnant women treated with thyroid hormone replacement will require a 30 – 50% increase in the dose throughout the course of their pregnancy and for several months after giving birth. Aggressive control of hypothyroidism in pregnancy is recommended. Treatment should ideally be started prior to the pregnancy.

PREGNANCY AND HYPERTHYROIDISM

Poor control of hyperthyroidism in pregnancy is associated with pregnancy loss, prematurity and low birth weight, like hypothyroidism, as well as thyroid storm, maternal hypertension and congestive heart failure. There can be lasting effects in the baby, including seizure disorders and neurobehavioral disorders. Pregnancy should be postponed until a stable euthyroid state is reached. If a woman with hyperthyroidism becomes pregnant, she should be evaluated to see if treatment can be stopped (mild disease). If treatment is needed, it should be with antithyroid drugs based on the trimester. For the first trimester, PTU should be used (due to fetal toxicity with methimazole). After that, the decision is individualized, as both PTU and methimazole carry potential risks. Historically, the patient would be switched to methimazole for the remainder of the pregnancy.

Select Guidelines/References

2016 American Thyroid Association Guidelines for Diagnosis and Management of Hyperthyroidism and Other Causes of Thyrotoxicosis. Thyroid. 2016;26(10):1343-1422.

Guidelines for the Treatment of Hypothyroidism: Prepared by the American Thyroid Association Task Force on Thyroid Hormone Replacement. Thyroid. 2014;24(12):1670-1751.

2017 Guidelines of the American Thyroid Association for the Diagnosis and Management of Thyroid Disease During Pregnancy and the Postpartum. Thyroid. 2017;27(3):315-389.

CONTENT LEGEND

 ☀ = Study Tip Gal　　 ⚷ = Key Drug Guy

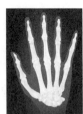  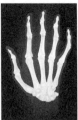 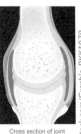

Hand normal joint　　Cross section of joint　　Hand with Rheumatoid arthritis　　Cross section of joint with Rheumatoid arthritis

iStock.com/Graphic_BKK1979

CHAPTER 46
SYSTEMIC STEROIDS & AUTOIMMUNE CONDITIONS

SYSTEMIC STEROIDS

There are several drug classes that can be used to treat inflammation, including drugs that target the chemical pathway of inflammation (e.g., biologics), cancer drugs that have strong anti-inflammatory properties, steroids and NSAIDs. Steroids and NSAIDs are used commonly; of these two classes, steroids are stronger anti-inflammatory drugs. Both have serious adverse effects, but chronic use of NSAIDs is considered to be safer than chronic use of steroids. See the Pain chapter for a review of NSAIDs.

Steroids are used for a variety of conditions, such as inflammatory conditions (e.g., rheumatoid arthritis, psoriasis, acute asthma exacerbation) and immune suppression post-transplant. They can also be used to treat adrenal insufficiency; when the adrenal gland fails to produce sufficient amounts of naturally occurring (i.e., endogenous) steroids, systemic steroids can be given as replacement therapy. Two primary endogenous steroids that can require replacement are:

- Cortisol: replaced by giving any of the steroids.
- Aldosterone: replaced by giving fludrocortisone.

Hydrocortisone, cortisone and prednisolone are commonly used as adrenal hormone replacement therapy. These have more glucocorticoid activity (i.e., more anti-inflammatory effects) than fludrocortisone, which has mineralocorticoid activity (i.e., it helps maintain water and electrolyte balance). Fludrocortisone mimics aldosterone and is used to treat Addison's disease and sometimes orthostatic hypotension.

The rest of this section discusses only the commonly used glucocorticoids, which will be referred to simply as "steroids." Systemic steroids can cause the adrenal gland to stop producing cortisol through feedback inhibition. This is called suppression of the hypothalamic-pituitary-adrenal (HPA) axis (see diagram on the next page). When long-term steroids are discontinued, they need to be tapered off to give the adrenal gland time to resume cortisol production.

CUSHING'S SYNDROME

Cushing's syndrome can develop when the adrenal gland produces too much cortisol, or if exogenous (i.e., taken as a drug) steroids are taken in doses higher than the normal amount of endogenous cortisol. See the diagram below for the adverse effects of long-term steroids and Cushing's syndrome.

Addison's disease can be thought of as the opposite of Cushing's. In Addison's disease, the adrenal gland is not making enough cortisol. If exogenous steroids are suddenly stopped, it can cause an adrenal crisis (also known as an "Addisonian Crisis)." Hallmarks of an adrenal crisis are volume depletion and hypotension, which can be fatal.

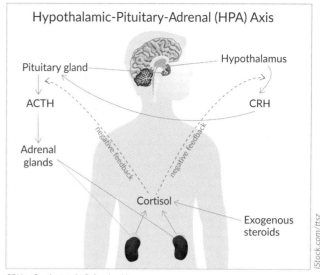

CRH = Corticotropin Releasing Hormone;
ACTH = Adrenocorticotropic Hormone, also called corticotropin

Long-Term Effects of Steroids (e.g., Cushing's Syndrome)

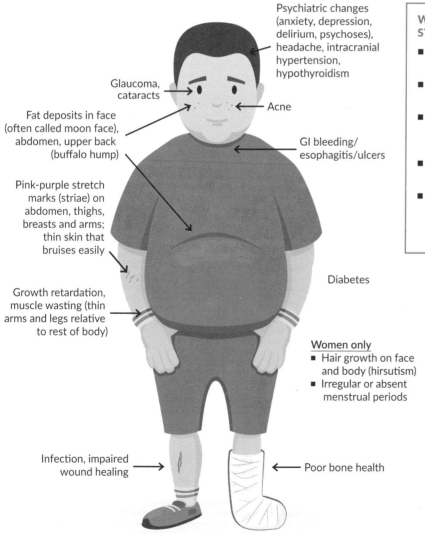

Psychiatric changes (anxiety, depression, delirium, psychoses), headache, intracranial hypertension, hypothyroidism

Glaucoma, cataracts

Acne

Fat deposits in face (often called moon face), abdomen, upper back (buffalo hump)

GI bleeding/ esophagitis/ulcers

Pink-purple stretch marks (striae) on abdomen, thighs, breasts and arms; thin skin that bruises easily

Growth retardation, muscle wasting (thin arms and legs relative to rest of body)

Diabetes

Infection, impaired wound healing

Poor bone health

Women only
- Hair growth on face and body (hirsutism)
- Irregular or absent menstrual periods

WAYS TO REDUCE SYSTEMIC STEROID RISKS

- Use every other day dosing; this decreases Cushing-like side effects.

- For joint inflammation, use intra-articular injections (i.e., inject into the joint).

- For GI conditions, use a steroid with low systemic absorption [e.g., delayed-release budesonide (Entocort EC)].

- For treatment of asthma, use inhaled steroids that mainly stay in the lungs.

- For conditions that require long-term steroids (e.g., transplant, a severe autoimmune condition), use the lowest effective dose for the shortest possible time.

iStock.com/ttsz

SYSTEMIC STEROIDS (PO, IV) DOSE EQUIVALENCE

Cortisone	25 mg	Short-acting
Hydrocortisone	20 mg	
Prednisone	5 mg	Intermediate-acting
Prednisolone	5 mg	
Methylprednisolone	4 mg	
Triamcinolone	4 mg	
Dexamethasone	0.75 mg	Long-acting & highest potency
Betamethasone	0.6 mg	

STEROIDS: LEAST POTENT TO MOST POTENT

Remember: **C**ute **H**elpful **P**harmacists and **P**hysicians **M**arry **T**ogether & **D**eliver **B**abies

iStock.com/aleksey-martynyuk

GLUCOCORTICOIDS (SYSTEMIC STEROIDS)

DRUG	DOSING	SAFETY/SIDE EFFECTS/MONITORING
Dexamethasone (**Decadron***, DexPak 6, 10 or 13 day*, Dexamethasone Intensol, others)	Dosing varies by condition Many formulations: liquids, ODT (children), injections [fast-acting, long-acting (usually for joints)], tablets, others If once daily, take between 7-8 AM to mimic the natural diurnal cortisol release Take oral doses with food to decrease GI upset	**CONTRAINDICATIONS** Live vaccines, serious systemic infections **WARNINGS** Adrenal suppression – HPA axis suppression may lead to adrenal crisis and death; if taking longer than 14 days, must taper slowly Immunosuppression, psychiatric disturbances, Kaposi sarcoma; can worsen heart failure, diabetes, hypertension and osteoporosis
Hydrocortisone (**Solu-Cortef**, Cortef, Alkindi Sprinkle)		
Methylprednisolone (**Medrol, Solu-Medrol**, Depo-Medrol)		**SIDE EFFECTS** **Short-term side effects (used < 1 month)** Fluid retention, stomach upset, emotional instability (euphoria, mood swings, irritability), insomnia, ↑ appetite, weight gain, acute ↑ blood glucose/pressure (with higher doses)
Prednisone (Deltasone*, Prednisone Intensol, Rayos)		**Long-term side effects** See previous Long-Term Effects of Steroids figure
Prednisolone (**Millipred***, **Orapred ODT**, Pediapred)		**MONITORING** BP, weight, appetite, mood, growth (children/adolescents), bone mineral density, blood glucose, electrolytes, infection, IOP if > 6 weeks
Triamcinolone (**Kenalog**, Pro-C-Dure kits)		**NOTES** Cortisone is a prodrug of cortisol Prednisone is a prodrug of prednisolone
Betamethasone (Celestone Soluspan)		Methylprednisolone is available in a therapy pack (commonly called a "Medrol Dose Pack," see Study Tip Gal on next page) and as an injection
Cortisone		Prednisolone is used commonly in children (many formulations)

Topical steroids are discussed in the Common Skin Conditions chapter.
*Brand discontinued but name still used in practice.

CASE SCENARIO

AS is a 30-year-old female who came to the hospital with an acute flare of Crohn's disease. She was started on *Solu-Medrol* 40 mg IV BID. The medical team is now ready to transition her to oral prednisone at an equivalent dose. Assuming the IV:PO ratio of *Solu-Medrol* is 1:1, what is the equivalent daily dose?

$$\frac{\text{Methylprednisolone 4 mg}}{\text{Prednisone 5 mg}} = \frac{\text{Methylprednisolone 80 mg}}{\text{Prednisone X mg}}$$

X = 100 mg Prednisone

IMMUNOSUPPRESSION FROM STEROIDS

A patient is immunosuppressed when using ≥ 2 mg/kg/day or ≥ 20 mg/day of prednisone or prednisone equivalent (see potency table) for > 2 weeks.

For these patients:

- Avoid live vaccines due to a high risk of infection.

- Taper when discontinuing steroids due to HPA axis suppression (to allow the adrenal gland to resume normal cortisol production); otherwise, the patient is at risk for adrenal crisis.

There are many ways to taper steroids; one method is to reduce the dose by ~10-20% every few days. Taper lengths vary depending on the condition being treated.

TREATING ACUTE INFLAMMATION WITH STEROIDS

Give a high dose initially (to quickly reduce inflammation), then taper the dose down to treat the remaining inflammation while preventing a rebound attack.

The *Medrol* **therapy pack*** provides a convenient taper kit, with 21 x 4 mg tablets:

DAY	BEFORE BREAKFAST	LUNCH	DINNER	BEDTIME
Day 1	2 tablets	1 tablet	1 tablet	2 tablets
Day 2	1 tablet	1 tablet	1 tablet	2 tablets
Day 3	1 tablet	1 tablet	1 tablet	1 tablet
Day 4	1 tablet	1 tablet	---	1 tablet
Day 5	1 tablet	---	---	1 tablet
Day 6	1 tablet	---	---	---

*Will not be appropriate for all patients (e.g., may need a longer taper or higher starting dose)

AUTOIMMUNE CONDITIONS

Autoimmune diseases are conditions that occur when the body's immune system attacks and destroys healthy body tissue. The immune system is a complex organization of cells and antibodies designed to "seek and destroy" invaders of the body, particularly infections. Symptoms vary based on the type of autoimmune disease and the location of the immune response. Common symptoms of most autoimmune diseases include fatigue, weakness and pain. Nonspecific laboratory blood tests that can be useful in detecting inflammation include erythrocyte sedimentation rate (ESR), C-reactive protein (CRP), rheumatoid factor (RF) and anti-nuclear antibody (ANA).

Rheumatoid arthritis (RA), systemic lupus erythematosus (SLE), multiple sclerosis (MS), celiac disease, Sjögren's syndrome, Raynaud's, myasthenia gravis and psoriasis are discussed in this chapter. Other autoimmune diseases covered elsewhere in the book include type 1 diabetes (see the Diabetes chapter) and Hashimoto's thyroiditis and Graves' disease (see the Thyroid Disorders chapter).

TREATMENT

Treatment of autoimmune diseases typically involves drugs that suppress the immune system (e.g., steroids, disease-modifying antirheumatic drugs); these decrease the immune response (see Study Tip Gal for steroid immunosuppression overview). The use of strong immunosuppressants can increase the risk of certain conditions, including:

- Reactivation of tuberculosis or hepatitis (B or C): testing and treatment (if needed) must be done prior to starting immunosuppressive drugs.

- Viruses: if required, live vaccines should be given prior to starting immunosuppressive drugs.

- Lymphomas and certain skin cancers: these cancer types are normally suppressed by a competent immune system.

- Infections of various types (e.g., bacterial, fungal): this requires monitoring of symptoms (by the patient), complete blood counts (CBC) and may require infection control measures.

RHEUMATOID ARTHRITIS

Rheumatoid arthritis (RA) is a <u>chronic, progressive</u> autoimmune disorder that primarily affects <u>joints</u>. Other organs in the body, including the kidneys, eyes, heart and lungs can be affected. Like many other autoimmune conditions, RA varies in severity, with some patients having more aggressive disease than others.

CLINICAL PRESENTATION

RA typically results in warm, tender, swollen and painful joints. Articular (i.e., joint) pain usually presents in the smaller joints of the fingers, wrist, ankles and feet first. <u>Bilateral, symmetrical</u> inflammation with pain is consistent with an <u>RA diagnosis</u>, in contrast to osteoarthritis (OA), which presents unilaterally (e.g., right hand only).

The classic symptoms of RA are shown in the box to the right. RA is a systemic disease and has systemic symptoms (e.g., fever, weakness, loss of appetite). Stiffness and pain are <u>worse after rest</u>, which is why "<u>morning stiffness</u>" is a common complaint. In contrast, <u>OA does not cause prolonged stiffness</u>. Diagnosis depends on a combination of signs, symptoms, lab tests and x-rays.

Joint pain and swelling are common to both types of arthritis, making it challenging to identify the specific type of arthritis causing the symptoms. Joint erosion and rheumatoid nodules can be absent in early RA. <u>Anti-citrullinated peptide antibody</u> (ACPA) and <u>rheumatoid factor (RF)</u> are useful laboratory tests for diagnosing RA. RF has a lower specificity for RA (see the Biostatistics chapter) and can be positive due to another autoimmune disorder.

NON-DRUG TREATMENT

Non-drug treatments include rest, physical therapy, occupational therapy, exercise, diet modifications, weight control and surgical intervention (e.g., joint replacement).

DRUG TREATMENT

RA is classified as low, moderate or high disease activity. Patients with <u>symptomatic RA</u> should be started on a disease-modifying antirheumatic drug (<u>DMARD), regardless of the severity</u> of disease. DMARDs work via various mechanisms to <u>slow the disease process</u> and help <u>prevent further joint damage</u>; remission or low disease activity is the treatment goal. <u>Methotrexate (MTX)</u> is the <u>preferred initial therapy</u> for most patients. For patients with moderate or high disease activity despite MTX (with or without a systemic steroid), a combination of DMARDs, a tumor necrosis factor (TNF)

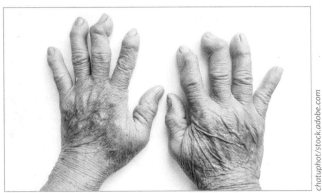
Hands with rheumatoid arthritis

chatuphot/stock.adobe.com

CLASSIC ARTICULAR SYMPTOMS OF RA	
<u>Joint swelling</u>	Weakness
<u>Pain</u>	Difficult to move
<u>Stiffness</u>	Edema
<u>Bone deformity</u>	Redness

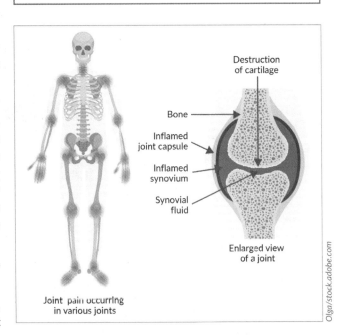

Destruction of cartilage

Bone

Inflamed joint capsule

Inflamed synovium

Synovial fluid

Enlarged view of a joint

Joint pain occurring in various joints

Olga/stock.adobe.com

inhibitor biologic or a non-TNF biologic, with or without MTX, is recommended. <u>Never use two biologic DMARDs in combination</u> due to the risk of serious (fatal) infections.

For patients with moderate or high disease activity, low-dose steroids (i.e., ≤ 10 mg/day of prednisone or equivalent) can be added as a "bridging" option while waiting for the DMARD to take effect, or in the case of DMARD failure. <u>Steroids</u> are commonly used in RA flares and should be used at the <u>lowest dose</u> and for the <u>shortest duration</u> possible. NSAIDs are a less toxic, weaker option than steroids for bridging, but high doses are necessary for their anti-inflammatory effect and their toxicity (e.g., GI bleeding, CVD risk) must be considered.

Traditional (Non-Biologic) Disease-Modifying Antirheumatic Drugs (DMARDs)

DRUG	DOSING	SAFETY/SIDE EFFECTS/MONITORING
Methotrexate *(Trexall, Otrexup, Rasuvo, Xatmep)* Trexall is an oral tablet *Otrexup* and *Rasuvo* are single-dose (needle included) SC auto-injectors *Xatmep* is an oral solution for use in pediatric patients Injection (IV/IT) – for oncology use Irreversibly binds and inhibits dihydrofolate reductase, inhibiting folate, thymidylate synthetase and purine; has immune modulator and anti-inflammatory activity	7.5-20 mg once weekly (PO, SC, IM) Low weekly doses are used for RA; to avoid error, it is safest to take as a single dose (rather than divided oral dosages of 2.5 mg Q12H x 3 doses per week – see below) Never dose daily for RA; numerous incidences of adverse events (e.g., mouth sores, intestinal bleeding, liver damage) have occurred due to patients taking daily	**BOXED WARNINGS** Hepatotoxicity, myelosuppression, mucositis/stomatitis, pregnancy (teratogenic), acute renal failure, pneumonitis, GI toxicity, dermatologic reactions, malignant lymphomas, potentially fatal opportunistic infections; renal and lung toxicity are more likely when using higher oncology doses **CONTRAINDICATION** Pregnancy, breastfeeding, alcohol use disorder, chronic liver disease, blood dyscrasias, immunodeficiency syndrome **SIDE EFFECTS** Vary by route and dosage N/V/D, ↑ LFTs, stomatitis, alopecia, photosensitivity, arthralgia, myalgia **MONITORING** CBC, LFTs (at baseline, every 2-4 weeks for first 3 months or following dose increases, every 8-12 weeks for 3-6 months, then less frequently), chest X-ray, hepatitis B and C serologies (if at high risk), SCr, PFTs (if lung-related symptoms), TB test **NOTES** Folate can be given to ↓ hematological, GI and hepatic side effects; give 5 mg PO weekly on the day following MTX administration (some take 1 mg daily on non-MTX days) *Xatmep* requires no preparation; eliminates the need for needles, crushing or splitting tablets, or compounding tablets into a liquid formulation
Hydroxychloroquine *(Plaquenil)* Tablet +/- MTX Immune modulator	400-600 mg/day initially, then 200-400 mg/day for maintenance dose Take with food or milk	**WARNINGS** Irreversible retinopathy, cardiomyopathy and QT prolongation, myopathy and neuropathy, hypoglycemia, psychiatric events (including suicidal behaviors), renal toxicity (possibly related to phospholipidosis) **SIDE EFFECTS** Vision changes (dose-related), N/V/D, abdominal pain, rash, pruritus, headache, pigmentation changes of the skin and hair (rare), bone marrow suppression (anemia, leukopenia, thrombocytopenia) and hemolysis in patients with G6PD deficiency, hepatotoxicity **MONITORING** CBC, LFTs and ECG at baseline and periodically; eye exam and muscle strength at baseline and every 3 months during prolonged therapy **NOTES** Lower risk of liver toxicity than MTX, can use as an alternative when there is a concern for liver disease Monotherapy: if low disease activity and symptoms < 24 months If inadequate or no response after 6 months, consider alternative
Sulfasalazine *(Azulfidine, Azulfidine EN-tabs)* Tablet (immediate and delayed release) +/- MTX Immune modulator	500-1,000 mg/day initially, then 1,000 mg BID (max is 3 grams/day) Take with food and 8 oz. of water to prevent crystalluria	**CONTRAINDICATION** Patients with a sulfa or salicylate allergy, GI or GU obstruction, porphyria **WARNINGS** Blood dyscrasias, severe skin reactions (SJS/TEN), hepatic failure and pulmonary fibrosis; use caution in patients with G6PD deficiency **SIDE EFFECTS** Headache, rash, anorexia, dyspepsia, N/V/D, oligospermia (reversible), folate deficiency, arthralgia, crystalluria **MONITORING** CBC and LFTs (baseline, then every other week for first 3 months, then monthly for 3 months, then once every 3 months), renal function **NOTES** Can cause yellow-orange coloration of skin/urine Impairs folate absorption, can give 1 mg/day folate supplement

DRUG	DOSING	SAFETY/SIDE EFFECTS/MONITORING
Leflunomide (*Arava*) Tablet +/- MTX Inhibits pyrimidine synthesis resulting in anti-proliferative and anti-inflammatory effects Prodrug of teriflunomide	100 mg PO x 3 days, then 20 mg PO daily (can use 10 mg PO daily if unable to tolerate 20 mg) May omit loading dose if at higher risk of liver toxicity or myelosuppression	**BOXED WARNINGS** Do not use in pregnancy (teratogenic); must test for and rule out pregnancy prior to starting therapy Hepatotoxicity: avoid in pre-existing liver disease or ALT > 2x upper limit of normal (ULN) **CONTRAINDICATION** Pregnancy, severe hepatic impairment, current teriflunomide therapy **WARNINGS** Severe infections, serious skin reactions (SJS/TEN), peripheral neuropathy, interstitial lung disease, hypertension Upon discontinuation of treatment, use accelerated drug elimination procedure (see Notes) to reduce levels of active metabolite, teriflunomide **SIDE EFFECTS** ↑ LFTs, nausea, diarrhea, respiratory infections, rash, headache **MONITORING** LFTs and CBC at baseline and monthly for first 6 months, BP at baseline and regularly, screen for TB and pregnancy prior to starting therapy **NOTES** Accelerated drug elimination options: 1. Cholestyramine 8 grams PO TID x 11 days (use 4 g if 8 g dose not tolerated) 2. Activated charcoal suspension 50 grams PO Q12H x 11 days Must have negative pregnancy test prior and use 2 forms of birth control during treatment; if pregnancy is desired, must wait 2 years after discontinuation or use accelerated drug elimination procedure

Janus kinase inhibitors: inhibits janus kinase (JAK) enzymes, which stimulate immune cell function

DRUG	DOSING	SAFETY/SIDE EFFECTS/MONITORING
Tofacitinib (*Xeljanz, Xeljanz XR*) Tablet +/- non-biologic DMARDs (MTX)	5 mg PO BID XR: 11 mg PO daily Dose adjustments with moderate-strong CYP 450 3A4 inducers and hepatic or renal impairment Do not start if: absolute lymphocyte count < 500 cells/mm^3, Hgb < 9 g/dL, or ANC < 1,000 cells/mm^3	**BOXED WARNINGS** Serious infections including tuberculosis (TB), fungal, viral, bacterial or other opportunistic infections; screen for active and latent TB and treat before starting Malignancy: ↑ risk for lymphomas and other malignancies Thrombosis: ↑ risk of serious (sometimes fatal) blood clots, including pulmonary embolism (PE), deep vein thrombosis (DVT) and arterial thrombosis Mortality and major adverse cardiovascular events: ↑ risk in patients ≥ 50 years of age with ≥ 1 cardiovascular risk factor **WARNINGS** GI perforation, ↑ LFTs, hematologic toxicities, avoid live vaccines
Baricitinib (*Olumiant*) Tablet +/- non-biologic DMARDs (MTX)	2 mg PO daily GFR < 30 mL/min/1.73m^2: not recommended Do not start if: absolute lymphocyte count < 500 cells/mm^3, Hgb < 8 g/dL, or ANC < 1,000 cells/mm^3	**SIDE EFFECTS** Upper respiratory tract infections (URTIs), urinary tract infections (UTIs), diarrhea, HA, hypertension, ↑ lipids **MONITORING** CBC (for lymphopenia, neutropenia and anemia) and lipids at baseline, then 4-8 weeks later, then every 3 months, LFTs (at baseline and periodically thereafter), new-onset abdominal pain, signs of infection
Upadacitinib (*Rinvoq*) Tablet +/- non-biologic DMARDs (MTX)	15 mg daily Do not start if: absolute lymphocyte count < 500 cells/mm^3, Hgb < 8 g/dL, or ANC < 1,000 cells/mm^3	**NOTES** Do not use with biologic DMARDs or potent immunosuppressants Caution in patients of Asian descent (↑ frequency of side effects)

Methotrexate Drug Interactions

- MTX should <u>not</u> be taken <u>with alcohol</u> due to an ↑ risk of liver toxicity.

- Renal elimination is ↓ by <u>aspirin/NSAIDs</u>, beta-lactams and probenecid, resulting in MTX toxicity; caution if using together.

- Sulfonamides and topical tacrolimus ↑ adverse effects of MTX. Avoid using together.

- MTX can ↓ effectiveness of loop diuretics; loop diuretics can ↑ the MTX concentration. Use caution if using together.

- MTX and cyclosporine levels will both ↑ when used together, leading to toxicity; avoid using together.

Anti-TNF Biologic DMARDs

<u>Tumor necrosis factor (TNF) alpha inhibitors</u> (also called anti-TNF biologics) are used for a variety of diseases. Dosing for RA is provided below. Recommended dosing for psoriatic arthritis, plaque psoriasis, Crohn's disease, ulcerative colitis and other indications may vary. Each drug has a <u>pregnancy registry</u> for tracking potential risks to the fetus.

DRUG	DOSING	SAFETY/SIDE EFFECTS/MONITORING
Etanercept (*Enbrel*) Biosimilars: *Erelzi, Eticovo* Single-dose prefilled syringe or auto-injector, multidose vial +/- MTX	50 mg <u>SC weekly</u>	**BOXED WARNINGS** <u>Serious infections</u>, some fatal, including TB, fungal, viral, bacterial or opportunistic; screen for <u>latent TB</u> (and <u>treat</u> if needed) prior to therapy Lymphomas and other <u>malignancies</u>
Adalimumab (*Humira*, Humira Pen) Biosimilars: *Abrilada, Amjevita, Cyltezo, Hadlima, Hulio, Hyrimoz, Idacio, Yuflyma, Yusimry* Single-dose prefilled syringe or auto-injector +/- MTX	40 mg <u>SC every other week</u> (if not taking MTX, can ↑ dose to 40 mg SC weekly)	**CONTRAINDICATIONS** Active systemic infection, doses > 5 mg/kg in moderate-severe heart failure (infliximab), sepsis (etanercept) **WARNINGS** Can cause <u>demyelinating</u> disease, <u>hepatitis B reactivation</u>, <u>heart failure, hepatotoxicity, lupus-like syndrome</u>, seizures, myelosuppression and severe infections <u>Do not use with other biologic DMARDs or live vaccines</u>
Infliximab (*Remicade*) Biosimilars: *Avsola, Renflexis, Inflectra, Ixifi* Injection (IV) + MTX	3 mg/kg <u>IV</u> at weeks 0, 2 and 6, then every 8 weeks (can ↑ dose to 10 mg/kg or treat as often as every 4 weeks based on need, but infection risk will ↑) Requires a filter and is stable in <u>NS only</u> <u>Infusion reactions</u>: hypotension, fever, chills, pruritus (can premedicate with acetaminophen, antihistamine, steroids) <u>Delayed hypersensitivity reaction</u> 3-12 days after administration (fever, rash, myalgia, HA, sore throat)	**SIDE EFFECTS** Infections and injection site reactions (redness, rash, swelling, itching, or bruising), positive anti-nuclear antibodies, headache, nausea, ↑ CPK (adalimumab) **MONITORING** Prior to initiation: <u>TB test</u> and <u>treat</u> if positive <u>before starting therapy</u> (see the Infectious Disease II chapter); test for <u>HBV</u> (HBsAg and anti-HBc) Routine: <u>signs of infection</u>, CBC, LFTs, HBV, TB (annually if risk factors for TB are present), symptoms of heart failure, malignancies, vitals (during infliximab infusion)
Certolizumab pegol (*Cimzia*, Cimzia Starter Kit) Single-dose prefilled syringe and vial starter kit +/- MTX	400 mg SC at weeks 0, 2 and 4, then 200 mg <u>SC every other week</u> (can consider 400 mg every 4 weeks)	**NOTES** <u>Do not shake or freeze</u>; requires <u>refrigeration</u> (biologics will denature if hot); allow to reach room temperature before injecting (15-30 minutes); etanercept and adalimumab can be stored at room temperature for a maximum of 14 days; do not refrigerate once warmed MTX is used 1st line and anti-TNF biologics are <u>add-on therapy</u>; however, if the initial presentation is <u>severe</u>, they can be started as <u>initial therapy</u> (with or without MTX)
Golimumab (*Simponi*, Simponi Aria) Single-dose prefilled syringe or auto-injector (SC), injection (IV) + MTX	<u>SC</u> (*Simponi*): 50 mg <u>monthly</u> IV (*Simponi Aria*): 2 mg/kg infused over 30 minutes at weeks 0 and 4, then every 8 weeks IV golimumab requires a <u>filter</u>	Antibody induction can occur and will ↓ usefulness of the drug Rotate injection sites

Other Biologic DMARDs (Non-TNF Inhibitors)

The following drugs are biologics that affect the immune system by mechanisms other than TNF inhibition. Safety data on the use of non-TNF biologics in pregnancy is limited. Pregnant patients exposed to these drugs are encouraged to register in a <u>pregnancy exposure registry</u> so that pregnancy can be monitored.

DRUG	DOSING	SAFETY/SIDE EFFECTS/MONITORING
Rituximab (Rituxan) Biosimilars: *Riabni, Ruxience, Truxima* Injection (IV) <u>+ MTX</u> <u>Depletes CD20 B cells</u> believed to have a role in RA development and progression	1,000 mg <u>IV</u> on day 1 and day 15 (in combination with MTX for both doses) Can repeat treatment if needed at 16-24 weeks Premedicate with a <u>steroid, acetaminophen and an antihistamine</u> Start infusion at 50 mg/hr; can ↑ by 50 mg/hr every 30 minutes if no reaction (max 400 mg/hr) Gently invert the bag to mix the solution, do not shake	**BOXED WARNINGS** Serious, and fatal, <u>infusion-related reactions</u> (usually with the first infusion), progressive multifocal leukoencephalopathy (PML) due to JC virus infection (can be fatal), serious skin reactions (SJS/TEN) <u>HBV</u> reactivation, some cases resulting in fulminant hepatitis, hepatic failure and death; <u>screen high-risk groups for HBV and HCV</u> prior to initiating therapy; monitor patients for clinical and laboratory signs (HBsAg and anti-HBc) several months after treatment **WARNINGS** Infections; <u>do not give with other biologic DMARDs or live vaccines</u> **SIDE EFFECTS** In patients treated for RA: infusion-related reactions, URTIs, UTIs, N/V/D, peripheral edema, weight gain, hypertension, headache, angioedema, fever, insomnia, pain **MONITORING** ECG, vitals, infusion reactions, CBC, SCr, electrolytes, screen for HBV before treatment
Anakinra *(Kineret)* Single-dose prefilled syringe +/- MTX IL-1 receptor antagonist; IL-1 mediates immunologic reactions in RA; not recommended first-line per guidelines	100 mg SC daily (same time each day) Give only after failure of one or more DMARDs CrCl < 30 mL/min: 100 mg SC every other day	**WARNINGS** <u>Malignancies and serious infections</u>, discontinue if a serious infection develops, screen for TB prior to initiating therapy, do not give with other biologics or live vaccines **SIDE EFFECTS** URTIs, headache, N/D, abdominal pain, injection site reactions, antibody development, arthralgias **MONITORING** CBC, SCr, signs of infection **NOTES** Do not shake or freeze; refrigerate and protect from light
Abatacept *(Orencia, Orencia ClickJect)* Single-dose prefilled syringe or auto-injector (SC), injection (IV) +/- MTX Inhibits T-cell activation by binding to CD80 and CD86 on antigen presenting cells (blocking interaction with CD28)	IV: 500-1,000 mg (based on TBW) at 0, 2 and 4 weeks, then every 4 weeks Infuse over 30 minutes SC: 125 mg weekly SC with IV loading dose: give first IV dose as above, then 125 mg SC within 24 hours, then 125 mg SC weekly	**WARNINGS** Same warnings as above for anakinra plus: caution in patients with COPD – may worsen symptoms **SIDE EFFECTS** Headache, nausea, injection site reactions, infections, nasopharyngitis, antibody development **MONITORING** Signs of infection, hypersensitivity **NOTES** Stable in NS only Requires a filter and light protection during administration; do not shake

DRUG	DOSING	SAFETY/SIDE EFFECTS/MONITORING
Tocilizumab (*Actemra, Actemra ACTPen*) Single-dose prefilled syringe (SC), injection (IV) +/- MTX IL-6 receptor antagonist; IL-6 mediates immunologic reactions in RA	IV: 4 mg/kg every 4 weeks given over 60 minutes (can ↑ to 8 mg/kg) Max dose per infusion: 800 mg SC: If < 100 kg: 162 mg every other week (can ↑ to weekly) If ≥ 100 kg: 162 mg weekly	**BOXED WARNING** Serious <u>infections</u>, discontinue if a serious infection develops, <u>screen for TB</u> prior to initiating therapy **WARNINGS** ↑ LFTs, neutropenia and thrombocytopenia, GI perforation, can cause demyelinating diseases, hypersensitivity reactions, lipid abnormalities, <u>do not give with other biologic DMARDs or live vaccines</u>
Sarilumab (*Kevzara*) Single-dose prefilled syringe +/- MTX IL-6 receptor antagonist	200 mg SC every 2 weeks	**SIDE EFFECTS** URTIs, headache, hypertension, injection site reactions, ↑ LDL and total cholesterol **MONITORING** LFTs, CBC (baseline, 4-8 weeks after start of therapy, and every 3 months thereafter), lipid panel, signs of infection **NOTES** Do not use SC injection for IV infusion; SC products contain polysorbate 80 Do not start if: ALT or AST are > 1.5 times ULN, ANC < 2,000 cells/mm³, or platelets < 100,000 cell/mm³

KEY COUNSELING POINTS

See the Drug Formulations and Patient Counseling chapter for counseling language/layman's terminology.

METHOTREXATE

- Dosed once weekly for rheumatoid arthritis and psoriasis. Do not use daily or double-up doses. Choose a day of the week to take your medication that you can remember.

- Can cause:

  ❑ Liver damage.

  ❑ Infection.

  ❑ Mouth sores.

  ❑ Stomach bleeding, when used with aspirin/NSAIDs.

- Avoid in pregnancy (teratogenic). Use an effective form of birth control, whether you are male or female.

- Avoid alcohol.

- Take folic acid to decrease side effects.

Rasuvo and *Otrexup* single-use auto-injectors:

- Administer by subcutaneous injection into the <u>abdomen</u> (two inches away from the navel) or <u>upper thigh</u> only. Do not inject in the arms or any other areas of the body.

- Pinch the skin and inject at a 90° angle. Press firmly until you hear a click. Hold three seconds for *Otrexup* and five seconds for *Rasuvo*.

- Needles are included with single-dose subcutaneous auto-injector products and do not need to be purchased separately.

ADALIMUMAB, ETANERCEPT AND GOLIMUMAB

- Administer by subcutaneous injection as prescribed (once weekly for etanercept, every 1 – 2 weeks for adalimumab, monthly for golimumab).

- Can cause:

  ❑ Injection site reactions.

  ❑ Infection.

  ❑ Liver damage.

  ❑ Heart failure.

- Store the medication (single-dose syringes or multidose vials) in the refrigerator with protection from light and sources of heat. <u>Etanercept</u> and <u>adalimumab</u> can be stored at <u>room temperature</u> for a maximum <u>of 14 days</u>. Allow the medication to warm to room temperature before injecting.

- For <u>adalimumab (*Humira*)</u>: inject SC into the <u>abdomen or thigh</u>.

- For <u>etanercept (*Enbrel*)</u> syringe or auto-injector: inject SC into the <u>abdomen, thigh or upper arm</u>.

- For <u>golimumab (*Simponi*)</u>: inject SC into the <u>abdomen, thigh or upper arm</u>.

- Needles are included with single-dose subcutaneous auto-injector products and do not need to be purchased separately.

SYSTEMIC LUPUS ERYTHEMATOSUS

BACKGROUND

Systemic lupus erythematosus (SLE) is an autoimmune disease commonly referred to as lupus. SLE primarily affects young women, with a female-to-male ratio of 10:1.

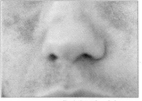
velimir/stock.adobe.com

SLE predominantly occurs in people 15 – 45 years old and is more common in women of African-American and Asian descent. Patients experience flare-ups of varying degrees, as well as periods of disease remission. The exact cause of SLE is unknown, but sunlight, certain drugs and viral infections can cause the disease. As the disease progresses, it can affect almost every organ system, with the heart, lungs, kidneys and brain being most affected. Drug-induced lupus erythematosus (DILE) can have similar clinical and laboratory features as SLE, but usually resolves within weeks after drug discontinuation. A few common DILE drugs are listed in the Key Drugs Guy.

CLINICAL PRESENTATION

More than half of individuals with SLE develop a distinct, flat, red rash on their face, across the nose bridge and cheeks. This is called a malar rash, commonly known as a "butterfly rash" because of its shape, and is not usually painful or itchy. Exposure to sunlight can aggravate the facial rash and worsen the inflammation in other organs. Other common symptoms include fatigue, depression, anorexia, weight loss, muscle pain, discoid rash, photosensitivity and joint pain and stiffness (e.g., arthritis).

Arthritis and cutaneous manifestations are most common, but renal, hematologic and neurologic manifestations contribute largely to morbidity and mortality. Lupus nephritis (kidney disease) develops in over 50% of patients with SLE. Common laboratory findings may include positive autoantibodies, such as:

- Antinuclear antibodies (ANA)
- Anti-single stranded DNA (anti-ssDNA)
- Anti-double stranded DNA (anti-dsDNA)
- Antiphospholipid antibodies

Patients may also have low complement (C3, C4, CH50) and elevated acute phase reactants (such as ESR, CRP).

SELECT DRUGS THAT CAN CAUSE DRUG-INDUCED LUPUS ERYTHEMATOSUS (DILE)	
Methimazole	Anti-TNF agents
Propylthiouracil	Terbinafine
Methyldopa	Isoniazid
Minocycline	Quinidine
Procainamide	Remember: **M**y **P**retty **M**alar **M**arking **P**robably **H**as **A** **T**ransient **Q**uality
Hydralazine (alone, and in BiDil)	

NON-DRUG TREATMENT

Non-drug treatment consists of rest and proper exercise to manage the fatigue. Smoking cessation is encouraged since tobacco smoke can be a trigger for disease flares. Photosensitivity is common with the condition and is also a risk with some treatments; sunscreens and sun protection/avoidance are required.

DRUG TREATMENT

Treatment approaches emphasize using a combination of drugs to minimize chronic exposure to steroids. Patients with mild disease may do well on an NSAID prescribed at anti-inflammatory doses, but use caution since the doses are high and these patients are more sensitive to the GI and renal side effects. Use with a proton pump inhibitor is generally recommended to reduce GI risk.

Many patients with SLE will require one or more immunosuppressants or cytotoxic agents to control the disease. Hydroxychloroquine, cyclophosphamide, azathioprine, mycophenolate mofetil and cyclosporine are all options for chronic therapy. In some cases, it may take up to six months to see maximal benefit from treatment. Except for hydroxychloroquine, these drugs do not have an FDA indication for SLE and are discussed in detail in other chapters (see the Transplant, Oncology and Inflammatory Bowel Disease chapters). Anifrolumab *(Saphnelo)* is FDA-approved for lupus and works by inhibiting type 1 interferons. Belimumab is approved for the treatment of lupus and lupus nephritis; voclosporin, a drug related to cyclosporine, is approved only for the treatment of lupus nephritis.

DRUG	DOSING	SAFETY/SIDE EFFECTS/MONITORING
IgG1-lambda monoclonal antibody: prevents the survival of B lymphocytes by blocking the binding of soluble human B lymphocyte stimulator protein (BLyS) to receptors on B lymphocytes; this reduces the activity of B-cell mediated immunity and the autoimmune response		
Belimumab (Benlysta) Single-dose prefilled syringe or auto-injector (SC), injection (IV)	IV: 10 mg/kg every 2 weeks x 3 doses, then every 4 weeks thereafter; infuse over 1 hour Consider giving pre-medication for infusion reactions and hypersensitivity reactions SC: 200 mg once weekly	**WARNINGS** Serious (sometimes fatal) <u>infections</u>, PML, acute hypersensitivity reactions, malignancy, psychiatric events, <u>do not give with other biologic DMARDs or live vaccines</u> **SIDE EFFECTS** Nausea, diarrhea, fever, depression (including suicidal ideation), insomnia **NOTES** Crosses the placenta - caution with use in pregnancy African-American patients may have a lower response rate; use with caution
Calcineurin inhibitor: suppresses immune system by inhibiting T-lymphocyte activation		
Voclosporin (Lupkynis) Capsule	23.7 mg BID in combination with steroids and mycophenolate	**BOXED WARNINGS** Serious (sometimes fatal) <u>infections; malignancies</u> **WARNINGS** <u>Nephrotoxicity</u>, neurotoxicity, <u>hypertension</u>, hyperkalemia, QT prolongation, red cell aplasia, <u>do not give with live vaccines</u> **SIDE EFFECTS** <u>Hypertension, diarrhea, headache</u>, anemia, cough, UTI, abdominal pain, dyspepsia, fatigue, <u>renal impairment</u> **NOTES** Avoid use in pregnancy; breastfeeding is not recommended by the manufacturer

MULTIPLE SCLEROSIS

BACKGROUND

Multiple sclerosis (MS) is a <u>chronic, progressive</u> autoimmune disease in which the patient's immune system <u>attacks the myelin sheath</u>, the fatty substance that surrounds and insulates nerve fibers of the brain and spinal cord axons. As demyelination progresses, nerves can no longer properly conduct electrical impulses, leading to impaired motor and autonomic function.

CLINICAL PRESENTATION

The presentation of MS is highly variable, with some patients having a much more aggressive course while others have occasional discrete attacks. Similar to other autoimmune conditions, most patients experience periods of disease activity followed by intervals of remission (i.e., relapsing-remitting MS). Others can have a progressive decline in function (i.e., primary or secondary progressive MS).

Early symptoms include <u>fatigue</u>, weakness, tingling, <u>numbness</u> and <u>blurred vision</u>. As the condition worsens, a variety of physical and psychological issues can make life very challenging, including <u>cognitive decline, muscle</u>

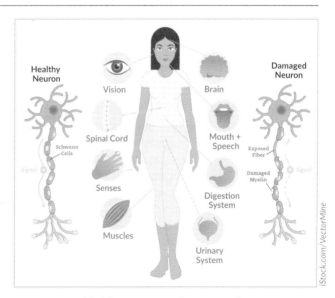

spasms, pain, bladder spasticity, depression, heat sensitivity, sexual dysfunction, difficulty walking with <u>gait instability</u> and visual disturbances.

If left untreated, about 30% of patients will develop significant physical disability. Up to 10% of patients have no significant physical disability, although these patients may develop mild cognitive dysfunction. Patients with primary progressive MS (PPMS) generally have the worst prognosis. Symptoms are characterized as:

- Primary: muscle weakness
- Secondary: result from primary symptoms, such as incontinence due to muscle impairment
- Tertiary: involve psychological and social concerns, such as depression

MS occurs in both men and women, but as with other autoimmune conditions, it is more common in women (ratio 2:1); however, males are more likely to have more progressive illness. The typical onset is between 20 – 40 years of age. Frequency of symptoms, spinal or brain lesions on magnetic resonance imaging (MRI), spinal fluid analysis and evoked potentials (tests that measure electrical conduction of the brain) are used to diagnose MS. A primary goal of therapy is prevention of disease progression; what is lost in neuronal function cannot be regained. Drugs that can modify disease progression are costly, ranging from approximately $65,000 – $80,000/year.

TREATMENT

Treating MS requires a holistic approach, including functional rehabilitation, an anti-inflammatory diet and supporting emotional health at all stages. Programs exist to support cognitive and vocational rehabilitation. Physical and occupational therapy programs are available for motor functions, speech and swallowing. Medications are used to modify disease, treat relapses and manage symptoms.

Steroids are used to treat relapses. Usually, 3 – 7 days of IV methylprednisolone is given, with or without an oral steroid taper afterwards.

Disease-Modifying Therapies

Disease-modifying therapies (DMTs) are used to reduce the frequency and severity of relapses. Many different drugs are used for the treatment of MS (see the Drug Tables below), though the mechanism of these drugs in treating MS is often not well defined. The selection of a drug is based on patient factors (e.g., disease severity, insurance, comorbidities), the route of administration, efficacy and adverse effects.

Interferon beta formulations (*Betaseron, Avonex, Rebif, Extavia, Plegridy*) and glatiramer acetate (*Copaxone, Glatopa*) are parenteral drugs that were once the mainstay of treatment for patients with relapsing forms of MS, and both are still preferred treatments in patients of childbearing potential who are actively trying to conceive. Pegylated interferon beta (*Plegridy*) allows for more convenient SC dosing every 14 days. When the medication is supplied as a single-dose prefilled syringe, auto-injector or vial kit for SC injection, needles are included with the device and do not require a separate purchase.

Oral DMTs, such as fingolimod (*Gilenya*), diroximel fumarate (*Vumerity*) and ozanimod (*Zeposia*) are often used as initial treatments for patients with relapsing remitting MS. Other options include certain monoclonal antibodies (e.g., ofatumumab, ocrelizumab) and chemotherapy drugs (e.g., cladribine). Mitoxantrone is a chemotherapeutic agent approved for MS, though it is rarely used due to its risks and wide availability of alternative drugs; a review of mitoxantrone can be found in the Oncology chapter. Monoclonal antibodies and chemotherapy drugs are considered second- or third-line options for most relapsing remitting MS patients due to the risk of significant toxicities, though these may be used first-line for patients with more aggressive MS.

A few injectable drugs are supplied as a powder that requires reconstitution, and some of these contain albumin. Some patients will not wish to use, or cannot use, albumin-containing products.

DRUG	DOSING	SAFETY/SIDE EFFECTS/MONITORING
Glatiramer acetate: an immune modulator thought to induce and activate T-lymphocyte suppressor cells in relapsing forms of MS		
Glatiramer acetate (***Copaxone**, Glatopa*) Prefilled syringes 20 and 40 mg/mL concentrations are not interchangeable	20 mg SC daily or 40 mg SC 3 times per week (at least 48 hours apart) If increasing dose to 40 mg, start 48 hrs after the 20 mg dose	**WARNINGS** Chest pain, immediate post-injection reaction, lipoatrophy **SIDE EFFECTS** Injection site reactions (inflammation, erythema, pain, pruritus, residual mass), flushing, diaphoresis, dyspnea, infection, pain, weakness, anxiety, rash, nausea, nasopharyngitis, vasodilation, antibody development **NOTES** Preferred agent if treatment is necessary during pregnancy Check solution for discoloration and discard if present Can be kept at room temperature for up to one month, or in the refrigerator (preferred); if cold, let it stand at room temperature for 20 minutes prior to injecting

DRUG	DOSING	SAFETY/SIDE EFFECTS/MONITORING
Interferon beta products: alter the expression and response to surface antigens, enhancing immune cell function		
Interferon beta-1a (*Avonex, Avonex Pen, Rebif, Rebif Rebidose*) Powder (for reconstitution), prefilled syringe and auto-injector	*Avonex*: 30 mcg IM weekly *Rebif*: 22 mcg or 44 mcg SC three times per week (at least 48 hours apart)	**WARNINGS** Psychiatric disorders (depression/suicide), injection site necrosis, myelosuppression, ↑ LFTs, thyroid dysfunction (hyper and hypo-), infections, anaphylaxis, worsening cardiovascular disease, seizure risk **SIDE EFFECTS** Flu-like symptoms following administration (lasting minutes to hours); ↓ with continued treatment – can use acetaminophen or NSAIDs prior to injection or start with lower doses and titrate weekly to target dose
Interferon beta-1b (*Betaseron, Extavia*) Powder (for reconstitution), and auto-injector	SC: 0.25 mg every other day (use within 3 hrs of reconstitution)	Visual disturbances, fatigue, depression, pain, urinary tract infections, HA **MONITORING** LFTs, CBC (at 1, 3 and 6 months, then periodically); thyroid function every 6 months (in patients with thyroid dysfunction or as clinical necessary)
Peginterferon beta-1a (*Plegridy, Plegridy Starter Pack*) Prefilled syringe and auto-injector	SC: 63 mcg on day 1, 94 mcg on day 15, then 125 mcg every 14 days starting on day 29	**NOTES** Refrigerate all except *Betaseron* and *Extavia* (which can be stored at room temperature). If refrigerated, let stand at room temperature prior to injection. Do not expel the small air bubble in prefilled syringes due to loss of dose. Do not shake *Avonex, Betaseron* or *Extavia* Some formulations contain albumin which can increase the risk of Creutzfeldt-Jakob disease transmission (rare); avoid in albumin-sensitive patients

DRUG	SAFETY/SIDE EFFECTS/MONITORING
Sphingosine 1-phosphate (S1P) receptor modulators: block lymphocytes from exiting lymph nodes, reducing lymphocytes in the periphery; may limit lymphocyte migration into the CNS	
Fingolimod (*Gilenya, Tascenso ODT*) Capsule, ODT	**CONTRAINDICATIONS** Some arrhythmias, or any of the following in the past 6 months: MI, unstable angina, stroke/TIA or some HF (decompensation requiring hospitalization, or Class III/IV) Ozanimod: severe untreated sleep apnea, concomitant use of an MAO inhibitor
Ozanimod (*Zeposia*) Capsule	Siponimod: CYP2C9*3/*3 genotype (testing required before use) **WARNINGS** Can cause bradycardia or other bradyarrhythmias – use caution with other drugs that slow HR; patients starting fingolimod must be monitored for at least 6 hours after the first dose (ECG required at baseline and at end of initial observation period or if treatment course is interrupted)
Ponesimod (*Ponvory*) Tablet	↑ risk for infection (monitor CBC), screen for VZV antibodies before starting; vaccinate if negative (or no history of chickenpox) Other side effects: malignancies, macular edema (monitor with eye exams), hepatotoxicity (monitor LFTs), ↑ BP, ↓ lung function, fetal risk [use contraception during and for some time after stopping therapy if of childbearing potential (duration varies from 7-90 days based on the drug)]
Siponimod (*Mayzent*) Tablet	**NOTES** MS can become much worse when treatment is stopped Unopened *Mayzent* is stored in the refrigerator, once opened it can be stored at room temperature
Fumarates or Nuclear factor (erythroid-derived 2)-like 2 (Nrf2) activators: anti-inflammatory and cytoprotective	
Dimethyl fumarate (*Tecfidera*) Capsule	Hepatotoxicity (monitor LFTs), neutropenia (reversible, but monitor CBC), PML Can cause flushing (prevent with aspirin 30 minutes prior to dose and administer with food), GI side effects (less with *Vumerity*)
Diroximel fumarate (*Vumerity*) Capsule	Do not crush, chew or sprinkle capsule contents on food Monomethyl fumarate is the active metabolite of diroximel fumarate and dimethyl fumarate
Monomethyl fumarate (*Bafiertam*) Capsule	

DRUG	SAFETY/SIDE EFFECTS/MONITORING
Pyrimidine synthesis inhibitor: anti-inflammatory; may reduce the number of activated lymphocytes in the CNS	
Teriflunomide (*Aubagio*) Tablet	Severe hepatotoxicity and teratogenicity – <u>contraindicated in pregnancy</u> and with severe hepatic impairment Can use accelerated elimination to remove drug - see leflunomide Active metabolite of leflunomide
CD20-directed monoclonal antibodies	
Ofatumumab (*Kesimpta*) Injection (SC) *Arzerra* – for CLL Ublituximab-xiiy (*Briumvi*) Injection (IV) Ocrelizumab (*Ocrevus*) Injection (IV)	**CONTRAINDICATIONS** Active hepatitis B infection, screen before starting therapy **WARNINGS** ↑ risk of serious and potentially fatal infections (including PML), avoid live vaccinations during treatment, fetal risk, infusion reactions, reduction in immunoglobulin levels *Ocrevus:* immune-mediated colitis **NOTES** *Briumvi* and *Ocrevus:* indicated for relapsing forms of MS, premedicate with a steroid, antihistamine and/or acetaminophen *Ocrevus* requires a 0.22-micron in-line filter, has similar safety issues as other CD20-directed MABs (e.g., rituximab)
Other monoclonal antibodies (various mechanisms)	
Alemtuzumab (*Lemtrada*) Injection (IV) *Campath* – for CLL CD52-directed cytolytic monoclonal antibody	**BOXED WARNINGS** <u>REMS</u> program required; serious, sometimes fatal, autoimmune conditions, infusion reactions, malignancies, stroke **CONTRAINDICATIONS** HIV (causes prolonged ↓ in CD4 count) **NOTES** Indicated when there is an inadequate response to ≥ 2 MS drugs Complete all vaccinations 6 weeks before treatment Premedicate with a steroid, an antihistamine and/or acetaminophen (varies by drug)
Natalizumab (Tysabri) <u>Injection</u> (IV) Monoclonal antibody that binds to the alpha-4 subunit of integrin molecules	See Inflammatory Bowel Disease chapter (used for treatment of <u>Crohn's Disease</u>) **BOXED WARNINGS** Progressive multifocal leukoencephalopathy (PML); only available through the <u>REMS</u> TOUCH Prescribing Program
Oral anti-neoplastic	
Cladribine (*Mavenclad*) Tablet	Boxed warning for malignancies, teratogenicity Contraindicated in patients with current malignancy, HIV or active chronic infections Contraception must be used for males and females of reproductive potential during treatment and for 6 months after the last dose
Potassium channel blocker: may increase nerve signal conduction	
Dalfampridine (*Ampyra*) Tablet	Contraindicated in patients with a history of seizures Not a disease modifying agent, only increases walking speed Takes up to 6 weeks to show efficacy; most patients do not respond

Drugs Used for Symptom Control

Patients with MS may need <u>a variety of medications for symptom control</u>. The individual drugs used can be found in different chapters in this book. Drugs commonly used for symptom control in MS include <u>anticholinergics for incontinence, laxatives for constipation</u> (or loperamide if diarrhea), skeletal <u>muscle relaxants</u> for muscle spasms/spasticity, or <u>analgesics</u> for muscle spasms and pain. For localized pain and spasms, botulinum toxin (*Botox*) injections can provide relief for up to three months. <u>Propranolol</u> can help with <u>tremor</u>. Dalfampridine (*Ampyra*) is used to increase walking speed but should be avoided in patients with a history of seizures. For depression, many antidepressants can be used. An SNRI may be chosen to help with neuropathic pain. Fatigue is often treated with modafinil or stimulants used for ADHD (e.g., methylphenidate). Meclizine and scopolamine are used for dizziness and vertigo. Acetylcholinesterase inhibitors, including donepezil, can be used to help cognitive function. Erectile dysfunction can be treated with phosphodiesterase-5 inhibitors.

Notice that <u>drugs used for symptom control can worsen other symptoms</u>. For example, anticholinergics can worsen cognitive function (not all of them do; it is patient-specific), as can drugs for vertigo and propranolol. Propranolol has added concerns for worsening depression and causing problems with sexual performance. The SSRI and SNRI antidepressants can worsen sexual dysfunction. Opioids, if used for pain, will worsen constipation, can decrease cognition and have dependence concerns. Pharmacists play a major role in managing the various medications used for MS.

KEY COUNSELING POINTS

See the Drug Formulations and Patient Counseling chapter for counseling language/layman's terminology.

GLATIRAMER ACETATE

- Subcutaneous injection. Rotate injection sites.

- Available in two different doses; depending on your dose, inject daily or three times a week ≥ 48 hours apart. Administer consistently on the same three days each week.

- Can cause:

  - Injection site reactions.

  - Chest pain.

  - Shortness of breath and flushing.

- Store in the refrigerator before use; can be kept at room temperature for up to one month. Allow to warm to room temperature before injecting.

S1P RECEPTOR MODULATORS

- Can cause:

  - Liver damage.

  - Vision problems.

  - Serious infections.

  - Slowed heart rate.

- MS can become worse after stopping treatment.

INTERFERON BETA PRODUCTS

- Injected subcutaneously except for *Avonex* (IM).

- Can cause:

  - Injection site reactions.

  - Flu-like symptoms (e.g., fever, chills, myalgias); can use acetaminophen or NSAIDs for prevention prior to injecting.

  - New or worsening depression.

- *Betaseron* and *Extavia* may be stored at room temperature. All other interferons should be stored in the refrigerator prior to use. Allow drug to reach room temperature before injecting.

RAYNAUD'S PHENOMENON

Raynaud's is a common condition that is triggered by exposure to <u>cold and/or stress</u>, leading to <u>vasospasm</u> in the extremities (most commonly in the <u>fingers and/or toes</u>). The vasospasm causes the skin to turn <u>white</u> and then <u>blue</u>, which is followed by painful swelling when the affected areas warm and can result in amputation in severe cases. Laboratory findings that can signify other autoimmune conditions are generally absent.

Prevention and treatment involve <u>vasodilation</u> to improve blood flow to the affected areas. The <u>calcium channel blocker</u> (CCB) <u>nifedipine</u> is commonly used for prevention but other CCBs can be used. Additional drugs used for vasodilation include iloprost, topical nitroglycerin and the phosphodiesterase-5 inhibitors. See <u>Study Tip Gal</u>.

DRUG-INDUCED RAYNAUD'S

↓ **blood flow to fingers causes ↑ cyanosis (bluish fingers) and pain**

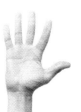 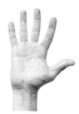 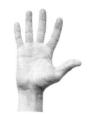

Fingers become white due to lack of blood flow. *Fingers turn blue as vessels dilate to keep blood in tissues.* *Fingers finally turn red as blood flow returns.*

iStock.com/filistimlyanin

Drugs that cause or worsen Raynaud's:

Beta-blockers

Bleomycin, cisplatin

Sympathomimetics (from vasoconstriction): amphetamines (e.g., *Concerta, Vyvanse*), pseudoephedrine and illicit drugs (e.g., cocaine and methamphetamine)

CELIAC DISEASE

BACKGROUND

Celiac disease (celiac sprue) is an immune response to eating gluten, a protein found in wheat, barley and rye. The primary and most effective treatment is to avoid gluten entirely. Gluten is present in many foods, food additives and many drug excipients. Pharmacists can assist patients in avoiding gluten-containing drugs completely, as even a small exposure will trigger a reaction. The FDA permits food products to be labeled "gluten-free" only if the food contains less gluten than 20 parts per million.

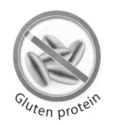
Gluten protein
iStock.com/ttsz

CLINICAL PRESENTATION

The common symptoms of celiac disease are diarrhea, abdominal pain, bloating and weight loss. Constipation (rather than diarrhea) can be present and is more common in children. In celiac disease, antibodies attack and damage the lining of the small intestine, which can lead to vitamin and nutritional deficiencies as a result of decreased absorption. Other complications include small bowel ulcers, amenorrhea and infertility, as well as an increased risk of cancer (primarily lymphomas). 95% of cases will respond well to dietary changes, although avoiding gluten entirely is not a simple task.

Dermatitis herpetiformis is an extremely itchy, blistery skin rash with chronic eruptions that occurs in 20 – 25% of patients with celiac disease, more often in males. The rash can be present with or without overt intestinal symptoms and is often mistaken for eczema or psoriasis, which leads to a delay in diagnosis and treatment.

GLUTEN IN MEDICATIONS

The FDA has strict regulations on active ingredients in drug formulations, but there is little oversight for the excipients, making the identification of gluten difficult. Active drugs are gluten-free, but excipients may contain gluten. Do not assume that generic formulations will have the same excipients as the brand, since there is no legal requirement to match the excipients.

Package inserts might contain information on the excipient components. Look for the keyword "starch," which will be either corn, potato, tapioca or wheat. If the package insert lists "starch" alone, the manufacturer must be consulted to determine if the starch is wheat. The manufacturer might report that they do not use gluten in the manufacturing process, but they cannot state whether the excipients purchased from outside vendors are gluten-free. The risk of cross-contamination is low but not absent, and this information should be provided to the patient. It is ultimately up to the patient, hopefully in consultation with the prescriber, whether to take the drug or not.

MYASTHENIA GRAVIS

BACKGROUND

Myasthenia gravis (MG) is an autoimmune condition that attacks the connections between nerves and muscles, often leading to weakness in the muscles that control the eyes, face, neck and limbs. In most cases, the immune system targets acetylcholine (ACh) receptors. Common symptoms include eye/vision changes [e.g., double vision (diplopia), drooping eyelid (ptosis)], difficulty chewing/swallowing and jaw or neck weakness.

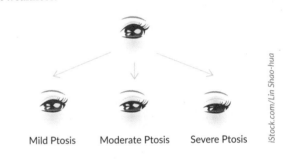
Mild Ptosis   Moderate Ptosis   Severe Ptosis
iStock.com/Lin Shao-hua

DRUGS THAT CAN WORSEN MYASTHENIA GRAVIS

Many drugs can worsen or unmask MG. These drugs should be avoided or used cautiously in patients with MG:

- Select antibiotics (e.g., aminoglycosides, quinolones, macrolides)
- Magnesium salts
- Select antiarrhythmics
- Beta-blockers and calcium channel blockers
- Select antipsychotics
- Muscle relaxants
- Botulinum toxin

TREATMENT

Pyridostigmine (*Mestinon*), a cholinesterase inhibitor, is the mainstay of treatment for MG. Immunotherapy (e.g., steroids, azathioprine, cyclosporine, methotrexate) may be used for patients who remain symptomatic on pyridostigmine or who need long-term MG treatment. Some cases may require a thymectomy (removal of the thymus gland), plasmapheresis or intravenous immunoglobulin (IVIG).

Eculizumab *(Soliris)* is an injectable complement inhibitor approved for the treatment of MG in adults who are ACh receptor-antibody positive; this drug can increase the risk of meningococcal infections and has a REMS program that must be followed (e.g., patients must be up to date on meningococcal vaccinations).

DRUG	DOSING	SAFETY/SIDE EFFECTS/MONITORING
Cholinesterase inhibitors: block the breakdown of acetylcholine by acetylcholinesterase, which improves neuromuscular transmission and increases muscle strength		
Pyridostigmine *(Mestinon)* Tablet IV and IM forms used for myasthenia gravis crisis, nerve gas exposure and reversal of nondepolarizing muscle relaxants	60-1,500 mg/day (usually 600 mg/day) divided into 5-6 doses	**CONTRAINDICATIONS** Mechanical intestinal or urinary obstruction **WARNINGS** Cholinergic effects: symptoms of excess ACh can occur (e.g., salivation, lacrimation, excessive urination, diarrhea); refer to the Basic Science Concepts chapter CVD, glaucoma, bronchospastic respiratory disease (e.g., COPD or asthma)

SJÖGREN'S SYNDROME

Sjögren's syndrome is an autoimmune disease most often characterized by severe dry eyes and dry mouth. Many other symptoms can be associated with Sjögren's (e.g., thyroiditis, Raynaud's phenomenon, neuropathy, lymphadenopathy). Sjögren's syndrome can be primary or secondary (e.g., associated with another autoimmune disease, such as RA or SLE). Dry mouth and dry eyes are a source of significant morbidity for these patients and can lead to complications, such as dental caries, corneal ulceration and chronic oral infections. There is no known cure for Sjögren's; treatment focuses on reducing the symptoms of dry eyes and dry mouth.

DRY EYES TREATMENT

The use of artificial teardrops is the primary treatment for xerophthalmia (i.e., dry eyes). Popular OTC artificial teardrops available are *Systane, Refresh, Clear Eyes* and *Liquifilm*. It may be necessary to try a couple of different OTC eye drops before finding one that provides the most comfort. If the preservative (e.g., benzalkonium chloride) is irritating, preservative-free artificial tear drops packaged in individual use containers are available. If the eyes dry out while sleeping, an ointment is preferable.

Cyclosporine eye drops *(Restasis)* can be used in patients who do not have satisfactory relief from other measures, including ductal occlusion (lacrimal duct plugs). *Restasis* provides benefit for a small percentage of users, but it is expensive. Patients should be instructed to monitor for a reduction in symptoms and a reduction in the use of OTC eye drops. Counsel patients to use *Restasis* properly to avoid infection and that it may take up to 3 – 6 months to notice an increase in tear production. Lifitegrast *(Xiidra)*, a first-in-class drug, is approved for the treatment of signs and symptoms of dry eye disease. Refer to the Drug Formulations and Patient Counseling chapter for detailed patient counseling information for eye drops.

Eye Drops for Dry Eyes

DRUG	DOSING	SAFETY/SIDE EFFECTS/MONITORING
Cyclosporine Emulsion (Restasis, *Cequa, Verkazia)* Ophthalmic	1 drop in each eye Q12H	**SIDE EFFECTS** Ocular (burning, stinging, redness, pain, blurred vision, foreign body sensation, discharge, itching eye) **NOTES** Prior to use, invert the vial several times to make the emulsion uniform
Lifitegrast *(Xiidra)* Ophthalmic	1 drop in each eye Q12H	**SIDE EFFECTS** Unusual taste, eye irritation, discomfort, blurred vision **NOTES** Store in the original foil pouch to protect from light

DRY MOUTH TREATMENT

Non-drug treatment for xerostomia (i.e., dry mouth) includes salivary stimulation, using sugar-free chewing gum (with xylitol) or lozenges, and daily rinses with antimicrobial mouthwash. Salivary substitutes are available in lozenges, rinses, sprays and swabs (*Aquoral, Mouth Kote, Biotene Oral Balance*). These contain carboxymethylcellulose or glycerin. If OTC treatments do not provide sufficient relief, prescription oral muscarinic agonists, such as pilocarpine (*Salagen*) or cevimeline (*Evoxac*), can be used. These drugs are contraindicated in patients with uncontrolled asthma and narrow-angle glaucoma, due to cholinergic properties and associated side effects.

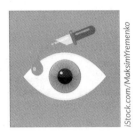

iStock.com/MaksimYremenko

PSORIASIS

BACKGROUND

Psoriasis is a chronic, autoimmune disease that appears on the skin. There are several types of psoriasis. The most common is plaque psoriasis, which appears as raised, red patches covered with a silvery-white buildup of dead skin cells on any part of the body. Treatments can be divided into three main types: light therapy, topical and systemic medications. Most psoriasis is treated with topical medication and UV light therapy. Soaking can also help loosen and remove the plaques.

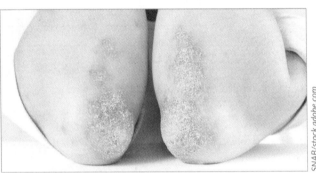

SNAB/stock.adobe.com

NON-DRUG TREATMENT

Ultraviolet (UV) light exposure causes activated T-cells in the skin to die. This slows skin turnover and decreases scaling and inflammation. Brief, daily exposures to small amounts of sunlight can improve psoriasis, but intense sun exposure can worsen symptoms and cause skin damage. UVB phototherapy, in controlled doses from an artificial source, can improve mild to moderate psoriasis symptoms. Other non-drug treatments include photochemotherapy (ultraviolet A light with psoralen, a light sensitizer) and laser light therapy.

DRUG TREATMENT

There are many topical options for treating psoriasis, including steroids, a vitamin D analog (calcipotriene), anthralin, retinoids (some of the same drugs used for acne), salicylic acid (primarily in medicated shampoo), coal tar, tapinarof and moisturizers. Calcipotriene, tazarotene and salicylic acid are used in combination with topical steroids. If these fail, topical calcineurin inhibitors (*Protopic, Elidel*) can be tried; these are the preferred agents when applying to the face. Treatment for more severe symptoms can require immunosuppressants, including methotrexate, cyclosporine, hydroxyurea or immunomodulators (e.g., etanercept, infliximab, adalimumab, certolizumab). Newer systemic drugs approved for plaque psoriasis include *Otezla* and monoclonal antibodies that have interleukin receptor antagonist actions.

Topical Psoriasis Treatment

DRUG/DRUG CLASS	COMMENTS
Steroids	Use high-potency steroids only short-term due to risk of side effects
	Can be used as monotherapy or with other therapies
	See Common Skin Conditions chapter
Coal Tar products (many, including *DHS Tar, Ionil-T, Psoriasin, Pentrax Gold*)	Coal tar products are messy, time-consuming and can stain clothing and bedding, but some patients get relief at a reasonable cost
+ salicylic acid (*Tarsum*) OTC	There are many topical formulations available (cream, foam, emulsion, ointment, oil, shampoo) and bath products (e.g., bar soap)
Also used for dandruff and dermatitis	Do not use salicylic acid products with other salicylates as systemic absorption can occur
	Can cause skin irritation and photosensitivity

DRUG/DRUG CLASS	COMMENTS
Tazarotene (Tazorac) – a topical retinoid + halobetasol (Duobrii)	See Common Skin Conditions chapter
Anthralin (Zithranol)	Keratolytic containing salicylic acid with irritant potential, ↑ contact time as tolerated up to 30 min
Calcipotriene (Dovonex, Sorilux) Cream, foam, ointment, solution + betamethasone (Taclonex ointment, Enstilar foam)	Vitamin D analog – contraindicated and should be avoided in hypercalcemia or vitamin D toxicity If using a suspension, shake well Do not apply to face, axillae or groin
Tapinarof (VTAMA) Cream	Most common side effects include folliculitis, nasopharyngitis, contact dermatitis, and pruritis Wash hands after use

Systemic Psoriasis Treatment

DRUG/DRUG CLASS	COMMENTS
Retinoid	
Acitretin Tablet	Boxed warning for hepatotoxicity and pregnancy (female must sign informed consent before dispensing) Used only in severe cases when patient is unresponsive to other therapies due to numerous contraindications and side effects
Phosphodiesterase-4 inhibitor	
Apremilast (Otezla) Tablet	Warnings: weight loss, depression and suicidal ideation Most common side effects are diarrhea, N/V, headache
Interleukin receptor antagonists: monoclonal antibodies that bind to and interfere with proinflammatory cytokines	
Brodalumab (Siliq) Bimekizumab (Bimzelx) Guselkumab (Tremfya) Ixekizumab (Taltz) Risankizumab (Skyrizi) Secukinumab (Cosentyx) Tildrakizumab (Ilumya) Ustekinumab (Stelara) All available in single-dose prefilled syringes, auto-injectors or vials for subcutaneous injection	Like other monoclonal antibodies, these can cause serious infections (including active TB); screen for latent TB (and treat if needed) before starting; avoid live vaccines, may exacerbate Crohn's disease, latex hypersensitivity Other common side effects include diarrhea and URTIs Brodalumab: boxed warning for suicidal ideation and behavior; REMS program required
Selective tyrosine kinase 2 inhibitor	
Deucravacitinib (Sotyktu) Tablet	FDA-approved for moderate to severe plaque psoriasis Warnings: may increase risk for infections, screen for latent TB (and treat if needed) before starting, avoid live vaccines; malignancy (including lymphomas); rhabdomyolysis and laboratory abnormalities (elevated triglycerides and liver enzymes) Most common side effects include upper respiratory infections, elevated CPK, mouth ulcers and acne Not recommended for use in combination with other potent immunosuppressants

Select Guidelines/References

American College of Rheumatology Clinical Practice Guidelines. https://www.rheumatology.org/Practice-Quality/Clinical-Support/Clinical-Practice-Guidelines (accessed 2023 Dec 14).

Narayanaswami P, Sanders DB, Wolfe G, et al. International consensus guidance for management of myasthenia gravis. Neurology. 2021;96(3):114-122.

Sanders DB, Wolfe GI, Benatar M, et al. International consensus guidance for management of myasthenia gravis. Neurology. 2016;87(4):419-425.

American Academy of Dermatology. Psoriasis Clinical Guidelines. Section 1-6. https://www.aad.org/practicecenter/quality/clinical-guidelines/psoriasis (accessed 2023 Dec 14).

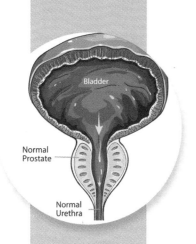

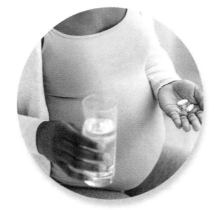

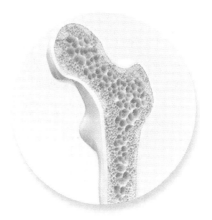

MALE & FEMALE HEALTH

CONTENTS

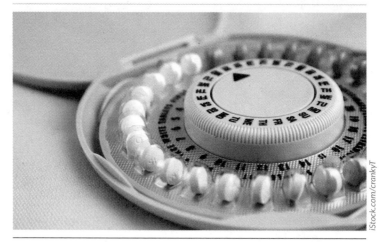

iStock.com/crankyT

CHAPTER 47
CONTRACEPTION & INFERTILITY

BACKGROUND

The majority of women between the ages of 15 and 49 have used contraception, which is available in many different forms, including OTC and prescription options. Proper use is essential to prevent unintended pregnancy. With so many forms of contraception available, patient-specific factors should drive product selection. Pharmacists are in a unique position to increase the appropriate use of contraceptive methods, access to contraception and prevention of unintended pregnancies. In some states, pharmacists are authorized to prescribe contraception.

On the other hand, many people struggle with becoming pregnant. Infertility treatments can be invasive and expensive. Pharmacists (usually in specialty settings) play an essential role in gaining access to and assisting with the appropriate use of infertility treatments.

MENSTRUAL CYCLE PHASES

A normal menstrual cycle ranges from <u>23 – 35 days</u> (average <u>28</u> days). <u>The start of bleeding (menses)</u> indicates that the <u>next cycle has begun and is counted as day 1 of the cycle</u>; the remnants of the previous cycle (the thick, bloody endometrial lining) are sloughing off. Menstruation typically lasts a few days. Changes in hormone levels cause the events that characterize the different phases of the menstrual cycle (see next page). The follicular phase begins with the onset of menses, when the estrogen and progesterone levels start off low.

CONTENT LEGEND

 = Study Tip Gal

PHASES OF THE MENSTRUAL CYCLE

Follicular	Each follicle in an ovary contains an oocyte (immature egg). Follicle stimulating hormone (FSH) spurs follicle development and causes estrogen to surge. Estrogen peaks by the end of this phase.* The surge in estrogen causes luteinizing hormone (LH) and FSH to increase.
Ovulatory	The LH surge triggers ovulation 24-36 hours later. Ovulation is the release of the egg (ova) from the ovary.
Luteal	The start of ovulation begins the luteal (last) phase, during which the corpus luteum develops in the ovaries, and lasts ~14 days. Progesterone is dominant in this phase.*

Estrogen and progesterone cause the endometrium (the lining of the uterus) to thicken to prepare for an embryo, and progesterone causes the cervical mucus to thicken and body temperature to increase. When estrogen and/or progesterone are low during the cycle, blood can drip off the lining, causing spotting (which can require an increase in estrogen or progesterone in birth control pills).

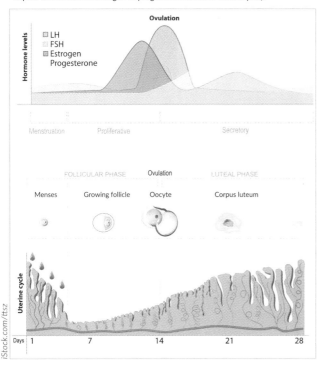

FERTILITY AWARENESS

The mid-cycle luteinizing hormone (LH) surge results in release of the oocyte (egg) from the ovary into the fallopian tube. The oocyte lives for 24 hours once released, while sperm can survive for ~3 days. Ovulation kits predict the best time for intercourse based on ovulation in order to try to conceive (get pregnant). These kits test for LH in the urine and are positive if LH is present. A person wishing to conceive should have intercourse when the LH surge is detected, and for the following 2 days (as the LH surge typically occurs 24 – 36 hours prior to ovulation).

Alternative methods to test for ovulation include monitoring body temperature and cervical mucus (discussed on the next page).

PREGNANCY

Human chorionic gonadotropin (hCG) is released when a fertilized egg attaches to the lining of the uterus (called implantation). Detecting hCG in the urine or blood indicates pregnancy. A home urine test can detect pregnancy sooner if the woman tests the first urine in the morning, when the hCG level is highest.

PRECONCEPTION HEALTH

Preconception health focuses on steps to take to protect the health of a baby in the future. Any woman planning to conceive (and all women of childbearing age) should:

- Increase their folic acid (folate, vitamin B9) consumption from a combination of dietary supplements and fortified foods (e.g., dried beans, leafy green vegetables, oranges). Folate deficiency can cause birth defects of the brain and spinal cord (neural tube defects), which occur very early in pregnancy before many women know they are pregnant. Adults are recommended to take 400 mcg of dietary folate equivalents (DFE) per day, and this folate requirement increases during pregnancy to 600 mcg DFE/day.

- Stop smoking, using illicit drugs and drinking excessive amounts of alcohol.

- Keep vaccinations current. Attempt to avoid illnesses that will adversely affect the baby (e.g., toxoplasmosis).

- Avoid toxic chemicals, including drugs on the Hazardous Drugs List developed by NIOSH; see the Compounding chapters.

- Consult with a healthcare provider to evaluate the teratogenic potential of all current medications. Some may need to be stopped or switched to a safer alternative (See Drug Use in Pregnancy & Lactation chapter).

The general health of the male partner is also important.

CONTRACEPTION

Contraception can be used until ready to conceive. A prompt return to fertility occurs when most contraceptives are discontinued. The only reversible contraceptive method that has a delay in return to fertility is the medroxyprogesterone injection.

Contraceptive preferences vary markedly with age. For women in their teens and 20s, hormonal contraception is preferred. Women ≥ 35 years of age often rely on sterilization, which can be performed immediately postpartum (following a birth). Male contraception options are limited. Presently, male condoms and vasectomy are the only options.

EFFECTIVENESS OF CONTRACEPTIVE METHODS

The figure below provides a comparison of the efficacy of contraceptive methods that are available as OTC or prescription products. Contraceptive methods, except for condoms, do not provide protection from sexually transmitted infections (STIs). Both male and female condoms provide protection from some STIs, including HIV.

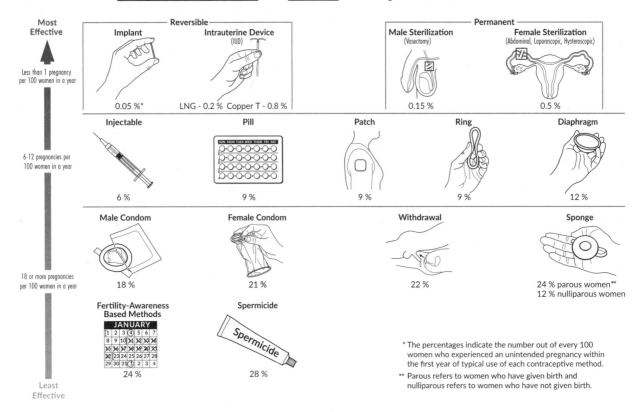

CDC, March 2021

NON-PHARMACOLOGIC AND OTC CONTRACEPTIVE METHODS

Abstinence is the only 100% effective way to prevent pregnancy and STIs. Other non-pharmacologic methods of contraception include temperature and cervical mucus tracking and the use of barrier methods.

TEMPERATURE AND CERVICAL MUCUS METHODS

Keeping track of body temperature and cervical mucus can be used primarily to avoid pregnancy by abstaining from intercourse on days when a woman is fertile. Tracking basal body temperature is used to predict ovulation. The temperature needs to be taken first thing each morning, prior to any other activity. The typical temperature prior to ovulation is 96 – 98°F and increases to 97 – 99°F during ovulation. The changes are recorded on a calendar and used to predict ovulation (i.e., fertility) in the following months. There is an FDA-approved app, *Natural Cycles*, which can aid in tracking and predicting ovulation.

Because a small (~1°) increase can be missed, temperature methods work best when done in conjunction with tracking changes in the cervical mucus (i.e., vaginal discharge), which has slight changes in color, texture and volume during ovulation.

BARRIER METHODS

Barrier methods of contraception include condoms, diaphragms and caps. These are non-pharmacologic options that form a physical barrier preventing passage of sperm to the egg.

Diaphragms and Caps

These options are soft latex or silicone barriers that cover the cervix and prevent sperm passage. They should be used with spermicide. Many diaphragms and caps require a prescription for fitting; the *Caya* diaphragm is available as a single size and does not require fitting.

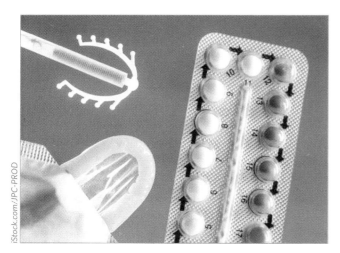

iStock.com/JPC-PROD

Condoms

Male condoms are a thin latex or plastic sheath worn on the penis. Female condoms are inserted into the vagina. Both are available OTC. Condoms help protect against many STIs [only if they are latex or polyurethane (plastic), not "natural" sheepskin].

- Use with nonoxynol-9 spermicide can cause irritation and increase risk of HIV transmission.

- Lubricant makes condoms less likely to break by reducing dry friction. Never recommend oil-based lubricant for use with a latex or non-latex synthetic condom; only recommend water or silicone-based lubricants. These products are discussed in the Osteoporosis, Menopause and Testosterone Use chapter.

OTHER CONTRACEPTIVE METHODS

Other OTC contraceptive methods include foams, films, creams, suppositories, sponges and jellies. These contain the spermicide nonoxynol-9. Do not use spermicide with anal sex. It is irritating and can increase the risk of STIs. The sponge is a round piece of plastic foam that is inserted prior to intercourse. It covers the cervix, continuously releases spermicide and is removed and discarded after use.

A prescription-only option is *Phexxi*, a vaginal gel that maintains an acidic pH (range 3.5 – 4.5), which is inhospitable to sperm and reduces their mobility. It should not be used with vaginal rings or in those with a history of recurrent UTIs or urinary tract abnormalities.

HORMONAL CONTRACEPTIVES

Hormonal contraceptives work by inhibiting the production of FSH and LH, which prevents ovulation. They also alter cervical mucus, which inhibits the sperm from penetrating the egg. If implantation of the fertilized egg in the uterus has already taken place, none of these methods are effective, and the pregnancy will proceed normally.

Available treatments include progestin-only options (pill, injectable, implant and IUD) or estrogen/progestin combinations (pill, patch and vaginal ring). All contraceptives containing both estrogen and progestin are referred to as combined hormonal contraceptives (CHC). This includes combination oral contraceptives (COCs), as well as non-oral contraceptives (e.g., patch, ring). The patch and the ring have unique considerations (such as instructions for use) but contain hormones similar to pill formulations. Contraindications are the same for all CHCs.

Hormonal contraceptives provide health benefits, including a decrease in menstrual pain, menstrual irregularity, endometriosis pain, acne, and decreased risk of ectopic pregnancy, noncancerous breast cysts/lumps and endometrial/ovarian cancer.

The FDA requires that the Patient Package Insert (PPI) be dispensed with oral contraceptives – it will be in the product packaging. The PPI has important safety information, instructions on proper use and what to do if pills are missed.

ESTROGEN AND PROGESTIN COMBINATION ORAL CONTRACEPTIVES

Most COCs contain the estrogen ethinyl estradiol (EE) and a progestin [e.g., norethindrone, levonorgestrel (LNG), drospirenone]. There are different formulations of COCs.

- Monophasic COCs have the same dose of estrogen and progestin throughout the pill pack.

- Biphasic, triphasic and quadriphasic pill packs mimic the estrogen and progesterone levels during a menstrual cycle. The type of formulation (e.g., triphasic) refers to the number of times the amount of the hormones change (e.g., three times). The name of the pill can reflect the type (e.g., *Tri-Sprintec* is triphasic, with three different hormone "cycles").

Drospirenone is a unique progestin that is used in some COCs to reduce adverse effects commonly seen with oral contraceptives. It is a mild potassium-sparing diuretic due to its antimineralocorticoid activity, which decreases bloating, premenstrual syndrome (PMS) symptoms and weight gain; drospirenone-containing products are also associated with less acne, as they have anti-androgenic activity. Other progestins with low androgenic activity include norgestimate, desogestrel and dienogest.

Treatment of Other Indications

COCs are used for other indications besides pregnancy prevention, including dysmenorrhea (menstrual cramps), PMS, acne (in females), anemia (by reducing blood loss), peri-menopausal symptoms (hot flashes, night sweats) and menstrual migraine prophylaxis. The use of COCs to regulate menses is first-line treatment for polycystic ovary syndrome (PCOS), a condition where infrequent, irregular or prolonged menstrual periods are common. Some women with PCOS will experience infertility, hirsutism, acne, weight gain and insulin resistance.

COCs are used as first-line treatment for endometriosis (10% of women) in which endometrial tissue grows outside of the uterus. COCs reduce the symptoms of dysmenorrhea and heavy bleeding. Elagolix (*Orilissa*), a gonadotropin-releasing hormone antagonist which suppresses LH and FSH, is FDA-approved for moderate to severe pain associated with endometriosis.

Natazia (a COC) and *Mirena* (a levonorgestrel-releasing IUD) are indicated for heavy menstrual bleeding (menorrhagia). *Oriahnn*, which contains estradiol, norethindrone and elagolix, is indicated for heavy menstrual bleeding associated with uterine fibroids, but is not a contraceptive (not intended to prevent pregnancy). The oral formulation of tranexamic acid (antifibrinolytic) is a nonhormonal treatment for menorrhagia.

PROGESTIN-ONLY PILLS

Progestin-only pills (POPs, mini-pills) contain no estrogen and have 28 days of active pills in each pack. POPs prevent pregnancy by suppressing ovulation, thickening the cervical mucus to inhibit sperm penetration and thinning the endometrium. POPs are primarily used in women who are lactating (breastfeeding), because estrogen decreases milk production. They can be started soon after delivery (3 – 6 weeks postpartum). It is not safe to use estrogen this soon after delivery because of an increased risk of thrombosis. POPs can also be useful for women with a contraindication or intolerance to estrogen. POPs require good adherence; the pill must be taken daily within three hours of the scheduled time. POPs are sometimes used for migraine prophylaxis and are safe in women who have migraines with aura; estrogen cannot be used with this type of migraine due to the risk of stroke.

NON-ORAL HORMONAL CONTRACEPTIVES

Contraceptive Patches

Patches have the same side effects, contraindications and drug interactions as COCs, but patches cause a higher systemic estrogen exposure. This leads to an even higher risk of thromboembolism, making it critical to avoid their use in anyone with a high clotting risk (e.g., patients > 35 years old who smoke, patients with cerebrovascular disease or past blood clots, postpartum patients). They should also be avoided in women with a BMI ≥ 30 kg/m^2 [due to an increased risk

of thromboembolism (*Xulane, Zafemy*) or decreased efficacy (*Twirla*)]. *Xulane* and *Zafemy* may also be less effective in women who weigh ≥ 198 pounds (90 kg).

Vaginal Contraceptive Rings

The vaginal rings have the same side effects, contraindications and drug interactions as COCs, as they contain estrogen and progestin. These are small, flexible rings that are inserted into the vagina once a month. The exact position of the ring in the vagina does not matter.

Injectable Contraception

The injection (*Depo-Provera, Depo-subQ Provera 104*) is depot medroxyprogesterone acetate (DMPA), a progestin. It suppresses ovulation, thickens cervical mucus and causes thinning of the endometrium. DMPA is given by IM (150 mg) or SC (104 mg) injection every 3 months.

Intrauterine Devices (IUDs)

IUDs are long-acting, reversible forms of contraception. Some IUDs contain levonorgestrel, a progestin, to enhance their effects; others are hormone free. IUDs are discussed in more detail later in the chapter, in the Long-Acting Reversible Contraceptives section.

CONTRACEPTION AND MENSTRUAL PERIODS

Most COC formulations involve 28 days (4 weeks) of pills, with 21 – 24 pills containing active hormone and the remaining pills containing no hormone (many use placebo pills, some contain iron or folate). During week 4 (the inactive pills), bleeding (menses) occurs for 3 – 7 days. Fewer inactive pills results in a shorter hormone-free interval and shorter bleeding time. Women who take COCs often have lighter bleeding because the endometrium remains relatively thin. For the contraceptive patch or vaginal ring, bleeding occurs during the patch-free or ring-free interval (week 4). About half of medroxyprogesterone acetate users will be amenorrheic (no menses) after 1 year of use; likelihood increases with increased duration of use.

Extended-cycle COCs involve 84 days of active hormonal pills followed by 7 days of inactive or very low-dose estrogen pills. With this schedule, bleeding occurs every 3 months rather than every month. By taking continuous contraception, it is possible to suppress menses altogether. This involves taking hormonal pills only (no placebo pills). *Amethyst* is approved for this; other CHCs are used off-label in this way. With continuous use, it can be difficult to tell if a woman becomes pregnant. Spotting (breakthrough bleeding) occurs commonly with continuous contraception, which can lead to discontinuation. It is important to counsel patients that this typically resolves after 3 – 6 months. There are benefits to continuous use, such as less anemia and menstrual migraines.

SELECT CONTRACEPTIVE TYPES

This is not a comprehensive list. For exam purposes, consider patient-specific factors that help in selecting a medication and understand the counseling points that are unique to each formulation.

PRODUCT TYPE	DESCRIPTION
General tips for contraceptive names:	

- "Lo" indicates ≤ 35 mcg of estrogen; less estrogen causes less estrogenic side effects. Ex: *Loestrin*
- "Fe" indicates an iron supplement is included. Ex: *Microgestin Fe 1/20*
- "24" indicates a shorter placebo time: 24 active + 4 placebo = 28 day cycle. Ex: *Minastrin 24 Fe*
- "Pro" indicates a progestin in the product. Ex: *Depo-Provera*

Combination Oral Contraceptive (COC) Pills

PRODUCT TYPE	DESCRIPTION
Monophasic Formulations	Provides the same dose of progestin and estrogen throughout the active pill days. Example: *Junel 1/20* contains 1 mg norethindrone and 20 mcg EE
Junel Fe 1/20, Microgestin Fe 1/20, Sprintec 28, Loestrin 1/20, Yasmin 28, *Apri, Aviane, Cryselle-28, Levora-28, Nortrel 1/35, Ocella, Portia-28, Zovia 1/35*	21/7 pill pack contains 21 active hormonal pills, 7 inactive pills
Yaz, *Loestrin 24 Fe*,* **Beyaz,** *Minastrin 24 Fe,* **Nikki**	24/4 pill pack contains 24 active hormonal pills, 4 inactive pills
Lo Loestrin Fe	24/2/2 pill pack contains 24 active combined hormonal pills, 2 pills of just EE, and 2 inactive pills (with iron); very low dose estrogen used (EE 10 mcg)
Biphasic, Triphasic Formulations	"Phasic" in the name refers to the differing hormone dose being delivered in phases. The beginning of the name indicates the number of phases throughout the cycle (e.g., biphasic has two phases)
Tri-Sprintec, *Ortho Tri-Cyclen Lo*, Nortrel 7/7/7, Trivora-28, Velivet*	3 different weeks (7/7/7) or "tri" indicates a triphasic formulation
Quadriphasic Formulations *Natazia*	Hormone doses change over 26 days (four phases of estradiol valerate and dienogest) followed by 2 placebo pills to mimic menstrual cycle and minimize menstrual bleeding
Extended Cycle Formulations	Period occurs every 3 months
Jolessa	84 days of EE + LNG followed by 7 days of placebo
Seasonique, *Camrese, Camrese Lo, Amethia*	84 days of EE + LNG followed by 7 days of low dose EE
Continuous Formulations	No inactive pills (taken continuously); no period occurs
Amethyst	28 days of EE + LNG with no placebo pills
Drospirenone Containing Formulations	Mild potassium-sparing diuretic effect to reduce bloating and other effects
Yasmin 28, Yaz, *Loryna, Ocella, Nextstellis, Nikki, Safyral, Syeda, Beyaz (Safyral & Beyaz contain folate)*	Contraindicated in renal or liver disease Monitor potassium, kidney function during use

Patches (contain estrogen and progestin)

Transdermal patch	Higher estrogen exposure than pills
Xulane, *Zafemy, Twirla*	Weeks 1-3: apply once weekly; week 4: off

Rings (contain estrogen and progestin)

Vaginal ring	Lower estrogen exposure than pills
NuvaRing, *EluRyng, Haloette, Annovera*	Insert monthly: leave in x 3 weeks; remove x 1 week
	Annovera: reusable vaginal ring; wash and store when it is removed, then reinsert; used for 1 year

Progestin-Only Pills (Mini-Pill/POP)

Errin, Camila, Nora-BE, *Incassia*	*Errin, Camila, Nora-BE* contain a fixed dose of <u>norethindrone</u>; take active tablet daily (no placebo days)
Slynd	*Slynd* is drospirenone-only
Opill	*Opill* is approved for use <u>without a prescription</u>

Injection (contains progestin only)

Depo-Provera	Contains depot medroxyprogesterone (DMPA); injected every 3 months (150 mg IM or 104 mg SC)

*Brand discontinued but name still used in practice.

ADVERSE EFFECTS OF HORMONAL CONTRACEPTIVES

Estrogen
Side effects of estrogen can include:

- Nausea

- Breast tenderness/fullness, bloating, weight gain and increased blood pressure (which can all be partially due to fluid retention)

- Melasma (dark skin patches, most often on the face)

Reducing the estrogen dose reduces the side effects, but a dose that is too low will cause breakthrough bleeding (spotting), especially during the early to mid-part of the cycle.

Serious adverse effects are rare, but can include thrombosis, including heart attack, stroke, deep vein thrombosis (DVT) or pulmonary embolism (PE); see Study Tip Gal. The risk for clots increases as the woman ages, if she smokes, if she has diabetes or hypertension, if she requires prolonged bed rest and if she is overweight. The higher the estrogen dose or exposure (e.g., with a transdermal patch), the higher the clotting risk. When evaluating thrombotic risk from use of CHCs, also consider risks of an unintended pregnancy if CHCs are not used; the thrombotic risk during pregnancy and postpartum is higher than that of CHCs.

SEVERE & RARE ADVERSE EFFECTS OF ESTROGEN

The dose of estrogen in birth control pills used to be much higher – with a higher risk of clotting. Current formulations have lower estrogen doses and lower risk of clotting. To be safe, patients should be able to recognize symptoms of a DVT, PE and less common clots.

Remember: **ACHES**

Abdominal pain that is severe
- ❏ Can indicate a mesenteric or pelvic vein thrombosis.

Chest pain
- ❏ Sharp, crushing, or heavy pain can indicate a heart attack. Shortness of breath with chest pain can indicate a PE (a blood clot in the lungs).

Headaches
- ❏ Sudden and severe with vomiting or weakness/numbness on one side of the body can indicate a stroke.

Eye problems
- ❏ Blurry vision, flashing lights or partial/complete vision loss can indicate a blood clot in the eye.

Swelling or sudden leg pain
- ❏ Can indicate a DVT (a blood clot in the leg).

Progestin
Progestin can cause breast tenderness, headache, fatigue and depression.

Drospirenone has a slightly higher risk of clotting, and should not be used in women with clotting risk. It can also ↑ potassium levels; do not use with kidney, liver or adrenal gland disease (as these can ↑ potassium levels) or in those with ↑ potassium levels at baseline.

The injectable depot medroxyprogesterone acetate can cause a loss in bone mineral density. This can be especially important for teens and young women who are still accumulating bone mass. Minimally, women should be taking adequate calcium and vitamin D (see recommendations in the Osteoporosis, Menopause & Testosterone Use chapter).

Breakthrough Bleeding
Breakthrough bleeding (i.e., spotting) usually resolves within 2 – 3 months. Continuous contraception has more breakthrough bleeding, especially during the first few months.

Always check adherence; spotting can be due to a fast drop in estrogen from missing a pill.

If spotting persists:

- And currently taking < 30 mcg estrogen daily: increase estrogen dose.

- And currently taking ≥ 30 mcg estrogen daily: try a different progestin.

RISKS OF HORMONAL CONTRACEPTIVES

BOXED WARNINGS

All CHC products (pills, ring, patch)
- Do not use in women ≥ 35 years old who smoke due to risk of serious cardiovascular events

Estrogen + progestin transdermal patch
- Do not use in women with a BMI ≥ 30 kg/m² [due to increased risk of thromboembolism *(Xulane, Zafemy)* or decreased efficacy *(Twirla)*]

Depo-Provera
- Loss of bone mineral density with long-term use

DO NOT USE ESTROGEN WITH THESE CONDITIONS
History of DVT/PE, stroke, CAD, thrombosis of heart valves or acquired hypercoagulopathies

History of breast, ovarian, liver or endometrial cancer; liver disease; uncontrolled hypertension (e.g., > 160/100 mmHg); severe headaches or migraines with aura (especially if > 35 years of age); diabetes with vascular disease; unexplained uterine bleeding; others (vary by formulation)

CONSIDERATIONS FOR DRUG SELECTION

TYPE OF PATIENT	PRODUCT SELECTION CONSIDERATIONS
Acne or hirsutism	Use COC with a progestin that has lower androgenic activity [e.g., norgestimate (Sprintec 28)] or no androgenic activity [e.g., drospirenone (Yaz, Yasmin)].
Breastfeeding	Choose progestin-only (e.g., POPs) or nonhormonal method. See Postpartum below.
Estrogen contraindication (including clotting risk)	Choose progestin-only (e.g., POPs) or nonhormonal method.
Migraine	If with aura, choose progestin-only or nonhormonal method; do not use estrogen. If no aura, choose any method.
Fluid retention/bloating	Choose a product containing drospirenone.
Heavy menstrual bleeding (menorrhagia)	Natazia (a COC) and Mirena (a levonorgestrel-releasing IUD) are indicated for this condition. COCs with only 4 placebo pills (rather than 7) or continuous/extended regimens will minimize bleeding time.
Hypertension	If BP uncontrolled, some estrogen formulations are contraindicated. Choose progestin-only or nonhormonal method.
Mood changes/disorder	Use monophasic COC – extended cycle or continuous with drospirenone is preferred.
Nausea	Take at night, with food; consider decreasing estrogen dose or switching to a progestin-only method (e.g., POPs), vaginal ring or nonhormonal method (ideally after a 3 month trial).
Overweight	Choose any method. Counsel patient about the possibility of reduced effectiveness with the contraceptive patch [and do not use the patch in obesity (BMI ≥ 30 kg/m^2)]. Do not use DMPA if trying to avoid weight gain.
Postpartum	Do not use CHCs for 3 weeks, or for 6 weeks if patient has additional risk factors for VTE. Can use progestin-only (e.g., POPs) or nonhormonal method during this time.
Premenstrual dysphoric disorder	Choose a product containing drospirenone (e.g. Yaz). An SSRI antidepressant may be needed; see Depression chapter.
Spotting/"breakthrough bleeding"	Common when initiating extended cycles or continuous regimens; usually resolves within 3-6 months. When starting conventional formulations, wait 3 cycles before switching. If early or mid-cycle spotting occurs, the estrogen dose may need to be increased. If later in the cycle, the progestin dose may need to be increased.
Wishes to avoid monthly cycle/menses	Use extended (91-day) or continuous formulations. Alternative: monophasic 28-day formulation & skip placebo pills.

DRUG INTERACTIONS WITH HORMONAL CONTRACEPTIVES

Efficacy of contraception may be ↓ by other drugs so the package insert of new medications should always be checked for potential interactions. A back-up contraception method, such as condoms/spermicide, may be required; an IUD or injectable may also be considered. The injectable contraceptive bypasses first-pass metabolism and achieves higher serum concentrations, which ↓ drug interactions. If in doubt, it is safest to use a back-up method.

Drug Interactions that Decrease Hormonal Contraception Efficacy

- Some antibiotics (e.g., rifampin, rifabutin, rifapentine; these are all strong CYP450 inducers) and antifungals (e.g., griseofulvin).

  ❑ With rifampin, the induction can be prolonged; a back-up contraception method is needed for 6 weeks after rifampin has been discontinued.

- Anticonvulsants (carbamazepine, oxcarbazepine, phenytoin, primidone, topiramate, barbiturates and perampanel).

- St. John's wort.

- Smoking tobacco.

- Ritonavir-boosted protease inhibitors, bosentan (Tracleer), mycophenolate (CellCept, Myfortic).

- Colesevelam: separate by at least 4 hours.

- Mounjaro (for COCs): use back-up contraception (non-oral or barrier) for 4 weeks after initiation and dose increases.

Risks with Hepatitis C Treatment

- Mavyret use is not recommended with any formulation containing > 20 mcg of ethinyl estradiol due to the risk of liver toxicity.

- With all new hepatitis C drugs being dispensed to a patient using contraception, the package insert should be checked to avoid missing an interaction that could cause toxicity.

Drospirenone Drug Interactions

- Risk of ↑ potassium; caution must be used with other drugs that ↑ potassium, including aldosterone antagonists, potassium supplements, salt substitutes (KCl), ACE inhibitors, angiotensin receptor blockers, heparin, canagliflozin and calcineurin inhibitors (see hyperkalemia discussion in Renal Disease chapter).

STARTING BIRTH CONTROL PILLS

Combination Oral Contraception

In general, it takes 7 days of hormonal pills to achieve contraceptive efficacy. Therefore, back-up (nonhormonal) contraception is required for 7 days, unless the COC is started within 5 days after the start of a period.

- Start today (also called "quick start"). Best practice recommendation. Maximizes time protected from unintended pregnancy.
- Sunday start. Starts the Sunday after onset of menstruation. This is commonly used if the patient prefers that menstruation occur during the week and is complete before the following weekend. It can lead to missed doses if the patient inadvertently runs out of refills over the weekend.
- First day start. Starts on the first day of menses. Because the COC is started within 5 days after the start of the period, no back-up method of birth control is needed; protection is immediate.

Progestin-Only Pills

- Start at any time. Use another method of birth control for the first 48 hours of progestin-pill use (unless within 5 days of the start of menses); protection begins after two days. All come in 28-day packs and all pills are active.

LATE OR MISSED PILLS – INSTRUCTIONS FOR TYPICAL FORMULATIONS

Missed pills are a common cause of contraceptive failure, particularly if the hormone-free interval is extended. These are the standard instructions from the CDC; when answering questions in practice, check the package insert for the individual product. For the exam, you should know the general approach to missed doses:

- Start as soon as remembered.
- If more than one COC pill is missed, back-up contraception is required for 7 days.
- If missed pills/days are in the third week of the cycle, omit the hormone-free week and start the next package of pills right away without skipping any days; back-up contraception should be used for 7 days.

Missed Doses for Standard Cycle (28 days)

		WEEK 1	WEEK 2	WEEK 3	WEEK 4
COCs	**1 late or missed pill** (< 48 hours since last dose)	Take missed pill as soon as possible and take next dose on schedule (even if that makes 2 pills in 1 day).			
		Back-up contraception required? No			
		EC*: Not usually needed. Consider if missed doses earlier in the same cycle or in week 3 of the previous cycle.			
	2 missed pills (≥ 48 hours since last dose)	Take the most recent missed pill as soon as possible (discard any other missed pills). Take next dose on schedule (even if that makes 2 pills in 1 day).			
				Omit hormone-free week: start next pack of pills right after finishing current pack.**	
		Back-up contraception required? Yes, x 7 days			
		EC*: Consider if unprotected sex in last 5 days.	EC*: Can be considered.		
POPs	**If > 3 hours past scheduled time**	Take pill as soon as possible and take next dose on schedule.			
		Back-up contraception required? Yes, x 48 hours			
		EC*: Consider if unprotected sex in last 5 days.			

*EC = emergency contraception (with the exception of ulipristal acetate)
**If unable to start a new pack right away, use back-up contraception until 7 days of hormonal pills have been taken

LONG-ACTING REVERSIBLE CONTRACEPTIVES

These devices are generally not dispensed from community pharmacies. They must be placed and removed by trained healthcare professionals. They are the most effective forms of reversible contraception, and are as effective as sterilization.

- Intrauterine devices *(Mirena, Skyla, Kyleena, Liletta)* are hormonal IUDs that contain the progestin levonorgestrel. These cause lighter menstrual bleeding and minor or no cramping. *Mirena* and *Liletta* are FDA-approved for heavy menstrual bleeding. After insertion, the IUD can be left in place for several years (i.e., 3 – 8 years) before it needs to be replaced; the specific timing is product-dependent. About half of women will become amenorrheic after 2 years of use.

- The copper-T IUD *(Paragard)* can be used for emergency contraception (EC) and/or regular birth control. It can be used for up to 10 years, but causes heavier menstrual bleeding and cramping. Some women prefer this nonhormonal method.

- The implant *(Nexplanon)* is a plastic rod placed subdermally in the arm. It releases the progestin etonogestrel for three years.

CASE SCENARIO

KL is a 37-year-old female (G2 P2)* with antiphospholipid syndrome, diagnosed 2 years ago after a second DVT. She takes aspirin daily. Her last pregnancy was difficult. She requests contraception that is highly effective.

KL is 5 feet, 4 inches; 145 pounds; BP 111/77 mmHg

- Assess her medical history:
  - ❑ Estrogen is contraindicated with antiphospholipid syndrome or any clotting condition. She cannot use COCs, a vaginal ring or transdermal patch.
  - ❑ She could use POPs (the mini-pill), but the risk of unplanned pregnancy is high with missed or even late pills.
  - ❑ Another hormonal option is the *Depo-Provera* injection. Her bone health should be considered prior to use.
  - ❑ IUD placement or sterilization may be acceptable to KL.

*G2 P2 is an abbreviation for gravida and para. She has been pregnant twice and has had 2 deliveries after 24 weeks gestation.

EMERGENCY CONTRACEPTION (EC)

Emergency contraception (EC) is a form of contraception that prevents pregnancy after unprotected intercourse. Formulations include an IUD (copper IUD) and oral options (levonorgestrel and ulipristal acetate), which are also known as the "morning after pill." The sooner EC is used, the higher the efficacy. The use of higher doses of COCs is no longer a common practice as it is less effective than these options, leads to more nausea/vomiting and has more contraindications.

EMERGENCY CONTRACEPTIVE	EFFECTIVENESS	TIMING	CONSIDERATIONS
Copper IUD *(Paragard)*	Most effective (99.9%)	Within 5 days	Must be placed in the uterus by a healthcare professional Lasts for up to 10 years
Ulipristal acetate *(Ella)*	More effective than levonorgestrel Less effective if > 195 pounds or BMI > 30 kg/m² (consider IUD)	ASAP, within 5 days	Prescription required Must be taken after every episode of unprotected sex
Levonorgestrel *(Plan B One-Step* or a generic)	Less effective if > 165 pounds or BMI > 25 kg/m² (consider *Ella* or IUD)	ASAP, within 3 days*	Available OTC Must be taken after every episode of unprotected sex

*Remains moderately effective within 5 days; use may be considered

EC can be an important resource after unprotected sex, such as from missed pills, a condom breaking, a diaphragm or cap moving out of place during intercourse or if a female has been sexually assaulted. If sexual assault has occurred, empiric STI treatment (chlamydia, gonorrhea, trichomoniasis), HIV post-exposure prophylaxis, HBV and HPV vaccines may be required. Pharmacists should have referrals for other providers available to assist patients.

LEVONORGESTREL

Plan B One-Step and generics are packaged as <u>one 1.5 mg tab of levonorgestrel</u>. This EC formulation reduces the risk of pregnancy by up to 89% if started <u>within 72 hours (3 days)</u> after unprotected intercourse. <u>The sooner it is taken, the higher the efficacy.</u>

Plan B One-Step and generics (*Take Action, Aftera, My Way, React*) are available <u>OTC with no age or other restrictions.</u> These products can be sold in stores without a pharmacy. Per the FDA, these should be placed in the OTC aisles with the other family-planning products, such as condoms and spermicide. There is no reason to use a prescription with the formulations available OTC, except to use insurance coverage.

If the EC is purchased OTC, there is no requirement for purchasers to sign a registry. They can <u>purchase multiple doses</u> and the American College of Obstetrics and Gynecologists (ACOG) recommends an additional dose for future use, if needed, since EC is more effective the sooner it is used.

- Mechanism of action: primarily works by <u>preventing or delaying ovulation</u> and thickens cervical mucus.
- Preferred regimen is 1.5 mg as a single dose (*Plan B One-Step*).
- The primary side effect is <u>nausea</u>, which occurs in 23% of women, and 6% have vomiting. If the woman is easily nauseated, an <u>OTC antiemetic</u> should be recommended to avoid losing the dose. If a patient <u>vomits within two hours</u> of taking the medication, she should consider repeating the dose.

ULIPRISTAL ACETATE *(ELLA)*

Some patients may not wish to use ulipristal because it is a chemical cousin to mifepristone (*Mifeprex*), also known as the "abortion pill" or <u>RU-486</u>. They are not the same drug and are used differently.

- Mechanism of action: <u>prevents or delays ovulation</u> and may alter the endometrium to impair implantation (which may be controversial for some patients).
- Given as a single 30 mg dose. Requires a <u>prescription</u>.
- Indicated for up to <u>five days after unprotected intercourse</u>. More effective than levonorgestrel if 72 – 120 hours since unprotected intercourse or if the woman is overweight.
- Progestin-containing contraceptives should not be used in combination or within 5 days of ulipristal administration due to concern for decreased efficacy of ulipristal.
- Primary side effects are headache, nausea and abdominal pain. Some women have changes in their menstrual cycle, but the menstrual period typically restarts within one week of the expected date. Can only use once per cycle. Use a barrier method of contraception the rest of the cycle as ovulation may occur later than normal.

KEY COUNSELING POINTS

See the Drug Formulations and Patient Counseling chapter for counseling language/layman's terminology.

OTC CONTRACEPTIVE METHODS

Diaphragm

- Wash hands thoroughly. Place one tablespoon of spermicide in the diaphragm and disperse inside and around the rim.
- Pinch the ends of the cup and insert the pinched end into the vagina.
- Leave in for six hours after intercourse. Diaphragms should not be in place greater than 24 hours.
- Reapply spermicide if intercourse is repeated or diaphragm is in place for more than two hours before sex, by inserting jelly with applicator.
- Wash with mild soap and warm water after removal, air dry.
- Can be used for 2 – 5 years, depending on material. Check frequently for holes between uses.

Foams, Creams, Suppositories and Jellies
- Place deep into the vagina 10 – 15 minutes before intercourse where they melt (except for foam, which bubbles).
- Reinsert if more than 1 hour passes before intercourse.

Sponge
- Wet the sponge and squeeze to activate the spermicide.
- Place deep into the vagina right before intercourse.
- Leave in place for at least six hours after intercourse, but it can be used for up to 24 hours. Remove and discard after use.

COMBINATION ORAL CONTRACEPTIVES

- Can increase risk of blood clots.

- Can cause nausea, weight gain and breast tenderness. Side effects often improve after three months of use. Taking the pill with food or at night helps to reduce nausea.

- Take the pill at the same time each day; pick a time of day that you will remember.

- Many drug interactions.

Drospirenone Formulations
- Can increase potassium.

NON-ORAL FORMULATIONS

Contraceptive Patch
- Apply to clean, dry skin of buttocks, stomach, upper arm or upper torso once a week for 21 out of 28 days. Do not apply to breasts.

- Start on either day 1 (no back-up needed) or Sunday (back-up seven days if not day 1).

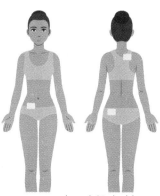

sudowoodo/stock.adobe.com

- If the patch becomes loose or falls off for > 24 hours during the three weeks of use, or if > 7 days have passed during the fourth week where no patch is required, there is a risk of pregnancy. A back-up method should be used for one week after starting a new patch.

NuvaRing Vaginal Contraceptive Ring
- The ring is inserted into the vagina once a month. It is kept in place for three weeks and taken out for one week before replacement with a new ring. The ring is effective for up to four weeks and, though not FDA-approved, can be kept in place to prevent a period. If the ring is kept in place for > 4 weeks: remove the ring, confirm no pregnancy, then insert a new ring and use back-up contraception until the new ring has been in place for seven continuous days.

- The exact position of the ring in the vagina does not matter.

- Starting therapy and no hormonal contraceptive use in preceding cycle: insert the ring the first day of menstrual bleeding. If inserted on days 2 – 5 of cycle, back-up contraception should be used for the first seven days in the first cycle.

- If the ring is expelled or removed:
  - ❏ Weeks 1 and 2: if ring is out > 3 hours, rinse with cool to lukewarm water and reinsert. Use back-up contraception for seven days while the ring is in place, consider EC if intercourse within last five days.
  - ❏ Week 3: discard and insert a new ring. Use back-up contraception for seven days while the ring is in place.

- Store for up to four months at room temperature (refrigerate prior to dispensing).

Injectable Contraception (Medroxyprogesterone)
- Can decrease bone density. Take the recommended daily intake of calcium and vitamin D.

- You might experience a change in your normal menstrual cycle.

EMERGENCY CONTRACEPTION

- Can cause nausea/vomiting. OTC antiemetics can help. If you vomit after taking the dose, contact your healthcare provider (may need to take another dose).

- If you do not get your period in three weeks (or it is more than a week late), a pregnancy test should be taken. Severe abdominal pain or irregular bleeding requires immediate medical attention.

- Visit your healthcare provider for a regular birth control method and information about preventing STIs. If you may have contracted an infection, you should get care right away.

- You may wish to get a package of EC for future use, if needed.

- Regular hormonal contraceptives (COCs, injection, ring, patch) should be started on the same or the following day as taking the EC (with the exception of ulipristal; hormonal contraception should be started after 5 days with this).

- You should only use one type of oral EC pill. Do not use two different types together.

INFERTILITY

Infertility is defined as not being able to get pregnant (conceive) after <u>one year</u> or longer of unprotected sex. Infertility can be due to either the male or female. This section covers drugs used in females.

The treatment choice for females depends on the cause of the infertility (e.g., absent ovulation). <u>Clomiphene</u>, a <u>selective estrogen receptor modulator</u> (SERM), and letrozole, an aromatase inhibitor, are oral tablets used to induce ovulation. Drugs that are SERMs act as estrogen <u>agonists</u> in some tissues and estrogen <u>antagonists</u> in other tissues. Clomiphene, like estrogen, causes LH and FSH to surge, which triggers ovulation. The surge in LH commonly causes <u>hot flashes</u>. SERMs have <u>clotting risks</u>. Letrozole impacts ovulation primarily through estrogen negative feedback (estrogen production is suppressed resulting in an initial FSH surge that leads to follicle development and ovulation).

<u>Gonadotropins</u> trigger ovulation by acting similar to the endogenous (naturally produced) gonadotropins <u>FSH</u> or <u>LH</u>. Gonadotropins are used after a poor response to clomiphene or letrozole, or to spur egg release for procedures such as intrauterine insemination and *in vitro* fertilization.

Alternatively, exogenous hCG or gonadotropin releasing hormone agonists (GnRHA), such as leuprolide (*Lupron*), can be used to trigger ovulation. The hCG hormone is important in pregnancy <u>and</u> in ovulation, where it binds to the LH receptor with a similar effect. Leuprolide and other GnRHAs are more commonly used to decrease hormone levels in breast or prostate cancer treatment.

Fertility medications, including <u>gonadotropins</u> and <u>clomiphene</u>, can cause multiple eggs to be released, which causes a <u>risk</u> of <u>multiple births</u> (see Study Tip Gal). Gonadotropins, similar to the majority of drugs that are hormones, cannot be taken orally. They are administered by <u>SC</u> or <u>IM injection</u>. This is one of the rare times a patient (or their partner) could be injecting IM, which is more painful than SC administration.

INFERTILITY DRUGS ACT LIKE ENDOGENOUS HORMONES TO TRIGGER OVULATION

↑ LH/FSH → ovulation (release of eggs)

- Clomiphene acts as estrogen to ↑ LH/FSH
- Aromatase inhibitors suppress estrogen to ↑ FSH → cause ovulation
- Gonadotropin drugs act as LH, FSH or hCG (similar to LH)

GOOD: Infertility drugs trigger ovulation (egg release)

GOOD? They can trigger the release of multiple eggs and ↑ risk of multiple births

---

GONADOTROPIN DRUG NAMES

<u>Generic</u> names include chorionic gonadotropin-recombinant, follicle stimulating hormone-recombinant, human chorionic gonadotropin-recombinant and menotropin, which contains LH and FSH extracted from the urine of menopausal females.

<u>Brand</u> names can include parts of the words <u>reproduce</u>, men(strual), <u>follicle</u>, <u>gonadotropin</u>, <u>pregnancy</u> and <u>ovary</u>, including *Menopur, Follistim AQ, Gonal-f, Pregnyl, Novarel* and *Ovidrel*.

Select Guidelines/References
US Selected Practice Recommendations (US SPR) for Contraceptive Use, 2016 https://www.cdc.gov/reproductivehealth/contraception/mmwr/spr/combined.html (accessed 2024 Jan 11).

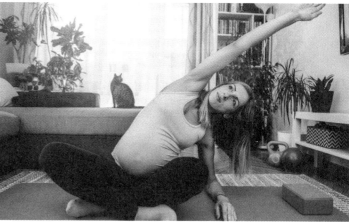

iStock.com/microgen

CHAPTER 48

DRUG USE IN PREGNANCY & LACTATION

PREGNANCY

BACKGROUND

Pregnancy typically lasts 37 – 40 weeks and is divided into three trimesters. High levels of human chorionic gonadotropin (hCG) in the urine or blood confirms pregnancy. The first trimester (0 – 12 weeks) is when most organ development occurs, making the embryo most susceptible to birth defects caused by teratogens during this time (though they can also occur later). For a drug to be teratogenic, the drug has to cross the placenta into the fetal circulation. Teratogenic drugs should be discontinued prior to pregnancy, if possible.

Pharmacokinetic changes during pregnancy can require dose and regimen changes. For example, in women being treated for hypothyroidism, an increased dose of levothyroxine will be required in order to keep thyroid hormones within normal ranges. The American College of Obstetricians and Gynecologists (ACOG) is an organization that publishes guidelines for safe and effective drug use in conditions impacting women, including pregnancy.

A patient's obstetric history can be described using gravida and para. Gravida (G) is the number of times the person has been pregnant. Para (P) is the number of times a patient has given birth. For example, a patient that is gravida 2, para 1 (or G2, P1 for short), has been pregnant twice and given birth once.

LIFESTYLE MANAGEMENT

Lifestyle modifications should always be considered first when treating pregnant patients. This includes encouragement to stop using recreational drugs, alcohol and tobacco, each of which is teratogenic. Behavioral intervention is a safe and sometimes effective strategy for prenatal smoking cessation. See the Tobacco Cessation chapter for more information.

Vitamin and Mineral Supplementation

Folate deficiency can cause birth defects of the brain and spinal cord (neural tube defects). Folate (folic acid, vitamin B9) is found in many healthy foods, including fortified flour and cereals, dried beans, green leafy vegetables and orange juice.

Adults should consume 400 mcg of dietary folate equivalents (DFE) per day. During pregnancy, folate requirements increase to 600 mcg DFE/day. Females of childbearing potential should increase their folic acid consumption from a combination of dietary supplements, fortified foods and their diet.

The baby's skeleton requires adequate calcium and vitamin D. If deficient in calcium, the mother's bone health will be sacrificed to provide for the baby. Pregnant women from 19 – 50 years old require 1,000 mg/day of calcium and 15 mcg/day (600 IU/day) of vitamin D. Iron is also vital to ensure adequate oxygenation for fetal development; 27 mg/day of iron is recommended for pregnancy.

Prenatal vitamins are available by prescription and OTC. Most contain 800 – 1,000 mcg DFE, 15 – 25 mcg (600 – 1,000 IU) vitamin D, 100 – 200 mg calcium and 27 mg iron, though composition varies. Calcium is bulky and the prenatal vitamin would be too large if it contained more calcium. If the woman's dietary intake is insufficient, a separate calcium supplement may be needed.

CHANGES TO FDA PREGNANCY CATEGORIES

The old pregnancy categories were viewed as confusing and overly simplistic. Categories were difficult to interpret, leading physicians to unintentionally apply the provided information incorrectly. The updated labeling is intended to provide patients and clinicians with more detailed benefit/risk data on prescription drugs in order to make informed decisions. See the previous categories and new pregnancy package insert requirements in the tables to the right.

The deadline for the transition to the new pregnancy and lactation labeling format was June 2020. Drugs approved before 2001 are exempt from adopting the new labeling requirements but are required to remove the old categories. The manufacturers of these older drugs are not required to replace the old categories with new information.

Despite the updated labeling, prescribers will likely continue to use the previous terminology in practice. For this reason, it is important to remain familiar with the traditional categories. Drugs with known risk from the old categories should be considered to have the same risk unless noted otherwise. If a drug was Pregnancy Category X, it is contraindicated in pregnancy, which means it cannot be used in pregnancy for any reason.

Previous Pregnancy Categories & Interpretation

A	Controlled studies in animals & women show no risk in the first trimester. Risk of fetal harm is remote.
B	Animal studies have not demonstrated a fetal risk, but no well-controlled studies are available in pregnant women.
C	Animal studies have shown harm to the fetus, but there are no well-controlled studies in pregnant women. Use only if potential benefit outweighs the risk.
D	Positive evidence of risk to the human fetus is available, but the benefits may outweigh the risk with life-threatening or serious diseases.
X	Studies in animals or humans show fetal abnormalities. The risks involved clearly outweigh potential benefits; use in pregnancy is contraindicated.

Updated Pregnancy Sections in Package Inserts

8.1 Pregnancy	A pregnancy risk summary is required for all medications that includes the risk of adverse developmental outcomes based on human and animal data and the drug's pharmacology. Includes any dose adjustments, maternal/fetal adverse reactions and disease risks.
	Includes pregnancy exposure registry information. Pregnant women should be encouraged to participate in registries, which exist for select disease states and drugs. The registries collect health information from women who take prescription drugs and vaccines when pregnant and breastfeeding. Information is also collected on the newborn baby.
8.2 Lactation	Includes whether the drug/metabolites are present in human milk, the effects on the breastfed infant, and the effects on milk production. If applicable, ways to minimize exposure and monitor for adverse reactions are included.
8.3 Females & Males of Reproductive Potential	Includes any effects on fertility and requirements for pregnancy testing and contraception.

DRUG TREATMENT

If possible, use lifestyle measures to treat medical conditions in pregnant women. When this is impossible or ineffective, choose drugs carefully.

Common Teratogens

Teratogenic drugs should be discontinued prior to pregnancy, if possible, but many pregnancies are not planned. Once pregnancy is confirmed, medical providers should switch patients from teratogenic drugs to safer options.

Throughout the UWorld RxPrep course book, medications with boxed warnings and contraindications associated with teratogenicity are noted in the drug tables. A summary of many commonly used drugs with teratogenic risk is shown in the Key Drugs Guy to the right and should be known for the exam. Some are well-documented teratogens, and use in a pregnant patient is rarely, if ever, appropriate. Drugs with significant teratogenic risk may have REMS requirements due to potential harm to the fetus (see the Drug Allergies & Adverse Drug Reactions chapter).

Teratogens are hazardous drugs according to the National Institute for Occupational Safety and Health (NIOSH) and require special handling to avoid risk to healthcare workers; see the Compounding with Hazardous Drugs chapter.

Use of some medications in pregnant patients is debatable, and many medications have limited data regarding safety in pregnancy. With any medication, the drug's potential harm must be weighed against the risk of the condition not being adequately treated. For example, the use of lamotrigine in pregnancy carries a risk of congenital malformations, but seizures cause damage to both the mother and child. In some cases, a switch to a safer drug is possible, while in other situations the risk of switching is high. A pregnant woman may need to remain on lamotrigine if she has a history of poor seizure control before being placed on the drug.

Always check reputable, up-to-date resources when prescribing/dispensing to pregnant women. *Briggs' Drugs in Pregnancy and Lactation* and other resources are reviewed in the Drug References chapter.

Immunizations

There are several immunizations that are routinely recommended for pregnant patients. The inactivated influenza vaccine (not live) is recommended during any trimester at the beginning of flu season. A single dose of Tdap should be administered during each pregnancy, ideally between weeks 27 and 36. All pregnant individuals are recommended to be vaccinated against COVID-19 during any trimester. The RSV vaccine *(Abrysvo)* is also recommended if the patient will be between weeks 32 and 36 during

TERATOGENS: DANGER IN PREGNANCY

KEY DRUGS

Acne
Isotretinoin, topical retinoids

Antibiotics*
Quinolones, tetracyclines

Anticoagulants
Warfarin**

Dyslipidemia, Heart Failure and Hypertension
Statins, RAAS inhibitors (ACE inhibitors, ARBs, aliskiren, sacubitril/valsartan)

Hormones
Most, including estradiol, progesterone (including megestrol), raloxifene, *Duavee*, testosterone, contraceptives

Migraine
Dihydroergotamine, ergotamine

Other important teratogens

Hydroxyurea	Ribavirin
Lithium	Thalidomide
Methotrexate	Topiramate
Misoprostol	Weight loss drugs
NSAIDs	
Paroxetine	Valproic Acid/ Divalproex

Others:
Amiodarone
Dronedarone
Aminoglycosides
Atenolol
Benzodiazepines
Dutasteride
Finasteride
Fluconazole
Voriconazole
Griseofulvin
ERAs (e.g., bosentan)
Leflunomide
Lenalidomide
Lomitapide
Methimazole
Propylthiouracil
Mycophenolate
Radioactive iodine
Carbamazepine
Phenobarbital
Phenytoin

*See Infectious Diseases I chapter for information on metronidazole, nitrofurantoin, sulfamethoxazole/ trimethoprim and telavancin.
**See Anticoagulation chapter for details.*

September to January. All live vaccines are contraindicated in pregnant patients. See the Immunizations chapter for more information on vaccination in pregnancy.

Preeclampsia

Preeclampsia is a complication of pregnancy that presents with elevated blood pressure and evidence of organ damage (e.g., proteinuria), most often to the kidneys or liver. It typically occurs after 20 weeks gestation and can occur in women with previously normal blood pressure. If not treated, preeclampsia can progress to eclampsia, which can lead to seizures and death. The only cure for preeclampsia is delivery of the baby.

To prevent preeclampsia, ACOG and American Diabetes Association (ADA) guidelines recommend adding daily low-dose aspirin at the end of the first trimester for pregnant women at risk for preeclampsia (e.g., diabetes, renal disease, history of preeclampsia, chronic hypertension). See the Hypertension chapter for more information.

Select Conditions and Preferred Management During Pregnancy

CONDITION	PREFERRED MANAGEMENT	NOTES
Morning Sickness, Nausea, Vomiting	Lifestyle first: avoid an empty stomach, eat smaller, more frequent meals, drink plenty of water, avoid spicy or odorous foods and avoid environmental triggers. If lifestyle measures fail, ACOG recommends pyridoxine (vitamin B6) +/- doxylamine first line. Rx: doxylamine/pyridoxine (Bonjesta, Diclegis).	Ginger is rated "possibly effective" for treating morning sickness. Hyperemesis gravidarum is severe N/V, causing weight loss, dehydration and electrolyte imbalance. It will be treated under the care of an obstetrician and may require hospitalization.
GERD/Heartburn	Lifestyle first: eat smaller, more frequent meals, avoid foods that worsen GERD. If symptoms occur while sleeping, recommend elevating the head of the bed and not eating 3 hours prior to sleep. If lifestyle measures fail, recommend antacids. Calcium antacids, such as calcium carbonate (Tums), are a good choice to also supplement calcium intake.	If heartburn symptoms are not relieved by antacids, H2 receptor antagonists or PPIs can be considered for add-on therapy.
Flatulence	Simethicone (Gas-X, Mylicon).	
Constipation	Lifestyle first: ↑ fluid intake, ↑ dietary fiber intake and ↑ physical activity. If lifestyle measures fail, fiber (psyllium, calcium polycarbophil, methylcellulose), with adequate amounts of fluids, is preferred. Docusate and polyethylene glycol can also be used to prevent and treat constipation.	Many prenatal vitamins contain iron, which can worsen constipation.
Cough, Cold, Allergies	First line: cromolyn. Second line: First-generation antihistamines [e.g., chlorpheniramine (drug of choice), diphenhydramine] are recommended due to a history of safety but cause sedation. The non-sedating second-generation agents (loratadine and cetirizine) are now often recommended by obstetricians. If nasal steroids are needed for chronic allergy symptoms, all intranasal steroids are considered to be safe. Budesonide is preferred.	Oral decongestants (e.g., pseudoephedrine) should not be recommended during the first trimester. The cough-suppressant dextromethorphan and the mucolytic guaifenesin have limited safety data in pregnancy/lactation, but are sometimes used. Avoid liquid formulations that contain alcohol.
Pain	Non-drug options such as hot/cold packs, light massage or physical therapy can help limit or avoid the use of analgesics. ACOG recommends acetaminophen first-line for mild pain during pregnancy because it has a better safety profile than NSAIDs and opioids.	Avoid NSAIDs, including aspirin (except for low-dose aspirin for preeclampsia prevention), especially at 20 weeks gestation or later. During pregnancy, NSAID use can cause premature closure of the fetal ductus arteriosus and kidney problems in the fetus (leading to low amniotic fluid). Opioids should only be used during pregnancy if there are no alternatives.
Asthma	Maintenance therapy: budesonide is preferred but all inhaled corticosteroids (ICS) are considered safe for use in pregnancy. Long-acting beta-agonists can be continued with ICS if needed. Rescue therapy: ICS-formoterol or albuterol (short-acting beta agonist).	Budesonide Respules are used in a nebulizer.
Iron Deficiency Anemia	Supplemental iron, prenatal vitamins with iron.	Iron worsens constipation.
Hypertension*	Labetalol, nifedipine extended-release, methyldopa.	ACE inhibitors, ARBs, aliskiren and Entresto are contraindicated in pregnancy. Low-dose aspirin is recommended for preeclampsia prevention in patients with chronic hypertension.
Diabetes*	Insulin is preferred if not controlled with lifestyle. Metformin and glyburide are sometimes used.	Low-dose aspirin is recommended for preeclampsia prevention in both type 1 and 2 diabetes. If diabetes develops during pregnancy it is called gestational diabetes.

CONDITION	PREFERRED MANAGEMENT	NOTES
Infection*	**Generally considered safe to use:** penicillins (including amoxicillin and ampicillin), cephalosporins, erythromycin and azithromycin. **VAGINAL FUNGAL INFECTIONS** Topical antifungals (creams, suppositories) x 7 days. **URINARY TRACT INFECTIONS** Cephalexin 500 mg PO Q6H x 7 days. Amoxicillin 500 mg PO Q8H x 7 days. Alternatives: nitrofurantoin, SMX/TMP and fosfomycin. Must treat bacteriuria, even if asymptomatic. Untreated bacteriuria can lead to pyelonephritis, premature birth and perinatal mortality. **TOXOPLASMOSIS** Many people who are infected with toxoplasmosis are asymptomatic. If a woman contracts toxoplasmosis during pregnancy, it can cause miscarriage, stillbirth or damage to the baby's brain and eyes. Women can be tested prior to pregnancy with an IgM and IgG test. Pregnant women should avoid dirty food and water (uncommon in the U.S.), unpasteurized dairy products and cat feces (including contact with cat litter boxes), which can contain the parasite.	Do not use: quinolones (due to cartilage damage) and tetracyclines (due to teeth discoloration). **VAGINAL FUNGAL INFECTIONS** Avoid fluconazole. **URINARY TRACT INFECTION** Nitrofurantoin and SMX/TMP should be considered last line during the 1st trimester, and should not be used in the last 2 weeks of pregnancy.
Conditions requiring anticoagulation	**VENOUS THROMBOEMBOLISM (VTE)** Treatment: low molecular weight heparin (LMWH) is preferred over unfractionated heparin (UFH) due to ease of administration. Prophylaxis: pneumatic compression devices ± LMWH (preferred over UFH). **MECHANICAL VALVE** Women who require chronic warfarin therapy for mechanical heart valves or inherited thrombophilias are generally converted to LMWH during pregnancy. They may be switched back to warfarin after the 13th week of pregnancy, then back to LMWH close to delivery.	The risk of developing a VTE is increased during pregnancy and for the first six weeks postpartum. Warfarin is teratogenic. The oral factor Xa inhibitors and direct thrombin inhibitors have not been adequately studied in pregnancy and are not recommended. Monitor peak anti-Xa levels, drawn 4 hours post-dose (LMWH), or aPTT (UFH).
Hypothyroidism	Levothyroxine (will require a 30-50% dose increase during pregnancy).	Hypothyroidism must be treated during pregnancy; if left untreated, severe consequences could include miscarriage or stillbirth, preeclampsia, low birth weight, cognitive impairment and growth retardation.
Hyperthyroidism	Mild cases will not require treatment. It is preferable to normalize the mother's thyroid function prior to pregnancy. Contraception should be used until the condition is controlled. If drugs are necessary (i.e., Graves' disease), both methimazole and propylthiouracil (PTU) carry potential fetal risks. Methimazole is generally preferred over PTU, except for early in pregnancy. In the 1st trimester, patients should receive PTU if therapy is needed.	Both PTU and methimazole have a high risk for liver damage. Uncontrolled maternal hyperthyroidism can cause premature delivery and low birth weight. Radioactive iodine is teratogenic and not used in pregnancy.

Managing hypertension, diabetes, HIV and certain infections during pregnancy are discussed in detail in the respective chapters.

LACTATION

The American Academy of Pediatrics (AAP) recommends that babies be exclusively breastfed for the first six months of life, as long as it is mutually desired by the mother and baby and if safety risks are not present. After this, it is recommended to continue breastfeeding with complimentary foods for at least two years if feasible. Mothers who are breastfeeding should increase their diet by 330 – 400 kcal/day and continue prenatal vitamins and omega-3 supplements. Babies receiving breast milk partially or exclusively should receive 10 mcg (400 IU) of vitamin D supplementation daily.

Human milk contains very little iron (unlike formula), but most newborns have adequate iron stores in the body for at least the first 4 months of life. Iron supplementation (1 mg/kg daily) may be needed after 4 months of age for breastfed babies until the infant can obtain adequate iron from eating iron-rich solid foods, which usually occurs at 6 months old. See the Dietary Supplements, Natural & Complementary Medicine chapter for more information.

Excretion into breast milk is higher with drugs that are non-ionized, have a small molecular weight, a low volume of distribution and high lipid solubility. The majority of medications have low excretion into breast milk and can be taken safely while breastfeeding. Additionally, breastfeeding can continue when the mother has a cold, influenza and with the majority of other infections. *LactMed* (https://www.ncbi.nlm.nih.gov/books/NBK501922/) or *Briggs' Drugs in Pregnancy and Lactation* can be used to check for drug safety during breastfeeding. Refer to the Drug References chapter for more information.

TREATING PAIN

Postpartum pain can often be adequately treated with acetaminophen or ibuprofen, which are safe to use while breastfeeding. Codeine and tramadol should not be used by breastfeeding mothers due to risk of excessive sleepiness, breathing difficulty and/or death in the infant. Breastfed infants have died, especially in mothers taking codeine who were CYP450 2D6 ultra-rapid metabolizers. Because of the importance, this is discussed further in the Drug Interactions, Pharmacogenomics and Pain chapters. Even small doses of opioids taken by the mother can cause serious side effects for the infant.

KNOWN OR SUSPECTED HIV

Breastfeeding is not recommended for women with documented HIV infection in the United States, especially for those who are not on antiretroviral therapy (ART) or do not have sustained viral suppression while on ART. Any woman with suspected HIV infection should stop breastfeeding until HIV is ruled out with proper testing.

SPECIFIC MEDICATIONS

Drugs that should be avoided completely during lactation include chemotherapy, illicit drugs and radioactive compounds used for treatment and diagnostic studies (e.g., iodine).

Some medications should be avoided during lactation, if possible. Use of these drugs while breastfeeding is not without significant risk and a decision must be made based on a discussion between patient and provider. In some cases, patients may be able to pump and dispose of the breastmilk when drug concentrations are at the highest. Examples of these medications include amphetamines, amiodarone, ergotamines, lithium, metronidazole, phenobarbital and statins. Most often, safer alternatives are available.

For all drugs taken during lactation, the infant should be monitored for adverse effects caused by maternal medication use.

Select Guidelines/References

American College of Obstetricians and Gynecologists (ACOG) Practice Guidelines, available at www.acog.org (accessed 2024 Jan 22).

CDC Recommendations for Breastfeeding, available at www.cdc.gov (accessed 2024 Jan 22).

CONTENT LEGEND

 * = Study Tip Gal

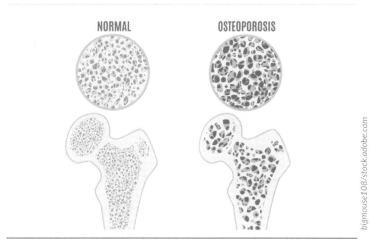

NORMAL   OSTEOPOROSIS

bigmouse108/stock.adobe.com

CHAPTER 49

OSTEOPOROSIS, MENOPAUSE & TESTOSTERONE USE

OSTEOPOROSIS

BACKGROUND

Osteoporosis ("porous bones") is a condition that causes bones to become weak and fragile. It is estimated that more than one-quarter of all adults in the U.S., and over half of those > 50 years of age, have osteoporosis, low bone density or low bone mass. Osteoporosis can occur in both men and women of all races. It is most common in postmenopausal females. About one in two women and one in five men will have an osteoporosis-related fracture during their lifetime. Falls are the most common cause of fractures, but with extremely porous bones, they can be caused by coughing or rolling over in bed.

The most common locations for fractures are the vertebrae (spine), proximal femur (hip) and distal forearm (wrist). Vertebral fractures can occur without a fall and can initially be painless (the only clue may be a gradual loss of height). Hip fractures are the most devastating type of fractures, with higher costs, disability and mortality than all other fractures combined. Hip fractures are more common after the age of 75 years. Wrist fractures, and other types of fractures, appear in younger people and serve as an early indicator of poor bone health.

RISK FACTORS

Osteoporosis can occur as a result of normal age-related bone loss. Bone accumulates until approximately age 30. After that, men lose bone at a rate of 0.2 – 0.5% per year, and women lose bone at a similar rate, except in the 10 years after menopause when bone loss is accelerated (1 – 5% per year). Patient-specific characteristics that can contribute to osteoporosis risk include lifestyle habits, diseases and medications (see the Study Tip Gal on the following page).

SELECT FACTORS AND CONDITIONS WITH OSTEOPOROSIS RISK

Patient Characteristics
Advanced age

Ethnicity (Caucasian and Asian are at ↑ risk)

Family history

Sex (females > males)

Low body weight

Medical Diseases/Conditions
Diabetes

Eating disorders (e.g., anorexia nervosa)

Gastrointestinal diseases (e.g., IBD, celiac disease, gastric bypass, malabsorption syndromes)

Hyperthyroidism

Hypogonadism in men

Menopause

Rheumatoid arthritis, autoimmune diseases

Others (e.g., epilepsy, HIV/AIDS, Parkinson disease)

Lifestyle Factors
Smoking

Excessive alcohol intake (≥ 3 drinks per day)

Low calcium intake

Low vitamin D intake

Physical inactivity

Medications
Antiseizure medications (e.g., carbamazepine, phenytoin)

Aromatase inhibitors

Depo-medroxyprogesterone

GnRH (gonadotropin-releasing hormone) agonists

Lithium

PPIs (↑ gastric pH decreases Ca absorption)

Steroids* (≥ 5 mg daily of prednisone or prednisone equivalent for ≥ 3 months)

Thyroid hormones (in excess)

Others (e.g., loop diuretics, SSRIs, TZDs, tenofovir)

Long-term use of steroids is the major drug-contributing factor to poor bone health.

DIAGNOSIS

Bone Mineral Density

Bone is not "dead tissue"; it is living and undergoes constant remodeling. Osteoblasts are the cells involved in bone formation. Osteoclasts are the cells involved in bone resorption; they break down tissue in the bone. Bone health is evaluated by measuring bone mineral density (BMD). The gold standard to measure BMD and diagnose osteoporosis is a dual-energy X-ray absorptiometry (DEXA or DXA) scan. This measures BMD of the spine and hip and calculates a T-score or a Z-score. See the Study Tip Gal for interpreting T-scores for the diagnosis of osteoporosis and osteopenia.

All women ≥ 65 years and men ≥ 70 years should have BMD measured. BMD can be checked earlier if there is a history of a fragility fracture (e.g., a fall from standing height or lower that results in a fracture) after age 50, risk for disease or drug-induced bone loss, a parental history of hip fracture or other clinical risk factors (e.g., smoking, alcoholism, low body weight).

If a DXA scan is unavailable, an ultrasound may be performed. Ultrasounds are less expensive, portable and do not emit radiation, but they are less than optimal. Ultrasound readings provide bone density in one location, such as the heel. If low, the patient should be encouraged to get a DXA scan. Since vertebral fractures are so common in older adults and usually lack symptoms, vertebral imaging may be performed if height loss is observed or if BMD testing indicates osteopenia.

Fracture Risk Assessment Tool (FRAX)

The FRAX tool is a computer-based algorithm developed by the World Health Organization (WHO) that estimates the risk

DIAGNOSIS OF OSTEOPOROSIS

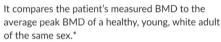

WHAT IS A T-SCORE?
It compares the patient's measured BMD to the average peak BMD of a healthy, young, white adult of the same sex.*

A DEXA (or DXA) measures BMD so a T-score can be determined.

T-scores are negative: a score at or above -1 correlates with stronger (denser) bones, which are less likely to fracture.**

WHO SHOULD HAVE BMD MEASURED?
Women ≥ 65 years and men ≥ 70 years.

Younger patients at high risk for fracture (see text).

INTERPRETING T-SCORE RESULTS
Normal: ≥ -1

Osteopenia (low bone mass): -1 to -2.4***

Osteoporosis: ≤ -2.5

A Z-score is calculated the same way, but compares the patient's measured BMD to the mean BMD of an age, sex and ethnicity-matched population.
Scores less than -1 reflect the standard deviation from the comparator group (e.g., a T-score of < -2.5 means the patient's BMD is at least 2.5 standard deviations below the average BMD for healthy, young, white adults).
Repeat DXA scanning (every 2 years) is recommended for patients with T-scores < -2.0 but > -2.5 or with ongoing risk of bone loss (including diabetes).

of osteoporotic fracture in the next 10 years (available at www.bonesource.org/frax-tool or https://frax.shef.ac.uk/FRAX/). It has been well-validated, and the U.S. tool has adapted versions available for White, Black, Asian and Hispanic women. Clinical risk factors included in the tool are age, sex, weight, height, previous fracture, parental hip fracture, femoral neck BMD, smoking status, steroid use, alcohol intake, disorders strongly associated with osteoporosis (e.g., type 1 diabetes, chronic liver disease, premature menopause) and diagnosis of rheumatoid arthritis. The tool is intended for postmenopausal women and men > 50 years of age.

PREVENTION

Fall Prevention Measures

If the bone density is low, care must be taken to avoid falls. Factors that put a patient at increased fall risk include a history of recent falls, medications that cause sedation or orthostasis (e.g., antihypertensives, sedatives, hypnotics, narcotic analgesics, psychotropics), neurologic disorders, conditions causing physical instability or poor coordination (e.g., Parkinson disease, dementia, prior stroke, peripheral neuropathy), impaired vision or hearing, poor health/frailty and urinary or fecal urgency. A home safety assessment should ensure that lighting is appropriate, floors are safe (throw rugs/clutter/cords have been removed), storage is at reasonable heights, bathrooms have safety bars and non-skid floors, handrails are present on all stairs and the stairs are well-lit with non-skid treads or carpet.

Preventing falls requires measures to improve muscle strength, balance and vision. Adequate corrective lenses, safe shoes and appropriate clothing (that will not cause falls) are required. If a disability is present, canes or walkers should be strongly recommended.

Lifestyle Measures

Patients with low bone density should perform regular weight-bearing exercise (e.g., walking, jogging, Tai-Chi) and muscle-strengthening exercise (e.g., weight training, yoga). They should be encouraged to stop smoking and avoid secondhand smoke, reduce alcohol intake and adopt fall prevention strategies, as described above.

Calcium and Vitamin D Intake

Adequate calcium intake is required throughout life. It is critically important in children (who can build bone stores), in pregnancy (when the fetus can deplete the mother's stores) and during the years around menopause when bone loss is rapid. Dietary intake of calcium is preferred, with supplements used if needed. Intake in excess of the recommended allowances may contribute to kidney stones, cardiovascular disease and stroke, though the evidence remains controversial.

Vitamin D is required for calcium absorption, and low levels contribute to various health conditions, including autoimmune conditions and cancer. Vitamin D deficiency in children causes rickets, and in adults, it causes osteomalacia (softening of the bones). The Bone Health and Osteoporosis Foundation recommends 20 – 25 mcg [800 – 1,000 international units (IU)] of vitamin D daily for adults age ≥ 50 years. Other organizations recommend 15 mcg (600 IU) daily for people ≥ 71 years. Many endocrinologists suggest a higher intake of 25 – 50 mcg (1,000 – 2,000 IU) daily. The National Academy of Medicine considers a safe upper limit to be 100 mcg (4,000 IU) daily for adolescents and adults. Higher doses are needed if a vitamin D deficiency is present (see the Study Tip Gal below).

Calcium and Vitamin D Supplementation

Calcium obtained through the diet is generally not enough; most women need an additional 600 – 900 mg daily (2 to 3 servings of dairy products) to reach recommended levels.

Calcium absorption is saturable; doses above 500 – 600 mg of elemental calcium should be divided. Calcium products are available in many forms (e.g., capsules, tablets, chewables, liquids, granules/powder).

- Calcium carbonate has more elemental calcium per unit compared to calcium citrate, but requires an acidic environment for absorption

- Calcium citrate has better absorption with an increased gastric pH (e.g., elderly patients, use of PPIs)

Vitamin D deficiency can be treated with high doses of vitamin D2 (ergocalciferol) or vitamin D3 (cholecalciferol) for 8 to 12 weeks, followed by maintenance therapy. Maintenance therapy is 25 – 50 mcg (1,000 – 2,000 IU) daily, or dosed to maintain target levels. See the Renal Disease chapter for information on vitamin D analogs (e.g., calcitriol).

Sunlight is another source of vitamin D3 but is not ideal due to the risk of skin cancer. Dietary intake and supplements are the preferred sources of vitamin D.

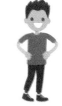

CALCIUM AND VITAMIN D

CALCIUM
- Recommended daily intake for most adults is 1,000-1,200 mg elemental calcium
  - ❑ Do not exceed 500-600 mg of elemental calcium per dose
- Calcium carbonate (e.g., *Tums*)
  - ❑ 40% elemental calcium
  - ❑ Absorption: acid-dependent
  - ❑ Must take with meals
- Calcium citrate (e.g., *Cal-Citrate*)
  - ❑ 21% elemental calcium
  - ❑ Absorption: not acid-dependent
  - ❑ Can take with or without food

Avoid low bone density later in life by building strong bones in children

VITAMIN D
- Required for calcium absorption
- Deficiency: serum vitamin D [25(OH)D] < 30 ng/mL
- Treat deficiency with cholecalciferol (vitamin D3) or ergocalciferol (vitamin D2)
  - ❑ Cholecalciferol: 125-175 mcg (5,000-7,000 IU) daily
  - ❑ Ergocalciferol: 1,250 mcg (50,000 IU) weekly

DRUG	DOSING	SAFETY/SIDE EFFECTS/MONITORING
Calcium Supplements		
Calcium Carbonate (Tums, *Oysco, Os-Cal*,* others) + cholecalciferol **(Caltrate)** <u>40% elemental calcium</u>	Calcium 500 mg PO TID with meals (can vary with formulation used) Total daily dose of elemental calcium should be < 2,000 mg (diet and supplements)	**SIDE EFFECTS** <u>Constipation</u>, hypercalcemia, nausea **MONITORING** Ca, PO4, PTH **NOTES** Hypercalcemia is especially problematic with concomitant use of vitamin D (due to increased calcium absorption)
Calcium Citrate (Cal-Citrate, others) + cholecalciferol **(Citracal)** <u>21% elemental calcium</u>	<u>1 g calcium carbonate = 400 mg elemental calcium</u> <u>1 g calcium citrate = 210 mg elemental calcium</u>	Calcium carbonate: take <u>with food</u>; <u>do not use with PPIs</u> Calcium citrate: take <u>with or without food</u>

*Brand discontinued but name still used in practice

DRUG TREATMENT

There are a number of FDA-approved options for the treatment and prevention of osteoporosis. Medications approved for <u>prevention</u> include <u>bisphosphonates</u> (except IV ibandronate) and the <u>estrogen-based therapies, raloxifene</u> and *Duavee*. <u>Bisphosphonates, denosumab</u>, parathyroid hormone analogs (e.g., <u>teriparatide</u>, abaloparatide) and <u>calcitonin</u> are indicated for <u>treatment</u>. These medications have primarily been studied in postmenopausal women with osteoporosis, and there is limited data in men or in those with glucocorticoid-induced osteoporosis. Regardless of drug selection, treatment must include <u>adequate calcium</u> and <u>vitamin D</u> intake, with levels evaluated before initiating therapy. See the <u>Study Tip Gal</u> below for important facts about each drug/drug class.

Criteria for Initiating Treatment*

Osteoporosis	■ T-score ≤ -2.5* in the spine, femoral neck, total hip or 1/3 radius, OR ■ Presence of a fragility fracture, regardless of BMD
Osteopenia, if high risk	■ Low bone density (T-score between -1 and -2.5) AND ■ FRAX score indicates a 10-year probability of a major osteoporosis-related fracture ≥ 20% or a 10-year hip fracture probability ≥ 3%

*For patients with diabetes, consider treatment for a T-score ≤ -2.0.

DRUG SUMMARY FOR OSTEOPOROSIS TREATMENT AND PREVENTION

BISPHOSPHONATES
- First-line for treatment or prevention in most patients
- PO administration: must stay upright for 30 minutes (60 minutes for ibandronate) and drink 6-8 oz of plain water
- Side effects: esophagitis, hypocalcemia, GI effects
- Rare (but serious) side effects:
  - ❏ Atypical femur fractures
  - ❏ Osteonecrosis of the jaw (ONJ): jaw bone becomes exposed and cannot heal due to decreased blood supply
- Formulations:
  - ❏ PO: given daily, weekly or monthly
  - ❏ IV: given quarterly/yearly (if GI side effects or adherence issues with PO formulation)
- Treatment duration: 3-5 years in patients with a low risk of fracture (due to the risk of femur fractures and ONJ)

DENOSUMAB (PROLIA)
- Alternative to bisphosphonates
- SC administration every 6 months
- Side effect: hypocalcemia

TERIPARATIDE (FORTEO), ABALOPARATIDE (TYMLOS)
- Recommended for very high-risk patients only (e.g., history of severe vertebral fractures)
- SC administration daily
- Side effect: hypercalcemia

RALOXIFENE (EVISTA), CONJUGATED ESTROGENS/BAZEDOXIFENE (DUAVEE)
- Alternative to bisphosphonates if high risk of vertebral fractures
- Increased risk for VTE and stroke
- Raloxifene can be used if low VTE risk or high breast cancer risk
  - ❏ Side effect: vasomotor symptoms
- *Duavee* can be used in women with an intact uterus for prevention of osteoporosis
  - ❏ Also used as treatment for vasomotor symptoms
  - ❏ Side effect: increased risk of breast cancer

LAST LINE OR NOT RECOMMENDED
- Estrogen (with or without progestin) for prevention only in postmenopausal women with vasomotor symptoms; use lowest possible dose for shortest duration of time
- Calcitonin for treatment only if other options are not suitable (less effective and has a risk of cancer with long-term use)

Bisphosphonates

Bisphosphonates increase bone density by <u>inhibiting osteoclast activity and bone resorption</u>. They reduce vertebral and hip fracture risk (<u>except ibandronate</u>, which only reduces vertebral fractures). Bisphosphonates are <u>first-line</u> for most patients for the <u>prevention or treatment</u> of osteoporosis. A <u>drug holiday</u> (i.e., time off of the drug) should be considered for low-risk patients <u>after 3 – 5 years</u> of treatment. Bisphosphonates are also used to treat Paget's disease, glucocorticoid-induced osteoporosis (in patients taking ≥ 7.5 mg daily of prednisone or prednisone equivalent) and <u>hypercalcemia of malignancy</u>.

DRUG	DOSING	SAFETY/SIDE EFFECTS/MONITORING
Oral Bisphosphonates		
Alendronate **(Fosamax,** Binosto) Tablet, oral solution, effervescent tablet (Binosto) + cholecalciferol (Fosamax Plus D) Tablet	**Prevention (postmenopausal females)** 5 mg PO daily or 35 mg PO weekly **Treatment (males and postmenopausal females)** 10 mg PO <u>daily</u> or 70 mg PO <u>weekly</u> Fosamax Plus D: 70 mg/2,800 IU or 70 mg/5,600 IU PO weekly **Glucocorticoid-Induced Osteoporosis** 5 mg PO daily Postmenopausal women not on estrogen: 10 mg PO daily	**CONTRAINDICATIONS** <u>Hypocalcemia; inability to stand or sit upright for at least 30 minutes</u> (60 minutes for ibandronate); abnormalities of the esophagus (e.g., stricture, achalasia); high risk of aspiration (effervescent tablet or oral solution) **WARNINGS** ONJ: ↑ risk with invasive dental procedures, poor dental hygiene, cancer diagnosis, use with chemotherapy or corticosteroids and duration of exposure Atypical <u>femur fractures</u>; bone, joint or muscle pain (may be severe) Esophagitis, esophageal ulcers, erosions, stricture or perforation (rare): <u>follow administration instructions</u> (see Key Counseling Points section) <u>Hypocalcemia</u> must be corrected prior to use <u>Renal impairment</u>: do not use if CrCl < 35 mL/min (alendronate) or CrCl < 30 mL/min (ibandronate, risedronate)
Risedronate (Actonel, Atelvia) Tablet, delayed-release tablet (Atelvia)	**Prevention and Treatment (postmenopausal females)** 5 mg PO <u>daily</u>, 35 mg PO <u>weekly</u>, or 150 mg PO <u>monthly</u> **Treatment (males)** 35 mg PO weekly **Glucocorticoid-Induced Osteoporosis** 5 mg PO daily	**SIDE EFFECTS** <u>Dyspepsia, dysphagia, heartburn, N/V, hypocalcemia</u>, hypophosphatemia (mild, transient), abdominal pain, musculoskeletal pain Risedronate: headache, hypertension, skin rash, UTI, infection **NOTES** Check calcium and vitamin D levels prior to initiating treatment Due to the risk of jaw decay/necrosis, <u>dental work</u> should be completed <u>prior to starting treatment</u> Use caution with aspirin or NSAIDs (can worsen GI irritation)
Ibandronate (Boniva*) Tablet	**Prevention and Treatment (postmenopausal females)** 150 mg PO <u>monthly</u> (on the same date every month)	<u>Separate</u> from <u>calcium, antacids, iron and magnesium</u> by at least <u>2 hours</u> Separate at least 30 minutes from food and beverages (except water) Atelvia (delayed-release): requires an <u>acidic gut</u> for absorption; <u>do not use with H2RAs and PPIs</u>
Injectable Bisphosphonates		
Ibandronate (Boniva*) Injection	**Treatment (postmenopausal females)** 3 mg IV <u>every 3 months</u> Administer over 15-30 seconds	**CONTRAINDICATIONS** <u>Hypocalcemia</u> Zoledronic acid: CrCl < 35 mL/minute or evidence of acute renal impairment
Zoledronic Acid **(Reclast)** **Zometa** – for hypercalcemia of malignancy	**Prevention (postmenopausal females)** 5 mg IV every 2 years **Treatment (males and postmenopausal females)** 5 mg IV <u>once yearly</u> **Glucocorticoid-Induced Osteoporosis** 5 mg IV once yearly Administer over ≥ 15 minutes	**WARNINGS** Same as oral bisphosphonates (except no GI problems) plus: <u>Renal impairment</u>: monitor SCr before each dose; use caution if dehydrated and with comorbid conditions or medications that can cause renal impairment Ibandronate: do not use if CrCl < 30 mL/min Zoledronic acid: use caution in aspirin-sensitive asthma (risk of bronchoconstriction), avoid in pregnancy (teratogenic) **SIDE EFFECTS** Same as oral bisphosphonates (except no esophageal problems) plus: Acute-phase reaction (flu-like symptoms: fever, achiness, runny nose, headache) Zoledronic acid: edema, hypotension, fatigue, dehydration, ↓ PO4, K and Mg **NOTES** <u>Preferred if esophagitis is present</u> (due to <u>risk for esophageal cancer</u>)

*Brand discontinued but name still used in practice.

Estrogen Agonist/Antagonist-Containing Products

Raloxifene is an estrogen agonist/antagonist [a selective estrogen receptor modulator (SERM)] that ↓ bone resorption. Conjugated estrogens/bazedoxifene (*Duavee*) is an equine (horse) estrogen/SERM combination indicated for osteoporosis prevention in postmenopausal women with a uterus.

DRUG	DOSING	SAFETY/SIDE EFFECTS/MONITORING
Raloxifene (*Evista*) Tablet	**Prevention and Treatment (postmenopausal females)** 60 mg PO daily	**BOXED WARNINGS** ↑ risk of VTE (DVT/PE); ↑ risk of death due to stroke in women with CHD or at risk for coronary events **CONTRAINDICATIONS** Pregnancy, history of or current VTE, **SIDE EFFECTS** Hot flashes, peripheral edema, arthralgia, leg cramps/muscle spasms, flu symptoms, infection **NOTES** Separate raloxifene and levothyroxine by several hours Discontinue 72 hours prior to and during prolonged immobilization
Conjugated Estrogens/Bazedoxifene (*Duavee*)	**Prevention (postmenopausal females with a uterus)** 1 tablet (0.45/20 mg) PO daily Other indications: treatment of moderate-severe vasomotor symptoms associated with menopause (same dose)	**BOXED WARNINGS** Endometrial cancer (due to unopposed estrogen); ↑ risk of DVT and stroke in postmenopausal women 50-79 years of age (do not use to prevent CVD); dementia (women ≥ 65 years); use lowest effective dose for shortest duration possible **CONTRAINDICATIONS** Breast cancer (any history); pregnancy; undiagnosed uterine bleeding; history of or active VTE, MI or stroke; protein C, S or antithrombin deficiency; hepatic impairment **WARNINGS** ↑ risk of breast cancer (due to unopposed estrogen) and ovarian cancer; ↑ risk of retinal vascular thrombosis; lipid effects (↑ HDL, ↑ TG, ↓ LDL) **SIDE EFFECTS** Nausea, diarrhea, dyspepsia, abdominal pain, muscle spasms **NOTES** Not recommended for women > 75 years of age Use estrogen-containing products for the shortest duration possible

Calcitonin

Calcitonin inhibits bone resorption by osteoclasts. It is less effective than other agents for the treatment of osteoporosis and, with long-term use, the risk of cancer is increased. It is rarely used for this indication.

DRUG	DOSING	SAFETY/SIDE EFFECTS/MONITORING
Calcitonin (*Miacalcin*) Nasal spray, injection	**Treatment (females > 5 years postmenopause)** Nasal spray: 1 spray (200 units) in one nostril daily (alternate nostril daily) SC or IM: 100 units daily	**WARNINGS** Hypocalcemia (associated with tetany and seizures); ↑ risk of malignancy with long-term use; hypersensitivity reactions to salmon-derived products (e.g., bronchospasm, anaphylaxis, swelling of the tongue or throat); antibody formation Nasal spray: can cause nasal ulceration, epistaxis and rhinitis; nasal exams are recommended **SIDE EFFECTS** Back pain, myalgia, nausea, dizziness Injection: flushing, injection site reactions **NOTES** Keep the injection and unopened nasal spray bottles refrigerated Can be used in the management of hypercalcemia of malignancy (see the Oncology chapter)

Parathyroid Hormone 1-34

Teriparatide and abaloparatide are analogs of human parathyroid hormone, which stimulates osteoblast activity and increases bone formation. They are used to treat osteoporosis when there is a very high risk of fracture (e.g., previous history of vertebral fracture). Due to safety issues, the cumulative lifetime treatment duration is restricted to two years or less.

DRUG	DOSING	SAFETY/SIDE EFFECTS/MONITORING
Teriparatide (Forteo) Injection (prefilled multi-dose pen; needles not included)	**Treatment (males and postmenopausal females)** 20 mcg SC daily **Glucocorticoid-Induced Osteoporosis** 20 mcg SC daily	**WARNINGS** Osteosarcoma (bone cancer): risk dependent on dose and duration of use, do not use in bone malignancy or metabolic bone diseases Hypercalcemia; orthostatic hypotension; use caution with urolithiasis (urinary stones) **SIDE EFFECTS** Arthralgias, leg cramps, nausea, orthostasis/dizziness
Abaloparatide (Tymlos) Injection (prefilled multi-dose pen; needles not included)	**Treatment (males and postmenopausal females)** 80 mcg SC daily	Tymlos: ↑ uric acid, antibody development, erythema at injection site (58%) **NOTES** Keep refrigerated Forteo: protect from light

Receptor Activator of Nuclear Factor kappa-B Ligand (RANKL) Inhibitor

Denosumab is a monoclonal antibody that binds to RANKL and blocks its interaction with RANK (a receptor on osteoclasts) to prevent osteoclast formation; this leads to ↓ bone resorption and ↑ bone mass. It is used for the treatment of osteoporosis when there is a high risk of fracture.

DRUG	DOSING	SAFETY/SIDE EFFECTS/MONITORING
Denosumab (Prolia) Injection **Xgeva** – hypercalcemia of malignancy, bone cell tumor, prevention of bone metastasis Other indications: treatment of bone loss in men on androgen deprivation therapy for prostate cancer and women on aromatase inhibitor therapy for breast cancer	**Treatment (males and postmenopausal females)** 60 mg SC every 6 months Must be administered by a healthcare professional	**BOXED WARNING** Risk for severe hypocalcemia in patients with advanced kidney disease (e.g., dialysis) **CONTRAINDICATIONS** Hypocalcemia (correct prior to using); pregnancy **WARNINGS** ONJ: ↑ risk with invasive dental procedures, poor dental hygiene, cancer diagnosis, use of chemotherapy or steroids and a longer duration of exposure Atypical femur fractures; bone, joint or muscle pain (may be severe) Hypocalcemia: use caution in predisposed patients (e.g., hypoparathyroidism, thyroid surgery, malabsorption syndromes, CrCl < 30 mL/min) Infections (e.g., skin, urinary tract); skin reactions (e.g., dermatitis, eczema, rash) **SIDE EFFECTS** Hypertension, fatigue, edema, N/V/D, ↓ PO4, dyspnea, headache **NOTES** If discontinued, bone loss can be rapid; consider alternative agents to maintain BMD

Romosozumab

Romosozumab is indicated for postmenopausal females with a history of an osteoporotic fracture or multiple risk factors. It is recommended as an alternative to other treatments. It inhibits sclerostin, a protein that blocks bone formation.

DRUG	DOSING	SAFETY/SIDE EFFECTS/MONITORING
Romosozumab (Evenity) Injection	**Treatment** 210 mg SC (administered in two separate injections) once a month Duration of therapy is limited to 12 months (due to decreased efficacy after this time)	**BOXED WARNINGS** Increased risk of MI, stroke and cardiovascular death **CONTRAINDICATIONS** Hypocalcemia **SIDE EFFECTS** Arthralgia, headache, injection site reactions **NOTES** Keep refrigerated; let sit at room temperature for 30 min before administration

OSTEOPOROSIS KEY COUNSELING POINTS

See the Drug Formulations and Patient Counseling chapter for counseling language/layman's terminology.

All Osteoporosis Medications

- Must supplement with calcium and vitamin D.
  - ❏ Do not take calcium carbonate with proton pump inhibitors (acidic gut is needed for absorption).
  - ❏ Switch to calcium citrate if use of a proton pump inhibitor is required.

Bisphosphonates

- Oral formulations (except *Atelvia*): take in the morning with 6 – 8 oz of plain water at least 30 minutes before first food. Take *Atelvia* with ≥ 4 oz of water immediately after breakfast.
  - ❏ Must stay sitting or standing upright for at least 30 minutes after taking (at least 60 minutes with *Boniva*) and until after first food of the day.
  - ❏ Separate from calcium, iron, magnesium, antacids and multivitamin supplements.
- Dissolve *Binosto* in 4 oz of plain water (room temperature). Wait five minutes to dissolve, then stir for 10 seconds.
- Do not take *Atelvia* with acid-suppressing medications.
- Can cause dyspepsia.
- Missed dose:
  - ❏ Daily dosing: skip missed dose; take next dose at regularly scheduled time.
  - ❏ Weekly dosing: take missed dose the next morning; do not take two doses on the same day.
  - ❏ Monthly dosing: take missed dose the morning after you remember, unless it is less than one week from the next dose, then skip it; do not take two doses in the same week.

Raloxifene

- Can cause blood clots.
- Discontinue at least 72 hours prior to and during prolonged immobilization (e.g., surgery requiring bed rest).

Teriparatide and Abaloparatide

- Can cause:
  - ❏ Dizziness.
  - ❏ Orthostasis.
- Generally, treatment duration should not exceed 2 years.

Calcitonin Nasal Spray

- Refrigerate unused bottles.
- Allow bottle to reach room temperature prior to use, then store at room temperature. Discard after 30 doses.
- Prime the pump before first use by pressing the two white side arms toward the bottle, releasing at least five sprays, until a full spray is produced.
- Alternate nostrils each day.

MENOPAUSE

BACKGROUND

Menopause is reached when the last menstrual period was over 12 months ago. Menopause usually occurs between the ages of 40 – 58 years (average age is 52 years). A decrease in estrogen and progesterone causes an increase in follicle stimulating hormone (FSH), resulting in vasomotor symptoms. Many women experience these symptoms during the menopause transition period (perimenopause) as estrogen production by the ovaries declines. These are often described as hot flashes (transient episodes of flushing and a sensation of heat in the upper body and face, sometimes followed by chills) and night sweats (hot flashes that occur during sleep). Sleep can be disturbed, and mood changes may be present. Due to a decline in estrogen in the vaginal mucosa, vaginal dryness, burning and dyspareunia (painful intercourse) can occur (called the genitourinary syndrome of menopause).

Some women remain largely asymptomatic during menopause, while others suffer from severe symptoms that significantly impact quality of life. Vasomotor symptoms can last up to seven years. Women who have both ovaries removed, or receive chemotherapy or radiation for cancer, will experience induced menopause. The symptoms are similar but often more acute initially due to a sudden decline in estrogen (rather than a natural, gradual decline).

ESTROGEN-PROGESTIN PRODUCTS

The most effective treatment for vasomotor symptoms is systemic hormone therapy with estrogen. Estrogen causes a decrease in luteinizing hormone (LH) and more stable temperature control. It improves bone density as well, but has a number of safety issues to consider before initiating. The North American Menopause Society (NAMS) and the American Association of Clinical Endocrinologists (AACE) provide criteria for the use of estrogen to control vasomotor symptoms. See the Study Tip Gal below for the appropriate use and health risks associated with hormone therapy.

Formulation Considerations

Transdermal, local (topical) and low-dose oral estrogen products are associated with a lower risk of venous thromboembolism (VTE) and stroke than standard doses of oral estrogen. Estrogen is generally well tolerated but can cause nausea, dizziness, headaches, mood changes, vaginal bleeding, bloating and breast tenderness/fullness. Topical formulations (e.g., patch, gel, emulsion) bypass first-pass metabolism and lower doses can be used. They may decrease systemic exposure, resulting in fewer side effects.

Local estrogen products are preferred for patients who have vaginal symptoms only (vaginal dryness and/or painful intercourse). Any of the vaginal products in this chapter (creams, tablets, rings) or OTC lubricants (discussed later in the products for dyspareunia section) can be helpful for localized symptoms.

HORMONE THERAPY: HEALTH RISKS AND APPROPRIATE USE

Estrogen
- Most effective treatment for vasomotor symptoms.

- Women with a uterus: use in combination with a form of progesterone (e.g., a progestin). Unopposed estrogen increases the risk of endometrial cancer.

- Associated with significant safety risks (see the drug table on the following page), including boxed warnings for VTE, stroke, dementia and breast cancer (bigger concern in the elderly).

Progestin
- Progestins (e.g., norethindrone, levonorgestrel, drospirenone) can be given as part of a combination pill (with estrogen) or as a separate tablet, most commonly medroxyprogesterone (MPA).

- Can cause mood disturbances, which may be intolerable; if taken intermittently (e.g., for two weeks per month as with *Premphase)*, spotting can occur.

- Micronized progestins (e.g., *Prometrium)* are considered to be safer than synthetic progestins (e.g., medroxyprogesterone).

CRITERIA FOR USE OF HORMONE THERAPY
- Healthy, symptomatic women who are within 10 years of menopause, ≤ 60 years of age and have no contraindications to use.

- Extending treatment beyond age 60 years may be acceptable (e.g., patient has osteoporosis) if the lowest possible dose is used and the woman is advised of the safety risks.

- Consider quality-of-life priorities and personal risk factors (e.g., age, time since menopause, risk of blood clots, heart disease, stroke, breast cancer) before use. Patients with risk factors should use non-hormonal treatments (e.g., SSRIs, SNRIs, fezolinetant).

Common Hormone Therapy Products

Estradiol-containing products and conjugated estrogens are used primarily for vasomotor symptoms, vaginal atrophy and osteoporosis prevention. Oral contraceptives, used for contraception, contain ethinyl estradiol (discussed in the Contraception & Infertility chapter).

COMPONENTS	FORMULATION	SAFETY/SIDE EFFECTS/MONITORING
Local Hormone Therapies		
17-Beta-Estradiol	Vaginal cream (*Estrace*) Vaginal ring (*Estring*) Vaginal tablet (*Vagifem*) Vaginal insert (*Imvexxy*)	**NOTES** Topical (vaginal) hormone products may have lower systemic absorption, but some may still occur; the safety issues below should be considered
Conjugated Equine Estrogens	Vaginal cream (*Premarin*): 0.625 mg/gram	
Systemic Hormone Therapies		
Estradiol	Topical gel (*Elestrin*) Transdermal patch (*Climara, Vivelle-Dot, Menostar, Minivelle, Alora**) Vaginal ring (*Femring*)	**BOXED WARNINGS** Endometrial cancer (if estrogen used without progestin in women with a uterus); dementia (women ≥ 65 years); ↑ risk of VTE and stroke in postmenopausal women 50-79 years of age (do not use to prevent CVD); breast cancer; use lowest effective dose for shortest duration possible
17-Beta-Estradiol	Oral tablet, micronized Topical gel (*Divigel, Estrogel*) Topical spray (*Evamist*)	*Evamist*: secondary exposure can cause breast budding and breast masses in prepubertal females, and gynecomastia and breast masses in prepubertal males; keep children away from spray/application site
Estradiol and Levonorgestrel	Transdermal patch (*ClimaraPro*) "Pro" indicates it contains a progestin	**CONTRAINDICATIONS** Estrogen-containing products: breast cancer (any history); undiagnosed uterine bleeding; active VTE, arterial thromboembolic disease, or known protein C, S or antithrombin deficiency; hepatic impairment; pregnancy
Estradiol and Norethindrone	Transdermal patch (*CombiPatch*) Oral tablet (*Activella, Amabelz*)	
Estradiol and Drospirenone	Oral tablet (*Angeliq*)	**WARNINGS** ↑ risk of breast cancer (from use of estrogen alone) and ovarian cancer; ↑ risk of retinal vascular thrombosis; lipid effects (↑ HDL, ↑ TG, ↓ LDL)
Conjugated Equine Estrogens	Oral tablet (*Premarin*): 0.3, 0.45, 0.625, 0.9, 1.25 mg Injection (*Premarin*)	**SIDE EFFECTS** Edema, hypertension, headache, weight gain, depression, nausea, abdominal pain
Conjugated Equine Estrogens and Medroxyprogesterone (MPA)	Oral tablet (*Prempro*): 0.3/1.5, 0.45/1.5, 0.625/2.5, 0.625/5 mg Oral tablet (*Premphase*): phasic dosing – 0.625 mg on days 1-14, then 0.625/5 mg on days 15-28	Patch: redness/irritation of the skin Remove transdermal patches prior to an MRI *CombiPatch*: store in the refrigerator prior to dispensing; once dispensed, it can be kept at room temperature for up to 6 months
Medroxyprogesterone *Depo-Provera* – SC or IM for contraception	Oral tablets (*Provera*): 2.5, 5, 10 mg	*Vivelle-Dot*, and *Minivelle* patches are applied twice weekly; *Climara* and *Menostar* patches are once weekly
Micronized progesterone	Oral tablet (*Prometrium*)	Gels and *Evamist* spray are flammable
Conjugated Estrogens/ Bazedoxifene	Oral tablet (*Duavee*)	Micronized progestin (in combination with estrogen) may have a lower risk of breast cancer and cardiovascular events than synthetic progestin, medroxyprogesterone (in combination with estrogen)

Brand discontinued but name still used in practice.

"Bioidentical" Nomenclature

Some females prefer to use bioidentical hormones to treat symptoms, including commercially available products approved by the FDA or compounded preparations. *Bijuva* is an oral capsule and the first FDA-approved bioidentical estradiol and progesterone combination for the treatment of moderate-severe hot flashes. The term "bioidentical" has different meanings; some use it to refer to hormones that have an identical structure to those found in the female body, while others use it to refer to plant-derived hormones that are compounded.

There are no well-designed studies to confirm risk or benefit of bioidentical hormone therapy, and the AACE does not recommend bioidentical hormones to treat menopausal symptoms.

ESTROGEN-PROGESTIN KEY COUNSELING POINTS

See the Drug Formulations and Patient Counseling chapter for counseling/layman's terminology.

- Topical gels for systemic absorption: apply once daily; wash hands after applying.
  - ❏ Apply *Divigel* to the upper thigh (alternate legs daily).
  - ❏ Apply *Elestrin* to the upper arm and shoulder.
  - ❏ Apply *Estrogel* to the entire arm from wrist to shoulder.
- *Evamist* spray: spray on the inside of the forearm (between elbow and wrist) every morning.
- Patch: apply to the lower abdomen, below the waistline.

PRODUCTS FOR DYSPAREUNIA

Ospemifene *(Osphena)* is an oral estrogen agonist/antagonist indicated for dyspareunia and moderate-severe vaginal dryness, which are symptoms of vulvar and vaginal atrophy due to menopause. It is not indicated for mild symptoms (other topical vaginal products are safer for this purpose). Ospemifene should be used short-term for moderate-severe symptoms. *Intrarosa* (prasterone), a vaginally inserted steroid, is another treatment for moderate-severe dyspareunia.

Common OTC lubricants and moisturizers can also help with local symptoms, such as *Replens* and *Luvena*. *Astroglide* is a lubricant marketed specifically for dyspareunia. Oil-based lubricants should not be used with condoms as they can cause the condom to tear. *Astroglide* or silicone-based lubricants are safe to recommend with condoms.

DRUG	DOSING	SAFETY/SIDE EFFECTS/MONITORING
Estrogen Agonist/Antagonist		
Ospemifene *(Osphena)* Tablet	60 mg PO daily Take with food	**BOXED WARNINGS/CONTRAINDICATIONS** Same as for other estrogen-containing products (see the Common Hormone Therapy Products table on the previous page) **WARNING** Should not be used in women with severe hepatic impairment **SIDE EFFECTS** Hot flashes, vaginal discharge, hyperhidrosis, muscle spasms

NONHORMONAL PRODUCTS FOR MENOPAUSAL VASOMOTOR SYMPTOMS

While hormone therapy is the most effective treatment for menopausal vasomotor symptoms, some patients may choose to avoid hormone therapy or have contraindications. There are several nonhormonal options for these patients.

SSRIs and SNRIs

Paroxetine *(Brisdelle)* is approved for the treatment of moderate-severe vasomotor symptoms associated with menopause. The dose of paroxetine used is lower than the recommended dose for depression. *Brisdelle* should not be used with tamoxifen or warfarin. Paroxetine is a CYP450 2D6 inhibitor, and it will block the effectiveness of tamoxifen (a prodrug). Other SSRIs (e.g., citalopram, escitalopram) and SNRIs (e.g., venlafaxine, desvenlafaxine) have shown efficacy in treating vasomotor symptoms related to menopause, but they are not FDA-approved for this indication. Fluoxetine and sertraline are not recommended because of studies showing negligible improvement in vasomotor symptoms. See the Depression chapter for important safety issues and side effects of SSRIs and SNRIs.

Neurokinin B Antagonist

Fezolinetant *(Veozah)* is a neurokinin B antagonist that works to modulate neuronal activity in the thermoregulatory center and is FDA-approved for the treatment of moderate to severe vasomotor symptoms associated with menopause (see the drug table on the next page).

DRUG	DOSING	SAFETY/SIDE EFFECTS/MONITORING
Neurokinin B Antagonist		
Fezolinetant (*Veozah*) Tablet	45 mg PO daily Take with liquids at about the same time each day	**CONTRAINDICATIONS** Known cirrhosis, severe renal impairment (including ESRD), concomitant use with CYP1A2 inhibitors (check for drug interactions) **SIDE EFFECTS** Hot flashes, abdominal pain, diarrhea, elevated ALT/AST, back pain

Other Drugs

Gabapentin (an antiseizure medication) and oxybutynin (an anticholinergic drug used for urinary incontinence) have shown benefit in reducing vasomotor symptoms, however, side effects associated with each may make other options preferable. Neither gabapentin nor oxybutynin are FDA-approved for this indication.

While clonidine and pregabalin have some evidence for use for vasomotor symptoms, due to greater risk of side effects, they are not recommended.

Natural Products

Natural products used for vasomotor symptoms include black cohosh, evening primrose oil, red clover, soy, flaxseed, dong quai, St. John's wort and chasteberry. The mild "plant estrogens" found in soy and red clover are called phytoestrogens; phyto means plant. While use of these products may be popular among patients, evidence of efficacy is lacking (or very limited) and they are not recommended over other available products.

Non-Pharmacologic Interventions

Cognitive behavioral therapy, clinical hypnosis and weight loss have shown efficacy in reducing vasomotor symptoms and are recommended. Other lifestyle modifications (e.g., cooling techniques, avoiding triggers, dietary modifications, yoga, exercise) have not been shown to be effective in reducing menopausal vasomotor symptoms and are not recommended.

HYPOGONADISM IN MALES

Hypogonadism in older males can be due to a normal age-related decline in testosterone, or it can be secondary to a medical condition, surgical procedure or medications that lower testosterone. Medications that can lower testosterone include opioids (especially methadone when used for opioid dependence), chemotherapy drugs used for prostate cancer (see the Oncology chapter), cimetidine and spironolactone.

TESTOSTERONE USE

In recent years, the increased use of testosterone is largely due to older males requesting treatment for "Low T" symptoms to increase sexual interest (libido), sexual performance, muscle mass, bone density, energy, memory and concentration. The use of testosterone replacement for conditions other than accepted medical uses is controversial, and a clear benefit of improved sexual function has not been established. The FDA has released a warning about the cardiovascular risks associated with testosterone use, and they recommend treatment only in men with low testosterone levels caused by certain medical conditions and confirmed by laboratory tests.

There have been reports of increased clotting risk in men using testosterone therapy. Most men who experienced clotting may have had a higher risk at baseline, and the link to testosterone use is unclear. Testosterone increases hematocrit, which can cause polycythemia and an increase in clotting risk.

Testosterone can cause noncancerous prostate growth and use is restricted in men with severe BPH. If dispensing a 5 alpha-reductase inhibitor for BPH (e.g., finasteride) that blocks the conversion of testosterone to an active form, it would not make sense to dispense another drug that provides testosterone directly. Common side effects of testosterone include increased male pattern baldness, acne and gynecomastia.

Testosterone and anabolic androgenic steroids (AAS) carry a warning for abuse potential and risk of serious adverse events. When used at higher than prescribed doses, serious adverse outcomes can occur, including myocardial infarction, heart failure, stroke, depression, hostility, aggression, liver toxicity and male infertility. Individuals abusing high doses of testosterone can have withdrawal symptoms, such as depression, fatigue, irritability, loss of appetite, decreased libido and insomnia.

Testosterone Formulations

Testosterone comes in many formulations, including parenteral (IM or SC) injections, topical gels and solutions. The injections are painful, and patients may report feeling symptomatic when it is getting close to the time for the next dose. The injections can increase hematocrit more than topical formulations. *Testopel* is a small SC pellet that is implanted under the skin. Oral formulations of testosterone undecanoate (e.g., *Jatenzo*) are FDA-approved for hypogonadism due to medical conditions (and not age-related hypogonadism).

The gel formulations (*AndroGel* and other topical gels) are popular and relatively well tolerated. *AndroGel* is applied to the upper body. Men who use the gel need to let it dry prior to dressing and be careful not to let others touch the application area, as this increases the risk of drug transfer. If the drug transfers to a female or male child, it can cause "early virilization," and depending on the dose received, the child could have enlarged genital organs, aggressive behavior and premature pubic hair growth. The risk of early virilization is a boxed warning and requires counseling (see the Testosterone Key Counseling Points section). There are new formulations that reduce accidental exposure risk (e.g., *Fortesta* and *Natesto*).

Testosterone Products: C-III

TESTOSTERONE	DOSING/COUNSELING	SAFETY/SIDE EFFECTS/MONITORING
Topical Gels and Solutions		**BOXED WARNINGS** Topical gel/solution: secondary exposure to testosterone in children can result in virilization; children should avoid contact with any unwashed or unclothed application sites in men using topical testosterone
Testosterone gel [*AndroGel* (1%, 1.62%), *AndroGel* Pump (1.62%)]	*AndroGel* 1%: apply daily to upper arms, shoulders and/or abdomen	
	1.62%: apply to upper arms or shoulders (not the abdomen)	Oral testosterone undecanoate and SC testosterone ethanate: can increase blood pressure which increases the risk of major adverse cardiovascular events
Testosterone gel 1% (*Vogelxo, Vogelxo Pump*)	Apply to upper arms and shoulders daily	*Aveed*: pulmonary oil microembolism reactions (cough, dyspnea, throat tightening, anaphylaxis) can be life-threatening; observe in a healthcare setting for 30 minutes after each injection; only available by restricted access through the *Aveed* REMS Program
Testosterone gel 1% (*Testim*)	Apply to arms and shoulders daily	
Testosterone gel 2% (*Fortesta*)	Apply to front and inner thighs daily	**CONTRAINDICATIONS** Breast cancer, prostate cancer, pregnancy, breastfeeding
Testosterone solution	Apply to armpits daily	*Aveed*: allergy to castor oil or benzyl benzoate
Testosterone nasal gel (*Natesto*)	1 spray per nostril TID	*Depo-Testosterone*: serious cardiac, hepatic or renal disease
Alternative Formulations		**WARNINGS** ↑ risk of breast cancer, prostate cancer, cardiovascular events, VTE, dyslipidemia, gynecomastia, polycythemia, priapism; use caution in hepatic impairment; may worsen BPH (↑ PSA)
Injections:		
Testosterone cypionate (*Depo-Testosterone*)	IM every 4 weeks (2 doses), then every 10 weeks	**SIDE EFFECTS** ↑ appetite, acne, edema, hepatotoxicity, reduced sperm count, ↑ SCr, sensitive nipples, sleep apnea
Testosterone undecanoate (*Aveed*)	IM every 2-4 weeks	*Natesto*: nasal irritation
Testosterone enanthate	IM every 2-4 weeks	Injections: pain at the site of injection
Testosterone enanthate (*Xyosted*)	SC auto-injector every week	**MONITORING** Testosterone levels, PSA, liver function, cholesterol, hematocrit (some products)
Implantable pellets (*Testopel*)	SC every 3-6 months	**NOTES** Gels: apply at the same time each morning; flammable until dry
Testosterone undecanoate oral capsule (*Jatenzo, Kyzatrex, Tlando*)	Administered BID	*Xyosted* contains sesame oil

TESTOSTERONE KEY COUNSELING POINTS

See the Drug Formulations and Patient Counseling chapter for counseling/layman's terminology.

- Topical gels/solutions: do not let others come in contact with the application site (can cause secondary exposure, leading to adverse effects). Keep application site covered by clothing.

- For maximal absorption, wait at least 2 – 6 hours after applying gels/solutions before showering or swimming.

- Gels are flammable while wet; do not smoke or go near an open flame until dry.

- Apply deodorant prior to applying solutions to the underarms.

- *AndroGel Pump:* before first use, prime the device by pushing the pump down three times. Do not apply the gel released during priming.

- *Natesto:* prime the pump ten times, then insert the actuator into the nostril, depress slowly until the pump stops, remove from the nose while wiping the tip to transfer gel to the lateral side of the nostril, then press on the nose and lightly massage. Do not blow your nose or sniff for one hour after administration.

Select Guidelines/References

American Association of Clinical Endocrinologists/American College of Endocrinology Clinical Practice Guidelines for the Diagnosis and Treatment of Postmenopausal Osteoporosis. *Endocrine Practice.* 2020;26(1).

Management of Osteoporosis in Postmenopausal Women: the 2021 Position Statement of the North American Menopause Society. *Menopause.* 2021;28(9).

The North American Menopause Society (NAMS) 2023 Position Statement on Nonhormone Therapy. *Menopause.* 2023;30(6).

American Association of Clinical Endocrinologist and American College of Endocrinology Clinical Position Statement on Menopause-2017 Update. *Endocr Practice.* 2017;23(7).

Testosterone Therapy in Men With Hypogonadism: An Endocrine Society Clinical Practice Guideline. *J Clin Endocrinolo Metab.* 2018;103(5).

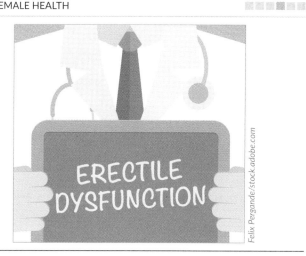

Felix Pergande/stock.adobe.com

CHAPTER 50

SEXUAL DYSFUNCTION

BACKGROUND

This chapter focuses on erectile dysfunction in males and hypoactive sexual desire disorder in females. Erectile dysfunction (impotence) refers to difficulty getting or sustaining an erection that is firm enough for sex. This is a common type of sexual dysfunction in males and can generally be treated with phosphodiesterase-5 inhibitors (PDE-5 inhibitors). Males can experience other types of sexual dysfunction, including problems with ejaculation and low libido, which is sometimes due to low testosterone levels. Testosterone treatment is discussed in the Osteoporosis, Menopause & Testosterone Use chapter.

In women, sexual dysfunction can be due to either an inability to reach orgasm (anorgasmia), painful intercourse or hypoactive (i.e., lower than normal) sexual desire disorder (HSDD). Flibanserin (*Addyi*) and bremelanotide (*Vyleesi*) are FDA-approved to treat HSDD for premenopausal women only.

In both males and females, sexual dysfunction can be due to the use of an SSRI or SNRI, or less commonly, another antidepressant. An alternate antidepressant can be tried that does not cause sexual side effects, such as bupropion.

ERECTILE DYSFUNCTION

The most common cause of erectile dysfunction (ED) is reduced blood flow to the penis. This can be common in patients with cardiovascular diseases, such as hypertension and atherosclerosis, and conditions that cause neuropathy, such as diabetes. Since the arteries supplying blood to the penis are smaller than those supplying blood to the heart, they can become restricted sooner than the larger vessels. ED can be considered an early warning indicator of cardiovascular disease, and males with ED who have cardiovascular disease risk factors should be referred for cardiac evaluation. Psychological issues (including depression and stress) and neurological illness (spinal cord injury, stroke) can be contributory. Medications used for other conditions, including blood pressure lowering drugs used in cardiovascular diseases, can contribute to erectile dysfunction (see Key Drugs Guy).

DRUGS THAT CAN CAUSE ERECTILE/ SEXUAL DYSFUNCTION

KEY DRUGS

Alcohol

Antidepressants
Especially SSRIs and SNRIs (including ↓ libido)

Antihypertensives
Beta-blockers, clonidine, thiazides

Antipsychotics
First-generation (e.g., chlorpromazine)

Prolactin-raising second-generation (e.g., risperidone, paliperidone)

BPH medications
Finasteride, dutasteride, and silodosin (mostly retrograde ejaculation)

Others

Anticancer drugs:
Leuprolide, flutamide

Anticholinergics

Atomoxetine

Digoxin

H2RAs:
Cimetidine, ranitidine

Nicotine

Opioids (chronic use, especially methadone)

NON-DRUG TREATMENT

Lifestyle changes, including weight loss, quitting tobacco and reducing alcohol intake, can improve ED. Underlying diseases that can contribute to the condition should be properly managed, and any offending agents should be discontinued, if possible. Non-drug options that are beneficial in some males are vacuum erection devices, penile implants and surgery.

NATURAL PRODUCTS

Natural products used to treat ED include yohimbe, L-arginine and panax ginseng. *The Natural Medicines Database* rates L-arginine (taken in high doses) and panax ginseng as "possibly effective" for this purpose. L-arginine can cause dizziness, headaches and flushing. The same side effects are caused by PDE-5 inhibitors, and the additive effects should be avoided. Yohimbe is rated as "insufficient evidence to date." Yohimbe causes gastrointestinal side effects, anxiety and more severe health concerns, including tachycardia and arrhythmias. Ginseng can increase the risk of bleeding.

There are many products marketed to "treat" ED. It is important to recognize that the majority of these products contain a false list of ingredients, have not been tested and are not regulated by the FDA.

DRUG TREATMENT

PDE-5 inhibitors (sildenafil, vardenafil, tadalafil and avanafil) are first-line for the treatment of ED. These are often started at a low dose, then titrated as tolerated and to desired effect. Treatment success is defined by the patient and partner. Treatment failure could be due to a number of factors, such as lack of sexual stimulation, timing of the dose and eating a large meal with the dose. Efficacy appears to be similar among the most common PDE-5 inhibitors (sildenafil, vardenafil and tadalafil), but patients could consider switching between drugs if they do not achieve desired effect. See the PDE-5 Inhibitor table on the next page for details.

If a patient cannot tolerate or has a contraindication to PDE-5 inhibitors, alprostadil can be used instead. Alprostadil is either injected into the penis or inserted into the penis with a urethral suppository. This treatment is invasive, painful and short-acting.

Two of the PDE-5 inhibitors used for ED are indicated for other conditions. Tadalafil *(Cialis)* is used for benign prostatic hyperplasia (BPH) at a dose of 5 mg daily, which could treat concurrent ED. Sildenafil *(Revatio)* and tadalafil *(Adcirca, Alyq)* are indicated for pulmonary arterial hypertension (PAH). Patients should not be using two PDE-5 inhibitors concurrently due to the risk of additive side effects.

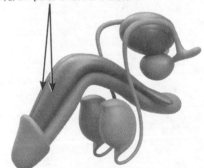

The corpora cavernosa (plural) are the two spongy tubular vessels that run down the length of the penis. When the vessels are filled with blood, the penis is hard and erect.

Nitric oxide (NO) → guanylate cyclase → ↑ cGMP → relaxes the smooth muscle in the arteries → blood flows into the vessels → erection.

Phosphodiesterase type 5 (PDE-5) degrades cGMP.

MYKOLA/stock.adobe.com

Phosphodiesterase Type 5 (PDE-5) Inhibitors

Following sexual stimulation, there is a local release of nitric oxide, which increases cGMP and causes smooth muscle relaxation. This permits blood to flow in, resulting in an erection (see figure on previous page). PDE-5 inhibitors block PDE-5 from degrading cGMP. PDE-5 inhibitors do not increase libido (sexual interest), which must be present for the drugs to work.

DRUG	DOSING	SAFETY/SIDE EFFECTS/MONITORING
Sildenafil (*Viagra*) ***Revatio*** – PAH	On-demand dosing: 25-100 mg daily PRN Start at 50 mg, take ~1 hr before sexual activity Start at 25 mg in select conditions (see Study Tip Gal)	**CONTRAINDICATIONS** Do not use with nitrates or riociguat (a guanylate cyclase stimulator). **WARNINGS** Impaired color discrimination (dose-related) – patients with retinitis pigmentosa may have higher risk.
Vardenafil (*Levitra, Staxyn*)	On-demand dosing: 5-20 mg daily PRN Start at 10 mg, take ~1 hr before sexual activity Start with a lower dose of *Levitra* in select conditions (see Study Tip Gal) *Staxyn* is an ODT and only available as 10 mg (max dose)	Hearing loss, with or without tinnitus/dizziness. Vision loss – rare, but can be due to nonarteritic anterior ischemic optic neuropathy (NAION). Risk factors: low cup-to-disc ratio, CAD and other vascular conditions, age > 50 yrs, Caucasian ethnicity. Avoid with retinal disorders. Hypotension, due to vasodilation. Higher risk with fluid depletion, resting BP < 90/50 mmHg or autonomic dysfunction.
Tadalafil (*Cialis*) ***Cialis*** – also used for BPH ***Adcirca*, Alyq –** PAH Lasts the longest – known as the "weekend pill"	Daily dosing: 2.5-5 mg daily Start at 2.5 mg; do not use daily dosing with severe renal or liver impairment On-demand dosing: 5-20 mg daily PRN Start at 10 mg, at least 30 min before sexual activity Start at 5 mg in select conditions (see Study Tip Gal) CrCl 30-50 mL/min: 5 mg PRN CrCl < 30 mL/min: 5 mg PRN Q72H	Priapism, seek emergency medical care if erection lasts > 4 hrs. CVD, caution with low or very high BP or recent cardiac events. If chest pain occurs, seek immediate medical help. **SIDE EFFECTS** Headache, flushing, dizziness, dyspepsia, blurred vision, difficulty with color discrimination, increased sensitivity to light, epistaxis, diarrhea, myalgia, muscle/back pain (mostly with tadalafil). **NOTES** Take with or without food. Sildenafil and vardenafil can have decreased efficacy if taken with a high-fat or large meal (common cause of treatment failure per guidelines).
Avanafil (*Stendra*)	On-demand dosing: 50-200 mg daily PRN Start at 100 mg, take 15-30 min before sexual activity Start at 50 mg in select conditions (see Study Tip Gal)	For ED, no more than one dose per day is recommended. *Stendra* can be taken closest to sexual activity.

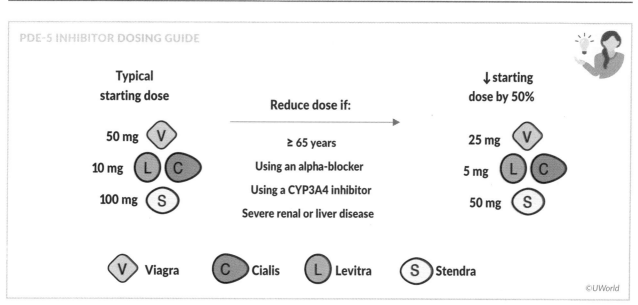

PDE-5 INHIBITOR DOSING GUIDE

Typical starting dose

50 mg V

10 mg L C

100 mg S

Reduce dose if:

≥ 65 years

Using an alpha-blocker

Using a CYP3A4 inhibitor

Severe renal or liver disease

↓ **starting dose by 50%**

25 mg V

5 mg L C

50 mg S

V Viagra   C Cialis   L Levitra   S Stendra

©UWorld

PDE-5 Inhibitor Drug Interactions

- It is an <u>absolute contraindication</u> to use <u>nitrates</u> or riociguat with PDE-5 inhibitors. These combinations can cause <u>severe hypotension</u>. This includes any prescription nitrates (e.g., *Nitrostat, Nitrolingual Pumpspray,* and *BiDil*) or illicit alkyl nitrates ("poppers" such as amyl nitrate and butyl nitrate).

  - Avoid long-acting nitrates completely. If a patient with ED has taken a PDE-5 inhibitor and develops angina, short-acting nitroglycerin should not be used until after 12 hours for avanafil, after 24 hours for sildenafil or vardenafil, and after 48 hours for tadalafil. Occasionally, if needed, nitrates are used in an acute emergency with careful monitoring.

  - Riociguat should not be administered within 24 hours of sildenafil, or within 24 hours before or 48 hours after tadalafil.

- Use caution with other agents that cause hypotension, including <u>alpha-blockers</u> and <u>antihypertensive drugs</u>.

  - PDE-5 inhibitors can enhance the hypotensive effects of alpha-1 blockers. The patient should be <u>stable on the alpha-1 blocker</u> (without excessive dizziness/hypotension) <u>before</u> starting the <u>PDE-5 inhibitor</u>. If *Cialis* is being used to treat BPH, do not use alpha-1 blockers concurrently.

  - Alcohol can enhance hypotension with PDE-5 inhibitors.

- Moderate and strong CYP450 <u>3A4 inhibitors</u> (e.g., grapefruit juice, protease inhibitors, azole antifungals) increase the drug levels of PDE-5 inhibitors; <u>lower starting doses</u> and/or extended dosing intervals are required. Strong CYP3A4 <u>inducers decrease drug levels; monitor effectiveness</u>.

Alprostadil (Prostaglandin E1)

Alprostadil is <u>prostaglandin E1</u>, a <u>vasodilator</u> that allows blood to flow into the cavernosal arteries, which then enlarges the penis. It is either <u>injected into the penis, or a pellet is inserted</u> through the urethra. This treatment is invasive, painful and does not last as long as the PDE-5 inhibitors. Alprostadil is used in some men who cannot tolerate or have contraindications to PDE-5 inhibitors.

DRUG	DOSING	SAFETY/SIDE EFFECTS/MONITORING
Alprostadil (*Caverject, Caverject Impulse, Edex*) Intracavernous injection Reconstitute prior to use	Inject 1.25-2.5 mcg into the base of the penis; titrate until desired response is achieved Appropriate dose should cause erection 5-10 min after injection; lasts ~1 hr Max 1x/day, 3x/week	**CONTRAINDICATIONS** Conditions that predispose the patient to priapism (e.g., sickle cell anemia, multiple myeloma, leukemia) Intracavernous injection: anatomical deformation or fibrotic conditions of the penis, penile implants Urethral pellets: urethral stricture, balanitis, severe hypospadias and curvature, urethritis, venous thrombosis
Alprostadil (*Muse*) Urethral pellets	Insert 125-250 mcg pellet into urethra Urinate before administration Max 2x/day Refrigerate	**SIDE EFFECTS** <u>Penile pain, priapism</u>, headache, dizziness Intracavernous injection: hematoma, bruising at injection site Urethral pellets: urethral burning or bleeding

HYPOACTIVE SEXUAL DESIRE DISORDER

Hypoactive sexual desire disorder (HSDD) is characterized by a low sexual desire that causes marked distress or interpersonal difficulty. The low sexual desire is not due to a health condition or drug.

DRUG TREATMENT

Flibanserin exhibits agonist activity at 5-HT1A and antagonist activity at 5-HT2A receptors. Bremelanotide is a nonselective melanocortin receptor agonist. The exact mechanism of how either of these medications treat HSDD is unknown. They are both indicated for use in premenopausal females only.

DRUG	DOSING	SAFETY/SIDE EFFECTS/MONITORING
Flibanserin (Addyi)	100 mg QHS Discontinue if no benefit after 8 weeks	**BOXED WARNINGS** Contraindicated: with alcohol due to an ↑ risk of severe hypotension and syncope (REMS program required); in combination with moderate or strong CYP3A4 inhibitors; in patients with hepatic impairment **WARNINGS** Hypotension, syncope, CNS depression **SIDE EFFECTS** Dizziness, somnolence, nausea, fatigue, insomnia, dry mouth **NOTES** Avoid in pregnancy or if breastfeeding
Bremelanotide (Vyleesi) Injection	1.75 mg SC PRN, injected ≥ 45 minutes before sexual activity Maximum dose: 1.75 mg/24 hours; no more than 8 doses per month Discontinue if no benefit after 8 weeks	**CONTRAINDICATIONS** Do not use with uncontrolled hypertension or known cardiovascular disease **WARNINGS** ↑ BP and ↓ HR after each dose, skin hyperpigmentation, nausea, delayed gastric emptying **NOTES** Avoid in pregnancy; effective contraception should be used

Flibanserin Drug Interactions

- Use with CNS depressants will ↑ the risk of hypotension and syncope.
- Flibanserin is a major substrate of CYP3A4 and inhibits P-glycoprotein. Concurrent moderate-strong CYP3A4 inhibitors are contraindicated.

KEY COUNSELING POINTS

See the Drug Formulations and Patient Counseling chapter for counseling language/layman's terminology.

ALL PDE-5 INHIBITORS

- Take approximately 15 minutes (avanafil), 30 minutes (tadalafil, when taken as needed) or 1 hour (sildenafil and vardenafil) before sexual activity.
- Sexual activity can put an extra strain on your heart. Stop sexual activity and get medical help right away if you have chest pain, dizziness or nausea during sexual activity.
- Can cause:
  - Priapism.
  - Orthostasis and decreased blood pressure. Do not take with nitrates; they worsen this effect.
  - Dizziness, headache, flushing and indigestion.
  - Ringing in the ears (tinnitus) or loss of hearing in one or both ears.
  - Vision changes, including blurry vision and changes to the look of colors (blue color tinge). Sudden vision loss in one or both eyes is a rare but serious side effect. Get medical help right away if this occurs.

Tadalafil (Cialis)

- Can cause muscle or back pain. This usually occurs 12 to 24 hours after taking, and can last up to two days.

Select Guidelines/References
Erectile Dysfunction: AUA Guideline (2018). http://www. auanet.org/guidelines/male-sexual-dysfunction-erectile-dysfunction-(2018).

Normal Prostate   **Prostate Cancer**

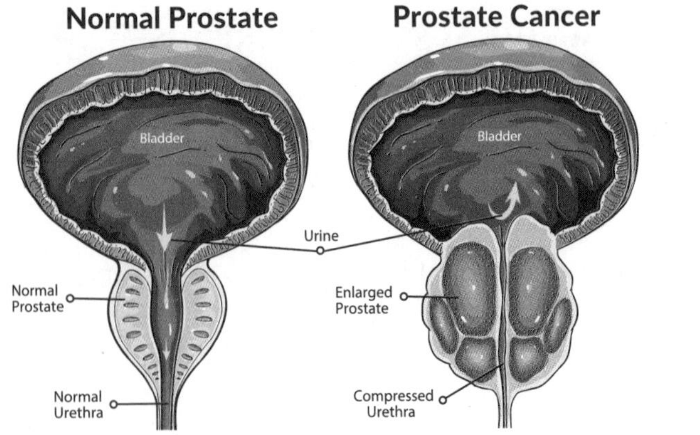

corbacserdar/stock.adobe.com

CHAPTER 51

BENIGN PROSTATIC HYPERPLASIA (BPH)

BACKGROUND

The prostate is a walnut-sized gland that surrounds the male urethra at the base of the bladder. As part of the male reproductive system, the main function of the prostate is to secrete fluid that becomes part of the seminal fluid carrying sperm.

The prostate is dependent on androgens (mainly testosterone) for development, maintenance of size and function. Testosterone is metabolized to dihydrotestosterone (DHT) by 5 alpha-reductase. DHT is responsible for normal and hyperplastic growth (increase in the number of cells). Benign prostatic hyperplasia (BPH) results from overgrowth of the stromal and epithelial cells of the prostate gland.

The layer of tissue surrounding the enlarged prostate stops it from expanding, causing the gland to press against or pinch the urethra. This contributes to lower urinary tract symptoms (LUTS) via direct bladder outlet obstruction and increased smooth muscle tone and resistance. The bladder wall becomes thicker and irritated. It begins to contract even when it contains small amounts of urine, causing frequent urination. Eventually, the bladder weakens and loses the ability to empty itself.

Prostate gland enlargement does not typically cause problems until after 65 years of age. Diagnosis requires assessment of the medical history (surgeries, trauma and medications, including herbal and OTC drugs) and a physical exam. The physical exam should

DRUGS THAT CAN WORSEN BPH

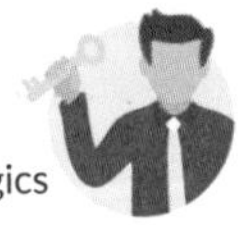

Centrally-acting anticholinergics (e.g., benztropine)

Drugs with anticholinergic effects:
Antihistamines (e.g., diphenhydramine)
Decongestants (e.g., pseudoephedrine)
Phenothiazines (e.g., prochlorperazine)
TCAs (e.g., amitriptyline)

Caffeine

Diuretics

SNRIs

Testosterone products

CONTENT LEGEND

  = Key Drug Guy

include a digital rectal exam (DRE) to determine the size of the prostate and identify any lumps or nodules. A urinalysis and serum prostate-specific antigen (PSA) are used to rule out conditions other than BPH. PSA, a protein produced by prostate cells, is frequently increased in prostate cancer. It can increase when the prostate becomes larger due to BPH, though BPH is a benign (non-cancerous) condition and does not increase prostate cancer risk.

SYMPTOMS AND COMPLICATIONS

The signs and symptoms of BPH are mainly LUTS, which include:

- Hesitancy, intermittent urine flow, straining or a weak stream of urine.
- Urinary urgency and leaking or dribbling.
- Urinary frequency, especially nocturia (urination at night).
- Incomplete emptying of the bladder (bladder feels full).
- Bladder outlet obstruction.

Symptoms can significantly impact quality of life. BPH rarely causes more severe symptoms, but if the blockage is severe, the urine could back up into the kidneys and result in acute renal failure. Urinary tract infections can also be present but are uncommon. Symptoms can be similar to prostate cancer, so all patients should be referred to a physician for an appropriate evaluation prior to starting treatment.

TREATMENT PRINCIPLES

The severity of reported BPH symptoms guides selection of treatment. Questionnaires, such as the American Urological Association Symptom Score (AUASS) or the International Prostate Symptom Score (I-PSS), are used to quantify symptoms. The scoring systems rate how bothersome the symptoms are, with higher scores indicating more severe symptoms. Treatment options can include watchful waiting, pharmacologic therapy or surgical intervention. Mild disease is generally treated with watchful waiting and yearly reassessments. Moderate/severe disease is generally treated with medications or a minimally invasive procedure or surgery, such as transurethral resection of the prostate (TURP).

NATURAL PRODUCTS

The American Urological Association (AUA) guidelines do not recommend natural products for the treatment of BPH symptoms, though various natural products have been investigated. Saw palmetto has been used for BPH, but it is unlikely to be effective based on contradictory and inconsistent data. Pygeum, pumpkin seed (beta-sitosterol) and rye pollen are other natural products that have shown

some improvement in BPH symptoms. Lycopene is used for prostate cancer prevention, but there is no good evidence for use in BPH. Pharmacists should not recommend natural products until the patient has seen a healthcare provider, as prostate cancer symptoms present similarly to BPH.

DRUG TREATMENT

Medications include alpha-blockers (selective and non-selective), used alone or in combination with a 5 alpha-reductase inhibitor. The 5 alpha-reductase inhibitors work by decreasing prostate size, but they have a delayed onset. They should not be used in men who have bladder outlet obstruction symptoms without prostate enlargement. Alpha-blockers work quickly, but do not shrink the prostate. The two classes are often used together to get the benefits of each.

Peripherally-acting anticholinergic drugs (e.g., tolterodine) or beta-3 receptor agonists (e.g., mirabegron) in combination with alpha-blockers are sometimes a reasonable option for men without an elevated post void residual (PVR) urine and when LUTS are predominately irritative. If anticholinergics are used, the PVR should be < 250 – 300 mL. These medications are used for overactive bladder and discussed in the Urinary Incontinence chapter.

Another treatment option is the phosphodiesterase-5 (PDE-5) inhibitor tadalafil, with or without finasteride. This can be used in men with BPH alone, and can be an attractive option for men with both BPH and erectile dysfunction (ED).

ALPHA-BLOCKERS

Alpha-1 blockers are first-line treatment for moderate-to-severe symptoms. They inhibit alpha-1 adrenergic receptors, causing relaxation of smooth muscle in the prostate and bladder neck. This reduces bladder outlet obstruction and improves urinary flow. There are three types of alpha-1 receptors. Alpha-1A receptors are primarily found in the prostate. Alpha-1B and alpha-1D receptors are dominant in the heart and arteries. The non-selective alpha-1 blockers (terazosin, doxazosin) have more side effects (e.g., orthostasis, dizziness, headache) than the selective alpha-1A blockers (tamsulosin, alfuzosin, silodosin).

Intraoperative Floppy Iris Syndrome
Alpha-blockers relax the smooth muscle of the prostate and bladder neck. The same receptors are present on the iris dilator muscle in the eye. Patients using alpha-blockers are at risk of developing intraoperative floppy iris syndrome (IFIS) during cataract surgery. With alpha-1 blockade, the iris becomes floppy, has a risk of prolapse and the pupils do not dilate well, complicating the procedure. If cataract surgery is planned, alpha-blocker treatment should be delayed until the surgery has been completed.

DRUG	DOSING	SAFETY/SIDE EFFECTS/MONITORING
Non-Selective Alpha-1 Blockers		**CONTRAINDICATIONS** Concurrent use of silodosin or alfuzosin with strong CYP3A4 inhibitors; hepatic impairment (Child-Pugh class C for silodosin, class B/C for alfuzosin); severe renal impairment (silodosin)
Doxazosin (Cardura, Cardura XL)	IR: start 1 mg at bedtime; titrate slowly up to 4-8 mg at bedtime XL: start 4 mg daily with breakfast; max 8 mg daily	**WARNINGS** Orthostatic hypotension/syncope, typically with the first dose, if therapy is interrupted for several days, if the dosage is increased too rapidly, or if another antihypertensive drug or PDE-5 inhibitor is started
Terazosin	Start 1 mg at bedtime; titrate slowly to a max of 20 mg at bedtime (10 mg generally effective)	Intraoperative floppy iris syndrome (IFIS) can occur in cataract surgery if currently on or previously treated with an alpha-1 blocker Priapism, seek medical attention if an erection lasts > 4 hours Angina, discontinue if symptoms of angina begin or worsen
Selective Alpha-1A Blockers		**SIDE EFFECTS** Dizziness, fatigue, headache, abnormal ejaculation (especially with tamsulosin and silodosin), fluid retention, rhinitis (tamsulosin)
Tamsulosin (Flomax) + dutasteride (Jalyn)	0.4 mg daily, 30 min after the same meal each day; max 0.8 mg daily	**MONITORING** BP, PSA, urinary symptoms **NOTES** The non-selective drugs are often given at bedtime to help minimize the initial "first-dose" effect of orthostasis/dizziness. This requires careful counseling, as nocturia is common, and getting up at night to use the bathroom can be dangerous if dizziness and orthostasis occur.
Alfuzosin (Uroxatral)	10 mg daily, immediately after the same meal each day CrCl < 30 mL/min: use with caution	Alpha-blockers work quickly on LUTS, but 4-6 weeks may be required to assess whether beneficial effects have been achieved; they do not shrink the prostate and do not change PSA levels. *Cardura XL* is an OROS formulation (see Drug Formulations and Patient Counseling chapter) and can leave a ghost tablet (empty shell) in the stool.
Silodosin (Rapaflo)	8 mg daily with a meal CrCl 30-50 mL/min: 4 mg daily CrCl < 30 mL/min: do not use	Silodosin can cause retrograde ejaculation in ~30% of patients. It is reversible upon drug discontinuation. Do not use alfuzosin if at risk for QT prolongation. Alpha-blockers can be used for bladder outlet obstruction in women (off-label).

Alpha-Blocker Drug Interactions

- Use caution when co-administered with PDE-5 inhibitors used for erectile dysfunction (sildenafil, tadalafil, vardenafil, avanafil) due to additive hypotensive effects. See the Sexual Dysfunction chapter. If tadalafil (*Cialis*) is being used to treat BPH, do not use in combination with alpha-1 blockers.

- Use caution with other drugs that lower BP.

- Tamsulosin, alfuzosin and silodosin are major CYP450 3A4 substrates; do not use with strong CYP3A4 inhibitors.

- Silodosin cannot be used with strong P-gp inhibitors, such as cyclosporine.

- Alfuzosin can cause QT prolongation; do not use with other QT-prolonging drugs. Use with caution in patients with cardiovascular disease.

5 ALPHA-REDUCTASE INHIBITORS

These medications inhibit the 5 alpha-reductase enzyme, which blocks the conversion of testosterone to dihydrotestosterone (DHT). Finasteride is selective for the 5 alpha-reductase type II enzyme (the more prevalent type within the prostate), while dutasteride inhibits both type I and type II. This class of medications is indicated for the treatment of symptomatic BPH in men with an enlarged prostate. They are used in combination with alpha-blockers to improve symptoms, decrease the risk of acute urinary retention and decrease the need for surgery (e.g., TURP, prostatectomy).

DRUG	DOSING	SAFETY/SIDE EFFECTS/MONITORING
Finasteride (Proscar) **Propecia** – for alopecia (hair loss) at lower doses (1 mg daily) + tadalafil (Entadfi)	5 mg daily	**CONTRAINDICATIONS** Women of child-bearing potential, pregnancy, children **WARNINGS** May ↑ risk of high-grade prostate cancer **SIDE EFFECTS** Impotence, ↓ libido, ejaculation disturbances, breast enlargement and tenderness, rash; sexual SEs ↓ with time and return to baseline at one year of use in some men
Dutasteride (Avodart) + tamsulosin (Jalyn)	0.5 mg daily Take Jalyn 30 min after the same meal each day	**MONITORING** PSA, urinary symptoms **NOTES** Pregnant women should not take or handle these medications, as the active ingredient can be absorbed through the skin from broken or crushed tablets and can be detrimental to the fetus. They are on the NIOSH list of hazardous drugs. Delayed onset, treatment for 6 months (or longer) may be required for maximal efficacy. 5 alpha-reductase inhibitors shrink the prostate and ↓ PSA levels. Swallow dutasteride whole. Do not chew or open as contents can cause oropharyngeal irritation.

5 Alpha-Reductase Inhibitor Drug Interactions

- Finasteride and dutasteride are minor CYP3A4 substrates; strong CYP3A4 inhibitors can ↑ levels.
- Do not use *Proscar* if using *Propecia* for hair loss.

PHOSPHODIESTERASE-5 INHIBITORS

The mechanism of action of PDE-5 inhibitors in treating BPH symptoms is not well known. They likely decrease smooth muscle and endothelial cell proliferation, decrease nerve activity, increase smooth muscle relaxation and tissue perfusion of the prostate and bladder. Tadalafil is the only PDE-5 inhibitor that is FDA-approved for the treatment of BPH with or without erectile dysfunction. It has been studied alone and in combination with finasteride. Due to the risks for hypotension, tadalafil should not be used in combination with an alpha-blocker for the treatment of BPH.

DRUG	DOSING	SAFETY/SIDE EFFECTS/MONITORING
Tadalafil (*Cialis*) *Cialis* – also for ED **Adcirca,** *Alyq* – for pulmonary arterial hypertension (PAH) + finasteride (*Entadfi*)	5 mg daily, at the same time each day CrCl 30-50 mL/min: 2.5 mg initially, max of 5 mg daily CrCl < 30 mL/min: do not use Use 2.5 mg if taking a strong CYP3A4 inhibitor	**CONTRAINDICATIONS** Do not use with nitrates or riociguat (a guanylate cyclase stimulator) **WARNINGS** Impaired color discrimination (dose-related), higher risk with retinitis pigmentosa Hearing loss, with or without tinnitus/dizziness Vision loss, rare, can be due to nonarteritic anterior ischemic optic neuropathy (NAION); risk factors: low cup-to-disc ratio, CAD, vascular conditions, age > 50 yrs, Caucasian ethnicity; avoid with retinal disorders Hypotension, due to vasodilation; higher risk with resting BP < 90/50 mmHg, fluid depletion or autonomic dysfunction CVD, caution with low or very high BP or recent CV events; seek immediate medical help for chest pain Priapism, seek emergency medical care if an erection lasts > 4 hrs **SIDE EFFECTS** Headache, flushing, dizziness, dyspepsia, muscle/back pain, myalgia, blurred vision, increased sensitivity to light, epistaxis, diarrhea **MONITORING** BP, PSA, urinary symptoms

- For drug interactions and key counseling points for tadalafil, see the Sexual Dysfunction chapter.

KEY COUNSELING POINTS

See the Drug Formulations and Patient Counseling chapter for counseling language/layman's terminology.

ALPHA-BLOCKERS

- Can cause orthostasis.
- Tell your healthcare provider about the use of this medication if having cataract surgery.

Doxazosin and Terazosin (Non-Selective)

- Take at bedtime.
- Ghost tablet in stool (*Cardura XL*).

Silodosin

- Can cause sexual dysfunction (retrograde ejaculation).

5 ALPHA-REDUCTASE INHIBITORS

- Can cause sexual dysfunction (decreased libido, ejaculation disturbances and erectile dysfunction).
- Avoid in pregnancy (teratogenic). Women who are or may become pregnant should not handle the tablets.

Select Guidelines/References
AUA Management of Lower Urinary Tract Symptoms Attributed to Benign Prostatic Hyperplasia. J Urol 2021;206. https://www.auanet.org/guidelines-and-quality/guidelines/benign-prostatic-hyperplasia-(bph)-guideline.

Normal Bladder
detrusor muscle
contracting when
bladder is full

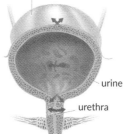

urine

urethra

Overactive Bladder
detrusor muscle
contracting before
bladder is full

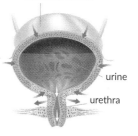

urine

urethra

iStock.com/Graphic_BKK1979

CHAPTER 52

URINARY INCONTINENCE

BACKGROUND

Urinary incontinence is a common and debilitating urinary disorder that affects many people. It is not a normal sign of aging. Overactive bladder (OAB) is a syndrome of bothersome urinary symptoms, including:

- Urinary urgency: a sudden feeling of needing to urinate. This is the primary symptom of OAB; it can occur with or without incontinence and is usually accompanied by urinary frequency and nocturia.

- Urinary frequency: voiding ≥ 8 times during waking hours.

- Nocturia: ≥ 2 awakenings in the night to urinate.

- Urinary incontinence: involuntary leakage of urine (see table for different forms).

About 1/3 of patients with OAB have incontinent episodes (OAB wet) and the other 2/3 of patients do not (OAB dry). Urge incontinence is a form of OAB wet that can be treated with the medications discussed in this chapter.

FORMS OF URINARY INCONTINENCE

Urge	A sudden and unstoppable urge to urinate. Associated with neuropathy and often present in those with diabetes, strokes, dementia, Parkinson disease or multiple sclerosis (although people without comorbidities can be affected).
Stress	Urine leaks out during any form of exertion (e.g., exercise, coughing, sneezing, laughing) as a result of pressure on the bladder.
Mixed	Combination of urge and stress incontinence.
Functional	There is no abnormality in the bladder, but the patient may be cognitively, socially or physically impaired thus hindering access to a toilet (e.g., patients in wheelchairs).
Overflow	Leakage that occurs when the quantity of urine stored in the bladder exceeds its capacity. Often occurs without the urge to urinate (BPH is the most common cause).

Many comorbidities exist in patients with OAB, including falls and fractures, skin breakdown and skin infections, UTIs, depression and sexual dysfunction. Due to the embarrassment of the condition, there are many social implications of OAB, including low self-esteem, lack of sexual intimacy, social and physical isolation, sleep disturbances, limits on travel and dependence on caregivers. These can lead to a reduced quality of life. Many patients become dehydrated because they limit fluid intake. The cost of pads and adult diapers can cause a financial burden.

PATHOPHYSIOLOGY AND ETIOLOGY

The bladder is commonly referred to as a "balloon" with an outer muscular layer known as the detrusor muscle. The detrusor muscle and the bladder outlet functions are neurologically coordinated to store and expel urine. The detrusor muscle is innervated mainly by the parasympathetic nervous system (acetylcholine acting on muscarinic receptors), while the bladder neck is innervated by the sympathetic nervous system. The internal sphincter is innervated by the sympathetic nervous system and the external sphincter is innervated by the somatic nervous system. Both voluntary and involuntary contractions of the detrusor muscle are mediated by acetylcholine activation of muscarinic receptors.

In OAB, there is inappropriate stimulation of the muscarinic receptors on the detrusor muscle causing involuntary contractions and the feeling of urinary urgency. This is a contraction of the bladder even when it is not full. Of the five known muscarinic receptor subtypes, the human bladder is comprised of M2 and M3 receptors in a 3:1 ratio. The M3 receptor is responsible for both emptying contractions as well as involuntary bladder contractions. Anticholinergic drugs inhibit the effects of acetylcholine on the M2 and M3 receptors. Similar to anticholinergics, the other drug used for OAB, mirabegron, causes relaxation of the detrusor muscle (prevents contraction) but it does so by acting as a beta-3 receptor agonist.

RISK FACTORS FOR OVERACTIVE BLADDER

Age > 40 years	Drugs that increase incontinence (e.g., alcohol, cholinesterase inhibitors, diuretics, sedatives)
Diabetes	
Prior vaginal delivery	Restricted mobility
Obesity	Hysterectomy
Neurologic conditions (e.g., Parkinson disease, stroke, dementia)	Pelvic injury

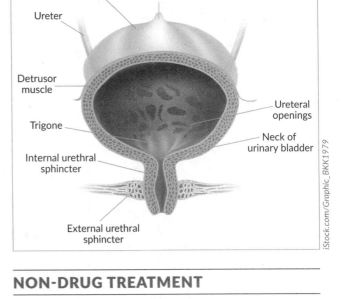

iStock.com/Graphic_BKK1979

NON-DRUG TREATMENT

Behavioral therapies are considered first-line to improve OAB symptoms. These include bladder training, delayed or scheduled voiding, pelvic floor muscle exercises (Kegel exercises), urge control techniques (distraction, self-assertions), fluid management, dietary changes (avoiding bladder irritants, such as caffeine), weight loss and other lifestyle measures (e.g., stopping medications that can worsen OAB; or with diuretics, changing the time of administration to avoid nocturia).

Behavioral therapies can be combined with other treatment modalities, such as medications. Surgical intervention should be reserved for the rare non-neurogenic patient who has failed all other therapeutic options and whose symptoms are intolerable.

Proper technique of Kegel exercises is key. Instruct the patient to imagine that they are trying to stop urination midstream. Squeeze the muscles they would use. If they sense a "pulling" feeling, those are the correct muscles for pelvic exercise. Pull in the pelvic muscles and hold for a count of three, then relax for a count of three. Patients should work up to three sets of ten exercises per day to reduce wetting episodes.

DRUG TREATMENT

A step-wise approach is recommended that begins conservatively with behavioral therapy (see previous section). Treatment depends on the degree of severity felt by the patient; with severe symptoms, treatment can begin at a higher level (see algorithm). Drugs are added to the behavioral recommendations (e.g., Kegel exercises, bladder training, weight loss), when needed.

URGE INCONTINENCE/MIXED INCONTINENCE

Mixed incontinence has an urge incontinence component and is treated in a similar manner. First-line drugs include anticholinergics (e.g., oxybutynin) or a beta-3 receptor agonist (e.g., mirabegron). OnabotulinumtoxinA *(Botox)* has higher efficacy but is not first-line due to cost and the route of administration through the urethra and into the detrusor muscle. Nerve stimulation or surgical intervention is used last.

Women with postmenopausal symptoms of vulvar and vaginal atrophy can use vaginal estrogen in a cream or a ring, which may provide modest relief of symptoms. Estrogen is not FDA-approved for this purpose. See the Osteoporosis, Menopause & Testosterone Use chapter.

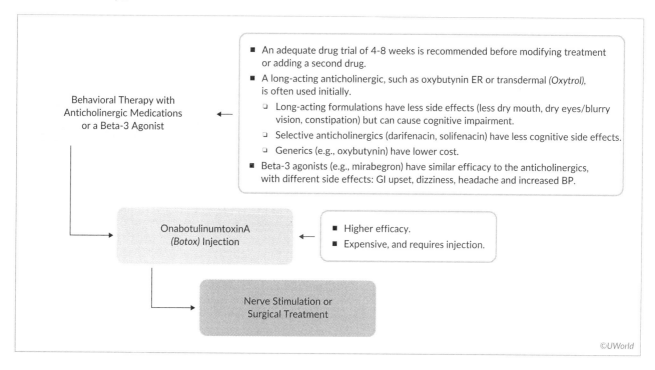

Behavioral Therapy with Anticholinergic Medications or a Beta-3 Agonist

- An adequate drug trial of 4-8 weeks is recommended before modifying treatment or adding a second drug.
- A long-acting anticholinergic, such as oxybutynin ER or transdermal *(Oxytrol)*, is often used initially.
  - Long-acting formulations have less side effects (less dry mouth, dry eyes/blurry vision, constipation) but can cause cognitive impairment.
  - Selective anticholinergics (darifenacin, solifenacin) have less cognitive side effects.
  - Generics (e.g., oxybutynin) have lower cost.
- Beta-3 agonists (e.g., mirabegron) have similar efficacy to the anticholinergics, with different side effects: GI upset, dizziness, headache and increased BP.

OnabotulinumtoxinA *(Botox)* Injection

- Higher efficacy.
- Expensive, and requires injection.

Nerve Stimulation or Surgical Treatment

©UWorld

STRESS INCONTINENCE

The medications used for stress incontinence are not FDA-approved for this use and have minimal efficacy, but there is a lack of more effective options. Pseudoephedrine, an agonist of norepinephrine (NE) and epinephrine (Epi), causes adrenaline-type effects, including tachycardia, palpitations, nervousness/anxiety, headache and insomnia. Duloxetine is commonly chosen when it is possible to treat two conditions with one drug (e.g., incontinence/depression), though it has little efficacy for incontinence (see the Depression chapter).

ANTICHOLINERGIC DRUGS

Anticholinergic drugs, also called antimuscarinic drugs, competitively bind to muscarinic receptors and block acetylcholine from binding. This limits contractions of the detrusor muscle. Extended-release formulations are preferred over immediate-release formulations due to a lower risk of dry mouth. Drugs that are more selective for the M3 receptor (solifenacin, darifenacin and fesoterodine) have fewer CNS side effects than the older, non-selective drugs, such as oxybutynin. The Beers Criteria recommend avoiding anticholinergics in patients aged 65 years and older, due to a risk of delirium and cognitive impairment.

DRUG	DOSING	SAFETY/SIDE EFFECTS/MONITORING
Oxybutynin IR	5 mg PO BID-QID	**CONTRAINDICATIONS** Uncontrolled narrow angle glaucoma, urinary retention, gastric retention, decreased gastric motility
Oxybutynin ER (Ditropan XL)	5-30 mg PO daily	
Oxybutynin patch (Oxytrol – Rx, Oxytrol for Women – OTC)	Apply one patch (3.9 mg/day) twice weekly (every 3-4 days; OTC patch is changed every 4 days)	*Oxytrol for Women* OTC: pain or burning when urinating, blood in urine, unexplained lower back or side pain, cloudy or foul-smelling urine, male sex, age < 18 years, urinary or gastric retention, glaucoma, accidental urine loss only due to coughing, sneezing or laughing
Oxybutynin 10% topical gel (*Gelnique*)	Apply contents of 1 sachet (or 1 pump) daily	**WARNINGS** Agitation, confusion, drowsiness, dizziness, blurred vision, hallucinations, and/or headache, which may impair physical or mental abilities; use caution if performing tasks which require mental alertness (e.g., operating machinery, driving)
Tolterodine (*Detrol*)	1-2 mg PO BID	Angioedema of the face, lips, tongue and/or larynx
Tolterodine ER (*Detrol LA*)	2-4 mg PO daily	**SIDE EFFECTS** Dizziness and drowsiness (greatest with oxybutynin and less with the newer, selective drugs), xerostomia (dry mouth), constipation, dry eyes/blurred vision, urinary retention, application site reactions (with topical gel and patch)
Trospium IR	20 mg PO BID	
Trospium XR	60 mg PO daily	
	Take on an empty stomach	**NOTES** ↓ dose in renal impairment (CrCl < 30 mL/min) with fesoterodine, solifenacin, tolterodine, and trospium (do not use trospium XR)
Solifenacin (*Vesicare*)	5-10 mg PO daily	*Ditropan XL* is an OROS formulation (see the Drug Formulations and Patient Counseling chapter) and can leave a ghost shell (empty shell) in the stool
Darifenacin	7.5-15 mg PO daily	Oxybutynin patch and gel cause less dry mouth and constipation than oral forms *Oxytrol* patch should be placed on dry, intact skin on the abdomen, hips or buttocks; avoid reapplication to the same site within 7 days; available OTC for women ≥ 18 years
Fesoterodine (*Toviaz*)	4-8 mg PO daily	Package labeling is not clear if metals may be present in *Oxytrol* patch (Rx and OTC); consider removing before MRI *Gelnique* should be applied to dry, intact skin on the abdomen, thighs or upper arms/shoulders; rotate application sites (do not use same site on consecutive days)

ANTICHOLINERGIC SIDE EFFECTS

Peripheral:	Central:
Dry mouth	Sedation
Dry eyes/blurred vision	Dizziness
Urinary retention	Cognitive impairment
Constipation	
Tachycardia	

Anticholinergic Drug Interactions

- Additive effects can be seen when used with other medications that have anticholinergic side effects.

- The lowest dose of tolterodine, solifenacin, darifenacin and fesoterodine should be used if the patient is taking strong CYP450 3A4 inhibitors.

- Acetylcholinesterase inhibitors used for dementia (e.g., donepezil) increase acetylcholine in the CNS. Although

DECREASING RISK OF DRY MOUTH

Dry mouth is a major reason that patients fail to comply with anticholinergic treatment.

Choosing a treatment that minimizes dry mouth can improve adherence.

- Try extended-release formulations (lower risk than IR formulations).

- Try oxybutynin gel or patch (lower risk than oral formulations).

- Beta-3 agonists have a lower incidence of dry mouth and can be helpful in patients who cannot tolerate anticholinergics.

- Try non-drug options to help with symptoms: avoid mouthwashes with alcohol, use ice chips, water, sugar-free candy or gum.

OAB drugs primarily stay in the periphery (outside the CNS), some patients can experience CNS side effects (e.g., memory impairment). While this is not a drug interaction, use of anticholinergic drugs can worsen dementia symptoms. The risk versus benefit must be considered.

BETA-3 AGONISTS

Beta-3 agonists <u>relax the detrusor muscle</u> and increase bladder capacity by <u>activating beta-3 receptors</u>. Mirabegron and vibegron have similar efficacy to anticholinergic drugs but cause <u>less dry mouth</u>. They can be used in combination with anticholinergic drugs or as monotherapy.

DRUG	DOSING	SAFETY/SIDE EFFECTS/MONITORING
Mirabegron (Myrbetriq)	25-50 mg PO daily CrCl 15-29 mL/min: 25 mg daily CrCl < 15 mL/min: not recommended	**WARNINGS** Urinary retention in patients with BPH and when used with anticholinergic drugs Mirabegron: ↑ BP, angioedema of the face, lips, tongue and/or larynx **SIDE EFFECTS** Nasopharyngitis, headache, constipation, diarrhea, dizziness
Vibegron (Gemtesa)	75 mg PO daily	Mirabegron: UTI **MONITORING** Urinary symptoms Mirabegron: BP **NOTES** Efficacy seen within 8 weeks

Beta-3 Agonist Drug Interactions

- Mirabegron is a moderate CYP2D6 inhibitor. Use caution in combination with narrow therapeutic drugs metabolized by CYP2D6. Levels of metoprolol are increased when co-administered with mirabegron. Levels of tamoxifen are decreased when co-administered with mirabegron. Use caution in combination with digoxin (use lowest digoxin dose and monitor levels).

ONABOTULINUMTOXINA (BOTOX)

Botox is a <u>third-line treatment</u> for patients who are <u>refractory</u> to first- and second-line treatment options. It affects the detrusor activity by inhibiting the release of acetylcholine.

DRUG	DOSING	SAFETY/SIDE EFFECTS/MONITORING
OnabotulinumtoxinA (Botox)	100 units total dose, administered as 0.5 mL (5 units) injections, across 20 sites (given intradetrusor) – repeat no sooner than 12 weeks from previous administration In adults treated with Botox for more than one indication, do not exceed a total dose of 360 units in a 3-month interval	**BOXED WARNING** All botulinum toxin products may spread from the area of injection to produce symptoms consistent with botulinum toxin effects; swallowing and breathing difficulties can be life-threatening **CONTRAINDICATIONS** Infection at the targeted injection site, urinary tract infection, urinary retention **SIDE EFFECTS** Urinary tract infection, urinary retention, dysuria **MONITORING** Post void residual volume, symptoms of OAB **NOTES** Potency units of Botox are not interchangeable with other preparations of botulinum toxin products Prophylactic antimicrobial therapy (excluding aminoglycosides) should be administered 1-3 days prior to, on the day of, and for 1-3 days following Botox administration

Botox Drug Interactions

- Aminoglycosides and drugs affecting neuromuscular transmission can increase the side effects of Botox.

NOCTURIA TREATMENT

The only medication FDA-approved for the treatment of nocturia in adults is desmopressin, an antidiuretic hormone analog that temporarily decreases urine production. It is administered before bed to prevent patients from having to urinate during the night.

DRUG	DOSING	SAFETY/SIDE EFFECTS/MONITORING
Desmopressin tablet *(DDAVP)* SL tablet *(Nocdurna)* Nasal spray *(DDAVP)* Injection *(DDAVP)* Diabetes insipidus – *DDAVP* tablet, nasal spray, injection Hemophilia A – *DDAVP* injection, *Stimate* von Willebrand's disease – *DDAVP* injection, *Stimate*	0.2-0.6 mg at bedtime Females: 27.7 mcg 1 hour before bedtime Males: 55.3 mcg 1 hour before bedtime	**BOXED WARNING** Severe, life-threatening hyponatremia can develop **CONTRAINDICATIONS** Patients with increased risk of severe hyponatremia (e.g., excessive fluid intake, illnesses or drugs that can cause fluid or electrolyte imbalances, including chronic kidney disease, SIADH, loop diuretics, systemic or inhaled glucocorticoids) and patients with increased risk of fluid retention (e.g., uncontrolled hypertension, heart failure) **WARNINGS** Do not use with nasal conditions (nasal spray) **SIDE EFFECTS** Hyponatremia, headache, hypertension, xerostomia *(Nocdurna)* **MONITORING** Serum Na (baseline, 1 week and 1 month)

KEY COUNSELING POINTS

See the Drug Formulations and Patient Counseling chapter for counseling language/layman's terminology.

ANTICHOLINERGICS

- Can cause:
  - ❑ Dry mouth.
  - ❑ Constipation.
  - ❑ Dizziness.
- Avoid mouthwashes with alcohol, and use ice chips, sugar-free candy or gum to help with dry mouth symptoms.

Oxybutynin XL *(Ditropan XL)*
- Ghost tablet in stool.

Oxytrol Patch

- Open one pouch and apply one patch to clean, dry, intact skin on the abdomen, hips or buttocks. Avoid applying the patch on your waistline, since tight clothing can rub the patch off.
- Apply a new patch twice weekly. Select a new site for each new patch (avoid reapplication to the same site within seven days).

DESMOPRESSIN

- Can cause low sodium.

Select Guidelines/References
AUA/SUFU Guideline: Diagnosis and Treatment of Overactive Bladder (Non-Neurogenic) In Adults. J Urol 2019;202:55. https://www.auanet.org/guidelines-and-quality/guidelines/overactive-bladder-(oab)-guideline.

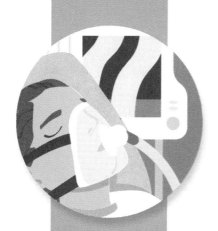
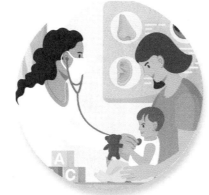
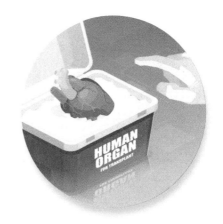

SPECIAL POPULATIONS

CONTENTS

CONTENT LEGEND

= Study Tip Gal   = Required Formula

iStock.com/shironosov

CHAPTER 53
ACUTE & CRITICAL CARE MEDICINE

BACKGROUND

When a patient is sick enough to require an advanced level of care, they are assessed for risk and admitted to either the hospital general medical unit (acute care) or the critical care/intensive care unit (ICU). If their illness has a high probability of imminent or life-threatening deterioration, treatment in the ICU is needed. The goal of critical care treatment is stabilization. If the illness is not as life-threatening, treatment in a general medical (acute care) unit is acceptable. The goal of acute care treatment is to diagnose and treat the illness, and return the patient to their normal state of health.

Common conditions and associated medications used in hospitalized general medical and critically ill patients are addressed in this chapter.

FLUIDS

CRYSTALLOIDS VS. COLLOIDS

Intravenous (IV) fluids, used to replace fluid losses and treat various conditions, are categorized as crystalloids or colloids. Crystalloids contain various concentrations of sodium and/or dextrose that pass freely between semipermeable membranes. Most of the administered volume does not remain in the intravascular space (inside the blood vessels), but moves into the extravascular or interstitial space. Crystalloids are less costly and generally have fewer adverse reactions than colloids. Balanced solutions (e.g., Lactated Ringer's) may be preferred in certain disease states, such as sepsis, since the chloride load from a sodium chloride solution can be high enough to contribute to cellular injury, including renal damage.

Colloids are large molecules (typically protein or starch) dispersed in a solution; they primarily remain in the intravascular space and ↑ oncotic pressure. Colloids provide greater intravascular volume expansion than equal volumes of crystalloids, but are more expensive and have not shown a clear clinical benefit over crystalloids.

Many different crystalloid and colloid products are available, including combination formulations (e.g., D5NS). Dextrose-containing products contain "free water" and are used when water is needed intracellularly. Lactated Ringer's and normal saline are the most common fluids used for volume resuscitation in shock states (see the Types of Shock section). Albumin is the most commonly used colloid and is particularly useful when there is significant edema (e.g., cirrhosis); albumin should not be used for nutritional supplementation when serum albumin is low. Hydroxyethyl starch should only be used if other treatments are unavailable due to its boxed warning for mortality, renal injury and coagulopathy (bleeding).

CLASS	COMMON FLUIDS
Crystalloids	**5% Dextrose (D5W)***
	0.9% NaCl (normal saline, NS)*
	Lactated Ringer's (LR) – contains NaCl, KCl, CaCl$_2$, Na-lactate (lactate is converted to bicarbonate)
	Multiple electrolyte injection (**Plasma-Lyte A,** others)
Colloids	**Albumin 5%, 25% (Albutein, AlbuRx,** others)
	Dextran
	Hydroxyethyl starch (Hespan, Hextend)

There are various crystalloid concentrations and combinations including: D50, D5NS, D5½NS, ½NS

ELECTROLYTE DISORDERS

Electrolyte abnormalities are common in hospitalized general medical and critically ill patients, though they can also occur in nonhospitalized patients. There are many causes (see specific electrolyte sections that follow). Electrolyte abnormalities can lead to severe complications (e.g., seizures, cardiac arrhythmias, coma, death). Electrolyte replacement protocols, used to correct deficiencies, should be followed to avoid toxicity. Electrolytes and their reference ranges are discussed in the Lab Values & Drug Monitoring chapter.

SODIUM

Hyponatremia

Hyponatremia (Na < 135 mEq/L) is usually not symptomatic until the sodium is ≤ 120 mEq/L, unless the serum level falls rapidly (e.g., acute hyponatremia). Symptoms most often result from cerebral edema and increased intracranial pressure, and can range from mild-moderate (e.g., headache, confusion, lethargy, gait disturbances) to severe (e.g., seizures, coma, respiratory arrest).

Hyponatremia is classified according to serum osmolality and volume status:

- Hypotonic hypervolemic hyponatremia is caused by fluid overload (e.g., cirrhosis, heart failure, renal failure). Diuresis with fluid restriction is the preferred treatment.

- Hypotonic isovolemic (euvolemic) hyponatremia can be caused by the syndrome of inappropriate antidiuretic hormone (SIADH). Treatment includes diuresis, restricting fluids and stopping drugs that can induce SIADH. Demeclocycline can be used off-label for SIADH.

- Hypotonic hypovolemic hyponatremia can be caused by diuretics, salt-wasting syndromes, adrenal insufficiency, blood loss or vomiting/diarrhea. The treatment is to correct any underlying causes and stop intake of hypotonic solutions; patients with acute hyponatremia, severe symptoms and/or Na < 120 mEq/L are candidates for hypertonic (3%) sodium chloride IV (see correction goals and risks below).

Hyponatremia should not be corrected too quickly (a typical goal is 4 – 8 mEq/L/24 hours). Correcting sodium more rapidly than 12 mEq/L/24 hours can cause osmotic demyelination syndrome (ODS) or central pontine myelinolysis, which can cause paralysis, seizures and death. Administration of desmopressin reduces water diuresis and can help avoid overcorrection.

The arginine vasopressin (AVP) receptor antagonists (conivaptan and tolvaptan) may be used to treat SIADH and hypervolemic hyponatremia. They increase excretion of free water while maintaining sodium. The role of these drugs is still being determined, as they are more expensive than 3% saline and use beyond 30 days with the oral product, tolvaptan, is not recommended.

Arginine Vasopressin Receptor Antagonists

DRUG	DOSE	SAFETY/SIDE EFFECTS/MONITORING
Conivaptan *(Vaprisol)* Injection Dual AVP antagonist [vasopressin 1A (V1A) and vasopressin 2 (V2)]	LD: 20 mg IV over 30 minutes MD: 20 mg continuous IV infusion over 24 hours; can ↑ to 40 mg IV daily if Na does not ↑ at desired rate; do not use > 4 days CrCl < 30 mL/min: avoid ↓ dose in moderate and severe hepatic impairment	**CONTRAINDICATIONS** Hypovolemic hyponatremia, concurrent use with strong CYP450 3A4 inhibitors, anuria **WARNING** Overly rapid correction of hyponatremia (> 12 mEq/L/24 hours) is associated with ODS (life-threatening) **SIDE EFFECTS** Orthostatic hypotension, fever, hypokalemia, infusion site reactions (> 60%) **MONITORING** Rate of Na increase, BP, volume status, urine output
Tolvaptan (*Samsca*, *Jynarque)* Tablet Selective AVP antagonist [vasopressin 2 (V2) only]	15 mg PO daily; max 60 mg PO daily; limited to ≤ 30 days due to hepatotoxicity CrCl < 10 mL/min: avoid Avoid fluid restriction in the first 24 hours of therapy	**BOXED WARNINGS** Should be initiated and re-initiated in a hospital with close monitoring of serum Na Overly rapid correction of hyponatremia (> 12 mEq/L/24 hours) is associated with ODS (life-threatening); consider slower correction with severe malnutrition, alcoholism or advanced liver disease **CONTRAINDICATIONS** Patients who are unable to sense or respond appropriately to thirst, urgent need to raise Na, hypovolemic hyponatremia, use with strong CYP3A4 inhibitors, anuria **WARNINGS** Hepatotoxicity (avoid use > 30 days and in liver disease/cirrhosis) **SIDE EFFECTS** Thirst, nausea, dry mouth, polyuria, weakness, hyperglycemia, hypernatremia **MONITORING** Rate of Na increase, BP, volume status, urine output, signs of drug-induced hepatotoxicity

LD = loading dose, MD = maintenance dose

Hypernatremia

Hypernatremia (Na > 145 mEq/L) is associated with a water deficit and hypertonicity.

- Hypovolemic hypernatremia is caused by dehydration, vomiting or diarrhea and is treated with fluids.

- Hypervolemic hypernatremia is caused by intake of hypertonic fluids and is treated with diuresis.

- Isovolemic (euvolemic) hypernatremia is frequently caused by diabetes insipidus (DI), which can ↓ antidiuretic hormone (ADH). It is treated with desmopressin.

POTASSIUM

Hyperkalemia is often due to chronic kidney disease, discussed in the Renal Disease chapter. This section discusses hypokalemia.

Hypokalemia, or potassium (K) < 3.5 mEq/L, is a common occurrence in hospitalized patients. In general, a drop of 1 mEq/L in serum K below 3.5 mEq/L represents a total body deficit of 100 – 400 mEq. Management includes treating the underlying cause [e.g., metabolic alkalosis, overdiuresis, medications (such as amphotericin, insulin)] and administering oral or IV potassium. The oral route is preferred for potassium replacement when feasible. Oral potassium salt formulations are reviewed in the Chronic Heart Failure chapter. Some hospitals use potassium sliding scales that allow a healthcare provider (usually a nurse) to administer a certain dose of potassium based on the serum potassium level in patients with normal kidney function (see example protocol below).

EXAMPLE POTASSIUM REPLACEMENT PROTOCOL

Step 1: check phosphate level. If > 2.5 mg/dL, proceed to step 2. If ≤ 2.5 mg/dL, use separate potassium phosphate replacement protocol.

Step 2: provide replacement doses as follows.

SERUM POTASSIUM (MEQ/L)	INSTRUCTION
< 2.6	100 mEq KCl IV; contact MD
2.6-2.9	80 mEq KCl IV; contact MD
3.0-3.2	60 mEq KCl PO/IV
3.3-3.5	40 mEq KCl PO/IV

Step 3: order follow-up labs. For K < 3.2 mEq/L, recheck immediately and with AM labs. For K ≥ 3.2 mEq/L, recheck with AM labs only.

Potassium chloride premixed IV solutions are generally used for IV replacement. Safe recommendations for administration of IV potassium through a peripheral line include a maximum infusion rate ≤ 10 mEq/hr and a maximum concentration of 10 mEq/100 mL. More rapid infusions and higher concentrations may be warranted in severe or symptomatic hypokalemia; these require a central line and cardiac monitoring. IV potassium can be fatal if administered undiluted or via IV push. When hypokalemia is resistant to treatment, serum magnesium should be checked. Magnesium is necessary for potassium uptake; hypomagnesemia can worsen and/or prevent correction of hypokalemia. Magnesium should be replaced first when both hypokalemia and hypomagnesemia are present.

MAGNESIUM

Hypomagnesemia, or magnesium (Mg) < 1.3 mEq/L, is more common than hypermagnesemia, which is most often due to renal insufficiency. Common causes of hypomagnesemia include chronic alcohol use, diuretics, amphotericin B, vomiting and diarrhea. When serum Mg is ≤ 1 mEq/L with life-threatening symptoms (e.g., seizures, arrhythmias), IV magnesium sulfate replacement is recommended. When serum Mg is < 1 mEq/L without life-threatening symptoms, therapy can be administered IV or IM. When serum Mg is > 1 mEq/L and < 1.5 mEq/L, magnesium is replaced orally, most commonly with magnesium oxide. Magnesium replacement regimens should continue for 5 days to fully replace body stores.

PHOSPHORUS

Hyperphosphatemia is often due to chronic kidney disease, and is discussed in the Renal Disease chapter. This section discusses hypophosphatemia.

Hypophosphatemia is considered severe and is usually symptomatic when serum phosphate (PO4) is < 1 mg/dL. Symptoms can include muscle weakness and respiratory failure. Hypophosphatemia can be caused by phosphate-binding drugs (e.g., calcium salts, sevelamer), chronic alcohol intake and hyperparathyroidism. When serum PO4 is ≤ 1 mg/dL, IV phosphorus is used for replacement. Many regimens can be used, but 0.08 – 0.16 mmol/kg in 500 mL of NS or D5W over 6 hours is common. Patients must be carefully monitored and additional doses may be necessary. Patients with hypophosphatemia often have hypokalemia and hypomagnesemia that will require correction. Less severe hypophosphatemia can be treated orally and full replacement often takes one week or longer.

OTHER TREATMENTS IN HOSPITALIZED PATIENTS

VTE PROPHYLAXIS

People in the hospital often have limited mobility and other risk factors for developing a venous thromboembolism (VTE). For this reason, the need for VTE prophylaxis should be evaluated in all inpatients. Refer to the Anticoagulation chapter for a discussion on VTE prophylaxis treatment.

INCENTIVE SPIROMETRY

Incentive spirometry is a technique used to facilitate lung expansion in patients with atelectasis (i.e., completely or partially collapsed lung with reduced lung volume). Atelectasis is a common complication in hospitalized patients, especially post-operatively, and can lead to retained airway secretions, dyspnea, hypoxemia and other pulmonary complications (e.g., pneumonia). An incentive spirometer is a mechanical device that facilitates deep breathing (with use of a visual indicator that provides feedback on breathing quality); deep breathing, along with other interventions (e.g., head of bed elevation, coughing, ambulation), helps keep lung alveoli open and promotes secretion removal.

INTRAVENOUS IMMUNOGLOBULIN

Intravenous immune globulin (IVIG or IGIV) contains pooled immunoglobulin (IgG) that is administered intravenously. The IgG is extracted from the plasma of a thousand or more blood donors (this is the FDA's minimum; typically the IVIG is derived from between 3,000 – 10,000 donors). IVIG is given as plasma protein replacement therapy for immune-deficient patients who have decreased or abolished antibody production capabilities. Initially, IVIG was used only for immunodeficiency conditions. Currently, IVIG has several FDA-approved indications and is used for a variety of off-label indications (e.g., multiple sclerosis, myasthenia gravis, Guillain-Barré syndrome) with varying results. IVIG treatment can impair the response to vaccination (refer to the Immunizations chapter for a discussion on the timing of vaccinations and antibody-containing products).

DRUG	DOSING	SAFETY/SIDE EFFECTS/MONITORING
Intravenous immunoglobulin (*Gammagard, Gamunex-C, Octagam, Privigen,* others)	Indication and product specific IBW or AdjBW is usually used to calculate the dose Use a slower infusion rate in renal and CV disease patients Do not freeze, shake or heat	**BOXED WARNINGS** Acute renal dysfunction can occur (rare) and has been associated with fatalities; it usually occurs within 7 days (more likely with products stabilized with sucrose); use caution in the elderly, those with renal disease, diabetes, volume depletion, sepsis, paraproteinemia or taking nephrotoxic medications Thrombosis can occur even without risk factors; for patients at risk, administer the minimum dose **CONTRAINDICATIONS** IgA deficiency (use the product with the lowest amount of IgA) **WARNINGS** Use with caution in CV disease (use isotonic products and a lower infusion rate) **SIDE EFFECTS** Headache, nausea, diarrhea, injection site reaction, infusion reaction (facial flushing, chest tightness, fever, chills, hypotension – slow/stop infusion), renal failure or blood dyscrasias (both rare) **MONITORING** Renal function, urine output, volume status, Hgb **NOTES** Patients should be asked about past IVIG infusions, including product used and any reactions that occurred; a slower titration and premedication may be needed Lot numbers of administered IVIG products must be tracked (it is a blood product)

CRITICAL CARE

For life-threatening injuries or illnesses that require specialized care, treatment is often initiated pre-hospital or in an emergency department and continued in the ICU. Large hospitals have specialized ICUs for different types of care (e.g., medical, surgical, cardiovascular, trauma, pediatric, neonatal). Many medications in the ICU are administered IV with an infusion pump, which bypasses gut/absorption issues and allows for a rapid onset of effect, easy titration and continuous administration. Often, a central line is used; this is especially important with vesicants and IV solutions that can contribute to phlebitis.

The ICU mortality rate in the U.S. is ~15%. The Acute Physiologic Assessment and Chronic Health Evaluation II (APACHE II) is a scoring tool used to determine prognosis and estimate ICU mortality risk. With adequate care, most patients will recover and return home. Conditions that commonly require ICU care are addressed in the rest of this chapter.

ICU MEDICATIONS THAT TARGET THE SYMPATHETIC NERVOUS SYSTEM

VASOPRESSORS

Most vasopressors work by stimulating alpha receptors; this causes peripheral vasoconstriction (think "pressing down on the vasculature") and increases systemic vascular resistance (SVR), which increases blood pressure (BP). Vasopressors that stimulate beta receptors can increase heart rate (HR) and cardiac output (CO). Phenylephrine is a pure alpha-agonist that increases SVR without increasing HR. Epinephrine and norepinephrine are mixed alpha- and beta-agonists, causing an increase in SVR, CO and HR. Dopamine is a natural precursor of norepinephrine and has dose-dependent receptor effects.

> **DOPAMINE DOSING**
>
> Dopamine stimulates different receptors depending on the dose.
>
> - Low (renal) dose: 1-4 mcg/kg/min
>   - ❑ Dopamine-1 agonist
> - Medium dose: 5-10 mcg/kg/min
>   - ❑ Beta-1 agonist
> - High dose: 10-20 mcg/kg/min
>   - ❑ Alpha-1 agonist

Vasopressin and angiotensin II both increase SVR by unique mechanisms. Vasopressin acts directly on vasopressin receptors. Angiotensin II *(Giapreza)* raises blood pressure by vasoconstriction and aldosterone release, which results in sodium and water retention; due to a lack of robust evidence and clinical experience, it is not considered a first-line agent. Angiotensin II, a natural hormone produced in the renin-angiotensin-aldosterone system, is discussed in detail in the Hypertension chapter. A review of the nervous system and receptor pharmacology can be found in the Basic Science Concepts chapter.

DRUG	MOA	SAFETY/SIDE EFFECTS/MONITORING
Dopamine	Dose-dependent, see Study Tip Gal	**BOXED WARNING** Dopamine and norepinephrine have a boxed warning regarding extravasation; all vasopressors are vesicants when administered IV; treat extravasation with phentolamine
Epinephrine (Adrenalin) **EpiPen,** others – for anaphylaxis	Alpha-1, beta-1, beta-2 agonist	**WARNINGS** Use extreme caution in patients taking an MAO inhibitor; prolonged hypertension may result (dopamine, epinephrine and norepinephrine) **SIDE EFFECTS** Arrhythmias, tachycardia (especially dopamine, epinephrine), necrosis (gangrene), bradycardia (phenylephrine), hyperglycemia (epinephrine), tachyphylaxis, peripheral and gut ischemia
Norepinephrine (Levophed)	Alpha-1 agonist activity > beta-1 agonist activity	**MONITORING** Continuous BP monitoring (with continuous infusions), HR, mean arterial pressure (MAP), ECG, urine output, infusion site for extravasation
Phenylephrine	Alpha-1 agonist	**NOTES** Solutions should not be used if they are discolored or contain a precipitate All vasopressors are Y-site compatible with each other (except angiotensin II) Some institutions use non-weight-based infusions (mcg/min) instead of weight-based infusions (mcg/kg/min)
Vasopressin *(Vasostrict)* Known as arginine vasopressin (AVP) and antidiuretic hormone (ADH)	Vasopressin receptor agonist Vasoconstrictor, no inotropic or chronotropic effects	All vasopressors should be administered via central IV line There is no clear evidence that low dose dopamine (renal dosing) provides benefit Epinephrine used for IV push is 0.1 mg/mL (1:10,000 ratio strength); epinephrine used for IM injection or compounding IV products is 1 mg/mL (1:1,000 ratio strength); ratio strength has been removed from labeling per the FDA

Extravasation

Many drugs used in the ICU, including vasopressors, are vesicants that cause severe tissue damage/necrosis with extravasation (leakage of drug from the blood vessel into the surrounding tissue). This is a medical emergency. To reduce the risk, every attempt should be made to infuse vasopressors through a central line. Vasopressor extravasation should be treated with phentolamine, an alpha-1 blocker that antagonizes the effects of the vasopressor. If extravasation occurs with norepinephrine, epinephrine or phenylephrine, stop the infusion but do not disconnect the needle/cannula and do not flush the line; instead, gently aspirate (remove) the drug. Nitroglycerin ointment is sometimes used topically as an alternative if phentolamine is unavailable.

VASODILATORS

Vasodilators administered by continuous IV infusion include nitroglycerin (NTG) and nitroprusside. Frequent or continuous BP monitoring is required when using IV vasodilators, and doses must be decreased if there is hypotension or worsening renal function. NTG is often used when there is active myocardial ischemia or uncontrolled hypertension, but effectiveness may be limited to 24 – 48 hours due to tachyphylaxis (tolerance).

Nitroprusside is a mixed (equal) arterial and venous vasodilator at all doses. It has a greater effect on BP than NTG. It should not be used in active myocardial ischemia because it can cause blood to be diverted away from the diseased coronary arteries ("coronary steal"). The metabolism of nitroprusside results in thiocyanate and cyanide formation, which can cause toxicity in patients with renal or hepatic insufficiency, respectively. Hydroxocobalamin can be administered to reduce the risk of thiocyanate toxicity or to treat cyanide toxicity. Sodium thiosulfate + sodium nitrite (*Nithiodote*) is used for cyanide toxicity (see the Toxicology & Antidotes chapter).

DRUG	MOA	SAFETY/SIDE EFFECTS/MONITORING
Nitroglycerin See the Stable Ischemic Heart Disease chapter for other formulations	Low doses: venous vasodilator High doses: arterial vasodilator	**CONTRAINDICATIONS** SBP < 90 mmHg, use with PDE-5 inhibitors or riociguat **WARNINGS** Severe hypotension and ↑ intracranial pressure (ICP) **SIDE EFFECTS** Headache, tachycardia, tachyphylaxis (within 24-48 hours of continuous administration), lightheadedness **MONITORING** BP, HR **NOTES** Requires a non-PVC container (e.g., glass, polyolefin); use administration sets (tubing) intended for NTG
Nitroprusside *(Nipride)*	Mixed (equal) arterial and venous vasodilator	**BOXED WARNINGS** Metabolism produces cyanide (use the lowest dose for the shortest duration necessary), excessive hypotension (continuous BP monitoring required), not for direct injection (must be further diluted; D5W preferred) **WARNINGS** ↑ ICP **SIDE EFFECTS** Headache, tachycardia, thiocyanate/cyanide toxicity (risk ↑ in renal and hepatic impairment) **MONITORING** BP (continuous), HR, renal/hepatic function, urine output, s/sx of thiocyanate/cyanide toxicity, acid-base status, venous oxygen concentration **NOTES** Requires light protection during administration; use only clear solutions, a blue color indicates degradation to cyanide – do not use

INOTROPES

Intravenous inotropes <u>increase the contractility</u> of the heart. <u>Dobutamine</u> is a <u>beta-1 agonist</u> that increases HR and the force of myocardial contraction, which increases CO. It has weak beta-2 (vasodilation) and alpha-1 agonist activity. <u>Milrinone</u> is a selective <u>phosphodiesterase-3 inhibitor</u> in cardiac and vascular tissue. It produces inotropic effects with <u>significant vasodilation</u>. Dobutamine and milrinone should only be used when BP is adequate because they produce vasodilation.

DRUG	MOA	SAFETY/SIDE EFFECTS/MONITORING
Dobutamine	<u>Beta-1 agonist</u> with some beta-2 and alpha-1 agonism	**SIDE EFFECTS** Dobutamine: hyper/hypotension, ventricular arrhythmias, tachycardia, angina Milrinone: ventricular arrhythmias, hypotension **MONITORING** Continuous BP and ECG monitoring, HR, central venous pressure (CVP), MAP, urine output, LFTs and renal function (with milrinone)
Milrinone	<u>Phosphodiesterase-3 (PDE-3) inhibitor</u>	**NOTES** Milrinone: dose must be reduced for renal impairment Dobutamine may turn <u>slightly pink due to oxidation</u>, but potency is not lost Dobutamine and milrinone are often referred to as "inodilators" Risk of hypotension; use for inotropic effect only after adequate perfusion is achieved

TYPES OF SHOCK

Shock is a medical emergency common in ICU patients. It is characterized by <u>hypoperfusion</u>, usually in the setting of <u>hypotension</u>, defined as SBP < 90 mmHg or MAP < 70 mmHg. There are four main types of shock:

- Hypovolemic (e.g., hemorrhagic)
- Distributive (e.g., septic, anaphylactic)
- Cardiogenic (e.g., post-myocardial infarction)
- Obstructive (e.g., massive pulmonary embolism)

The diagnosis of shock is based on hemodynamic parameters, and more than one type of shock can occur at the same time. Drugs used for shock may also be used for advanced cardiac life support (ACLS)/cardiac arrest, hypotension during surgery/anesthesia, acute decompensated heart failure (ADHF) and other critical conditions.

HYPOVOLEMIC SHOCK

To treat hypovolemic shock, restore intravascular volume, and improve oxygen-carrying capacity. <u>Fluid resuscitation</u> with <u>crystalloids</u> is generally recommended <u>first-line</u> for <u>hypovolemic shock</u> that is <u>not caused by hemorrhage</u>. Blood products (e.g., packed red blood cells, fresh frozen plasma) should be administered in hypovolemic shock with intravascular depletion due to bleeding. If the patient does not respond to the initial crystalloid or blood product therapy ("fluid challenge"), then vasopressors may be indicated. <u>Vasopressors</u> will not be effective unless the <u>intravascular volume</u> is <u>adequate</u>.

DISTRIBUTIVE SHOCK

Distributive shock is characterized by low SVR, and initially high CO followed by low or normal CO. <u>Septic</u>, anaphylactic and neurogenic shock are examples of distributive shock.

Sepsis and Septic Shock

<u>Sepsis</u> is defined as <u>life-threatening organ dysfunction</u> caused by a <u>dysregulated host response to infection</u> (see the Study Tip Gal on the next page for common causes of ICU infections). Several screening tools, each using some different combination of criteria (e.g., tachypnea, tachycardia, hypotension, fever, decreased mental status), are available to evaluate for sepsis and infection-induced organ dysfunction. Tools such as the National Early Warning Score (NEWS) and systemic inflammatory response syndrome (SIRS) criteria are recommended over the quick Sequential Organ Failure Assessment (qSOFA).

GENERAL PRINCIPLES FOR TREATING SEPTIC SHOCK

Target a mean arterial pressure (MAP) of ≥ 65 mmHg

$$MAP = [(2 \times DBP) + SBP]/3$$

FILL THE TANK
Optimize preload with IV crystalloids (balanced fluids such as Lactated Ringer's preferred)

SQUEEZE THE PIPE AND KICK THE PUMP
Alpha-1 agonist activity (peripheral vasoconstriction) to ↑ SVR

Beta-1 agonist activity to ↑ myocardial contractility and CO

> **TWO COMMON CAUSES OF ICU INFECTIONS**
>
> **Mechanical ventilation: pushes air into the lungs for patients who cannot breathe on their own.**
>
> Mechanical ventilators are called respirators. Air flows into the trachea through an endotracheal tube (ET tube) placed through the mouth or nose. This is called intubation. "Weaning" refers to the process of getting the patient off the ventilator when they are ready to breathe on their own again.
>
> **↑ time on ventilator = ↑ risk of infection, including lung infections**
>
> *Pseudomonas* (and a few other organisms) thrive in the moist air in the ventilator.
>
> **Indwelling urinary catheter.**
>
> Intubated patients have an indwelling catheter that is inserted into the bladder to drain urine.
>
> Foley catheters are the most common type.
>
> **↑ time with Foley catheter = ↑ risk of bladder infection**

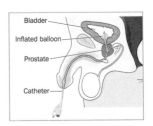

Septic shock is sepsis with persistent hypotension requiring a vasopressor to maintain MAP ≥ 65 mmHg and a serum lactate level ≥ 2 mEq/L, despite adequate fluid resuscitation.

The Surviving Sepsis Campaign is an initiative that prompts the use of selected evidence-based interventions (called "bundles") to reduce mortality from sepsis and septic shock. These bundles include early administration of broad-spectrum antibiotics and fluid resuscitation with IV crystalloids. When combined with additional measures, this is associated with lower overall mortality. If adequate perfusion cannot be maintained with IV crystalloids, vasopressors are used. Norepinephrine is considered the vasopressor of choice in septic shock. Vasopressin is commonly used in addition to norepinephrine.

ACUTE DECOMPENSATED HEART FAILURE AND CARDIOGENIC SHOCK

Patients with heart failure may experience episodes of worsening symptoms, such as sudden weight gain, an inability to lie flat without becoming short of breath, decreasing functionality (e.g., unable to perform their daily routine), increasing shortness of breath and fatigue. This is called acute decompensated heart failure (ADHF); when hypotension and hypoperfusion are also present, it is called cardiogenic shock.

Clinical Presentation and Assessment

ADHF is caused by worsening HF, a cardiac event (e.g., MI, arrhythmia, valvular disease, uncontrolled hypertension) or a non-cardiac cause (e.g., non-adherence with medications or dietary restrictions, worsening renal function, infection, illicit drug use). Negative inotropes (e.g., non-DHP CCBs), drugs that cause fluid retention (e.g., NSAIDs) and cardiotoxic drugs can worsen cardiac function and cause/exacerbate HF.

ADHF presents with volume overload, hypoperfusion or both. Some patients require invasive monitoring with a catheter that is guided through the right side of the heart into the pulmonary artery, called a Swan-Ganz or pulmonary artery catheter. The catheter provides hemodynamic measurements of congestion (pulmonary capillary wedge pressure, or PCWP), hypoperfusion (cardiac output) and other measurements (e.g., SVR, CVP) useful for guiding treatment. Treatment of ADHF generally consists of diuretics, inotropes and vasodilators, used in various combinations depending on the patient's symptoms (see the Study Tip Gal below). Beta-blockers should only be stopped in an ADHF episode if hypotension or hypoperfusion is present.

Treating Volume Overload

ADHF most commonly presents with volume overload. Volume overload is treated with diuretics and possibly IV vasodilators. Loop diuretics are initially given IV since volume overload also affects the vessels of the gut and can decrease oral drug absorption. If diuretic resistance develops, the dose can be increased or a thiazide-type diuretic (e.g., metolazone, chlorothiazide) can be added to the loop diuretic.

> **TREATING ADHF**
>
>
>
> Patients with edema (pulmonary or lower extremity), jugular venous distention (JVD) and/or ascites are **VOLUME OVERLOADED**; treatment options include:
>
> - Loop diuretics
> - Vasodilators can be added (NTG, nitroprusside)
>
> Patients with ↓ renal function, altered mental status and/or cool extremities have **HYPOPERFUSION***; treatment options include:
>
> - Inotropes (dobutamine, milrinone)
> - If the patient becomes hypotensive, consider adding a vasopressor (dopamine, norepinephrine, phenylephrine)
>
> Some patients experience both **VOLUME OVERLOAD** and **HYPOPERFUSION**; treatment options include:
>
> - A combination of agents above
>
> **Avoid vasodilators; these can ↓ BP and worsen hypoperfusion*

Treating Hypoperfusion

The most common cause of cardiogenic shock (or ADHF with hypoperfusion) is an MI, with resulting failure of the left ventricle. Cardiogenic shock requires treatment with vasopressors and/or inotropes. The vasodilatory and inotropic properties of dobutamine and milrinone make them uniquely suited to treat ADHF in patients with adequate BP and symptoms of both congestion and hypoperfusion. If BP is inadequate, inotropes will often be used in combination with vasopressors. Inotropes are associated with worse heart failure outcomes and should be stopped as soon as the patient is stabilized.

OTHER COMMON ICU CONDITIONS

PAIN

IV opioids (e.g., morphine, hydromorphone, fentanyl) are first-line for analgesia (to reduce pain) in the ICU (see the Pain chapter for a full discussion of opioids). The pharmacokinetic properties of the drug and the renal/hepatic function of the patient will dictate the choice of agent because all IV opioids exhibit similar analgesic efficacy when dosed correctly. Adjuvants (e.g., acetaminophen, NSAIDs) may be appropriate depending on the type of pain. An assessment of pain (with a validated pain scale) should be performed at least every 2 – 4 hours in the ICU, and all ICU patients should be evaluated for pain at rest. Analgesia-based sedation or "analgosedation" is a sedation strategy that uses analgesia first to relieve pain and discomfort, which are the primary causes of agitation. Compared to benzodiazepines, analgosedation is associated with less time on the ventilator and shorter ICU length of stay (LOS).

AGITATION

Sedation is necessary for some ICU patients to maintain synchronized breathing with the ventilator (prevent "bucking" the ventilator) and to limit suffering in the harsh ICU environment. Agitation is managed with benzodiazepines (lorazepam, midazolam) and/or non-benzodiazepine hypnotics (propofol, dexmedetomidine). Non-benzodiazepines (propofol and dexmedetomidine) are preferred for sedation and are associated with improved ICU outcomes, shorter mechanical ventilation duration and decreased LOS. Dexmedetomidine (Precedex) is the only sedative approved for use in intubated and non-intubated patients. Benzodiazepines have an important role in sedation in the presence of seizures or alcohol/benzodiazepine withdrawal. Benzodiazepines are discussed in the Anxiety chapter.

Sedatives are used with validated sedation scales that allow for titration to light sedation (preferred) or deep sedation. Common sedation scales include the Richmond Agitation Sedation Scale (RASS – see table below), the Ramsay Agitation Scale (RAS) and the Riker Sedation-Agitation Scale (SAS). The Glasgow Coma Scale is used to determine the level of consciousness (often after traumatic brain injury). Sedated patients should be monitored every 2 – 3 hours to make sure they are receiving the least amount of drug to keep them calm and pain-free. Daily interruptions ("sedation vacations") of continuous sedative infusions are used to assess readiness to wean off/stop the sedative as soon as possible.

DELIRIUM

Delirium assessment is required, as it affects up to 80% of ventilated ICU patients and is associated with increased mortality and LOS. Early mobilization and control of the patient's environment (light, noise, stimuli) are recommended to decrease delirium incidence, but no medications are recommended for prevention. Providing sedation with non-benzodiazepines may reduce the incidence of delirium and/or shorten the duration in patients who already have it. There is little evidence to support the use of haloperidol for treatment of ICU delirium, although this is common in practice. Atypical antipsychotics, primarily quetiapine, which is mildly sedating and has little risk for movement disorders, can be useful (see the Schizophrenia/Psychosis chapter).

RICHMOND AGITATION AND SEDATION SCALE (RASS)

SCORE	TERM	DESCRIPTION
+4	Combative	Overtly combative, violent, immediate danger to staff
+3	Very agitated	Pulls or removes tube(s) or catheter(s); aggressive
+2	Agitated	Frequent, non-purposeful movement, fights ventilator
+1	Restless	Anxious, but movements not aggressive or vigorous
0	Alert and calm	
-1	Drowsy	Not fully alert, but has sustained awakening (eye opening/eye contact) to voice (≥ 10 seconds)
-2	Light sedation	Briefly awakens with eye contact to voice (< 10 seconds)
-3	Moderate sedation	Movement or eye opening to voice (but no eye contact)
-4	Deep sedation	No response to voice, but movement or eye opening to physical stimulation
-5	Unarousable	No response to voice or physical stimulation

DRUG	SAFETY/SIDE EFFECTS/MONITORING
Pain/Analgesia	
Fentanyl (Sublimaze)	See the Pain chapter for additional information
	In critical care patients, monitor BP, HR, respiration, pain and sedation
Hydromorphone (Dilaudid)	Fentanyl: less hypotension (no histamine release) than morphine; 100x more potent than morphine; rapid onset and short duration of action (half-life increases with duration of infusion); can accumulate in hepatic impairment; CYP3A4 substrate and potential for numerous drug interactions
Morphine (Duramorph, Infumorph)	
Remifentanil (Ultiva)	Hydromorphone: very potent, dose carefully
Oliceridine (Olinvyk)	
Agitation/Sedation	
Dexmedetomidine (Precedex) Alpha-2 adrenergic agonist *Igalmi* – sublingual film indicated for agitation associated with schizophrenia or bipolar disorder	**WARNINGS** Use with caution in patients with hepatic impairment, diabetes, heart block, bradycardia, severe ventricular dysfunction, hypovolemia or chronic hypertension **SIDE EFFECTS** Hypo/hypertension, bradycardia, dry mouth, nausea, constipation **MONITORING** BP, HR, sedation scale **NOTES** Does not require refrigeration Duration of infusion should not exceed 24 hours per FDA labeling Used for sedation in intubated and non-intubated patients; patients are arousable and alert when stimulated (less respiratory depression than other sedatives)
Propofol (Diprivan) Short-acting general anesthetic	**CONTRAINDICATIONS** Hypersensitivity to egg, egg product, soy or soy product **SIDE EFFECTS** Hypotension, apnea, hypertriglyceridemia, green urine/hair/nail beds, propofol-related infusion syndrome (PRIS – rare, but can be fatal), myoclonus, pancreatitis, pain on injection (particularly peripheral vein), QT prolongation **MONITORING** BP, HR, RR, sedation scale, triglycerides (if administered longer than 2 days), signs and symptoms of pancreatitis **NOTES** Shake well before use; do not use if there is separation of phases in the emulsion Use strict aseptic technique due to potential for bacterial growth; discard vial and tubing within 12 hours of use If transferred to a syringe prior to administration, must discard syringe within 6 hours Do not use a filter < 5 microns for administration Does not require refrigeration Oil-in-water emulsion (opaque, white solution); provides 1.1 kcal/mL
Lorazepam (Ativan, *Lorazepam Intensol***)** Benzodiazepine	**NOTES** Injection is formulated in propylene glycol; total daily dose as low as 1 mg/kg/day can cause propylene glycol toxicity (acute renal failure and metabolic acidosis) In critical care patients, monitor BP, HR, RR, sedation scale, s/sx of propylene glycol toxicity (BUN, SCr, lactate, anion gap) if receiving continuous infusion; limit use for delirium See the Anxiety chapter for additional information

DRUG	SAFETY/SIDE EFFECTS/MONITORING
Midazolam *(Versed*, Nayzilam)* Benzodiazepine Used specifically in acute care settings	**BOXED WARNINGS** Respiratory depression, respiratory arrest, apnea; start at lower end of dosing range in debilitated patients and geriatric population; do not administer by rapid IV injection in neonates **CONTRAINDICATIONS** Intrathecal or epidural administration (benzyl alcohol in formulation), acute narrow-angle glaucoma, <u>do not use with potent CYP3A4 inhibitors</u> **SIDE EFFECTS** Hypotension **MONITORING** BP, HR, RR, sedation scale **NOTES** Shorter acting than lorazepam if patient has normal organ function (no hepatic or renal impairment or HF) Can accumulate in obese patients (highly lipophilic) and <u>renal impairment (active metabolite)</u> – caution with continuous infusion
Etomidate *(Amidate)* Nonbarbiturate hypnotic Ultra short-acting; used as an induction agent for intubation	**WARNING** Inhibits 11-B-hydroxylase which can lead to ↓ cortisol production for up to 24 hours **MONITORING** S/sx of <u>adrenal insufficiency</u> (hypotension, hyperkalemia), respiratory status, BP, HR, infusion site, sedation scale
Ketamine *(Ketalar)* NMDA receptor antagonist Used as an induction agent for intubation; used off-label for continuous sedation, pain and other indications	**WARNINGS** <u>Emergence reactions</u> (vivid dreams, hallucinations, delirium), cerebrospinal fluid (CSF) pressure elevation, respiratory depression/apnea, dependence/tolerance **MONITORING** BP, HR, respiratory status, emergence reactions, sedation scale **NOTES** Pretreatment with benzodiazepine can ↓ incidence of emergence reactions (see warnings) by 50%

Delirium

Haloperidol *(Haldol*)*	See the Schizophrenia/Psychosis chapter
	Commonly used, but not recommended for treatment of delirium in current guidelines
Quetiapine (Seroquel)	See the Schizophrenia/Psychosis chapter
	May decrease duration of delirium

Brand discontinued but name still used in practice.

STRESS ULCERS

In patients with critical illness, blood flow is diverted to the body's major organs and there is reduced blood flow to the gut. This results in a breakdown of gastric mucosal defense mechanisms, including prostaglandin synthesis, bicarbonate production and cell turnover, which can lead to stress ulcers.

RISK FACTORS FOR THE DEVELOPMENT OF STRESS ULCERS	
Mechanical ventilation > 48H	Major burns
Coagulopathy	Acute renal failure
Sepsis	High dose systemic steroids
Traumatic brain injury	

Histamine-2 receptor antagonists (H2RAs) and proton pump inhibitors (PPIs) are recommended to prevent stress-related mucosal damage in patients with risk factors (see box). H2RAs can cause thrombocytopenia and mental status changes in the elderly or those with renal impairment. Tachyphylaxis has also been reported. PPIs are associated with an increased risk of GI infections (*C. difficile*), fractures and nosocomial pneumonia. These drugs are discussed further in the Gastroesophageal Reflux Disease (GERD) & Peptic Ulcer Disease (PUD) chapter.

ADDITIONAL DRUGS USED IN THE ICU AND OPERATING ROOM

ANESTHETICS

Anesthetics are used for a variety of effects, including to numb an area (local anesthesia), block pain (regional anesthesia) or cause a reversible loss of consciousness and sleepiness during surgery (general anesthesia). Anesthetics can be given via several routes of administration: topical, inhaled, intravenous, epidural or spinal.

Increasingly, anesthetics are being used with opioids to reduce the opioid requirement for pain control. They work by decreasing the neuronal permeability to sodium ions, which blocks the initiation and conduction of nerve impulses. Most patients receiving anesthetics must have vital signs

COMMONLY USED ANESTHETICS

LOCAL
- Lidocaine *(Xylocaine)*, benzocaine, liposomal bupivacaine *(Exparel)*

INHALED
- Desflurane *(Suprane)*, sevoflurane *(Ultane)*, isoflurane *(Forane)*, nitrous oxide

INJECTABLE
- Bupivacaine *(Marcaine, Sensorcaine)*, lidocaine *(Xylocaine)*, ropivacaine *(Naropin)*

(especially respiration) continuously monitored. The main side effects of anesthetics include hypotension, bradycardia, nausea, vomiting and a mild drop in body temperature that can cause shivering. Overdose can cause respiratory depression. Allergic reactions are possible, and though rare, inhaled anesthetics can cause malignant hyperthermia.

It is important to verify use of the correct anesthetic product, concentration and route of administration. Bupivacaine, commonly used in epidurals, can be fatal if administered intravenously. Lidocaine should not be given by dual routes of administration (e.g., IV and topical). Lidocaine/epinephrine combination products are used for some local procedures that require an anesthetic, such as inserting an IV line. The epinephrine is added for vasoconstriction, which keeps the lidocaine localized to the area where the numbing is needed. Deaths have occurred due to mix-ups with epinephrine products and lidocaine/epinephrine products.

NEUROMUSCULAR BLOCKING AGENTS

Patients can require the use of a neuromuscular blocking agent (NMBA) in surgery conducted under general anesthesia, to facilitate mechanical ventilation, to treat muscle spasms (tetany) or to prevent shivering when undergoing therapeutic hypothermia after cardiac arrest. The use of NMBAs is typically recommended when other methods have proven ineffective; they are not routinely used in all critically ill patients. NMBAs cause paralysis of the skeletal muscle, including those used for respiration (e.g., the diaphragm), and patients must be mechanically ventilated. Since they have no effect on pain or sedation, patients should receive adequate sedation and analgesia prior to starting an NMBA. NMBAs are considered high-risk medications by ISMP; all agents should be labeled with a colored auxiliary label stating "WARNING, PARALYZING AGENT" and care should be taken to separate NMBAs from other solutions to avoid confusion and inadvertent administration to a patient for whom it was not intended.

There are two types of NMBAs: depolarizing and non-depolarizing. Succinylcholine is the only available depolarizing agent; resembling acetylcholine (ACh), succinylcholine binds to and activates the ACh receptors and desensitizes them. It is typically reserved for intubation and is not used for continuous neuromuscular blockade. Succinylcholine has been associated with causing malignant hyperthermia (particularly when used with inhaled anesthetics).

The non-depolarizing NMBAs work by binding to the ACh receptor, blocking the actions of endogenous ACh. Patients receiving NMBAs are unable to breathe, move, blink or cough. Special care must be taken to protect the skin, lubricate the eyes and suction the airway frequently to clear secretions while NMBAs are being used. Glycopyrrolate is an anticholinergic drug that can be used to reduce secretions. Numerous medications can enhance the neuromuscular blocking activity of the NMBAs, leading to toxicity (e.g., aminoglycosides, polymyxins, calcium channel blockers, cyclosporine, inhaled anesthetics, lithium, quinidine, vancomycin). Monitoring for the appropriate depth of paralysis is recommended (see the Toxicology & Antidotes chapter for NMBA antidotes).

DRUG	SAFETY/SIDE EFFECTS/MONITORING
Depolarizing NMBA	
Succinylcholine *(Anectine, Quelicin)*	Short-acting, fast onset (30-60 seconds)
Non-Depolarizing NMBAs	
For all non-depolarizing NMBAs	**SIDE EFFECTS** Flushing, bradycardia, hypotension, tachyphylaxis, acute quadriplegic myopathy syndrome (long-term use) **MONITORING** Peripheral nerve stimulator to assess depth of paralysis during continuous infusions [also called train-of-four (TOF)], vital signs (BP, HR, RR)
Atracurium	Short t½; intermediate-acting; metabolized by Hofmann elimination (independent of renal and hepatic function)
Cisatracurium *(Nimbex)*	Short t½; intermediate-acting; metabolized by Hofmann elimination (independent of renal and hepatic function)
Pancuronium	Long-acting; can accumulate in renal or hepatic dysfunction; ↑ HR
Rocuronium	Intermediate-acting
Vecuronium	Intermediate-acting; can accumulate in renal or hepatic dysfunction

HEMOSTATIC AGENTS

The term hemostasis means causing bleeding to stop. Hemostatic methods include simple manual pressure with one finger, electrical tissue cauterization, or the systemic administration of blood products (transfusions) and hemostatic agents. The systemic hemostatic drugs work by inhibiting fibrinolysis or enhancing coagulation and may be beneficial in select critical care scenarios (e.g., intracerebral hemorrhage due to traumatic brain injury). Several factor products are available to treat hemorrhage in patients with hemophilia or rare factor deficiencies *(Feiba, Coagadex, Adynovate)*. Some hemostatic drugs (e.g., *Praxbind, Andexxa)* have been approved as reversal agents for specific anticoagulants (see the Anticoagulation chapter).

There are many topical hemostatic agents, most of which are used surgically. These include thrombin in bandages, liquids and sprays, fibrin sealants, acrylates and a few others (names often include "throm": *Recothrom, Thrombin-JMI)*. A few topical hemostatics are OTC.

DRUG	SAFETY/SIDE EFFECTS/MONITORING
Aminocaproic acid *(Amicar)* Tablet, solution, injection	**CONTRAINDICATIONS** Disseminated intravascular coagulation (without heparin); active intravascular clotting process **SIDE EFFECTS** Injection-site reactions, thrombosis **NOTES** FDA-approved for excessive bleeding associated with cardiac surgery, liver cirrhosis and urinary fibrinolysis. Do not use in patients with active clots, and do not give with factor IX complex concentrates due to ↑ risk for thrombosis.
Tranexamic acid *(Cyklokapron,* injection) *(Lysteda,* tablet)	**CONTRAINDICATIONS** IV: acquired defective color vision, active intravascular clotting, subarachnoid hemorrhage Oral: previous or current thromboembolic disease, current use of combination hormonal contraception **SIDE EFFECTS** Injection: vascular occlusion, thrombosis Oral: retinal clotting **NOTES** Oral tranexamic acid is approved for heavy menstrual bleeding (menorrhagia). The injection is approved for bleeding with hemophilia and is often used off-label to control surgical bleeding and trauma-associated hemorrhage (e.g., traumatic brain injury).
Recombinant Factor VIIa **(NovoSeven RT,** *Sevenfact)* Injection	**BOXED WARNING** Risk of thrombotic events, particularly when used off-label **NOTES** FDA-approved for hemophilia and factor VII deficiency; has been used successfully off-label for patients with hemorrhage from trauma and warfarin-related bleeding events.

Select Guidelines/References

Singer M, Deutschman CS, Seymour CW, et al. The Third International Consensus Definitions for Sepsis and Septic Shock (Sepsis-3). *JAMA.* 2016;315(8):801-10.

Evans LE, Rhodes A, Alhazzani W, et al. Surviving Sepsis Campaign: International Guidelines for Management of Severe Sepsis and Septic Shock: 2021. *Crit Care Med.* 2021;49(11):e1063-e1143.

Devlin J, Skrobik, Y, Gelinas C et al. Clinical Practice Guidelines for the Prevention and Management of Pain, Agitation/Sedation, Delirium, Immobility, and Sleep Disruption in Adult Patients in the ICU. Crit Care Med. 2018;46(9):1532-48.

PEDIATRIC TOPIC	CHAPTER
Vaccines	Immunizations
Infections (e.g., acute otitis media)	Infectious Diseases
Cough and cold	Allergic Rhinitis, Cough & Cold
Pediculosis (lice) and diaper rash	Common Skin Conditions
Asthma	Asthma
Diabetes	Diabetes
Seizures	Seizures/Epilepsy
Iron and vitamin D recommendations	Dietary Supplements, Natural & Complementary Medicine

CONTENT LEGEND

 = Study Tip Gal

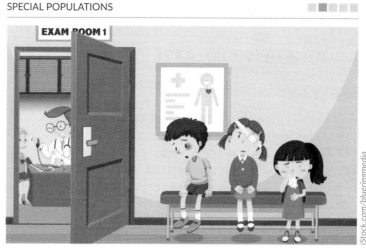

iStock.com/blueringmedia

CHAPTER 54
PEDIATRIC CONDITIONS

BACKGROUND

Pediatric patients have unique, age-related physiologic characteristics (e.g., metabolism) that require patient-specific dosing of medications.

PEDIATRIC AGE CLASSIFICATIONS

Neonate	0 – 28 days
Infant	1 month – < 2 years
Child	2 – 11 years
Adolescent	12 – 18 years

Young children (especially infants) can become seriously ill very quickly and must be referred for medical care in certain situations (see box below). Often the first sign of illness is an elevated temperature. Various methods (e.g., oral, axillary, rectal, ear, forehead) can be used to measure temperature, but rectal measurements are most accurate, especially in infants < 3 months old.

Several common pediatric conditions are covered in this chapter; the table to the left shows topics that are covered in other chapters.

WHEN TO SEEK MEDICAL CARE FOR A PEDIATRIC PATIENT

- Temperature ≥ 100.4°F (rectally) in patients < 3 months old
- Temperature ≥ 101°F (rectally) in patients ≥ 3 months old
- Allergic reactions
- Blood in the urine or stool
- Dehydration (e.g., limited/no urine output) or unable to tolerate oral liquids
- Difficulty breathing
- Limping or unable to move an extremity
- Head injury
- Ingestions
- Seizure
- Severe rash or any rash with fever

ROUTINE NEWBORN CARE

APGAR SCORING

A newborn's ability to adapt to extrauterine life is assessed at one and five minutes after birth with an Apgar score. The Apgar score measures performance in five categories: appearance (color), pulse (heart rate), grimace (reflex irritability, the newborn's response to stimulation), activity (muscle tone) and respiratory effort.

A score ≥ 7 indicates that the newborn is adapting well to extrauterine life and can receive routine newborn care. A score < 7 is a sign that the newborn is experiencing distress and prompt medical intervention (e.g., respiratory resuscitation) is needed.

MEDICATIONS AND SCREENING

Routine medications administered shortly after birth include intramuscular vitamin K (to prevent bleeding), ophthalmic erythromycin (to prevent conjunctivitis) and the first dose of the hepatitis B vaccine series. Other treatments may be given for select conditions, such as analgesia (if being circumcised) or phototherapy (i.e., light therapy) for jaundice.

Newborn screening tests (e.g., heel blood sample, hearing test, pulse oximetry) are conducted prior to discharge to detect congenital illnesses, such as phenylketonuria, cystic fibrosis and heart defects.

SELECT NEONATAL CONDITIONS

There are select conditions that present within (and are often limited to) the neonatal period (i.e., ≤ 28 days after delivery), and their likelihood can be influenced by the length of gestation (i.e., time in utero). A neonate is classified as premature if delivery occurs before 37 weeks of gestation.

Premature neonates have a higher risk of experiencing conditions such as patent ductus arteriosus (PDA) and respiratory distress syndrome (RDS). However, persistent pulmonary hypertension of the newborn (PPHN) is more often observed in term neonates (i.e., gestation ≥ 37 weeks). These conditions typically result in low Apgar scores, indicating there is an issue related to an immature pulmonary or cardiovascular system.

PATENT DUCTUS ARTERIOSUS

The ductus arteriosus is a normal opening between the aorta and pulmonary artery in an unborn fetus. It is maintained by maternal prostaglandin and allows blood (oxygenated via the placenta) to bypass the immature lungs. The ductus arteriosus should close naturally after delivery (as prostaglandin levels decrease in the neonate).

A patent ductus arteriosus (PDA), which occurs when the ductus arteriosus remains open (patent) after birth, requires medical observation and/or intervention; interventions can include surgery or drugs. NSAIDs (such as IV indomethacin or ibuprofen) can help the PDA close via their mechanism of blocking cyclooxygenase and inhibiting prostaglandin synthesis. This mechanism of NSAIDs is why they should not be used in the third trimester of pregnancy (because they can cause the PDA to close prematurely).

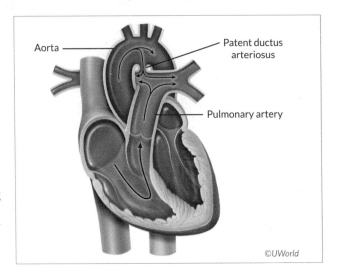

©UWorld

RESPIRATORY DISTRESS SYNDROME

The fetus begins to produce lung surfactant around week 20 of gestation and is producing an adequate amount by week 35. A deficiency of surfactant production in lungs that are not fully developed causes the alveoli to collapse, which causes respiratory distress syndrome (RDS), followed by respiratory failure and death.

For this reason, most neonates born before 35 weeks of gestation will receive surfactant immediately after birth or within the first few days of life. Surfactant products can be recognized by either "surf" or "actant" in the name, such as poractant alfa (Curosurf) and calfactant (Infasurf).

PERSISTENT PULMONARY HYPERTENSION OF THE NEWBORN

When an infant is born, blood vessels in the lungs (which have a high resistance in utero) relax, allowing blood to begin circulating through the pulmonary vasculature. When the blood vessels fail to relax (i.e., vascular resistance remains elevated), it can lead to persistent pulmonary hypertension of the newborn (PPHN). PPHN may be linked to in utero exposure to selective serotonin reuptake inhibitors (SSRIs).

In addition to supportive care, inhaled nitric oxide (NO), to dilate the pulmonary vasculature, is the standard treatment. Some drugs used to treat pulmonary arterial hypertension, such as sildenafil (a PDE-5 inhibitor), can be used for PPHN.

NEONATAL SEPSIS

Any full term, previously healthy neonate (i.e., age ≤ 28 days, gestation ≥ 37 weeks) with a temperature ≥ 100.4°F (38°C) should be evaluated for bacterial infection because a delay in treatment can cause rapid progression to bacteremia, sepsis and/or meningitis, which can be fatal.

A sepsis evaluation generally involves obtaining blood and urine cultures, a lumbar puncture (to diagnose meningitis), a chest X-ray (if respiratory symptoms are present) and laboratory tests (e.g., CBC, C-reactive protein, complete metabolic panel). Signs of neonatal meningitis can include fever (or hypothermia), lethargy, poor feeding, irritability and seizures. Bulging fontanelles (swelling between the bones of the skull) occur rarely. Other classic signs of meningitis (e.g., headache, nuchal rigidity) are uncommon in neonates.

Common neonatal bacterial pathogens differ from other age groups due to the vertical transmission of organisms from the mother to the neonate via contaminated amniotic fluid or during vaginal delivery. *Escherichia coli* is a common cause of bacteremia, while meningitis (discussed fully in the Infectious Diseases II chapter) is most often caused by Group B *Streptococcus* (GBS) and (rarely) *Listeria*. Because pregnant women may be colonized with GBS, universal GBS screening is performed during pregnancy and those who test positive receive antibiotic prophylaxis (e.g., penicillin G aqueous) during labor to decrease the risk of transmission to the neonate.

Empiric antibiotic treatment in neonates with a fever consists of ampicillin plus ceftazidime, cefepime or gentamicin. Ceftriaxone, which is commonly used in adults, is generally avoided in neonates. Ceftriaxone displaces bilirubin from albumin, which can cause bilirubin-induced brain damage (kernicterus). In addition, ceftriaxone and calcium-containing solutions can precipitate, causing an embolus and death; concurrent use of these products in neonates is contraindicated.

SELECT PEDIATRIC CONDITIONS

BRONCHIOLITIS

Bronchiolitis is a common lower respiratory tract condition that nearly all children experience by two years of age. It is the most frequent cause of hospitalization in children < 6 months. Neonates and premature infants have a higher risk for severe disease, complications and death.

Respiratory syncytial virus (RSV) infection is responsible for the majority of bronchiolitis cases, but co-infection with other viruses (e.g., rhinovirus, human metapneumovirus) is possible in up to 30% of cases. RSV invades via the nasopharynx, enters the lower respiratory tract and causes increased mucus production and sloughing of cells that line the bronchi. This can lead to significant swelling within the airway and respiratory distress.

Bronchiolitis symptoms typically peak on days 3 – 5 of illness and include rhinitis, cough, wheezing, tachypnea and nasal flaring. Hypoxemia can occur due to mucus plugging. Apnea is a greater concern in younger infants and those with a history of prematurity. Similar to other viral infections, the treatment is primarily supportive (suction of secretions, hydration, supplemental oxygen and fever management). Bronchodilators and systemic steroids are not used routinely. Inhaled ribavirin *(Virazole)* can be considered for immunocompromised patients with severe RSV infection.

Respiratory Syncytial Virus Infection Prophylaxis

The recombinant RSV vaccine *(Abrysvo)* is recommended for pregnant patients between 32 – 36 weeks gestation to prevent RSV infection in infants < 6 months old. Alternatively (i.e., if the mother was not vaccinated), RSV prophylaxis is recommended in the infant during RSV season (late fall, winter, early spring), although prophylaxis may be considered outside of this window. Two monoclonal antibodies are available for this purpose: nirsevimab *(Beyfortus)* and palivizumab *(Synagis)*.

DRUG	DOSING*	RECOMMENDED USE
Nirsevimab *(Beyfortus)* IM injection Prefilled syringe	Single IM dose for RSV season < 5 kg: 50 mg ≥ 5 kg: 100 mg Second RSV season: 200 mg	■ Indicated for the following patients: ❑ Neonates and infants ≤ 8 months old born during or entering their first RSV season ❑ Children ≤ 20 months who are vulnerable to severe RSV disease
Palivizumab *(Synagis)* IM injection Vial	15 mg/kg IM once monthly through RSV season Maximum of 5 doses unless the season is extended Discontinue if breakthrough infection occurs requiring hospitalization	■ Recommended in the following patients (list not all-inclusive): ❑ Premature infant born at < 29 weeks of gestation and age ≤ 12 months ❑ Premature infant born at ≤ 35 weeks of gestation and age ≤ 6 months ❑ Age ≤ 24 months with select congenital heart conditions or chronic lung disease

Doses are administered in the anterolateral thigh muscle; the deltoid can be used once the muscle mass is adequate (generally at ≥ 3 years old).

CROUP

Croup, or laryngotracheobronchitis, is usually due to a viral infection that causes significant inflammation of the upper airway, larynx and trachea. The inflammation results in the hallmark signs of inspiratory stridor (a high-pitched breathing sound), barking cough and hoarseness. Croup is most common in children < 6 years old and is often worse at night. The illness is classified and treated based on the severity of symptoms.

Drug Treatment

- Systemic steroids (e.g., dexamethasone 0.6 mg/kg) are a mainstay of treatment for mild to severe croup cases.

- In an acute care setting, a patient with difficulty breathing may be given nebulized racemic epinephrine in addition to the systemic steroid. Epinephrine is an adrenergic agonist that eases symptoms via decreased airway edema and

obstruction. When administered using a nebulizer, the onset of action is fast but the duration of action is short (~2 hours) and the child should be monitored for symptom recurrence.

- ❏ Nebulized racemic epinephrine is a 1:1 mixture of dextro (D) and levo (L) isomers (the L-isomer is the active component).

- ❏ If racemic epinephrine is not available, L-epinephrine is used; this is half of the drug (one of the isomers) and the dose is half of the racemic formulation.

- Severe symptoms (e.g., stridor at rest, respiratory distress, severe retractions, mental status changes) can require respiratory support, such as intubation.

- Antibiotics are used only if a bacterial infection is also present.

Key Differences Between Bronchiolitis and Croup

	BRONCHIOLITIS	CROUP
Cause	Viral (especially RSV)	Viral (especially parainfluenza)
Age of onset	≤ 2 years	≤ 6 years
Pathophysiology	Lower respiratory tract mucus plugging, swelling in bronchioles	Upper respiratory tract edema, inflammation in larynx
Symptoms	Nasal flaring, rhinitis, tachypnea, apnea, hypoxemia	Inspiratory stridor, barking cough, hoarseness
Treatment	Supportive care (especially suctioning of secretions and supplemental oxygen)	Dexamethasone ± racemic epinephrine

NOCTURNAL ENURESIS

Nocturnal enuresis, or bed-wetting, is a normal part of a child's development and is not generally treated before age 5 years. Boys (more often than girls) can be developing nighttime bladder control until 7 years of age.

Non-Drug Treatment

Behavioral approaches should be attempted first for up to three months. These include positive reinforcement and establishing a normal daytime voiding pattern, bowel pattern and hydration pattern. Fluid intake should be limited prior to bedtime.

If behavioral methods do not result in dryness, alarm therapy can be tried. There are numerous alarms available that attach to underwear or pajamas and sound an alarm when wet. The child may sleep through the alarm, but generally stops voiding. When the alarm sounds, a caregiver should wake the child and escort them to the bathroom.

Drug Treatment

Desmopressin oral tablet is the preferred treatment for enuresis. It is a synthetic analog of antidiuretic hormone (ADH); simulating ADH will ↓ nocturnal urine production. Desmopressin can be used in combination with alarm therapy.

DRUG	DOSING	SAFETY/SIDE EFFECTS/MONITORING
Desmopressin (*DDAVP*) Tablets used for enuresis Tablets, nasal spray or injection used for diabetes insipidus and hemophilia A (to control bleeding)	Start 0.2 mg PO QHS, can titrate to 0.6 mg max	**BOXED WARNINGS** Severe, life-threatening hyponatremia can develop **CONTRAINDICATIONS** Hyponatremia, history of hyponatremia, CrCl < 50 mL/min **SIDE EFFECTS** Headache, fatigue, possible ↓ Na due to water retention **NOTES** Limit fluid intake starting 1 hour before dose and until the next morning

PEDIATRIC SAFE MEDICATION PRACTICES

Pediatric patients have an increased risk of adverse drug events compared to the adult population; this is due to various factors that increase the risk of errors, such as age-related pharmacokinetic differences, off-label prescribing and weight-based dosing calculations.

Improved communication between caregivers and pharmacists can decrease the incidence of preventable adverse drug events. In addition, pharmacists play an essential role in safe medication use for pediatric patients.

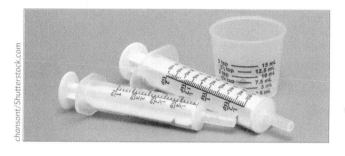

chansont/Shutterstock.com

Select measures that can be used to decrease the risk of errors include:

- For liquid pediatric medications that utilize weight-based dosing (which is most), verify that the dose is appropriate for the patient's weight.

  ❑ Transcribe the dose in milliliters only on the label.

  ❑ Dispense the prescription with an oral measuring device (dosing syringe or cup) appropriate for the age of the patient and the dose volume, and instruct caregivers on correct use, ideally using demonstration and the teach-back counseling method.

  ❑ Household spoons should not be used for measuring medication because they are highly variable in size and cause dosing inaccuracies.

- Counsel caregivers to store all medications in a safe, secure location.

OVER-THE-COUNTER PRODUCTS FOR CHILDREN

The FDA does not recommend OTC cough and cold medications in children < 2 years old, but most manufacturers include product labeling to avoid in children under age 4. Some combination products have additional labeling restrictions for use only in children ≥ 6 years old.

MILD PAIN AND FEVER

Aspirin and salicylate-containing products (e.g., bismuth subsalicylate) are associated with Reye's syndrome when used in children recovering from a viral infection (especially influenza and chickenpox). Because a viral infection may not be apparent in this patient population, these products are not recommended in patients ≤ 18 years old.

Acetaminophen infant drops and children's suspension are the same concentration to help reduce dosing errors. Use of acetaminophen in doses above the recommended amount is the most common cause of liver failure. Accidental overdose can be due to the inadvertent use of multiple acetaminophen-containing combination products; caregivers should be counseled about this danger.

Ibuprofen for pain/fever should be avoided in infants < 6 months old due to the risk of nephrotoxicity. To prevent dosing errors in patients ≥ 6 months old, caregivers should be aware that ibuprofen drops and suspension are supplied in different dosage strengths for infants and children, respectively.

In children ≥ 6 months old, acetaminophen or ibuprofen are appropriate for treating pain and fever. Some physicians may recommend giving them together in alternating doses (e.g., acetaminophen first, then ibuprofen three hours later).

Select OTC Analgesics and Antipyretics

DRUG	DOSING	SAFETY/SIDE EFFECTS/MONITORING	
Fever and/or Pain			
Acetaminophen (Tylenol Children's, FeverAll Children's, others)	10-15 mg/kg/dose every 4-6 hours (max 75 mg/kg/day) Acetaminophen oral liquid formulations (infants and childrens) are the same concentration: 160 mg/5 mL	For simplicity, age and weight-based dosing is on the side of the container Caution caregivers regarding incorrect dosing or overdose due to the use of multiple acetaminophen-containing products	
Ibuprofen (Infants' Advil Drops, Motrin Infants' Drops, Children's Motrin, Children's Advil, others)	5-10 mg/kg/dose every 6-8 hours (max 40 mg/kg/day) Infant drops: 50 mg/1.25 mL Children's suspension: 100 mg/5 mL	Indicated for infants ≥ 6 months old Can cause nausea	

Sheila Fitzgerald/Shutterstock.com

CASE SCENARIO

The father of LC, a 9-month-old female, comes to a community pharmacy stating that his daughter has a rectal temperature of 102°F. The pediatrician recommended OTC treatment and the father asks for assistance with products to purchase and dosing. LC weighs 18.5 lbs.

What medications and doses would be appropriate?
Acetaminophen and ibuprofen (based on her age and no past medical history) are both appropriate and can be used together (in alternating doses).

To calculate the dose, convert LC's weight to kg: 18.5 lbs / 2.2 = 8.409 kg

Next, calculate LC's dose range for each medication.

Acetaminophen: 10-15 mg/kg/dose every 4-6 hours	Ibuprofen: 5-10 mg/kg/dose every 6-8 hours
LC's dose: 84.09-126.14 mg every 4-6 hours	LC's dose: 42.05-84.09 mg every 6-8 hours

How should the father be instructed to give these medications?
Determine a dose within the range that can easily be administered based on the products available.

Acetaminophen: 160 mg/5 mL	Ibuprofen Infant Drops: 50 mg/1.25mL
LC's dose: 96 mg (3 mL) every 4-6 hours	LC's dose: 80 mg (2 mL) every 6-8 hours

The father can alternate the two medications every 3 hours as needed, keeping at least 6 hours between doses of the same medication.

NASAL CONGESTION

Nasal congestion is very common in infants and small children and can be especially problematic if a viral illness is present. Children < 6 months old breathe mostly through their nose; they have not yet learned to breathe through their mouth. Gentle suction with intranasal saline drops or spray (e.g., Ocean for Kids, Little Remedies) to loosen and remove mucus is the primary treatment.

INTESTINAL GAS

Intestinal gas is a common neonatal and infant condition that causes distress after feedings. The associated crying and fussiness generally dissipate when the child is ~6 – 8 months old and the digestive tract has grown. Simethicone drops (20 mg, 1 – 4 times daily PRN) can offer mild, if any, benefit. Simethicone is not absorbed and is safe to use.

DIARRHEA

Dehydration can occur as a result of significant diarrhea and can be dangerous in infants. Fluid and electrolytes can be replaced with OTC oral rehydration solutions, such as Pedialyte and Enfamil Enfalyte. Bismuth subsalicylate should not be used due to the risk of Reye's syndrome. Loperamide is not recommended for OTC use in children ≤ 6 years old.

CONSTIPATION

There are a variety of treatment options to treat children with constipation. Product selection depends on patient age. In addition, prunes or pears (as fruit or juice) or kiwi fruit can be helpful. Any child with ongoing constipation issues should be seen by a pediatrician.

- Age < 6 months: OTC pediatric glycerin suppositories are commonly used for quick relief (off-label, the FDA-approved indication is for children ≥ 2 years).

- Age ≥ 6 months: oral polyethylene glycol 3350 (MiraLax) 0.2 – 1.5 g/kg/day is the preferred treatment for most cases of intermittent constipation.

- Age ≥ 2 years: additional options include magnesium hydroxide, docusate, senna and rectal enemas.

  ❑ OTC rectal enemas [e.g., sodium phosphate (Fleet Pedia-Lax Enema)] should not be used in children < 2 years old due to the risk of severe dehydration and electrolyte abnormalities that could lead to serious complications (e.g., arrhythmia, acute kidney injury, death).

- Children ≥ 6 years: additional options include bisacodyl suppositories or oral mineral oil.

  ❑ Mineral oil should be used with caution in children at risk for aspiration (e.g., neurologic impairment) or with significant gastrointestinal reflux, nausea or vomiting; unintentional aspiration can cause respiratory distress or pneumonitis.

DRUGS NOT GENERALLY RECOMMENDED FOR PEDIATRIC PATIENTS

The Key Potentially Inappropriate Drugs in Pediatrics: The KIDs List is a useful resource to determine which medications are considered unsafe for use in children and reasons why they should be avoided. Select examples of medications to avoid in pediatric patients are listed below.

- Topical teething products containing benzocaine increase the risk of methemoglobinemia. The FDA recommends against their use in children < 2 years old.

- Promethazine is contraindicated in children ≤ 2 years old due to the risk of severe or fatal respiratory depression.

- Codeine is metabolized to morphine by the CYP2D6 enzyme; children who over-express this enzyme produce a higher than expected amount of morphine. This can result in respiratory depression and possibly death. There is a similar risk (and boxed warning) for tramadol (also metabolized to an active metabolite by CYP2D6).

  ❑ Codeine and tramadol are contraindicated in all patients < 12 years old and in those ≤ 18 years old after tonsillectomy/adenoidectomy.

  ❑ Prescription cough and cold medications that contain codeine or hydrocodone are no longer indicated in patients ≤ 18 years old.

- Quinolones are generally not recommended in pediatric patients due to the possibility of cartilage, bone and muscle adverse effects. However, for select conditions (e.g., anthrax, complicated urinary tract infections, cystic fibrosis), the benefits may outweigh the risks.

- Tetracyclines are not recommended in children < 8 years of age because they stain teeth and deposit into mineralizing (i.e., growing) bone and cartilage, which slows bone growth.

  ❑ One notable exception is the treatment of tick-borne Rickettsial diseases (e.g., Rocky Mountain spotted fever). Doxycycline is the most effective treatment (see the Infectious Diseases II chapter) and is recommended in pediatric patients, because the risk to the teeth and bone is outweighed by the risk of severe illness or death.

DRUGS TO AVOID IN PEDIATRIC PATIENTS

Contraindicated
- Neonates (age 0-28 days):
  ❑ Ceftriaxone
- Age < 2 years:
  ❑ Promethazine
  ❑ OTC teething medications containing benzocaine
- Age < 12 years:
  ❑ Codeine
  ❑ Tramadol

Not generally recommended
- Aspirin
- Quinolones
- Tetracyclines
- OTC cough and cold preparations

VACCINE-PREVENTABLE CHILDHOOD DISEASES

Vaccine-preventable diseases occur more commonly than in previous years due to lower immunization rates in some areas (see the Immunizations chapter for vaccine information). The symptoms of the more common vaccine-preventable diseases are noted in the table below. Each of the conditions included can lead to severe, permanent damage. Although chickenpox (an acute illness) generally dissipates without serious consequences, any person who has had chickenpox is at risk for developing shingles (a painful condition that results from reactivation of the virus in some nerves) later in life (see the Infectious Diseases III chapter for more information).

ILLNESS	CLASSIC SYMPTOMS	NOTES
Measles	Koplik spots (small white spots on the inside of the mouth that appear 2-5 days prior to the rash), maculopapular rash, fever, malaise, cough, rhinitis, conjunctivitis _phichet chaiyabin/Shutterstock.com_	Transmission is airborne and measles is highly contagious. If not immune, 90% of people who are in contact with an infected person will also become infected. Prevention: MMR vaccine.
Mumps	Swollen salivary glands under the ears (parotitis), fever, headache, myalgia, fatigue, loss of appetite; up to 50% of patients have mild or no symptoms _airdone/Shutterstock.com_	Prevention: MMR vaccine
Rubella	Rash (fine, pink, begins on the face and quickly spreads to the rest of the body), fever, swollen glands, cold-like symptoms, aching joints; up to 50% of patients have mild or no symptoms _Akkalak Aiempradit/Shutterstock.com_	Can cause birth defects if contracted by a pregnant woman. Prevention: MMR vaccine

ILLNESS	CLASSIC SYMPTOMS	NOTES
Polio	Fever, sore throat, fatigue, nausea, headache, abdominal pain; can cause severe nerve damage (paralytic polio) and post-polio syndrome (progressive weakness and cognitive issues) *podsy/Shutterstock.com*	Prevention: IPV vaccine
Pertussis (Whooping cough)	Sudden cough outbursts ("whoop" sounding cough), fever, rhinitis, bluish skin (cyanosis), vomiting, fatigue	Can cause respiratory failure and death, especially in infants. Prevention: DTaP vaccine
Rotavirus	Severe, watery diarrhea, fever, vomiting	Can lead to dehydration and death. Most likely to occur in the winter and spring (December through June). Prevention: rotavirus vaccine
Chickenpox (Varicella)	Itchy rash, fever, malaise The rash appears as crops of sores (head, then trunk, then arms and legs), that turn into blisters, burst, then form crusts *John-Kelly/Shutterstock.com*	Long-term implications include shingles (herpes zoster) with risk of ophthalmic involvement and postherpetic neuralgia (severe pain after the infection). Prevention: varicella vaccine

Select Guidelines/References

Smith DK, McDermott AJ, Sullivan JF. Croup: diagnosis and management. *Am Fam Physician.* 2018; 97:575-1073.

Lu H, Rosenbaum R. Developmental pharmacokinetics in pediatric populations. *J Pediatr Pharmacol Ther.* 2014;19(4):262-276.

Meyers R, Thackray J, Matson K, et al. Key potentially inappropriate drugs in pediatrics: the KIDs list. *J Pediatr Pharmacol Ther.* 2020;25(3):175-191.

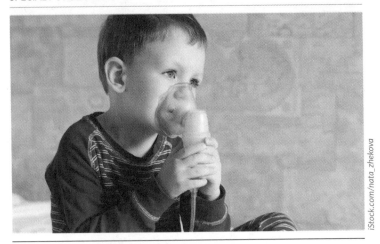

iStock.com/nata_zhekova

CHAPTER 55

CYSTIC FIBROSIS

BACKGROUND

Cystic fibrosis (CF) is an incurable, hereditary disease caused by a mutation in the gene for the protein cystic fibrosis transmembrane conductance regulator (CFTR). The mutation causes abnormal transport of chloride, bicarbonate and sodium ions across the epithelium, leading to thick, viscous secretions. The thick mucus affects the lungs, pancreas, liver and intestines, which causes difficulty breathing, lung infections and digestive complications. The name cystic fibrosis refers to the characteristic scarring (fibrosis) and cyst formation that occurs within the pancreas. The average life expectancy of a person with CF is 35 – 40 years with more than 75% of patients being diagnosed by 2 years of age. The disease is progressive, with some eventually qualifying for lung transplantation.

DIAGNOSIS

Newborn screening is performed in the U.S. in the first 2 – 3 days after a baby is born and includes testing for CF and other conditions. If the initial screening identifies a risk of CF, then a sweat chloride test (or "sweat test") is performed to confirm the diagnosis. The sweat test measures the amount of salt (chloride) in the sweat, which is high in patients with CF.

SIGNS AND SYMPTOMS

The classic symptoms of CF are salty tasting skin, poor growth and poor weight gain (despite adequate food intake), thick and sticky mucus production, frequent lung infections, coughing and shortness of breath. Patients experience obstruction of pancreatic ducts causing steatorrhea (fatty stools) and poor absorption of nutrients, including fat-soluble vitamins. Clubbing of the fingers may be present. Malnutrition and a failure to thrive can result if CF is not treated.

DRUG TREATMENT

The primary goals of therapy include preventing/treating lung infections, maintaining adequate nutrition and optimizing quality of life. Most patients will receive airway clearance therapies (see drug table on the next page), inhaled antibiotics targeting *Pseudomonas aeruginosa* and pancreatic enzyme replacement. Targeted CFTR modulators reduce the frequency of exacerbations and may be appropriate for some patients. Early diagnosis and a comprehensive treatment plan can improve survival and quality of life. Specialty clinics for CF can be found in many communities.

LUNG COMPLICATIONS

Multiple medications are used to help manage the thick mucus in the lungs and reduce the risk of infections. Administering the inhaled medications in the correct order is critical to maximize absorption and effect. Airway clearance therapies (e.g., bronchodilators, hypertonic saline and dornase alfa) are given before inhaled antibiotics (see Study Tip Gal to the right).

Inhaled therapies are the foundation of treatment for CF. The drug is delivered directly to the lungs, resulting in minimal systemic absorption (reducing the risk of toxicity). Although inhaled medications are an effective form of drug delivery, the average patient with CF receives up to 10 doses of inhaled medications daily, which can take 2 – 3 hours to administer. This requires lifestyle modification since dosing must be scheduled around work, school and other activities.

INFECTIONS

Intermittent Infection

Impaired mucus clearance causes bacterial colonization and lung infections. The most common organisms seen early in the disease are *Staphylococcus aureus* and *Haemophilus influenzae*, followed by *Pseudomonas aeruginosa* in adolescents and adults. Acute pulmonary exacerbations are characterized by an increase in cough, sputum production with a change in sputum color (greenish), shortness of breath and a rapid decline in FEV1. Treatment often includes an extended course of antibiotics (2 – 4 weeks) and modalities to increase airway clearance.

For infections caused by *Pseudomonas aeruginosa*, two IV drugs are recommended to provide potential synergy and prevent resistance. These include aminoglycosides, beta-lactams, quinolones and others that cover *Pseudomonas aeruginosa*. See the Infectious Diseases I chapter for a complete discussion of treatment options for *Pseudomonas aeruginosa*. Doses tend to be larger than normal to address altered pharmacokinetics in patients with CF, to obtain therapeutic drug concentrations in lung tissue, and to overcome reduced susceptibility of the bacteria chronically colonizing the airways.

INHALED MEDICATIONS FOR CF

ORDER	INTERVENTION	PURPOSE
1st	Inhaled bronchodilators (e.g., albuterol)	Opens the airways
2nd	Hypertonic saline (e.g., *HyperSal*)	Mobilizes mucus to improve airway clearance
3rd	Dornase alfa (*Pulmozyme*)	Decreases viscosity of (thins) mucus to promote airway clearance
4th	Chest physiotherapy	Mobilizes mucus to improve airway clearance
5th	Inhaled antibiotics	Controls airway infection

Most patients will require oral medications (e.g., pancreatic enzyme products, azithromycin). These can be given at any time.

Chronic Infection

Lung infections occur intermittently at first, but eventually become chronic. Chronic lung infections with *Pseudomonas aeruginosa* are associated with a more rapid decline in pulmonary function. Inhaled antibiotics are recommended for patients with chronic *Pseudomonas aeruginosa* lung infections to reduce the bacterial burden. Treatment is cycled with 28 days on therapy, followed by 28 days off. This is associated with an improvement in lung function and a reduction in the frequency of acute pulmonary exacerbations. If a patient is using a bronchodilator and/or mucolytic (e.g., dornase alfa), these should be given prior to the antibiotic inhalation (see Study Tip Gal above).

Inhaled antibiotics should be taken as prescribed in order to reduce the risk of developing antibiotic resistance. Inhaled aztreonam (*Cayston*), an antibiotic used for chronic suppression (see drug table on the next page), is dosed TID and should be scheduled as close to every 8 hours as possible. This dosing provides optimal bacterial killing around the clock, while minimizing the time when the antibiotic concentration is low (which can worsen resistance). Dosing every 8 hours requires waking up in the middle of the night, so it is usually more convenient to give doses during waking hours (e.g., before school, after school and before bed). The doses must be at least 4 hours apart to provide adequate drug concentrations throughout the day. Similarly, inhaled tobramycin (*TOBI, TOBI Podhaler*) is dosed every 12 hours and should be scheduled as close to every 12 hours as possible with at least 6 hours in between doses.

A six month trial of oral azithromycin can be considered for patients with chronic infection who are worsening on conventional treatment. Azithromycin has no direct bactericidal activity against *Pseudomonas*, but disrupts biofilm formation by the bacteria which can improve lung function and decrease exacerbations.

Treatment for Lung Complications and Infections

DRUG	DOSING	SAFETY/SIDE EFFECTS/MONITORING
Airway Clearance Therapies (Inhaled)		
Bronchodilator (e.g., albuterol)	2-4 times daily	See Asthma chapter
Hypertonic saline (*HyperSal, PulmoSal*) 4 mL unit-dose vial	4 mL via nebulizer twice daily	Hypertonic saline is supplied as small ready-to-use vials that are <u>delivered via a nebulizer</u> *PulmoSal* is buffered to match physiologic pH of the airway surface Hypertonic saline is a high-alert drug, especially with IV administration
Dornase alfa (*Pulmozyme*) 2.5 mg single-use ampule	2.5 mg daily with recommended nebulizer and compressor system	<u>Decreases viscosity of mucus</u> (i.e., thins the mucus) **CONTRAINDICATIONS** Hypersensitivity to Chinese hamster ovary (CHO) products **SIDE EFFECTS** Chest pain, fever, rash, rhinitis, laryngitis, voice alteration, throat irritation **NOTES** <u>Store ampules in the refrigerator</u> (do not expose to room temperature ≥ 24 hours) <u>Protect from light</u> <u>Do not mix with any other drug in the nebulizer</u>
Antibiotics (Inhaled): target *Pseudomonas aeruginosa* colonization to ↓ infections/hospitalization		
Tobramycin (*TOBI, TOBI Podhaler*, *Bethkis, Kitabis Pak*) Solution for inhalation: *TOBI, Kitabis*: 300 mg/ 5 mL single-use ampule *Bethkis*: 300 mg/4 mL single-use ampule <u>Capsule for inhalation:</u> *TOBI Podhaler*: 28 mg capsules in blister card	Age ≥ 6 years: **Solution for inhalation** *TOBI, Bethkis, Kitabis Pak:* 300 mg via nebulizer Q12H **Capsule for inhalation** *TOBI Podhaler:* 112 mg (4 x 28 mg caps) via inhalation Q12H	**SIDE EFFECTS** <u>Ototoxicity, tinnitus, voice alteration, mouth and throat pain</u>, dizziness, bronchospasm **NOTES** Give for <u>28 days, followed by 28 days off</u> cycle Dosed every 12 hours, but must be at least <u>6 hours apart</u> *TOBI, Bethkis, Kitabis:* <u>refrigeration recommended</u> (can be kept at <u>room temperature up to 28 days</u>); store in foil pouch to protect from light; <u>do not mix with any other drug in the nebulizer</u> *TOBI:* use with *PARI LC Plus* nebulizer and *DeVilbiss Pulmo-Aide* air compressor *Bethkis:* use with *PARI LC Plus* nebulizer and *PARI Vios* air compressor *TOBI Podhaler:* store capsules at <u>room temperature</u> in a dry place; <u>use with *Podhaler*</u> (device dispensed with the capsules); <u>do not swallow</u> capsules
Aztreonam (*Cayston*) Solution for inhalation **Azactam** (IV) – for acute infection	Age ≥ 7 years: 75 mg via nebulizer TID	**SIDE EFFECTS** <u>Allergic reactions (may be severe), bronchospasm, fever, wheezing, cough, chest discomfort</u> **NOTES** Give for <u>28 days, followed by 28 days off</u> cycle Dosed every 8 hours, but must be at least <u>4 hours apart</u> <u>Refrigeration recommended</u> (can be kept at <u>room temperature</u> up to <u>28 days</u>) <u>Do not mix with any other drug in the nebulizer</u> Use with *Altera* nebulizer system Protect from light
Antibiotic (Oral): to ↓ inflammation and ↓ exacerbations		
Azithromycin (*Zithromax*) Off-label	Age ≥ 6 years: < 40 kg: 250 mg 3 times/week ≥ 40 kg: 500 mg 3 times/week	**SIDE EFFECTS** In CF: tinnitus, nausea, risk of QT prolongation **NOTES** Do not use as monotherapy in individuals with nontuberculous mycobacteria lung infections

WHAT'S IN A NAME?

Enzymes are proteins that break bonds and speed up chemical reactions (in addition to other functions). You can spot an enzyme because the generic name usually ends in "-ase."

Lungs: Dornase alfa / *Pulmozyme* indicates that it is an enzyme

- Breaks DNA strands into smaller pieces, thinning the mucus to make it easier to cough up

GI Tract: Pancrelipase

- Pancrelipase contains the enzymes lipase, protease and amylase that are needed to break down fats, proteins and starches

  ❏ *Zenpep* identifies that it is a pancreatic enzyme product (PEP)

  ❏ *Creon* comes from the generic name pancrelipase

  ❏ *Viokace* indicates that it is an enzyme by the suffix (slightly different spelling)

PANCREATIC ENZYME PRODUCTS

The thick mucus in CF obstructs pancreatic enzyme flow, resulting in a lack of these enzymes reaching the gastrointestinal tract and subsequent malabsorption. Frequent, greasy, oily, foul-smelling stools are manifestations of pancreatic insufficiency. Most patients with CF need to supplement their diet with pancreatic enzyme products (PEPs) to help break down fat, starches and protein. This is called pancreatic enzyme replacement therapy (PERT).

Pancrelipase is a natural product harvested from porcine pancreatic glands which contains a combination of lipase, amylase and protease. PEPs are formulated to dissolve in the more basic pH of the duodenum. The dose is individualized for each patient and is based on the lipase component. Once PEP therapy is started, the dose is adjusted every 3 – 4 days until stools are normalized.

DRUG	DOSING	SAFETY/SIDE EFFECTS/MONITORING
Pancrelipase **(Creon, Viokace, Zenpep**, Lip-Prot-Amyl, Pancreaze, Pertzye)	**Initial** Age < 1 year: varies by product Age 1-3 years: lipase 1,000 units/kg/meal Age ≥ 4 years: lipase 500 units/kg/meal **Max (all ages)** Lipase ≤ 2,500 units/kg/meal or ≤ 10,000 units/kg/day; doses > 6,000 units/kg/meal are associated with colonic stricture	**WARNINGS** Fibrosing colonopathy advancing to colonic strictures (rare: higher risk with doses > 10,000 lipase units/kg/day), mucosal irritation, hyperuricemia **SIDE EFFECTS** Abdominal pain, flatulence, nausea, HA, neck pain **MONITORING** Abdominal symptoms, nutritional intake, weight, height (children), stool, fecal fat **NOTES** See Study Tip Gal below

COMMON ISSUES WITH PANCREATIC ENZYME PRODUCTS

Pancreatic enzyme replacement helps patients with CF digest food, maintain weight and improve nutrient absorption.

- PEP formulations are not interchangeable. Commonly used products are *Creon, Viokace* and *Zenpep*.
- *Viokace* is the only PEP that is a tablet. It is non-enteric coated and must be given with a PPI.
- All other PEPs are capsules.

  ❏ Do not crush or chew the contents of the capsules.

  ❏ Delayed-release capsules with enteric-coated microspheres or microtablets may be opened and sprinkled on soft, acidic foods (pH ≤ 4.5) like applesauce. Avoid foods with high pH such as dairy.

  ❏ Do not retain the capsule contents in the mouth. Swallow immediately and follow with water to avoid mucosal irritation and stomatitis.

- Take PEPs before or with all meals and snacks. High-fat meals may require higher doses.

  ❏ Use 50% of the mealtime dose with snacks.

- Protect from moisture; dispense in original container (exceptions: *Zenpep* and some *Creon* strengths). Do not refrigerate.

CYSTIC FIBROSIS TRANSMEMBRANE CONDUCTANCE REGULATOR (CFTR) MODULATORS

Ivacaftor works by increasing the time the CFTR channels remain open, which enhances chloride transport activity. Lumacaftor, tezacaftor and elexacaftor help correct the CFTR folding defect, which increases the amount of CFTR delivered to the cell surface. Because each drug is approved for very specific mutations, genotype testing must be performed prior to initiation.

The most common mutation in the CFTR gene is a homozygous F508del mutation (two copies of the same allele). Combination products (Orkambi, Symdeko and Trikafta) are approved for the most common CF mutation.

DRUG	APPROVED MUTATION	SAFETY/NOTES
Ivacaftor (Kalydeco) Tablet, oral granules	Not approved for use in homozygous F508del mutation; approved for use in other responsive mutations	**WARNINGS** ↑ LFTs, cataracts in children **NOTES** Take with high-fat containing food Minimum age cut-off for use varies by product; confirm with package labeling
Lumacaftor/ivacaftor (Orkambi) Tablet, oral granules Tezacaftor/ivacaftor (Symdeko) Co-packaged tablets Elexacaftor/tezacaftor/ivacaftor (Trikafta) Co-packaged tablets, oral granules	Approved for use in homozygous F508del mutation and additional responsive mutations	

CFTR Modulator Drug Interactions

- Ivacaftor is a substrate of CYP450 3A4 (major) and should be avoided with strong CYP3A4 inducers. Dosage adjustments may be required when CFTR modulators are used with CYP3A4 inhibitors.

OTHER CONCERNS

CF is usually diagnosed in very young children. Appropriate measures to address the patient's growth, nutrition, bone health and other CF complications are critical.

- A high-fat and calorically dense diet is recommended to help with nutrition, normal weight and growth, increased energy needs and to prolong survival.
- Vitamin supplements are required, especially the fat-soluble vitamins A, D, E and K for normal cellular function. Calcium and vitamin D intake/absorption should be monitored to maximize bone health.
- Many patients with CF will eventually require insulin for treatment of CF-related diabetes mellitus.
- If the patient maintains good health, the chances of qualifying for a lung transplant are improved.

KEY COUNSELING POINTS

See the Drug Formulations and Patient Counseling chapter for counseling language/layman's terminology.

TOBI Podhaler

- Do not swallow capsules.
- Use only the provided Podhaler device.
- Take doses as close to 12 hours but no less than six hours apart.

Pancreatic Enzyme Products

- Take at the beginning of a meal or snack. Take half of the meal-time dose with snacks.
- Swallow whole.
- Contents can be sprinkled on a spoonful of soft food (e.g., applesauce, pureed bananas or pears). Use right away.
- Do not mix with dairy products.
- Drink plenty of non-caffeinated liquids every day.

Select Guidelines/References
ECFS Best Practice Guidelines: The 2018 Revision. *J Cyst Fibros* 2018;17:153-78.

Cystic Fibrosis Foundation: Clinical Care Guidelines. https://www.cff.org/Care/Clinical-Care-Guidelines/ (accessed 2023 Nov 7).

CONTENT LEGEND

 = Study
       Tip Gal

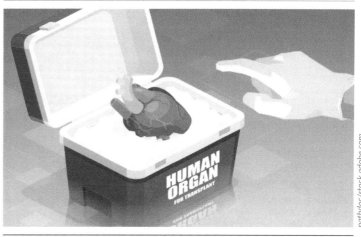

pathdoc/stock.adobe.com

CHAPTER 56

TRANSPLANT

BACKGROUND

Transplantation is one of the most challenging and complex areas of modern medicine. The main goal of transplantation is to prolong patient and graft (i.e., the transplanted organ or tissue) survival. United Network for Organ Sharing (UNOS) is the organization responsible for organ allocation in the U.S. Organs that have been successfully transplanted include the kidney, liver, pancreas, heart and lungs, with kidney and liver transplants being most common. Bone marrow transplantation has been used successfully for certain hematological and immunodeficiency conditions.

PREVENTION OF GRAFT REJECTION

An allograft is the transplant of an organ or tissue from one individual to another of the same species with a different genotype. This can also be called an allogenic transplant. A transplanted organ from a genetically identical donor (such as an identical twin) is called an isograft. An autograft (also called autologous transplant) is a transplant in the same patient, from one site to another (e.g., autologous stem cell transplant or skin grafting).

Rejection occurs when the body has an immune response to the allograft. This response may lead to transplant failure, the need for organ failure support (e.g., dialysis) or removal of the transplanted organ. Immunosuppressant medications prevent or stop the patient's immune system from attacking the new organ. These drugs are given before or at the time of transplant (induction immunosuppression), chronically after transplant (maintenance immunosuppression) or in the event of an acute rejection episode. Immunosuppressants drugs share many significant risks and warnings (see Study Tip Gal on the next page).

Prior to any transplant, tissue typing or crossmatching is performed to assess donor-recipient compatibility for human leukocyte antigen (HLA) and ABO blood group. A mismatch in either instance would lead to a fast, acute rejection (see Study Tip Gal).

A panel reactive antibody (PRA) test can be used to gauge the degree to which the recipient is "sensitized" to foreign (or "non-self") proteins. A high PRA correlates with the likelihood of graft rejection and could necessitate a desensitization protocol before the transplant.

AVOIDING AN "ABO MISMATCH" OR INCOMPATIBILITY REACTION

BLOOD GROUP	CAN GIVE BLOOD TO	CAN RECEIVE BLOOD FROM
AB Universal receiver	AB	AB A B O
A	A AB	A O
B	B AB	B O
O Universal donor	AB A B O	O

BOXED WARNINGS FOR TRANSPLANT DRUGS OVERLAP

Infection Risk

Transplant drugs suppress the immune system and prevent organ rejection. Unfortunately, an immunosuppressed state increases the risk of different types of infections. Prophylaxis for infections is often required and can include some of the same drugs used for opportunistic infection in HIV when the CD4+ count is low.

Cancer Risk

A healthy immune system suppresses some types of cancers, including lymphomas, melanoma and non-melanoma skin cancers. Transplant drugs blunt these processes making sun protective measures and cancer screening essential for transplant patients.

"Only Experienced Prescribers..."

Transplant drugs require experienced prescribers. This is especially important when the drugs are started. The transplant team includes several types of highly skilled practitioners, including pharmacists who have specialized in managing transplant drugs.

INDUCTION IMMUNOSUPPRESSION

Induction immunosuppression is given immediately before or at the time of transplant to prevent acute rejection during the early post-transplant period. It consists of a short course of effective intravenous (IV) medication, either a polyclonal or monoclonal antibody (these end in "-mab"), most often combined with high-dose IV steroids. In some cases, high-dose IV steroids may be given alone.

A commonly used induction drug is basiliximab, an interleukin-2 (IL-2) receptor antagonist (see figure on the next page). The IL-2 receptor is expressed on activated T-lymphocytes and is a critical pathway for activating T-lymphocytes to attack and reject the organ. Basiliximab does not deplete immature T-lymphocytes and therefore cannot be used to treat rejection (only for prevention). Because the protein is humanized, infusion-related reactions are unlikely, and pre-medication is not necessary.

As an alternative to basiliximab, patients at higher risk of rejection can receive a lymphocyte-depleting medication, antithymocyte globulin. These drugs are made by injecting human T-lymphocytes into animals, allowing the animals to make antibodies against the T-lymphocytes, and then administering the animal's purified antibodies back to the human transplant recipients. Because they deplete both mature and immature T-lymphocytes, they can be used for both induction and treatment of rejection. Alemtuzumab, a monoclonal antibody usually used for leukemia and multiple sclerosis, can also be used off-label for induction (only available through a restricted distribution program). Induction immunosuppression may not be required if the transplant is from an identical twin.

DRUG	DOSING	SAFETY/SIDE EFFECTS/MONITORING

Interleukin-2 (IL-2) receptor antagonist – Chimeric (murine/human) monoclonal antibody that inhibits the IL-2 receptor on the surface of activated T-lymphocytes.

Basiliximab (Simulect) Injection	20 mg IV on the day of transplant (day 0) then repeat dose on post-operative day 4	**BOXED WARNINGS** Administer under the supervision of a physician experienced in immunosuppressive therapy. **SIDE EFFECTS** ↑ BP, fever, stomach upset/nausea/vomiting/cramping, peripheral edema, dyspnea, upper respiratory irritation/infection, tremor, painful urination. **MONITORING** Signs and symptoms of hypersensitivity (within 24 hours) and infection.

Antithymocyte globulins – Bind to antigens on T-lymphocytes and interfere with their function.

Antithymocyte Globulin (Atgam – Equine) **(Thymoglobulin** – Rabbit) Injection	Atgam: 5-15 mg/kg/day IV Thymoglobulin: 1-1.5 mg/kg/day IV Normal equine doses are approximately 10-fold greater than the rabbit product	**BOXED WARNINGS** Administer under the supervision of a physician experienced in immunosuppressive therapy. Anaphylaxis can occur; intradermal skin testing recommended prior to the 1st dose of Atgam. **SIDE EFFECTS** Infusion-related reactions/cytokine release syndrome (fever, chills, pruritus, rash, ↓ BP; particularly common with the first dose), infections, leukopenia, thrombocytopenia, chest pain, ↑ BP, edema. **MONITORING** CBC with differential, vital signs during administration, lymphocyte profile (T-cell count). **NOTES** Premedicate (diphenhydramine, acetaminophen and steroids) to lessen infusion-related reactions. Epinephrine and resuscitative equipment should be nearby. Administer over at least 4 hours (6 hours for the first dose of Thymoglobulin) to minimize infusion reactions. Infuse with an in-line filter.

MAINTENANCE IMMUNOSUPPRESSION

Maintenance immunosuppression is generally provided by the combination of:

- A calcineurin inhibitor (CNI) such as cyclosporine or tacrolimus. Tacrolimus is the first-line CNI.

  ❑ Belatacept may be used as an alternative to a CNI.

- An antiproliferative agent such as mycophenolate or azathioprine. Mycophenolate is first-line in most protocols.

  ❑ Mammalian target of rapamycin (mTOR) inhibitors (everolimus and sirolimus) may be used as an alternative.

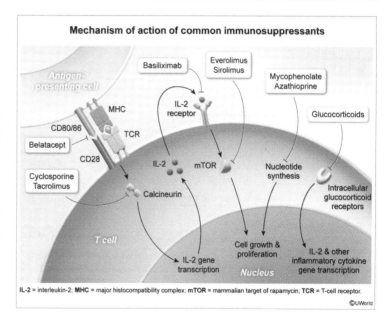

Mechanism of action of common immunosuppressants

IL-2 = interleukin-2; **MHC** = major histocompatibility complex; **mTOR** = mammalian target of rapamycin; **TCR** = T-cell receptor.

©UWorld

- With or without steroids (typically prednisone). If the patient is low immunological risk, the steroids can be discontinued; otherwise, the long-term adverse effects need to be considered.

Suppressing the immune system via multiple mechanisms with different drug classes (see figure) is designed to both lower toxicity risk of the individual immunosuppressants and reduce the risk of graft rejection. Doses and goal blood levels of maintenance immunosuppression vary depending on the type of transplant, drug interactions, time from transplant, risk for rejection and specific transplant center protocols. The following drug tables contain general dosing and blood level information.

DRUG	DOSING	SAFETY/SIDE EFFECTS/MONITORING
Calcineurin inhibitors – Suppress cellular immunity by inhibiting T-lymphocyte activation.		
Cyclosporine (modified: *Gengraf*, *Neoral;* non-modified: *Sandimmune*) Capsule, Oral Solution, Injection *Restasis*, *Cequa*, *Verkazia* – ophthalmic for dry eyes	Dosing is individualized to achieve goal trough level of 100-400 ng/mL Cyclosporine (modified): 4-8 mg/kg/day, PO divided Q12H Cyclosporine (non-modified): 3-10 mg/kg/day, PO divided Q12H IV cyclosporine (*Sandimmune*) dose is ⅓ of the PO dose	**BOXED WARNINGS** Increased risk of malignancy (lymphoma, skin cancer); ↑ risk of infection; nephrotoxicity (can occur at any trough level); ↑ BP; due to differences in bioavailability, cyclosporine (modified) and cyclosporine (non-modified) are not interchangeable. Should only be prescribed by healthcare providers experienced in immunosuppressive therapy. **SIDE EFFECTS** ↑ BG, hyperlipidemia, hyperkalemia, hypomagnesemia, hirsutism, gingival hyperplasia, neurotoxicity (tremor, headache, paresthesia), hyperuricemia, edema, abdominal discomfort/nausea/diarrhea, viral infections, viral associated nephropathy. **MONITORING** Trough levels, serum electrolytes (K and Mg), renal function, LFTs, BP, blood glucose, lipid profile. **NOTES** Numerous drug interactions: CYP3A4 inhibitor, and a CYP3A4 and P-gp substrate. Do not administer oral liquid from a plastic or Styrofoam cup. Use the syringe provided and do not rinse before or after use (see Key Counseling Points). IV: non-PVC sets should be used to minimize leaching of DEHP.
Tacrolimus (*Prograf*) Capsule, Granules for Oral Solution, Injection Extended-Release Capsule – *Astagraf XL* Extended-Release Tablet – **Envarsus XR** *Protopic* – topical for eczema	Dosing is individualized to achieve goal trough level of 3-15 ng/mL *Prograf*: 0.1-0.2 mg/kg/day, PO divided Q12H *Astagraf XL* and *Envarsus XR* are given as a single dose, every 24 hours PO IR doses are 3-4 times that of IV; start oral dosing 8-12 hours after last IV dose	**BOXED WARNINGS** Increased risk of malignancy (lymphoma, skin cancer); ↑ risk of infection. Extended-release tacrolimus (*Astagraf XL*) associated with ↑ mortality in female liver transplant recipients. **SIDE EFFECTS** ↑ BP, ↑ BG, hyperlipidemia, nephrotoxicity, hypomagnesemia, hypo/hyperkalemia, alopecia, neurotoxicity (tremor, headache, dizziness, paresthesia), edema, hypo/hyperphosphatemia, QT prolongation, diarrhea, urinary tract infection, anemia, leukopenia, leukocytosis, thrombocytopenia, elevated liver enzymes, arthralgia. **MONITORING** Trough levels, serum electrolytes (K, Phos and Mg), renal function, LFTs, BP, blood glucose, lipid profile. **NOTES** Administer under the supervision of a physician experienced in immunosuppressive therapy. Do not interchange XL/XR to immediate-release (IR) without prescriber approval. Numerous drug interactions: CYP3A4 and P-gp substrate. Food decreases absorption. Avoid alcoholic beverages with *Astagraf XL* and *Envarsus XR* (↑ rate of release and risk of side effects). IV is administered as a continuous infusion; must use non-PVC bag and tubing.
Antiproliferative agents – Inhibit T- and B-lymphocyte proliferation by altering purine nucleotide synthesis.		
Azathioprine (*Azasan*, *Imuran*) Tablet, Injection	1-3 mg/kg PO daily CrCl < 50 mL/min: adjustment required	**BOXED WARNINGS** Increased risk of malignancy (lymphoma, skin cancer). **WARNINGS** Myelosuppression, either dose-related, or with conventional doses due to a genetic deficiency of thiopurine methyltransferase (TPMT), both requiring dose adjustment; ↑ risk of infection. **SIDE EFFECTS** GI (severe N/V/D), acute pancreatitis, rash, hepatotoxicity. **MONITORING** LFTs, CBC, renal function.

DRUG	DOSING	SAFETY/SIDE EFFECTS/MONITORING
Mycophenolate Mofetil (CellCept) Tablet, Capsule, Suspension, Injection **Mycophenolic Acid (Myfortic)** Delayed-Release Tablet	*CellCept*: 1-1.5 g PO/IV Q12H *Myfortic*: 360-720 mg PO Q12H	**BOXED WARNINGS** Increased risk of malignancy (lymphoma, skin cancer); ↑ risk of infection; ↑ risk of congenital malformations and spontaneous abortions when used during pregnancy. Should only be prescribed by healthcare providers experienced in immunosuppressive therapy. **SIDE EFFECTS** Diarrhea, abdominal pain, nausea, vomiting, leukopenia, anemia, thrombocytopenia, ↑ or ↓ BP, edema, tachycardia, pain, ↑ BG, hypo/hyperkalemia, hypomagnesemia, hypocalcemia, hypercholesterolemia, infections. **MONITORING** CBC, intolerable diarrhea, pregnancy tests, renal function, LFTs, signs of infection. **NOTES** REMS drug. *CellCept* and *Myfortic* are not interchangeable due to differences in absorption (*CellCept* 500 mg ≅ to *Myfortic* 360 mg). Interchange requires provider approval. *Myfortic* is enteric coated to decrease diarrhea. Tablets must be protected from light; dispense in a light-resistant container, such as the manufacturer's original container. *CellCept* IV is stable in D5W only. Do not use IV if allergy to polysorbate 80. Begin infusion within 4 hours of reconstitution. Decreases efficacy of oral contraceptives.

Mammalian target of rapamycin (mTOR) kinase inhibitors – Inhibit T-lymphocyte activation/proliferation; may be synergistic with CNIs.

DRUG	DOSING	SAFETY/SIDE EFFECTS/MONITORING
Everolimus (*Zortress*) Tablet *Afinitor* – for certain cancers	Dosing is individualized to achieve goal trough level of 3-8 ng/mL 0.5-1.5 mg PO Q12H	**BOXED WARNINGS** Increased risk of malignancy (lymphoma, skin cancer); ↑ risk of infection. Should only be prescribed by healthcare providers experienced in immunosuppressive therapy. Everolimus: When used with cyclosporine, reduced doses of cyclosporine are recommended; ↑ risk of renal artery thrombosis can result in graft loss; not recommended in heart transplant. Sirolimus: Not recommended for use in liver (hepatic artery thrombosis) or lung transplantation. **WARNINGS** Hyperlipidemia, impaired wound healing, pneumonitis (discontinue drug if this develops), angioedema, fluid accumulation (surgical site), proteinuria, male infertility. Everolimus: ↑ risk hepatic artery thrombosis can result in graft loss (do not use within 30 days of transplant).
Sirolimus (*Rapamune*) Tablet, Oral Solution	Dosing is individualized to achieve goal trough level of 4-12 ng/mL 1-5 mg PO daily	Sirolimus: Decline in renal function (when used long-term with cyclosporine), latent viral infections, ↑ risk of hemolytic uremic syndrome when used with a CNI. **SIDE EFFECTS** Peripheral edema, ↑ BP, ↑ BG, constipation, N/V/D, abdominal pain, headache, fatigue, fever, rash/pruritus, acne, anemia, leukopenia, thrombocytopenia, stomatitis. **MONITORING** Trough levels, renal function, LFTs, lipids, blood glucose, BP, CBC, urine protein, signs of infection. **NOTES** Numerous drug interactions: CYP3A4 and P-gp substrate. Everolimus: Protect from light and moisture. Sirolimus: Tablets and oral solution are not bioequivalent.

DRUG	DOSING	SAFETY/SIDE EFFECTS/MONITORING

Belatacept – Inhibits T-lymphocyte activation and production of inflammatory mediators by binding to CD80 and CD86 on antigen presenting cells, blocking costimulation with CD28 on T-lymphocytes.

Belatacept (*Nulojix*) Injection	Initial: 10 mg/kg on days 1, 5 and then at the end of weeks 2, 4, 8, and 12 after transplantation Maintenance: 5 mg/kg at the end of week 16 after transplantation and then monthly thereafter Dose using TBW and round dose to the nearest 12.5 mg	**BOXED WARNINGS** Increased risk of post-transplant lymphoproliferative disorder (PTLD) with the highest risk in recipients without immunity to Epstein-Barr Virus (EBV); use in EBV seropositive patients only. Increased risk of infection and malignancies; avoid use in liver transplant patients due to risk of graft loss and death. Administer under the supervision of a physician experienced in immunosuppressive therapy. **WARNINGS** Increased risk of opportunistic infections, sepsis and/or fatal infections, ↑ risk of tuberculosis (TB); test for latent TB prior to initiation and treat latent TB prior to use. **SIDE EFFECTS** Headache, anemia, leukopenia, constipation, diarrhea, nausea, peripheral edema, ↑ or ↓ BP, cough, photosensitivity, insomnia, urinary tract infection, pyrexia, ↑ or ↓ K, hypophosphatemia. **MONITORING** Neurological, cognitive or behavioral signs/symptoms [consider progressive multifocal leukoencephalopathy (PML), PTLD or CNS infection]; signs/symptoms of infection, TB screening prior to initiation, EBV seropositive verification prior to initiation. **NOTES** Use silicone-free disposable syringe (comes with drug).

Systemic steroids – Naturally occurring hormones that prevent or suppress inflammatory and cytokine gene expression.

Prednisone Tablet, Oral Solution	2.5-20 mg PO daily, or on alternate days	**SHORT-TERM SIDE EFFECTS** Fluid retention, stomach upset, emotional instability (euphoria, mood swings, irritability), insomnia, ↑ appetite, weight gain, acute rise in blood glucose and blood pressure with high doses. **LONG-TERM SIDE EFFECTS** Adrenal suppression/Cushing's syndrome, impaired wound healing, ↑ BP, diabetes, acne, osteoporosis, impaired growth in children. See Systemic Steroids & Autoimmune Conditions chapter for further information on chronic steroid use.

TRANSPLANT DRUGS: WHAT'S USED, WHEN

Immunosuppression protocols vary by center and type of transplant.

Induction Immunosuppressants
- Basiliximab, an interleukin-2 (IL-2) receptor antagonist
- Antithymocyte globulin in patients at higher risk of rejection
- High-dose IV steroids

Maintenance Immunosuppressants
- The calcineurin inhibitors (CNIs) [tacrolimus (primarily) or cyclosporine]
  - ❏ Belatacept as an alternative to a CNI
- Adjuvant medications given with a CNI (to achieve adequate immunosuppression while decreasing the dose and toxicity of the individual agents)
  - ❏ Antiproliferative agents [mycophenolate (primarily) or azathioprine]
  - ❏ mTOR inhibitors (everolimus or sirolimus)
- Steroids at lower or tapering doses

DRUG INTERACTIONS

Pharmacokinetic Interactions

- Cyclosporine inhibits CYP3A4. Both cyclosporine and tacrolimus are CYP3A4 and P-glycoprotein (P-gp) substrates. Inducers of either enzyme (e.g., carbamazepine, nafcillin, rifampin) decrease the CNI concentration, and inhibitors (e.g., azole antifungals, diltiazem, erythromycin) increase the CNI concentration. Both interact with the majority of drugs.

- Cyclosporine can ↑ sirolimus, everolimus and some statins (which transplant patients often require).

- Mycophenolate can ↓ levels of hormonal contraception; mycophenolate levels can be ↓ by antacids (containing aluminum/magnesium), multivitamins, metronidazole, PPIs, quinolones, sevelamer, bile acid resins and rifampin and derivatives.

- Azathioprine is metabolized by xanthine oxidase. <u>Avoid using azathioprine with xanthine oxidase inhibitors</u> (<u>allopurinol or febuxostat</u>). Febuxostat is contraindicated. If allopurinol is used, reduce the azathioprine dose by 75% and monitor for myelosuppression and GI side effects.

Pharmacodynamic Interactions

Maintenance immunosuppressants have a high incidence of certain adverse effects that require monitoring and likely intervention (e.g., nephrotoxicity, diabetes, hyperlipidemia). Caution with additive drugs that:

- Are <u>nephrotoxic with CNIs</u> (e.g., NSAIDs).
- <u>Raise blood glucose with steroids, CNIs</u> and mTOR inhibitors.
- <u>Worsen lipids with mTOR inhibitors</u>, steroids and cyclosporine.
- <u>Raise blood pressure</u> with CNIs and steroids.
- Are <u>myelosuppressive with azathioprine</u> and mycophenolate.

Drug-Food and Natural Product Interactions

- Avoid <u>grapefruit juice and St. John's wort</u> with CNIs.
- Tacrolimus absorption is decreased by food.

ORGAN TRANSPLANT COMPLICATIONS

MONITORING BY PATIENT & HEALTH CARE TEAM

In addition to symptoms of drug toxicity, patients should monitor for symptoms of organ rejection.

Monitoring Questions
Is it a symptom of drug **toxicity**?
Is it a symptom of **organ rejection**?
Is it a symptom of an **infection**?

Common symptoms of acute rejection include <u>flu-like symptoms</u>, such as chills, body aches, nausea, cough, shortness of breath and organ-specific symptoms that depend on the transplant type.

Examples include:

- Heart failure symptoms or a new arrhythmia could be due to heart transplant rejection.

- A <u>decrease in urine output, fluid retention</u>, blood pressure elevation or graft tenderness could be due to kidney transplant rejection.

Immunosuppressive medications require <u>careful monitoring</u> (including drug <u>trough levels</u> for some) to minimize toxicities and the incidence of rejection. Trough levels should be drawn <u>30 minutes</u> before a scheduled dose.

All transplant recipients must self-monitor for <u>symptoms of infection</u>:

- Fever of 100.4°F (38°C) or higher (lower if elderly), chills
- Cough, more sputum or change in color of sputum, sore throat
- Pain with passing urine, ear or sinus pain
- Mouth sores or a wound that does not heal

ACUTE REJECTION

<u>Acute rejection</u> of the transplanted organ arises from either <u>T-cell (cellular)</u> or <u>B-cell (humoral or antibody)</u> mediated mechanisms. Both types can occur simultaneously (mixed rejection). Distinguishing the type and severity of rejection <u>via biopsy</u> is essential to determine treatment.

An <u>initial</u> approach to treating acute cellular rejection (ACR) is the administration of <u>high-dose steroids</u> and optimizing maintenance immunosuppression (e.g., increasing the trough level). Antithymocyte globulin is usually reserved for steroid-resistant or a more aggressive ACR.

Antibody-mediated rejection (AMR), sometimes referred to as humoral rejection, is more challenging to treat as the antibodies against the graft must be removed and then suppressed from recurring. This is accomplished with plasmapheresis and administration of intravenous immunoglobulin (IVIG) and steroids, and can be followed by a dose of rituximab (see the Acute & Critical Care Medicine chapter for more information on IVIG). Rituximab, a monoclonal antibody against the CD20 antigen on B-cells, may prevent further antibody development. See the Systemic Steroids & Autoimmune Conditions and Oncology chapters.

REDUCING INFECTION RISK

The effective use of immunosuppressants increases successful outcomes in organ transplantation but comes at the cost of an increased risk of infections. These infections are a major cause of morbidity and mortality in transplant recipients, and can be:

- Bacterial (e.g., surgical site)
- Viral (e.g., HSV reactivation)
- Opportunistic (e.g., fungal, protozoal)

Infection prophylaxis is essential, especially in the first six months post-transplant, when immunosuppression is highest, and after receiving treatment for acute rejection. The drugs used for infection prophylaxis are often the same as those used for treatment, but treatment usually requires larger doses, IV administration and a combination of drugs (see the Infectious Diseases IV chapter).

Routine infection control must include reducing risk from transmission, such as proper hand-washing techniques (see the Medication Safety & Quality Improvement chapter), air filtration systems, keeping the mouth clean and keeping away from dusty, crowded areas and sick people. Vaccine-preventable illness is an important consideration pre-transplant since live vaccines cannot be given post-transplant (see Study Tip Gal).

CANCER

Cancer risk is higher in transplant recipients compared to the general population. The cancer risk is similar to that seen with the use of immunosuppressant medications used for autoimmune conditions.

Some cancer types are viral-mediated and related to immunosuppression, which causes increased cancer incidence. For example, the Epstein-Barr virus infects most people without serious consequences. In transplant recipients, there is a marked increase in the risk of malignancies associated with the infection.

Age-appropriate cancer screening is performed as part of the transplant candidate work-up. Screening for common cancers is routine, along with lifestyle measures known to reduce risk. Skin cancer is common following a transplant. Sunscreen must be used routinely, along with sun avoidance or sun protection with clothing. The skin should be assessed professionally at least annually.

CARDIOVASCULAR DISEASE

Many of the medications used to prevent transplant rejection can cause metabolic syndrome. These patients are among the highest risk for cardiovascular disease (CVD), so blood pressure, blood glucose, cholesterol and weight must be tightly controlled. Specific goals based on transplant protocols are managed by specialists, including pharmacists, who have received transplant medicine training. Blood glucose and post-transplantation diabetes mellitus (PTDM) are managed according to the ADA guidelines, and cholesterol according to the ACC/AHA guidelines. Weight is measured at each visit, and weight loss programs are used as-needed. Refer to the individual chapters for treatment of these conditions, but keep in mind that drug interactions and adverse effects may limit the use of standard first-line therapies in some transplant patients.

VACCINE-PREVENTABLE ILLNESS IN TRANSPLANT RECIPIENTS

Required vaccines are given pre-transplant if not up-to-date (see the Immunizations chapter for additional information).

Inactivated vaccines can be given 3-6 months post-transplant (once the immune system recovers from induction immunosuppression), except for the influenza vaccine, which can be administered 1 month post-transplant.

Live vaccines cannot be given post-transplant.

Important vaccines for transplant recipients:
- Influenza (inactivated, not live) annually
- Pneumococcal vaccine in adults ≥ 19 years. Give one of the following:
  - PCV20 (*Prevnar 20*) x 1 or
  - PCV15 (*Vaxneuvance*) x 1 followed by PPSV23 (*Pneumovax 23*) x 1 ≥ 8 weeks later.

- Varicella vaccine
  - High risk for serious varicella infections, with a very high risk of disseminated disease if infection occurs.
  - Vaccinate pre-transplant.
  - Vaccinate close contacts. Although there is a small risk that transmission could occur (from the vaccine recipient to the transplant recipient), ACIP states that the benefits outweigh the risk of transmission.
  - If a vaccinated close contact develops a rash they are considered contagious, and must avoid contact with the transplant recipient and contact their physician.
  - If the transplant patient develops a rash, they need to be seen right away.
- Hepatitis B vaccine
  - Vaccinate pre-transplant or post-transplant (if indicated).

KEY COUNSELING POINTS

See the Drug Formulations and Patient Counseling chapter for counseling language/layman's terminology.

See the Drug Interactions section.

ALL IMMUNOSUPPRESSANTS

- Take the medication <u>exactly as prescribed</u> by your healthcare provider, at the same time every day. <u>Stay consistent on how you take your medication</u>.

- If getting a blood test to measure the drug level, take your medication after you have your blood drawn (not before). It is important to measure the <u>lowest (trough) level</u> of drug in your blood (<u>30 minutes before</u> a scheduled dose).

- Can increase risk of:
  - ❑ Infection.
  - ❑ Cancer, particularly lymphoma and skin cancer.

- Many drug interactions (including natural products and OTC medications).

- Live vaccines must be avoided. Check with your transplant team before getting any vaccines.

Tacrolimus

- Take <u>every 12 hours, or once daily in the morning for XL or XR formulations</u>.

- Food decreases absorption, but many patients take this with meals to improve adherence. However it is taken (with food or without), <u>consistency</u> is most important.

- Can cause:
  - ❑ Nephrotoxicity.
  - ❑ Increased blood pressure.
  - ❑ Hyperglycemia.
  - ❑ Headache.
  - ❑ Alopecia.

- Avoid grapefruit.

Mycophenolate

- Requires a MedGuide.

- Mycophenolic acid (Myfortic) and mycophenolate mofetil (CellCept) are not interchangeable. Do not switch between products unless directed by your prescriber.

- Can cause stomach upset (e.g., diarrhea).

- Avoid in pregnancy (teratogenic). Birth control pills do not work as well with this drug.

- Drug interactions due to binding. Avoid taking antacids and vitamins at the same time.

Cyclosporine

- Different brands deliver different amounts of medication; do not switch brands of cyclosporine unless directed by your prescriber.

- Can cause:
  - ❑ Nephrotoxicity.
  - ❑ Increased blood pressure.
  - ❑ Hyperglycemia.
  - ❑ Gingival hyperplasia.
  - ❑ Hirsutism.

- Avoid grapefruit.

- Follow instructions for proper oral cyclosporine solution administration (see <u>Study Tip Gal</u>).

ADMINISTRATION OF CYCLOSPORINE ORAL SOLUTION[1]

 Use the syringe provided by the manufacturer to measure the dose.

 Do not rinse the syringe before or after use.

 Use a compatible diluent[2] (e.g., orange juice) at room temperature.

 Mix the dose and diluent thoroughly in a glass container. Do not administer from a plastic or Styrofoam cup.

 Administer or drink immediately. Rinse the container with extra diluent to ensure the total dose is taken.

1 Modified and non-modified.
2 Consistently use the same diluent. Refer to the specific product package insert for guidance on compatible diluents.

©UWorld

Select Guidelines/References

Kidney Disease: Improving Global Outcomes (KDIGO) Transplant Work Group. KDIGO Clinical Practice Guideline for the Care of Kidney Transplant Recipients. *Am J Transplant*. 2009; 9 (Suppl 3):S1-155.

Danziger-Isakov L, Kumar D; AST ID Community of Practice. Vaccination of solid organ transplant candidates and recipients: Guidelines from the American society of transplantation infectious diseases community of practice. Clin Transplant. 2019 Sep;33(9):e13563.

Nelson, J, Alvey, N, Bowman, L, et al. Consensus recommendations for use of maintenance immunosuppression in solid organ transplantation: Endorsed by the American College of Clinical Pharmacy, American Society of Transplantation, and the International Society for Heart and Lung Transplantation. *Pharmacotherapy*. 2022; 42: 599- 633.

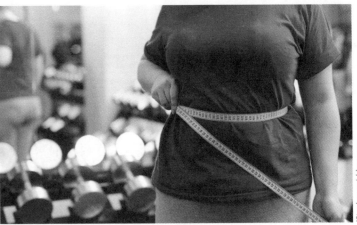

iStock.com/shironosov

CHAPTER 57

WEIGHT LOSS

BACKGROUND

The conditions of overweight and obesity are national health threats and a major public health challenge. Data from the CDC estimates that ~74% of U.S. adults and ~40% of children and adolescents are overweight (BMI 25 – 29.9 kg/m²) or obese (BMI ≥ 30 kg/m²). A person who is overweight is at a higher risk for coronary heart disease, hypertension, stroke, type 2 diabetes, certain types of cancer and premature death. In addition to the health risks, being overweight can reduce quality of life and cause social stigmatization and discrimination.

Weight loss must involve an "energy deficit." Calories must be decreased and/or energy expenditure increased to force the body to use fat as an energy source. If someone is hungry, it is difficult not to eat. Many weight loss drugs work by increasing satiety (feeling full) or decreasing appetite.

MEDICAL CONDITIONS, DRUGS AND WEIGHT

Prior to starting a weight loss treatment plan, other causes of weight gain should be evaluated and managed, as appropriate. Select drugs and medical conditions can cause weight gain (see Key Drugs Guy on top of the following page). Weight will increase when a medication known to cause weight loss is discontinued, when a medication that causes weight gain is started or if a condition with weight gain is left untreated. Weight will decrease when a condition known to cause weight gain is treated.

When treating other medical conditions in patients who are overweight or obese, medications that cause weight gain should be avoided (if able) and preference should be given to medications that can cause weight loss (see Key Drugs Guy on the bottom of the following page).

CONTENT LEGEND

 = Study Tip Gal    = Key Drug Guy

SELECT DRUGS/CONDITIONS THAT CAN CAUSE WEIGHT GAIN

KEY DRUGS

Antipsychotics (e.g., clozapine, olanzapine, risperidone, quetiapine)

Diabetes drugs (insulin, sulfonylureas, meglitinides, thiazolidinediones)

Divalproex/valproic acid

Gabapentin, pregabalin

Lithium

Mirtazapine

Steroids

TCAs (e.g., amitriptyline, nortriptyline)

Conditions:
Hypothyroidism

Others:

Beta-blockers

Dronabinol

Hormones (e.g., estrogen, megestrol)

MAO inhibitors

SSRIs (paroxetine, others may be weight neutral)

Vasodilators (e.g., minoxidil)

TREATMENT PRINCIPLES

The American Association of Clinical Endocrinologists/American College of Endocrinology (AACE/ACE) obesity guidelines recommend various eating plans that are either reduced-calorie (daily deficit ~500 – 750 kcal) or individualized, based on personal and cultural preferences. These include Mediterranean, DASH, low-carbohydrate, low-fat, volumetric, high protein and vegetarian diets. Select patients may be candidates for very low-calorie diets.

Physical activity should increase to ≥ 150 minutes per week, performed on three to five separate days. This should include resistance exercises two or three times weekly. Behavioral interventions should be used to assist patients, depending on factors that are hindering successful weight loss. These can include self-monitoring (of food intake, exercise, weight), goal setting, stress reduction, stimulus control, use of social support structures and/or guidance by trained educators.

Weight loss medications should only be added when lifestyle measures alone have failed to achieve adequate weight loss, maintain weight loss or prevent continued weight gain. In patients with weight-related complications (e.g., diabetes, dyslipidemia, hypertension, sleep apnea), weight loss medications may be started at the same time as lifestyle measures. As weight decreases, these conditions can improve. Treatment may need to be reevaluated and possibly decreased to prevent adverse effects (e.g., hypoglycemia, hypotension).

DRUG TREATMENT

OTC SUPPLEMENTS

OTC weight loss supplements commonly contain stimulants, such as bitter orange (see the Dietary Supplements, Natural & Complementary Medicine chapter) and/or excessive amounts of caffeine, which can be packaged under different names (e.g., yerba mate, guarana, concentrated green tea powder). OTC supplements are generally ineffective and are not recommended as they can be harmful, especially in patients with cardiovascular disease.

PRESCRIPTION WEIGHT LOSS MEDICATIONS

Prescription drugs are not appropriate for patients with small amounts of weight to lose. They are indicated with a BMI ≥ 30 kg/m², or a BMI ≥ 27 kg/m² with at least one weight-related condition, such as dyslipidemia, hypertension or diabetes. Weight loss medications are only used in addition to a dietary plan and increased physical activity. Selection of a medication is based on the patient's comorbid conditions. Some treatments can worsen other conditions and must be avoided in certain populations (see Study Tip Gal on the following page).

Older stimulant drugs (e.g., phentermine, diethylpropion) are only used short-term to "jump-start" a diet. The newer drugs *Qsymia, Contrave, Saxenda, Wegovy, Zepbound* and the orlistat formulations can be continued long-term for weight maintenance. Weight loss drugs should be discontinued if they do not produce at least a 5% weight loss at 12 weeks.

SELECT DRUGS/CONDITIONS THAT CAN CAUSE WEIGHT LOSS

KEY DRUGS

ADHD drugs (e.g., amphetamine, methylphenidate)

Bupropion

GLP-1 agonists (e.g., exenatide, liraglutide)

Pramlintide

Roflumilast

SGLT2 inhibitors (e.g., canagliflozin, empagliflozin)

Topiramate

Tirzepatide

Conditions:
Hyperthyroidism
Celiac disease
Inflammatory bowel disease

Others:

Acetylcholinesterase inhibitors (e.g., donepezil, rivastigmine, galantamine)

Antiseizure medications (zonisamide, ethosuximide)

Interferons

Thyroid drugs (e.g., levothyroxine)

Conditions:
Cystic fibrosis
GERD or peptic ulcer disease
Lupus
Tuberculosis (active disease)

PRESCRIPTION WEIGHT LOSS DRUGS: AVOID OR USE CAUTION

PREGNANCY	HYPERTENSION	DEPRESSION	SEIZURES	TAKING OPIOIDS
Avoid all weight loss drugs	**Avoid** *Contrave* (contains bupropion) and stimulants (e.g., phentermine) – contraindicated with uncontrolled BP **Caution** *Qsymia* – monitor HR (contains phentermine)	**Caution in young adults and adolescents** *Contrave* – suicide risk (contains bupropion)	**Avoid** *Contrave* – lowers seizure threshold (contains bupropion) **Caution** *Qsymia* – must taper off slowly if used (contains topiramate)	**Avoid** *Contrave* – blocks opioid receptors (contains naltrexone)

WEIGHT LOSS DRUGS

DRUG	DOSING	SAFETY/SIDE EFFECTS/MONITORING
	**Phentermine: sympathomimetic (stimulant); release of norepinephrine stimulates the satiety center which ↓ appetite** **Topiramate: ↑ satiety and ↓ appetite, possibly by ↑ GABA, blocking glutamate receptors and/or inhibition of carbonic anhydrase**	
Phentermine/Topiramate ER (*Qsymia*) C-IV REMS drug due to teratogenic risk; pregnancy test needed before treatment and monthly thereafter; use effective contraception during treatment	Start: 3.75 mg/23 mg PO QAM x 14 days; titrate up based on weight loss Max dose: 15 mg/92 mg PO QAM CrCl < 50 mL/min: max dose is 7.5 mg/46 mg/day	**CONTRAINDICATIONS** Pregnancy, glaucoma, hyperthyroidism, MAO inhibitor use within past 14 days **SIDE EFFECTS** Tachycardia, CNS effects [e.g., insomnia (take in the morning to ↓ risk), depression, anxiety, suicidal thoughts, headache, paresthesias], vision problems, constipation, dry mouth, ↓ HCO3, upper respiratory tract infection, ↑ SCr **NOTES** Taper off due to seizure risk
	**Naltrexone: ↓ food cravings** **Bupropion: ↓ appetite**	
Naltrexone/Bupropion (*Contrave*)	ER tablet: 8 mg/90 mg Initial: 1 tab PO QAM, titrate weekly as tolerated Max dose: 2 tabs BID Do not cut, chew or crush; swallow whole Fatty food increases drug levels; do not take with high-fat meal	**BOXED WARNING** Not approved for treatment of major depressive disorder (MDD) or psychiatric disorders; antidepressants (bupropion) can increase the risk of suicidal thinking and behavior in children, adolescents and young adults; not approved for use in pediatric patients **CONTRAINDICATIONS** Pregnancy, chronic opioid use or acute opiate withdrawal, uncontrolled hypertension, seizure disorder, use of other bupropion-containing products, bulimia/anorexia, abrupt discontinuation of alcohol, benzodiazepines, barbiturates, or antiseizure medications, use of MAO inhibitors within 14 days **WARNINGS** Use caution with psychiatric disorders, discontinue with s/sx of hepatotoxicity, can ↑ HR and BP, glaucoma **SIDE EFFECTS** N/V, constipation, headache, dizziness, dry mouth, insomnia, ↑ SCr **NOTES** Naltrexone blocks opioids and buprenorphine, which blocks analgesia and can induce withdrawal; discontinue opioids or buprenorphine 7-14 days prior to use of *Contrave*

DRUG	DOSING	SAFETY/SIDE EFFECTS/MONITORING
Glucagon-Like Peptide 1 (GLP-1) Agonists: ↑ satiety		**BOXED WARNING** Risk of thyroid C-cell carcinomas – seen in animal studies; risk to humans unknown
Liraglutide (Saxenda) Injection **Victoza** – for diabetes	Start: 0.6 mg SC daily x 1 week, titrate up by 0.6 mg SC daily at weekly intervals Target dose: 3 mg SC daily	**CONTRAINDICATIONS** Personal or family history of medullary thyroid carcinoma (MTC) or patients with Multiple Endocrine Neoplasia syndrome type 2 (MEN 2) *Saxenda*: pregnancy
Semaglutide (Wegovy) Injection **Ozempic** and *Rybelsus* – for diabetes	Start: 0.25 mg SC weekly x 4 weeks, titrate up every 4 weeks Target dose: 2.4 mg SC weekly, or 1.7 mg SC weekly (if 2.4 mg dose is not tolerated)	**WARNINGS** Pancreatitis, hypoglycemia, acute kidney injury, gallbladder disease Not recommended in patients with severe GI disease, including gastroparesis (drug-induced ileus has been reported) **SIDE EFFECTS** Nausea (primary side effect), vomiting, diarrhea, constipation, hypoglycemia, injection site reactions
Dual GLP-1 and Glucose-Dependent Insulinotropic Polypeptide (GIP) Agonist: ↑ satiety		Tirzepatide: increased heart rate
Tirzepatide (Zepbound) Injection *Mounjaro* – for diabetes	Start: 2.5 mg SC weekly x 4 weeks, then ↑ to 5 mg SC weekly Can ↑ to 15 mg SC weekly	**NOTES** May need to ↓ insulin or sulfonylurea/meglitinide doses to ↓ risk of hypoglycemia Can reduce the absorption of orally administered drugs due to ↓ gastric emptying. Use caution with narrow therapeutic index drugs or drugs that require threshold concentrations for efficacy (e.g., antibiotics, oral contraceptives); see the Diabetes chapter.
Lipase Inhibitor: ↓ absorption of dietary fats by ~30%		
Orlistat Rx – **Xenical** OTC – **Alli**	*Xenical*: 120 mg PO w/ each meal containing fat; take with meal or up to 1 hr after eating *Alli*: 60 mg PO w/ each meal containing fat Must be used with a low-fat diet plan	**CONTRAINDICATIONS** Pregnancy, chronic malabsorption syndrome, cholestasis **WARNINGS** Liver damage (rare), cholelithiasis, ↑ urinary oxalate/kidney stones, hypoglycemia (in patients with diabetes) **SIDE EFFECTS** GI (flatus with discharge, fatty stool, fecal urgency) **NOTES** Take multivitamin with A, D, E, K and beta-carotene at bedtime or separated by ≥ 2 hours; do not use with cyclosporine or separate by ≥ 3 hours; separate levothyroxine by ≥ 4 hours Must stick to dietary plan for both weight improvement and to help lessen GI side effects (max 30% of kcals from fat)
Appetite Suppressants: sympathomimetics (stimulants), release of norepinephrine stimulates the satiety center which ↓ appetite		
Phentermine (Adipex-P, *Lomaira*) C-IV	15-37.5 mg PO daily, before or after breakfast, or in divided doses	**CONTRAINDICATIONS/WARNINGS** Cardiovascular disease (e.g., uncontrolled hypertension, pulmonary hypertension, arrhythmias, heart failure, CAD), hyperthyroidism, glaucoma, pregnancy, breast feeding, history of drug abuse, MAO inhibitors within the past 14 days
Diethylpropion C-IV	IR: 25 mg PO TID, 1 hour before meals and mid-evening SR: 75 mg PO once at mid-morning	**SIDE EFFECTS** Tachycardia, agitation, ↑ BP, pulmonary hypertension (use > 3 months), insomnia, dizziness, tremor, psychosis
Phendimetrazine C-III	IR: 35 mg PO BID-TID, 1 hr before meals ER: 105 mg PO daily, 30-60 minutes before the morning meal	**MONITORING** HR, BP, symptoms of pulmonary hypertension (e.g., dyspnea, edema) **NOTES** Used short-term, up to 12 weeks, to "jump-start" a diet Stimulants taken later in the day can cause insomnia
Benzphetamine C-III	25-50 mg PO daily to TID; avoid late afternoon administration	Potential for misuse/dependence

BARIATRIC SURGERY

Guidelines recommend weight loss or bariatric surgery for adults with:

- BMI ≥ 35 kg/m²
- BMI ≥ 30 kg/m² and type 2 diabetes
- BMI ≥ 30 kg/m² who cannot achieve or sustain a goal BMI or improvement in an obesity-related comorbidity with other methods

Traditional bariatric surgery restricts food intake, which leads to weight loss. Patients must commit to a lifetime of healthy eating and regular exercise to sustain the weight loss. Some common issues associated with bariatric surgery are described below.

COMMON NUTRIENT DEFICIENCIES

- Calcium is mostly absorbed in the duodenum, which may be bypassed. Calcium citrate supplementation is preferred as it has non-acid-dependent absorption.
- Anemia can result from vitamin B12 and iron deficiency; both may require supplementation.
- Iron and calcium supplements should be taken two hours prior or four hours after antacids.
- Patients may require life-long supplementation of the fat-soluble vitamins A, D, E and K due to fat malabsorption.

MEDICATION CONCERNS

- Medications may require dose reduction and may need to be crushed and put in liquid or used in transdermal form for up to two months post-surgery. Pharmacists need to assess which drugs can be safely crushed and provide alternatives to drugs that cannot be crushed (i.e., extended-release formulations).
- Rapid weight loss can cause gallstones. Ursodiol (*Actigall, Urso 250, Urso Forte*) dissolves gallstones and may be needed, unless the gallbladder has been removed.

KEY COUNSELING POINTS

See the Drug Formulations and Patient Counseling chapter for counseling language/layman's terminology.

ALL WEIGHT LOSS MEDICATIONS

- Weight loss can improve diabetes and hypertension. Monitor these conditions closely; dose reductions may be needed for medications.

Phentermine/Topiramate (*Qsymia*)

- Take this medication in the morning. Avoid taking this medication in the evening, to prevent insomnia.
- Phentermine can cause increased heart rate.

Naltrexone/Bupropion (*Contrave*)

- Do not take with opioids or with a history of seizures.
- Can cause increased blood pressure.

GLP-1 Agonists and GLP-1/GIP Agonists

- Subcutaneous injection (see Diabetes chapter for details).
- Can cause:
  - Nausea, diarrhea.
  - Pancreatitis and gallbladder disease.
  - Kidney damage, especially from dehydration due to severe vomiting or diarrhea.
  - Hypoglycemia.
- Do not take with other GLP-1 agonists (used for diabetes).

Orlistat (*Xenical* and *Alli*)

- Take one capsule at each main meal, or up to one hour after a meal that contains fat.
- You should be eating a healthy diet that is low in fat in order to reduce GI side effects.
- Can cause stomach issues (e.g., fatty/oily stool, oily spotting, intestinal gas with discharge, need to have a bowel movement right away, increased number of bowel movements or poor bowel control).

Appetite Suppressants

- Can cause:
  - Increased blood pressure.
  - Increased heart rate.

Select Guidelines/References
US DHHS/ODPHP's 2020 – 2025 Dietary Guidelines for Americans, 9th Ed. Available at https://health.gov/our-work/food-nutrition.

2022 American Society for Metabolic and Bariatric Surgery (ASMBS) and International Federation for the Surgery of Obesity and Metabolic Disorders (IFSO): Indications for Metabolic and Bariatric Surgery. Surg Obes Relat Dis. 2022 Dec;18(12):1345-1356.

AACE/ACE Comprehensive clinical practice guidelines for medical care of patients with obesity. Endoc Pract. 2016; 22(3):1-203.

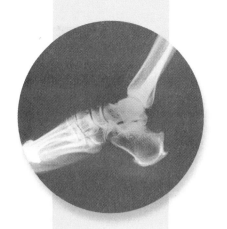
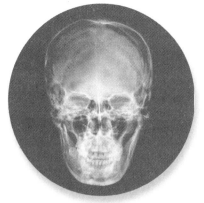
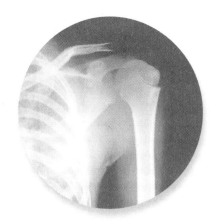

PAIN/RELATED CONDITIONS

CONTENTS

CONTENT LEGEND

Study
Tip Gal

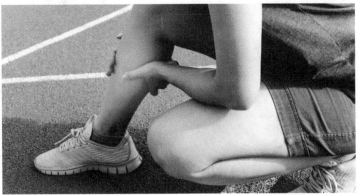

iStock.com/yaom

CHAPTER 58

PAIN

BACKGROUND

Pain can be defined as an unpleasant experience and physical suffering caused by an illness or injury. Pain can lead to a significant decrease in quality of life and ability to carry out daily tasks. It is one of the top reasons why adults seek medical care in the United States; approximately one in five adults have chronic pain.

PATHOPHYSIOLOGY

Pain is classified into two main categories (nociceptive pain and neuropathic pain) based on the underlying cause of the pain. Nociceptive pain occurs when tissue damage causes stimulation of sensory nerves (nociceptors). Injured tissue releases substances [e.g., prostaglandins (PGs), substance P, histamine] that cause nociceptors to send impulses to the brain; this results in feeling pain. Nociceptive pain can result from injury to internal organs (visceral pain) or from an injury to the skin, muscles, bones, joints or ligaments (musculoskeletal or somatic pain).

Neuropathic pain is different from nociceptive pain as it does not result from tissue injury or damage, but rather from damage or malfunction of the nervous system. Examples of neuropathic pain conditions include fibromyalgia, diabetic neuropathy, chronic headaches and certain drug-induced toxicities (e.g., vinca alkaloids).

ACUTE AND CHRONIC PAIN

Acute pain begins suddenly and usually feels sharp. It is typically nociceptive in nature, such as a fracture, burn, acute illness, surgery or childbirth. The pain can last just a few moments or longer, and usually goes away when the cause of the pain has resolved. Acute pain can cause anxiety and physical symptoms, including sweating and tachycardia. If left untreated, acute pain can increase the risk for development of chronic pain.

Chronic pain has been described as pain that persists for three months or longer. It can persist with a visible injury (such as crushed lumbar vertebrae, causing lower back pain) or when no visible injury is present, such as with osteoarthritis (OA) or diabetic neuropathy (see the Diabetes chapter). OA is a common type of chronic pain caused by cartilage breakdown within a joint, which results in stiffness, pain and/or swelling. Chronic pain is subdivided into cancer pain or chronic non-cancer pain, with each having separate treatment guidelines. Poorly managed chronic pain can cause depression and physical symptoms, (e.g., muscle tension, fatigue).

TREATMENT PRINCIPLES

Pain is subjective; it is primarily measured by the patient's own description, along with observations. Patients with chronic pain should be taught to monitor and document their pain by recording the pain level, the sensation or quality (e.g., burning, shooting, stabbing, aching), anything that worsens or lessens the pain and the time of day the pain improves or worsens. This helps to evaluate pain control and provides guidance on pain medication changes.

Pain scales are useful to assess pain severity and intensity. Pain is commonly rated using a numeric scale (0 = no pain, 10 = worst pain) or with the visual analog scale (see figure below). The Joint Commission (TJC) standards require that pain be assessed and managed while patients are hospitalized. Hospitals must inquire about, assess, treat and re-assess pain in a timely manner using non-pharmacologic and/or pharmacologic treatments. Pain scales are also used during outpatient clinic visits to evaluate any new pains and to help track changes in pain control over time.

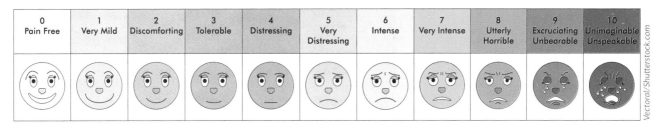

SELECTING AN ANALGESIC REGIMEN

Pain can be treated using a stepwise approach, where the choice of drug depends on the patient's self-reported pain severity. When initially using any class of analgesic (including opioids), start low and stop titrating at the lowest dose that adequately reduces the pain without causing intolerable adverse effects. Using medications with multiple mechanisms of action (i.e., multimodal pain control) often produces improved pain control via additive or synergistic effects.

Non-opioid analgesics [e.g., acetaminophen, non-steroidal anti-inflammatory drugs (NSAIDs)] are most commonly used for mild pain (acute or chronic) but can be added to an opioid-based regimen to reduce the total opioid dose required and provide better pain relief. Opioids are most appropriate for moderate to severe pain; use should be limited, as able, due to risks of abuse and dependence. Adjuvant treatments [e.g., antidepressants, antiseizure medications (ASMs), muscle relaxants] should be considered for any pain type and are especially beneficial for neuropathic pain; some treatments traditionally considered as adjuvants may be preferred as primary treatments in certain conditions (e.g., tricyclic antidepressants for fibromyalgia). If pain is not controlled after taking these steps, invasive or minimally invasive interventions (e.g., intrathecal drug administration) may be tried.

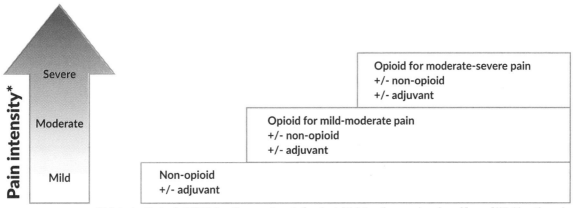

*Pain is classified as "mild" if 1-3 on the numeric scale, "moderate" if 4-6 on the numeric scale, and "severe" if 7-10 on the scale.

NON-OPIOID ANALGESICS

ACETAMINOPHEN

Acetaminophen reduces pain and fever (i.e., antipyretic) but does not provide an anti-inflammatory effect. The mechanism of action is not well defined but is thought to involve inhibition of PG synthesis in the central nervous system (CNS), resulting in reduced pain impulse generation.

DRUG	DOSING	SAFETY/SIDE EFFECTS/MONITORING
Acetaminophen (Tylenol, FeverAll, Ofirmev,* most "Non-Aspirin" pain relievers) Tablet/caplet, chewable tablet, ODT, suspension, suppository, injection **FeverAll:** rectal suppository Ofirmev*: injection (IV) Rx and OTC **+ hydrocodone** (Norco,* Vicodin*) **+ oxycodone (Endocet, Percocet)** **+ codeine** (Tylenol #3,* #4*) + tramadol **+ caffeine (Excedrin Tension Headache)** **+ aspirin/caffeine (Excedrin Extra Strength, Excedrin Migraine,** Goody's Powder) **+ caffeine/pyrilamine (Midol Complete)** + butalbital/caffeine (Fioricet) +/– codeine + diphenhydramine (Tylenol PM Extra Strength) + ibuprofen (Advil Dual Action) And in multiple cough & cold products and OTC combinations	**Adults** Maximum < 4,000 mg/day from all sources Maximum of 325 mg per prescription dosing unit in combo products, per the FDA Dosing ranges and maximum doses depend on the formulation 325 mg: max 2 tabs Q4H/10 tabs per 24 hr (3,250 mg) 500 mg: max 2 tabs Q6H/6 tabs per 24 hr (3,000 mg) 650 mg ER: max 2 tabs Q8H/6 tabs per 24 hr (3,900 mg) Rectal suppository 650 mg: max 1 PR Q4H/ 6 per 24 hr (3,900 mg) IV max: 650 mg Q4H or 1,000 mg Q6H/ 4-6 injections per 24 hr (4,000 mg) **Pediatrics (< 12 years)** 10-15 mg/kg Q4-6H Max: 5 doses/day OTC: use weight and age based dosing table on label Infant and children's suspension; use dosing syringe or dosing cup: 160 mg/5 mL	**BOXED WARNINGS** Severe hepatotoxicity (can require liver transplant or result in death) associated with doses ≥ 4 grams/day or use of multiple acetaminophen-containing products (see Study Tip Gal below) Risk of 10-fold dosing errors with injection **WARNINGS** Severe skin reactions including SJS, TEN (rare) Renal impairment: use cautiously **SIDE EFFECTS** Generally well-tolerated with oral administration **NOTES** Avoid using "APAP" abbreviation **Injection** Concentration is 10 mg/mL (in 100 mL vials); use caution with dosing Should always be ordered in mg, not mL All IV acetaminophen doses should be prepared in the pharmacy

*Brand discontinued but name still used in practice.

Acetaminophen Drug Interactions

- Acetaminophen can be used with warfarin, but if used chronically (doses > 2 grams/day), it can increase the INR.

- Avoid or limit alcohol use due to the risk of hepatotoxicity.

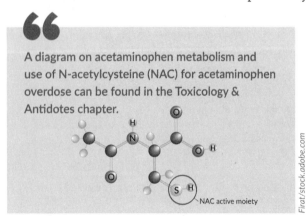

A diagram on acetaminophen metabolism and use of N-acetylcysteine (NAC) for acetaminophen overdose can be found in the Toxicology & Antidotes chapter.

NAC active moiety

Firat/stock.adobe.com

ACETAMINOPHEN OVERDOSE

The antidote for acetaminophen overdose is N-acetylcysteine (NAC, Acetadote).

- Glutathione precursor (↑ glutathione).

- Administered intravenously or orally (using the solution for inhalation or injectable formulation).

The Rumack-Matthew nomogram uses the serum acetaminophen level and the time since ingestion to determine whether hepatotoxicity is likely (and the need for NAC).

NON-STEROIDAL ANTI-INFLAMMATORY DRUGS

NSAIDs include the traditional non-selective agents (e.g., ibuprofen, aspirin) and the selective cyclooxygenase (COX) 2 inhibitors. The COX-1 and 2 enzymes catalyze the conversion of arachidonic acid to PGs and thromboxane A2 (TxA2). All NSAIDs decrease the formation of PGs, which results in decreased inflammation, alleviation of pain and reduced fever. Non-selective NSAIDs block the synthesis of both COX enzymes. COX-2 selective NSAIDs block the synthesis of COX-2 only, and therefore have less GI risks (because COX-1, which protects the gastric mucosa, is not affected). Blocking COX-1 decreases the formation of TxA2, which is required for both platelet activation and aggregation. Aspirin is an irreversible COX-1 and 2 inhibitor and is an antiplatelet agent that provides cardiovascular (CV) benefit (i.e., cardioprotection).

Non-Aspirin Boxed Warnings

All prescription non-aspirin NSAIDs require a MedGuide due to the risks listed below. These warnings are not repeated in the drug tables.

- GI Risk: NSAIDs can increase the risk of serious GI adverse events (e.g., bleeding, ulceration). Patients who are elderly, have a history of GI bleed or are taking systemic steroids, SSRIs or SNRIs are at the greatest risk. Aspirin also carries this risk.

- CV Risk: NSAIDs can increase the risk of MI and stroke. Avoid use in patients with CV disease or risk factors.

- Coronary Artery Bypass Graft (CABG) Surgery: NSAID use is contraindicated after CABG surgery. Antiplatelet therapy (typically aspirin) is recommended after CABG surgery.

Side Effects of All NSAIDs

All NSAIDs can cause:

- Decreased renal clearance by reducing blood flow to the glomerulus; additional nephrotoxic agents or dehydration increases this risk. All NSAIDs should be used cautiously (or avoided) in renal failure.

- Increased blood pressure. Use cautiously in controlled hypertension, and avoid in uncontrolled hypertension.

- Premature closure of the ductus arteriosus, which can lead to heart failure in the fetus. Do not use NSAIDs in the third trimester of pregnancy (≥ 30 weeks). See the Study Tip Gal below.

- Rare, but serious, renal impairment in the fetus if used around 20 weeks gestation or later in pregnancy.

- Nausea, especially salicylates. Nausea can be minimized by taking with food, switching to an enteric-coated or buffered product or changing to a different NSAID.

- Photosensitivity. Avoid the sun during mid-day hours, use sun-protective clothing and broad-spectrum sunscreen with an SPF of at least 30.

NSAIDS AND THE DUCTUS ARTERIOSUS

Before birth, the ductus arteriosus (DA) connects the pulmonary artery to the aorta, allowing oxygenated blood to flow to the fetus, bypassing the immature lungs.

Do not use NSAIDs in the third trimester of pregnancy. NSAIDs can prematurely close the DA.

After birth, the DA should close on its own. In some cases, it remains patent (open) and NSAIDs can be used to help it close.

IV NSAIDs (indomethacin, ibuprofen) can be used within 14 days after birth to close a patent ductus arteriosus (PDA).

Non-Aspirin NSAIDs

DRUG	DOSING	SAFETY/SIDE EFFECTS/MONITORING
COX-1 and COX-2 Non-selective NSAIDs: all agents have GI risk, CV risk and risk in post-operative CABG setting		
Ibuprofen (Advil, Motrin IB, Caldolor, NeoProfen) Tablet, capsule, chewable tablet, suspension, injection Rx and OTC	**Adults** OTC: 200-400 mg Q4-6H Max: 1.2 grams/day Rx: 400-800 mg Q6-8H Max: 3.2 grams/day **Pediatrics** 5-10 mg/kg/dose Q6-8H (as an antipyretic) Max: 40 mg/kg/day	**SIDE EFFECTS** All NSAIDs: dyspepsia, abdominal pain, nausea (see above text) **NOTES** NeoProfen injection is indicated for closure of PDA in premature infants OTC: limit self-treatment to < 10 days Severe skin reactions, including SJS/TEN
Indomethacin (Indocin) Capsule, oral suspension, suppository, injection	IR: 25-50 mg BID-TID CR: 75 mg daily-BID	**NOTES** High risk for CNS side effects (avoid in psych conditions) The IR formulation is an older NSAID approved for gout IV injection is indicated for closure of PDA in premature infants

DRUG	DOSING	SAFETY/SIDE EFFECTS/MONITORING
Naproxen (Aleve, Naprelan, Naprosyn) Tablet, capsule, suspension Rx and OTC + sumatriptan (Treximet) **+ esomeprazole (Vimovo)** And in OTC combos with diphenhydramine and pseudoephedrine	OTC (pain, fever): <u>220 mg Q8-12H</u> (1st dose can take 2 tabs) Max: 3 tabs in 24 hours (600 mg) Rx (inflammation, mild-mod pain): 500 mg Q12H (or 250 mg Q6-8H) Max: 1,000 mg/day (1,250 mg day 1)	**NOTES** Prescribers and patients may prefer naproxen since it can be <u>dosed BID</u> Naproxen base 200 mg = Naproxen Na 220 mg PPI in Vimovo is used to protect the GI tract
Ketorolac (Toradol,* Acular, Sprix) Tablet, injection, nasal spray, ophthalmic Acular: ophthalmic Sprix: nasal spray	Oral: 10-20 mg x 1, then 10 mg Q4-6H PRN (max: 40 mg/day) IV (≥ 50 kg): 30 mg x 1 or 30 mg Q6H (↓ dose if ≥ 65 yrs) IM (≥ 50 kg): 60 mg x 1 or 30 mg Q6H (↓ dose if ≥ 65 yrs) Nasal spray: < 65 yrs and ≥ 50 kg: 1 spray in <u>each</u> nostril Q6-8H ≥ 65 yrs or < 50 kg: 1 spray in <u>one</u> nostril Q6-8H	**BOXED WARNINGS** <u>Max combined duration IV/IM and PO/nasal is 5 days</u> in adults Oral ketorolac: for short-term moderate to severe acute pain only as continuation of IV or IM ketorolac Not for intrathecal or epidural use; avoid in advanced renal disease or those at risk for renal impairment due to volume depletion; hypersensitivity reactions to ketorolac or other NSAIDs; avoid use in labor and delivery and use with aspirin or NSAIDs; dose adjustments needed in ≥ 65 yrs or < 50 kg **WARNINGS** ↑ bleeding, acute renal failure, liver failure and anaphylactic shock **SIDE EFFECTS** Headache, injection site pain (often given IM) **NOTES** Usually used after surgery, never before Nasal spray: <u>prime five times before use</u>. No additional priming is needed if additional doses are used. Discard 24 hours after opening.
Piroxicam (Feldene)	10-20 mg daily	**NOTES** High risk for GI toxicity and severe skin reactions, including SJS/TEN; used when other NSAIDs have failed; may require GI protection (PPI, misoprostol)
Sulindac	150-200 mg BID	**NOTES** Sometimes used with reduced renal function, and in patients on lithium who require an NSAID

Other less commonly used NSAIDs include: meclofenamate, mefenamic acid, ketoprofen, fenoprofen, flurbiprofen, oxaprozin (Daypro – caution similar to piroxicam – higher risk of side effects)

Increased COX-2 Selectivity: lower risk for GI complications (but still present), ↑ risk MI/stroke (avoid with CV risk, avoid ↑ doses and longer duration in patients at risk for CV disease), same risk for renal complications

Celecoxib (Celebrex) Capsule, oral solution + tramadol (Seglentis)	OA: 100 mg BID or 200 mg daily RA: 100-200 mg BID Indications: OA, RA, juvenile RA, acute pain, primary dysmenorrhea, ankylosing spondylitis Seglentis: acute pain	**CONTRAINDICATIONS** <u>Sulfonamide allergy</u> **NOTES** <u>Highest COX-2 selectivity</u> Avoid in pregnancy; risk greatest at ≥ 30 weeks gestation Severe skin reactions, including SJS/TEN
Diclofenac (Voltaren, Cambia, Flector, Lofena, Pennsaid, Xrylix, Zipsor, Zorvolex) Tablet, capsule, cream, packet, gel (OTC), patch, topical solution, injection **Voltaren** (OTC): gel Rx and OTC + misoprostol (Arthrotec)	Oral tablets: 50-75 mg BID-TID Voltaren gel: 2-4 g to affected joint four times per day (<u>total body max 32 grams/day</u>) Flector: 1 patch (180 mg) to most painful area BID Cambia: 1 packet (50 mg) mixed in water for acute migraine Zipsor: 25 mg four times per day Zorvolex: 18 mg or 35 mg TID	**BOXED WARNINGS** Arthrotec: <u>avoid in females of childbearing potential</u> unless the female is capable of complying with effective contraceptive measures **SIDE EFFECTS** Topical: occasional application site reactions (rash/pruritus) **NOTES** Has <u>some COX-2 selectivity</u> Oral diclofenac formulations are not bioequivalent, even if same mg strength <u>Misoprostol</u> is used to replace the gut-protective prostaglandins to ↓ GI risk; can ↑ uterine contractions (which can terminate pregnancy) and causes cramping and diarrhea Remove Flector patch before an MRI

*Brand discontinued but name still used in practice.

DRUG	DOSING	SAFETY/SIDE EFFECTS/MONITORING
Meloxicam (Mobic) Tablet, capsule, ODT, oral suspension	7.5-15 mg once daily Capsule: 5-10 mg once daily	**NOTES** These agents have some COX-2 selectivity Meloxicam capsules and ODT are not interchangeable with other formulations
Etodolac Tablet, capsule, ER tablet	300-500 mg Q6-8H	
Nabumetone Tablet	1,000-2,000 mg daily (can be divided BID)	

Salicylate NSAIDs

DRUG	DOSING	SAFETY/SIDE EFFECTS/MONITORING
Aspirin/Acetylsalicylic Acid (Ascriptin, Bufferin, Ecotrin, Durlaza, Vazalore**)** Tablet, caplet, chewable tablet, liquid-filled capsule, suppository **Ascriptin, Bufferin, Ecotrin:** EC/buffered Durlaza (Rx): ER capsule Rx and OTC **+ acetaminophen/caffeine (Excedrin, Excedrin Migraine,** Goody's Powder**)** + antacid (Alka-Seltzer) + caffeine (BC Powder) + calcium (Bayer Women's Low Dose) + dipyridamole (Aggrenox*) for stroke + omeprazole (Yosprala) And in multiple other OTC combinations	Cardioprotection dosing: 81-162 mg once daily Durlaza: 162.5 mg once daily Analgesic dosing: 325-650 mg Q4-6H Goody's Powder: 520 mg per packet BC Powder: 845-1000 mg per packet	**WARNINGS** Avoid with NSAID hypersensitivity (past reaction with trouble breathing), nasal polyps, asthma Avoid aspirin in children and teenagers with any viral infection due to potential risk of Reye's syndrome (symptoms include somnolence, N/V, lethargy, confusion); other NSAIDs can be used in pediatrics Severe skin rash (rare) including SJS/TEN GI ulceration and bleeding can occur Avoid in the third trimester of pregnancy due to fetal harm **SIDE EFFECTS** Dyspepsia, heartburn, bleeding, nausea **NOTES** To ↓ nausea, use EC or buffered product or take with food PPIs may be used for GI protection with chronic NSAID use; consider the risks from chronic PPI use (↓ bone density, ↑ infection risk)
NON-ACETYLATED SALICYLATES		
Salsalate	Up to 3 grams/day, divided BID-TID	Do not use Durlaza or Yosprala when immediate effect is needed (e.g., acute myocardial infarction) Salicylate overdose can cause tinnitus Methyl salicylate is a popular OTC topical found in BenGay, IcyHot, Thera-Gesic, Salonpas; see Topical Adjuvants Aspirin has risk of gastritis/ulceration; the benefit of chronic (daily) use must outweigh the risk of GI bleeding
Magnesium Salicylate (Doan's Extra Strength)	580 mg ES tab: 2 tablets Q6H Max: 8 tablets/day	
Choline Magnesium Trisalicylate	1 gram BID-TID or 3 grams QHS	
Diflunisal	500 mg BID-TID Max 1.5 grams daily	
Salicylate salts	No longer commonly used	

*Brand discontinued but name still used in practice.

NSAID Drug Interactions

- Additive bleeding risk with other agents that can ↑ bleeding risk (e.g., steroids). See the Drug Interactions chapter.

- Caution using aspirin with other ototoxic agents (e.g., aminoglycosides, IV loop diuretics).

- Multiple NSAIDs should not be used together, except the addition of low dose aspirin for cardioprotection when indicated. If using aspirin for cardioprotection and ibuprofen for pain, take aspirin one hour before or eight hours after ibuprofen.

- NSAIDs can ↑ the levels of lithium and methotrexate.

OPIOID ANALGESICS

Opioid drugs interact in a variety of ways with the three primary types of opioid receptors: μ (mu), κ (kappa) and δ (delta). Opioids are mu receptor agonists within the CNS; this action primarily results in pain relief, but can also cause euphoria and respiratory depression. These drugs are used to treat moderate to severe acute pain and chronic pain.

Buprenorphine is a partial mu-opioid agonist. It is an agonist at low doses and an antagonist at higher doses. Buprenorphine is used in lower doses to treat pain and higher doses to treat opioid use disorder.

SAFETY CONCERNS

A Risk Evaluation and Mitigation strategy (REMS) exists for all opioid medications; this mainly includes prescriber education and specific counseling requirements. Opioid medications have several boxed warnings (see Study Tip Gal to the right); these are not repeated in the following drug tables. Patients should be periodically assessed and educated on opioid safety practices.

Elderly, debilitated or cachectic patients and patients with chronic pulmonary disease (i.e., conditions associated with hypoxia) or head injury/increased intracranial pressure should be monitored closely. All are at increased risk of respiratory depression. Opioids also have a risk of hypotension.

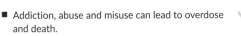

OPIOID BOXED WARNINGS

- Addiction, abuse and misuse can lead to overdose and death.
- Respiratory depression, which can be fatal.
- Use of any opioid with benzodiazepines or other CNS depressants, including alcohol, can increase the risk of respiratory depression and death.
- Morphine ER capsules, *Nucynta ER*, oxymorphone ER and hydrocodone ER capsules: do not consume alcohol with this medication. Alcohol can cause increased drug plasma levels, which can lead to a potentially fatal overdose.
- Accidental ingestion/exposure of even one dose in children can be fatal. Never give this medication to anyone else (includes patches).
- Crushing, dissolving or chewing the long-acting products can cause delivery of a potentially fatal dose.
- Life-threatening neonatal opioid withdrawal can occur with prolonged use during pregnancy.

TERMINOLOGY

TERM	DEFINITION
Physical Dependence	Almost all patients using chronic opioids, including those abusing opioids, become physiologically adapted to the opioid and experience physical withdrawal symptoms when the opioid is stopped or a dose is late or missed. The symptoms include anxiety, tachycardia, shakiness and shortness of breath. The withdrawal causes much suffering. Physical dependence is not addiction.
Addiction	A strong desire or compulsion to take the drug despite harm. Involves drug-seeking behavior (e.g., exaggerating pain or physical impairment, prescription forgery, obtaining similar prescriptions from multiple providers).
Opioid Use Disorder (OUD)	A problematic pattern of opioid use that causes significant impairment or distress. Specific criteria must be met for a diagnosis of OUD, including unsuccessful trials to reduce or control opioid use or opioid use resulting in a failure to fulfill obligations at work, school or home.
Tolerance	A higher opioid dose is needed to produce the same level of analgesia that a lower dose previously provided. Tolerance develops over time with chronic opioid use. It is important to distinguish whether the higher pain severity is due to a condition (e.g., cancer that has spread), or a decrease in the drug's effectiveness due to tolerance, or both. If tolerance develops, it may be preferable to switch to another opioid rather than increase the dose.
Opioid Hyperalgesia	When the opioid dose is increased to treat the pain, but the pain becomes worse rather than better. This occurs occasionally. If suspected, a different class of analgesic or a switch to another opioid should be tried.
Break-Through Pain [(BTP), end of dose pain]	Sharp spikes of severe pain that occur despite the use of an ER opioid. Must be treated with an immediate-release (IR) opioid or a fast-acting analgesic (e.g., an injection, transmucosal immediate release fentanyl for cancer BTP only). When multiple doses are required for BTP, a higher baseline dose can be required, or possibly a switch to a different opioid. BTP medication is dispensed with scheduled, long-acting opioids and may be adjusted or discontinued based on treatment response.
Opioid-Induced Respiratory Depression (OIRD)	Respiratory depression due to opioid use (i.e., the body's natural drive to breath is suppressed). The usual cause of fatality in opioid overdose. Hospitalized patients receiving IV opioids must be carefully monitored for sedation and oxygen saturation.
Centrally-Acting Opioid Antagonists	These drugs block opioids from binding to opioid receptors. Examples include naloxone (used to reverse opioid-induced respiratory depression) and naltrexone (used for opioid-use disorder to block the effects of opioids).

COMMON OPIOIDS

DRUG	DOSING	SAFETY/SIDE EFFECTS/MONITORING
ALL OPIOIDS		
C-II (except where noted otherwise)		
Risks include constipation, nausea/vomiting (especially with acute, high-dose use), somnolence, dizziness/lightheadedness, seizures, opioid-induced hyperalgesia, respiratory depression and overdose (risk ↑ as dose increases; see Study Tip Gal on previous page). Pruritus is common, especially in opioid-naïve patients; diphenhydramine can be used (especially with morphine) to reduce rash and itching.		
Neonatal opioid withdrawal syndrome can occur with prolonged use in a pregnant patient.		

DRUG	DOSING	SAFETY/SIDE EFFECTS/MONITORING
Codeine C-II (single-entity tablets) **+ acetaminophen** (Tylenol #3,* #4*) C-III (tablet/capsule combination products) Oral solution combination products (e.g., cough syrups): C-V + chlorpheniramine/ pseudoephedrine + promethazine + promethazine/ phenylephrine (Promethazine VC/ Codeine)	15-60 mg Q4H PRN Tylenol #3: codeine 30 mg + acetaminophen 300 mg Tylenol #4: codeine 60 mg + acetaminophen 300 mg Q4-6H PRN, range 15-120 mg codeine	**BOXED WARNINGS** Respiratory depression and death have occurred in children who were found to be ultra-rapid metabolizers of codeine (due to a CYP450 2D6 polymorphism) after tonsillectomy and/or adenoidectomy; use with CYP3A4 inducers/inhibitors or CYP2D6 inhibitors should be carefully considered due to variable effects **CONTRAINDICATIONS** Do not use in children < 12 years (any indication) and < 18 years following tonsillectomy/adenoidectomy surgery; FDA recommends to avoid codeine-containing cough and cold products for children < 18 years of age **WARNINGS** Adolescents between 12-18 years who are obese or have sleep apnea or severe lung disease are at ↑ risk of breathing problems; breastfeeding **SIDE EFFECTS** Codeine has a high degree of GI side effects including constipation **NOTES** Codeine, a prodrug, is metabolized to morphine via CYP2D6 (see Drug Interactions chapter); deaths have occurred in nursing infants after being exposed to high concentrations of morphine because the mothers were ultra-rapid metabolizers
Fentanyl (Sublimaze, Duragesic*, others) Injection, patch, oral transmucosal lozenge on a stick ("lollipop") Fentora: buccal tabs Subsys: spray, SL	**Patch** Apply 1 patch Q72H (can be Q48H) Available in different strengths ranging from 12-100 mcg/hr 12 mcg patch delivers 12.5 mcg/hr **Lozenge** Always start with 200 mcg, can titrate to 4 BTP episodes/day	**BOXED WARNINGS** Potential for medication errors when converting between dosage forms, use with strong or moderate CYP3A4 inhibitors can result in ↑ effects and potentially fatal respiratory depression, avoid exposing transdermal fentanyl to external heat **SIDE EFFECTS** Hyperhidrosis (excessive sweating), dry mouth, asthenia, loss of appetite, application site redness/erythema (patch) **NOTES** Outpatient use of fentanyl is for chronic pain management only Patch and lozenge: not used in opioid-naïve patients; a patient who has been using equivalent to morphine 60 mg/day or more for at least 7 days can be converted to a fentanyl patch Lozenge: cut off stick and flush unused/unneeded doses Short t½ when given IV (boluses given Q1-2H); continuous infusion or PCA are most common Similar drugs (IV only) include alfentanil (Alfenta), remifentanil (Ultiva), sufentanil (Dsuvia) REMS program for transmucosal immediate-release fentanyl (e.g., lozenge, buccal tabs, SL) requires documentation of patient's opioid tolerance with each prescription; for cancer BTP **Fentanyl Patch** Analgesic effect can be seen 8-16 hrs after application; discontinue all around-the-clock opioid drugs when the patch is applied Do not apply > 1 patch at a time; apply to hairless skin (cut hair short if necessary) Can be covered only with the permitted adhesive film dressings Bioclusive or Tegaderm Do not cover with a heating pad or any other bandage Some patches need to be removed before an MRI (specific to each formulation and manufacturer); check the individual manufacturer package insert Dispose of patch by flushing down the toilet; keep away from children and pets

Brand discontinued but name still used in practice.

DRUG	DOSING	SAFETY/SIDE EFFECTS/MONITORING
Buprenorphine C-III For pain management: **Belbuca:** buccal film **Butrans:** patch Buprenex: injection Used for treatment of pain and for opioid use disorder	*Belbuca* (opioid-naïve): 75 mcg daily or Q12H *Butrans* (opioid-naïve): 5 mcg/hr patch once weekly **Film application** Insert between gum and cheek tissue (must be wet from saliva or water); do not eat or drink for 30 minutes **Patch application** Apply to chest, upper outer arm or upper back; do not use the same site for at least 3 weeks	**BOXED WARNINGS** *Butrans*: QT prolongation (do not exceed one 20 mcg/hr patch at a time) **WARNINGS** CNS depression, severe dental adverse events with buccal formulations **SIDE EFFECTS** Dizziness, sedation, headache, confusion, mental and physical impairment, diaphoresis, QT prolongation, respiratory depression (dose-dependent) Patch: application site reactions (pruritus/erythema/rash), nausea/vomiting, constipation, somnolence, dry mouth **NOTES** *Butrans*: can only be covered with *Bioclusive* or *Tegaderm* (medical adhesive coverings); do not expose to heat; to dispose, fold sticky sides together and flush down the toilet or put in disposal unit included in the drug packaging
Hydrocodone IR (combination products only) Select combo products: **+ acetaminophen** (*Norco,* Vicodin**) + chlorpheniramine + chlorpheniramine/ pseudoephedrine + homatropine (*Hycodan, Hydromet*) + ibuprofen	2.5, 5, 7.5, 10 mg hydrocodone + 325 mg acetaminophen Usual starting dose: 5/325 mg Q4-6H PRN	**BOXED WARNINGS** Initiation of CYP3A4 inhibitors (or stopping CYP3A4 inducers) can cause fatal overdose **WARNINGS** Acetaminophen and opioids: respiratory and/or CNS depression, constipation, hypotension, skin reactions (rare), caution in liver disease (avoid or limit alcohol intake) and in CYP2D6 poor metabolizers **SIDE EFFECTS** Pruritus, dry mouth **NOTES** Hydrocodone containing cough and cold preparations are no longer indicated in patients < 18 years of age – do not use
Hydrocodone ER (*Hysingla ER*) Tablet, capsule	Capsule: start at 10 mg Q12H (opioid-naïve), range 10-50 mg Tablet: start at 20 mg Q24H (opioid-naïve), range 20-120 mg	**BOXED WARNINGS** Initiation of CYP3A4 inhibitors (or stopping CYP3A4 inducers) can cause fatal overdose **NOTES** Substrate of CYP3A4 (major) and CYP2D6 (minor) Preferably avoid use if breastfeeding Available in abuse-deterrent formulations *Hysingla ER*: QT prolongation has occurred at doses > 160 mg/day
Hydromorphone (Dilaudid) Tablet, injection, solution, suppository	Initial (opioid-naïve): Oral: 2-4 mg Q4-6H PRN IV: 0.2-1 mg Q2-3H PRN	**BOXED WARNINGS** Risk of medication error with high potency (HP) injection (use in opioid-tolerant patients only); HP injection (10 mg/mL) is more concentrated than standard hydromorphone (e.g., 1 mg/mL, 2 mg/mL) **SIDE EFFECTS** Pruritus, dry mouth, hyperhidrosis **NOTES** Potent: start low, convert carefully; high risk for overdose Commonly used in PCAs and epidurals ER tablet: abuse-deterrent formulation (crush and extraction resistant) contraindicated in opioid-naïve patients Two-week washout required between hydromorphone and MAO inhibitors

Brand discontinued but name still used in practice.

DRUG	DOSING	SAFETY/SIDE EFFECTS/MONITORING
Methadone (*Methadose, Methadone Intensol*) Tablet, soluble tablet, solution, oral concentrate Used for treatment of pain and for detox and maintenance treatment of opioid use disorder	Initial: 2.5-10 mg Q8-12H	**BOXED WARNINGS** Life-threatening QT prolongation and serious arrhythmias (e.g., Torsades de Pointes) have occurred during treatment (most involve large, multiple daily doses); should be prescribed by professionals who know requirements for safe use; initiation of CYP450 inhibitors (or stopping inducers) can cause fatal overdose **WARNINGS** Combination with other serotonergic drugs or MAO inhibitors can ↑ the risk of serotonin syndrome, methadone also blocks reuptake of norepinephrine Caution in elderly and those with seizure history **SIDE EFFECTS** Hyperhidrosis **NOTES** Due to variable half-life, methadone is hard to dose safely Can ↓ testosterone and contribute to sexual dysfunction Methadone is a major CYP3A4 substrate; avoid use with inhibitors or ↓ the dose of methadone
Meperidine (*Demerol*) Tablet, solution, injection Used off-label for post-operative rigors (shivering)	Oral/IM/SC: 50-150 mg Q3-4H PRN	**WARNINGS** Renal impairment/elderly at risk for CNS toxicity, avoid with or within 2 weeks of MAO inhibitor **SIDE EFFECTS** Hyperhidrosis **NOTES** No longer recommended as an analgesic (especially in elderly and renally impaired); avoid for chronic pain and even short-term in elderly; if use for acute pain cannot be avoided, use short-term or single use (e.g., sutures in ER) Short duration of action (pain controlled for max 3 hrs) Normeperidine (metabolite) is renally cleared and can accumulate and cause CNS toxicity, including seizures In combination with other drugs, it is serotonergic and can ↑ risk of serotonin syndrome
Morphine ER: **MS Contin** Injection: **Duramorph, Infumorph** Tablet (IR/ER), ER capsule, injection, solution, suppository	IR (including solution): 10-30 mg Q4H PRN ER: 15, 30, 60, 100, 200 mg Q8-12H IV (opioid-naïve): 2.5-5 mg Q3-4H PRN	**BOXED WARNINGS** Medication errors with oral solution (note strength), appropriate staff and equipment needed for intrathecal/epidural administration **SIDE EFFECTS** Pruritus, dry mouth, hyperhidrosis **NOTES** Do not use MSO4 or MS abbreviations for morphine or magnesium Do not crush or chew any ER products; morphine ER capsules can be opened and sprinkled on applesauce or soft food Renal impairment: start at a lower dose, or avoid morphine, due to accumulation of parent drug and/or active metabolite Diphenhydramine or similar can be given to block histamine-induced pruritus

DRUG	DOSING	SAFETY/SIDE EFFECTS/MONITORING
Oxycodone IR: ***Roxicodone***, *Oxaydo* CR: ***OxyContin*** ER: *Xtampza ER* Tablet (IR/ER), capsule (IR/ER), solution **+ acetaminophen (*Endocet, Percocet*)**	IR: 5-20 mg Q4-6H CR: 10-80 mg Q12H (60, 80 mg only for opioid-tolerant patients)	**BOXED WARNINGS** Initiation of CYP3A4 inhibitors (or stopping CYP3A4 inducers) can cause fatal overdose; caution with oxycodone oral solution and oral concentrate (confusion between mg and mL and different concentrations) **SIDE EFFECTS** Pruritus, dry mouth, hyperhidrosis **NOTES** Abuse-deterrent formulations: *Oxaydo, OxyContin* and *Xtampza ER* *Xtampza ER* capsules can be opened and contents administered with soft food or through a gastric tube Avoid high fat meals with higher doses (except re-formulated *OxyContin*) Renal impairment: start at a lower dose, or avoid oxycodone, due to accumulation of parent drug and/or active metabolite
Oxymorphone Tablet (IR/ER), injection	IR (opioid-naïve): 5-10 mg Q4-6H PRN	**NOTES** Do not use with moderate-to-severe liver impairment; use low doses in elderly, renal or mild liver impairment (due to higher drug concentrations in these patients) Take on empty stomach

Opioid Drug Interactions

- Caution with other CNS depressants: can have additive somnolence, dizziness, confusion and increased risk of respiratory depression. These include alcohol, hypnotics, benzodiazepines and muscle relaxants. Avoid alcohol with all opioids, especially ER formulations.

- Increased risk of hypoxemia with underlying respiratory disease (e.g., COPD, sleep apnea).

- Methadone: caution with agents that worsen cardiac function or increase arrhythmia risk, including those with QT prolongation. Caution with other serotonergic agents. Caution with agents that worsen renal function.

- Hydrocodone, fentanyl, methadone and oxycodone are CYP3A4 substrates. Avoid use with CYP3A4 inhibitors. Analgesic effect is decreased with CYP3A4 inducers.

DOSING CONVERSIONS

The correct opioid dose is the lowest dose that provides effective pain relief without producing intolerable or dangerous adverse effects. If the medicine is effective, but wears off too quickly, do not increase the dose. Rather, give the same dose more frequently. It is appropriate to consider switching to a different agent if:

- The dose has been increased or the interval shortened and the pain relief is not adequate

- The side effects are intolerable (patients react differently to different opioids)

- The drug is unaffordable or not included on formulary

- Changing formulations from IV to PO

For opioid conversions (except for methadone), you can use a ratio conversion (see table below). When converting one opioid to another, round down (do not round up) and use breakthrough doses. A patient may develop a tolerance or could respond better to one drug over another; rounding the dose down will reduce the risk of overdose.

DRUG	IV/IM (MG)	ORAL (MG)
Morphine	10	30
Hydromorphone	1.5	7.5
Oxycodone	–	20
Hydrocodone	–	30
Codeine	130	200
Fentanyl	0.1	–
Meperidine	75	300
Oxymorphone	1	10

Steps to Convert

- Calculate the total 24-hour dose of the current drug.

- Use the ratio conversion to calculate the dose of the new drug (refer to the Calculations I chapter for a review).

- Calculate the 24-hour dose of the new drug and reduce the dose ≥ 25% for cross-tolerance (if the exam does not specify to reduce, calculate the equivalent dose and do not reduce).

- Divide for the new drug's appropriate interval and dose.

- Always have medication available for BTP while making changes; dosing ranges from 5 – 17% (typically 10 – 15%) of the total daily baseline opioid dose, typically Q1 – 2H PRN. For the elderly, ~5% of the total daily baseline opioid dose is administered Q4H PRN.

Whenever possible, use an IR version of the long-acting opioid for BTP. Any drug that requires oral absorption will take time for the onset of action. For cancer pain (which can cause severe BTP), a sublingual form of fentanyl may be preferred due to faster onset. Combination products, such as hydrocodone/acetaminophen, can be used for BTP. Monitor the total acetaminophen intake from all sources (given alone or in combination). In an inpatient setting, injectable pain medications can be given. Injections have a faster onset and can be preferred for severe BTP. However, if the patient does not have an existing IV line, the injection itself will cause discomfort.

CASE SCENARIO

A hospice patient has been receiving 12 mg/day of IV hydromorphone. The pharmacist will convert the hydromorphone to morphine ER to be given Q12H. The hospice policy for opioid conversion is to reduce the new dose by 50%, and to use 5 – 17% of the total daily dose for BTP.

The conversion factors (the left side of the ratio conversion) are taken from the table on the previous page. The right side of the ratio conversion has the patient's current total daily hydromorphone IV dose in the denominator, and the total daily dose of morphine in the numerator:

$$\frac{30 \text{ mg oral morphine}}{1.5 \text{ mg IV hydromorphone}} = \frac{X \text{ mg oral morphine}}{12 \text{ mg IV hydromorphone}} \qquad X = 240 \text{ mg of oral morphine}$$

Reduce by 50%, as instructed in the case:

50% of 240 mg = 120 mg, the correct dose of morphine ER would be 60 mg BID

Using the BTP range provided by the hospice policy in the example, a dose of 15 mg IR morphine Q1 – 2H as needed for BTP could be used with morphine ER 60 mg BID.

Exception: Fentanyl Patches

Converting to a fentanyl patch is most commonly done using a dosing table provided in the package insert (see next table and example). If converting to fentanyl using the previous chart, remember that you are finding the total daily dose in mg, and will then need to convert it to mcg (multiply by 1,000) and then divide by 24 to get the patch dose; the fentanyl patch is dosed in mcg per hour (no oral dose conversion is listed on the conversion chart because fentanyl is not absorbed orally). Some clinicians use this estimation: morphine 60 mg total daily dose = 25 mcg/hr fentanyl patch. These methods can provide different answers. For the exam, follow the specific instructions given when converting to or from fentanyl patches.

CASE SCENARIO

MJ is a 52-year-old male who has been taking *OxyContin* 40 mg BID and *Endocet* 5/325 mg PRN for BTP. He uses the BTP medication 2 – 3 times weekly. Using the *OxyContin* dose only, select the fentanyl patch strength that should be chosen for this patient, using the following table:

FENTANYL PATCH CONVERSION

Current Analgesic	Daily Dosage (mg/day)			
Oral morphine	60–134	135–224	225–314	315–404
Intramuscular or Intravenous morphine	10–22	23–37	38–52	53–67
Oral oxycodone	30–67	67.5–112	112.5–157	157.5–202
Oral codeine	150–447			
Oral hydromorphone	8–17	17.1–28	28.1–39	39.1–51
Intravenous hydromorphone	1.5–3.4	3.5–5.6	5.7–7.9	8–10
Intramuscular meperidine	75-165	166-278	279-390	391-503
Oral methadone	20–44	45–74	75–104	105–134
	↓	↓	↓	↓
Recommended fentanyl patch dose	25 mcg/hour	50 mcg/hour	75 mcg/hour	100 mcg/hour

This table should not be used to convert from fentanyl patches to other medications because these conversions are conservative. Use of the above table for conversion to other analgesic therapies can overestimate the dose of the new agent (with a possible risk of overdosage).

Answer: oxycodone 80 mg daily is in the range of 67.5 – 112 mg daily which correlates to the 50 mcg/hr patch.

Exception: Methadone Conversion

Morphine to methadone conversion ranges from 3:1 – 20:1; this is due to methadone's highly variable half-life. There are separate conversion charts for pain specialists to estimate methadone dosing. This should be done only by specialists with experience in using methadone.

Methadone is used both for the treatment of opioid addiction (opioid use disorder) and for chronic pain. When used for chronic pain syndromes, it is typically administered 2 – 3 times per day. It should be started at very low doses of no more than 2.5 mg PO BID or TID in opioid naïve patients, and escalated slowly.

OPIOIDS & CHRONIC NON-CANCER PAIN

Opioids are not first-line for chronic pain treatment and should not be used routinely. When used, follow safe use recommendations:

- Establish and measure goals for pain and function. Reaching low pain rather than no pain may be reasonable.

- If using opioids, start with immediate release. *Start low and go slow.*

- Evaluate risk factors for opioid-related harm routinely.

- Pharmacists should check their state's Prescription Drug Monitoring Program (PDMP) database. *Look for high dosages, dangerous combinations and multiple prescribers.*

- Use adjunctive medications to enable a lower opioid dose.

- Avoid benzodiazepines and opioids given together, except in rare cases. *This quadruples the risk of overdose death.*

- Follow-up, taper the dose, consider discontinuation.

ALLERGY

True opioid allergies are rare. Most complaints of itching or rash are not a true allergic reaction. Symptoms of an opioid allergy (rare but dangerous if present) include difficulty breathing, severe drop in blood pressure, serious rash and swelling of the face, lips, tongue or larynx. In a true opioid allergy, use an agent in a different chemical class (see Study Tip Gal below).

OPIOID ALLERGY

The common drugs in the same chemical class that cross-react with each other have **cod** or **morph** in the name. Buprenorphine has **norph** instead of **morph**.

Codeine	**Morph**ine	Bupre**norph**ine
Hydro**cod**one	Hydro**morph**one	Heroin (diacetyl-morphine)
Oxy**cod**one	Oxy**morph**one	

What to do if a morphine-type allergy is reported? In practice, make sure it is an actual allergy, and not nausea or itching. If it seems to be accurate, choose a drug in a different chemical class, such as methadone or fentanyl. Meperidine is also in a different class, but is no longer recommended as an analgesic.

Tramadol package labeling warns of increased risk of reactions to tramadol in those with previous anaphylactic reactions to opioids. Tapentadol does not have this warning in the U.S., though tramadol and tapentadol are structurally similar. If allergic to tramadol, an allergy to tapentadol is likely, and vice versa.

SIDE EFFECTS AND MANAGEMENT

Opioid-induced respiratory depression (OIRD) is one of the greatest risks of opioid use, and the usual cause of fatality in opioid overdose. However, it rarely occurs when opioids are prescribed and taken according to accepted guidelines, especially if doses are appropriately titrated. Certain patients have a greater risk of OIRD (see Study Tip Gal below); screening for risk factors is essential for prevention.

OPIOID-INDUCED RESPIRATORY DEPRESSION (OIRD) RISKS

An opioid prescription requires a risk/benefit assessment, and monitoring.

OIRD risk factors include:

- History of previous overdose

- Substance use disorder

- Using large doses (≥ 50 mg morphine or equivalent)

- Use with benzodiazepines, gabapentin or pregabalin

- Comorbid illnesses, such as respiratory or psychiatric disease

An opioid antagonist (e.g., naloxone) should be readily available to patients with elevated risk for OIRD.

Most opioid side effects usually lessen over time, except constipation (see Study Tip Gal on next page). If a patient has a problem that persists or is bothersome despite treatment (e.g., hydroxyzine or diphenhydramine for pruritus), switching to another opioid is reasonable. Postoperative nausea and vomiting (PONV) occurs in surgical patients due primarily to the use of anesthesia and opioids. PONV is treated in the hospital with a 5-HT3 receptor antagonist, such as ondansetron, or a phenothiazine, such as prochlorperazine. All oral opioids (except oxymorphone) should be taken with food to lessen nausea.

Sedation and cognitive effects occur when an opioid is started, or when the dose is increased, and generally lessen over time. Seizures can also be caused by opioids. Pharmacists should advise patients not to drive or do anything potentially hazardous until they are accustomed to the medication. The use of other CNS depressants should be minimized. Alcohol should not be used with opioids.

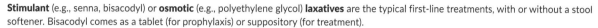

OPIOID-INDUCED CONSTIPATION

All opioids cause constipation, referred to as opioid-induced constipation (OIC).

Opioids reduce GI tract peristalsis, making it difficult to have a bowel movement.

Unlike CNS depression, OIC does not improve over time without treatment; it **must be anticipated and treated**.

Stimulant (e.g., senna, bisacodyl) or **osmotic** (e.g., polyethylene glycol) **laxatives** are the typical first-line treatments, with or without a stool softener. Bisacodyl comes as a tablet (for prophylaxis) or suppository (for treatment).

If laxatives are not sufficient, specific medications for OIC that counteract the effects of the opioid receptor in the gut **(PAMORAs)** can be used.

Lubiprostone, which is used for different types of constipation, could be considered following a trial of laxatives or PAMORAs.

TREATMENT OF OPIOID-INDUCED CONSTIPATION

DRUG	DOSING	SAFETY/SIDE EFFECTS/MONITORING
Peripherally-acting mu-opioid receptor antagonists (PAMORAs): block opioid receptors in the gut to reduce constipation without affecting analgesia. PAMORAs are indicated for OIC and are only effective when constipation is secondary to use of an opioid.		
Methylnaltrexone (Relistor) Injection, tablet	OIC with chronic non-cancer pain: 12 mg SC daily or 450 mg PO once daily OIC with advanced illness: weight-based dose SC every other day CrCl < 30 mL/min: ↓ dose	**CONTRAINDICATIONS** GI obstruction Naloxegol: do not use with strong CYP3A4 inhibitors (e.g., grapefruit juice) **WARNINGS** Risk of GI perforation (rare reports; monitor for severe abdominal symptoms), risk of opioid withdrawal (evaluate risk vs benefit and monitor) Methylnaltrexone: use > 4 months has not been studied, discontinue if opioid is discontinued or if severe/persistent diarrhea **SIDE EFFECTS** Abdominal pain, flatulence, diarrhea, nausea, dizziness **NOTES** Stay close to toilet after injecting Discontinue all laxatives prior to use Only for patients on opioids who have failed OTC laxatives
Naloxegol (Movantik) Tablet	OIC with chronic non-cancer pain: 25 mg once daily in the morning on empty stomach CrCl < 60 mL/min: 12.5 mg once daily	
Naldemedine (Symproic) Tablet	OIC with chronic non-cancer pain: 0.2 mg daily	
Chloride channel activator: approved for other indications in addition to OIC		
Lubiprostone (Amitiza) Capsule	OIC: 24 mcg BID	See the Constipation & Diarrhea chapter

CENTRALLY ACTING ANALGESICS

Both tramadol and tapentadol are mu-opioid receptor agonists and inhibitors of norepinephrine reuptake. Tramadol also inhibits reuptake of serotonin. Both tapentadol and tramadol have the same boxed warnings as opioids (see Opioid Analgesics, Safety Concerns).

DRUG	DOSING	SAFETY/SIDE EFFECTS/MONITORING
Tramadol (Ultram,* ConZip) C-IV Tablet (IR/ER), ER capsule, solution + acetaminophen + celecoxib (Seglentis)	IR: 50-100 mg Q4-6H, max 400 mg/day ER: 100 mg once daily, max 300 mg/day CrCl < 30 mL/min: IR: increase dosing interval to Q12H ER: do not use	**BOXED WARNINGS** Respiratory depression and death have occurred in children following tonsillectomy and/or adenoidectomy found to have evidence of being ultra-rapid metabolizers of tramadol due to a CYP450 2D6 polymorphism; use with CYP3A4 inducers/inhibitors or CYP2D6 inhibitors should be carefully considered due to variable effects **WARNINGS** Seizure risk (avoid in patients with seizure history, head trauma), risk of serotonin syndrome when used alone or with other serotonergic drugs or inhibitors of CYP2D6 or 3A4, CNS depression, hypoglycemia, respiratory depression (rare), avoid in patients who are suicidal, risk of serious breathing problems in adolescents age 12-18 years with obesity, sleep apnea or lung disease, breastfeeding mothers should avoid due to ↑ risk of serious breathing problems in breastfed infants **CONTRAINDICATIONS** Do not use in children < 12 years of age; or in children < 18 years of age following tonsillectomy/adenoidectomy surgery Do not use with concurrent MAO inhibitors or within 14 days **SIDE EFFECTS** Dizziness, constipation, nausea, somnolence or insomnia, dry mouth, pruritus, flushing, headache, asthenia Lower severity of GI side effects versus strong opioids On the Beers list: postmarketing reports of hyponatremia and SIADH **NOTES** Tramadol requires conversion to active metabolite by CYP2D6; use with CYP2D6 inhibitors has variable effects due to mixed mechanism of action of tramadol
Tapentadol (Nucynta, Nucynta ER) C-II Tablet (IR/ER)	IR: 50-100 mg Q4-6H ER: 50-250 mg BID CrCl < 30 mL/min: Use not recommended (not studied)	**CONTRAINDICATIONS** Do not use with concurrent MAO inhibitors or within 14 days **WARNINGS** Can increase seizure risk (avoid in patients with seizure history or seizure risk), risk of serotonin syndrome when used with other serotonergic drugs **SIDE EFFECTS** Dizziness, constipation, nausea, somnolence or insomnia, dry mouth, pruritus Lower severity of GI side effects versus strong opioids **NOTES** Tapentadol is a stronger analgesic than tramadol

Brand discontinued but name still used in practice.

Centrally Acting Analgesic Drug Interactions

- Caution with other agents that lower seizure threshold.
- Caution with other serotonergic drugs.
- Avoid tramadol with CYP2D6 inhibitors.
- Possibility of increased INR with warfarin; monitor.
- Tapentadol can enhance the adverse/toxic effect of MAO inhibitors; avoid use with MAO inhibitors.

OPIOID OVERDOSE

Opioid-related deaths have more than quadrupled since 1999. The U.S. government has created five strategies to prevent overdose death:

- Educate providers and the general public about how to prevent and manage opioid overdose (see Study Tip Gal).

- Ensure access to treatment for patients addicted to opioids.

- Ensure widely available and immediate access to naloxone. Encourage providers to discuss the availability of naloxone with all patients prescribed opioids or medications to treat opioid use disorder (OUD).

- Encourage the public to call 911 if an overdose is suspected.

- Encourage prescribers to use state Prescription Drug Monitoring Programs (PDMPs).

There have been a number of FDA-approved opioids designed to help mitigate abuse and misuse. It is important to note that these formulations do not eliminate the ability to abuse or misuse opioids. Some opioid combination products, such as Suboxone, are formulated with the abuse-deterrent medication naloxone, while others such as OxyContin and Hysingla ER are manufactured using specific technology designed to deter crushing, dissolving or other modifications.

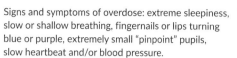

OPIOID OVERDOSE MANAGEMENT

Signs and symptoms of overdose: extreme sleepiness, slow or shallow breathing, fingernails or lips turning blue or purple, extremely small "pinpoint" pupils, slow heartbeat and/or blood pressure.

If overdose is suspected, give naloxone and call 911.

If an individual is not breathing or struggling to breathe, life support measures should be performed.

If there is a question about whether to give naloxone, give it, because fatality could result from not giving it.

After administering naloxone, monitor for signs of respiratory depression as opioids stay in the body longer than naloxone. Provide repeat doses as needed (i.e., after 20-60 minutes).

Naloxone is available in two options:

- Naloxone (nasal spray): available as OTC (3-4 mg/spray) and prescription (4-8 mg/spray) single-use devices; spray is administered in 1 nostril and may be repeated every 2-3 minutes in alternating nostrils until emergency medical assistance arrives; onset of action is slower than injection

- Naloxone (injection): generic formulation provided in multiple size vials, separate syringe will be needed, may need to repeat doses every 2-3 minutes until emergency medical assistance arrives

TREATMENT OF OPIOID OVERDOSE

Naloxone can be given if opioid overdose is suspected due to respiratory symptoms and/or symptoms of CNS depression. All approved naloxone formulations can be administered for prevention of opioid overdose death and to help reverse OIRD. Narcan (4 mg/spray) and RiVive (3 mg/spray) are nasal sprays available over-the-counter (OTC) and can be purchased by anyone to have it readily available in the event of a suspected opioid overdose. Nalmefene is another option for opioid overdose; it is available as a nasal spray and an injection.

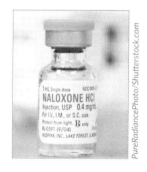

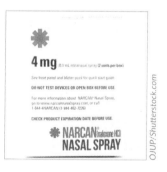

DRUGS FOR OPIOID OVERDOSE

DRUG	DOSING	SAFETY/SIDE EFFECTS/MONITORING
Naloxone Injection, nasal spray **Narcan** (OTC), **RiVive** (OTC), Kloxxado, Rextovy: nasal spray Zimhi: injection	IV/IM/SC: 0.4-2 mg Q2-3 min or IV infusion at 0.4 mg/hr Nasal spray: 1 spray (3-8 mg), can repeat Repeat dosing may be required (opioid can last longer than blocking agent)	**SIDE EFFECTS** Opioid-dependent: acute withdrawal symptoms (pain, anxiety, tachypnea) Injection: site reactions (erythema/irritation) Nasal: nasal dryness/congestion/swelling
Nalmefene Injection, nasal spray Opvee: nasal spray	IV (preferred)/IM/SC: Opioid-dependent: give 0.1 mg; if no evidence of withdrawal, administer 0.5 mg Non-opioid dependent: give 0.5 mg IV (preferred) After 2-5 minutes, can give a 1 mg dose if needed Nasal spray: 1 spray (2.7 mg), can repeat	**SIDE EFFECTS** Opioid-dependent: acute withdrawal symptoms (pain, anxiety, tachypnea, diarrhea, agitation)

OPIOID USE DISORDER

Opioid use disorder (OUD) is a pattern of problematic opioid use that causes significant impairment or distress (e.g., failure to fulfill obligations at home, school or work). OUD can affect anyone; approximately 2.7 million people in the U.S. report having OUD.

TREATMENT OF OPIOID USE DISORDER

Naloxone is an opioid antagonist; it replaces the opioid on the mu receptor. Given by itself, naloxone (injection or nasal spray) is used for opioid overdose. At high doses, buprenorphine acts as an opioid antagonist, making it an effective treatment for OUD. Buprenorphine/naloxone combination products are used as alternatives to methadone for OUD (buprenorphine suppresses withdrawal symptoms and naloxone helps prevent misuse).

Naltrexone is an opioid antagonist normally used to help treat alcohol and opioid use disorders because it blocks the effects of alcohol and opioids that may be taken inappropriately. It is available as a daily oral formulation and a monthly IM injection (*Vivitrol*). Lofexidine (*Lucemyra*), a non-opioid, alpha-2 adrenergic agonist, is not specifically indicated for OUD, but is approved to treat withdrawal symptoms in patients who wish to abruptly stop use of opioids altogether.

DRUGS FOR OPIOID USE DISORDER

DRUG	DOSING	SAFETY/SIDE EFFECTS/MONITORING
Buprenorphine C-III Injection, sublingual tablet/film *Sublocade*: once-monthly subcutaneous injection *Brixandi*: weekly or monthly subcutaneous injection **+ naloxone (*Suboxone*:** sublingual film, ***Zubsolv*:** sublingual tablets) Used for treatment of pain and for opioid use disorder	*Suboxone, Zubsolv*: used daily for opioid use disorder and used off-label for pain	**BOXED WARNINGS** Refer to the opioid boxed warnings Serious harm (e.g., thromboembolic events, tissue damage) or death when extended-release subcutaneous injection is administered intravenously (these formulations have a REMS program to decrease risk) **WARNINGS** CNS depression, QT prolongation, severe dental adverse events with sublingual formulations **SIDE EFFECTS** Dizziness, sedation, headache, confusion, mental and physical impairment, diaphoresis, QT prolongation, respiratory depression (dose-dependent) *Suboxone* SL film: constipation, nausea, hyperhidrosis **NOTES** *Sublocade*: patients must have been taking a stable dose of transmucosal buprenorphine for 7 days prior to initiation
Methadone		Used for treatment of pain and opioid use disorder See opioid drug table for details
Naltrexone (*Vivitrol*) Tablet, ER injection	Tablet: 25 mg daily for 1-3 days, then increase to 50 mg once daily Injection: 380 mg IM every 4 weeks	**NOTES** Do not initiate until patient is opioid free for at least 7-10 days (or longer for long-acting opioids)
Lofexidine (*Lucemyra*) Tablet For mitigation of withdrawal symptoms	Initial: 0.54 mg four times daily in 5 to 6 hour intervals; maximum duration of treatment 14 days	**WARNINGS** Risk of hypotension, bradycardia and syncope, QT prolongation, ↑ CNS depression, ↑ risk of opioid overdose after discontinuation, must taper when discontinuing **NOTES** Can reduce efficacy of oral naltrexone; paroxetine and other CYP2D6 inhibitors can ↑ risk of orthostatic hypotension and bradycardia, monitor closely

COMMON ADJUVANTS FOR PAIN MANAGEMENT

Adjuvants [e.g., muscle relaxants, antiseizure medications (ASMs), antidepressants, topical anesthetics] are useful in pain management though they are not classified as analgesics. They can be added to opioid or non-opioid analgesics (i.e., multimodal treatment).

Adjuvants are commonly used for pain associated with neuropathy (from diabetes or spinal cord injury), postherpetic neuralgia (PHN), fibromyalgia and osteoarthritis (OA). ASMs (e.g., pregabalin, gabapentin), tricyclic antidepressants (TCAs) and SNRIs are useful for neuropathic pain. TCAs and SNRIs block norepinephrine uptake, which has shown to be beneficial in neuropathic pain; SSRIs do not have this effect. Some adjuvants are developed and labeled for specific indications. For example, a lidocaine 1.8% patch formulation, *ZTlido*, was developed and approved for PHN. In severe cases, other classes of agents, including opioids, can provide benefit.

Muscle relaxants have various, poorly understood mechanisms of action. Some work predominantly by CNS depression leading to relaxation of skeletal muscles (e.g., carisoprodol, chlorzoxazone, metaxalone, methocarbamol), while others work by decreasing transmission of reflexes at the spinal level.

Injectable adjuvants can be used in specific cases by pain specialists. For example, clonidine injection can be added to opioids in intrathecal (epidural) pain infusion pumps for patients with cancer pain when other agents are insufficient. Only analgesics approved by the FDA for intrathecal administration should be used. Some other common injectable adjuvants include anesthetics like lidocaine injected locally to provide pain relief to a small area, such as before a dental procedure or before placing stitches (see a list of these agents in the Acute & Critical Care Medicine chapter) or steroid injections for temporary relief in some conditions. Triamcinolone acetonide extended-release *(Zilretta)* was approved for OA knee pain and is administered by injection into the knee joint (intra-articular) to provide 12 weeks of pain relief without opioids.

ORAL ADJUVANTS FOR NEUROPATHIC PAIN

DRUG	DOSING	SAFETY/SIDE EFFECTS/MONITORING
Antiseizure medications (ASMs)		
Gabapentin *(Neurontin)* Capsule, tablet, solution, suspension *Gralise:* tablet – for PHN Gabapentin enacarbil *(Horizant)*: ER tablet – for PHN and restless legs syndrome	Initial: 300 mg TID Max 3,600 mg/day CrCl < 60 mL/min: ↓ dose and/or extend interval	**WARNINGS** Angioedema/anaphylaxis, multiorgan hypersensitivity (DRESS) reactions, suicidal thoughts or behavior (all ASMs), ↑ seizure frequency if rapidly discontinued in those with seizures, CNS depression (if possible, avoid other CNS depressants; if prescribed with an opioid, use the lowest possible dose) **SIDE EFFECTS** Dizziness, somnolence, peripheral edema/weight gain, ocular effects (diplopia, blurred vision), ataxia, nystagmus, tremor, dry mouth, mild anxiolytic (scheduled in some states) **NOTES** Used most commonly off-label for fibromyalgia, pain (neuropathic), headache, alcohol use disorder, alcohol withdrawal Take ER formulation with food IR, ER and gabapentin enacarbil are not interchangeable
Pregabalin *(Lyrica)* C-V Capsule, solution, ER tablet	Initial: 75 mg BID or 50 mg TID Max 450 mg/day CrCl < 60 mL/min: ↓ dose and/or extend interval	**WARNINGS** Angioedema, hypersensitivity reactions, risks of suicidal thoughts or behavior (all ASMs), ↑ seizure frequency if rapidly discontinued in those with seizures; can cause peripheral edema, CNS depression such as dizziness and somnolence (if possible, avoid other CNS depressants; if prescribed with an opioid, use the lowest possible dose) **SIDE EFFECTS** Dizziness, somnolence, peripheral edema/weight gain, mild anxiolytic, diplopia, ataxia **NOTES** Approved for use in fibromyalgia, PHN and neuropathic pain associated with diabetes and spinal cord injury

DRUG	DOSING	SAFETY/SIDE EFFECTS/MONITORING
Carbamazepine (Tegretol, Tegretol XR, Carbatrol, Epitol, Equetro) Tablet (IR/ER), ER capsule, chewable tablet, suspension, injection	Initial: 100 mg BID Max 1,200 mg/day	**NOTES** FDA-approved for the treatment of trigeminal neuralgia See the Seizures/Epilepsy chapter

SNRIs and TCAs

DRUG	DOSING	SAFETY/SIDE EFFECTS/MONITORING
Milnacipran (Savella, Savella Titration Pack) Tablet	Day 1: 12.5 mg daily Days 2-3: 12.5 mg BID Days 4-7: 25 mg BID Then 50 mg BID CrCl < 30 mL/min: Max dose is 25 mg BID	**BOXED WARNINGS** Milnacipran is an SNRI; antidepressants ↑ the risk of suicidal thoughts and behavior in children, adolescents and young adults with depression and other psychiatric disorders (do not use in pediatric patients) **CONTRAINDICATIONS** Use with or within 2 weeks of MAO inhibitors, avoid with linezolid or IV methylene blue **SIDE EFFECTS** Nausea, headache, constipation, dizziness, insomnia, hot flashes **NOTES** Indicated for fibromyalgia only (not approved for depression) Do not use IV digoxin with milnacipran; milnacipran can ↑ the toxic effect of digoxin including postural hypotension and tachycardia (particularly IV digoxin) Increased bleeding risk with anticoagulants or antiplatelets
Amitriptyline Tablet Desipramine (Norpramin) Tablet **Duloxetine (Cymbalta,** Drizalma Sprinkle) Capsule	10-50 mg QHS, sometimes higher Initial: 25 mg daily Max 150 mg/day 30-60 mg/day	**NOTES** See the Depression chapter Desipramine: titrate every 3-7 days Duloxetine approved for the treatment of neuropathic and musculoskeletal pain

ORAL ADJUVANTS FOR MUSCULOSKELETAL PAIN/SPASMS

DRUG	DOSING	SAFETY/SIDE EFFECTS/MONITORING
Antispasmodics (muscle relaxants) with analgesic effects; use caution with other CNS depressants (e.g., alcohol, benzodiazepines and opioids) due to the additive risk of CNS depression		
Baclofen (Lioresal) Tablet, solution, injection, oral suspension, granules	5-20 mg TID-QID PRN Injection given via intrathecal pump for severe spasticity	**BOXED WARNINGS** Abrupt withdrawal of intrathecal baclofen has resulted in severe effects (high fever, lethargy, rebound/↑ spasticity, muscle rigidity and rhabdomyolysis), leading to organ failure and death **SIDE EFFECTS** All muscle relaxants: excessive sedation, dizziness, confusion, asthenia (muscle weakness) Baclofen: nausea, headache, constipation, hypotension, seizures **NOTES** Do not over dose in elderly (e.g., start low, titrate carefully), watch for additive side effects
Cyclobenzaprine (Amrix, Fexmid, Flexeril*) Tablet, capsule	IR: 5-10 mg TID PRN ER: 15-30 mg once daily	**SIDE EFFECTS** Dry mouth **NOTES** Can have efficacy with fibromyalgia Serotonergic: do not combine with other serotonergic agents Can precipitate or exacerbate cardiac arrhythmias; caution in elderly or those with heart disease (chemically similar to a tricyclic antidepressant; almost identical to amitriptyline)

Brand discontinued but name still used in practice.

DRUG	DOSING	SAFETY/SIDE EFFECTS/MONITORING
Tizanidine (Zanaflex) Tablet, capsule	2-4 mg Q6-8H PRN (max 36 mg/day)	**CONTRAINDICATIONS** Use with strong CYP1A2 inhibitors (e.g., fluvoxamine, ciprofloxacin) **SIDE EFFECTS** Hypotension, dry mouth, ↑ LFTs **NOTES** Centrally acting alpha-2 agonist
Antispasmodics (muscle relaxants) that exert their effects by sedation		
Carisoprodol (Soma, Vanadom) C-IV	250-350 mg QID PRN	**NOTES** Poor CYP2C19 metabolizers will have ↑ carisoprodol concentrations (up to 4-fold) Rapid CYP2C19 metabolizers will convert to the active metabolite (meprobamate) faster (↑ toxicity/sedation)
Metaxalone (Skelaxin)	800 mg TID-QID PRN	**SIDE EFFECTS** Hepatotoxicity
Methocarbamol (Robaxin)	1,500-2,000 mg QID PRN	**SIDE EFFECTS** Sedation

Rarely used muscle relaxants include dantrolene (Dantrium used for malignant hyperthermia), chlorzoxazone (Lorzone) and orphenadrine.

TOPICAL ADJUVANTS

DRUG	DOSING/NOTES	SAFETY/SIDE EFFECTS/MONITORING
Lidocaine topical Cream, gel, patch Rx and OTC **Lidocaine 5% [Lidoderm (Rx)]: patch** **Lidocaine viscous** (Rx): **gel** Lidocaine 1.8% [ZTlido (Rx)]: patch for PHN Lidocaine 4% and lower strengths [Salonpas Pain Relieving, Lidocare, others (OTC)]: patch	*Lidoderm:* Apply to painful area 1-3 patches/day and worn for up to 12 hrs/day Approved for PHN (shingles) pain	**SIDE EFFECTS** Patch: minor application site reactions (slight burning/pruritus/rash) **NOTES** Can cut into smaller pieces (before removing backing) *Lidoderm:* do not apply more than 3 patches at one time Caution with used patches; can harm children and pets; fold patch in half and discard safely Do not cover with heating pads/electric blankets Do not use on broken, abraded, severely burned skin or skin with open lesions (can significantly increase amount absorbed)
Capsaicin topical Cream, gel, patch, stick, lotion Rx and OTC **Capsaicin 0.025% and 0.075% [Zostrix, Zostrix HP (OTC)]:** cream Capsaicin 8% [Qutenza (Rx)]: patch	Apply to affected area TID-QID	**SIDE EFFECTS** Topical burning, which dissipates with continued use **NOTES** ↓ TRPV1-expressing nociceptive nerve endings (↓ substance P) Onset of pain relief takes 2-4 weeks of continuous application for OTC products and 1 week for *Qutenza* Do not touch genitals, nasal area, mouth or eyes after application; wash hands after application *Qutenza* is applied in the healthcare provider's office for PHN pain. It works in ~40% of patients to reduce pain. Causes topical burning and requires pre-treatment with lidocaine. Applied for 1 hour and effect lasts for months.
Methyl salicylate topical Patch, cream, stick OTC **BenGay, IcyHot, Salonpas, Thera-Gesic**, store brands Methyl salicylate plus other ingredients **Trolamine (Aspercreme)**	Apply to affected area TID-QID	**NOTES** Occasionally, topicals have caused first to third-degree burns, mostly in patients with pre-existing neuropathic damage; discontinue use and seek medical attention if signs of skin injury (pain, swelling, or blistering) occur following application

KEY COUNSELING POINTS

See the Drug Formulations and Patient Counseling chapter for counseling language/layman's terminology.

ACETAMINOPHEN

- The total daily dose of all products containing acetaminophen should not exceed 4,000 mg.
- Can cause hepatotoxicity.

NSAIDS

- Requires a MedGuide.
- Can cause:
  - ❏ Stomach bleeding.
  - ❏ Increased blood pressure.
  - ❏ Swelling.
  - ❏ Photosensitivity.
- Do not use this medicine if you have experienced breathing problems or allergic-type reactions after taking aspirin or other NSAIDs.
- Avoid in pregnancy (teratogenic).

Diclofenac Gel

- Use the reusable dosing card inside the package to correctly measure each dose. Apply diclofenac gel onto the dosing card evenly up to the correct dosing line.
  - ❏ The dose for hands, wrists or elbows is 2 grams applied four times daily. Do not exceed 8 grams each day to these areas.

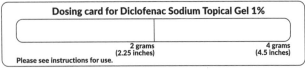

❏ The dose for feet, ankles or knees is 4 grams applied four times daily. Do not exceed more than 16 grams each day to these areas.
- Do not shower, bathe or wash your treated hands for at least one hour after application.

OPIOIDS

- Can cause:
  - ❏ Drowsiness.
  - ❏ Constipation.
- Take with food or milk if stomach upset occurs. Exception: oxymorphone should be taken on an empty stomach.
- Do not consume alcohol , especially with morphine ER capsules, *Nucynta ER,* oxymorphone ER or hydrocodone ER capsules.
- Morphine ER capsules can be opened and the contents sprinkled on applesauce immediately before ingestion.

MUSCLE RELAXANTS

- Can cause drowsiness.

CAPSAICIN TOPICAL

- Unless treating hand pain, wash hands thoroughly with soap and water immediately after use.
- If treating hands, leave on for 30 minutes, then wash hands as above.
- Do not touch genitals, nasal area, mouth or eyes with the medicine; it will burn the sensitive skin.
- The burning pain should dissipate with continual use; starting at the lower strength will help.
- Do not cover with heating pads/electric blankets or bandages; serious burning can occur.

Select Guidelines/References

CDC Clinical Practice Guideline for Prescribing Opioids for Pain. Nov 2022. *MMWR* 71(3);1-95.

SAMHSA Opioid Overdose Prevention Toolkit. https://store.samhsa.gov/system/files/sma18-4742.pdf (accessed 2023 Nov 21).

American Academy of Neurology. Oral and Topical Treatment of Painful Diabetic Polyneuropathy Practice Guideline Update. Jan 2022. Neurology 98;31-43.

CHAPTER CONTENT

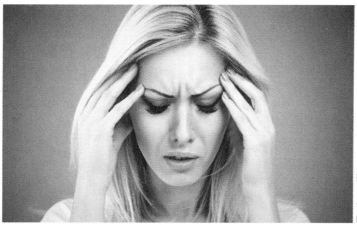

iStock.com/Sjphotography

CHAPTER 59

MIGRAINE

BACKGROUND

Headache treatment is a common concern in the community pharmacy. It is one of the most frequent complaints in neurologists' offices and a common pain complaint seen in family practice. Most headaches are migraine or tension-type headaches.

Migraines are chronic headaches that cause significant pain for hours or days. Most migraines cause nausea, vomiting and sensitivity to light and sound. In about one-third of patients, migraines are preceded or accompanied by sensory warning symptoms or signs (auras), such as flashes of light, blind spots or tingling in the arms or legs. Tension-type headaches are not typically associated with these symptoms; they are described as a pressure or tightness around the head.

A headache accompanied by fever, stiff neck, rash, confusion, seizures, double vision, weakness, numbness, chest pain, shortness of breath or aphasia (trouble speaking) could indicate a serious cardiovascular, cerebrovascular or infectious event. Patients with these symptoms should seek immediate medical attention.

CAUSES

The cause of migraines is not well understood. They may be caused by increased neuronal activity, which results in an imbalance of neurotransmitters (including serotonin), and/or activation of the trigeminal nerve [which leads to the release of calcitonin gene-related peptide (CGRP)]. These neurotransmitter and neuropeptide changes ultimately lead to neurogenic inflammation and vasodilation in cranial blood vessels.

Patients should identify and avoid "triggers" to reduce migraine incidence (see Study Tip Gal on the following page). A common trigger in women is fluctuating hormone levels. A menstrual migraine (MM) occurs close to the onset of menstruation and does not occur at other times of the month.

CONTENT LEGEND

Study
Tip Gal

COMMON MIGRAINE TRIGGERS

Hormonal Changes in Women
Fluctuations in estrogen can trigger headaches. Continuous or extended-cycle oral contraceptives can keep estrogen levels more constant and help reduce MM.

Migraine with aura is associated with ↑ risk of stroke. Progestin-only or nonhormonal contraceptives are recommended for migraine with aura to avoid additive stroke risk with estrogen-containing contraceptives.

Foods
Common offending agents include alcohol, especially beer and red wine, aged cheeses, chocolate, aspartame, overuse of caffeine, monosodium glutamate (MSG), salty foods and processed foods.

Stress

Sensory Stimuli
Bright lights, sun glare, loud sounds and certain scents (which may be pleasant or unpleasant odors).

Changes in Wake-Sleep Pattern
Either missing sleep or getting too much sleep (including jet lag).

Changes in the Environment (e.g., weather, barometric pressure)

DIAGNOSIS

Migraines can be diagnosed when an adult has at least five attacks (not attributed to another disorder) fulfilling the following criteria:

1. Headaches last 4 – 72 hours.

2. Headaches have ≥ 2 of the following characteristics: unilateral location, pulsating, moderate-severe pain and aggravated by (or causing avoidance of) routine physical activity.

3. One of the following occurs during the headache: nausea and/or vomiting, photophobia (sensitivity to light) and phonophobia (sensitivity to sound).

NON-DRUG TREATMENT

A headache diary can help patients identify triggers. Non-pharmacologic interventions involve avoiding triggers, stress management, aerobic exercise, massage, physical therapy, spinal manipulation or applying cold compresses/ice to the head. Acupuncture can be helpful for reducing migraines in some patients.

There are several neuromodulation devices approved for the prevention and/or treatment of migraines. These include transcutaneous electrical nerve stimulation (TENS) units (e.g., *Cefaly, Relivion)* and remote electrical neuromodulation (REN) devices (e.g., *Nerivio*). These devices are worn by the patient and provide small electrical pulses that ultimately block pain signals. The *gammaCore Sapphire* device is approved for both migraines and cluster headaches.

TREATMENT PRINCIPLES

NATURAL PRODUCTS

Riboflavin (vitamin B2), magnesium, butterbur, feverfew, peppermint (applied topically) and coenzyme Q10 (either alone or in combination) have been used for the prevention of migraines.

ACUTE VS. PROPHYLACTIC TREATMENT

Acute (abortive) treatment is taken only as needed for a headache that is already present. Drugs used to stop an active migraine will not prevent future migraines (the exception is rimegepant, discussed later in the chapter).

Prophylactic (preventive) treatment decreases the frequency and/or severity of migraines. Medication is taken routinely (even when the patient feels well), but will not be effective for treating an acute migraine.

MEDICATION OVERUSE HEADACHES

Medication overuse ("rebound") headaches (MOH) can result from the overuse of acute headache medications. MOH are headaches that occur ≥ 15 days per month in a patient with a preexisting headache disorder. All patients should be educated to limit acute headache treatment medications (limit depends on the drug being used). Patients with MOH should stop the "over-used" medication; if the drug is an opioid or contains butalbital (e.g., *Fioricet*), a slow taper is needed.

ACUTE DRUG TREATMENT

OTC options include acetaminophen, aspirin, *Advil Migraine* (which contains only ibuprofen), naproxen and combination products such as *Excedrin Migraine* (aspirin, acetaminophen and caffeine). OTC drugs can be tried for migraines that are mild to moderate. Refer to the Pain chapter for a more detailed discussion of these medications.

Prescription options for acute treatment include NSAIDs (higher doses or alternate options than those available OTC), serotonin receptor agonists (triptans), select CGRP receptor antagonists, ergotamine drugs and lasmiditan.

Butalbital-containing products, opioids, tramadol and tapentadol are not recommended due to decreased efficacy, abuse/dependence potential and risk of rebound headache (i.e., MOH).

Some patients get more relief from OTC products, some from triptans and others from a combination of medications. Always ask the patient what they have tried in the past, and if it was useful. Patients with nausea/vomiting may benefit from adjunctive treatment with an antiemetic.

TRIPTANS

Triptans are selective agonists for the 5-HT1 (serotonin) receptor (1B/1D subtypes); they vasoconstrict cranial blood vessels, inhibit neuropeptide release and decrease pain transmission. They are first line for acute treatment. Triptans should be taken at the first sign of a migraine for best results. Triptans should not be used for more than 10 days per month to avoid MOH.

DRUG	DOSING	SAFETY/SIDE EFFECTS/MONITORING
Almotriptan Tablet	Initial: 6.25-12.5 mg, can repeat x 1 after 2 hrs (max 25 mg/day)	**CONTRAINDICATIONS** Cerebrovascular disease (stroke/TIA), uncontrolled hypertension, ischemic heart disease, coronary artery vasospasm, peripheral vascular disease, history of hemiplegic or basilar migraine, use within 24 hrs of another triptan or ergotamine-type medication.
Eletriptan *(Relpax)* Tablet	Initial: 20-40 mg, can repeat x 1 after 2 hrs (max 80 mg/day)	See Drug Interactions section for triptans contraindicated with MAO inhibitors and CYP450 3A4 inhibitors.
Frovatriptan *(Frova)* Tablet	Initial: 2.5 mg, can repeat x 1 after 2 hrs (max 7.5 mg/day)	**WARNINGS** Risk of ↑ BP, serotonin syndrome, cardiac and cerebrovascular events, arrhythmias, MOH, seizures (sumatriptan only); caution in hepatic or renal impairment (product specific).
Naratriptan Tablet	Initial: 1-2.5 mg, can repeat x 1 after 4 hrs (max 5 mg/day)	**SIDE EFFECTS** Paresthesia (tingling/numbness), dizziness, hot/cold sensations, chest pain/tightness, dry mouth, somnolence, nausea, unpleasant taste, vision loss
Rizatriptan (Maxalt-MLT, *Maxalt, RizaFilm)* Tablet, ODT, oral film	Initial: 5-10 mg, can repeat x 1 after 2 hrs (max 30 mg/day) *RizaFilm:* 10 mg on tongue	Triptan sensations (pressure or heaviness in the chest or pressure in the neck region) usually dissipate after administration.
Sumatriptan Tablet, SC (autoinjector, prefilled syringe and solution), nasal spray **Imitrex** Tablet, nasal spray, SC injection **Imitrex STATdose System, Zembrace SymTouch** SC autoinjector **Onzetra Xsail** Nasal powder *Tosymra* Nasal spray	**Oral:** 25, 50 or 100 mg, can repeat x 1 after 2 hrs (max 200 mg/day) **Subcutaneous:** *Imitrex, Imitrex STATdose System:* 4 or 6 mg, can repeat x 1 after 1 hr (max 12 mg/day) *Zembrace SymTouch:* 3 mg, can repeat up to 4 times per day [wait a minimum of 1 hr between doses or 1 hr following use of another sumatriptan product (max 12 mg/day)] **Intranasal:** Spray *(Imitrex):* 5, 10, or 20 mg in one nostril can repeat x 1 after 2 hrs (max 40 mg/day) Spray *(Tosymra):* 10 mg in one nostril can repeat x 1 after 1 hr (max 30 mg/day) Powder *(Onzetra Xsail):* 11 mg in each nostril using nosepiece, can repeat x 1 after 2 hrs (max 44 mg/day)	**NOTES** ODTs, oral films, nasal sprays and injections are useful if nausea is present. No water is required for ODTs and oral film. Nasal sprays and injections work faster. Nasal sprays contain only 1 dose (do not prime). *Treximet:* protect from moisture; dispense in original container. *Treximet* carries all warnings associated with naproxen (see Pain chapter). *Maxalt-MLT* ODT contains phenylalanine and should not be used in patients with phenylketonuria. **Children and Adolescents** Almotriptan tablets, zolmitriptan nasal spray, *RizaFilm* and *Treximet* are approved for children and adolescents ≥ 12 years of age; rizatriptan tablets and ODT are approved for children and adolescents ≥ 6 years of age. **Duration of Action** Frovatriptan has the longest half-life (26 hrs). Both frovatriptan and naratriptan are considered long-acting, but onset is slower. These can be chosen if headache recurs after dosing, lasts a long time or can be anticipated (e.g., MM). All other triptans have a shorter half-life with a faster onset.
+ naproxen *(Treximet)* Tablet (85/500 mg)	**Treximet:** Adults: 1 tab, can repeat x 1 after 2 hrs (max 2 tabs/24 hrs)	
Zolmitriptan *(Zomig, Zomig ZMT*)* Tablet, ODT, nasal spray	PO: 1.25-5 mg, can repeat x 1 after 2 hrs Intranasal: 2.5-5 mg in one nostril, can repeat x 1 after 2 hrs Max 10 mg/day (all formulations)	**Sumatriptan Injections** All are injected SC. Preferred site is lateral thigh or upper arm. Protect from light. Needle shield of the prefilled syringe contains a latex derivative. This has the potential to cause allergic reactions in latex-sensitive individuals.

Brand discontinued but name still used in practice.

TRIPTAN FORMULATIONS

TABLET	ODT	NASAL SPRAY/POWDER	SC INJECTION
All triptans	Rizatriptan (Maxalt-MLT) Zolmitriptan	**Spray** Sumatriptan (Imitrex) Zolmitriptan (Zomig) **Powder** Sumatriptan (Onzetra Xsail)	**Prefilled Syringe and Vial** Sumatriptan **AutoInjector** Sumatriptan (Imitrex STATdose System, Zembrace SymTouch)

Triptan Drug Interactions

- The risk of <u>serotonin syndrome</u> may be increased when combining a triptan with other serotonergic drugs, such as SSRIs, SNRIs or MAO inhibitors (see the Drug Interactions chapter). Many patients take both safely since triptans are only used as needed, but there is an FDA warning regarding this combination.

- <u>Sumatriptan, rizatriptan and zolmitriptan</u> are <u>contraindicated with MAO inhibitors (or within two weeks of stopping)</u> due to increased triptan concentrations when used together.

- Use with strong CYP3A4 inhibitors: eletriptan is contraindicated; reduce the dose of almotriptan.

ERGOTAMINE DRUGS

Ergotamine, a <u>nonselective agonist of serotonin receptors</u>, causes cerebral vasoconstriction. Ergotamine may be an option for patients who do not find benefit with a triptan.

DRUG	DOSING	SAFETY/SIDE EFFECTS/MONITORING
Dihydroergotamine (Migranal, *Trudhesa, D.H.E. 45*)* <u>Injection (IM/SC/IV), nasal spray</u>	IM/SC/IV: 1 mg at first sign of headache, repeat hourly to a max dose of 2 mg/day (IV) or 3 mg/day (IM/SC) Weekly max: 6 mg **Intranasal** *Migranal:* 1 spray (0.5 mg) into each nostril, can repeat after 15 minutes, up to a total of 4 sprays (2 mg/day) *Trudhesa:* 1 spray (0.725 mg) into each nostril, can repeat after 1 hour, up to 2 doses/day or 3 doses/week	**BOXED WARNING** Contraindicated with <u>potent CYP3A4 inhibitors (protease inhibitors, macrolides)</u> due to serious and <u>life-threatening peripheral ischemia</u>. **CONTRAINDICATIONS** <u>Uncontrolled hypertension, ischemic heart disease</u> (e.g., angina, MI), coronary artery vasospasm, peripheral vascular disease, <u>pregnancy</u>, hemiplegic or basilar migraine, renal/hepatic impairment, sepsis, use with pressors/vasoconstrictive drugs, <u>use within 24 hours of serotonin agonists (triptans) or other ergotamine-type drugs</u>. **WARNINGS** <u>Cardiovascular effects</u> (avoid with baseline risk), <u>cerebrovascular events</u>, ergotism (intense vasoconstriction resulting in peripheral vascular ischemia and possible gangrene), cardiac valvular fibrosis, MOH, potentially serious <u>drug interactions</u>.
Ergotamine (Ergomar) Sublingual tablet	2 mg single dose, may repeat after at least 30 min, up to 6 mg/day or 10 mg/week	
Ergotamine + caffeine (Migergot, *Cafergot**) Tablet, suppository	PO (1 mg ergotamine + 100 mg caffeine): take 2 tablets at onset of migraine, then 1 tablet every 30 min PRN to a max of 6 tablets per attack Suppository (Migergot): 1 suppository at first sign of migraine, may repeat x 1 after 1 hr to a max of 2 suppositories per attack	**SIDE EFFECTS** Nausea, vomiting. Nasal spray: rhinitis, dysgeusia, local irritation. **NOTES** Nasal spray: <u>prime</u> by pumping 4 times. Do not inhale deeply (to let drug absorb into skin in nose). Recommended to use at first sign of attack, but can be used at any time during migraine.

Brand discontinued but name still used in practice.

OTHER ABORTIVE AGENTS

Rimegepant *(Nurtec)*, ubrogepant *(Ubrelvy)* and zavegepant *(Zavzpret)* are CGRP receptor antagonists. CGRP contributes to vasodilation and neurogenic inflammation in the pathogenesis of migraines; blocking the CGRP receptor helps reduce or eliminate migraine pain. Ubrogepant and zavegepant are approved to treat acute migraine attacks, and rimegepant is approved to both prevent and treat acute migraine attacks.

Lasmiditan *(Reyvow)* is a first-in-class serotonin agonist that is selective for the 5-HT1F receptor subtype. Unlike the triptans and ergotamine drugs, lasmiditan does not cause vasoconstriction, therefore it is not contraindicated in patients with CVD.

DRUG	DOSING	SAFETY/SIDE EFFECTS/MONITORING
CGRP Receptor Antagonists		
Rimegepant *(Nurtec)* ODT	75 mg PO once Max dose 75 mg/24 hours	**CONTRAINDICATIONS** Do not use with strong CYP3A4 inhibitors (ubrogepant only, but caution with rimegepant)
Ubrogepant *(Ubrelvy)* Tablet	50-100 mg PO, can repeat x 1 after 2 hrs Max dose 200 mg/24 hours Child-Pugh Class C: 50 mg (can repeat x 1) CrCl 15-29 mL/min: 50 mg (can repeat x 1) CrCl < 15 mL/min: do not use	**WARNINGS** Rimegepant: hypersensitivity reactions, including delayed serious reactions **SIDE EFFECTS** Nausea, somnolence, taste disorder (zavegepant)
Zavegepant *(Zavzpret)* Nasal spray	1 spray (10 mg) in 1 nostril Max dose 10 mg/day CrCl < 30 mL/min or Child-Pugh Class C: do not use	**NOTES** The safety of treating > 8 migraines/month (ubrogepant, zavegepant) or using > 18 doses/month (rimegepant) has not been established
Serotonin Receptor (5-HT1F) Agonist		
Lasmiditan *(Reyvow)* C-V	50-200 mg PO as a single dose Max 1 dose/24 hours	**WARNINGS** CNS depression, including significant driving impairment (should not be used if the patient cannot wait at least 8 hrs after dose to drive or operate heavy machinery); use caution if patient is taking other CNS depressants May cause serotonin syndrome with or without other serotonergic drugs May ↓ HR; use with caution if using other drugs that ↓ HR **SIDE EFFECTS** Dizziness, fatigue, paresthesia **NOTES** The safety of treating > 4 migraines/month has not been established

CGRP Receptor Antagonist Drug Interactions

- Rimegepant and ubrogepant are major substrates of CYP3A4 and minor substrates of P-gp. Strong 3A4 inhibitors and inducers should be avoided with both drugs; moderate 3A4 inducers should also be avoided with rimegepant.
  - ❑ The starting dose of ubrogepant is 50 mg in patients taking a moderate or weak 3A4 inhibitor or a P-gp inhibitor.
  - ❑ The starting dose of ubrogepant is 100 mg in patients is taking a moderate or weak 3A4 inducer.
  - ❑ Avoid using a second dose of rimegepant within 48 hours in patients taking a moderate 3A4 inhibitor or a P-gp inhibitor.

BUTALBITAL-CONTAINING PRODUCTS

Butalbital is a barbiturate. Acetaminophen/butalbital/caffeine *(Fioricet)* and aspirin/butalbital/caffeine (previously *Fiorinal*) are both available in combinations with codeine (e.g., *Fioricet with Codeine*). All of these products are federally classified as schedule III, except *Fioricet* (which is exempt). *Fioricet* remains a popular drug, but butalbital-containing products are not recommended for treating acute migraines due to abuse/dependence issues and lower efficacy. If discontinuing these products in patients who have used them regularly and long-term, they must be tapered off or the patient will have worsening of headache, tremors and be at risk for delirium and seizures.

PROPHYLACTIC DRUG TREATMENT

Preventive treatment should be considered in patients who have ≥ 4 migraines per month, have migraines that decrease quality of life, if acute treatments are ineffective, contraindicated, overused, or not tolerated or if patients request it.

Selection of a prophylactic drug is based on patient characteristics and the medication side effect profile; efficacy data is similar for all options (~50% reduction in headache days). A full trial, at a reasonable dose, is a minimum of 8 weeks. If no response after this trial, consider switching to a different drug. Consider continuing for 6 – 12 months if partial response is noted. Many patients try more than one drug before finding one that works well for them. Oral prophylactic therapies include:

- Antihypertensives: beta-blockers (best evidence is with propranolol, timolol and metoprolol, though others have been used). Lisinopril and candesartan are alternatives.
- Antiseizure medications: topiramate (*Topamax* and other brands) and valproic acid. Topiramate causes weight loss in many patients, making it a popular choice for patients also interested in weight loss.
- CGRP receptor antagonists: more options for prophylaxis (see table on following page) than for acute migraine treatment.
- Antidepressants: tricyclic antidepressants (most evidence with amitriptyline); venlafaxine (an SNRI) is an alternative.
- MM: extended-cycle or continuous oral contraceptives or the vaginal ring can be used (if no aura). NSAIDs or a triptan [specifically those with a longer half-life: frovatriptan (preferred) or naratriptan] can be started prior to menses and continued for 5 – 7 days.
- Natural products (discussed at the beginning of the chapter).

BETA-BLOCKERS AND ANTISEIZURE MEDICATIONS

DRUG	TYPICAL DOSING	COMMENTS/SIDE EFFECTS
Beta-Blockers (see Hypertension chapter for complete discussion)		
Propranolol (*Inderal LA*)	IR: 80-240 mg, divided in 2-4 doses LA: 80-240 mg once daily	**WARNINGS** Use caution with bronchospastic diseases (e.g., asthma, COPD), especially with non-selective agents (propranolol and timolol)
Metoprolol tartrate (*Lopressor*) **Metoprolol succinate (*Toprol XL*,** Kapspargo Sprinkle**)**	50-200 mg, divided in 2 doses (for tartrate only)	**SIDE EFFECTS** Bradycardia, hypotension, CNS effects (e.g., fatigue, dizziness, depression) (more so with propranolol, the most lipophilic), impotence, cold extremities (can exacerbate Raynaud's)
Timolol	5-15 mg twice daily	**NOTES** Propranolol XL formulations (*Inderal XL, InnoPran XL*) are not FDA-approved for migraine prophylaxis Metoprolol is beta-1 selective
Antiseizure Medications (see Seizures/Epilepsy chapter for complete discussion)		
Divalproex (*Depakote, Depakote ER, Depakote Sprinkle*) **Valproic acid**	*Depakote*: 250-500 mg twice daily *Depakote ER*: 500-1,000 mg once daily	**BOXED WARNINGS** Fetal harm, hepatic failure, pancreatitis **WARNINGS AND SIDE EFFECTS** Weight changes (gain > loss), thrombocytopenia, ↑ ammonia, alopecia, N/V, somnolence, tremor
Topiramate (*Topamax*, Topamax Sprinkle, Eprontia**)** Topiramate extended release (*Qudexy XR, Trokendi XR*)	*Topamax*: start 25 mg QHS, titrate to 50 mg BID	**WARNINGS** Fetal harm, metabolic acidosis, nephrolithiasis, ↑ ammonia, secondary angle-closure glaucoma and visual field defects, oligohidrosis **SIDE EFFECTS** Weight loss, somnolence, cognitive impairment, paresthesia, reduced efficacy of oral contraceptives

CGRP RECEPTOR ANTAGONISTS

There are two <u>oral</u> CGRP receptor antagonists approved for the <u>prevention</u> of migraines: atogepant (*Qulipta*) and <u>rimegepant</u> (*Nurtec*), which is also approved for the treatment of migraines (see Other Abortive Agents section earlier in the chapter). The remaining CGRP antagonists used for migraine prevention are <u>injectable monoclonal antibodies</u>.

DRUG	TYPICAL DOSING RANGE	COMMENTS/SIDE EFFECTS
Atogepant (*Qulipta*) Tablet	10, 30 or 60 mg <u>PO</u> daily	**WARNINGS** *Aimovig*: new or worsening hypertension Rimegepant: hypersensitivity reactions, including delayed serious reactions
Eptinezumab-jjmr (*Vyepti*) Injection	100 mg <u>IV</u> once <u>every 3 months</u>; some patients benefit from 300 mg	**SIDE EFFECTS** Injection site reaction, antibody development, constipation
Erenumab-aooe (*Aimovig*) SC autoinjector	70-140 mg <u>SC</u> once <u>monthly</u>	Atogepant, rimegepant: nausea, somnolence
Fremanezumab-vfrm (*Ajovy*) SC autoinjector, prefilled syringe	225 mg <u>SC</u> once <u>monthly</u> or 675 mg <u>SC</u> <u>every 3 months</u>	**NOTES** SC injection: self-administer in the abdomen, thigh or upper arm; store refrigerated in the original carton prior to use; allow to sit at room temperature for at least 30 min before injecting
Galcancezumab-gnlm (*Emgality*) SC autoinjector, prefilled syringe	240 mg SC as loading dose, then 120 mg <u>SC</u> once <u>monthly</u>	Atogepant: dose adjustments depend on concurrent use with CYP3A4 inhibitors or inducers or OATP inhibitors
Rimegepant (*Nurtec*) ODT	75 mg <u>PO</u> every other day	Rimegepant: do not use with moderate-strong CYP3A4 inducers or strong CYP3A4 inhibitors Galcancezumab: also approved for cluster headache prevention

BOTULINUM TOXIN

<u>Botulinum toxin type A</u> (*Botox*) injections are used for prophylaxis of <u>chronic</u> migraines <u>only</u> (≥ 15 headache days per month).

KEY COUNSELING POINTS

See the Drug Formulations and Patient Counseling chapter for counseling language/layman's terminology and for instructions on self-administered injections, nasal sprays/powder and ODTs.

ALL TRIPTANS

- Can cause serotonin syndrome if taken with other medications that can increase serotonin.
- If your symptoms are only partly relieved, or if your headache comes back, you may take a second dose in the time period explained to you by the pharmacist.
- If you use migraine treatments frequently or if your migraines are severe, discuss using a daily medication for prevention with your healthcare provider.

Imitrex STATdose System

- Includes a carrying case, a *STATdose* pen and two syringe cartridges.

Maxalt-MLT ODT

- Contains phenylalanine. Do not use if you have phenylketonuria (PKU).

Onzetra Xsail Nasal Powder

- Open the pouch and remove the first nosepiece. Insert the nosepiece into the device until you hear it click.
- Press and release the white button to pierce the medication capsule.
- Insert the nosepiece deeply into the nose (first nostril). Rotate the device to <u>place the mouthpiece into your mouth</u>.
- <u>Blow into the device with your mouth for 2 – 3 seconds to deliver medication into your nose</u>. A vibration (or rattling noise) may occur.
- Press the clear tab to remove the first nosepiece. Check the capsule to be sure the medication is gone. Discard the first nosepiece.
- Insert the second nosepiece into the device and repeat the steps above using the second nostril.

Select Guidelines/References

The American Headache Society Position Statement on Integrating New Migraine Treatments into Clinical Practice. https://doi.org/10.1111/head.13456 (accessed 2024 Jan 19).

CONTENT LEGEND

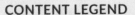

 Study Tip Gal    Key Drug Guy

uric acid crystals

iStock.com/colematt

CHAPTER 60

GOUT

BACKGROUND

Gout is a type of arthritis caused by a buildup of uric acid (UA) crystals, primarily in the joints. UA is produced as an end-product of purine metabolism (see adenosine metabolism later in the chapter). Purines are present in many foods, and they make up one of the base pairs of DNA. Under normal conditions, UA is excreted renally (mainly) and via the GI tract.

A normal serum UA level is 2 – 6.5 mg/dL in females and 3.5 – 7.2 mg/dL in males. When UA accumulates in the blood, some patients remain asymptomatic (i.e., hyperuricemic without developing gout) while others may develop UA crystals in the joints (i.e., tophi), causing a painful gout attack with burning and swelling of the affected joint. Gout attacks have a sudden onset. Gout typically occurs in one joint, most often the metatarsophalangeal joint (MTP, the big toe). If left untreated, the attacks can occur repeatedly and damage the joints, tendons and other tissues.

In addition to a UA level, a sample of synovial (joint) fluid can be evaluated to identify if UA crystals are present. Certain imaging studies (e.g., X-ray, US, MRI, CT) can be used to view the affected joint.

RISK FACTORS

Risk factors for gout include male sex, obesity, excessive alcohol consumption (particularly beer), hypertension, chronic kidney disease (CKD), lead intoxication, advanced age and using medications that increase UA (see Key Drugs Guy below).

DRUGS THAT INCREASE URIC ACID

Aspirin (lower doses)
Cyclosporine
Diuretics (loops and thiazides)
Niacin
Pyrazinamide
Select chemotherapy (with tumor lysis syndrome)
Select pancreatic enzyme products

Changing the diet can lower the risk of gout. Foods to avoid include organ meats, high-fructose corn syrup and alcohol. Foods that should be limited include fruit juices, table sugar, sweetened drinks, desserts, salt, beef, lamb, pork and seafood with high purine content (e.g., sardines, shellfish). A healthy diet, including low-fat dairy products and vegetables, reduces gout risk. Weight control, smoking cessation, exercise and hydration are other ways to reduce risk.

Tumor lysis syndrome (TLS) is a condition that can result from the use of certain chemotherapy drugs and can cause acute gout attacks (see the Oncology chapter for details).

DRUG TREATMENT

Asymptomatic hyperuricemia is not treated with drugs. Once a gout attack occurs, anti-inflammatory drugs are used to treat the acute attack. Gout develops as a result of either an underexcretion or an overproduction of UA; ideal treatment options include drugs that increase UA excretion or decrease UA production. If certain criteria are met, drugs may be started to prevent future attacks. Preventative medications are considered after multiple/frequent gout attacks have occurred, if there is radiographic evidence of advanced disease or if there are tophi present. See Study Tip Gal for an overview of treatments.

The drugs used for acute attacks target pain and inflammation (e.g., colchicine, NSAIDs and steroids). Prophylactic drugs are used to lower UA levels, with a goal UA level of ≤ 6 mg/dL.

GOUT TREATMENT BASICS

Treat acute pain with anti-inflammatory drugs:
- Colchicine
- Steroids (including intra-articular injections)
- NSAIDs (often with a high starting dose)
- Interleukin-1 antagonists (reserved for refractory disease or intolerance to other treatments)

Treat chronically to prevent future attacks:
- Xanthine oxidase inhibitor (XOI): allopurinol (preferred) or febuxostat

An acute gout flare can occur when an XOI is started, so give initially with colchicine or an NSAID

If XOI didn't work well enough and UA remains > 6 mg/dL:
- Add on probenecid to daily XOI
- Replace the XOI with IV pegloticase (*Krystexxa*)

ACUTE GOUT ATTACK TREATMENT

Gout attacks are extremely painful; acute treatment should begin as soon as possible. A single drug is recommended, which is either an NSAID, a systemic steroid or colchicine. In more severe disease, combination treatment usually includes colchicine with either an NSAID or an oral steroid. If the gout attack is localized to one or two joints, an intra-articular steroid injection into the affected joint can be helpful. For patients who cannot be treated with (or tolerate) NSAIDs, colchicine or steroids, or have an inadequate response, an interleukin-1 antagonist [e.g., canakinumab (*Ilaris*)] via subcutaneous injection can be used.

If an acute attack occurs in a patient using chronic urate-lowering therapy (ULT), such as allopurinol, they should continue the ULT during the acute attack. Applying topical ice to the affected joints can help alleviate pain and reduce inflammation.

Acute Gout Attack Therapy

DRUG	DOSING	SAFETY/SIDE EFFECTS/MONITORING
Colchicine		
Colchicine (*Colcrys*, *Gloperba*, *Mitigare*) Tablet, oral solution, capsule + probenecid *LoDoCo* is used for cardiovascular risk reduction (not gout)	**Treatment** 1.2 mg PO (i.e., two 0.6 mg tablets) followed by 0.6 mg in 1 hr (do not exceed 1.8 mg in 1 hr or 2.4 mg/day) CrCl < 30 mL/min: the treatment dose is the same, but do not give again for 2 weeks **Prophylaxis** 0.6 mg once or twice daily CrCl < 30 mL/min: ↓ to 0.3 mg/day	**CONTRAINDICATIONS** Do not use in combination with a P-gp or strong CYP3A4 inhibitor with renal and/or hepatic impairment **WARNINGS** Myelosuppression, neuromuscular toxicity (including rhabdomyolysis), if possible, do not use with cyclosporine, diltiazem, verapamil, gemfibrozil or statins as these drugs ↑ myopathy risk **SIDE EFFECTS** Diarrhea, nausea, myopathy, neuropathy (dose-dependent), ↓ vitamin B12 **NOTES** Start within 36 hours of symptom onset (for treatment) Wait 12 hours after a treatment dose before resuming prophylaxis dosing ↑ risk of myelosuppression, GI and neuromuscular adverse effects in elderly with CrCl < 30 mL/min; ↓ dose and monitor, or use steroid as an alternative Maintain adequate fluid intake

DRUG	DOSING	SAFETY/SIDE EFFECTS/MONITORING
NSAIDs		
Indomethacin (Indocin)	50 mg PO TID until attack resolved	*See Pain chapter for more information*
Naproxen (Aleve, Naprosyn, others)	500 mg PO BID until attack resolved	**NOTES** Avoid use in severe renal disease (UA is renally cleared and patients with gout often have renal insufficiency) and CVD risk, bleeding (risk is lower with short duration of use)
Sulindac	200 mg PO BID until attack resolved	
Celecoxib (Celebrex)	200 mg PO BID, discontinue 2-3 days after attack resolved	Indomethacin, naproxen and sulindac are approved for gout; other NSAIDs can be used
Steroids: given PO, IM, IV, intra-articular or as ACTH (adrenocorticotropic hormone), which triggers endogenous glucocorticoid secretion		
Prednisone/ Prednisolone	30-40 mg/day given daily or BID until attack resolved, then taper (reduce dose by 5 mg each day) over 7-10 days	*See Systemic Steroids & Autoimmune Disease chapter for more information* **NOTES** Acute side effects of steroids, including ↑ BG, ↑ BP, insomnia, ↑ appetite
Methylprednisolone (Medrol, Solu-Medrol)	Intra-articular: if 1-2 large joints involved Oral: methylprednisolone dose pack	Intra-articular steroid injections stay localized and do not cause systemic side effects; repeat injections can cause joint damage
Triamcinolone	If 1-2 joints: intra-articular 10-40 mg If ≥ 3 joints: IM 60 mg, may repeat once or twice Q48H	
Interleukin-1 Antagonist: for refractory gout or patients with contraindication/intolerance to other treatments		
Canakinumab (Ilaris) Injection	150 mg SC once (may be repeated in 12 weeks)	**SIDE EFFECTS** Nasopharyngitis, serious infections **NOTES** Must test for tuberculosis prior to initiation; avoid live vaccines Dosing varies by indication

Colchicine Drug Interactions

- Colchicine is a major substrate of CYP450 3A4 and P-gp. Fatal toxicity can occur if colchicine is combined with strong CYP3A4 inhibitors (e.g., clarithromycin), or a strong inhibitor of P-gp (e.g., cyclosporine); check for inhibitors prior to dispensing. If colchicine is used with a strong CYP3A4 inhibitor, the colchicine dose is reduced and repeated no earlier than three days. If using with a moderate CYP3A4 inhibitor, do not exceed 1.2 mg (2 tablets) of colchicine for acute treatment.

PROPHYLACTIC TREATMENT

Chronic ULT should be started in all patients with gout who have experienced multiple or frequent gout attacks, have evidence of joint damage or have tophi. When starting chronic ULT, colchicine, steroids or NSAIDs should be used as prophylaxis to reduce the risk of attacks, which can occur when UA is lowered rapidly (possibly due to mobilization of the urate crystals).

The first-line ULT is allopurinol, a xanthine oxidase inhibitor (XOI). Blocking the xanthine oxidase enzyme stops the production of UA and produces a non-toxic end product. Patients at high risk of a severe allopurinol hypersensitivity reaction (e.g., patients of Asian descent, African American patients) should be screened for the HLA-B*5801 allele prior to use. Febuxostat, another XOI, is available as an alternative treatment option. XOIs are titrated up slowly to lower the UA to a target level of < 6 mg/dL. Allopurinol is started at a lower dose with moderate or severe CKD.

If XOIs are contraindicated or not tolerated, probenecid (a uricosuric) is a second-line treatment that can be used; it can also be added when the UA level is not at goal despite maximal doses of XOIs. Probenecid inhibits reabsorption of UA in the proximal tubule of the nephron, which increases UA excretion. It requires adequate renal function to be effective, which many patients with gout do not have. Pegloticase is a recombinant uricase enzyme; it converts UA to an inactive metabolite that can be easily excreted and is reserved for severe, refractory gout.

Uric Acid Production and Drug Treatment

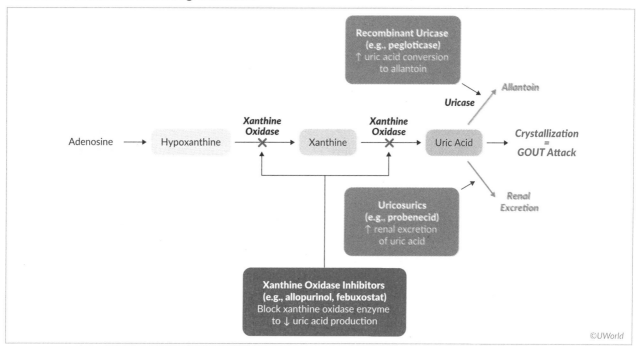

©UWorld

Chronic Urate Lowering Therapy

DRUG	DOSING	SAFETY/SIDE EFFECTS/MONITORING
Xanthine Oxidase Inhibitors: decrease uric acid production		
Allopurinol (Zyloprim, Aloprim) Tablet, injection	Start at 100 mg daily, then slowly titrate up until UA is < 6 mg/dL (doses > 300 mg can be necessary and should be divided BID) CrCl ≤ 30 mL/min: Start at 50 mg daily, increase gradually up 300 mg/day Take after a meal to ↓ nausea	**WARNINGS** Hypersensitivity reactions, including severe rash (SJS/TEN, DRESS); HLA-B*5801 testing prior to use if high risk (e.g., patients of Asian descent, African American patients) and do not use drug if positive; hepatotoxicity, bone marrow suppression, nephrotoxicity **SIDE EFFECTS** Rash, gout flare, nausea, diarrhea, ↑ LFTs **MONITORING** CBC, LFTs, renal function **NOTES** Higher doses used for tumor lysis syndrome (see Oncology chapter) Due to the high rate of gout attacks when beginning ULT, use with colchicine (0.6 mg once or twice daily) or an NSAID for the first 3-6 months
Febuxostat (Uloric) Tablet	Start at 40 mg daily, ↑ to 80 mg if UA not < 6 mg/dL at 2 weeks; max dose 120 mg/day CrCl < 30 mL/min: max dose 40 mg daily	**BOXED WARNING** Increased risk of cardiovascular (CV) death compared to allopurinol in patients with established CV disease; use should be limited to those who cannot tolerate allopurinol (e.g., hypersensitivity) or if allopurinol is not effective **CONTRAINDICATIONS** Do not use with mercaptopurine or azathioprine **WARNINGS** Hepatotoxicity, possible MI or stroke, gout flare, hypersensitivity and serious skin reactions (e.g., SJS/TEN, DRESS) **SIDE EFFECTS** Rash, nausea, ↑ LFTs, arthralgia **MONITORING** LFTs **NOTES** Due to the high rate of gout attacks when beginning ULT, use with colchicine (0.6 mg once or twice daily) or an NSAID for the first 3-6 months

DRUG	DOSING	SAFETY/SIDE EFFECTS/MONITORING
Uricosuric: inhibit reabsorption of uric acid in the kidneys, which ↑ uric acid excretion		
Probenecid Tablet + colchicine	Start 250 mg BID, can increase to 2 g/day CrCl < 30 mL/min: avoid use	**CONTRAINDICATIONS** Do not use with aspirin therapy, blood dyscrasias, UA kidney stones (nephrolithiasis), children < 2 years, initiation in acute gout attack **WARNINGS** ↓ effectiveness with CrCl < 30 mL/min (ACR guidelines: do not use if CrCl < 50 mL/min), do not use with G6PD deficiency **SIDE EFFECTS** Hypersensitivity reactions, hemolytic anemia **NOTES** Probenecid can be used to ↑ beta-lactam levels by ↓ beta-lactam renal excretion
Recombinant Uricase: converts uric acid to allantoin, which is excreted		
Pegloticase (Krystexxa) Injection	8 mg IV every 2 weeks	**BOXED WARNINGS** Anaphylactic reactions – monitor and premedicate with antihistamines and steroids, risk is greatest if UA is > 6 mg/dL; life-threatening hemolytic reactions and methemoglobinemia may occur with G6PD deficiency **CONTRAINDICATIONS** G6PD deficiency **WARNINGS** Acute gout flares can occur upon initiation; an NSAID or colchicine should be given 1 week prior to infusion and continued for at least 6 months **SIDE EFFECTS** Antibody formation, gout flare, infusion reactions, nausea, bruising, urticaria, erythema **NOTES** Do not use in combination with allopurinol, febuxostat or probenecid (↑ risk of anaphylaxis)

Xanthine Oxidase Inhibitor Drug Interactions

■ Allopurinol and febuxostat ↑ the concentration of mercaptopurine, the active metabolite of azathioprine. Do not use mercaptopurine or azathioprine with febuxostat, and use caution combining these with allopurinol (avoid or ↓ dose and monitor for toxicity).

■ Avoid use with didanosine; allopurinol and febuxostat can ↑ didanosine levels.

■ Antacids ↓ allopurinol absorption.

■ Avoid use with pegloticase (↑ risk of anaphylaxis)

Probenecid Drug Interactions

■ Probenecid reduces the renal clearance of other medications when taken together, including aspirin (do not use salicylates concurrently), methotrexate, penicillins, cephalosporins and carbapenems.

■ Probenecid is sometimes used with beta-lactams to ↑ the concentration of the antibiotic; this will ↑ the risk of adverse reactions. This is occasionally done with penicillin when treating neurosyphilis or other penicillin-treated infections.

■ Probenecid decreases the efficacy of loop diuretics but increases the risk of loop diuretic toxicity.

■ Avoid use with pegloticase (↑ risk of anaphylaxis)

KEY COUNSELING POINTS

See the Drug Formulations and Patient Counseling chapter for counseling language/layman's terminology.

COLCHICINE

- At the first sign of an attack, take two tablets. Take one more tablet in one hour.
    - Do not use more than three tablets in an hour, and do not use more than four tablets in 24 hours.
    - Do not take the second dose if you have upset stomach, nausea or diarrhea.
- Can cause:
    - Nausea and diarrhea.
    - Muscle damage.

ALLOPURINOL

- Can cause:
    - Mild or severe rash.
    - Liver damage.
    - Nausea.
- Take after a meal to reduce stomach upset (higher doses can be divided). Drink plenty of fluids.

Select Guidelines/References

Fitzgerald JD, Dalbeth N, Mikuls T, et al. 2020 American College of Rheumatology Guideline for the Management of Gout. *Arthritis Care & Research*. 2020;0:1-17.

Richette P, Doherty M, Pascual E, et al. 2016 updated EULAR evidence-based recommendations for the management of gout. Ann Rheum Dis. 2017;76:29-42.

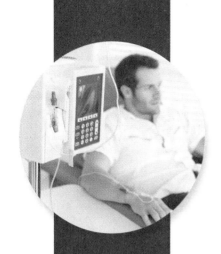
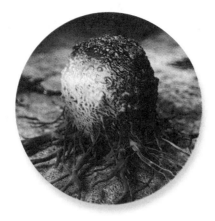
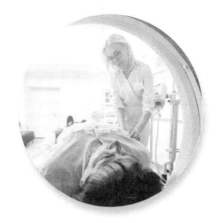

ONCOLOGY

CONTENTS

CONTENT LEGEND

 ☀ = Study Tip Gal   ⚙ = Required Formula

CHAPTER 61
ONCOLOGY

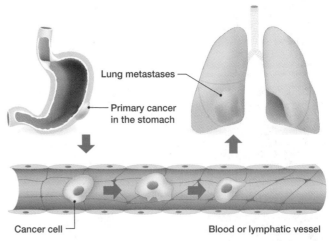

fotoyou/stock.adobe.com

BACKGROUND

Under normal conditions, human cells grow and divide to form new cells. Cancer is a group of diseases characterized by <u>abnormal cell proliferation</u>, whereby the process of cell division is disrupted and cells <u>divide uncontrollably</u>. Many cancers form a tumor (mass of cells), which can be <u>benign (non-cancerous)</u> or <u>malignant (cancerous)</u>.

■ Benign tumors are relatively harmless and stay in their primary location.

■ Malignant tumors can <u>travel</u> through the <u>lymphatic system</u> or <u>blood</u> to invade other tissues and form a <u>secondary tumor</u> with the <u>same cancerous cells</u> as the primary tumor.

■ The spread of cancer to a different part of the body is referred to as <u>metastasis</u>.

Lung metastases

Primary cancer in the stomach

Cancer cell

Blood or lymphatic vessel

Designua/Shutterstock.com

Cancer is caused by genetic mutations that are inherited, occur from errors during cell division, or result from DNA damage. The main types of genes involved in cancer include:

- Proto-oncogenes, which are involved in normal cell division. Mutated forms of proto-oncogenes, called oncogenes [e.g., human epidermal growth factor receptor 2 (HER2), epidermal growth factor receptor (EGFR)], promote cancer cell growth.

- DNA repair genes, which usually fix mistakes in DNA during replication. Mutations in these genes prevent cell repair, allowing more errors to accumulate within the cell.

- Tumor suppressor genes [e.g., breast cancer gene 1 (BRCA1), breast cancer gene 2 (BRCA2)], which normally regulate cell division; when these genes are inactivated by a mutation, cells can grow uncontrollably.

External factors, including lifestyle (e.g., tobacco use, excessive alcohol intake, poor diet, low physical activity) or environmental exposures (e.g., sunlight, chemicals, radiation, viruses), and internal factors (e.g., hormones, inherited genetic mutations, older age) can promote the development of cancer. However, in some cases, there is no identifiable cause.

CANCER PREVENTION

Certain cancers are more likely to occur following some type of exposure, such as lung cancer due to smoking or skin cancer caused by sun or ultraviolet (UV) light exposure.

General preventative measures that decrease external exposures or lower cancer risk by other means include:

- Avoiding tobacco (encourage enrollment in a tobacco cessation program if needed).

- Limiting alcohol intake.

- Maintaining a healthy lifestyle (e.g., achieving an ideal weight, exercising regularly, eating a balanced diet).

- Receiving certain vaccinations [e.g., human papillomavirus (HPV) vaccine].

- Low-dose aspirin (in select patients) to prevent colorectal cancer.

- Skin protection and screening for abnormal spots (see Skin Protection box and ABCDE image below).

- Regular check-ups to assess cancer risk, family history and individual history.

- Following cancer screening recommendations (see table on following page).

LOWERING SKIN CANCER RISK

Skin cancer is one of the most common cancers in the United States. Most skin cancers start in the epidermis or top layer of the skin, which contains squamous cells, basal cells and melanocytes. Basal cell carcinoma is the most common type, followed by squamous cell carcinoma. Melanoma is less prevalent but is often invasive and more likely to spread.

Risk factors for skin cancer include a history of UV light exposure (from sun or tanning beds), light skin that burns easily, light hair color, a skin cancer history and immunosuppressive drugs (e.g., post-transplant medications) or diseases (because the immune system can eliminate some early cancers, suppressing the immune system can increase skin cancer risk).

SKIN PROTECTION

- Seek shade, especially between 10 AM and 4 PM.

- Wear a shirt; tightly woven fabrics are best.

- Use a broad-spectrum sunscreen, at least SPF 30, and reapply every 2 hours.

- Wear a hat with at least a 2-3" brim.

- Wear sunglasses to protect the skin around the eyes.

ABCDE – Warning Signs of Melanoma

The "ABCDE" mnemonic below is used to educate patients about suspicious skin spots. A spot that is changing over time or looks different from other spots should be examined.

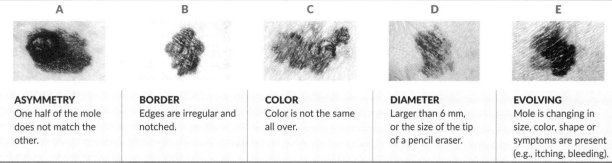

A	B	C	D	E
ASYMMETRY One half of the mole does not match the other.	**BORDER** Edges are irregular and notched.	**COLOR** Color is not the same all over.	**DIAMETER** Larger than 6 mm, or the size of the tip of a pencil eraser.	**EVOLVING** Mole is changing in size, color, shape or symptoms are present (e.g., itching, bleeding).

Skin Cancer Foundation, National Cancer Institute

CANCER SCREENING GUIDELINES FOR AVERAGE RISK PATIENTS

CANCER	SEX	AGE	SCREENING
Breast	F	40-44 years	Annual mammogram is optional
		45-54 years	Yearly mammogram
		≥ 55 years	Mammogram every 2 years or continue yearly
Cervical	F	25-65 years	Cervical cell analysis: ■ Pap smear every 3 years ■ HPV DNA test every 5 years ■ Pap smear + HPV DNA test every 5 years
Colorectal	M/F	≥ 45 years	Stool-based tests: ■ Highly sensitive fecal immunochemical test (FIT) yearly ■ Highly sensitive guaiac-based fecal occult blood test (gFOBT) yearly ■ Multi-targeted stool DNA test (MT-sDNA) every 3 years Visual exams of the colon and rectum: ■ Colonoscopy every 10 years (and as needed to confirm a positive result from any other test) ■ CT colonography (virtual colonoscopy) every 5 years ■ Flexible sigmoidoscopy (FSIG) every 5 years
Lung	M/F	≥ 50 years	Annual low-dose CT scan of chest if both of the following criteria are met: ■ Has at least a 20 pack-year smoking history ■ Still smoking or quit smoking within the past 15 years
Prostate	M	Individualized decision	If a patient chooses to be tested: ■ Prostate-specific antigen (PSA) blood test ■ +/– digital rectal exam (DRE)

CANCER EVALUATION

WARNING SIGNS OF CANCER

There are several signs and symptoms of cancer; most are nonspecific (e.g., unexplained weight loss), but referral to a physician is warranted if any of these CAUTION warning signs are present:

Change in bowel or bladder habits

A sore that does not heal

Unusual bleeding or discharge

Thickening or lump in the breast or elsewhere

Indigestion or difficulty swallowing

Obvious change in a wart or mole (see ABCDE warning signs on previous page)

Nagging cough or hoarseness

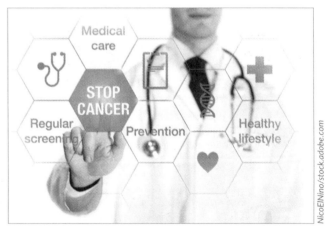

CANCER DIAGNOSIS

A cancer diagnosis requires a complete evaluation of the patient, including a thorough history and physical and various tests based on the type of cancer suspected. The assessment of cancer also includes staging to determine the extent of disease. Cancer stages can be indicated by numbers, where stage I is early-stage cancer and stage IV indicates advanced disease. The TNM staging system is also applicable to the majority of cancer types in which T describes the primary tumor size and location, N refers to lymph node involvement and M represents evidence of metastasis.

EVALUATION OF CANCER

History and physical

Complete blood count

Comprehensive metabolic panel

Biopsy: removal of a tissue sample to identify cancer cells

Imaging tests (e.g., X-ray, MRI, PET scan, CT scan): visualizes internal body structures

Biomarker (tumor marker) tests: detects genes, proteins or other substances released by cancer cells

Genetic tests: identifies specific cancer genes or mutations

SELECT CANCER TYPES

There are hundreds of cancer types. Cancers are classified by the organs or tissues where they originated or can be described by the type of cell that formed them (e.g., epithelial cell, squamous cell). The table below describes some of the more common cancer types.

NAME	CHARACTERISTICS
Carcinoma	Forms from epithelial cells that line internal and external surfaces of the body.
Leukemia	Originates in the bone marrow and usually affects leukocytes.
Lymphoma	Begins in the cells of the lymphatic system.
Multiple myeloma	Arises from plasma cells of the bone marrow.
Sarcoma	Develops in connective or supportive tissue (e.g., muscle, bone, cartilage).

TREATMENT OVERVIEW

Cancer treatment decisions are based on:

- Cancer type and characteristics (e.g., a breast tumor that is estrogen receptor-positive will receive different treatment than a breast tumor that is estrogen receptor-negative).

- Cancer stage (i.e., the size and how far it has metastasized, or spread).

- Patient characteristics, such as age, comorbidities, past treatments and physical functioning (i.e., performance status), which can be assessed with the Karnofsky or Eastern Cooperative Oncology Group (ECOG) rating scales.

- Risks and benefits of each treatment option (i.e., efficacy vs. tolerability of chemotherapy and/or surgery).

Each patient's treatment goals should be discussed with their healthcare team. Treatment options with curative intent are used to eradicate cancerous cells and prevent recurrence.

If cure is not possible, palliative treatment can help control symptoms and provide comfort. A patient's quality of life may lead the clinician and family to choose palliative measures over a more aggressive treatment plan that could have intolerable side effects.

TREATMENT TYPES

Cancer can be treated with surgery, radiation (high-energy X-rays to destroy cancer cells), chemotherapy, hormone therapy, targeted therapy and/or immunotherapy. Primary cancer treatment aims to completely remove or eliminate cancer cells; any treatment modality can be used, but surgery (to remove the bulk of the tumor) is a common primary treatment for resectable cancers.

Neoadjuvant therapy (e.g., radiation, chemotherapy) can be used before surgery to shrink the tumor and make complete resection more likely.

Adjuvant therapy is additional cancer treatment given after the primary treatment (i.e., surgery) to eradicate residual disease and decrease recurrence.

TREATMENT RESPONSE

- Complete response, or complete remission: the cancer responded to treatment and cannot be detected.

- Partial response, or partial remission: there is a substantial reduction in the cancer burden, but it is still present.

- Progressive disease: the cancer has grown or is worsening.

- Stable disease: the cancer is not improving or worsening.

CHEMOTHERAPY

Traditional chemotherapy drugs kill cancer cells (i.e., they are <u>cytotoxic</u>) by <u>interfering</u> with cell division and <u>DNA replication</u>. Cell cycle nonspecific agents kill cancer cells at all phases of the cell cycle, whereas cell cycle specific agents kill cancer cells during a specific phase of the cell cycle (see figure below).

Regardless of cell cycle specificity, traditional cytotoxic cancer drugs are <u>more effective</u> at <u>killing</u> actively dividing cells; therefore, cancers that are characterized by rapid cell growth are more susceptible to their cytotoxic effects.

Noncancerous cells in the body that are <u>rapidly dividing</u>, including cells in the <u>gastrointestinal tract, hair follicles</u> and <u>bone marrow</u>, are also susceptible to the damaging effects of cytotoxic drugs. This is why common chemotherapy side effects include <u>diarrhea, mucositis, nausea/vomiting, alopecia</u> and <u>myelosuppression</u>, and why supportive care measures (e.g., an antiemetic regimen) are used in conjunction with chemotherapy.

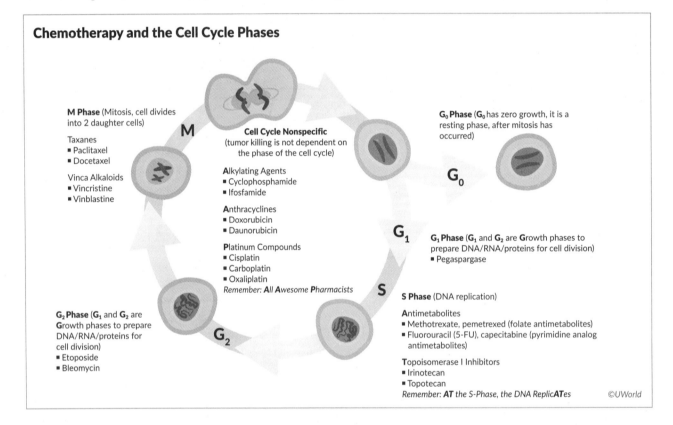

Chemotherapy and the Cell Cycle Phases

M Phase (Mitosis, cell divides into 2 daughter cells)

Taxanes
- Paclitaxel
- Docetaxel

Vinca Alkaloids
- Vincristine
- Vinblastine

Cell Cycle Nonspecific
(tumor killing is not dependent on the phase of the cell cycle)

Alkylating Agents
- Cyclophosphamide
- Ifosfamide

Anthracyclines
- Doxorubicin
- Daunorubicin

Platinum Compounds
- Cisplatin
- Carboplatin
- Oxaliplatin
*Remember: **A**ll **A**wesome **P**harmacists*

G_0 Phase (G_0 has zero growth, it is a resting phase, after mitosis has occurred)

G_1 Phase (G_1 and G_2 are **G**rowth phases to prepare DNA/RNA/proteins for cell division)
- Pegaspargase

S Phase (DNA replication)

Antimetabolites
- Methotrexate, pemetrexed (folate antimetabolites)
- Fluorouracil (5-FU), capecitabine (pyrimidine analog antimetabolites)

Topoisomerase I Inhibitors
- Irinotecan
- Topotecan
*Remember: **AT** the S-Phase, the DNA Replic**AT**es*

G_2 Phase (G_1 and G_2 are **G**rowth phases to prepare DNA/RNA/proteins for cell division)
- Etoposide
- Bleomycin

©UWorld

CHEMOTHERAPY REGIMENS

Chemotherapy regimens typically include a <u>combination</u> of drugs, which increases efficacy via <u>synergistic</u> effects (e.g., by targeting cells at <u>different stages of replication</u>). Regimens are usually administered in 2 – 6 week <u>cycles</u>, followed by days or weeks without treatment to allow for <u>recovery</u> from any <u>adverse effects</u> (e.g., myelosuppression, nausea/vomiting).

Example Breast Cancer Regimen

AC is a combination of two drugs given on day one of a 2- or 3-week treatment cycle and repeated for 4 cycles:

- Doxorubicin [**A**driamycin (a discontinued brand name)], an anthracycline.
- **C**yclophosphamide, an alkylating agent.

CHEMOTHERAPY CALCULATIONS

Most chemotherapy is dosed using body surface area (BSA), except carboplatin, which is dosed using the Calvert formula. The BSA formulas used most commonly are the Mosteller and Du Bois and Du Bois equations. Use the patient's actual body weight for dose calculations, unless instructed otherwise.

Mosteller Equation

$$BSA\ (m^2) = \sqrt{\frac{Ht\ (cm) \times Wt\ (kg)}{3{,}600}}$$

Example

A patient has a weight of 175 pounds and a height of 6' 1". Calculate the patient's BSA using the Mosteller equation. Round to the nearest hundredth.

Convert weight to kilograms: 175 lbs/2.2 = 79.5 kg
Convert height to centimeters: 73 inches x 2.54 = 185.4 cm

$$BSA\ (m^2) = \sqrt{\frac{185.4\ cm \times 79.5\ kg}{3{,}600}} = 2.02\ m^2$$

Calculate the dose of paclitaxel in milligrams for a patient with a BSA of 2.02 m² and a prescribed paclitaxel dose of 175 mg/m². Round to the nearest whole number.

$$175\ mg/m^2 \quad \times \quad 2.02\ m^2 \quad = \quad 354\ mg$$

Du Bois and Du Bois Equation

$$BSA\ (m^2) = 0.007184 \times [Ht\ (cm)]^{0.725} \times [Wt\ (kg)]^{0.425}$$

Example

A patient has a weight of 165 pounds and a height of 5' 6". Calculate the patient's BSA using the Du Bois and Du Bois equation. Round to the nearest hundredth.

Convert weight to kilograms: 165 lbs/2.2 = 75 kg
Convert height to centimeters: 66 inches x 2.54 = 167.6 cm

$$BSA\ (m^2) = 0.007184 \times (167.6\ cm)^{0.725} \times (75\ kg)^{0.425}$$

$$BSA\ (m^2) = 1.84\ m^2$$

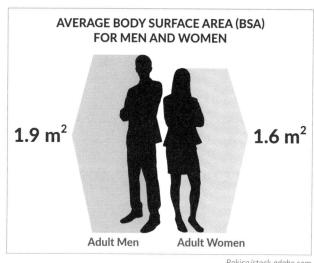

AVERAGE BODY SURFACE AREA (BSA) FOR MEN AND WOMEN

1.9 m²   1.6 m²

Adult Men   Adult Women

Bokica/stock.adobe.com

Calvert Formula

In the formula below (used for carboplatin dosing):

- AUC can range from 2 – 8 mg/mL x min
- GFR is commonly capped at 125 mL/min/1.73 m²
- Creatinine clearance may be used to estimate GFR (if GFR is not available)

$$Total\ carboplatin\ dose\ (mg) = (Target\ AUC) \times (GFR + 25)$$

Example

CA is a 55-year-old female with newly diagnosed ovarian cancer. She arrives at the clinic to start her first cycle of chemotherapy. Her laboratory values are within normal limits, and her GFR is 80 mL/min/1.73 m². Her regimen for day 1 of chemotherapy is:

Paclitaxel 175 mg/m² IV, followed by carboplatin (target AUC 5 mg/mL x min) IV

CA's carboplatin dose using the Calvert formula is:

$$(5\ mg/mL \times min) \times (80\ mL/min/1.73\ m^2 + 25) = 525\ mg$$

TRADITIONAL CYTOTOXIC CHEMOTHERAPY DRUGS

The following tables include commonly encountered "prototype drugs" from the major chemotherapy drug classes. The monitoring, prevention and/or treatment of their unique safety concerns are described, including the use of available chemoprotectants (i.e., medications that reduce toxicity without compromising the chemotherapeutic effect) when appropriate. Management of some safety concerns may also include the need to modify chemotherapy doses or stop/interrupt treatment.

Common chemotherapy-related adverse effects (e.g., myelosuppression, nausea/vomiting) and safety issues (e.g., extravasation) that require special management are discussed later in the chapter and are not included in the tables below.

CELL CYCLE NONSPECIFIC AGENTS

ALKYLATING AGENTS

Alkylating agents work by cross-linking DNA strands, which inhibits DNA and protein synthesis and results in cell death.

SELECT DRUGS*	SAFETY CONCERNS	MONITORING	MANAGEMENT
Cyclophosphamide **Ifosfamide** (Ifex)	Hemorrhagic cystitis, caused by the toxic metabolite acrolein, which concentrates in the bladder	Hematuria, urinalysis (for RBCs), lower urinary tract symptoms (e.g., urinary urgency, dysuria, incomplete bladder emptying)	**Prevention** ▪ Adequate hydration ▪ Mesna (a chemoprotectant) with all ifosfamide doses and high doses (e.g., > 1 gram/m^2) of cyclophosphamide **Treatment** ▪ Bladder irrigation with normal saline
	Ifosfamide: neurotoxicity, including encephalopathy and cerebellar dysfunction	S/sx of neurotoxicity (e.g., confusion, incoordination, imbalance)	**Prevention/Treatment** ▪ Methylene blue
Busulfan (Busulfex, Myleran)	Pulmonary toxicity (e.g., pulmonary fibrosis)	S/sx of pulmonary toxicity (e.g., dyspnea, cough), pulmonary function tests	**Treatment** ▪ Symptomatic care (e.g., oxygen)
	Seizures	S/sx of seizures (e.g., tonic-clonic movements, lack of awareness)	**Prevention/Treatment** ▪ Antiseizure medication (e.g., levetiracetam)
Carmustine (BiCNU, Gliadel Wafer)	Neurotoxicity (e.g., seizures, cerebral edema), particularly with the wafer implant	S/sx of seizures, headache	**Prevention/Treatment** ▪ Antiseizure medication
	Pulmonary toxicity (e.g., pulmonary fibrosis)	S/sx of pulmonary toxicity, pulmonary function tests	**Treatment** ▪ Symptomatic care (e.g., oxygen)

*Other drugs in class: bendamustine, dacarbazine, lomustine, mechlorethamine, melphalan, mitomycin, procarbazine, temozolomide.

PLATINUM-BASED COMPOUNDS

Platinum-based compounds are alkylating agents that cross-link DNA, interfering with DNA synthesis and cell replication, which results in cell death.

DRUGS	SAFETY CONCERNS	MONITORING	MANAGEMENT
Cisplatin* Carboplatin (Paraplatin) Oxaliplatin	Hypersensitivity reactions	S/sx of anaphylaxis (e.g., dyspnea, angioedema, urticaria), vital signs (e.g., BP, HR)	**Treatment** ■ Symptomatic care (e.g., oxygen, bronchodilators, systemic steroids)
	Nephrotoxicity	Renal function (e.g., BUN, SCr, intake/output), electrolytes (e.g., Mg, K, Na, Ca)	**Prevention** ■ Adequate hydration ■ Amifostine (Ethyol), a chemoprotectant that reduces cumulative renal toxicity with cisplatin ■ Limit cisplatin dose per cycle to ≤ 100 mg/m²
	Ototoxicity	S/sx of hearing loss or tinnitus, audiogram at baseline	**Prevention** ■ Avoid concomitant ototoxic medications (e.g., aminoglycosides)
	Peripheral neuropathy	S/sx of neuropathy (e.g., extremity numbness, paresthesia, pain)	**Treatment** ■ Symptomatic care (e.g., neuropathic pain medications)
	Oxaliplatin: acute sensory neuropathy exacerbated by cold	S/sx of acute sensory neuropathy [e.g., abnormal sensations (in hands, feet, perioral area, or throat), jaw spasm, chest pressure]	**Prevention** ■ Avoid cold exposure (e.g., cold temperatures, consumption of cold food/beverages)

*Greatest incidence of nephrotoxicity and ototoxicity.

ANTHRACYCLINES

Anthracyclines work by several mechanisms, including intercalation into DNA, inhibition of topoisomerase II and creation of oxygen-free radicals that damage cells.

SELECT DRUGS*	SAFETY CONCERNS	MONITORING	MANAGEMENT
Doxorubicin (Adriamycin**) **NAME TIP...** Generic name contains "-**rubi**-" (remember ruby red body fluids)	Cardiotoxicity (e.g., heart failure, cardiomyopathy)	Left ventricular ejection fraction (LVEF), s/sx of heart failure (e.g., edema, shortness of breath)	**Prevention** ■ Limit total lifetime cumulative dose to 450-550 mg/m² ■ Administer dexrazoxane (a chemoprotectant) in select patients ■ See Study Tip Gal below for further details
	Red discoloration of bodily fluids	S/sx (e.g., red urine)	**Prevention** ■ None
Mitoxantrone (an anthracenedione, related to the anthracyclines)	Blue discoloration of sclera and bodily fluids	S/sx (e.g., blue urine)	**Prevention** ■ None

*Other drugs in class: daunorubicin, epirubicin, idarubicin.
**Brand discontinued but name still used in practice.

REDUCE DOXORUBICIN CARDIOTOXICITY

1. Keep track of the lifetime cumulative doxorubicin dose for each patient

   (doxorubicin dose in mg/m²/cycle) x (total number of cycles received) = cumulative doxorubicin dose in mg/m²

   Example: (doxorubicin 50 mg/m²/cycle) x (6 cycles) = 300 mg/m²

2. When the doxorubicin cumulative dose is ≥ 300 mg/m² with planned continued treatment, consider dexrazoxane

3. When the doxorubicin cumulative dose reaches 450-550 mg/m², treatment must be stopped (the lower end of the dose range is used if CV risk or previous mediastinal radiation)

4. Monitor LVEF before and after treatment (using an echocardiogram or MUGA scan)

CELL CYCLE SPECIFIC AGENTS

TOPOISOMERASE I INHIBITORS

Topoisomerase I inhibitors block the coiling and uncoiling of the double-stranded DNA helix during the S phase of the cell cycle. This causes single and double-strand breaks in the DNA and prevents religation (sealing the DNA strands back together again) of single-strand breaks.

SELECT DRUG*	SAFETY CONCERNS	MONITORING	MANAGEMENT
Irinotecan (*Camptosar*) NAME TIP... "I run to the can"	Acute diarrhea, during or immediately after infusion, plus cholinergic symptoms (e.g., abdominal cramping, lacrimation, salivation) Delayed diarrhea (> 24 hours after infusion)	Frequency of bowel movements, electrolytes (e.g., K, Mg), dehydration (e.g., dizziness, decreased skin turgor)	**Prevention** ■ Acute diarrhea: atropine (an anticholinergic) **Treatment** ■ Acute diarrhea: atropine ■ Delayed diarrhea: antidiarrheal agent (e.g., loperamide) ■ Both: symptomatic care (e.g., hydration, electrolyte replacement)

Other drug in class: topotecan.

TOPOISOMERASE II INHIBITORS

Similar to topoisomerase I inhibitors, topoisomerase II inhibitors block the coiling and uncoiling of double-stranded DNA, but during the G2 phase of the cell cycle; this causes single and double-strand breaks in the DNA and prevents religation of single-strand breaks.

DRUG	SAFETY CONCERNS	MONITORING	MANAGEMENT
Etoposide	Infusion rate-related hypotension	Vital signs (e.g., BP)	**Prevention** ■ Infuse over at least 30-60 minutes **Treatment** ■ IV hydration, decrease infusion rate upon reinitiation

VINCA ALKALOIDS

Vinca alkaloids inhibit microtubule formation during the M phase of the cell cycle. Microtubules play a role in axonal transport, which is why neuropathies are a common side effect of these medications.

> **NAME TIP...**
> ■ Vin**C**ristine causes more **C**NS toxicity (neuropathy) than other vinca alkaloids
> ■ Vin**B**lastine and vinorel**B**ine cause more **B**one marrow suppression (myelosuppression) than vincristine

DRUGS	SAFETY CONCERNS	MONITORING	MANAGEMENT
Vincristine* Vinblastine Vinorelbine	Peripheral neuropathy	S/sx of neuropathy (e.g., extremity numbness, paresthesia, pain)	**Prevention** ■ Limit single vincristine doses to 2 mg (regardless of BSA-calculated dose) **Treatment** ■ Symptomatic care (e.g., neuropathic pain medications)
	Autonomic neuropathy (e.g., constipation)	S/sx of constipation (e.g., bowel movement frequency, hard stools)	**Prevention/Treatment** ■ Symptomatic care (e.g., diet modifications, laxatives)
	Paralysis and death if given intrathecally FOR INTRAVENOUS USE ONLY. FATAL IF GIVEN BY OTHER ROUTES.	Double check appropriate preparation of product	**Prevention** ■ Prepare in small IV bag (i.e., a piggyback) that cannot be used for intrathecal administration ■ Label products to prevent accidental intrathecal administration

Major CYP3A4 substrate; avoid interacting drugs (e.g., azole antifungals).

TAXANES

Taxanes <u>inhibit</u> the <u>depolymerization of tubulin</u> (which stabilizes microtubules) during the <u>M phase</u> of the cell cycle.

DRUGS	SAFETY CONCERNS	MONITORING	MANAGEMENT
Paclitaxel Cabazitaxel (Jevtana) Docetaxel Use <u>non-PVC</u> bag and tubing* Use <u>0.22 micron filter</u> (cabazitaxel and paclitaxel)	<u>Peripheral neuropathy</u>	S/sx of neuropathy (e.g., <u>extremity numbness, paresthesia, pain</u>)	**Treatment** ■ Symptomatic care (e.g., neuropathic pain medications)
	<u>Hypersensitivity reactions</u> (due to solvent systems)*	S/sx of <u>anaphylaxis</u> (e.g., dyspnea, angioedema, urticaria), vital signs (e.g., BP, HR)	**Prevention** ■ <u>Premedication</u> with a systemic steroid (e.g., dexamethasone), diphenhydramine and an H2RA (e.g., famotidine) **Treatment** ■ Stop/interrupt therapy; do not rechallenge if reaction is severe ■ Symptomatic care (e.g., oxygen, epinephrine)
	<u>Docetaxel: severe fluid retention</u>	S/sx of fluid retention (e.g. edema, dyspnea at rest, abdominal distension)	**Prevention** ■ Premedication with a systemic steroid (e.g., dexamethasone) **Treatment** ■ Symptomatic care (e.g., diuretics)

*Except albumin-bound paclitaxel (Abraxane).

CASE SCENARIO

LK is a 34-year-old male with testicular cancer, hypertension and chronic back pain. His current medications include hydrochlorothiazide 25 mg PO daily, naproxen 500 mg PO BID and hydrocodone/acetaminophen 5/325 mg PO Q4H PRN pain. He received his 3rd cycle of chemotherapy with:

> Paclitaxel 250 mg/m^2 IV on day 1
> Ifosfamide 1,500 mg/m^2 IV on days 2-5 (along with mesna)
> Cisplatin 25 mg/m^2 IV on days 2-5

He returns to the clinic to receive his 4th cycle of chemotherapy and complains of numbness and tingling pain in his fingertips. His laboratory values are within normal limits with the exception of: BUN = 22 mg/dL, SCr = 2.4 mg/dL. His vital signs are within normal limits and stable.

■ **How would you characterize the type of pain LK describes?** It is consistent with sensory peripheral neuropathy.

■ **What could be causing his new pain symptoms?** Paclitaxel and cisplatin are associated with sensory peripheral neuropathy.

■ **Dehydration is ruled out based on the BUN/SCr ratio and normal vital signs. What is the likely cause of LK's elevated SCr?**
Cisplatin-induced nephrotoxicity should be suspected. No further cisplatin should be given at this time. Naproxen and hydrochlorothiazide should be held, as NSAIDs can decrease renal blood flow and diuretics can cause dehydration and potentiate further kidney damage. An alternative medication can be chosen for BP control.

PYRIMIDINE ANALOG ANTIMETABOLITES

These agents inhibit pyrimidine DNA synthesis during the S phase of the cell cycle. Leucovorin or its L-isomer (levoleucovorin) is given with fluorouracil to ↑ efficacy.

SELECT DRUGS*	SAFETY CONCERNS	MONITORING	MANAGEMENT
Fluorouracil (also referred to as 5-FU) **Capecitabine** (Xeloda) Oral prodrug of fluorouracil	Hand-foot syndrome (palmar plantar erythrodysesthesia), caused by capillary drug leakage into the palms of the hands and soles of the feet	S/sx of hand-foot syndrome (e.g., painful erythema, skin peeling)	**Prevention/Treatment** ■ See Hand-Foot Syndrome Management box below
	Diarrhea	Frequency of bowel movements, electrolytes (e.g., K, Mg), dehydration (e.g., dizziness, decreased skin turgor)	**Treatment** ■ Antidiarrheal agents (e.g., loperamide) ■ Symptomatic care (e.g., hydration, electrolyte replacement)
	Mucositis	S/sx of mucositis (e.g., painful mouth ulcers, difficulty eating/drinking) S/sx of infection (e.g., thrush)	**Prevention/Treatment** ■ See Mucositis Management box on following page
	Dihydropyrimidine dehydrogenase (DPD) deficiency: ↑ risk of severe toxicity (e.g., myelosuppression, GI toxicity)	S/sx of toxicities	**Prevention** ■ Pharmacogenomic testing (not routine) **Treatment** ■ Antidote: use uridine triacetate (Vistogard) within 96 hours for overdose or early-onset toxicity ■ Symptomatic care (specific to the toxicity)
	Drug interaction with warfarin (can significantly ↑ INR)	INR, s/sx of bleeding	**Prevention** ■ Frequent INR monitoring
Cytarabine	Neurotoxicity (e.g., acute cerebellar toxicity with high doses)	S/sx of neurotoxicity (e.g., seizure, slurred speech, confusion, incoordination)	**Prevention** ■ Dose modifications for select patients (e.g., older age, pre-existing renal/hepatic dysfunction)
	Cytarabine syndrome occurring hours following administration	S/sx of cytarabine syndrome (e.g., fever, weakness, bone pain, chest pain)	**Prevention/Treatment** ■ Systemic steroids (e.g., dexamethasone)

Other drug in class: gemcitabine.

HAND-FOOT SYNDROME MANAGEMENT

■ Limit or modify daily activities to reduce friction and pressure to hands and feet (e.g., wear loose-fitting shoes, avoid tools that require squeezing hands).

■ Avoid heat exposure to hands and feet (e.g., take shorter showers in lukewarm water).

■ Cold compresses may provide temporary relief of pain and tenderness.

■ Use emollients (e.g., ammonium lactate, urea cream, Aquaphor) to retain moisture in the hands and feet.

■ Topical steroids (e.g., clobetasol) and pain medications can help lessen inflammation and pain.

■ Dose modifications or therapy interruptions may be required for severe cases.

FOLATE ANTIMETABOLITES

Folate antimetabolites interfere with the enzymes involved in the folic acid cycle, blocking purine and pyrimidine biosynthesis during the S phase of the cell cycle.

SELECT DRUG*	SAFETY CONCERNS	MONITORING	MANAGEMENT
Methotrexate**	Nephrotoxicity (with high doses ≥ 500 mg/m²)	Renal function (e.g., BUN, SCr, urine output), weight gain (edema), urine pH, methotrexate levels	**Prevention** ■ Leucovorin or levoleucovorin "rescue" (see Study Tip Gal below) ■ Hydration with IV sodium bicarbonate to alkalinize the urine (improves methotrexate solubility) ■ Avoid interacting medications (e.g., NSAIDs, salicylates, beta-lactams, proton pump inhibitors, sulfonamide antibiotics, probenecid) ■ Caution in patients with third spacing (e.g., ascites, pleural effusions), which delay drug clearance **Treatment** ■ Antidote: glucarpidase (Voraxaze) rapidly lowers methotrexate levels in patients with methotrexate-induced acute kidney injury and delayed methotrexate clearance
	Gastrointestinal toxicity (e.g., diarrhea, mucositis)	Same as pyrimidine analog antimetabolites (see diarrhea and mucositis sections in table on prior page)	**Prevention/Treatment** ■ Same as pyrimidine analog antimetabolites (see table on prior page and Mucositis Management box below) PLUS ■ Leucovorin or levoleucovorin "rescue" for high-dose methotrexate (see Study Tip Gal below)

*Other drugs in class: pemetrexed, pralatrexate.
**Can also cause hepatotoxicity and photosensitivity, especially with prolonged use for chronic conditions (e.g., rheumatoid arthritis, psoriasis).

MUCOSITIS MANAGEMENT

PREVENTION
■ Good oral hygiene (e.g., brushing with a soft toothbrush)

■ Hold ice chips in the mouth (can cause local vasoconstriction, leading to decreased delivery of mucotoxic agents)

■ Frequent rinsing with bland rinses (e.g., sodium bicarbonate or sodium chloride solutions)

TREATMENT
■ Continue good oral hygiene and frequent rinsing

■ Symptomatic care (e.g., viscous lidocaine 2%, magic mouthwash, systemic analgesics for pain)

■ Parenteral nutrition or IV hydration may be needed in some cases

■ Thrush treatment (e.g., nystatin oral suspension, clotrimazole troches) if indicated

---

WHICH FOLATE PRODUCT TO USE WITH METHOTREXATE

IN AUTOIMMUNE DISEASES
■ The dose of methotrexate is much lower (5-25 mg WEEKLY)

■ Folic acid (folate) 1-5 mg daily is recommended prophylactically to reduce methotrexate side effects (GI, hematologic, hepatic)

■ Leucovorin is NOT used unless unresponsive to folic acid

IN ONCOLOGIC DISEASES
■ Methotrexate doses are much higher (e.g., ≥ 40 mg/m² per dose)

■ Leucovorin or levoleucovorin "rescue" is required for doses ≥ 500 mg/m² to reduce toxicities (e.g., mucositis, diarrhea, nephrotoxicity, myelosuppression)

  ❑ Allows DNA synthesis to begin again by competing with methotrexate for transport into tissues and replenishing the supply of folate metabolites displaced by methotrexate

■ Folic acid is NOT effective for high-dose methotrexate rescue

MISCELLANEOUS CHEMOTHERAPY AGENTS

DRUGS	SAFETY CONCERNS	MONITORING	MANAGEMENT
Retinoic Acid Derivative: ↓ proliferation and ↑ differentiation of acute promyelocytic leukemia (APL) cells.			
Tretinoin (also referred to as all-*trans* retinoic acid, or ATRA)	Differentiation syndrome, previously known as retinoic acid-acute promyelocytic leukemia (RA-APL) syndrome	S/sx of differentiation syndrome (e.g., fever, dyspnea, weight gain, edema, pulmonary infiltrates, pericardial or pleural effusions)	**Prevention/Treatment** ■ Systemic steroids (e.g., dexamethasone) ■ Interrupt therapy for severe cases
Arsenic Trioxide: ↑ apoptosis of APL cells and damages the fusion protein promyelocytic leukemia-retinoic acid receptor alpha (PML-RARA).			
Arsenic trioxide (*Trisenox*)	QT prolongation	Electrocardiogram to assess QTc interval, electrolytes (e.g., K, Mg)	**Prevention** ■ Maintain K > 4 mEq/L and Mg > 1.8 mEq/L ■ Avoid concurrent QT-prolonging drugs
	Differentiation syndrome	S/sx of differentiation syndrome	**Prevention/Treatment** ■ Same as for tretinoin (see above)
Antitumor Antibiotic: inhibits DNA synthesis via DNA strand breaks.			
Bleomycin	Pulmonary toxicity (e.g., pulmonary fibrosis)	S/sx of pulmonary toxicity (e.g., dyspnea, cough), pulmonary function tests	**Prevention** ■ Limit lifetime cumulative dose to 400 units
	Hypersensitivity reactions	S/sx of anaphylaxis (e.g., dyspnea, angioedema, urticaria), vital signs (e.g., BP, HR)	**Prevention** ■ Can consider a test dose for the first 2 doses and/or premedication (e.g., acetaminophen, diphenhydramine)
Proteasome Inhibitors: inhibit proteasomes, which help regulate intracellular protein homeostasis by inhibiting cell cycle progression and inducing apoptosis.			
Bortezomib (*Velcade*) Carfilzomib (*Kyprolis*)	Herpes reactivation (zoster and simplex)	S/sx of herpes infection (e.g., rash)	**Prevention/Treatment** ■ Antiviral agents (e.g., acyclovir, valacyclovir)
	Peripheral neuropathy	S/sx of neuropathy (e.g., extremity numbness, paresthesia, pain)	**Prevention** ■ Administer bortezomib SC (less neuropathy than IV administration) **Treatment** ■ Symptomatic care (e.g., neuropathic pain medications)
Immunomodulators: block angiogenesis (i.e., the formation of new blood cells) and kill abnormal cells in the bone marrow while stimulating the bone marrow to produce normal healthy cells.			
Lenalidomide (*Revlimid*) Pomalidomide (*Pomalyst*) Thalidomide (*Thalomid*)	Severe birth defects	Pregnancy test (2 negative test results required before treatment initiation)	**Prevention** ■ Only available under a restricted distribution program: patient, prescriber and pharmacist must be registered with the REMS program ■ Two forms of contraception or abstain from sex
	Thrombosis (DVT/PE)	S/sx of thromboembolism (e.g., shortness of breath, chest pain, leg swelling)	**Prevention** ■ Prophylactic anticoagulation (choice based on patient's underlying risk factors)
Asparaginase Product: inhibits protein synthesis by depleting asparagine in leukemic cells.			
Pegaspargase (*Oncaspar*) Modified form of L-asparaginase (derived from *E. coli*) conjugated with polyethylene glycol	Hypersensitivity reactions (pegylated form allows for less frequent dosing and less allergic reactions)	S/sx of anaphylaxis (e.g., dyspnea, angioedema, urticaria), vital signs (e.g., BP, HR)	**Prevention** ■ Premedication with acetaminophen, an antihistamine (e.g., diphenhydramine) and an H2RA (e.g., famotidine) **Treatment** ■ Symptomatic care (e.g., oxygen, epinephrine)

SUMMARY OF CHEMOTHERAPY TOXICITIES

CHEMOMAN AND MAJOR TOXICITIES OF COMMON CHEMOTHERAPY DRUGS

Chemoman helps with learning the major toxicities of some of the common chemotherapy drugs. Use the blank version below to practice by filling in the body parts with the drugs, associated toxicities and prevention measures.

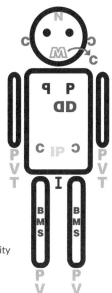

N   **Neurotoxicity:** carmustine

C   **Cisplatin:** ototoxicity, high emetogenicity, nephrotoxicity
- Prevention (nephrotoxicity):
  - Amifostine
  - Limit dose per cycle to ≤ 100 mg/m²

M   **Mucositis:** methotrexate, fluorouracil, capecitabine
- Prevention (high-dose methotrexate): leucovorin

P   **Pulmonary toxicity** (e.g., pulmonary fibrosis): bleomycin, busulfan, carmustine
- Prevention (bleomycin): limit lifetime cumulative dose to 400 units

D   **Doxorubicin & other anthracyclines:** cardiotoxicity (e.g., cardiomyopathy)
- Prevention (doxorubicin):
  - Dexrazoxane
  - Limit lifetime cumulative dose to 450-550 mg/m²

IP   **Ifosfamide & cyclophosphamide:** hemorrhagic cystitis
- Prevention (all doses of ifosfamide & high doses of cyclophosphamide): mesna

I   **Irinotecan:** diarrhea
- Prevention: atropine

PVT   **Platinum-based compounds** (e.g., oxaliplatin), **vinca alkaloids** (e.g., vincristine) & **taxanes** (e.g., paclitaxel): peripheral neuropathy
- Prevention (oxaliplatin): avoid cold exposure
- Prevention (vincristine): limit single doses to 2 mg

BMS   **Bone marrow suppression:** most chemotherapy EXCEPT bleomycin, pegaspargase & vincristine

©UWorld

CHEMOMAN AND MAJOR TOXICITIES OF COMMON CHEMOTHERAPY DRUGS

TEST YOURSELF!

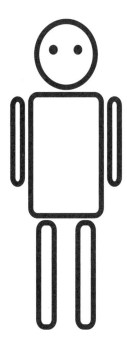

LABEL (on Chemoman)	DRUGS/TOXICITY	PREVENTION
N		
C		
M		
P		
D		
IP		
I		
PVT		
BMS		

©UWorld

CHEMOTHERAPY-RELATED ISSUES AND SUPPORTIVE CARE

MYELOSUPPRESSION OVERVIEW

Within the bone marrow, the process of hematopoiesis generates blood cells of all lineages. The main blood cells (see the Blood Cell Lines section in the Lab Values & Drug Monitoring chapter) produced in the myeloid lineage include:

- White blood cells (WBCs) (or granulocytes)
- Platelets (or thrombocytes)
- Red blood cells (RBCs) (or erythrocytes)

Myelosuppression (i.e., bone marrow suppression) is a common complication of many chemotherapy regimens; it is characterized by a decrease in blood cell production, resulting in fewer WBCs (neutropenia), platelets (thrombocytopenia) and RBCs (anemia). Almost all chemotherapy drugs can cause myelosuppression, except bleomycin, pegaspargase and vincristine. Most monoclonal antibodies (mAbs) also do not cause myelosuppression.

Myelosuppression Recovery

The lowest point that WBCs and platelets reach is called the nadir, which typically occurs about 7 – 14 days after chemotherapy. The RBC nadir occurs much later, generally after several months of treatment, due to the long life span (~120 days) of RBCs.

Patients are at the greatest risk of complications during the nadir period, after which, blood cell counts will start to recover. WBCs and platelets generally recover 3 – 4 weeks after treatment. However, in instances of prolonged myelosuppression, the next cycle of chemotherapy may need to be delayed, to allow more time for recovery, or doses may need to be reduced. The next cycle of chemotherapy is started after the WBCs and platelets have returned to a safe level. The image below summarizes the nadir and recovery of WBCs.

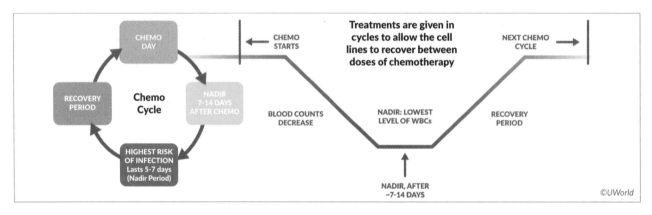

NEUTROPENIA

The major function of white blood cells, including neutrophils, is to prevent infection. Neutropenia (a type of leukopenia) is a low neutrophil count; it is assessed by calculating an absolute neutrophil count (ANC), the formula for which can be found in the Calculations IV chapter. The more significant the neutropenia (i.e., the lower the ANC), the higher the risk of infection.

Neutropenia Definitions (American Society of Clinical Oncology)

CATEGORY	ABSOLUTE NEUTROPHIL COUNT (ANC)
Neutropenia	< 1,000 cells/mm³
Severe neutropenia	< 500 cells/mm³
Profound neutropenia	< 100 cells/mm³

Granulocyte Colony-Stimulating Factors

Granulocyte colony-stimulating factors (G-CSFs, or simply CSFs) stimulate WBC production in the bone marrow. They are given prophylactically after chemotherapy to reduce the duration and severity of neutropenia (and therefore the risk of infection) and to enable delivery of more intensive chemotherapy when indicated.

Patients with a high risk of developing febrile neutropenia (e.g., based on their chemotherapy regimen or comorbidities) should receive G-CSF prior to their first cycle of chemotherapy and should have their risk re-evaluated with each subsequent cycle.

DRUGS*	DOSING	SAFETY/SIDE EFFECTS/MONITORING
Filgrastim (Neupogen) Biosimilars: *Nivestym, Releuko, Zarxio* tbo-filgrastim *(Granix)*	5 mcg/kg IV/SC daily until post-nadir recovery (round to the nearest 300 mcg or 480 mcg vial size)	**SIDE EFFECTS** Bone pain, rash, hypersensitivity/allergic reaction (including anaphylaxis), glomerulonephritis, splenic rupture, respiratory distress syndrome **MONITORING** CBC with differential, vital signs, upper abdominal pain
Pegfilgrastim (Neulasta, Neulasta Onpro) Pegylated form of filgrastim (extended half-life) Biosimilars: *Fulphila, Fylnetra, Nyvepria, Stimufend, Udenyca, Ziextenzo*	6 mg SC once per chemotherapy cycle	**NOTES** Store in refrigerator; protect vials and syringes from light Administer first dose no sooner than 24 hours after chemotherapy (can be up to 96 hours after) *Neulasta Onpro:* on-body injector applied to abdomen or back of arm after chemotherapy (delivers dose of pegfilgrastim ~27 hours after application)
Eflapegrastim-xnst *(Rolvedon)*	13.2 mg SC once per chemotherapy cycle	Pegfilgrastim/eflapegrastim-xnst: do not administer within 14 days before the next chemotherapy cycle

Sargramostim (Leukine) is a granulocyte macrophage colony-stimulating factor primarily used following bone marrow transplantation.

Febrile Neutropenia

If neutropenia occurs, the ability to fight infections is limited, and the risk of death from sepsis increases. Infection can be difficult to diagnose; fever may be the only sign of infection in a neutropenic patient (i.e., the usual increase in WBC count will not be present).

Febrile Neutropenia Diagnostic Criteria

FEVER	NEUTROPENIA
Oral temperature ≥ 38.3°C (101°F) x 1 reading, or	ANC < 500 cells/mm³, or
Oral temperature ≥ 38.0°C (100.4°F) sustained for > 1 hour	ANC < 1,000 cells/mm³ and expected to ↓ to < 500 cells/mm³ over the next 48 hours

Empiric antibiotics should be started immediately if a fever occurs in a neutropenic patient. Patients receiving cytotoxic chemotherapy have an increased risk for hospital-acquired infections (e.g., pneumonia) and bacteremia, from translocation of enteric bacteria into the bloodstream or use of a central venous access device (i.e., central line). Although gram-positive and gram-negative bacteria can both cause infection in patients with febrile neutropenia, gram-negative bacteria have the highest risk of causing sepsis and death.

The initial empiric antibiotic regimen must provide adequate activity against gram-negative bacteria, including *Pseudomonas aeruginosa*. Treatment modifications can be considered based on culture results or if the clinical situation does not improve (e.g., persistent fever). Antibiotics should be continued until the WBC count has recovered or for an appropriate treatment course if a source of infection is identified.

PATIENT RISK	RISK DEFINITION	INITIAL EMPIRIC ANTIBIOTICS
Low risk	Expected ANC ≤ 100 cells/mm³ for < 7 days No comorbidities	**Oral anti-pseudomonal antibiotics** Ciprofloxacin or levofloxacin, PLUS Amoxicillin/clavulanate (for adequate gram-positive coverage) or clindamycin (if allergic to penicillin)
High risk	Expected ANC ≤ 100 cells/mm³ for ≥ 7 days Presence of comorbidities Evidence of renal or hepatic impairment (CrCl < 30 mL/min or LFTs > 5x ULN)	**Intravenous anti-pseudomonal beta-lactams** Cefepime or Ceftazidime or Imipenem/cilastatin or Meropenem or Piperacillin/tazobactam

THROMBOCYTOPENIA

Low platelets can result in spontaneous, uncontrolled bleeding. The normal platelet range is 150,000 – 450,000 cells/mm³. The risk for spontaneous bleeding is increased when the platelet count is < 10,000 cells/mm³, which is the threshold at which a platelet transfusion (the primary thrombocytopenia treatment) is indicated. In addition to chemotherapy dose reduction or delaying therapy until platelets recover, management of chemotherapy-induced thrombocytopenia includes avoiding intramuscular injections and medications that affect platelet functioning (e.g., NSAIDs).

ANEMIA

Anemia is a decrease in RBCs and hemoglobin (Hgb), the oxygen-carrying component of RBCs. Normal Hgb levels are 12 – 16 g/dL for females and 13.5 – 18 g/dL for males. Patients with anemia should have levels of folate, vitamin B12 and iron evaluated to assess for other possible causes of anemia.

Anemia can resolve without treatment or, in patients with symptoms (e.g., fatigue, weakness), it can be treated with an RBC transfusion. An erythropoiesis-stimulating agent (ESA), including epoetin alfa (*Epogen, Procrit*) or the longer-acting darbepoetin alfa (*Aranesp*), can be considered in select patients. ESAs can shorten survival and ↑ tumor progression (i.e., they can contribute to cancer growth). Therefore, they are for palliation only and are not recommended in patients receiving chemotherapy with curative intent.

To minimize the risks of ESAs, the following requirements must be met:

- Patient has a non-myeloid malignancy (e.g., carcinoma, sarcoma) and anemia is due to the effect of myelosuppressive chemotherapy.
- Hgb is < 10 g/dL and there is a minimum of two additional months of planned chemotherapy.
- The lowest dose needed to maintain a Hgb level sufficient to avoid RBC transfusions is used.
- The ESA is discontinued following completion of chemotherapy.

Serum ferritin, transferrin saturation (TSAT) and total iron-binding capacity (TIBC) must be assessed (and iron replacement therapy provided, if needed) since ESAs will not correct the anemia if iron levels are inadequate. For further information regarding ESAs, see the Anemia chapter.

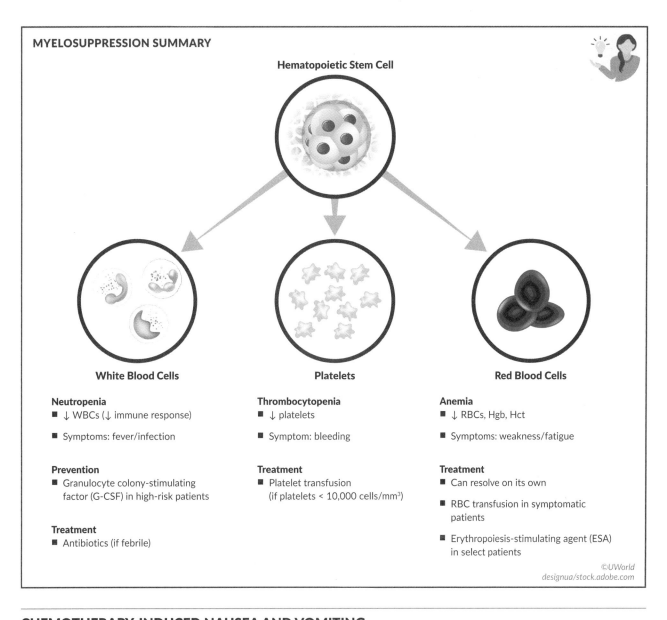

MYELOSUPPRESSION SUMMARY

Hematopoietic Stem Cell

White Blood Cells

Platelets

Red Blood Cells

Neutropenia
- ↓ WBCs (↓ immune response)
- Symptoms: fever/infection

Prevention
- Granulocyte colony-stimulating factor (G-CSF) in high-risk patients

Treatment
- Antibiotics (if febrile)

Thrombocytopenia
- ↓ platelets
- Symptom: bleeding

Treatment
- Platelet transfusion (if platelets < 10,000 cells/mm³)

Anemia
- ↓ RBCs, Hgb, Hct
- Symptoms: weakness/fatigue

Treatment
- Can resolve on its own
- RBC transfusion in symptomatic patients
- Erythropoiesis-stimulating agent (ESA) in select patients

©UWorld
designua/stock.adobe.com

CHEMOTHERAPY-INDUCED NAUSEA AND VOMITING

Chemotherapy-induced nausea and vomiting (CINV) is one of the most common adverse effects associated with cancer treatment. If poorly managed, it can lead to patient discomfort, reduced quality of life, medical complications (e.g., esophageal tears, dehydration) and potential treatment nonadherence.

CINV occurs most commonly with cisplatin, carboplatin, cyclophosphamide and anthracyclines. Patient factors that increase the risk of CINV include female sex, younger age, pretreatment anxiety, a history of motion sickness or morning sickness during pregnancy, and a history of nausea and vomiting with previous chemotherapy cycles.

CINV can be classified as:

- Acute: occurs within 24 hours after chemotherapy and peaks around 5 – 6 hours.
- Delayed: occurs > 24 hours after chemotherapy.
- Anticipatory: occurs before treatment and develops as a conditioned response from a previous negative experience.
- Breakthrough: occurs at any time after chemotherapy, despite the use of prophylaxis, and requires rescue antiemetics.
- Refractory: occurs when prophylaxis and/or rescue treatment is not effective.

Types of Antiemetics for CINV

The major neurotransmitters responsible for CINV include serotonin, substance P, neurokinin, dopamine and gamma-aminobutyric acid (GABA). The table below represents the most common drug classes used for CINV.

NEUROKININ-1 RECEPTOR ANTAGONISTS (NK1 RAs)	SEROTONIN RECEPTOR ANTAGONISTS (5-HT3 RAs)	DOPAMINE RECEPTOR ANTAGONISTS	OTHER
Aprepitant	Dolasetron	Olanzapine	Dexamethasone
Fosaprepitant	Granisetron	Haloperidol	Dronabinol
Rolapitant	Ondansetron	Metoclopramide	Lorazepam
	Palonosetron*	Prochlorperazine	
		Promethazine	

Combination products available: netupitant/palonosetron, fosnetupitant/palonosetron.

Antiemetic Regimens for Acute/Delayed Nausea & Vomiting

The primary goal of antiemetic therapy is to prevent nausea and vomiting (emesis). Therefore, antiemetic regimens (i.e, one dose of each drug in the regimen) are given at least 30 minutes before chemotherapy; if the patient is receiving a multi-day chemotherapy regimen, antiemetics are continued for the full period of emetic risk (i.e., select drugs are repeated each day chemotherapy is administered).

Chemotherapy regimens are divided into risk groups based on emetogenic potential, and the antiemetic regimen recommended is based on this risk (see table below). Lorazepam can be added to the antiemetic regimen if needed for anticipatory nausea and/or vomiting; it is started the night before treatment and repeated the day of treatment.

INTRAVENOUS CHEMOTHERAPY RISK	ANTIEMETIC REGIMEN (DAY 1)*
High emetic risk: 90% frequency of acute emesis (e.g., cisplatin, any regimen containing both an anthracycline and cyclophosphamide)	**3 or 4 drugs** ■ Preferred: NK1 RA + 5-HT3 RA + olanzapine + dexamethasone ■ NK1 RA + 5-HT3 RA + dexamethasone ■ Palonosetron + olanzapine + dexamethasone
Moderate emetic risk: 30-90% frequency of acute emesis	**2 or 3 drugs** ■ NK1 RA + 5-HT3 RA + dexamethasone ■ 5-HT3 RA + dexamethasone ■ Palonosetron + olanzapine + dexamethasone
Low emetic risk: 10-30% frequency of acute emesis	**1 drug** ■ 5-HT3 RA (dolasetron, granisetron or ondansetron) ■ Dexamethasone ■ Metoclopramide ■ Prochlorperazine
Minimal emetic risk: < 10% frequency of acute emesis (the majority of mAbs)	**No routine prophylaxis**

Can add H2RA or PPI for reflux symptoms.

Breakthrough CINV

Despite receiving antiemetic prophylaxis for acute and/or delayed CINV, some patients may experience breakthrough nausea and vomiting. The drug of choice for breakthrough CINV is based on an assessment of the current prophylaxis regimen and typically involves adding one or more drugs (often every 4 – 6 hours PRN) with a different mechanism of action.

Patient-specific factors also need to be considered, such as the preferred route of administration (e.g., ability to tolerate PO, active vomiting) and individual risk factors (e.g., age). Various medications may be beneficial, including 5-HT3 RAs (except palonosetron), dopamine receptor antagonists (e.g., prochlorperazine, promethazine, metoclopramide, haloperidol, olanzapine), cannabinoids, dexamethasone, lorazepam and scopolamine.

Antiemetics Used for CINV

DRUG	DOSING	SAFETY/SIDE EFFECTS/MONITORING
Substance P/Neurokinin-1 Receptor Antagonists (NK1 RAs): inhibit the substance P/neurokinin-1 receptor, thereby augmenting the antiemetic activity of 5-HT3 receptor antagonists and corticosteroids.		
Aprepitant (Emend, Emend Tri-Pack, Cinvanti)	PO: 80-125 mg IV (Cinvanti): 130 mg	**CONTRAINDICATIONS** Rolapitant: do not use with thioridazine or pimozide (CYP2D6 substrates)
Fosaprepitant (Emend)	<u>IV</u>: 150 mg	**SIDE EFFECTS** Abdominal pain, dizziness, dyspepsia, fatigue, hiccups, infusion-site reactions
Netupitant/Palonosetron (Akynzeo)	PO: 300/0.5 mg	**NOTES** Aprepitant, fosaprepitant, netupitant: inhibit the metabolism of dexamethasone (↑ dexamethasone levels)
Fosnetupitant/Palonosetron (Akynzeo)	IV: 235/0.25 mg	Fosaprepitant IV: converted to aprepitant within 30 minutes after the end of the infusion
Rolapitant (Varubi)	PO: 180 mg	Rolapitant: do not administer at less than 2-week intervals
<u>5-HT3 Receptor Antagonists</u>: block serotonin, both peripherally on vagal nerve terminals and centrally in the chemoreceptor trigger zone.		
Ondansetron (Zofran)	PO: 8-24 mg IV: 8-16 mg	**CONTRAINDICATIONS** <u>Do not use</u> with <u>apomorphine</u> (Apokyn) due to severe hypotension
Granisetron (Sancuso, Sustol)	PO: 2 mg IV: 10 mcg/kg (max dose 1 mg) SC (Sustol): 10 mg Patch (Sancuso): 3.1 mg/24 hour, apply 24-48 hours before chemotherapy; may leave in place up to 7 days	**WARNINGS** Dose-dependent <u>QT prolongation</u> (Torsades de Pointes) – more common with IV administration; <u>limit IV dose</u> of <u>ondansetron</u> to <u>16 mg</u>; the lowest risk is with palonosetron <u>Serotonin syndrome</u> when used in combination <u>with other serotonergic agents</u> (see Drug Interactions chapter) Hypersensitivity reactions
Palonosetron (Aloxi*)	IV: 0.25 mg	**SIDE EFFECTS**
+ netupitant (Akynzeo)	PO: 0.5/300 mg	<u>Headache, constipation</u>, fatigue, dizziness, injection site reactions
+ fosnetupitant (Akynzeo)	IV: 0.25/235 mg	
Dolasetron (Anzemet)	PO: 100 mg	**NOTES** Sustol: extended-release SC formulation; do not administer more than once every 7 days
Corticosteroid: mechanism of action as an antiemetic unknown.		
Dexamethasone (Decadron*)	PO/IV: 8-12 mg	**CONTRAINDICATIONS** Systemic fungal infections **SIDE EFFECTS** Short-term side effects include ↑ <u>appetite</u>/weight gain, <u>fluid retention</u>, emotional instability (euphoria, mood swings, irritability, acute psychosis), <u>insomnia</u>, GI upset/dyspepsia Higher doses ↑ <u>BP and blood glucose</u> (especially in patients with diabetes)
Benzodiazepine: <u>enhances GABA</u> (an inhibitory neurotransmitter), which decreases neuronal excitability and results in the alleviation of anxiety and suppression of <u>anticipatory nausea and vomiting</u>.		
Lorazepam (Ativan) C-IV	PO/SL/IV: 0.5-1 mg Start the <u>evening prior</u> to chemotherapy if used for anticipatory N/V	See the Anxiety Disorders chapter for details

DRUG	DOSING	SAFETY/SIDE EFFECTS/MONITORING
Dopamine Receptor Antagonists: <u>block dopamine receptors</u> in the CNS, including in the <u>chemoreceptor trigger zone</u>.		
Olanzapine (Zyprexa, *Zyprexa Zydis)*	PO: 5-10 mg	**BOXED WARNINGS** Olanzapine, prochlorperazine, haloperidol: ↑ mortality in elderly patients with dementia-related psychosis Promethazine: <u>do not use in children < 2 years</u> of age (risk of respiratory depression); can cause <u>serious tissue injury</u> due to <u>extravasation if administered intra-arterially, SC or IV</u> Metoclopramide: <u>tardive dyskinesia (TD) that can be irreversible</u>; discontinue if signs or symptoms of TD occur; risk ↑ with renal impairment, longer duration of treatment and total cumulative dose (avoid treatment > 12 weeks) **WARNINGS** Avoid use in patients with <u>Parkinson disease</u> (can <u>exacerbate</u> symptoms) **SIDE EFFECTS** <u>Sedation, lethargy, acute EPS</u> (antidote is diphenhydramine or benztropine), ↓ seizure threshold, hypotension, neuroleptic malignant syndrome (NMS), <u>QT prolongation</u> Strong anticholinergic side effects (e.g., constipation) except with metoclopramide (prokinetic effect causes diarrhea) **NOTES** Haloperidol/olanzapine: see the Schizophrenia chapter for details
Prochlorperazine *(Compro)*	PO/IV: 10 mg PR: 25 mg	
Promethazine *(Phenergan*, Promethegan)*	PO: 12.5-25 mg PR: 25 mg May cause severe tissue injury if administered parenterally	
Metoclopramide (Reglan)	PO/IV: 10-20 mg <u>CrCl < 60 mL/min: decrease dose 50%</u> (to avoid side effects)	
Haloperidol *(Haldol*, Haldol Decanoate)*	PO/IV: 0.5-2 mg	
Cannabinoid: activates cannabinoid receptors within the CNS and/or inhibits the vomiting control mechanism in the medulla oblongata.		
Dronabinol *Marinol* capsules: C-III *Syndros* solution: C-II <u>Refrigerate</u>	Capsules: 5-10 mg Solution: 2.1-4.2 mg/m²	**WARNINGS** Use caution in patients with a history of substance use disorder or psychiatric conditions **SIDE EFFECTS** <u>Somnolence, euphoria, ↑ appetite</u>, seizure **NOTES** Dronabinol oral solution contains 50% alcohol
Anticholinergic Agent: inhibits the actions of acetylcholine at central and peripheral muscarinic receptors.		
Scopolamine (Transderm Scop)	Transdermal patch: 1.5 mg/72 hours	See the Motion Sickness chapter for details

Brand discontinued but name still used in practice.

PREGNANCY AND BREASTFEEDING

Most chemotherapy is highly teratogenic. All patients must avoid conceiving during treatment. Contraception should include barrier methods to prevent a partner from having contact with body fluids. Pregnant females should not handle chemotherapy drugs. All patients should be informed when a medication can cause long-term sterility.

CHEMOTHERAPY HANDLING

All chemotherapy drugs are hazardous, which means they are carcinogenic, genotoxic or teratogenic. Because chemotherapy can cause harm to those exposed to the drug, healthcare staff (e.g., pharmacists, technicians, nurses) must use protective measures to limit exposure. The Compounding with Hazardous Drugs chapter provides detailed information on USP 800 requirements for handling hazardous drugs, the compounding environment and necessary equipment.

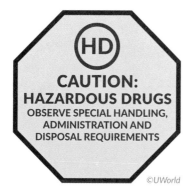

CHEMOTHERAPY ADMINISTRATION AND EXTRAVASATION

Many intravenous chemotherapy agents are vesicants that can cause tissue necrosis if the drug accidentally leaks from the vein into the surrounding tissue (also called extravasation).

Vesicants can be further categorized according to their potential for causing damage. DNA-binding vesicants (e.g., anthracyclines, mitomycin) can cause more tissue injury than non-DNA binding vesicants (e.g., vinca alkaloids), which are more easily metabolized.

Care should be taken to avoid extravasation by administering these drugs through central venous catheters or freshly started peripheral IV lines with confirmed patency. The infusion site and symptoms (e.g., redness, burning) should be monitored closely. Extravasation should be treated as follows:

- Anthracyclines: apply cold compresses and administer dexrazoxane or topical dimethyl sulfoxide (DMSO)

- Vinca alkaloids: apply warm compresses and administer hyaluronidase

Although most chemotherapy is administered intravenously, a limited number of agents can be given intrathecally (i.e., administered into the cerebrospinal fluid); these products must be preservative-free. Accidental intrathecal administration of vinca alkaloids, including vincristine, is fatal (see Vinca Alkaloids section earlier in the chapter).

TIMING OF VACCINATIONS

All vaccinations (both inactivated and live-attenuated products) should be avoided during chemotherapy because the antibody response is suboptimal. When chemotherapy is planned, vaccination should precede chemotherapy by ≥ 2 weeks. Patients receiving chemotherapy may receive the inactivated seasonal influenza vaccine between chemotherapy cycles. Live vaccines should not be administered to immunocompromised patients; they can be administered ≥ 4 weeks prior or at least three months after discontinuation of chemotherapy.

TARGETED THERAPIES

Targeted therapies recognize specific biomarkers or molecular targets (e.g., gene mutations) present on cancer cells that are involved in tumor growth and progression. They work in a variety of ways, including:

- Helping the immune system destroy cancer cells (e.g., immunotherapy).
- Interrupting signals that cause cancer cells to grow.
- Inhibiting angiogenesis (i.e., blood supply to the tumor).
- Inducing apoptosis.
- Starving cancer cells of hormones needed to grow (e.g., hormone or endocrine therapy).

Most targeted therapies are monoclonal antibodies or small molecule drugs (e.g., tyrosine kinase inhibitors). Pharmacogenomic testing must be performed to identify patients likely to respond to these targeted therapies, except with vascular endothelial growth factor (VEGF) inhibitors.

MONOCLONAL ANTIBODIES

Monoclonal antibodies (mAbs) are used for cancer treatment and many other conditions. They are large proteins that bind to specific antigens or receptors on the cell surface and cause cell death. Some mAbs are conjugated to cytotoxic drugs or radioactive compounds, which helps enable the delivery and release of these compounds directly into the cancer cell while reducing damage to normal cells. Other mAbs (i.e., immunotherapy) help activate the immune system so that it recognizes and destroys tumor cells.

Because they are biologic products that can be recognized by the immune system as a foreign substance, mAbs are associated with infusion-related reactions, which typically occur within the first few hours of administration and are characterized by fever, flushing, dyspnea, rash and sometimes anaphylaxis. Most mAbs require the following premedications:

- Acetaminophen (usually 650 mg PO).
- Diphenhydramine (IV or PO) or another antihistamine.

Additional medications that may be needed based on the severity of the reaction include H2RAs, steroids and/or meperidine (for rigors).

Representative monoclonal antibody targets and associated drugs are included in the following table (not a complete list).

NAME TIP...

- "tu" = tumors (e.g., rituximab, cetuximab)
- "ci" = circulatory system (e.g., bevacizumab)
- "li" = immune system (e.g., ipilimumab, pembrolizumab)

DRUGS	KEY SAFETY CONCERNS
Anti-Cluster of Differentiation (CD) Agents: bind to specific antigens expressed on the cell surface, causing cell death.	
Rituximab (Rituxan) Target: CD20 Biosimilars: *Riabni, Ruxience, Truxima* Others: Blinatumomab (*Blincyto*): targets CD19 Brentuximab vedotin (*Adcetris*): targets CD30 Daratumumab (*Darzalex*): targets CD38	■ Rituximab: hepatitis B reactivation ❑ Check hepatitis B panel (e.g., hepatitis B surface antigen, hepatitis B core antibody) prior to treatment initiation ❑ Consider antiviral (e.g., entecavir) prophylaxis in select patients
Epidermal Growth Factor Receptor (EGFR) Inhibitors: inhibit pathways involved in cellular proliferation, differentiation and survival.	
Cetuximab (Erbitux) Target: EGFR gene expression Other pharmacogenetic considerations: KRAS mutation: predicts lack of response to anti-EGFR drugs (can use if KRAS wild type) BRAF V600E mutation: must use only in combination with BRAF inhibitor	■ Dermatologic toxicity (e.g., acneiform rash) occurs within the 1st two weeks of treatment and correlates with response to therapy (i.e., rash indicates the drug is working) ❑ Advise patients to adopt general skin care measures (e.g., avoid sunlight, use sunscreen, apply moisturizers) ❑ Consider prophylactic measures to reduce the risk of skin damage (e.g., topical steroids, antibiotics)

DRUGS	KEY SAFETY CONCERNS
Human Epidermal Growth Factor Receptor 2 (HER2) Inhibitors: bind to extracellular ligand domain of HER2 protein to stop signaling pathways and cell proliferation.	
Trastuzumab (Herceptin) Target: HER2 overexpression (see Breast Cancer section) Biosimilars: Kanjinti, Herzuma, Ogivri, Ontruzant, Trazimera Others: Ado-trastuzumab emtansine (Kadcyla) Fam-trastuzumab deruxtecan (Enhertu) Pertuzumab (Perjeta)	■ Cardiotoxicity (e.g., cardiomyopathy) ❑ Monitor LVEF (using echocardiogram or MUGA scan) at baseline and during treatment and s/sx of heart failure (e.g., edema, shortness of breath) ■ Conventional trastuzumab, ado-trastuzumab emtansine and fam-trastuzumab deruxtecan are not interchangeable
Vascular Endothelial Growth Factor (VEGF) Inhibitors: inhibit growth of blood vessels needed for tumor proliferation.	
Bevacizumab (Avastin) Target: none Biosimilars: Alymsys, Mvasi, Vegzelma, Zirabev	■ Impaired wound healing (due to decreased blood flow) ❑ Do not administer for 28 days before or after surgery ■ Thromboembolic events (e.g., venous thromboembolism) ■ Hemorrhage/fatal bleeding ■ GI perforation
Programmed Death Receptor-1 (PD-1) Inhibitors: bind to the PD-1 receptor on T-cells to block PD-1 ligands from binding, thereby increasing T-cell activation and antitumor response; a type of immunotherapy.	
Pembrolizumab (Keytruda) Nivolumab (Opdivo)	■ Immune-mediated toxicities (e.g., endocrinopathies, colitis, hepatotoxicity, pneumonitis, thyroid disorders) ❑ Treatment typically requires administration of a systemic steroid and/or management of the specific toxicity
Cytotoxic T-Lymphocyte Antigen-4 (CTLA-4) Inhibitor: binds to CTLA-4 receptor, which removes the "brake" from T-cell activation, increasing T-cell responsiveness and antitumor response; a type of immunotherapy.	
Ipilimumab (Yervoy)	■ Immune-mediated toxicities (see above)

TYROSINE KINASE INHIBITORS

A large number of tyrosine kinase proteins play a role in the intracellular signaling pathways that control the growth and differentiation of cells. Tyrosine kinase inhibitors (TKIs) are orally administered small molecules that alter signal transduction and cell growth.

The table below is not all-inclusive, but contains representative TKIs, the genetic target/mutation that the patient should test positive for in order to use the TKI, and their key safety concerns.

DRUGS	KEY SAFETY CONCERNS
BCR-ABL Inhibitors: block tyrosine kinase signaling protein produced by the BCR-ABL fusion gene (Philadelphia chromosome) that causes uncontrolled cell division.	
Imatinib (Gleevec) Dasatinib (Sprycel) Nilotinib (Tasigna) Target: BCR-ABL fusion gene	■ Fluid retention (e.g., edema, pleural effusion, ascites) ■ QT prolongation (greatest risk with nilotinib) ❑ Assess QT interval with an electrocardiogram prior to treatment initiation ❑ Correct preexisting electrolyte abnormalities ❑ Avoid concurrent QT-prolonging drugs and strong CYP3A4 inhibitors ■ GI upset (e.g., abdominal pain) ❑ Imatinib: must be taken with food or within 1 hr after a meal
BRAF Inhibitors: inhibit certain mutated forms of protein kinase BRAF, blocking tumor cell growth.	
Dabrafenib (Tafinlar) Vemurafenib (Zelboraf) Target: BRAF V600E or V600K mutation	■ New malignancies (e.g., basal cell carcinoma) ■ QT prolongation ■ Febrile reactions, hyperglycemia, skin rash

DRUGS	KEY SAFETY CONCERNS
Mitogen-Activated Extracellular Kinase (MEK) 1 and 2 Inhibitors: inhibit MEK, a cell signaling protein downstream from RAF.	
Cobimetinib (*Cotellic*) Trametinib (*Mekinist*) Target: BRAF V600E or V600K mutation (when used in combination with a BRAF inhibitor, which is typical)	▪ Retinopathy ▪ Rhabdomyolysis
Epidermal Growth Factor Receptor (EGFR) Inhibitors: inhibit pathways involved in cellular proliferation, differentiation and survival.	

Afatinib (*Gilotrif*)
 	
 Erlotinib (*Tarceva*)
 	
 Target: EGFR gene mutation (exon 19 deletion or exon 21 substitution)
	▪ Dermatologic toxicity (e.g., acneiform rash) occurs within 1st two weeks of treatment and correlates with response to therapy (i.e., rash indicates the drug is working)
	   ❑ Advise patients to adopt general skin care measures (e.g., avoid sunlight, use sunscreen, apply moisturizers)
	   ❑ Consider prophylactic measures to reduce the risk of skin damage (e.g., topical steroids, antibiotics)

TREATMENT OF SELECT CANCERS

Although cancer is still a leading cause of death in the U.S., mortality rates have declined due to improved screening, early detection of disease and improved treatments. This section of the chapter discusses the risk factors, prevention and treatment of breast and prostate cancer, both of which have treatment modalities (e.g., hormone therapies) that are administered orally and commonly encountered in the community pharmacy setting.

BREAST CANCER

After skin cancer, breast cancer is the most common cancer in women, accounting for ~30% of all new female cancers annually.

BREAST CANCER RISK

The biggest risk factor for developing breast cancer is female sex. Females produce more estrogen and progesterone than males, which enables certain breast cells to grow. Female breast cells are also more likely to mutate because they are more active than male breast cells (which are largely inactive). Increasing age, a family history of breast cancer and genetics (e.g., BRCA gene mutation) are other nonmodifiable risk factors for developing breast cancer.

Less than 1% of breast cancer occurs in males. The risk increases in men with a BRCA gene mutation and the presence of any condition that increases estrogen production, such as Klinefelter syndrome. Klinefelter syndrome is a congenital condition in which males have one Y chromosome and two or more X chromosomes (instead of one X and one Y chromosome), resulting in more estrogen production than is typical and lower levels of androgens (i.e., male sex hormones).

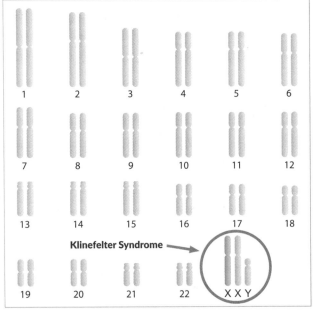

Klinefelter Syndrome

Ali/stock.adobe.com

BRCA1 and BRCA2 Gene Mutations

The BRCA1 and BRCA2 genes contain instructions for the production of proteins that repair damaged DNA. They normally suppress tumor growth; however, inherited mutations in either gene prevent cell repair and cause a dramatic increase in breast cancer incidence. BRCA mutations are also associated with an increased risk for ovarian and prostate cancer.

In a female without either mutation, the lifetime risk of developing breast cancer is ~12%; with either BRCA mutation, the risk can increase up to ~70%.

BREAST CANCER PREVENTION

Patients with an elevated risk of breast cancer may be candidates for prophylactic surgery (e.g., mastectomy) or a risk-reducing medication [e.g., selective estrogen receptor modulator (SERM), aromatase inhibitor (AI)]. Tamoxifen is a SERM that can be used in pre- or postmenopausal females. Raloxifene (another SERM) and the AIs, exemestane and anastrozole, are indicated for risk reduction in postmenopausal females only.

While tamoxifen and the AIs can be used for breast cancer prevention and treatment, raloxifene is for prevention only; raloxifene can be used for dual purposes since it increases bone density and is also indicated for the prevention and treatment of osteoporosis (which has a higher incidence post-menopause). Raloxifene is discussed further in the Osteoporosis, Menopause & Testosterone Use chapter.

IDENTIFYING BREAST CANCER

Breast Self-Exams
Breast self-exams are not used for screening, but can help identify a change in the look or feel of the breast or nipple, or nipple discharge, which would warrant follow-up screening.

Breast Imaging Studies
A mammogram uses low-dose X-rays to identify abnormal breast tissue. A few images are taken in a screening mammogram, and if they look suspicious, a diagnostic mammogram is performed. An ultrasound is useful to differentiate between a benign fluid-filled cyst and a solid mass that can be a cancerous tumor; it can also be used to guide a needle during a biopsy. A screening breast MRI in addition to an annual mammogram is recommended in high-risk females.

Following an abnormal imaging test (e.g., mammogram, MRI), a biopsy is performed to identify if cancer cells are present.

BREAST CANCER TREATMENT

Breast cancer treatment includes some combination of local (e.g., surgery, radiation) and/or systemic treatments (e.g., chemotherapy, hormone therapy) depending on the breast cancer type and stage. If the cancer expresses certain markers (e.g., HER2), the patient can benefit from targeted therapy.

Hormone Receptor-Positive Treatment (Endocrine Therapy)
About 75% of breast cancers have cells with receptors that attach estrogen and/or progesterone, which stimulate cell growth. Tumors that express either receptor type are referred to as hormone-sensitive or hormone receptor-positive (HR+). This is further classified as estrogen receptor-positive (ER+), progesterone receptor-positive (PR+) or both (ER+/PR+).

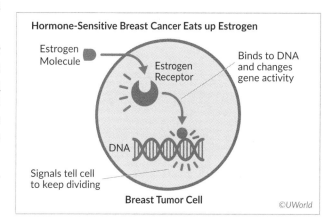

Patients with hormone-sensitive cancers are often prescribed adjuvant hormone (endocrine) therapy at diagnosis (to lower estrogen levels or stop estrogen from acting on breast cancer cells) and are treated for 5 – 10 years (to suppress cancer recurrence). The choice of treatment depends on the menopausal status of the patient.

- Premenopausal females produce estradiol (the most potent estrogen) in the ovaries. The first-line adjuvant treatment is tamoxifen, which prevents estrogen from binding to receptors.

  □ Aromatase inhibitors (AIs) block aromatase, an enzyme that catalyzes the peripheral conversion of androgens to estrogen. Because they do not block ovarian estrogen production, they are not useful as monotherapy in premenopausal females unless menopause is induced (i.e., ovarian suppression or ablation). This can be accomplished via surgery, radiation or a gonadotropin-releasing hormone (GnRH) agonist (goserelin or leuprolide), which decreases ovarian estradiol production via suppression of follicle stimulating hormone (FSH) and luteinizing hormone (LH).

- Postmenopausal females produce very little estradiol in the ovaries and instead obtain most of their estrogen from the peripheral conversion of androgens to estrogen. Postmenopausal females can be treated with tamoxifen or an AI.

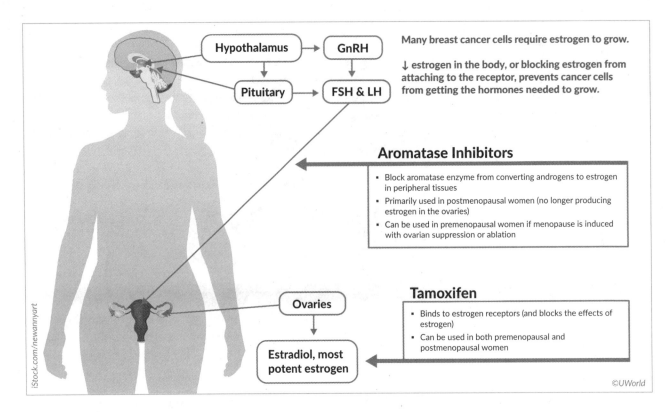

Many breast cancer cells require estrogen to grow.

↓ estrogen in the body, or blocking estrogen from attaching to the receptor, prevents cancer cells from getting the hormones needed to grow.

Aromatase Inhibitors

- Block aromatase enzyme from converting androgens to estrogen in peripheral tissues
- Primarily used in postmenopausal women (no longer producing estrogen in the ovaries)
- Can be used in premenopausal women if menopause is induced with ovarian suppression or ablation

Tamoxifen

- Binds to estrogen receptors (and blocks the effects of estrogen)
- Can be used in both premenopausal and postmenopausal women

iStock.com/newannyart

©UWorld

Hormone Receptor-Positive Treatment for Breast Cancer (Endocrine Therapy)

DRUGS	UNIQUE CONCERNS	SAFETY/SIDE EFFECTS/MONITORING
Selective Estrogen Receptor Modulators (SERMs): compete with estrogen at receptor binding sites in breast and other tissue.		
Tamoxifen (*Soltamox*) Toremifene (*Fareston*) Oral	Tamoxifen: a prodrug converted via CYP2D6 to the potent metabolite endoxifen Tamoxifen efficacy is decreased in slow CYP2D6 metabolizers or those taking CYP2D6 inhibitors Estrogen, and fluoxetine or paroxetine (CYP2D6 inhibitors), should not be used to treat hot flashes caused by tamoxifen; venlafaxine is preferred	**BOXED WARNINGS** Tamoxifen: ↑ risk of uterine or endometrial cancer and thromboembolic events Toremifene: QT prolongation **CONTRAINDICATIONS** Tamoxifen: do not use with warfarin or a history of DVT/PE Toremifene: QT prolongation, uncorrected hypokalemia/hypomagnesemia **SIDE EFFECTS** Hot flashes/night sweats, vaginal bleeding/discharge, arthralgia/myalgia, edema, hypertension Tamoxifen: ↓ bone density in premenopausal females (supplement with calcium/vitamin D), cataracts **NOTES** Tamoxifen is teratogenic; contraception should be used in premenopausal females
Selective Estrogen Receptor Degrader (SERD): estrogen receptor antagonist that causes receptor downregulation.		
Fulvestrant (*Faslodex*) IM injection		**SIDE EFFECTS** ↑ LFTs, injection site pain, hot flashes, arthralgia/myalgia, nausea, headache, cough, dyspnea
Aromatase Inhibitors: block peripheral conversion of androgens to estrogen.		
Anastrozole (*Arimidex*) Letrozole (*Femara*) Exemestane (*Aromasin*) Oral	Higher risk of osteoporosis due to ↓ bone mineral density (consider Ca and vitamin D supplementation, weight-bearing exercise, DEXA screening) Higher risk of CVD compared to SERMs	**SIDE EFFECTS** Hot flashes/night sweats, arthralgia/myalgia, lethargy/fatigue, N/V, rash, hepatotoxicity, hypertension, dyslipidemia

HER2-Positive Breast Cancer Treatment

Approximately 20% of breast tumors overexpress HER2/neu (an oncogene typically referred to as HER2) on the cell surface, which promotes rapid breast tumor growth. Although these tumors are aggressive malignancies, they respond well to drugs that target the HER2 protein. The HER2 proteins must be coupled (dimerized) to send signals that accelerate cell division and tumor growth. Trastuzumab (*Herceptin*), and other monoclonal antibodies (e.g., pertuzumab) in the same class, bind to the HER2 receptor, preventing dimerization (see Monoclonal Antibodies section earlier in the chapter).

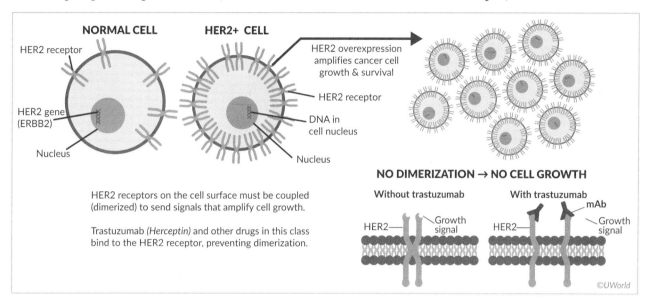

Triple-Negative Breast Cancer

Triple-negative breast cancers (i.e., ER-, PR- and HER2-negative) replicate and spread faster than most other types of breast cancer. Hormone therapy and HER2-directed therapy are not beneficial and outcomes (e.g., survival rates) are generally worse. Taxane or anthracycline-based chemotherapy regimens are preferred

Metastatic Breast Cancer

Breast cancer metastases are often located in the bone, lungs, liver and brain. In many patients, cure is unlikely and the goal of therapy is palliation (e.g., pain relief), prolongation of survival and maximizing quality of life. Chemotherapy (to shrink the tumor) and/or local palliation modalities (e.g., radiation, surgery) are common treatment options. Additional therapies include endocrine therapy (e.g., toremifene, fulvestrant) for HR+ cancers, and/or HER2-directed therapy for cancers with HER2 overexpression. Biomarker testing (e.g., PIK3CA, PD-L1) is recommended to identify patients eligible for targeted therapy.

PROSTATE CANCER

Prostate cancer is one of the most common cancers in males, affecting about 1 in 8 men. Fortunately, most prostate cancers are identified before the cancer has metastasized.

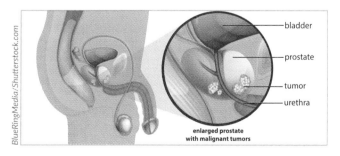

IDENTIFYING PROSTATE CANCER

Digital Rectal Exam

Most prostate cancers develop near the side of the prostate and can be felt with a digital rectal exam (DRE), where a healthcare provider inserts a gloved, lubricated finger into the rectum to palpate the prostate. If abnormal lumps or masses are felt, tissue from the prostate will be excised and sent to pathology to assess if cancerous cells are present.

Prostate-Specific Antigen

Prostate-specific antigen (PSA), produced in the prostate gland by normal and cancerous cells, increases with most prostate cancers. PSA is measured with a blood test (though screening is controversial, and false positives are common). Normal levels range from 0 – 4 ng/mL. A level above 4 ng/mL may indicate prostate cancer and requires further evaluation (i.e., with a biopsy); a PSA > 10 ng/mL likely indicates prostate cancer. Several factors can impact PSA levels, including benign prostatic hyperplasia (BPH), which increases PSA levels, and 5 alpha-reductase inhibitors (e.g., finasteride, dutasteride), which decrease PSA levels.

PROSTATE CANCER TREATMENT

For patients with localized disease and a low recurrence risk, observation or active surveillance is preferred; surgery, radiation or hormone therapy can be considered in those with intermediate or high recurrence risk.

Hormone Therapy (Androgen Deprivation Therapy)

Hormone therapy for prostate cancer blocks androgens (testosterone and the active metabolite dihydrotestosterone) and is referred to as androgen deprivation therapy (ADT), or sometimes chemical castration. The goal of ADT is to induce castrate levels of testosterone, which can be achieved with a GnRH antagonist (alone) or a GnRH agonist (initially taken with an antiandrogen).

Normally, the hypothalamus releases luteinizing hormone-releasing hormone (LHRH), which stimulates the GnRH receptor in the pituitary to release FSH and LH. FSH and LH stimulate testosterone production in the testes. Testosterone levels are controlled via feedback inhibition, whereby FSH and LH output are suppressed and testosterone production subsequently decreases. GnRH agonists initially cause the pituitary to release FSH and LH, increasing testosterone and causing a tumor flare. Because of this, GnRH agonists must be given with an antiandrogen to block the effects of the initial testosterone surge on the cancer cells. GnRH antagonists can be given alone (without an antiandrogen) because they decrease testosterone right away and do not cause a tumor flare.

Metastatic Prostate Cancer

Metastatic prostate cancer that has failed to respond to ADT is called "castration-resistant" and may be treated with a second-generation antiandrogen or chemotherapy.

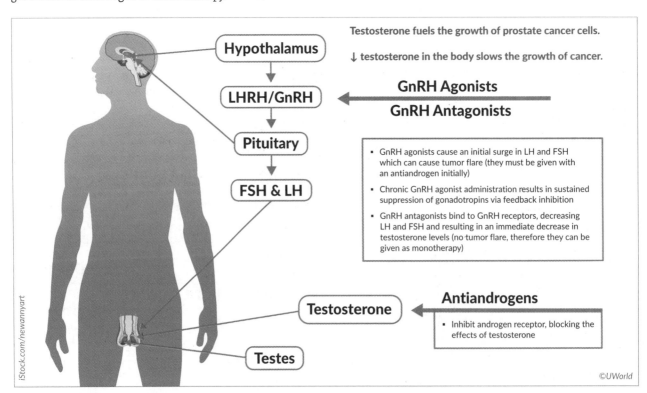

Hormone Therapies for Prostate Cancer (Androgen Deprivation Therapy)

DRUG	UNIQUE CONCERNS	SAFETY/SIDE EFFECTS/MONITORING
Gonadotropin-Releasing Hormone (GnRH) Agonists: also referred to as luteinizing hormone-releasing hormone (LHRH) agonists; cause an initial surge in testosterone, followed by a gradual reduction through a negative feedback mechanism.		
Leuprolide (Lupron Depot, *Eligard, Camcevi*) IM injection, SC injection **Goserelin (Zoladex)** SC injection Histrelin *(Supprelin LA)* SC injection Triptorelin *(Trelstar)* IM injection	Risk of osteoporosis due to ↓ bone mineral density (consider Ca and vitamin D supplementation, weight-bearing exercise, DEXA screening) Tumor flare: prevent with concurrent use of an antiandrogen (e.g., bicalutamide)	**CONTRAINDICATIONS** Pregnancy, breastfeeding **SIDE EFFECTS** Hot flashes, impotence, gynecomastia, bone pain, QT prolongation, injection site pain, dyslipidemia, hyperglycemia
Gonadotropin-Releasing Hormone (GnRH) Antagonists: block GnRH receptors directly causing a rapid decrease in testosterone production.		
Degarelix *(Firmagon)* SC injection Relugolix *(Orgovyx)* Oral	No tumor flare; antiandrogen not needed	**SIDE EFFECTS** Hot flashes, hypersensitivity reactions, QT prolongation, hyperglycemia
Antiandrogens, First-Generation: competitively inhibit testosterone from binding to prostate cancer cells.		
Bicalutamide *(Casodex)* Flutamide *(Eulexin)* Nilutamide *(Nilandron)* Oral		**CONTRAINDICATIONS** Bicalutamide: do not use in females Flutamide, nilutamide: severe hepatic impairment **SIDE EFFECTS** Hot flashes, gynecomastia, hepatotoxicity, ↑ risk of CVD Nilutamide: night blindness and disulfiram reactions (avoid alcohol)
Antiandrogen, Second-Generation		
Apalutamide *(Erleada)* Darolutamide *(Nubeqa)* Enzalutamide *(Xtandi)* Oral		**WARNINGS** Seizures, myocardial ischemia **SIDE EFFECTS** Hypertension, fatigue, ↑ LFTs, skin rash
Androgen Biosynthesis Inhibitor: interferes with CYP17 enzyme involved in the synthesis of steroid hormones in the testes and adrenal glands to decrease testosterone production.		
Abiraterone *(Zytiga, Yonsa)* Oral	Major CYP3A4 substrate; avoid concurrent use with strong CYP3A4 inducers or inhibitors	**WARNINGS** Hepatotoxicity Mineralocorticoid excess: fluid retention, ↑ BP, hypokalemia (reduce excess with concurrent prednisone) **SIDE EFFECTS** Edema, hypertension, hot flashes, hyperglycemia, ↑ TGs, hypophosphatemia

OTHER CANCER-RELATED ISSUES

TUMOR LYSIS SYNDROME

Tumor lysis syndrome (TLS) is an <u>oncologic emergency</u> that is most often caused by chemotherapy initiation; it can also occur spontaneously in patients with a high tumor burden or tumors with a high proliferative rate (e.g., leukemia, non-Hodgkin lymphoma). TLS results from the <u>rapid breakdown</u> (lysis) of <u>tumor cells</u> and the <u>release of intracellular components</u> into the bloodstream, including potassium, phosphate, purines and pyrimidines (the base pairs that compose DNA). This leads to:

- <u>Hyperkalemia</u>, which can cause <u>arrhythmias</u>.

- Hyperphosphatemia; phosphate can bind to calcium and precipitate in soft tissues.

- <u>Hypocalcemia</u>, which can cause anorexia, nausea and seizures.

- <u>Hyperuricemia</u>, which can <u>damage the kidneys</u> (see image).

- <u>Acute renal failure</u> (from uric acid crystallization or phosphate accumulation in the renal tubules).

Patients with, or at risk of developing, TLS should receive aggressive <u>IV hydration with normal saline</u> (to increase urine output and accelerate the excretion of excess intracellular components) and <u>urate lowering therapies</u>. If TLS occurs, additional management includes electrolyte correction (depending on the abnormality).

The xanthine oxidase enzyme is present in the blood and can readily convert large amounts of purines into uric acid. <u>Allopurinol</u> is a <u>xanthine oxidase inhibitor</u> that blocks this conversion. The usual initial dose of allopurinol for gout is ~100 mg daily, whereas higher doses (~400 – 800 mg/day) are indicated for TLS prevention and treatment. Allopurinol should be continued until TLS and any metabolic abnormalities have resolved. If allopurinol is not a reasonable option (e.g., risk of allopurinol-induced <u>rash/severe skin reactions</u>), febuxostat is an alternative agent. Allopurinol and febuxostat are reviewed in detail in the Gout chapter.

<u>Rasburicase</u> is used for the initial management of TLS in high-risk patients (e.g., WBCs > 100,000 cells/mm³, Burkitt lymphoma). It converts uric acid to a more water-soluble metabolite (allantoin), which is easily excreted. Rasburicase is <u>contraindicated in G6PD deficiency</u> and should be discontinued immediately and permanently in any patient who develops <u>hemolysis</u>.

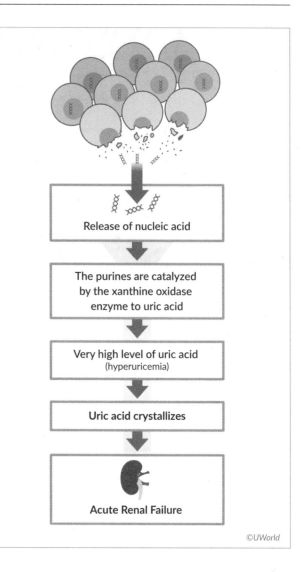

Release of nucleic acid

The purines are catalyzed by the xanthine oxidase enzyme to uric acid

Very high level of uric acid (hyperuricemia)

Uric acid crystallizes

Acute Renal Failure

©UWorld

HYPERCALCEMIA OF MALIGNANCY

Certain cancers cause calcium to leach from bone into the blood, which over time can lead to weak bones prone to fracture. It also leads to hypercalcemia which can range from mild to severe in presentation. Patients with mild hypercalcemia (corrected calcium 10.6 – < 12 mg/dL) do not require immediate treatment (though hydration can be considered).

Moderate (corrected calcium 12 – 13.9 mg/dL) or severe (corrected calcium > 14 mg/dL) hypercalcemia can be symptomatic, with nausea, vomiting, fatigue, dehydration and confusion. Treatment includes IV hydration with normal saline and medication to lower calcium levels. An IV bisphosphonate (e.g., pamidronate, zoledronic acid) is considered first line for moderate – severe hypercalcemia. In severe cases, calcitonin may be added (for up to 48 hours) to IV bisphosphonate therapy; the calcitonin treatment duration is short because tachyphylaxis (tolerance) develops quickly. Denosumab (a monoclonal antibody RANKL inhibitor) may be used for hypercalcemia refractory to IV bisphosphonates.

IV bisphosphonates and denosumab are common treatment options for osteoporosis (at different doses) and have the added benefit of building bone density and reducing fractures (see the Osteoporosis, Menopause & Testosterone Use chapter).

Hypercalcemia of Malignancy Treatment

TREATMENT	MECHANISM OF ACTION	NOTES
Hydration with normal saline	↑ renal calcium excretion	Onset: minutes to hours
IV Bisphosphonates **Zoledronic Acid (*Zometa*)** 4 mg IV once **Pamidronate** 60-90 mg IV over 2-24 hrs once	Inhibits bone resorption by stopping osteoclast function	Onset: 24-72 hours; may repeat dose in 7 days if needed Do not confuse *Zometa* with *Reclast*, which is dosed 5 mg IV yearly for osteoporosis
Calcitonin (*Miacalcin*) 4-8 units/kg IM/SC Q12H	Inhibits bone resorption, ↑ renal calcium excretion	Onset: 2-6 hours Nasal spray formulation is not effective for the treatment of hypercalcemia Limit duration of therapy to 48 hours due to tachyphylaxis
Denosumab (*Xgeva*) 120 mg SC once weekly for up to 3 doses, then monthly for persistent hypercalcemia	Prevents osteoclast formation by blocking the interaction between RANKL and RANK (a receptor on osteoclasts)	Onset: 24-72 hours Do not confuse with *Prolia*, which is dosed 60 mg SC every 6 months for osteoporosis

Select Guidelines/References
American Cancer Society. www.cancer.org (accessed 2023 Oct 18)
National Comprehensive Cancer Network (NCCN). www.nccn.org (accessed 2023 Oct 18)
American Society of Clinical Oncology (ASCO). www.asco.org (accessed 2023 Oct 18)

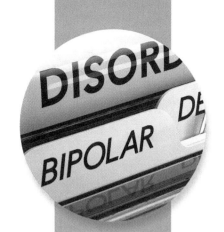 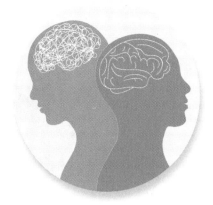 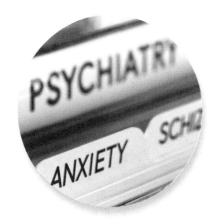

PSYCHIATRIC CONDITIONS

CONTENTS

CONTENT LEGEND

💡 = Study Tip Gal    🔑 = Key Drug Guy

CHAPTER 62
DEPRESSION

BACKGROUND

Major Depressive Disorder (MDD, referred to here as "depression") is one of the most common health conditions in the world. People with depression suffer greatly with persistent feelings of hopelessness, dejection, constant worry, poor concentration, a lack of energy, an inability to sleep and, sometimes, suicidal tendencies. The statistics are sobering. In 2021, approximately 21 million adults in the United States experienced a major depressive episode (about 8.3% of the population). About 61% of the adults with a major depressive episode received treatment.

About half of those with a first depression episode recover and experience no further episodes. The remaining patients will experience persistent or recurrent depression and the risk of recurrence increases with each episode. After three episodes, recurrence risk is nearly 100% without ongoing treatment.

Treatment problems that arise include discontinuation of medication without medical advice, or continuation of medication despite an inadequate response.

CAUSES

The causes of depression are poorly understood, but involve some combination of genetic, biologic and environmental factors. Neurotransmitters believed to be involved in depression include serotonin (5-HT), norepinephrine (NE), epinephrine (Epi), dopamine (DA), glutamate and acetylcholine (ACh). 5-HT may be the most important neurotransmitter (NT) involved with feelings of well-being. Certain drugs can cause or worsen depression (see Key Drugs Guy on the following page).

DIAGNOSIS

Diagnosis and treatment of depression is difficult since it is not possible to measure brain chemical imbalances. Diagnosis relies on symptom assessment according to the Diagnostic and Statistical Manual of Mental Disorders, 5th Edition (DSM-5-TR) (see Study Tip Gal). The Hamilton Depression Rating Scale (HDRS, also known as the Ham-D) is the most widely used depression assessment scale. It is designed to be used in a medical office. The patient rates their symptoms of depression on a numerical scale, and the total score indicates whether or not depression is present.

> **DEPRESSION DIAGNOSIS**
>
> **DSM-5 Criteria**
>
> At least 5 of the following symptoms present during the same two week period (must include depressed mood or diminished interest/pleasure):
>
> **M**ood - depressed
>
> **S**leep - increased/decreased
>
> **I**nterest/pleasure - diminished
>
> **G**uilt or feelings of worthlessness
>
> **E**nergy - decreased
>
> **C**oncentration - decreased
>
> **A**ppetite - increased/decreased
>
> **P**sychomotor agitation or retardation
>
> **S**uicidal ideation
>
> Remember: **M SIG E CAPS**

CONCURRENT BIPOLAR OR ANXIETY DISORDERS

It is necessary to rule out bipolar disorder prior to initiating antidepressant therapy to avoid inducing mania or causing rapid-cycling (cycling rapidly between bipolar depression and mania). Screening forms to assess mood and identify mania symptoms include questions such as "I get into moods where I feel very 'speeded-up' or irritable."

Benzodiazepines (BZDs) are often used to treat anxiety, though they are not first-line. When depression and anxiety occur together, BZDs should not be used alone; they can worsen and/or mask depression and can be problematic in patients with concurrent substance abuse disorders (called Dual Diagnosis). The risk for physiological dependence, withdrawal symptoms (e.g., tachycardia, anxiety) and respiratory depression and death (especially when given with opioids or other CNS depressants) is further discussed in the Anxiety Disorders chapter.

SELECT DRUGS THAT CAUSE OR WORSEN DEPRESSION

> **KEY DRUGS**
>
> **ADHD medications**
> Atomoxetine (*Strattera*)
>
> **Analgesics**
> Indomethacin
>
> **Antiretrovirals (NNRTIs)**
> Efavirenz (in *Atripla*)
> Rilpivirine (in *Complera, Odefsey*)
>
> **Cardiovascular medications**
> Beta-blockers (especially propranolol)
>
> **Hormones**
> Hormonal contraceptives
> Anabolic steroids
>
> **Other**
> Antidepressants: see Boxed Warnings & MedGuides Section
> Benzodiazepines
> Systemic steroids
> Interferons
> Varenicline
> Ethanol
>
> Medical conditions such as stroke, Parkinson disease, dementia, multiple sclerosis, hypothyroidism, low vitamin D levels, metabolic conditions (e.g., hypercalcemia), malignancy, overactive bladder and infectious diseases can contribute to depression.
>
> Others:
>
> Methylphenidate and other stimulants
>
> Methadone, and possibly other chronic opioid use that can lower testosterone or estrogen levels
>
> Clonidine
>
> Methyldopa
>
> Procainamide
>
> Cyclosporine
>
> Isotretinoin

NATURAL PRODUCTS

St. John's wort, SAMe (S-adenosyl-L-methionine), 5-HTP (5-hydroxytryptophan) or valerian may be helpful for treating depression, but there is less evidence of efficacy than with standard treatments. St. John's wort carries a weak recommendation for use in patients who are not pregnant or breastfeeding and prefer herbal treatment. St. John's wort, SAMe and 5-HTP can increase the risk of serotonin syndrome and should not be used with other serotonergic agents. St. John's wort is a broad-spectrum CYP450 enzyme inducer with many significant drug interactions, and it can cause phototoxicity.

DRUG TREATMENT

Treatment of depression can require one or more trials of medication/s. If a drug does not work after a suitable trial of at least 4 – 8 weeks, treatment should be reassessed (see Treatment-Resistant Depression). A thorough patient history is critical; what worked in the past, or did not work, should help guide therapy.

The initial treatment of depression (regardless of severity) can include psychotherapy alone [e.g., cognitive behavioral therapy (CBT)], medication alone or a combination of both. The effectiveness of the different antidepressant classes is generally comparable. The initial choice of medication should be based on the side effect profile, safety concerns and patient-specific symptoms. For most patients an SSRI or SNRI is preferred, or (with specific concurrent conditions) mirtazapine or bupropion.

DEPRESSION IN PREGNANCY AND POSTPARTUM DEPRESSION

Depression in pregnant women often goes unrecognized and untreated. Untreated depression, especially in the late second or early third trimesters, is associated with increased rates of adverse outcomes (e.g., premature birth, low birth weight, postnatal complications). Drug treatment carries a risk of adverse effects for the mother and unborn baby; the risks versus benefits of treatment must be considered carefully.

The American College of Obstetricians and Gynecologists (ACOG) has guideline recommendations for the treatment of depression during pregnancy and the postpartum period. Psychotherapy is the first-line treatment for mild to moderate depression during pregnancy. If a woman is taking antidepressants and wishes to become pregnant, the drug may be tapered off. In more severe cases, medications may be necessary and should consider the following:

- If the patient was successfully treated with an antidepressant before pregnancy, consideration should be given to continuing the same medication during pregnancy.

- If the patient is not taking antidepressants, SSRIs such as sertraline or escitalopram are first-line options. Paroxetine is avoided due to potential cardiac effects.
  - Although preferred, there is a warning regarding SSRI use during pregnancy and the potential risk of persistent pulmonary hypertension of the newborn (PPHN).

Postpartum depression can also have adverse outcomes for the mother, baby and family. Psychotherapy is advocated for mild to moderate cases. If medication treatment is necessary, the risks to a breastfed infant should be considered.

- SSRIs are preferred for treating postpartum depression.
- IV brexanolone (*Zulresso*) and oral zuranolone (*Zurzuvae*) are C-IV drugs indicated for postpartum depression. Both drugs can cause excessive sedation. Brexanolone can be considered for moderate to severe postpartum depression in select patients.

SAFETY ISSUES WITH ANTIDEPRESSANTS

Due to safety concerns (drug-drug and drug-food interactions) the use of oral nonselective monoamine oxidase inhibitors (MAO inhibitors) such as phenelzine, tranylcypromine and isocarboxazid is restricted to patients unresponsive to other treatments. Since many antidepressants increase serotonin levels, serotonin syndrome can occur with the administration of one or more serotonergic medications (e.g., SSRIs/SNRIs, mirtazapine, trazodone, opioids, tramadol, lithium, buspirone, triptans, dextromethorphan and St. John's wort). The risk is most severe when an MAO inhibitor is administered with another serotonergic medication. Higher doses increase the risk.

Symptoms of serotonin syndrome include severe nausea, dizziness, headache, diarrhea, agitation, tachycardia, hallucinations or muscle rigidity. Further discussion of MAO inhibitor drug interactions and serotonin syndrome can be found in the Basic Science Concepts and Drug Interactions chapters.

If an antidepressant is being discontinued, it should generally be tapered over several weeks to avoid withdrawal. Withdrawal symptoms include anxiety, agitation, insomnia, dizziness and flu-like symptoms. Paroxetine and venlafaxine carry a higher risk of withdrawal symptoms and must be tapered upon discontinuation. An exception to this rule is fluoxetine, which self-tapers because of its long half-life. Pharmacists must counsel patients on the risk of withdrawal symptoms and to not discontinue treatment without discussing with their healthcare provider.

BOXED WARNINGS & MEDGUIDES

All antidepressants carry a boxed warning of a possible increase in suicidal thoughts or actions in some children, teenagers or young adults within the first few months of treatment or when the dose is changed. MedGuides are required for all antidepressants. Patients and caregivers must be advised that mood may worsen and that they should contact a healthcare provider if changes in mood, behavior, thoughts or feelings are observed. This information is not included in the drug tables that follow.

LAG EFFECT AND SUICIDE PREVENTION

Antidepressant medication must be used daily, and will take time to work. Physical symptoms such as low energy improve within 1 – 2 weeks but psychological symptoms, such as low mood, may take a month or longer. Physicians and pharmacists must educate patients, family and caregivers about the risk of suicidality and screen for suicide risk. If a patient reports suicidal ideation, refer the patient to the emergency department, the suicide hotline or elsewhere for help. If someone has a plan to attempt suicide, it is more likely that the threat is immediate.

SELECTIVE SEROTONIN REUPTAKE INHIBITORS

Selective serotonin reuptake inhibitors (SSRIs) increase 5-HT by inhibiting its reuptake in the neuronal synapse. They weakly affect NE and DA. All SSRIs are approved for depression and a variety of anxiety disorders, except fluvoxamine which is only approved for obsessive-compulsive disorder (OCD).

DRUG	DOSING	SAFETY/SIDE EFFECTS/MONITORING
Citalopram (Celexa)	20-40 mg/day Max dose: 40 mg/day Max dose in elderly (> 60 years): 20 mg/day	**CONTRAINDICATIONS** Do not use with MAO inhibitors, linezolid, IV methylene blue or pimozide Fluoxetine, paroxetine: do not use with thioridazine Fluvoxamine: do not use with alosetron, thioridazine or tizanidine Sertraline solution: do not use with disulfiram
Escitalopram (Lexapro) – S-enantiomer of citalopram	10 mg/day Max dose: 20 mg/day Max dose in elderly: 10 mg/day	*Brisdelle*: pregnancy **WARNINGS** QT prolongation: do not exceed citalopram 20 mg/day in elderly (> 60 years), liver disease, with CYP2C19 poor metabolizers or on 2C19 inhibitors; do not exceed escitalopram 10 mg/day in elderly
Fluoxetine (Prozac) + olanzapine (Symbyax) – for treatment-resistant depression	10-60 mg/day Max dose: 80 mg/day; 90 mg/week (delayed release) To switch to fluoxetine delayed release 90 mg/weekly from fluoxetine 20 mg daily, start 7 days after last daily dose *Symbyax*: initial 6 mg/25 mg QHS	SIADH/hyponatremia, fall risk (Beers criteria: use caution in elderly, avoid if history of falls/fractures or use of CNS depressants) Bleeding (additive risk; see SSRI Drug Interactions) **SIDE EFFECTS** Sexual side effects: ↓ libido, ejaculation difficulties, anorgasmia, erectile dysfunction Somnolence, insomnia, nausea, dry mouth, diaphoresis (dose-related), weakness, tremor, dizziness, headache Most activating: fluoxetine; take dose in AM
Paroxetine (Paxil, Paxil CR) *Brisdelle* – for moderate-severe vasomotor symptoms associated with menopause	IR: 10-60 mg/day CR: 12.5-62.5 mg/day 10 mg IR = 12.5 mg CR *Brisdelle*: 7.5 mg QHS	Most sedating: paroxetine, fluvoxamine; take dose in the PM Others: take dose in the AM; if causing sedation, take in the PM Osteopenia/osteoporosis, restless leg syndrome (assess whether the onset coincided with initiation of treatment) **NOTES**
Sertraline (Zoloft)	50-200 mg/day	Fluoxetine, *Paxil CR* and sertraline are also approved for premenstrual dysphoric disorder (PMDD); dosing for PMDD can be continuous or intermittent [e.g., only during the luteal phase of the menstrual cycle (day 14 through menses), only when symptoms begin]
Fluvoxamine IR/ER	50-300 mg/day (daily doses > 100 mg/day should be divided BID)	All available in solution except fluvoxamine Sertraline is preferred in patients with cardiac risk

SSRI Drug Interactions

- MAO inhibitors and serotonin syndrome or hypertensive crisis:
  - Allow a two-week washout between MAO inhibitors and SSRIs. Fluoxetine is the exception; due to its long half life (4 – 6 days), a five-week washout period is required if switching from fluoxetine.
  - Do not initiate in patients receiving linezolid or IV methylene blue due to risk of serotonin syndrome.
- QT prolongation most consistently noted with citalopram and escitalopram (see max dose recommendations). Additive QT prolongation risk with SSRIs and other QT-prolonging drugs (see Arrhythmias chapter).
- ↑bleeding risk when used with anticoagulants, antiplatelets, NSAIDs, select natural products (e.g., ginkgo, garlic, ginger, ginseng, glucosamine, fish oils), thrombolytics.
- Fluoxetine, paroxetine and fluvoxamine are CYP2D6 inhibitors.
  - Tamoxifen requires conversion to its active form by CYP2D6. Decreased tamoxifen effectiveness occurs with fluoxetine and paroxetine. Venlafaxine (an SNRI) is preferred in combination with tamoxifen.
  - Some antipsychotic drugs (e.g., aripiprazole, olanzapine) are CYP2D6 substrates and may need a lower dose when given in combination with fluoxetine and paroxetine.
- Do not use with thioridazine, pimozide or cimetidine.
- Caution with drugs that cause orthostasis or CNS depression due to risk of falls.

SSRI COMBINED MECHANISM

DRUG	DOSING	SAFETY/SIDE EFFECTS/MONITORING
SSRI and 5-HT1A Partial Agonist		**CONTRAINDICATIONS** Do not use within 14 days of MAO inhibitors; do not use with linezolid or IV methylene blue
Vilazodone (*Viibryd, Viibryd Starter Pack*)	Start at 10 mg daily x 7 days, then 20 mg daily (dosing in patient starter kit); max 40 mg/day Take with food	**WARNINGS** Seizures; avoid in patients with seizure history
SSRI, 5-HT3 Receptor Antagonist and 5-HT1A Agonist		**SIDE EFFECTS** N/V/D, insomnia, ↓ libido (less sexual SEs compared to SSRIs and SNRIs) Vortioxetine: constipation
Vortioxetine (*Trintellix*)	5-20 mg/day, with or without food	**NOTES** Vortioxetine: decrease dose by 50% when used with strong CYP2D6 inhibitors (e.g., bupropion, fluoxetine, paroxetine or quinidine)

SEROTONIN AND NOREPINEPHRINE REUPTAKE INHIBITORS

Serotonin and norepinephrine reuptake inhibitors (SNRIs) have a similar mechanism as SSRIs, in that they increase 5-HT by inhibiting its reuptake in the neuronal synapse. SNRIs also inhibit reuptake of norepinephrine (NE). This explains the differences in indications and side effect profiles compared to SSRIs.

DRUG	DOSING	SAFETY/SIDE EFFECTS/MONITORING
Venlafaxine (*Effexor XR*) Depression, generalized anxiety disorder (GAD), panic disorder, social anxiety disorder	37.5-375 mg/day Max dose: 375 mg/day (IR), 225 mg/day (ER) Different generics; check *Orange Book*	**CONTRAINDICATIONS** SNRIs and MAO inhibitors can potentially cause a lethal drug interaction: hypertensive crisis (see SNRI Drug Interactions section) Do not initiate in a patient receiving linezolid or IV methylene blue
Duloxetine (*Cymbalta*) Depression, peripheral neuropathy (pain), fibromyalgia, GAD, chronic musculoskeletal pain	40-60 mg/day (or 20-30 BID) Max dose: 120 mg/day; doses > 60 mg/day not more effective	**WARNINGS** SIADH/hyponatremia, fall risk (Beers criteria: use caution in elderly, avoid if history of falls/fractures or use of CNS depressants) Bleeding (additive risk; see SNRI Drug Interactions)
Desvenlafaxine (*Pristiq*) Depression	50 mg/day (can ↑ to 400 mg/day, but no benefit > 50 mg)	**SIDE EFFECTS** Similar to SSRIs (due to ↓ 5-HT reuptake) Side effects due to ↑ NE: ↑ HR, dilated pupils (can lead to an episode of narrow angle glaucoma), dry mouth, excessive sweating and constipation
Levomilnacipran (*Fetzima*) Depression	Start 20 mg/day x 2 days then increase to 40 mg/day; can titrate by 40 mg/day no sooner than every 2 days Max dose: 120 mg/day Do not open, chew or crush capsules; do not take with alcohol	Can affect urethral resistance; caution when using SNRIs in patients prone to obstructive urinary disorders ↑ BP: risk is greatest with venlafaxine when dosed > 150 mg/day (all have risk, especially at higher doses); can ↓ dose, use antihypertensive/s or change therapy Osteopenia/osteoporosis, restless leg syndrome (assess whether the onset coincided with initiation of treatment) **NOTES** Do not use levomilnacipran with CrCl < 15 mL/min or duloxetine with CrCl < 30 mL/min *Pristiq* can leave a ghost tablet (empty shell) in the stool

SNRI Drug Interactions

- SNRIs and MAO inhibitors can cause hypertensive crisis or serotonin syndrome if used together.

  - ❏ A washout period is needed if changing between SNRIs and MAO inhibitors; 14 days are recommended.

  - ❏ Do not initiate in patients receiving linezolid or IV methylene blue due to risk of serotonin syndrome.

- Additive QT prolongation risk with venlafaxine.

- SNRIs can increase BP. Use caution, especially at higher doses, and monitor if on antihypertensive medications.

- Duloxetine is a moderate CYP2D6 inhibitor. Tamoxifen requires conversion to its active metabolite by CYP2D6. Decreased tamoxifen effectiveness occurs with duloxetine.

- ↑ bleeding risk with concurrent use of anticoagulants, antiplatelets, NSAIDs, select natural products (e.g., ginkgo, garlic, ginger, ginseng, glucosamine, fish oils), thrombolytics.

TRICYCLICS

Tricyclic antidepressants (TCAs) primarily inhibit NE and 5-HT reuptake. They also block ACh and histamine receptors, which contributes to the side effect profile. There are two main categories of TCAs: secondary amines and tertiary amines. Secondary amines are relatively selective for NE. Tertiary amines can be slightly more effective, but have a worse side effect profile.

DRUG	DOSING	SAFETY/SIDE EFFECTS/MONITORING
TERTIARY AMINES **Amitriptyline** **Doxepin** *Silenor* - for insomnia *Zonalon cream* - for pruritus Clomipramine Imipramine Trimipramine	**Amitriptyline:** 100-300 mg/day QHS or in divided doses **Doxepin:** 100-300 mg/day	**CONTRAINDICATIONS** Do not use with MAO inhibitors, linezolid, IV methylene blue; myocardial infarction; glaucoma and urinary retention (doxepin) **SIDE EFFECTS** **Cardiotoxicity** QT prolongation with overdose (monitor for suicidal ideation, as overdose can quickly cause fatal arrhythmias); obtain baseline ECG if cardiac risk factors or age > 50 years old Orthostasis, tachycardia
SECONDARY AMINES **Nortriptyline (*Pamelor*)** Amoxapine Desipramine Maprotiline Protriptyline	**Nortriptyline:** 25 mg TID-QID	**Anticholinergic** Dry mouth, blurred vision, urinary retention, constipation (taper off to avoid cholinergic rebound) Vivid dreams, weight gain (varies by agent and patient), sedation, sweating, myoclonus (muscle twitching – a symptom of drug toxicity) Beers criteria (use caution in elderly): risk of falls (avoid if history of falls/fractures or use of CNS depressants) **Seizures** High doses ↑ risk **NOTES** Low dose amitriptyline is commonly used and generally well tolerated Tertiary amines have increased anticholinergic properties, and are more likely to cause sedation and weight gain

Tricyclic Drug Interactions

- MAO inhibitors and hypertensive crisis: two-week washout if going to or from an MAO inhibitor.

- Additive QT prolongation risk with TCAs and other QT-prolonging drugs (see Arrhythmias chapter).

- Metabolized by CYP2D6; check for drug interactions.

DOPAMINE AND NOREPINEPHRINE REUPTAKE INHIBITOR

DRUG	DOSING	SAFETY/SIDE EFFECTS/MONITORING
Bupropion (Wellbutrin SR, Wellbutrin XL, Aplenzin, Forfivo XL, bupropion IR) + dextromethorphan (Auvelity) – ER Tablet for depression (dextromethorphan 45 mg/ bupropion 105 mg) **Wellbutrin XL** and Aplenzin – also approved for seasonal affective disorder (SAD) **Bupropion SR** (Zyban*) – for smoking cessation + naltrexone (Contrave) – for weight management	150-450 mg daily ■ Bupropion IR is TID ■ Wellbutrin SR is BID (Max: 200 mg/dose) ■ Wellbutrin XL is daily Do not exceed 450 mg/day (up to 522 mg/day with Aplenzin) due to seizure risk Auvelity: dextromethorphan 45 mg/bupropion 105 mg BID (at least 8 hours apart)	**CONTRAINDICATIONS** Seizure disorder; history of anorexia/bulimia, abrupt discontinuation of ethanol or sedatives; do not use with MAO inhibitors, linezolid, IV methylene blue or other forms of bupropion **WARNINGS** Neuropsychiatric adverse events possible when used for smoking cessation (can include mood changes, hallucinations, paranoia, aggression, anxiety) **SIDE EFFECTS** Dry mouth, CNS stimulation (insomnia, restlessness), tremors/seizures (dose-related), weight loss, headache/migraine, nausea/vomiting, constipation and possible blood pressure changes (more hypertension than hypotension) Sexual dysfunction is rare (no effect on 5-HT); can use if issues with other antidepressants Auvelity: dizziness, excessive sweating

Brand discontinued but name still used in practice

Bupropion Drug Interactions

■ Do not use multiple formulations of bupropion.

■ Increased risk of hypertensive crisis with MAO inhibitors. Allow 14-day washout when converting to an MAO inhibitor.

MONOAMINE OXIDASE INHIBITORS

Monoamine oxidase (MAO) inhibitors inhibit the enzyme monoamine oxidase, which breaks down catecholamines, including 5-HT, NE, Epi and DA. If these NTs increase dramatically, hypertensive crisis and death can result.

DRUG	DOSING	SAFETY/SIDE EFFECTS/MONITORING
Isocarboxazid (Marplan)	20 mg/day in divided doses Max dose: 60 mg/day	**CONTRAINDICATIONS** History of cardiovascular disease, cerebrovascular defect, headache, hepatic disease, pheochromocytoma Do not use with other sympathomimetics and related compounds (risk of hypertensive crisis – see Warnings and Drug Interactions below) Severe renal disease (isocarboxazid, phenelzine)
Phenelzine (Nardil)	15 mg TID Max dose: 60-90 mg/day	**WARNINGS** Not commonly used, but watch for drug-drug and drug-food interactions – if missed could be fatal Hypertensive crisis or serotonin syndrome can occur when taken with TCAs, SSRIs, SNRIs, many other drugs and tyramine-rich foods (see MAO Inhibitor Drug Interactions)
Tranylcypromine (Parnate)	30 mg/day in divided doses Max dose: 60 mg/day	**SIDE EFFECTS** Anticholinergic effects (taper upon discontinuation to avoid cholinergic rebound) Orthostasis Sedation (except tranylcypromine causes stimulation) Sexual dysfunction, weight gain, headache, insomnia
Selegiline transdermal patch (Emsam) MAO-B selective inhibitor Zelapar (ODT) is for Parkinson disease	Start at 6 mg patch/day, can ↑ by increments of 3 mg to 12 mg/day	**CONTRAINDICATIONS** Use with serotonergic drugs (see MAO Inhibitor Drug Interactions), pheochromocytoma **SIDE EFFECTS** Constipation, gas, dry mouth, loss of appetite, sexual dysfunction

MAO Inhibitor Drug Interactions

- To avoid hypertensive crisis, serotonin syndrome or psychosis, MAO inhibitors cannot be used with drugs or food that increase concentrations of epinephrine, norepinephrine, serotonin or dopamine.

  - Contraindicated drugs that increase serotonin: linezolid, lithium, tramadol, opioids, St. John's wort, SSRIs, SNRIs, mirtazapine, trazodone, triptans, buspirone and dextromethorphan.

  - Contraindicated drugs that increase epinephrine: bupropion, SNRIs, levodopa, linezolid, methylene blue, stimulants used for ADHD and OTC diet pills/herbal weight loss products.

  - Contraindicated to consume tyramine-rich foods that increase norepinephrine: aged cheese, pickled herring, yeast extract, air-dried meats, sauerkraut, soy sauce, fava beans and some red wines and beers (tap beer and any beer that has not been pasteurized - canned and bottled beers contain little or no tyramine). Foods can become high in tyramine when they have been aged, fermented, pickled or smoked.

MAO INHIBITORS – KEEP THEM SEPARATED

To avoid serotonin syndrome and hypertensive crisis*

- 2-week washout is required between MAO inhibitors and:
  - SSRIs (see fluoxetine, below)
  - SNRIs
  - TCAs
  - Bupropion
- 5-week washout is required when changing from:
  - Fluoxetine → MAO inhibitor (due to fluoxetine's long half-life)

See Drug Interactions chapter for more information on serotonin syndrome and hypertensive crisis with MAO inhibitors

MISCELLANEOUS ANTIDEPRESSANTS

DRUG	DOSING	SAFETY/SIDE EFFECTS/MONITORING
Tetracyclic antidepressant: has central presynaptic alpha-2 adrenergic antagonist effects, which results in ↑ release of NE and 5-HT		
Mirtazapine (Remeron, Remeron SolTab) Used commonly in oncology and skilled nursing facilities to help with sleep (dosed QHS) & to ↑ appetite (can ↑ weight gain in frail elderly)	15-45 mg QHS	**CONTRAINDICATIONS** Do not use with MAO inhibitors, linezolid or IV methylene blue **WARNINGS** Anticholinergic effects, QT prolongation, blood dyscrasias, CNS depression **SIDE EFFECTS** Sedation, ↑ appetite, weight gain, dry mouth, dizziness, agranulocytosis (rare)
Inhibits 5-HT reuptake, blocks H1 and alpha-1 adrenergic receptors		
Trazodone Rarely used as an antidepressant due to sedation; used primarily off-label for sleep	IR: 150-400 mg/day in divided doses ER: 150-375 mg QHS Sleep: dosed 50-100 mg QHS	**CONTRAINDICATIONS** Do not use with MAO inhibitors, linezolid or IV methylene blue **SIDE EFFECTS** Sedation (trazodone ER may be less sedating), orthostasis (risk in elderly for falls) Sexual dysfunction and risk of priapism (painful erection longer than 4 hours, medical emergency)
Inhibits 5-HT and NE reuptake, blocks 5-HT2 and alpha-1 adrenergic receptors		
Nefazodone Rarely used due to hepatotoxicity	200-600 mg/day divided BID	**BOXED WARNING** Hepatotoxicity **CONTRAINDICATIONS** Hepatic disease, concurrent use with MAO inhibitors, carbamazepine, cisapride, pimozide or triazolam **SIDE EFFECTS** Similar to trazodone, but less sedating

Drug Interactions

- Additive sedation; avoid use of any other sedating medications along with mirtazapine and trazodone.

- Mirtazapine, trazodone: additive QT prolongation risk. Use caution with other medications known to prolong the QT interval (see the Arrhythmias chapter).

- Avoid use with other serotonergic drugs, due to increased risk of serotonin syndrome.

- Avoid use with MAO inhibitors due to increased risk of hypertensive crisis.

SELECTING THE BEST ANTIDEPRESSANT

General Principles

The antidepressant selected should incorporate patient-specific information and history.

Did it work? If an antidepressant was taken at a reasonable dose for 4-8 weeks and did not work well, do not use it again.

Was it well-tolerated? Do not choose a treatment that was poorly tolerated in the past.

Does the patient have co-morbid conditions that make a drug a good or a poor choice?

- Cardiac/QT risk
  - Sertraline preferred
  - Do not choose a QT-prolonging drug/dose (e.g., high doses of citalopram or escitalopram)
  - Watch for additive QT effects when SSRIs, SNRIs, TCAs, mirtazapine or trazodone are used with other QT-prolonging drugs (see Arrhythmias chapter)
- Smoker
  - Bupropion SR is FDA-approved for smoking cessation
- Peripheral neuropathy or pain
  - Consider duloxetine
- Taking serotonergic antidepressants
  - Avoid multiple serotonergic medications due to risk of serotonin syndrome (See MAO Inhibitors section and Drug Interactions chapter)
  - ↑ bleeding risk with anticoagulants, antiplatelets, NSAIDs and some natural products (e.g., ginkgo, garlic, ginger, ginseng, glucosamine, fish oils)
- Seizure disorder or at risk for seizures (bulimia/anorexia, recent alcohol or sedative withdrawal)
  - Do not use bupropion

- Pregnant
  - Do not use paroxetine
  - Mild-to-moderate depression: psychotherapy is first-line
  - Certain SSRIs (e.g., escitalopram, sertraline) are first-line if using drug therapy
- Daytime sedation
  - Do not take a sedating drug early in the day (e.g., paroxetine, mirtazapine, trazodone)
  - Activating medications taken in the morning are preferred (e.g., fluoxetine, bupropion)
- Insomnia
  - Do not take an activating drug later in the day (e.g., bupropion, fluoxetine)
  - Sedating medications taken at night are preferred (e.g., paroxetine, mirtazapine, trazodone)
- Sexual dysfunction
  - High risk with SSRIs and SNRIs
  - Lower risk with bupropion and mirtazapine

TREATMENT-RESISTANT DEPRESSION

Depression that does not fully respond to two full treatment trials is considered treatment-resistant. The American Psychiatric Association (APA) guidelines state that patients should receive a 4 – 8 week trial of medication at a therapeutic dose before concluding that a drug is not working. If the patient is not improving (making progress toward the treatment goal of remission) or has an incomplete response, the following should be considered:

- Change to a new antidepressant.
- Increase the antidepressant dose.
- Use a combination of antidepressants with different mechanisms of action.

- Augment with buspirone or a low dose of an atypical antipsychotic. Agents approved as augmentation therapy with antidepressants are aripiprazole (Abilify), olanzapine + fluoxetine (Symbyax), quetiapine extended release (Seroquel XR), brexpiprazole (Rexulti) and cariprazine (Vraylar). Esketamine (Spravato) is an another option.
- Augmentation with lithium, thyroid hormone (i.e., T3), or in some cases, electroconvulsive therapy (ECT).

SELECT ADJUNCTIVE THERAPY IN TREATMENT-RESISTANT DEPRESSION

DRUG	DOSING	SAFETY/SIDE EFFECTS/MONITORING
Antipsychotics		
Aripiprazole (Abilify, Abilify Maintena, Abilify MyCite) Tablet, ODT, solution, injection Only oral formulations are indicated for treatment-resistant depression	Start 2-5 mg/day (QAM), can ↑ to 15 mg/day	**BOXED WARNING** Elderly patients with dementia-related psychosis treated with antipsychotic drugs are at ↑ risk of death Antidepressants increase the risk of suicidal thinking and behavior in children, adolescents, and young adults; see Boxed Warnings and MedGuides discussion
Olanzapine/fluoxetine (Symbyax)	Usually started at 6 mg/25 mg QHS (fluoxetine is activating, but olanzapine is more sedating), can ↑ cautiously	**CONTRAINDICATIONS** Olanzapine/fluoxetine (Symbyax): do not use with MAO inhibitors, linezolid, IV methylene blue, pimozide, thioridazine and caution with other drugs/conditions that cause QT prolongation **WARNINGS** Neuroleptic malignant syndrome, tardive dyskinesia (TD), falls, leukopenia, neutropenia
Quetiapine (Seroquel, Seroquel XR)	Start 50 mg QHS, ↑ to 150-300 mg QHS	Multiorgan hypersensitivity (drug reaction with eosinophilia and systemic symptoms, or DRESS) reactions with olanzapine (Symbyax) Pathological gambling and other compulsive behaviors (aripiprazole)
Brexpiprazole (Rexulti) Also approved for treatment of agitation associated with dementia due to Alzheimer's disease	Start 0.5-1 mg/day, can ↑ to 3 mg/day (titrate weekly)	**SIDE EFFECTS** Each of these drugs can cause metabolic issues, including dyslipidemia, weight gain, diabetes (less with aripiprazole) All can cause orthostasis/dizziness (can lead to falls) **Aripiprazole:** anxiety, insomnia, akathisia, constipation, agitation **Olanzapine:** sedation, weight gain, ↑ lipids, ↑ glucose, EPS, QT prolongation (lower risk)
Cariprazine (Vraylar)	Start 1.5 mg/day, can ↑ to 3 mg/day on day 15	**Quetiapine:** sedation, orthostasis, weight gain, ↑ lipids, ↑ glucose, EPS (lower risk) **Brexpiprazole:** weight gain, dyspepsia, diarrhea, agitation **Cariprazine:** EPS, dystonias, headache, insomnia
NMDA Receptor Antagonist		
Esketamine (Spravato) C-III Nasal spray Treatment-resistant depression and depression with suicidality	Start 56 mg intranasally twice weekly, can ↑ to 84 mg twice weekly if tolerated Must be administered under the supervision of a health care provider; monitor for adverse effects for at least 2 hours following administration	**BOXED WARNING** Sedation and dissociative or perceptual changes, potential for abuse and misuse Antidepressants increase the risk of suicidal thinking and behavior in children, adolescents, and young adults; see Boxed Warnings and MedGuides discussion **NOTES** Due to risks, only available through a restricted distribution system under the Spravato REMS program

KEY COUNSELING POINTS

See the Drug Formulations & Patient Counseling chapter for counseling language/layman's terminology.

All Antidepressants
- Can cause suicidal ideation.
- MedGuide required.
- Can take 1 – 2 weeks to feel a benefit from this drug and 6 – 8 weeks to feel the full effect on mood.

SSRIs
- Can cause:
  - ❏ Sexual dysfunction.
  - ❏ Serotonin syndrome.
- Fluoxetine: take in the morning.

SNRIs
- Can cause:
  - ❏ Increased blood pressure.
  - ❏ Increased sweating.
  - ❏ Sexual dysfunction.
  - ❏ Serotonin syndrome.
- Ghost tablet in stool (*Pristiq*).

Tricyclics
- Can cause:
  - ❏ Anticholinergic effects.
  - ❏ Orthostasis.

Bupropion
- Can cause insomnia.

MAO Inhibitors
- Can cause serotonin syndrome.
- Many drug interactions.

Other Antidepressants
- Trazodone: take at bedtime.
  - ❏ Can cause priapism.
- Mirtazapine: take at bedtime.

Select Guidelines/References

Practice Guideline for the Treatment of Patients with Major Depressive Disorder, 2010. https://psychiatryonline.org/pb/assets/raw/sitewide/practice_guidelines/guidelines/mdd.pdf (accessed 2023 Dec 20)

VA/DoD Clinical Practice Guideline for the Management of Major Depressive Disorder, 2022. https://www.healthquality.va.gov/guidelines/MH/mdd/VADoDMDDCPGFinal508.pdf (accessed 2023 Dec 20)

Treatment and Management of Mental Health Conditions During Pregnancy and Postpartum: ACOG Clinical Practice Guideline No. 5. *Obstet Gynecol* 2023;141(6):1262-1288.

Diagnostic and Statistical Manual of Mental Disorders, 5th Edition, Text Revision (DSM-5-TR).

Synaptic vesicle

Dopamine

Antipsychotics

Antipsychotics block the ability of dopamine to activate receptor

Synaptic cleft

Dopamine receptor

Designua/Shutterstock.com

DEFINITIONS: EXTRAPYRAMIDAL SIDE EFFECTS (EPS)

Extrapyramidal side effects (EPS) are a group of side effects related to irregular movements.

Dystonias: prolonged contraction of muscles during drug initiation, including painful muscle spasms; life-threatening if airway is compromised. Higher risk with younger males. Centrally-acting anticholinergics (diphenhydramine, benztropine) can be used for prophylaxis or treatment.

Akathisia: restlessness with anxiety and an inability to remain still; treated with benzodiazepines or propranolol.

Parkinsonism: looks similar to Parkinson disease, with tremors, abnormal gait and bradykinesia; treat with anticholinergics or propranolol if tremor is the main symptom.

Tardive dyskinesias (TD): abnormal facial movements, primarily in the tongue or mouth; higher risk with elderly females. TD can be irreversible. Must stop the drug and replace with a second-generation antipsychotic with low EPS risk (e.g., quetiapine, clozapine).

Dyskinesias: abnormal movements; more common with dopamine replacement for Parkinson disease.

CONTENT LEGEND

= Study Tip Gal

= Key Drug Guy

CHAPTER 63
SCHIZOPHRENIA/PSYCHOSIS

BACKGROUND

Schizophrenia is a chronic, severe and disabling <u>thought disorder</u> that occurs in ~1% of all societies regardless of class, color, religion or culture.

Common symptoms of schizophrenia include:

- <u>Hallucinations</u>: sensing something that is not present, such as imaginary voices.

- <u>Delusions</u>: a belief about something real that is not true, such as imagining that your family (which is real) wishes to hurt you (delusion).

- <u>Disorganized thinking/behavior</u>: inability to focus attention and communicate organized thoughts.

Schizophrenia ranges from relatively mild to severe. Some people can function adequately in daily life, while others need specialized, intensive care. <u>Treatment adherence</u> is important and <u>often difficult to achieve</u>, primarily due to a lack of insight (i.e., inability of the patient to recognize the illness). Schizophrenia can cause a life of torment and is associated with a high suicide rate.

The onset of symptoms usually begins in young adulthood. A diagnosis is not based on lab tests, but on behavior, which includes both <u>negative</u> and <u>positive</u> signs and symptoms (described on the following page). The <u>Diagnostic and Statistical Manual of Mental Disorders</u>, 5th Edition (<u>DSM-5</u>) sets the diagnostic criteria for psychiatric conditions.

PATHOPHYSIOLOGY

Schizophrenia's pathophysiology is multifactorial and includes altered brain structure and chemistry, primarily involving <u>dopamine</u>, <u>serotonin and glutamine</u>. Genetics (inherited susceptibility) and environmental factors (e.g., stress) contribute to disease risk. In addition to neurotransmitter imbalances and stressors, psychosis can be caused or exacerbated by drug use, including both recreational drugs and prescription drugs (see Key Drugs Guy below).

Medical conditions besides schizophrenia can cause psychosis. Dopamine is critical to many central nervous system functions, including movement. The motor symptoms characteristic of Parkinson disease are treated with medications that ↑ dopamine in the brain. Increased dopamine can worsen hallucinations or delusions in patients with Parkinson disease.

DSM-5 DIAGNOSTIC CRITERIA FOR SCHIZOPHRENIA

Note: delusions, hallucinations or disorganized speech must be present

Negative signs and symptoms	Positive signs and symptoms
Loss of interest in everyday activities	Hallucinations: can be auditory (hearing voices), visual or somatic
Lack of emotion (apathy)	Delusions: beliefs held by the patient that are without a basis in reality
Inability to plan or carry out activities	Disorganized thinking/behavior, incoherent speech, often on unrelated topics, purposeless behavior, or difficulty speaking and organizing thoughts, such as stopping in mid-sentence or jumbling together meaningless words
Poor hygiene	
Social withdrawal	
Loss of motivation (avolition)	
Lack of speech (alogia)	Difficulty paying attention

MEDICATIONS/RECREATIONAL DRUGS THAT CAN CAUSE PSYCHOTIC SYMPTOMS

Anticholinergics (centrally-acting, high doses)

Dextromethorphan

Dopamine or dopamine agonists (e.g., ropinirole, pramipexole, carbidopa/levodopa)

Interferons

Stimulants (including amphetamines), especially if already at risk

Systemic steroids (typically with lack of sleep – ICU psychosis)

Illicit/recreational substances
Cannabis

Cocaine

Lysergic acid diethylamide (LSD)

Methamphetamine

Phencyclidine (PCP)

Synthetic cathinones (bath salts, MDPV)

DRUG TREATMENT

Antipsychotics primarily block dopamine receptors. Newer antipsychotics also block serotonin and other receptors. Decreasing dopamine activity helps control psychosis, but negatively affects dopamine pathways involved in focus, attention and movement.

- Drugs can effectively treat positive symptoms (e.g., hallucinations, delusions).

- The negative symptoms (e.g., lack of motivation, cognitive and functional impairment) are more difficult to treat.

- Currently, second-generation antipsychotics (SGAs) are used first line due to a lower incidence of extrapyramidal symptoms (EPS), yet there are many patients who are stabilized on first-generation antipsychotics (FGAs) and in some initial cases, they may be preferable.

- FGAs have a high incidence of EPS (see expanded EPS definitions on the previous page), including painful dystonias (muscle contractions), dyskinesias (abnormal movements), tardive dyskinesias (repetitive, involuntary movements, such as grimacing and eye blinking) and akathisia (restlessness, inability to remain still).

- Tardive dyskinesia (TD) can be irreversible; the drug causing the TD should be discontinued.

FORMULATIONS

Adherence to antipsychotics is poor, primarily due to lack of insight (i.e., inability of the patient to recognize the illness). Various formulations can be used to increase adherence and help when dysphagia (i.e., difficulty swallowing) is present. See the Study Tip Gal (Formulation Considerations) later in the chapter.

- Long-acting injections [given intramuscularly (IM) or subcutaneously (SC)] eliminate daily oral dosing.

- Orally Disintegrating Tablets (ODTs) are useful with dysphagia (difficulty swallowing) and prevent cheeking (when tablets are hidden inside the cheek and spit out later). ODTs dissolve quickly in the mouth.

- Oral solutions/suspensions are useful for children and people with a feeding tube (e.g., PEG tube).

- Acute IM injections provide "stat" relief to calm down an agitated, psychotic patient for their own safety and the safety of others.

  - IM antipsychotics are often mixed with other drugs (in "cocktails"), such as benzodiazepines for anxiolytic/sedative effects, and anticholinergics to reduce dystonias (e.g., the "Haldol cocktail" contains haloperidol, lorazepam and diphenhydramine).

  - Olanzapine and benzodiazepines should not be given together (i.e., in an injection) due to risk of excessive sedation and breathing difficulty.

BOXED WARNINGS/OTHER WARNINGS

Antipsychotics are not indicated for agitation control in elderly patients with dementia-related psychosis. There is an increased risk of mortality when used for this purpose, mostly due to cardiovascular conditions (e.g., heart failure, sudden death) and infection. Several antipsychotics also carry a warning for an increased risk of stroke in patients with dementia. All antipsychotics carry a warning for falls.

FIRST-GENERATION ANTIPSYCHOTICS

First-generation antipsychotics (FGAs) work mainly by blocking dopamine-2 (D2) receptors, with minimal serotonin (5-HT2A) receptor blockade. Many of the FGAs are in the phenothiazine class; they can be easily recognized because their names end in "-azine" (e.g., thioridazine, fluphenazine).

First-Generation Antipsychotics (FGAs)

DRUG	DOSING	SAFETY/SIDE EFFECTS/MONITORING
Low Potency		**BOXED WARNINGS** Elderly patients with dementia-related psychosis: ↑ risk death from antipsychotics
Chlorpromazine	300-1,000 mg/day, divided	
		Thioridazine: QT prolongation
Thioridazine	300-800 mg/day, divided	*Adasuve*: bronchospasm (REMS program)
Mid Potency		**WARNINGS** Cardiovascular effects: QT prolongation (especially with thioridazine, haloperidol, chlorpromazine), orthostasis/falls, tachycardia
Loxapine (*Adasuve* - inhalation powder for acute agitation)	30-100 mg/day, divided	Anticholinergic effects: constipation, xerostomia, blurred vision, urinary retention
		CNS depression
Perphenazine	8-64 mg/day, divided	Extrapyramidal symptoms (EPS): including Parkinsonism, dystonic reactions, akathisia, tardive dyskinesia (↑ EPS with injections)
High Potency		Hyperprolactinemia: infertility, oligomenorrhea/amenorrhea (fewer or no menstrual periods), galactorrhea (abnormal breast discharge), erectile dysfunction/↓ libido
Haloperidol (*Haldol**, *Haldol Decanoate*) Tablet, oral solution, injection Class: butyrophenone Also used for Tourette syndrome (for tics and vocal outbursts)	Oral (tablet, solution): start 0.5-2 mg BID-TID, up to 30 mg/day IV: usually 5-10 mg Decanoate (monthly): IM only; for conversion from PO, use 10-20x the PO dose	Neuroleptic malignant syndrome (NMS): use may be associated with NMS; monitor for mental status changes, fever, muscle rigidity, autonomic instability Blood dyscrasias (leukopenia, neutropenia and agranulocytosis), ocular effects **SIDE EFFECTS** Sedation, dizziness, anticholinergic effects (see Warnings), ↑ prolactin (see Warnings)
Fluphenazine Tablet, elixir, injection	6-12 mg/day, divided Decanoate (every 2 weeks): IM only	EPS (see Warnings): can give anticholinergic (e.g., benztropine, diphenhydramine) to limit/avoid painful dystonic reactions *Adasuve*: dysgeusia (bad, bitter, or metallic taste in mouth)
Thiothixene	15-60 mg/day, divided	Injections (haloperidol, fluphenazine): injection site pain/redness
Trifluoperazine	15-50 mg/day, divided	**NOTES** Sedation and EPS: lower potency drugs have ↑ sedation and ↓ EPS, and higher potency drugs have ↓ sedation and ↑ EPS (all cause sedation and EPS)

Brand discontinued but name still used in practice.

SECOND-GENERATION ANTIPSYCHOTICS

Second-generation antipsychotics (SGAs) block dopamine (D2) and serotonin (5-HT2A) receptors. Aripiprazole, brexpiprazole and cariprazine are unique: they are D2 and 5-HT1A partial agonists, and brexpiprazole is also a 5-HT2A antagonist. SGAs are available in a variety of formulations to increase adherence (see the Study Tip Gal titled Formulation Considerations).

Second-Generation Antipsychotics (SGAs)

DRUG	DOSING	SAFETY/SIDE EFFECTS/MONITORING
Aripiprazole (Abilify, *Abilify MyCite, Abilify Maintena, Abilify Asimtufii, Aristada, Aristada Initio)* Tablet, ODT, oral solution, IM (prefilled syringe, suspension) Also approved for irritability with autism and Tourette syndrome	10-30 mg PO QAM **Intramuscular:** *Abilify Maintena* monthly *Aristada* every 4-8 weeks, depending on dose *Abilify Asimtufii* every 2 months	**SIDE EFFECTS** Akathisia, activating or sedating, headache, anxiety, constipation Lower risk of weight gain, some QT prolongation, EPS (in children) **NOTES** *Aristada Initio*: can be administered as a one-time IM loading dose (along with oral aripiprazole) when starting or restarting *Aristada* treatment *Abilify MyCite*: aripiprazole tablets (embedded with an ingestible sensor), along with a wearable sensor to help track drug compliance
Clozapine (Clozaril, *Versacloz* suspension) Only if failed to respond to 2 standard AP treatments, or had significant ADRs	300-900 mg/day, divided (start at 12.5 mg and titrate; titrate off since abrupt discontinuation can cause seizures) Clozapine is very effective and has ↓ risk of EPS/TD, but used no sooner than 3rd-line due to severe side effect potential (metabolic effects, neutropenia)	**BOXED WARNINGS** Significant risk of potentially life-threatening neutropenia/agranulocytosis (REMS program) Bradycardia, orthostatic hypotension, syncope and cardiac arrest; risk is highest during the initial titration period, especially with rapid dose increases; titrate slowly Myocarditis and cardiomyopathy; discontinue if suspected Seizures, dose related; start at no higher than 12.5 mg once or twice daily, titrate slowly, using divided doses; use with caution in patients at seizure risk (e.g., seizure history, head trauma, alcoholism or taking medications which lower seizure threshold) **SIDE EFFECTS** Agranulocytosis, seizures, constipation, somnolence, metabolic syndrome (↑ weight, ↑ BG, ↑ lipids), sialorrhea (hypersalivation), hypotension **MONITORING** REMS: prescribers and pharmacies must be certified and patients must be enrolled with the Clozapine REMS To start treatment, baseline ANC must be ≥ 1,500/mm^3 Check ANC weekly x 6 months, then every 2 weeks x 6 months, then monthly; stop therapy if ANC < 1,000/mm^3 **NOTES** Smoking reduces drug levels
Lurasidone (Latuda)	40-160 mg/day, divided Take with food ≥ 350 kcal	**CONTRAINDICATIONS** Use with strong CYP450 3A4 inducers and inhibitors **SIDE EFFECTS** Somnolence, EPS (dystonias), nausea, ↓ risk of metabolic syndrome compared to other SGAs
Olanzapine (Zyprexa, *Zyprexa Zydis ODT, Zyprexa Relprevv* injection) + fluoxetine *(Symbyax)* for treatment-resistant depression + samidorphan *(Lybalvi)* for treatment of schizophrenia and bipolar disorder	10-20 mg QHS IM injection (acute agitation) *Relprevv* injection suspension lasts 2-4 weeks; restricted use	**BOXED WARNING** *Zyprexa Relprevv*: sedation (including coma) and delirium (including agitation, anxiety, confusion, disorientation) have been observed following injection; must be administered in a registered healthcare facility and patients are monitored for 3 hours post-injection (*Zyprexa Relprevv* REMS program requirements). **SIDE EFFECTS** Somnolence, metabolic syndrome (↑ weight, ↑ blood glucose, ↑ lipids), orthostasis **NOTES** Smoking reduces drug levels *Lybalvi*: samidorphan is an opioid receptor antagonist that may help mitigate weight gain from olanzapine; use is contraindicated in anyone taking opioids or undergoing acute opioid withdrawal

DRUG	DOSING	SAFETY/SIDE EFFECTS/MONITORING
Paliperidone (*Invega*, *Invega Sustenna*, *Invega Trinza*, *Invega Hafyera*) Tablet, IM (prefilled syringe, suspension) Active metabolite of risperidone; SEs similar	PO: 3-12 mg daily CrCl < 50 mL/min: 3 mg daily CrCl < 10 mL/min: Not recommended **Intramuscular:** *Invega Sustenna* monthly *Invega **Tri**nza* every **3** months *Invega **Hafyer**a* every **6** months	**SIDE EFFECTS** ↑ prolactin – sexual dysfunction, galactorrhea, irregular/missed periods EPS, especially at higher doses Tachycardia, QT prolongation Metabolic syndrome (↑ weight, ↑ blood glucose, ↑ lipids) Somnolence **NOTES** *Invega* can leave a ghost tablet (empty shell) in the stool Adequate treatment with with IM paliperidone (monthly or every 3 months) must be established before starting *Invega Trinza* or *Hafyera* OROS delivery enables once daily dosing – do not break or crush
Quetiapine (*Seroquel*, *Seroquel XR*)	400-800 mg/day, divided BID or XR QHS	**SIDE EFFECTS** Somnolence, metabolic syndrome (↑ weight, ↑ blood glucose, ↑ lipids), orthostasis, possible ocular effects (cataracts) Low EPS risk – often used for psychosis in Parkinson disease **NOTES** Take XR at night, without food or with a light meal (≤ 300 kcal)
Risperidone (*Risperdal*, *Risperdal Consta*, *Rykindo*, *Perseris*, *Uzedy*) Tablet, ODT, oral solution, SC (prefilled syringe), IM (suspension) Also approved for irritability associated with autism	2-16 mg/day, divided **Intramuscular:** *Risperdal Consta* and *Rykindo*, 25-50 mg every 2 weeks **Subcutaneous:** *Perseris* monthly *Uzedy* every 1-2 months	**SIDE EFFECTS** ↑ prolactin – sexual dysfunction, galactorrhea, irregular/missed periods EPS, especially at higher doses Tachycardia, QT prolongation Metabolic syndrome (↑ weight, ↑ blood glucose, ↑ lipids) Somnolence
Ziprasidone (*Geodon*)	40-160 mg/day, divided BID Take with food Acute injection: *Geodon* IM 10 mg Q2H or 20 mg Q4H Max: 40 mg/day IM	**CONTRAINDICATIONS** QT prolongation; do not use with QT risk **SIDE EFFECTS** Somnolence, EPS, dizziness, nausea
Asenapine (*Saphris*, *Secuado*) *Saphris*: sublingual tablet *Secuado*: patch	10-20 mg/day, divided BID No food/drink for 10 min after dose *Secuado*: 3.8-7.6 mg applied daily	**CONTRAINDICATIONS** Severe hepatic impairment **SIDE EFFECTS** Somnolence, tongue numbness (sublingual tablet), EPS (5% more than placebo), QT prolongation
Cariprazine (Vraylar)	1.5-6 mg daily	**SIDE EFFECTS** EPS, dystonias, headache, insomnia
Brexpiprazole (*Rexulti*)	2-4 mg daily	**SIDE EFFECTS** Weight gain, dyspepsia, diarrhea, akathisia
Iloperidone (*Fanapt*)	12-24 mg/day, divided Titrate slowly due to orthostasis	**SIDE EFFECTS** Dizziness, somnolence, orthostasis, tachycardia, QT prolongation
Lumateperone (*Caplyta*)	42 mg daily	**SIDE EFFECTS** Somnolence, EPS

SELECTING AN ANTIPSYCHOTIC

Antipsychotics are chosen based on several considerations, including past medication history and side effects. SGAs have variable degrees of metabolic side effects, including weight gain, increased cholesterol, increased triglycerides (TGs) and increased blood glucose (BG). Drugs with higher metabolic risk should be monitored during treatment and avoided if diabetes or cardiovascular disease is present. Although at a lower incidence than FGAs, some of the SGAs can cause dose-related EPS. Prolactin levels can increase, causing gynecomastia (painful, swollen breast tissue), galactorrhea, sexual dysfunction and oligomenorrhea/amenorrhea. Clozapine has the highest efficacy, but has multiple boxed warnings (e.g., agranulocytosis, seizures, myocarditis). Clozapine can be tried after failure with at least two other antipsychotics (at least one SGA). Some experts suggest one of the two antipsychotics to be a long-acting injectable. The Study Tip Gal (Treatment Consideratons) lists the drugs most likely to cause major adverse effects; avoid using them in an at-risk patient.

TREATMENT CONSIDERATIONS

When assessing treatment resistance or evaluating the best option for a partial response, it is important to evaluate whether the patient has had an adequate trial (at least 6 weeks) of an antipsychotic, including whether the dose is adequate and whether the patient has been taking the medication as prescribed.

Did it work and was it well-tolerated?

If the drug was being taken (at a reasonable dose and for a long-enough trial period) and did not work well, do not use it again.

Do not choose a treatment that was poorly tolerated in the past (e.g., painful dystonia or tardive dyskinesia with haloperidol, painful gynecomastia with paliperidone/risperidone).

Cardiac risk/QT prolongation risk

Do not choose a QT-prolonging drug like ziprasidone, haloperidol, thioridazine or chlorpromazine.

History of movement disorder (e.g., Parkinson disease)

Do not choose a drug with high risk of EPS [e.g., FGAs, risperidone, paliperidone (at higher doses)]. Quetiapine is preferred.

Overweight/metabolic risk (e.g., ↑ TG)

Do not choose a drug that worsens metabolic issues like olanzapine or quetiapine. There is a lower metabolic risk with aripiprazole, ziprasidone, lurasidone and asenapine.

Nonadherence or unhoused patients

Choose a long-acting injection (see algorithm below).

FORMULATION CONSIDERATIONS

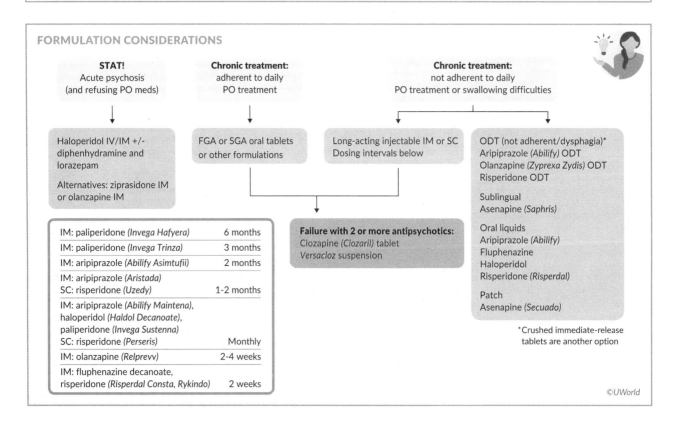

PSYCHOSIS IN PARKINSON DISEASE

Commonly, quetiapine is used to treat psychosis in Parkinson disease because it has a low risk of causing extrapyramidal effects. Pimavanserin *(Nuplazid)* is approved for psychosis with Parkinson disease. It is an inverse agonist and antagonist at serotonin 5-HT2A receptors and a lesser extent at serotonin 5-HT2C receptors. It does not affect dopamine receptors and does not worsen motor symptoms of Parkinson disease.

DRUG	DOSING	SAFETY/SIDE EFFECTS/MONITORING
Pimavanserin *(Nuplazid)*	34 mg PO daily (two 17 mg tablets)	**WARNINGS** Not approved for dementia-related psychosis. See Boxed Warnings discussion. QT prolongation; avoid use with drugs that also increase the QT interval and in patients with risk factors for prolonged QT interval. **SIDE EFFECTS** Peripheral edema, confusion.

ANTIPSYCHOTIC DRUG INTERACTIONS

- All antipsychotics can prolong the QT interval. Some are considered higher risk than others. The higher risk QT-prolonging SGAs are noted previously. Thioridazine, a FGA, is high-risk for QT prolongation (boxed warning). Use caution with other medications that increase risk.
- Smoking can reduce plasma levels of olanzapine and clozapine; patients who smoke can require higher doses.
- High plasma levels of risperidone and paliperidone can increase prolactin and cause EPS. Caution when using risperidone with CYP2D6 inhibitors, including paroxetine and fluoxetine.
- Avoid concurrent drugs that lower the seizure threshold with clozapine.
- Monitor for respiratory depression and hypotension when antipsychotics are given with benzodiazepines.
- Caution with other dopamine blocking agents (e.g., metoclopramide), as EPS and TD risk may be increased.

KEY COUNSELING POINTS

See the Drug Formulations and Patient Counseling chapter for counseling language/layman's terminology.

ALL ANTIPSYCHOTICS

- MedGuide required.
- Can cause:
  - Drowsiness.
  - Orthostasis.
  - Unusual body movements. Symptoms include shakiness, stiffness, or uncontrollable movements of the mouth, tongue, cheeks, jaw, arms or legs. Contact your healthcare provider immediately.
  - Fever, sweating, severe muscle stiffness (rigidity) and confusion. Contact your healthcare provider immediately.

Olanzapine, Risperidone, Paliperidone and Quetiapine

- Can cause hyperglycemia and weight gain.

Clozapine

- Can cause low white blood cell count; requires monitoring via REMS program.

Risperidone

- *Risperdal* oral solution: administered directly from the calibrated pipette, or mixed with water, coffee, orange juice or low-fat milk; it cannot be mixed with cola or tea.

Asenapine Sublingual

- Can cause tongue numbness.

TARDIVE DYSKINESIA

Tardive dyskinesia (TD) is a complication that can occur with dopamine receptor blockade, as with antipsychotics. TD can cause irreversible symptoms that include uncontrollable movements in the tongue, face, trunk and extremities and can interfere with walking, talking and breathing. Valbenazine and deutrabenazine reversibly inhibit vesicular monoamine transporter 2 (VMAT2), a transporter that regulates monoamine uptake from the cytoplasm to the synaptic vesicle for storage and release. Both medications are approved for the treatment of TD and chorea associated with Huntington's disease.

DRUG	DOSING	SAFETY/SIDE EFFECTS/MONITORING
Valbenazine (*Ingrezza*)	Start 40 mg PO daily, increase in 1 week to 80 mg PO daily; maintenance dose of 60-80 mg daily Moderate-severe hepatic impairment: adjustment required CYP2D6 poor metabolizer: consider dose reduction	**WARNINGS** Somnolence, QT prolongation (avoid in long QT syndrome)
Deutetrabenazine (*Austedo, Austedo XR*)	Start 6 mg PO BID, increase weekly based on response (max 48 mg/day) Concurrent strong CYP2D6 inhibitors or CYP2D6 poor metabolizer: max dose 36 mg/day	**CONTRAINDICATIONS** Hepatic impairment, administration with tetrabenazine or valbenazine, administration with an MAO inhibitor (within 14 days) **WARNINGS** Somnolence, QT prolongation (avoid in long QT syndrome)

Drug Interactions

- Avoid use with MAO inhibitors.

- Valbenazine and deutetrabenazine are substrates of CYP3A4 and 2D6. Dose reduction is required when given with strong inhibitors of CYP3A4 (e.g., itraconazole, clarithromycin) or 2D6 (e.g., paroxetine, fluoxetine).

- Valbenazine is a P-gp inhibitor and can increase digoxin concentrations. Dosage adjustment of digoxin may be required.

NEUROLEPTIC MALIGNANT SYNDROME

Antipsychotics used to be called neuroleptics. Neuroleptic malignant syndrome (NMS) is rare but is highly lethal. It occurs most commonly with the FGAs and is due to D2 blockade. NMS is less common with SGAs and with other dopamine blocking agents, including metoclopramide (*Reglan*). The majority of cases occur within two weeks of starting treatment or immediately following high doses of injectables given alongside multiple oral doses. Occasionally, patients develop NMS after years of antipsychotic use. NMS is a medical emergency. Intense muscle contractions can lead to acute renal injury (due to rhabdomyolysis from the destruction of muscle tissue), suffocation and death.

Signs

- Hyperthermia (high fever, with profuse sweating)

- Extreme muscle rigidity (called "lead pipe" rigidity), which can lead to respiratory failure

- Mental status changes

- Tachycardia, tachypnea and blood pressure changes

Laboratory Results

- ↑ creatine phosphokinase and ↑ white blood cells

Treatment

- Stop the antipsychotic and provide supportive care: cardiorespiratory and hemodynamic support and manage electrolytes

- Control the patient's temperature: cooling bed, antipyretics, cooled IV fluids

- Relax the muscles: benzodiazepines, dantrolene (*Ryanodex, Dantrium, Revonto*) or some cases may require a dopamine agonist (e.g., bromocriptine)

- After resolution of the symptoms, consider a different antipsychotic (e.g., quetiapine or clozapine)

Select Guidelines/References

Diagnostic and Statistical Manual of Mental Disorders, 5th Edition, Text Revision (DSM-5-TR).

The American Psychiatric Association Practice Guideline for the Treatment of Patients with Schizophrenia. Third Ed. American Psychiatric Association; 2021 (accessed 2024 Jan 8).

BIPOLAR CLASSIFICATIONS AND DEFINITIONS

BIPOLAR I

At least one episode of mania, and usually, bouts of intense depression (a depressive episode is not required for diagnosis).

Mania is associated with at least one of the following: significant impairment in social/work functioning, psychosis/delusions or requires hospitalization.

BIPOLAR II

At least one episode of hypomania (lasting ≥ 4 consecutive days) and at least one depressive episode (lasting ≥ 2 weeks).

Hypomania does not affect social/work functioning, does not cause psychosis nor require hospitalization.

BIPOLAR DEPRESSION

Predominant symptoms of a depressive episode include feelings of sadness or depressed mood and/or loss of interest in previously enjoyed activities (see Depression chapter).

PSYCHOSIS

Severe mental condition where there is a loss of contact with reality, involves abnormal thinking and perception (e.g., hallucinations and delusions).

CONTENT LEGEND

☀ = Study Tip Gal

---

iStock.com/Siphotography

CHAPTER 64

BIPOLAR DISORDER

BACKGROUND

Bipolar disorder occurs in ~2.8% of adults. It is characterized by fluctuations in mood from an extremely sad or hopeless state to an abnormally elevated, overexcited or irritable mood called mania or hypomania (a milder form of mania). Each mood episode represents a drastic change from an individual's usual mood and behavior. Some episodes include symptoms of both mania and depression, which is called a mixed state. Individuals may seek help during a depressive episode, which can lead to a misdiagnosis of depression only.

Bipolar disorder is classified as bipolar I or bipolar II, which differ primarily by the severity of mania experienced (see Bipolar Classifications and Definitions to the left). Cyclothymia is a related disorder consisting of periods of hypomanic and depressive symptoms without meeting criteria for a major depressive, manic or hypomanic episode. Bipolar disorder can reduce quality of life or cause problems with relationships and employment. It can also lead to drug abuse, anxiety disorders and suicide.

DIAGNOSTIC CRITERIA

Diagnostic and Statistical Manual of Mental Disorders, Fifth Edition (DSM-5) criteria are used to diagnose bipolar disorders. A toxicology screen should be done prior to starting treatment to rule out drug-induced mania.

WHAT IS MANIA?

Symptoms
- Inflated self-esteem
- Needs less sleep
- More talkative than normal
- Jumping from topic to topic
- Easily distracted
- Increase in goal-directed activity
- High-risk, pleasurable activities (e.g., buying sprees, sexual indiscretions, gambling)

Definition
Abnormally elevated or irritable mood for at least a week (or any duration if hospitalization is needed)

Diagnosis
Exhibits ≥ 3 symptoms (if mood is only irritable, exhibits ≥ 4 symptoms)

DRUG TREATMENT

Patients with bipolar disorder usually cycle between mania and depression. The goal of treatment is to stabilize the mood without inducing a depressive or manic state. The traditional mood stabilizers, such as lithium and antiepileptic drugs (valproate, lamotrigine and carbamazepine), treat both mania and depression without inducing either state. Antipsychotics, while not traditional mood stabilizers, can help stabilize the mood when mania occurs with psychosis. Antidepressants can induce or exacerbate a manic episode when used as monotherapy, so they should only be used in combination with a mood stabilizer.

To select treatment, consider the following:

- The side effect profile of the drug.
- The patient's medication history and first-degree relatives' medication history; if the patient or a family member responded well to a drug, the same drug might be a reasonable option.
- The drug formulations available and cost.

Note that the term "valproate" is used to refer to any formulation of valproic acid and/or valproic acid derivatives.

ACUTE TREATMENT

Acute treatment will depend on the type of episode (mania vs. depression).

- Manic episode: first-line treatment is an antipsychotic (e.g., olanzapine, risperidone), lithium or valproate. A combination of an antipsychotic + lithium or valproate is preferred for severe episodes.
- Depressive episode: first-line treatment is an antipsychotic (e.g., quetiapine, lurasidone). Lithium, valproate or lamotrigine can be added or used as alternatives.

MAINTENANCE

Medications that were effective for acute episodes should be continued as maintenance treatment to prevent relapse. These include lithium, antiepileptic drugs and second-generation antipsychotics (SGAs). Combination treatment might be more effective than monotherapy at preventing relapse.

MedGuides are required with all antidepressants (primarily due to suicide risk) and antipsychotics (due to increased risk of death in elderly patients with dementia-related psychosis).

ANTIEPILEPTIC DRUGS

Several anticonvulsants are used for the treatment of bipolar disorder. See the Seizures/Epilepsy chapter for a detailed review of these medications:

- **Lamotrigine (Lamictal, Lamictal ODT, Lamictal XR, Lamictal Starter Kit):** requires a slow titration due to the risk of a severe rash. Do not use for acute mania.
- **Valproate/Valproic Acid Derivatives (Depakote)**
- **Carbamazepine** (Equetro)

SECOND-GENERATION ANTIPSYCHOTICS

Antipsychotics can be used alone or in combination with one of the traditional mood stabilizers. A major concern with antipsychotics is the risk of extrapyramidal symptoms (EPS). The first-generation antipsychotics (e.g., haloperidol) have a higher incidence of EPS than SGAs, so SGAs are preferred. The following are the more common SGAs that can be used alone or in combination with mood stabilizers for acute mania and/or maintenance treatment:

- **Aripiprazole (Abilify,** Abilify Maintena)
- **Olanzapine (Zyprexa,** Zyprexa Relprevv, Zyprexa Zydis)
- **Quetiapine (Seroquel,** Seroquel XR)
- **Risperidone (Risperdal,** Risperdal Consta, Perseris)
- **Ziprasidone (Geodon)**

Other common SGAs used for bipolar disorders include:

- **Lurasidone (Latuda):** can use alone or in combination with mood stabilizers for bipolar depressive episodes.
- Olanzapine/Fluoxetine (Symbyax): can use alone for acute depressive episodes.

See the Schizophrenia/Psychosis chapter for a detailed review of the SGAs.

LITHIUM

Lithium is proposed to work by influencing the reuptake of serotonin and/or norepinephrine or by moderating glutamate levels in the brain. Glutamate is the primary excitatory neurotransmitter, so high levels could cause mania.

DRUG	DOSING	SAFETY/SIDE EFFECTS/MONITORING
Lithium (Lithobid) Tablet, capsule, syrup	Start: 300-900 mg/day, divided BID-TID Usual range: 900-1,800 mg/day, divided BID-TID Extended-release: take BID Titrate slowly, as tolerated Take with or after meals to reduce nausea **Therapeutic range** 0.6-1.2 mEq/L (trough level) Acute mania may require up to 1.5 mEq/L initially	**BOXED WARNING** Serum lithium levels should be monitored to avoid toxicity **WARNINGS** Renal impairment, hyponatremia and dehydration (↑ lithium toxicity) Serotonin syndrome (see Drug Interactions) **SIDE EFFECTS** **Within therapeutic range:** GI upset (nausea/diarrhea), cognitive effects, cogwheel rigidity, fine hand tremor, thirst, polyuria/polydipsia, weight gain, hypothyroidism, hypercalcemia, cardiac abnormalities, edema, anorexia, worsening psoriasis, blue-gray skin pigmentation, impotence **Toxicity:** > 1.5 mEq/L: ataxia, coarse hand tremor, vomiting, persistent diarrhea, confusion, sedation > 2.5 mEq/L: CNS depression, arrhythmia, seizure, coma **MONITORING** Serum lithium levels, renal function, thyroid function (TSH, FT4), electrolytes (calcium, potassium, sodium) **NOTES** Renally cleared; no CYP450 interactions Avoid in pregnancy; associated with cardiac malformations in first trimester; avoid in breastfeeding

Lithium Drug Interactions

- Lithium levels ↑ with:
  - ↓ salt intake, sodium loss (e.g., with ACE inhibitors, ARBs, thiazide diuretics)
  - NSAIDs: aspirin and sulindac are safer options
- Lithium levels ↓ with:
  - ↑ salt intake, caffeine and theophylline
- ↑ risk of serotonin syndrome if lithium is taken with:
  - SSRIs, SNRIs, triptans, linezolid and other serotonergic drugs (see Drug Interactions chapter)
- ↑ risk of neurotoxicity (e.g., ataxia, tremors, nausea) if lithium is taken with:
  - Verapamil, diltiazem, phenytoin and carbamazepine

CONVERTING BETWEEN LITHIUM FORMULATIONS

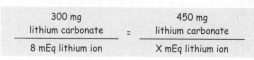

5 mL lithium citrate syrup = 8 mEq of lithium ion

8 mEq of lithium ion = 300 mg lithium carbonate tabs/caps

CASE SCENARIO

A patient is taking 450 mg lithium carbonate BID, but reports difficulty swallowing the capsules. How many milliliters of lithium citrate syrup should be given for each dose? (Round to the nearest TENTH.)

Determine how many milliequivalents of lithium are required for each dose.

$$\frac{300 \text{ mg lithium carbonate}}{8 \text{ mEq lithium ion}} = \frac{450 \text{ mg lithium carbonate}}{X \text{ mEq lithium ion}}$$

$$X = 12 \text{ mEq lithium ion}$$

Next determine how many milliliters of lithium citrate syrup are required.

$$\frac{12 \text{ mEq}}{X \text{ mL}} = \frac{8 \text{ mEq}}{5 \text{ mL}}$$

7.5 mL of lithium citrate syrup per dose

This problem can also be solved using the milliequivalent formula. Refer to the Calculations II chapter for additional examples.

PREGNANCY

Treating bipolar disease in pregnancy is complex since the common mood stabilizers have known teratogenic effects.

- Valproate exposure in pregnancy can increase the risk of fetal anomalies, including neural tube defects, fetal valproate syndrome and long-term adverse cognitive effects. Avoid in pregnancy, if possible, especially during the first trimester.

- Carbamazepine exposure in pregnancy can cause fetal carbamazepine syndrome, which can result in facial abnormalities and other significant issues. Avoid in pregnancy, if possible, especially during the first trimester.

- Lithium exposure in pregnancy can cause an increase in congenital cardiac malformations and other abnormalities.

During pregnancy, lamotrigine is a safer option relative to the other mood stabilizers mentioned in this section. SGAs are safer choices than valproate, carbamazepine or lithium. Lurasidone has the most favorable safety profile in pregnancy, but its use is limited since it is only approved for bipolar depression.

KEY COUNSELING POINTS

See the Drug Formulations and Patient Counseling chapter for counseling language/layman's terminology.

LITHIUM

- Take with food or at end of meal to reduce nausea.

- Maintain consistent salt intake. Changes in salt intake can alter lithium levels in the body.

- Maintain adequate hydration with non-caffeinated fluids.

- Avoid dehydration (e.g., excessive sweating, diarrhea, vomiting and prolonged heat/sun exposure). Can increase lithium levels and side effects.

- Avoid in pregnancy/breastfeeding.

- Notify healthcare provider immediately for worsening nausea or diarrhea, slurred speech or confusion.

- Can impair alertness, use caution while driving or during other tasks requiring you to be alert.

Select Guidelines/References

Diagnostic and Statistical Manual of Mental Disorders, 5th Edition, Text Revision (DSM-5-TR). Arlington VA, American Psychiatric Association, 2022.

Bobo WV. The Diagnosis and Management of Bipolar I and II Disorders: Clinical Practice Update. Mayo Clin Proc. 2017;92(10):1532-1551.

WFSBP: Update 2012 on the long-term treatment of bipolar disorder. The World Journal of Biological Psychiatry. 2013;14:154–219.

APA, Treatment of Patients with Bipolar Disorder. http://psychiatryonline.org/pb/assets/raw/sitewide/practice_guidelines/guidelines/bipolar.pdf (accessed 2023 Feb 21).

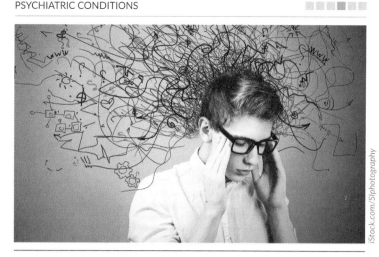

iStock.com/SIphotography

CHAPTER 65

ATTENTION DEFICIT HYPERACTIVITY DISORDER (ADHD)

BACKGROUND

ADHD is the most common neurodevelopmental disorder in children, with a higher prevalence in males compared to females. It is a chronic illness that can continue to cause symptoms throughout adolescence and adulthood.

ADHD is characterized by symptoms of inattention, hyperactivity and impulsivity. Patients often have difficulty focusing, are easily distracted, have trouble staying still and are frequently unable to control impulsive behavior. The primary presenting symptoms can vary; some individuals are more inattentive, and others are more impulsive. With increasing age, inattention and impulsivity can remain, and hyperactivity can decrease.

The pathogenesis of ADHD is not well defined, but an imbalance of catecholamine metabolism, with subsequent decreased dopaminergic activity, is thought to play a role. This is why stimulant medications (e.g., methylphenidate, amphetamine) are the primary treatment for ADHD, because they raise dopamine and norepinephrine levels.

Treatment of ADHD includes a combination of medication and behavioral therapy. The decision to medicate should be weighed against the risks, especially in young children. A child with untreated ADHD can have impaired academic standing, poor social skills and risky behavior. Medications are beneficial, but they have side effects. For this reason, first-line treatment for preschool-aged children (age 4 – 5 years) is parent training in behavior management and/or behavioral classroom intervention. Methylphenidate can be considered if moderate-severe symptoms persist despite behavioral interventions.

ADHD medications are first line in patients ≥ 6 years old and should be used with behavioral interventions when available.

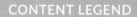

DIAGNOSTIC CRITERIA

The Diagnostic and Statistical Manual of Mental Disorders (DSM-5) provides definitions and diagnostic criteria for various mental disorders. The DSM-5 diagnostic criteria for ADHD are based on an assessment of the primary symptoms, inattention and/or hyperactivity and impulsivity, as described below.

INATTENTION

≥ 6 symptoms of inattention for children up to age 16 (≥ 5 symptoms for ages 17 and older); symptoms must have been present for at least 6 months and are inappropriate for the developmental level.

Symptoms:
Fails to pay attention, has trouble holding attention, does not pay attention when someone is talking, does not follow through on instructions, fails to finish schoolwork, has difficulty organizing tasks, avoids or dislikes tasks which require mental effort, loses things, is easily distracted, is forgetful.

HYPERACTIVITY & IMPULSIVITY

≥ 6 symptoms of hyperactivity-impulsivity for children up to age 16 (≥ 5 symptoms for ages 17 and older); symptoms must have been present for at least 6 months and are inappropriate for the developmental level.

Symptoms:
Often fidgets or squirms, leaves seat unexpectedly, runs about when not appropriate, unable to play quietly, is "on the go" as if "driven by a motor," talks excessively, blurts out answers, has trouble waiting his/her turn, interrupts or intrudes on others.

THE FOLLOWING CONDITIONS MUST BE MET:
- Several inattentive or hyperactive-impulsive symptoms were present before age 12.
- Symptoms must have been present in 2 or more settings (e.g., at home, school, work, with friends, relatives or caregivers).
- Symptoms interfere with functioning and are not caused by another disorder.

NATURAL PRODUCTS

Fish oils are increasingly used for various psychiatric conditions and may modestly improve cognitive function and behavior; however, data establishing their efficacy for ADHD is limited and they are not routinely recommended. Melatonin may be used for sleep onset insomnia in individuals taking stimulants.

DRUG TREATMENT

Stimulants are the first-line medications for ADHD. Some stimulant medications come in formulations that are easier for children to swallow (see Study Tip Gal to the right) or more difficult to abuse. Long-acting formulations are preferred for children, to help maintain more steady symptom control and avoid the need for a dose during the day at school.

A non-stimulant medication (e.g., atomoxetine, guanfacine ER) can be tried when stimulants do not work well enough (after 2 – 3 medication trials) or the side effects are intolerable. Non-stimulants can be used first line when prescribers are concerned about the possibility of stimulant abuse or diversion by the patient or family.

Almost all ADHD medications are approved for use in adults and children ≥ 6 years of age, with a few exceptions, as noted in the drug tables in this chapter.

PATIENT-FRIENDLY FORMULATIONS FOR STIMULANTS

Young children (and others) who cannot swallow capsules or tablets can use alternative long-acting formulations or capsules that can be opened, such as those listed below.

When putting capsule contents in food, use a small amount of food (do not warm the food). Eat the food right away, without chewing.

- Capsules that can be opened
  - ❑ Many long-acting capsules (e.g., *Adderall XR, Ritalin LA*) can be opened and the contents sprinkled on a small amount of applesauce
  - ❑ *Vyvanse* capsule contents can be mixed in water, orange juice or yogurt
- Chewable tablets (e.g., *Vyvanse*)
- Orally-disintegrating tablets
- Patches (e.g., *Daytrana*)
- Suspensions

RedlineVector, Kolonko/Shutterstock.com

TREATMENT OF ADHD

Stimulants are first line
(take in AM)

Methylphenidate* (e.g., *Concerta, Daytrana, Ritalin*)

Lisdexamfetamine *(Vyvanse)*

Dextroamphetamine/Amphetamine
(Adderall, Adderall XR)

Non-stimulants are second line
Atomoxetine *(Strattera)*
Viloxazine *(Qelbree)*

Add-on medications (or can be used alone)
Guanfacine ER *(Intuniv)*
Clonidine ER *(Kapvay)*

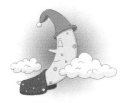

To help sleep at night
Clonidine IR
Diphenhydramine
Melatonin

Jornay PM is taken in the evening.

nicolaiivanovici/stock.adobe.com

STIMULANT SAFETY CONCERNS

All stimulants are C-II medications and must be dispensed with a MedGuide. The boxed warnings, contraindications and warnings discussed on this page are common to most stimulant drugs and will not be repeated in the stimulant drug tables that follow. Additional safety issues unique to specific products are noted in the drug tables.

Boxed Warning: Abuse, Misuse and Addiction

Stimulant medications have a high potential for abuse and dependence, which can contribute to the development of substance use disorder and addiction. The misuse of stimulants, especially unapproved administration methods (e.g., snorting, injecting), can lead to overdose and death. Risk for abuse (e.g., history of alcohol or other substance use disorder) should be assessed prior to prescribing, and symptoms of misuse (e.g., dilated pupils, increased heart rate and blood pressure, sweating, tremor, anxiety) should be monitored during treatment.

Contraindications

- Do not use within 14 days of an MAO inhibitor due to the risk of hypertensive crisis when used together.

Warnings

- The high risk of stimulant abuse and misuse (see boxed warning) can lead to drug diversion for non-medical, illicit use and/or distribution. Patients and caregivers should be counseled to store stimulant medications in a safe (ideally locked) place and properly dispose of unused drug.

- Increased levels of dopamine and norepinephrine can increase heart rate and blood pressure. This can cause serious cardiovascular events in children and adults with or without preexisting cardiac disease. Assess for cardiac disease at baseline and avoid stimulants when cardiac abnormalities are present, due to an increased risk of sudden death.

- Other vascular problems (e.g., priapism, Raynaud's disease) can occur and may require a dose reduction or discontinuation.

- New-onset psychosis or mania, or an exacerbation of preexisting psychosis (e.g., a mixed/manic episode in bipolar disorder) can occur. Caution should be used when prescribing stimulants in patients with a preexisting psychiatric condition.

- A loss of appetite is common. This is especially concerning in children, as it can contribute to a decrease in the child's growth trajectory.

- The risk of serotonin syndrome is increased when stimulants are used in combination with other serotonergic drugs (e.g., SSRIs, SNRIs, TCAs, buspirone). Refer to the Drug Interactions chapter.

- Some stimulants can lower the seizure threshold, which increases the risk for seizures.

- Visual disturbances (e.g., difficulty with accommodation and blurry vision) can occur.

STIMULANTS

Stimulants block the reuptake of norepinephrine and dopamine; they are highly effective for ADHD and are recommended first line. Most stimulants are dosed every morning (IR products and some others can be given in divided doses) with doses titrated up every seven days, as needed, to reduce adverse effects. Stimulants do not need to be tapered off when used as directed (i.e., not abused).

DRUG	DOSING	SAFETY/SIDE EFFECTS/MONITORING
Methylphenidate		
IR tablet: **Ritalin** IR oral solution: *Methylin* IR chewable tablet ER tablet ER tablet with OROS delivery: **Concerta**, *Relexxii*	Start 5 mg BID, 30 min before breakfast and lunch Max: 60 mg/day Start 18-36 mg QAM Max: 72 mg/day	See Stimulant Safety Concerns **WARNINGS** *Daytrana*: loss of skin pigmentation at application site and areas distant from the application site (can resemble vitiligo); allergic contact dermatitis with local reactions (e.g., edema, papules) *Concerta, Relexxii*: do not use with GI narrowing conditions (e.g., motility issues, small bowel disease)
ER capsule: **Ritalin LA**, *Aptensio XR, Jornay PM*	Ritalin LA: start 10-20 mg QAM Aptensio XR: start 10 mg QAM Max: 60 mg/day Jornay PM: start 20 mg QPM Max: 100 mg/day	**SIDE EFFECTS** Insomnia, ↓ appetite/weight loss, headache, irritability, nausea/vomiting, blurry vision, dry mouth **MONITORING** Consider ECG prior to treatment; monitor BP and HR, cardiac symptoms, CNS effects, abuse potential and height and weight (children)
ER oral suspension: *Quillivant XR* ER chewable tablet: *QuilliChew ER*	Start 20 mg QAM Start 20 mg QAM Max: 60 mg/day	**NOTES** OROS delivery: the outer coat dissolves fast to provide immediate action, and the rest is released slowly; can see a ghost tablet in stool; harder to crush, which decreases abuse potential
ER orally-disintegrating tablet: *Cotempla XR-ODT*	Start 17.3 mg QAM for ages 6-17 years Max: 51.8 mg/day	*Jornay PM*: outer coating delays initial drug release 10 hours to allow for evening dosing; inner coating controls the slow release of the drug during the day *Daytrana*: apply to the hip 2 hrs before desired effect (or as soon as the child awakens so it starts to deliver prior to school); remove after 9 hrs; alternate hips daily; discard used patches by flushing down the toilet
Transdermal patch: **Daytrana**	Start 10 mg/9 hr patch QAM Max: 30 mg/9 hr	Chewable tablets: contain phenylalanine (avoid with PKU)
Dexmethylphenidate		
Dexmethylphenidate (*Focalin, Focalin XR*) IR tablet, ER capsule	IR: start 2.5 mg BID, given at least 4 hrs apart Max: 20 mg/day ER: start 5 mg (children) or 10 mg (adults) QAM Max: 30 mg/day (children) or 40 mg/day (adults)	See Stimulant Safety Concerns **NOTES** Active isomer of methylphenidate; to convert from methylphenidate to dexmethylphenidate use one-half of the total daily dose of methylphenidate
Serdexmethylphenidate/Dexmethylphenidate (*Azstarys*) Capsule	Start 39.2 mg/7.8 mg QAM Max: 52.3 mg/10.4 mg daily	See Stimulant Safety Concerns **NOTES** Serdexmethylphenidate: prodrug to dexmethylphenidate, provides extended duration of action following faster-acting dexmethylphenidate

DRUG	DOSING	SAFETY/SIDE EFFECTS/MONITORING
Amphetamine, Dextroamphetamine and Combinations		
Dextroamphetamine/Amphetamine		See Stimulant Safety Concerns
IR tablet: **Adderall**	Start 5 mg QAM or BID, with 2nd dose 4-6 hrs after 1st dose Max: 40 mg/day	**NOTES** IR products approved for children ≥ 3 years of age (except *Evekeo ODT*) AAP guidelines do not recommend dextroamphetamine in children ≤ 5 years of age
ER capsules: **Adderall XR,** *Mydayis*	Start 5-10 mg (6-12 yrs), 10 mg (13-17 yrs) or 10-20 mg (adults) QAM Max: 30 mg/day (children) or 60 mg/day (adults)	ER formulations cannot be substituted for other amphetamine products on a mg-per-mg basis; follow dosing schedule provided by manufacturer *Dyanavel XR*: shake suspension prior to use Do not take with acidic foods such as juice or vitamin C (↓ absorption)
Amphetamine ER orally-disintegrating tablet: *Adzenys XR-ODT*	Start 6.3 mg (children) or 12.5 mg (adults) QAM Max: varies based on age	
ER tablet (can be chewed): *Dyanavel XR* ER oral suspension: *Dyanavel XR*	Start 2.5-5 mg QAM Max: 20 mg/day	
IR tablet: *Evekeo* IR orally-disintegrating tablet: *Evekeo ODT*	Start 5 mg QAM or BID, with 2nd dose 4-6 hrs after 1st dose (6-17 yrs) Max: 40 mg/day	
Dextroamphetamine ER capsule: *Dexedrine* IR oral solution: *ProCentra* IR tablet: *Zenzedi* ER patch: *Xelstrym*	Oral formulations: start 5 mg QAM or BID, with 2nd dose 4-6 hrs after 1st dose Max: 40 mg/day	
Lisdexamfetamine (prodrug of dextroamphetamine)		
Lisdexamfetamine (Vyvanse) Capsule, chewable tablet	Start 20-30 mg (children) or 30 mg (adults) QAM Max: 70 mg/day	See Stimulant Safety Concerns **NOTES** Low abuse potential; prodrug composed of l-lysine (amino acid) bonded to dextroamphetamine; it is hydrolyzed in the blood to active dextroamphetamine; if injected or snorted, the fast effect (rush) is muted
Methamphetamine		
Methamphetamine (*Desoxyn*) Tablet	Start 5 mg QAM or BID Max: 20-25 mg daily	See Stimulant Safety Concerns

NON-STIMULANTS

These medications are used <u>second line</u> if trials of <u>stimulant medications fail</u> or side effects are intolerable. They can be used first line if the prescriber is concerned about stimulant <u>abuse or diversion potential</u> (non-stimulant medications are not controlled and therefore do not have the same potential for abuse and dependence as stimulants).

<u>Clonidine ER</u> and <u>guanfacine ER</u> are antihypertensive drugs that are also marketed in longer-acting formulations for ADHD. They can be used <u>alone</u> or in <u>combination with stimulant</u> medications.

DRUG	DOSING	SAFETY/SIDE EFFECTS/MONITORING
Selective Norepinephrine Reuptake Inhibitors		
Atomoxetine (Strattera) Capsule	> 70 kg: start 40 mg daily ≤ 70 kg: start 0.5 mg/kg/day Max: 100 mg/day Can take in divided doses if needed (morning and late afternoon/early evening) Concurrent use of strong CYP450 2D6 inhibitors (e.g., paroxetine): max dose is 80 mg daily	**BOXED WARNINGS** Risk of <u>suicidal ideation</u>; monitor for suicidal thinking or behavior, worsening mood, or unusual behavior **CONTRAINDICATIONS** <u>MAO inhibitor use within the past 14 days</u> Atomoxetine: glaucoma, pheochromocytoma, severe cardiovascular disorders Viloxazine: concurrent use of major CYP1A2 substrates (or substrates with a narrow therapeutic index) **WARNINGS** Cardiovascular events, psychosis/mania: assess at baseline and as needed during treatment Atomoxetine: aggressive behavior, hepatotoxicity, priapism, urinary hesitancy and retention, growth delays
Viloxazine (Qelbree) Capsule	Start 100 mg daily (children < 12 years) or 200 mg daily (children ≥ 12 years and adults) Max: 400 mg/day (children < 18 years) or 600 mg/day (adults) Dose reductions required with severe renal impairment	**SIDE EFFECTS** ↓ appetite, insomnia, somnolence, dry mouth, ↑ BP, ↑ HR, headache, nausea, abdominal pain **MONITORING** BP, HR, ECG, mood, weight **NOTES** <u>Atomoxetine: do not open the capsule</u> – ocular irritant Viloxazine: capsule can be opened and contents sprinkled on 1 teaspoon of pudding or applesauce, which must be swallowed without chewing
Centrally-Acting Alpha-2 Adrenergic Receptor Agonists		
Clonidine ER (Kapvay) Tablet Clonidine IR, clonidine ER (Nexiclon XR), clonidine patch – for hypertension	Start 0.1 mg <u>QHS</u>, increase by 0.1 mg weekly and take BID (if uneven dosing, take the higher dose QHS) Max: 0.4 mg/day	**WARNINGS** <u>Dose-dependent cardiovascular effects</u> (bradycardia, hypotension, orthostasis, syncope), <u>sedation and drowsiness</u> <u>Do not discontinue abruptly</u> (can cause <u>rebound hypertension</u>) Guanfacine: skin rash (rare, discontinue if occurs); dose adjustments required with CYP3A4 inducers and inhibitors (see Drug Interactions section) **SIDE EFFECTS** <u>Dry mouth, somnolence, fatigue, dizziness, constipation, ↓ HR, hypotension,</u> headache, nausea, abdominal pain
Guanfacine ER (Intuniv) Tablet Guanfacine IR – for hypertension	Start 1 mg <u>daily</u> and increase by ≤ 1 mg weekly Max: varies based on age Do not take with high-fat meal (↑ absorption)	**MONITORING** BP, HR **NOTES** <u>Must be tapered</u> off to decrease the risk of rebound hypertension: decrease dose (≤ 0.1 mg/day for clonidine and ≤ 1 mg/day for guanfacine) every 3-7 days Do not substitute IR clonidine or guanfacine for ER formulations

Atomoxetine Drug Interactions

- Atomoxetine is a CYP2D6 substrate; CYP2D6 inducers or inhibitors can necessitate a change in atomoxetine dose.

Viloxazine Drug Interactions

- Viloxazine is a strong CYP1A2 inhibitor and a weak CYP2D6 and CYP3A4 inhibitor. Significant drug interactions can occur.

Clonidine and Guanfacine Drug Interactions

- Additive sedation can occur when used in combination with other CNS depressants.
- Use caution with other drugs that decrease blood pressure and heart rate (e.g., beta-blockers, non-DHP CCBs).
- Guanfacine:
  - ❏ Double the dose if used with strong CYP3A4 inducers.
  - ❏ Decrease the dose by 50% if used with strong CYP3A4 inhibitors.

KEY COUNSELING POINTS

See the Drug Formulations and Patient Counseling chapter for counseling language/layman's terminology and formulation-specific administration instructions.

STIMULANTS

- MedGuide required.
- Can cause abuse, misuse and addiction.
- Can cause:
  - ❏ Increased heart rate and blood pressure
  - ❏ Serious cardiovascular events
  - ❏ Insomnia
  - ❏ Psychosis
  - ❏ Priapism
- Decreased appetite: eat a larger breakfast to prevent weight loss; check height and weight regularly in children.
- Ghost tablet in stool (*Concerta*).
- Some formulations contain phenylalanine. Do not use if you have phenylketonuria (PKU).

ATOMOXETINE AND VILOXAZINE

- MedGuide required.
- Can cause:
  - ❏ Suicidal ideation
  - ❏ Increased blood pressure and heart rate

CLONIDINE ER AND GUANFACINE ER

- Do not discontinue abruptly.
- Can cause:
  - ❏ Decreased heart rate and blood pressure
  - ❏ Drowsiness
  - ❏ Dry mouth
  - ❏ Constipation

Select Guidelines/References

Diagnostic and Statistical Manual of Mental Disorders, Fifth Edition, Text Revision (DSM-5-TR). Arlington, VA, American Psychiatric Association, 2022.

Clinical Practice Guideline for the Diagnosis, Evaluation, and Treatment of Attention-Deficit/Hyperactivity Disorder in Children and Adolescents. Pediatrics 2019;144 (4):1-19.

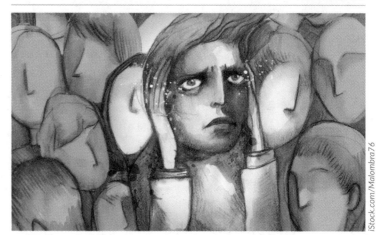

iStock.com/Malombra76

SELECT DRUGS THAT CAUSE ANXIETY

Albuterol (if used too frequently or incorrectly)

Antipsychotics (e.g., aripiprazole, haloperidol)

Bupropion

Caffeine, in high doses

Decongestants (e.g., pseudoephedrine)

Illicit drugs (e.g., cocaine, LSD, methamphetamine)

Levothyroxine (if therapeutic overdose occurs)

Steroids

Stimulants (e.g., amphetamine, methylphenidate)

Theophylline

CONTENT LEGEND

 = Study Tip Gal    = Key Drug Guy

CHAPTER 66

ANXIETY DISORDERS

BACKGROUND

The general population can experience occasional anxiety when faced with challenging issues at work, home or school. The symptoms of occasional anxiety (fear, worry) and any physical symptoms (tachycardia, palpitations, shortness of breath, stomach upset, chest pain or other pain, insomnia or fatigue) resolve once the issue is gone.

With an anxiety disorder, the symptoms are chronic, severe and cause great distress. The disorder can interfere with the ability to do well at school or work and can harm relationships. The major types of anxiety disorders are generalized anxiety disorder (GAD), panic disorder (PD) and social anxiety disorder (SAD). Other disorders that have symptoms of anxiety include obsessive-compulsive disorder (OCD) and posttraumatic stress disorder (PTSD). These are classified differently by the Diagnostic and Statistical Manual of Mental Disorders, Fifth Edition (DSM-5). OCD is categorized as "obsessive-compulsive and related disorders," and PTSD is categorized under "trauma and stressor-related disorders."

NON-DRUG TREATMENT

Patients with an anxiety disorder should be assessed for comorbid conditions (e.g., hyperthyroidism) or medications that could be contributing to the problem (see Key Drugs Guy). Comorbid conditions should be treated and medications that worsen anxiety should be discontinued if possible.

Lifestyle changes can improve symptoms. Increasing physical activity, helping others, community involvement, yoga and meditation are some of the methods that can reduce stress. Cognitive Behavioral Therapy (CBT) is a type of mental health treatment in which a trained clinician helps the patient explore patterns of thinking that lead to problem-solving, relaxation techniques, worry exposure and more. In some cases, CBT provides adequate relief without the need for chronic medications.

NATURAL PRODUCTS

Some natural products may provide benefit when treating anxiety, but their use is generally limited by safety issues. St. John's wort, used for depression and anxiety, is a strong CYP3A4 inducer and can decrease the concentration of other medications. St. John's wort also causes photosensitivity and is serotonergic, which increases the risk of serotonin syndrome when used in combination with other serotonergic medications. Valerian is used for anxiety and sleep, but some products may be contaminated with liver toxins; if used, liver function should be monitored. Passionflower appears to be safe and is rated as "possibly effective" by the *Natural Medicines Database*. Kava is a relaxant, but it can cause severe liver damage and is not recommended.

DRUG TREATMENT

A number of medications can be used long-term to manage anxiety. Some antidepressants are FDA-approved for anxiety and other drugs are used off-label. The selection of a drug is based on both the efficacy and the risk of adverse effects. The table below summarizes the first and second-line options to consider. Benzodiazepines (BZDs) should only be used short-term and are discussed in-depth later in the chapter.

Drugs Used for Anxiety

DRUG/DRUG CLASS	COMMENTS
First-Line: selective serotonin reuptake inhibitors (SSRIs) and serotonin and norepinephrine reuptake inhibitors (SNRIs)	
Escitalopram (*Lexapro*) **Fluoxetine (*Prozac*)** **Paroxetine (*Paxil*, Paxil CR, Pexeva)** **Sertraline (*Zoloft*)** **Duloxetine (*Cymbalta*, Drizalma Sprinkle)** **Venlafaxine XR (*Effexor XR*)**	Most drug dosing will start at half the initial dose used for depression and slowly titrate to minimize anxiousness and jitteriness (common during the first couple of weeks) Will not provide immediate relief; takes at least four weeks at higher doses for a noticeable effect Other SSRIs and SNRIs may be used off-label for anxiety disorder Refer to the Depression chapter for more information on antidepressants
Second-Line	
Buspirone	Can use in combination with antidepressants (e.g., when there is a poor response) Considered a more favorable add-on medication than benzodiazepines in elderly patients (less sedating) or if there is a risk for benzodiazepine abuse Does not provide immediate relief; takes 2-4 weeks for effect
Tricyclic Antidepressants **Amitriptyline** **Nortriptyline (*Pamelor*)** Imipramine	Not FDA-approved for anxiety Risk of adverse effects (e.g., anticholinergic side effects) limit use (see the Depression chapter)
Hydroxyzine (Vistaril)	Sedating antihistamine with anticholinergic activity FDA-approved for anxiety but does not treat the underlying condition Should not be used long-term; use only short-term, as needed, as an alternative to benzodiazepines See the Common Skin Conditions chapter for more information
Pregabalin (*Lyrica*, Lyrica CR) C-V **Gabapentin (*Neurontin*, Gralise)**	Not FDA-approved for anxiety but has shown benefit in patients with anxiety and neuropathic pain Has immediate anxiolytic effects similar to benzodiazepines
Special Situations	
Propranolol (*Inderal LA, Inderal XL*, others)	Not FDA-approved for anxiety but can reduce symptoms of stage fright or performance anxiety (e.g., tremor, tachycardia) Dose: 10-40 mg one hour prior to an event (such as a public speech) Can cause CNS side effects (e.g., dizziness, confusion) See Hypertension chapter for more information

BUSPIRONE

The mechanism of action of buspirone is unknown, but its effects may be due to its affinity for 5-HT1A and 5-HT2 receptors.

DRUG	DOSING	SAFETY/SIDE EFFECTS/MONITORING
Buspirone Tablet	Start 5-7.5 mg PO BID Can increase by 5 mg/day every 2-3 days, to a max dose of 30 mg PO BID Take with or without food, but must be consistent	**CONTRAINDICATIONS** Do not use with MAO inhibitors (or within 14 days of discontinuation), linezolid or IV methylene blue **WARNINGS** Risk of serotonin syndrome alone or in combination with other serotonergic drugs **SIDE EFFECTS** Dizziness, drowsiness, headache, lightheadedness, nausea, excitement **NOTES** No potential for abuse, tolerance or physiological dependence When switching from a benzodiazepine to buspirone, the benzodiazepine must be tapered off slowly Avoid use in severe kidney or liver impairment

Buspirone Drug Interactions

- Risk of serotonin syndrome is ↑ when used in combination with other serotonergic drugs. See the Drug Interactions chapter.

- Avoid grapefruit and grapefruit juice as they may ↑ buspirone levels.

- Buspirone is a major substrate of CYP3A4.

  ❑ Decrease the dose if used in combination with moderate and strong CYP3A4 inhibitors (e.g., erythromycin, diltiazem, verapamil, itraconazole).

  ❑ An increase in the buspirone dose may be required with CYP3A4 inducers (e.g., rifampin).

BENZODIAZEPINES

- BZDs enhance gamma-aminobutyric acid (GABA), an inhibitory neurotransmitter. This causes CNS depression, resulting in anxiolytic, anticonvulsant, sedative and/or muscle relaxant properties.

- They provide fast relief of symptoms (antidepressants have a longer onset of action), but they do not treat the underlying causes of anxiety.

- BZDs can be useful for short-term treatment of acute anxiety that is preventing restful sleep and disrupting life. This can be due to the recent death of a loved one, a natural disaster or another stressful situation.

- If taken long-term, patients can become addicted to BZDs and develop tolerance. Due to the risk of dependence, they should only be used for 1 – 2 weeks and then discontinued. If used for longer periods of time, they must be tapered off slowly to prevent withdrawal symptoms.

- Beers Criteria: BZDs are potentially inappropriate in patients ≥ 65 years old. BZDs have a high risk of confusion, dizziness and falls in the elderly, which is increased if used with other CNS depressants. The elderly also have a higher risk of having a "paradoxical" reaction (hyperactivity, aggression, agitation). If a BZD is used in an elderly patient, the L-O-T drugs (see Study Tip Gal) are preferred due to the lower risk of adverse reactions. Lorazepam and oxazepam are indicated for anxiety; temazepam is used for insomnia.

SAFE USE OF BENZODIAZEPINES

Benzodiazepines (BZDs) are highly sedating and often not preferred due to safety concerns

Anxiety
- Most anxiety is due to depression; SSRIs and SNRIs are preferred
- If used, consider a BZD with a longer half-life and less risk of abuse (e.g., clonazepam, lorazepam, diazepam)

Sleep
- First-line: non-pharmacologic treatment
- Second-line: non-BZD hypnotics, like zolpidem (fewer safety issues than BZDs)
- If used, consider temazepam

Elderly or Patients with Liver Impairment
- If used, consider BZDs that undergo glucuronidation; **L-O-T** drugs (**L**orazepam, **O**xazepam, **T**emazepam)

Seizures
- Injectable BZDs or diazepam rectal gel (*Diastat AcuDial*); diazepam rectal gel can be administered by a caregiver at home

DRUG	DOSING	SAFETY/SIDE EFFECTS/MONITORING
Alprazolam (Xanax, Xanax XR, Alprazolam Intensol) Tablet, ODT, oral solution	0.25-0.5 mg PO TID	**BOXED WARNING** Use with opioids can result in sedation, respiratory depression, coma and death Risk for abuse, misuse and addiction, which can lead to overdose or death
Clonazepam (Klonopin) Tablet, ODT	0.25-0.5 mg PO BID	Continued use can lead to physical dependence; abrupt discontinuation can cause withdrawal symptoms (taper off slowly)
Diazepam (Valium, Diastat AcuDial, Diazepam Intensol) Tablet, injection, oral solution, rectal gel, intranasal	2-10 mg PO BID-QID	**CONTRAINDICATIONS** Acute narrow-angle glaucoma, sleep apnea, severe respiratory insufficiency, severe liver disease (clonazepam and diazepam), myasthenia gravis (diazepam), not for use in infants < 6 months of age (diazepam oral), premature infants (lorazepam parenteral products)
Lorazepam (Ativan, Lorazepam Intensol, Loreev XR) Tablet, injection, oral solution	2-3 mg PO daily in divided doses	**WARNINGS** CNS depression, anterograde amnesia, potential for abuse, safety risks in patients age 65 years and older (impaired cognition, delirium, falls/fractures), extravasation with IV use, paradoxical reactions, severe renal or hepatic impairment Pregnancy: crosses placenta; can cause birth defects and neonatal withdrawal syndrome
Chlordiazepoxide Capsule	5-25 mg TID-QID	**SIDE EFFECTS** Somnolence, dizziness, ataxia, weakness, lightheadedness **NOTES** C-IV
Clorazepate (Tranxene) Tablet	30 mg PO daily in divided doses	Diazepam: lipophilic, fast onset, long half-life, high abuse potential Alprazolam: fast onset, often abused due to its quick action Commonly used for alcohol withdrawal syndrome: lorazepam, diazepam, chlordiazepoxide
Oxazepam Capsule	10-30 mg PO TID-QID	Midazolam (Versed) used in acute care (see the Acute & Critical Care Medicine chapter) Antidote: flumazenil (refer to the Toxicology & Antidotes chapter)

Benzodiazepine Drug Interactions

- Additive effects with CNS depressants (e.g., alcohol, anticonvulsants, antihistamines, antipsychotics, opioids, mirtazapine, skeletal muscle relaxants, trazodone).

- Diazepam, clonazepam, chlordiazepoxide and clorazepate: use cautiously with CYP3A4 inhibitors.

- Alprazolam is contraindicated with strong CYP3A4 inhibitors (e.g., ketoconazole, itraconazole). Use caution with moderate CYP3A4 inhibitors.

- Valproate increases the serum concentration of lorazepam.

KEY COUNSELING POINTS

See the Drug Formulations and Patient Counseling chapter for counseling language/layman's terminology.

BUSPIRONE

- The tablets are scored to easily break in half or into thirds.
- Can cause:
  - ❏ Dizziness.
  - ❏ Drowsiness.
  - ❏ Nausea.

- Do not use with opioid medications (can cause profound sedation, respiratory depression, coma and death).

- Do not use with alcohol (can increase risk of CNS depression).

BENZODIAZEPINES

- If used regularly for > 10 days, do not stop suddenly. Taper off slowly to avoid withdrawal symptoms (e.g., anxiety, shakiness, fast heart rate, difficulty sleeping, muscle pain).

- To reduce the risk of addiction, do not take doses more frequently or for a longer period than prescribed.

- Can cause drowsiness.

Select Guidelines/References
American Psychiatric Association: Diagnostic and Statistical Manual of Mental Disorders, Fifth Edition. Arlington VA, American Psychiatric Association, 2013.

Locke AB, Kirst N, Shultz CG. Diagnosis and management of generalized anxiety disorder and panic disorder in adults. *Am Fam Physician* 2015;91:617-624.

Anxiety and Depression Association of America. Clinical practice review for GAD. Revised 2015. https://adaa.org/resources-professionals/practice-guidelines-gad (accessed 2023 Feb 24).

iStock.com/OcusFocus

CHAPTER 67

SLEEP DISORDERS

BACKGROUND

There are several types of sleep disorders. This chapter discusses types managed with medications: chronic insomnia, restless legs syndrome (RLS) and narcolepsy. Another common sleep disorder is obstructive sleep apnea, which is primarily treated with non-drug measures, including continuous positive airway pressure (CPAP).

A lack of restful sleep contributes to poor health and is linked to the development of a number of chronic conditions, including cardiovascular disease, mood disorders, alcohol use disorder and depression. Patients who chronically use OTC medications for sleep should be referred to a healthcare provider.

CHRONIC INSOMNIA

Insomnia is characterized by difficulty falling asleep (sleep initiation or sleep latency), reduced sleep duration and/or poor sleep quality (e.g., awakenings after sleep onset). A diagnosis of chronic insomnia occurs when the patient has symptoms at least three times per week for at least three months, despite adequate opportunity to sleep. This often causes daytime impairment, such as being absent from work or experiencing accidents due to fatigue, somnolence, poor memory and decreased concentration.

NON-DRUG TREATMENT

Cognitive behavioral therapy for chronic insomnia (CBT-I) is preferred and includes changes to sleep hygiene that can reduce the need for drugs (see the flow diagram on the following page).

It is important to treat any underlying medical conditions that may be contributing (e.g., pain, shortness of breath due to heart failure, anxiety, bipolar disorder, depression, alcohol use disorder) and discontinue medications that can worsen insomnia (see Key Drugs Guy on next page), if possible.

NATURAL PRODUCTS

Melatonin (1 – 5 mg in the evening) is commonly used for insomnia and is also used for jet lag. It can cause additive adverse effects (e.g., drowsiness, daytime somnolence) if used with other CNS depressants. Melatonin is a substrate of CYP450 1A2, and prolonged effects may be observed with CYP1A2 inhibitors (e.g., ciprofloxacin, fluvoxamine). Valerian and kava are not recommended due to a risk of hepatotoxicity. Drinking chamomile tea in the evening to feel calmer can help some patients with insomnia.

DRUG TREATMENT

Sedative-hypnotics are the mainstay of treatment for chronic insomnia, though it is preferable to reserve use for when non-drug treatments have failed, and to select drugs with the best evidence for sleep onset and/or sleep maintenance depending on the problem identified (see diagram below).

SELECT DRUGS THAT CAN WORSEN INSOMNIA

Acetylcholinesterase inhibitors (e.g., donepezil)

Alcohol

Aripiprazole

Atomoxetine

Bupropion

Caffeine

Decongestants (e.g., pseudoephedrine)

Diuretics (due to nocturia)

Fluoxetine, if taken late in the day

Nicotine (including nicotine replacement therapy)

Integrase strand transfer inhibitors (INSTIs)

Steroids

Stimulants (e.g., methylphenidate, phentermine)

Varenicline

Guideline Recommendations for Chronic Insomnia

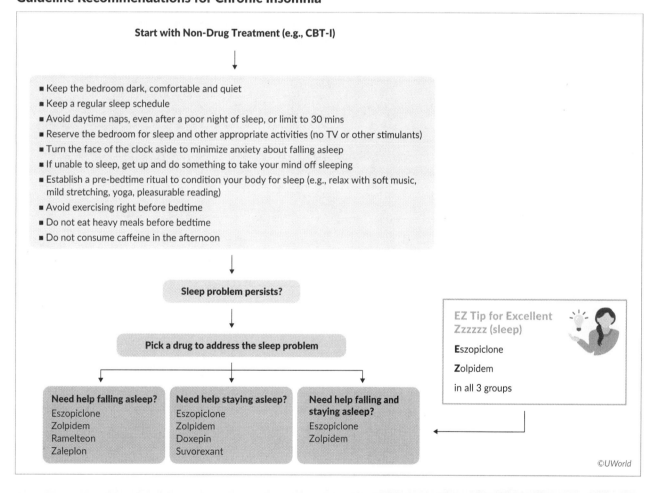

©UWorld

CASE SCENARIO

A 55-year-old female comes to the clinic and reports difficulty falling asleep, which impairs her ability to concentrate at work. She wakes up and stares at the clock throughout the night and takes extra naps during the day to compensate for lost sleep.

Patient Counseling: improve sleep hygiene by turning the face of the clock away and reducing naps. Consider additional CBT-I and follow up in 2–4 weeks to determine if pharmacotherapy is warranted.

In patients using pharmacotherapy long-term, non-benzodiazepines are preferred over benzodiazepines due to a decreased risk of physical dependence and fewer daytime cognitive effects. The lowest effective dose should be used for all medications to minimize adverse effects, and treatment should be limited to the shortest duration possible.

Patients may self-treat insomnia with OTC first-generation antihistamines, such as diphenhydramine or doxylamine. While these can help short-term, they should not be used long-term for the treatment of insomnia. The American Academy of Sleep Medicine (AASM) guidelines state that the following treatments are not recommended for chronic use: diphenhydramine, melatonin, trazodone and valerian.

Benzodiazepines (e.g., temazepam) can be used for short-term insomnia (e.g., caused by an acute trauma) if there is no substance abuse history or current use of opioids. According to the Beers Criteria, benzodiazepines, non-benzodiazepine hypnotics (e.g., zolpidem) and first-generation antihistamines are considered potentially inappropriate in patients aged 65 years and older. If benzodiazepines are used, lorazepam, oxazepam or temazepam (L-O-T) are preferred in older adults due to the lower risk of adverse reactions; see the Anxiety Disorders chapter for more details.

Hypnotics

Non-benzodiazepine hypnotics act selectively at benzodiazepine receptors to increase GABA, an inhibitory neurotransmitter. This causes CNS depression.

DRUG	DOSING	SAFETY/SIDE EFFECTS/MONITORING
Eszopiclone (Lunesta) C-IV	1-3 mg PO QHS	**BOXED WARNINGS** Complex sleep behavior (e.g., sleep-walking, sleep-driving, engaging in other activities while not fully awake) can lead to serious injury or death **CONTRAINDICATIONS** History of complex sleep behavior
Zolpidem C-IV **Ambien, Ambien CR** IR and ER tablets **Edluar** SL tablets	*Ambien, Edluar:* Female/older adult: 5 mg PO/SL QHS Male: 5-10 mg PO/SL QHS *Ambien CR:* Female/older adult: 6.25 mg PO QHS Male: 6.25-12.5 mg PO QHS	**WARNINGS** ↑ risk of CNS depression and next-day impairment with < 7-8 hours of sleep (especially with higher doses or coadministration of CNS depressants, including alcohol), abnormal thinking and behavioral changes, worsening depression, respiratory depression Potential for abuse and dependence (can cause withdrawal symptoms if used longer than 2 weeks) **SIDE EFFECTS** Somnolence, dizziness, ataxia, headache, lightheadedness, "pins and needles" feeling on the skin
Zaleplon (*Sonata*) C-IV	5-20 mg PO QHS	Eszopiclone: dysgeusia (altered sense of taste) **NOTES** Preferred over benzodiazepines for first-line treatment due to ↓ abuse, dependence and tolerance Do not take with fatty food, a heavy meal (delays onset of action) or alcohol

Eszopiclone, Zaleplon and Zolpidem Drug Interactions

- Use caution in combination with potent CYP3A4 inhibitors (e.g., protease inhibitors, ketoconazole, itraconazole, erythromycin, clarithromycin).
- Additive effects when used with other sedating drugs, including most pain medications, muscle relaxants, antihistamines, mirtazapine, trazodone and alcohol.

Orexin Receptor Antagonists

The orexin neuropeptide signaling system promotes wakefulness. Orexin receptor antagonists block the orexin neuropeptide signaling system, resulting in drowsiness. These medications are major CYP3A4 substrates; use caution and implement recommended dose reductions if used with CYP3A4 inhibitors.

DRUG	DOSING	SAFETY/SIDE EFFECTS/MONITORING
Daridorexant (Quviviq) C-IV	25-50 mg PO QHS	**CONTRAINDICATIONS** Narcolepsy **WARNINGS** Worsening depression/suicidal ideation, sleep paralysis, hallucinations, cataplexy-like
Lemborexant (DayVigo) C-IV	5-10 mg PO QHS	symptoms (sudden loss of muscle tone), complex sleep behavior, daytime impairment (risk ↑ if used with other CNS depressants) **SIDE EFFECTS** Somnolence, headache, dizziness, abnormal dreams
Suvorexant (Belsomra) C-IV	5-20 mg PO QHS	**NOTES** Onset of action delayed if taken with a meal Not recommended in patients with severe hepatic impairment Do not take if < 7 hours of sleep remaining

Melatonin Receptor Agonists

These drugs are agonists at MT1 and MT2 melatonin receptors. They promote sleepiness and regulate the circadian rhythm to coordinate the sleep-wake cycle.

DRUG	DOSING	SAFETY/SIDE EFFECTS/MONITORING
Ramelteon (Rozerem)	8 mg PO QHS	**WARNING** Ramelteon: complex sleep behavior **SIDE EFFECTS** Somnolence, dizziness
Tasimelteon (Hetlioz, Hetlioz LQ) Capsule, oral suspension	20 mg PO QHS	**NOTES** Not a controlled substance Do not take with fatty food Do not take with fluvoxamine (a strong CYP1A2 inhibitor that increases ramelteon and tasimelteon serum concentrations)

Tricyclic Antidepressant

Tricyclic antidepressants inhibit norepinephrine and serotonin reuptake. They also block acetylcholine and histamine receptors, which contributes to side effects (e.g., somnolence). *Silenor* is a branded formulation of doxepin that is FDA-approved for insomnia.

DRUG	DOSING	SAFETY/SIDE EFFECTS/MONITORING
Doxepin (Silenor)	3-6 mg PO QHS 3 mg if ≥ 65 years	**BOXED WARNING** Increase in suicidal thoughts or actions in some children, teenagers or young adults within the first few months of treatment or when the dose is changed (see the Depression chapter) **CONTRAINDICATIONS** Use within 2 weeks of an MAO inhibitor, narrow angle glaucoma, severe urinary retention **WARNING** Complex sleep behavior **SIDE EFFECTS** Seizures, somnolence, anticholinergic effects

Benzodiazepines

These drugs enhance GABA, an inhibitory neurotransmitter, causing CNS depression. A brief summary of the drugs that are FDA-indicated for insomnia is provided below; consult the Anxiety Disorders chapter for a full discussion of benzodiazepines.

DRUG	DOSING	SAFETY/SIDE EFFECTS/MONITORING
Temazepam (*Restoril*) C-IV	7.5-30 mg PO QHS	**BOXED WARNINGS** Use with opioids can result in sedation, respiratory depression, coma and death Risk for abuse, misuse and addiction, which can lead to overdose or death
Estazolam C-IV	0.5-2 mg PO QHS	Continued use can lead to physical dependence; abrupt discontinuation can cause life-threatening withdrawal symptoms (taper off slowly) **CONTRAINDICATIONS** Pregnancy, due to observed teratogenicity
Quazepam (*Doral*) C-IV	7.5-15 mg PO QHS	Triazolam: do not use with strong CYP3A4 inhibitors (e.g., azole antifungals, protease inhibitors)
Flurazepam C-IV	15-30 mg PO QHS	**WARNINGS** Complex sleep behaviors (e.g., sleep-driving), abnormal thinking and behavioral changes, worsening depression
Triazolam (*Halcion*) C-IV	0.125-0.5 mg PO QHS	**SIDE EFFECTS** Drowsiness, dizziness/↑ fall risk, cognitive impairment **NOTES** Lorazepam, oxazepam and temazepam (L-O-T) are preferred for older patients; temazepam can be used for sleep; lorazepam and oxazepam are indicated for anxiety

Antihistamines

These drugs block H1 histamine receptors.

DRUG	DOSING	SAFETY/SIDE EFFECTS/MONITORING
Diphenhydramine (*Benadryl*) Rx and OTC	25-50 mg PO QHS	**SIDE EFFECTS** Sedation (tolerance to sedative effects can develop after 10 days of use), confusion (can exacerbate memory/cognition difficulty), seizures (high dose, older adults) Paradoxical excitation in young children; do not use doxylamine in children < 12 years Peripheral anticholinergic side effects: dry mouth, urinary retention, dry eyes/blurry vision, constipation
Doxylamine (*Unisom SleepTabs*, Sleep Aid) OTC	25 mg PO QHS	**NOTES** Avoid use in BPH (can worsen symptoms) and glaucoma (can elevate IOP) Avoid in older adults (Beers Criteria) due to confusion, dizziness, risk of falls and hypotension Risk of mix-up; some OTC *Unisom* branded-products contain diphenhydramine

RESTLESS LEGS SYNDROME

Restless legs syndrome (RLS) is an urge to move the lower legs, which is sometimes described as a "creeping" sensation. It is worse at night and relieved with movement. RLS is thought to be due to a dysfunction of dopamine.

DRUG TREATMENT

The primary treatment of RLS includes dopamine agonists and the anticonvulsant gabapentin. Pramipexole and ropinirole are dopamine agonists primarily used for Parkinson disease (PD). For RLS, the immediate-release (IR) formulations are taken 1 – 3 hours before bedtime. Rotigotine (*Neupro*) is a dopamine agonist patch that is applied once daily.

Gabapentin enacarbil (*Horizant*) is an extended-release form of gabapentin approved for RLS. It is taken at ~5:00 PM daily. The IR formulation of gabapentin is used off-label as a less expensive alternative. Refer to the Parkinson Disease chapter for additional information on the dopamine agonists and the Seizures/Epilepsy chapter for additional information on gabapentin.

NARCOLEPSY

Narcolepsy is <u>excessive daytime sleepiness with cataplexy</u> (sudden loss of muscle tone) and sleep paralysis. Narcolepsy causes sudden daytime "sleep attacks" due to poor control of normal sleep-wake cycles. The sleep attacks last a few seconds to several minutes. Patients with narcolepsy have difficulty managing daily activities; they can fall asleep while at work, school or in the middle of a conversation. Sleep quality at night is poor.

DRUG TREATMENT

Narcolepsy is treated with <u>stimulants</u>, such as <u>modafinil</u> or armodafinil, and/or <u>sodium oxybate</u>. Several of the stimulants used for ADHD have an indication for narcolepsy, including <u>dextroamphetamine, dextroamphetamine/amphetamine</u> and various <u>methylphenidate</u> formulations.

Stimulants for Narcolepsy

DRUG	DOSING	SAFETY/SIDE EFFECTS/MONITORING
Modafinil (Provigil) C-IV	200 mg PO QAM	**WARNINGS** Use caution in patients with pre-existing cardiac, hepatic, renal or psychiatric conditions
Armodafinil (Nuvigil) R-isomer of modafinil C-IV	150-250 mg PO QAM	Severe <u>rash, can be life-threatening</u> (e.g., Stevens-Johnson syndrome) **SIDE EFFECTS** Headache, insomnia, anxiety, nausea

Sodium Oxybate

These drugs are <u>derived from GABA</u>. They help with sleep at night and are generally used with daytime stimulants.

DRUG	DOSING	SAFETY/SIDE EFFECTS/MONITORING
Sodium oxybate (Xyrem, Lumryz) Calcium, magnesium, potassium and sodium oxybates (Xywav) Oral liquid <u>C-III</u> (narcolepsy) C-I (illicit use)	Start 4.5 grams PO QHS; Xyrem and Xywav doses are divided into one dose QHS and one dose 2.5-4 hours later Titrate to effect; dosing range ~6-9 grams/night Dilute with water; take at least 2 hours after eating; lie down immediately after taking and stay in bed; sleep onset typically occurs within 5-15 minutes after the first dose	**BOXED WARNINGS** Strong CNS depressant; respiratory depression, coma and death can result; risk is increased when taken with other CNS depressants The active moiety of oxybate salts is the sedative GHB, which is used illicitly and sometimes to facilitate <u>sexual assault</u> (due to its rapid onset and amnestic effects); to reduce the risk of abuse, these drugs are only available <u>through REMS programs</u> **CONTRAINDICATIONS** Use with sedative-hypnotics or alcohol **WARNINGS** Depression, suicide, psychosis, anxiety, sleepwalking **SIDE EFFECTS** Dizziness, confusion, nausea **NOTES** Xyrem, Lumryz: high sodium content; limiting dietary sodium intake may be required

Other Oral Medications for Narcolepsy

DRUG	SAFETY/SIDE EFFECTS/MONITORING
Pitolisant *(Wakix)* Histamine-3 receptor antagonist/inverse agonist	**CONTRAINDICATIONS** Severe hepatic impairment **WARNINGS** QT prolongation **SIDE EFFECTS** Insomnia, nausea, anxiety, headache
Solriamfetol *(Sunosi)* Dopamine and norepinephrine reuptake inhibitor (DNRI)	**CONTRAINDICATIONS** Concomitant use with MAO inhibitors or within 14 days of discontinuation **WARNINGS** Increase in blood pressure and heart rate, psychiatric symptoms (e.g., anxiety, irritability) **SIDE EFFECTS** Headache, nausea, decreased appetite, insomnia, anxiety

KEY COUNSELING POINTS

See the Drug Formulations and Patient Counseling chapter for counseling language/layman's terminology.

Non-Benzodiazepine Hypnotics and Orexin Receptor Antagonists

- Can cause:
  - Drowsiness, lightheadedness, dizziness and headache. You may still feel drowsy the day after taking this medication. Use caution when driving a car or operating dangerous machinery.
  - Abnormal thoughts and behavior (e.g., more outgoing or aggressive behavior than usual, confusion, agitation, hallucinations, worsening depression, suicidal thoughts or actions).
  - Withdrawal symptoms (e.g., sweating, shakiness, cramps, nausea) if abruptly stopped.
- This medication is a federally controlled substance (C-IV) because it can be abused or lead to dependence. Keep the bottle in a safe place to prevent misuse and abuse.

Antihistamines

- Can cause anticholinergic effects.

Stimulants

- Take in the morning to avoid difficulty falling asleep at night.

Select Guidelines/References

Clinical practice guideline for the pharmacologic treatment of chronic insomnia in adults: an American Academy of Sleep Medicine clinical practice guideline. *J Clin Sleep Med.* 2017;13(2):307-349.

Practice guideline summary: Treatment of restless legs syndrome in adults: Report of the American Academy of Neurology. *Neurology.* 2016;87:2585-2593.

Treatment of central disorders of hypersomnolence: an American Academy of Sleep Medicine clinical practice guideline. *J Clin Sleep Med.* 2021;17(9):1881–1893.

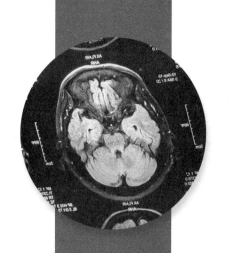
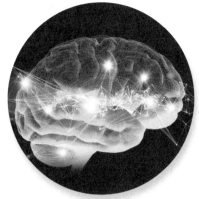
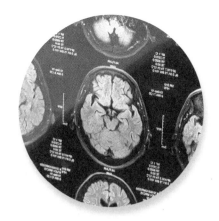

NEUROLOGIC CONDITIONS

CONTENTS

Stooped posture

Masked Face

Back rigidity

Forward tilt of trunk

Flexed elbows
and wrists

Reduced arm swing

Hand tremor

Tremors
in the legs

Slightly flexed
hip and knees

Shuffling, short
stepped gait

iStock.com/ttsz

CHAPTER 68
PARKINSON DISEASE

BACKGROUND

Parkinson disease (PD) is a degenerative neurological disorder. It usually develops after age 65, but 15% of cases are diagnosed under age 50. PD occurs when neurons die in the basal ganglia, which includes the substantia nigra, striatum and thalamus. The cause of neuronal death is multi-factorial but not well understood. These cells produce the neurotransmitter dopamine (DA), which enables smooth, coordinated muscle function and movement. PD motor symptoms appear when ~80% of the dopamine-producing cells are damaged (see Study Tip Gal).

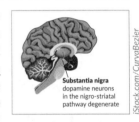

Substantia nigra
dopamine neurons
in the nigro-striatal
pathway degenerate

iStock.com/CurvaBezier

PARKINSON DISEASE SYMPTOMS

Pathophysiology:
Less dopamine → less instructions to the brain → movement problems referred to as "**TRAP**"

TRAP Major Symptoms:

Tremor: when resting

Rigidity: in legs, arms, trunk and face (mask-like face)

Akinesia/bradykinesia: lack of/ slow start in movement

Postural instability: imbalance, falls

Additional Symptoms:

Small, cramped handwriting (micrographia)

Shuffling walk, stooped posture

Muffled speech, drooling, dysphagia

Depression, anxiety (psychosis in advanced disease)

Constipation, incontinence

Tremor is often the first noticeable symptom, and usually starts in one hand or foot (on just one side, unilateral) and eventually spreads to both sides (bilateral). *Resting* tremor means it appears when the hand is not moving, such as when a person's hand is resting in their lap.

Medications can cause similar symptoms, and can mimic PD or make PD worse (see Key Drugs Guy on the following page). The Abnormal Involuntary Movement Scale (AIMS) can be used to measure involuntary movements (e.g., tardive dyskinesias) from medications.

CONTENT LEGEND

💡 = Study
     Tip Gal

⚷ = Key Drug
     Guy

834

DOPAMINE BLOCKING DRUGS THAT CAN WORSEN PD

- Phenothiazines (e.g., prochlorperazine) used for psychosis, nausea, agitation

- Butyrophenones (e.g., haloperidol, droperidol) used for psychosis and behavior disorders or nausea

- First and second-generation antipsychotics (e.g., risperidone at higher doses, paliperidone); lowest risk with quetiapine

- Metoclopramide, a renally-cleared drug that can accumulate in older adults

Non-motor symptoms can precede motor symptoms and may appear much earlier in the disease process. These include a loss of smell (anosmia), constipation, sleep difficulties, low mood/depression and orthostasis.

Even with high doses of PD drugs and various combinations, the disease will progress, including extended periods of "off time." This is when symptoms of the disease worsen before the next dose of medication is due. An "off" episode, with muscle stiffness, slow movements and difficulty starting movement, is one of the most frustrating aspects of living with the disease. Symptoms can progress to severe disability, and patients can lose the ability to walk, feed themselves and swallow food.

RELATED PSYCHIATRIC CONDITIONS

Patients with PD have a high incidence of depression. SSRIs or SNRIs are commonly used for treatment, though there is some concern that they may contribute to tremor or an increased risk of serotonin syndrome in patients who are taking other serotonergic drugs. Tricyclic antidepressants, preferably secondary amines (e.g., desipramine and nortriptyline), and the dopamine agonist pramipexole (reported to provide antidepressant effects) are other options.

Psychosis can occur with advanced disease or can be due to side effects of drug treatment. Quetiapine is the preferred antipsychotic due to a low risk of movement disorders, but it can cause metabolic complications (e.g., increased cholesterol and blood glucose). Clozapine has a low risk of worsening movement disorders but has a high risk of seizures, agranulocytosis (requires frequent monitoring and reporting of white blood cells) and other serious complications. Pimavanserin (Nuplazid), a 5-HT2A/2C receptor inverse agonist, is FDA-approved to treat hallucinations and delusions in PD. Refer to the Schizophrenia/Psychosis chapter for a discussion of antipsychotic drugs.

Abrupt withdrawal of levodopa or dopamine agonists can lead to a condition similar to neuroleptic malignant syndrome (NMS), which is a life-threatening condition sometimes seen with antipsychotics. These medications must be slowly tapered when discontinued to prevent NMS.

DRUG TREATMENT

Medications are used to improve movement, which also helps related issues (e.g., psychosis, constipation); these drug treatments either mimic dopamine, increase dopamine or decrease acetylcholine (since dopamine depletion triggers an excess of acetylcholine); see Study Tip Gal below. Levodopa, a prodrug of dopamine, is the most effective agent. Carbidopa is given with levodopa (such as in the combination product Sinemet) to prevent the breakdown of levodopa outside of the CNS (i.e., peripheral metabolism), which would destroy most of the drug before it crosses the blood-brain barrier. It is important to provide the right amount of carbidopa without causing excess side effects (see the drug table on the following page). Carbidopa/levodopa may be better tolerated than dopamine agonists for initial treatment in older adults.

Dopamine agonists are eventually used in most patients. As the disease progresses, treatment goals include reducing "off" periods and limiting dyskinesias (abnormal movement). This will require the use of multiple drug classes, such as catechol-o-methyltransferase (COMT) inhibitors and MAO-B inhibitors.

Centrally-acting anticholinergics (e.g., benztropine) treat PD by reducing acetylcholine activity within the CNS, which reduces motor symptoms; these are used for tremor-predominant disease in younger patients. The considerable side effects of these drugs make them difficult to use in older adults; the Beers criteria for potentially inappropriate medication use in older adults recommends to avoid use. Amantadine, or a selective monoamine oxidase (MAO) inhibitor, are other options for initial treatment of tremor. Note that for PD, selective MAO inhibitors are used; the non-selective inhibitors that are used for depression are contraindicated with dopaminergic drugs because they would block drug metabolism.

Amantadine can be useful to help with dyskinesias, in addition to tremor. Apomorphine treats severe "freezing" episodes that usually occur in more advanced disease, but it requires subcutaneous (SC) administration, has worrisome side effects and only improves movement ability for about an hour. Droxidopa (Northera) is a newer drug indicated for orthostatic hypotension, which can affect PD patients.

PARKINSON DISEASE TREATMENT PRINCIPLES

Primary treatment: replace dopamine
✓ Give a drug that mimics dopamine (e.g., dopamine agonist).
✓ Give a drug that increases dopamine (e.g., levodopa +/- COMT inhibitor).
✓ Give other drugs for specific symptoms (e.g., anticholinergics for resting tremor).

DOPAMINE REPLACEMENT DRUGS & AGONISTS

DRUG	DOSING	SAFETY/SIDE EFFECTS/MONITORING
Carbidopa/levodopa: levodopa is a <u>precursor</u> of <u>dopamine</u>. Carbidopa <u>inhibits the dopa decarboxylase enzyme</u>, preventing peripheral <u>metabolism</u> of levodopa.		

DRUG	DOSING	SAFETY/SIDE EFFECTS/MONITORING
Carbidopa/Levodopa IR tablet, ER tablet, ODT ***Sinemet*** Tablet ***Dhivy*** Scored IR tablet to facilitate titration ***Rytary*** ER capsule ***Duopa*** Enteral suspension given via J-tube ***Inbrija*** Levodopa capsule for oral inhaler, used as needed for symptoms during off periods	<u>Titrate cautiously</u> IR (starting dose): <u>25/100 mg PO TID</u> ER (starting dose): 50/200 mg PO BID <u>ER tab can be cut in half</u> – do not crush or chew *Rytary*: start at 23.75/95 mg PO TID if levodopa-naive; <u>take whole or sprinkle</u> on a small amount of applesauce *Inbrija*: 84 mg (2 capsules) inhaled up to 5 times daily as needed, max dose: 420 mg/day	**CONTRAINDICATIONS** <u>Non-selective MAO inhibitors</u> (e.g., phenelzine, isocarboxazid) within 14 days, narrow angle glaucoma **SIDE EFFECTS** <u>Nausea, dizziness, orthostasis, dyskinesias, hallucinations, psychosis</u>, xerostomia (dry mouth), dystonias (occasional, painful), confusion <u>Can cause brown, black or dark</u> discoloring of <u>urine</u>, saliva or sweat and can discolor clothing; positive <u>Coombs test: discontinue drug (hemolysis risk)</u>; <u>unusual sexual urges, priapism</u>; ↑ uric acid *Rytary*: suicidal ideation and attempts *Duopa*: GI complications **NOTES** <u>70-100 mg/day of carbidopa required</u> to inhibit dopa decarboxylase <u>Long-term</u> use can lead to <u>fluctuations</u> in response and <u>dyskinesias</u> Separate from oral iron and high protein foods <u>Do not discontinue abruptly</u>; must be tapered *Duopa* cassettes: store in freezer, thaw in refrigerator prior to dispensing (good for 12 weeks upon refrigeration)

DRUG	DOSING	SAFETY/SIDE EFFECTS/MONITORING
COMT inhibitors: <u>increase the duration of action of levodopa</u>; <u>inhibit the enzyme catechol-O-methyltransferase (COMT)</u> to prevent peripheral conversion of levodopa. COMT inhibitors should <u>only</u> be used <u>with levodopa</u>.		

DRUG	DOSING	SAFETY/SIDE EFFECTS/MONITORING
Entacapone (*Comtan*) + carbidopa/levodopa (*Stalevo*)	<u>200 mg PO with each dose</u> of carbidopa/levodopa (Max = 1,600 mg/day) *Stalevo*: carbidopa/levodopa in a ratio of 1:4 with 200 mg of entacapone in each tablet (example: 12.5/50/200 mg)	**SIDE EFFECTS** Similar to levodopa, due to extending its duration **NOTES** ↓ in levodopa dose of 10-30% is usually necessary when adding on a COMT inhibitor Dyskinesias can occur earlier with COMT inhibitors Tolcapone: rarely used due to hepatotoxicity risk
Opicapone (*Ongentys*)	50 mg PO QHS Dose ↓ needed in liver disease	
Tolcapone (*Tasmar*)		

DRUG	DOSING	SAFETY/SIDE EFFECTS/MONITORING
Dopamine agonists: act <u>similar to dopamine</u> at the <u>dopamine receptor</u>.		

DRUG	DOSING	SAFETY/SIDE EFFECTS/MONITORING
Pramipexole (*Mirapex*, Mirapex ER*) IR formulation also approved for restless legs syndrome (RLS)	IR: start with 0.125 mg PO TID, titrate weekly to max of 1.5 mg TID ER: start with 0.375 mg PO daily, titrate weekly to max of 4.5 mg daily ↓ dose if CrCl < 50 mL/min (90% renally excreted)	**WARNINGS** <u>Somnolence</u> (including <u>sudden daytime sleep attacks</u>), <u>orthostasis, hallucinations, dyskinesias</u>, impulse control disorders Rotigotine patch: <u>application site (skin) reactions</u> Pramipexole: postural deformity (e.g., bent spine, dropped head), rhabdomyolysis **SIDE EFFECTS** Dizziness, nausea, vomiting, dry mouth, peripheral edema, constipation Rotigotine: hyperhidrosis
Ropinirole (*Requip XL**) IR formulation also approved for RLS	IR: start with 0.25 mg PO TID, titrate weekly to max of 8 mg TID XL: start with 2 mg PO daily, titrate weekly to max of 24 mg daily	**NOTES** A slow titration (no more than weekly) is required to avoid withdrawal symptoms (e.g., anxiety, depression, insomnia, sweating); <u>do not discontinue abruptly</u> Ropinirole: CYP450 1A2 substrate; caution with CYP1A2 inhibitors Bromocriptine is another drug in the class that is no longer recommended
Rotigotine (*Neupro*) Patch Also approved for RLS	Patch: start with 2 mg/24 hrs (early PD) Max dose: 8 mg/24 hours	**Patch** Apply <u>once daily</u> at the same time each day to the stomach, thigh, hip, side of the body, shoulder or upper arm; do <u>not</u> use the <u>same site</u> for at least <u>14 days</u> Remove the patch before an MRI; avoid if sensitivity/allergy to <u>sulfites</u>

*Brand discontinued but name still used in practice.

DRUG	DOSING	SAFETY/SIDE EFFECTS/MONITORING
Dopamine agonist: used as a "rescue" movement drug for "off" periods.		
Apomorphine *Apokyn* SC injection Taken in addition to other PD medications	**Injection:** Start with 0.2 mL (2 mg) SC PRN (up to 5x/day); titrate by 1 mg every few days Max single dose: 0.6 mL (6 mg) Lasts 45-90 minutes Must be started with a test dose in a medical office	**CONTRAINDICATION** Do not use with 5-HT3 antagonists (e.g., ondansetron) due to severe hypotension and loss of consciousness **SIDE EFFECTS** Severe nausea/vomiting, hypotension, yawning, dyskinesias, somnolence, dizziness, QT prolongation **NOTES** Monitor supine and standing blood pressure For emesis prevention: give trimethobenzamide *(Tigan)* 300 mg PO TID, or a similar antiemetic, started 3 days prior to the initial dose

Carbidopa/Levodopa *(Sinemet)* Drug Interactions

- Contraindicated with non-selective MAO inhibitors (a two-week separation is required).

- Iron and protein-rich foods can ↓ absorption.

- Do not use with dopamine blockers, which will worsen Parkinson symptoms (e.g., phenothiazines, metoclopramide).

OTHER DRUGS FOR PARKINSON DISEASE

DRUG	DOSING	SAFETY/SIDE EFFECTS/MONITORING
Amantadine: blocks dopamine reuptake into presynaptic neurons and increases dopamine release from presynaptic fibers. Primarily used to treat dyskinesias associated with peak-dose of carbidopa/levodopa.		
Amantadine IR: tablet, capsule, syrup Extended-release (ER): *Gocovri, Osmolex ER*	IR: 100 mg PO BID *Osmolex ER:* 137 mg PO daily, increase after 1 week to 274 mg daily *Gocovri:* 129 mg daily, increase weekly to max dose of 322 mg daily ↓ dose in renal impairment eGFR < 15 mL/min/1.73 m²: ER products contraindicated	**WARNINGS** Somnolence (including falling asleep without warning during activities of daily living), compulsive behaviors, psychosis (hallucinations, delusions, paranoia) **SIDE EFFECTS** Dizziness, orthostatic hypotension, syncope, insomnia, abnormal dreams, dry mouth, constipation Cutaneous reaction called livedo reticularis (reddish skin mottling – can require drug discontinuation) **NOTES** *Gocovri* is indicated for the treatment of dyskinesia in patients receiving levodopa-based therapy Avoid live vaccines while on treatment
Selective MAO-B inhibitors: block the breakdown of dopamine which increases dopaminergic activity. Primarily used as adjunctive treatment to carbidopa/levodopa; rasagiline has an indication for monotherapy.		
Selegiline Capsule, tablet (generics) *Zelapar* – ODT *Emsam* – patch; only indicated for depression	Capsule, tablet: 5 mg PO BID, with breakfast and lunch ODT: 1.25-2.5 mg daily (not recommended if CrCl < 30 mL/min) Selegiline can be activating; do not take dose at bedtime; if dosed twice daily, take the 2nd dose at midday	**CONTRAINDICATIONS** Use in combination with other MAO inhibitors (including linezolid), opioids, SNRIs, TCAs, others (see Drug Interactions) *Xadago:* severe hepatic impairment **WARNINGS** Serotonin syndrome, hypertension, nausea, CNS depression, dyskinesias, impulse control disorders, caution in patients with psychotic disorders (may exacerbate) or ophthalmic disorders *(Xadago)* Rasagiline (monotherapy): headache, joint pain, indigestion
Rasagiline *(Azilect)*	0.5-1 mg PO daily	
Safinamide *(Xadago)*	Start with 50 mg once daily; after 2 weeks may increase to 100 mg once daily When stopping treatment: decrease the dose to 50 mg for one week before discontinuing	**MONITORING** BP, signs of serotonin syndrome, visual changes *(Xadago)* **NOTES** May need to reduce levodopa dose when beginning treatment with a selective MAO-B inhibitor

DRUG	DOSING	SAFETY/SIDE EFFECTS/MONITORING
Centrally-acting anticholinergics: have <u>anticholinergic</u> and antihistamine effects. Primarily used for tremor.		
Benztropine (*Cogentin**)	0.5-2 mg TID (start QHS)	**SIDE EFFECTS** High incidence of peripheral and central anticholinergic effects: <u>dry mouth</u>, <u>constipation</u>, <u>urinary retention</u>, <u>blurred vision</u>, <u>mydriasis</u>, <u>somnolence</u>, <u>confusion</u>, tachycardia
Trihexyphenidyl	1-5 mg TID (start 1 mg QHS)	**NOTES** Avoid use in older adults
Adenosine receptor antagonist: used in combination with carbidopa/levodopa to reduce "off" episodes.		
Istradefylline (*Nourianz*)	20 mg PO daily, can titrate to a max of 40 mg daily Dose must be adjusted if used with CYP3A4 inhibitors or tobacco smoking	**WARNINGS** Hallucinations, dyskinesias, impulse control disorders **SIDE EFFECTS** Nausea, constipation
Alpha/beta agonist: used for neurogenic orthostatic hypotension.		
Droxidopa (*Northera*)	Start at 100 mg PO TID, can titrate every 24-48 hour to a max of 1800 mg/day Take the last dose at least 3 hours prior to bedtime (to avoid supine hypertension during sleep)	**BOXED WARNING** Supine hypertension: monitor supine BP prior to and during treatment; elevate the head of the bed and measure BP in this position; if supine hypertension cannot be managed by elevation of the head of the bed, reduce dose or discontinue **SIDE EFFECTS** Syncope, falls, headache

*Brand discontinued but name still used in practice.

MAO-B Inhibitor Drug Interactions

- While taking, do not eat <u>foods high in tyramine</u>, including <u>aged or matured cheese</u>, <u>air-dried or cured meats</u> (e.g., sausages, salamis), <u>sauerkraut</u>, fava or broad bean pods, tap/draft beers, Marmite concentrate, soy sauce or other soybean condiments. Avoid these foods during and for two weeks after discontinuation of the medication.
- Do not use with products containing dopamine, tyrosine, phenylalanine, tryptophan or caffeine.
- Do not use with other drugs that increase the risk of <u>serotonin syndrome</u>. See the Drug Interactions chapter.
- Rasagiline is a CYP1A2 substrate; limit dose to 0.5 mg daily with ciprofloxacin or other CYP1A2 inhibitors.

KEY COUNSELING POINTS

See the Drug Formulations and Patient Counseling chapter for counseling language/layman's terminology.

ALL PARKINSON DISEASE PATIENTS

- Increased risk of:
  - Irregular movements, psychosis, suicidal ideation or depression.
- Treatments have many drug interactions.
- Avoid alcohol.

CARBIDOPA/LEVODOPA

- Can cause:
  - Nausea, dizziness, orthostasis or psychosis.
  - Body fluid discoloration (e.g., dark brown urine, saliva or sweat).
  - Priapism.
- Drug interactions due to binding or delayed absorption; specifically with iron and high-protein foods.

DOPAMINE AGONISTS

- Can cause orthostasis, drowsiness or psychosis.

Rotigotine (*Neupro*) Patch

- Can cause skin irritation.
- Patch application:
  - Wear for 24 hours. Rotate where you place the patch. Wait at least 14 days before applying in the same location. Remove patch before an MRI.

Select Guidelines/References

Pringsheim T, Day GS, Smith DB, et al. Dopaminergic therapy for motor symptoms in early parkinson disease practice guideline summary. *Neurology*. 2021;97(20):942-957.

Seppi K, Ray Chaudhuri K, Coelho M, et al. Update on Treatments for Nonmotor Symptoms of Parkinson's Disease-An Evidence-Based Medicine Review. *Movement Disorders*. 2019 Feb;34(2):180-198.

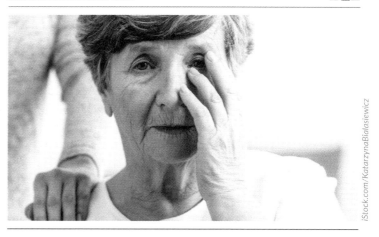

iStock.com//KatarzynaBialasiewicz

CHAPTER 69
ALZHEIMER'S DISEASE

BACKGROUND

Mild age-associated cognitive decline is normal and can cause bothersome symptoms, such as losing the car keys more often. If the decline is measurable, but is not severe enough to significantly interfere with daily functioning, the condition is called mild cognitive impairment (MCI).

With dementia, the decline in cognition is more severe. Intellectual and social abilities progressively worsen, and functioning becomes impaired. The most noticeable initial symptom is memory loss. As dementia progresses, patients develop difficulty with judgment, attention, planning and personal grooming. Agitation, aggression and depression can be present and are challenging for patients and caregivers.

SIGNS OF DEMENTIA

Memory loss

Difficulty planning and organizing

Getting lost in familiar places

Repeating words and information

Difficulty finding words for common objects

Inability to learn or remember new information

Apathy and social disengagement

Delusions and agitation

Poor coordination and motor function

DEMENTIA TYPES

A patient's clinical findings help characterize the dementia type (e.g., Alzheimer's disease, vascular dementia, Lewy body dementia). Alzheimer's disease is the most common type and has well-defined treatment, though the benefits are modest. The pathophysiology of Alzheimer's disease includes neuropathologic changes (e.g., amyloid beta plaques, tau tangles) that lead to the death of cholinergic neurons, resulting in decreased acetylcholine.

CONTENT LEGEND

 = Key Drug
Guy

SCREENING AND DIAGNOSIS

An early diagnosis of dementia provides a person with time to plan for the future while he or she can still participate in decision making. Common assessment tools include the Folstein Mini-Mental State Exam (MMSE, max score is 30, a score < 24 indicates a memory disorder), the Montreal Cognitive Assessment (MoCA) and Diagnostic and Statistical Manual of Mental Disorders, Fifth Edition (DSM-5) criteria. Functional abilities can be assessed using the Alzheimer's Disease Cooperative Study – Activities of Daily Living (ADCS-ADL) tool. These screening tools use various techniques to evaluate cognitive impairment (e.g., spelling a word backward, counting backward from 100 by sevens) and/or assess functional abilities with activities of daily living (e.g., bathing, dressing, using a telephone, housekeeping).

Initial screening should attempt to rule out reversible causes of memory impairment, such as vitamin D or B12 deficiency, depression and infection. In some patients, the use of medications can cause or exacerbate memory loss (see Key Drugs Guy). Anticholinergics are particularly concerning and are discussed below.

To determine which type of dementia a patient has, clinicians will use the pattern of neurological deficits (i.e., patient symptoms) and findings on brain imaging. For Alzheimer's disease, brain imaging, cerebrospinal fluid tests and blood tests that measure amyloid beta and tau concentrations are growing in use. If these tests correlate with the clinical picture of Alzheimer's disease, they increase the confidence of the diagnosis. Amyloid beta tests may also be used to qualify a patient for drugs that target amyloid beta plaques.

ANTICHOLINERGICS & MEMORY IMPAIRMENT

Anticholinergics are used to treat multiple conditions, including incontinence (e.g., oxybutynin), allergies or insomnia (e.g., diphenhydramine) and dystonic reactions (e.g., benztropine, diphenhydramine). A drug with high anticholinergic potency can cause acute cognitive impairment and, occasionally, psychosis and hallucinations.

The effects depend on the patient's baseline cognitive function, sensitivity to the drug, drug dosing and clearance, and the number of concurrent drugs with additive effects that the patient is taking. Anticholinergics are listed as drugs to avoid per the American Geriatrics Society Beers Criteria on potentially inappropriate medications in older adults.

KEY DRUGS THAT CAN WORSEN DEMENTIA

Antipsychotics (e.g., aripiprazole, chlorpromazine)

CNS Depressants
Barbiturates (e.g., phenobarbital)

Benzodiazepines (e.g., alprazolam, clonazepam)

Opioids (e.g., hydrocodone, morphine)

Hypnotics (e.g., eszopiclone, zolpidem)

Skeletal muscle relaxants (e.g., carisoprodol)

Drugs with Anticholinergic Effects
Antiemetics (e.g., prochlorperazine)

Antihistamines (e.g., diphenhydramine, doxylamine)

Central anticholinergics (e.g., benztropine)

Peripheral anticholinergics (e.g., oxybutynin, dicyclomine)

Tricyclic antidepressants (e.g., amitriptyline)

NON-DRUG TREATMENT

The health of the blood vessels in the brain is vital for cognitive function. Controlled blood glucose, blood pressure and cholesterol throughout life can decrease the likelihood of developing vascular dementia. Physical activity, a healthy diet and cognitive rehabilitation may also prevent dementia or improve symptoms.

NATURAL PRODUCTS

Vitamin E (2,000 IU daily) may minimally slow the rate of decline for patients with mild to moderate dementia. Other supplements used for Alzheimer's disease include acetyl-L-carnitine, ginkgo biloba and vinpocetine.

DRUG TREATMENT

Drug treatment for Alzheimer's disease provides modest benefits, but the patient may have a slower clinical decline than with no treatment. For family members and caregivers, this may mean that the patient can feed themselves for a little while longer or use the bathroom independently for several more months.

Acetylcholinesterase inhibitors (e.g., donepezil) are the primary treatment for all stages of Alzheimer's disease and are recommended first line in patients with mild to moderate disease. In moderate to severe disease, memantine may be added or used alone, but combination treatment is more effective at delaying disease progression than monotherapy with either agent. Drug discontinuation is advised if dementia has advanced to the point where drug treatment lacks clinical benefit or side effects become intolerable, though some patients will experience a noticeable deterioration when medication is stopped.

There are two amyloid beta-directed antibodies for the treatment of mild Alzheimer's disease, aducanumab (Aduhelm) and lecanemab (Leqembi). They reduce amyloid beta plaques, but the clinical benefit has yet to be demonstrated and their role in treatment is not well defined.

Depression, agitation and psychosis are challenging to diagnose and treat in patients with dementia. Antidepressants (e.g., sertraline) can be used to treat depression and anxiety. After addressing underlying causes (e.g., pain) and attempting non-pharmacologic interventions (e.g., reassurance, activities, stable environment), a trial of antipsychotic therapy may be used for agitation and psychosis if the patient remains in significant distress or poses harm to themselves or others. The antipsychotic should be discontinued when possible because of side effects, including a boxed warning for an increased risk of death in elderly patients. Brexpiprazole (Rexulti) is the only FDA-approved antipsychotic for the treatment of agitation associated with dementia due to Alzheimer's disease, though others (e.g., olanzapine, quetiapine) may be used off-label.

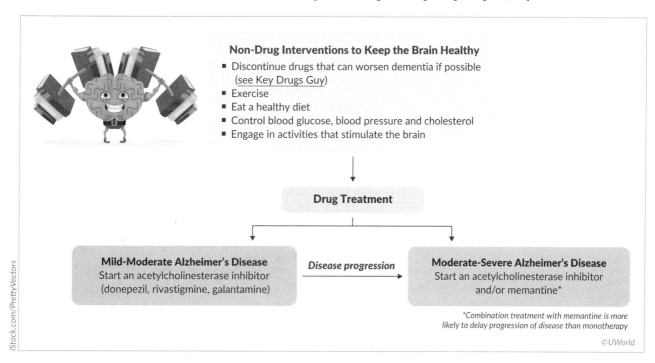

Non-Drug Interventions to Keep the Brain Healthy
- Discontinue drugs that can worsen dementia if possible (see Key Drugs Guy)
- Exercise
- Eat a healthy diet
- Control blood glucose, blood pressure and cholesterol
- Engage in activities that stimulate the brain

Drug Treatment

Mild-Moderate Alzheimer's Disease
Start an acetylcholinesterase inhibitor (donepezil, rivastigmine, galantamine)

Disease progression

Moderate-Severe Alzheimer's Disease
Start an acetylcholinesterase inhibitor and/or memantine*

*Combination treatment with memantine is more likely to delay progression of disease than monotherapy

iStock.com/PrettyVectors

©UWorld

ALZHEIMER'S DISEASE DRUGS

DRUG	DOSING	SAFETY/SIDE EFFECTS/MONITORING
Acetylcholinesterase inhibitors: inhibit centrally-active acetylcholinesterase, the enzyme responsible for hydrolysis (breakdown) of acetylcholine; this causes ↑ acetylcholine		
Donepezil *Aricept:* ODT, tablet *Adlarity:* patch **+ memantine (Namzaric)**	Oral: start 5 mg QHS, can increase to 10 mg QHS after 4-6 weeks Moderate-severe disease: can increase to 23 mg QHS after ≥ 3 months of 10 mg QHS *Adlarity* patch: start 5 mg/24 hrs once weekly, can increase to 10 mg/24 hrs once weekly after 4-6 weeks	**WARNINGS** Cardiac effects, including bradycardia, AV block, syncope Donepezil: QT prolongation GI effects, including nausea, vomiting, diarrhea, weight loss and/or anorexia; risk increased with higher doses and in patients with low body weight (e.g., < 55 kg) Skin reactions (all formulations), including allergic contact dermatitis (rivastigmine) and SJS (galantamine) **SIDE EFFECTS** Insomnia, dizziness
Rivastigmine (Exelon) Capsule, patch	Capsule: start 1.5 mg BID, can increase every 2 weeks to 6 mg BID Patch: start 4.6 mg/24 hrs once daily, can increase every 4 weeks to 13.3 mg/24 hrs once daily Hepatic impairment: max patch dose is 4.6 mg/24 hrs	**NOTES** Donepezil is dosed QHS to ↓ nausea; if insomnia occurs, morning dosing may be preferred Slower titration (e.g., every 6 weeks) may decrease GI side effects; if treatment is interrupted ≥ 3 days, retitrate from starting dose *Adlarity* patch: store in refrigerator; before use, remove patch from refrigerator and allow to reach room temperature (apply within 24 hrs of removal from fridge); if transitioning from oral donepezil, apply patch at the same time as the last oral dose
Galantamine Tablet, capsule, solution	IR tablet or solution: start 4 mg BID, can increase every 4 weeks to 12 mg BID ER capsule: start 8 mg daily, can increase every 4 weeks to 24 mg daily Severe hepatic/renal impairment: do not use	*Exelon* patch: if transitioning from oral rivastigmine, apply patch the day after the last oral dose; some products may contain metal (remove before MRI) Take oral rivastigmine and galantamine with food Galantamine solution can be mixed with liquid; drink immediately If stable on donepezil 10 mg, can switch to *Namzaric* (memantine 7 mg/donepezil 10 mg QHS) and titrate weekly
N-methyl-D-aspartate (NMDA) receptor blocker: prevents glutamate (an excitatory neurotransmitter) from binding to the NMDA receptor and causing overstimulation and neuronal death		
Memantine (Namenda, Namenda XR, Namenda Titration Pack) Tablet, capsule, oral solution **+ donepezil (Namzaric)**	IR: start 5 mg PO daily, titrate weekly to 10 mg PO BID ER: start 7 mg PO daily, titrate weekly to 28 mg PO daily Can switch IR 10 mg BID to ER 28 mg daily; begin ER the day after the last IR dose CrCl < 30 mL/min: max dose 5 mg PO BID (IR) or 14 mg PO daily (ER)	**WARNINGS** Caution with drugs (e.g., sodium bicarbonate, acetazolamide) or conditions (e.g., severe urinary tract infection) that ↑ urine pH, which ↓ clearance of memantine **SIDE EFFECTS** Generally well-tolerated, can cause dizziness, confusion, headache, constipation **NOTES** ER capsule and *Namzaric:* do not crush or chew; capsules can be opened and sprinkled on applesauce (swallow immediately) Oral solution: use provided dosing syringe and squirt into mouth The brand name NaMenDA has NMDA embedded in the name

Acetylcholinesterase Inhibitor Drug Interactions

- Use caution with other drugs that can lower heart rate (e.g., beta-blockers, diltiazem, verapamil, digoxin).

- Drugs that have anticholinergic effects can reduce the efficacy of acetylcholinesterase inhibitors.

- Acetylcholinesterase inhibitors can increase gastric acid secretion; use caution in patients at risk of GI bleeding (e.g., concurrent NSAID use, history of GI ulcers).

KEY COUNSELING POINTS

See the Drug Formulations and Patient Counseling chapter for counseling language/layman's terminology.

ALL ALZHEIMER'S DISEASE MEDICATIONS

- Tell your healthcare provider which prescription and over-the-counter medications you are taking; other drugs can worsen memory problems.

ACETYLCHOLINESTERASE INHIBITORS

- Can cause:
  - ❏ Nausea and vomiting. Take donepezil at bedtime.
  - ❏ Diarrhea.
  - ❏ Decreased heart rate.

Adlarity Patch

- Store the patch in the <u>refrigerator</u>. When ready to apply a patch, remove one pouch from the box and allow it to come to room temperature naturally (do not apply a heat source). The patch must be used within 24 hours of removal from the refrigerator.

- Apply a new patch at the same time <u>each week</u> to the <u>upper or lower back</u> (preferred site), <u>upper buttocks</u> or <u>upper outer thigh</u>.

- Rotate application sites. Do not use the same site within 14 days.

- After 7 days, remove the used patch. Do not touch the sticky side. Fold the patch in half with the sticky sides together and dispose of it in the trash.

Exelon Patch

- Apply a new patch at the same time <u>each day</u> to the <u>upper or lower back</u> (preferred sites if patient might remove patch), or the <u>upper arm or chest</u>.

- Rotate application sites. Do not use the same site within 14 days.

- After 24 hours, remove the used patch. Do not touch the sticky side. Fold the patch in half with the sticky sides together and dispose of it in the trash.

Select Guidelines/References

Rabins PV, Rovner BW, Rummans T, et al. APA Guideline Watch (October 2014): Practice Guideline for the Treatment of Patients with Alzheimer's Disease and Other Dementias. https://psychiatryonline.org/pb/assets/raw/sitewide/practice_guidelines/guidelines/alzheimerwatch.pdf.

CHAPTER CONTENT

CONTENT LEGEND

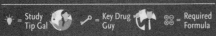

☀ = Study Tip Gal   ⚷ = Key Drug Guy   ⚙⚙ = Required Formula

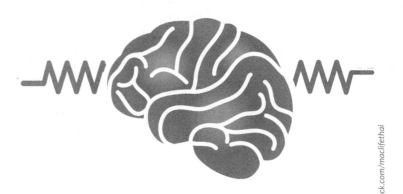

iStock.com/maclifethai

CHAPTER 70
SEIZURES/EPILEPSY

BACKGROUND

A seizure occurs when excitatory neurons produce a sudden surge of uncontrolled electrical activity in the brain. Seizures can be caused by temporary conditions such as fever (common in children), infection, alcohol withdrawal, hypoglycemia or electrolyte abnormalities; in these cases, treating the underlying cause stops the seizure. Some drugs can lower the seizure threshold, making a person more susceptible to a seizure. These drugs should be avoided in a person with a history of seizures. See the Key Drug Guy on the next page.

Epilepsy is a chronic seizure disorder. This is a complex condition with various types of seizures and a variety of drug treatments available. These drugs are known as antiseizure medications (ASMs), sometimes also referred to as antiepileptic drugs (AEDs). Seizure symptoms vary from uncontrolled jerking movements (e.g., tonic-clonic seizures) to a subtle momentary loss of awareness (e.g., absence seizures). Seizures can damage and destroy neurons, which causes brain damage and can be life-threatening.

The incidence of epilepsy is highest in the young and the elderly. One-third of new cases in the U.S. each year (50,000 of 150,000) are in children and adolescents. Seizures caused by a high fever in infants and young children do not usually lead to epilepsy. The elderly are at risk for seizures due to conditions that are more prevalent in the elderly, including dementia, brain tumors and, most commonly, damage from a stroke.

Severe head trauma from motor vehicle accidents, sports injuries, falls and other events can lead to brain damage and cause seizures; emergency room treatment for such injuries often includes prevention or treatment of seizures. Half of all seizure cases have no identifiable cause and are attributed to some combination of environmental exposures or genetic factors.

Individuals with epilepsy are evaluated for age of onset, seizure type, seizure frequency, description of witnessed seizure, identifiable causes or triggers and a thorough neurologic (brain and brain function) exam. An electroencephalogram (EEG), the most common test used to diagnose epilepsy, records electrical activity in the brain. An EEG can show abnormal patterns even when the patient is not having a seizure. Brain imaging with a CT or MRI can help identify conditions that can provoke seizures (e.g., brain tumors, damage from a stroke).

DRUGS THAT CAN CAUSE SEIZURES

KEY DRUGS

Analgesics
Opioids (esp. tramadol, meperidine)*

Anti-infectives
Quinolones
Carbapenems*
Cephalosporins*
Penicillins*
Mefloquine

Psychiatric medications
Bupropion
Antipsychotics (esp. clozapine)
Lithium*
Tricyclic antidepressants*

*High doses and/or renal impairment ↑ risk

Others:
Baclofen*
Diphenhydramine*
Metoclopramide
Metronidazole*
Theophylline
Varenicline
Stimulants (e.g., methylphenidate)*

CLASSIFICATION OF SEIZURE TYPES

Seizures are classified into three main types based on where the seizure starts in the brain: focal seizures, generalized seizures and unknown onset seizures.

Focal seizures start on one side of the brain but can spread to the other side. Generalized seizures start on both sides of the brain. Seizures are classified as unknown onset if the seizures are unwitnessed or occur during the night and the initial symptom presentation is not known.

Focal seizures are further classified based on the patient's level of awareness during the seizure:

- Focal aware seizure: the patient experiences no loss of consciousness (previously known as a simple partial seizure).

- Focal seizure with impaired awareness: the patient experiences loss of consciousness (previously known as a complex partial seizure).

Patients with generalized seizures experience loss of consciousness or are unaware during the seizure event.

All seizure types can be described based on the patient's symptoms. Motor symptoms include sustained rhythmical jerking movements (clonic), limp or weak muscles (atonic), muscle twitching (myoclonus) and rigid or tense muscles (tonic). Non-motor symptoms include changes in sensation, emotions, thinking or cognition. Generalized seizures with non-motor symptoms are called absence seizures, which typically present as staring spells.

ACUTE SEIZURE MANAGEMENT

Most seizures last less than two minutes and do not require medical intervention. Seizures that continue longer cause brain damage and can be fatal. Status epilepticus (SE) is a seizure that lasts five minutes or more; this is due to the normal mechanisms that terminate seizures not working. At 30 minutes, long-term damage can occur. This is a medical emergency; emergency treatment should begin with any seizure lasting longer than five minutes.

SE management is divided into phases (see figure below). Initial treatment is a benzodiazepine injection. Intravenous (IV) access can be difficult during a seizure; if it is not possible to insert an IV line, midazolam can be given intramuscularly (IM).

If the patient is not receiving urgent medical care (i.e., not in a medical facility), diazepam rectal gel (Diastat AcuDial), or intranasal or buccal midazolam are non-injectable options.

Status Epilepticus Treatment

0-5 minutes
Stabilization phase

Stabilize circulation, airway and breathing
Time the seizure, start ECG
Check ASM levels and electrolytes
If blood glucose is low, treat with dextrose

↓

5-20 minutes
Initial treatment phase

If seizures continue:
Give IV lorazepam, IM midazolam or IV diazepam
Alternatives: rectal diazepam, intranasal or buccal midazolam

↓

20-40 minutes
Second treatment phase

If seizures continue:
Give nonbenzodiazepine ASM:
IV fosphenytoin, valproic acid or levetiracetam
Alternative: IV phenobarbital

↓

Third treatment phase (refractory)

No clear evidence to guide therapy
Repeat second-line therapy or midazolam,
pentobarbital or propofol

©UWorld

Diastat AcuDial is prescribed for patients who are at risk of long-lasting seizures. It includes special dispensing and counseling requirements for pharmacists (see Study Tip Gal).

DIASTAT ACUDIAL DISPENSING

Each package contains two rectal syringes prefilled with diazepam rectal gel.

Each syringe MUST be dialed to the right dose and locked BEFORE DISPENSING. Syringes come in 2.5, 10 and 20 mg.

Pharmacist instructions for locking in the dose are included on a card in the package:

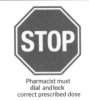

Pharmacist must dial and lock correct prescribed dose

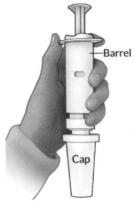
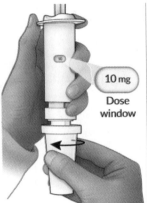
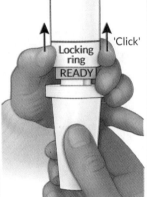
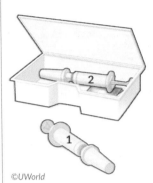

©UWorld

Hold the barrel of the syringe in one hand with the cap facing down and the dose window visible. Do not remove the cap.	Use the other hand to grab the cap firmly and turn to adjust the dose.	Confirm the correct dose shows in the window. Hold the locking ring at the bottom of the syringe barrel and push upward on both sides of the ring. Once locked, the green band should say "READY," and the syringe cannot be unlocked.	Repeat these steps with the second syringe in the case. When counseling, check both syringes with the patient before they leave the pharmacy to ensure they are dialed and locked. See the Key Counseling Points section for administration instructions.

FMStox/Shutterstock.com

CHRONIC SEIZURE MANAGEMENT

ASMs are first-line treatment for epilepsy. The initial one or two drugs will provide adequate control in approximately 70% of cases. Seizures that are resistant to ASMs need to be addressed another way; uncontrolled seizures cause brain damage and can be fatal. ASMs should not be stopped abruptly as this can lead to increased seizures.

ADJUVANT TREATMENTS

Adjuvant treatment options for chronic seizure management include medical marijuana (cannabis), a ketogenic diet, vagal nerve stimulation or surgical intervention.

Medical Marijuana (Cannabis)

There are patients with resistant seizures who receive some degree of seizure control with medical cannabis. _Epidiolex_, or cannabidiol (CBD), was the first cannabis-derived medication approved by the FDA to treat rare forms of epilepsy. _Epidiolex_ does not contain tetrahydrocannabinol (THC), but there are other CBD and medical marijuana products available that contain varying amounts of THC. Pharmacists should consider the impact of additive CNS side effects (e.g., somnolence, euphoria, anxiety, paranoia) and the potential for drug interactions.

Ketogenic Diet

A ketogenic diet can be used in patients with refractory seizures (not responding to medications). The diet contains high fats, normal protein and low carbohydrates (usually a 4:1 ratio of fats to combined protein and carbohydrates). This forces the body to break down fatty acids into ketone bodies as the primary energy source. Ketone bodies pass into the brain and replace glucose. This elevated ketone state is called ketosis and can lead to a reduction in seizure frequency.

ANTISEIZURE MEDICATIONS

Broad-spectrum ASMs (e.g., lamotrigine, levetiracetam, topiramate, valproic acid) treat both focal and generalized seizures. Narrow-spectrum ASMs primarily treat focal-onset seizures. A few ASMs are used for isolated conditions, such as ethosuximide for absence seizures.

The ASM drug tables in this chapter are organized by therapeutic spectrum and frequency of use. Pregabalin and gabapentin are not listed with common ASMs; they are mainly used to treat neuropathic pain, not epilepsy. The section on other ASMs includes drugs that are used less commonly but have important safety issues that must be known.

COMMON CONCERNS WITH ASMs

ASMs should be selected based on patient-specific factors, including seizure type, age, childbearing potential and daily activities. The best ASM for one patient may not be appropriate for another patient with the same seizure type. Below are factors to consider when selecting an ASM.

CNS and Psychiatric Effects

Regardless of the specific mechanism of action, all ASMs are designed to decrease electrical activity in the brain and must cross the blood-brain barrier to prevent seizures. Because of this, all ASMs increase the risk of CNS depression (e.g., dizziness, confusion, sedation, ataxia/coordination difficulties) and subsequently increase the risk for cognitive impairment, falls and injuries. The degree of CNS depression is an important consideration when selecting treatment for patients who need to perform cognitive tasks, such as driving or studying for school.

All ASMs also have a warning for suicide risk and require monitoring for changes in mood or behavior, especially in patients with psychiatric conditions.

Bone Loss

ASMs can cause bone loss and increase fracture risk. All patients on ASMs should be supplemented with calcium and vitamin D. Bone loss can occur as soon as two years after the start of an ASM. Modifiable factors that affect bone density should be addressed (see the Osteoporosis, Menopause & Testosterone Use chapter).

Rash

Many ASMs can cause serious skin rash, including an increased risk of Stevens-Johnson syndrome (SJS) and toxic epidermal necrolysis (TEN). Higher ASM blood levels increase this risk.

Drug reaction with eosinophilia and systemic symptoms (DRESS) is a multiorgan hypersensitivity reaction that includes skin manifestations (e.g., purpura, maculopapular rash) and can be caused by ASMs.

TAKE YOUR VITAMINS ON ASMs!

Supplement with:

- ALL ASMs: calcium and vitamin D
- Women of childbearing age: folate
- Valproic acid: possibly carnitine (see drug table)
- Lamotrigine and valproic acid: if alopecia develops, supplement with biotin, selenium and zinc

---

ASM MECHANISMS OF ACTION

DRUG/CLASS	MECHANISM OF ACTION	DESCRIPTION
Benzodiazepines	Enhances GABA effect	A seizure is an episode of sudden, uncontrolled neuronal firing within the brain. The sudden electrical activity is caused by a receptor malfunction or an imbalance of neurotransmitters (NTs).
Phenobarbital		Seizures can occur due to a deficiency of the inhibitory NT, gamma-aminobutyric acid (GABA), or an excess of the excitatory NT, glutamate.
Valproate	Blocks sodium channels and ↑ GABA	
Levetiracetam	Inhibits vesicle fusion by binding SV2A proteins	ASMs ↓ abnormal electrical activity by either:
Carbamazepine		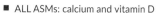 ↑ GABA
Phenytoin/ Fosphenytoin	Blocks sodium channels	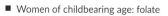 ↓ Glutamate
Topiramate		■ Blocking (or altering) Ca channels, which slows down or stops transmission of the electrical signal
Lamotrigine	Blocks sodium channels and ↓ glutamate	■ Blocking Na channels, which decreases the neuronal firing rate
Ethosuximide	Blocks T-type Ca channels	

NEURON — DENDRITES — NUCLEUS — CELL BODY — AXON — AXON TERMINALS — SYNAPSE

iStock.com/TefiM

COMMON BROAD-SPECTRUM ANTISEIZURE MEDICATIONS

Lamotrigine

DRUG	DOSING	SAFETY/SIDE EFFECTS/MONITORING
Lamotrigine (Lamictal, Lamictal ODT, Lamictal Starter Kit, Lamictal XR, Subvenite, Subvenite Starter Kit-Blue, Green, Orange) Tablet, chewable, ODT Also used for bipolar disorder	**Initial (standard dosing):** Weeks 1 and 2: 25 mg daily Weeks 3 and 4: 50 mg daily Week 5 and on: can ↑ by 50 mg daily every 1-2 weeks Can vary based on interacting drugs **Maintenance dose:** IR: 225-375 mg daily, divided BID XR: 300-400 mg daily	**BOXED WARNING** Serious skin reactions, including SJS/TEN (rate of rash is greater in pediatrics than adults); ↑ risk with higher than recommended starting doses, dose escalation or when used with valproic acid **WARNINGS** Multiorgan hypersensitivity reactions (DRESS), aseptic meningitis, blood dyscrasias, cardiac rhythm abnormalities, serious rare immune system reaction [hemophagocytic lymphohistiocytosis (HLH)] that can be fatal **SIDE EFFECTS** Alopecia (supplement biotin, selenium and zinc), N/V, somnolence, rash, tremor, ataxia, impaired coordination, dizziness, diplopia, blurred vision **MONITORING** Rash, fever **NOTES** Discontinue if there is any sign of hypersensitivity reaction or unspecified rash Use starter kit when initiating treatment to ensure correct dosing (see next Study Tip Gal) If discontinued for ≥ 5 half-lives (> 6 days for most patients), restart initial dosing titration

Lamotrigine Drug Interactions

- Drugs that induce or inhibit uridine diphosphate glucuronosyltransferase (UGT), the enzyme responsible for lamotrigine glucuronidation, can alter lamotrigine concentrations.

- Valproic acid ↑ lamotrigine concentrations more than two-fold; use lower dose starter kit (blue box).

- Oral estrogen-containing contraceptives ↓ lamotrigine; higher maintenance doses of lamotrigine may be needed.

- Carbamazepine, phenytoin, phenobarbital, primidone, lopinavir/ritonavir, atazanavir/ritonavir and rifampin ↓ lamotrigine levels by 40%. Use the higher dose starter kit (green box).

LAMICTAL STARTER KITS BY COLOR

Lamotrigine doses need to be just right.
- Too much leads to a higher risk of severe rash.

- Too little leads to seizures.

The colored starter kits are helpful to make sure the right dose is selected.

BLUE	ORANGE	GREEN
■ Lower starting dose ■ Use if taking valproic acid (enzyme inhibitor)	■ Standard starting dose ■ Use if no interacting medications	■ Higher starting dose ■ Use if taking an enzyme inducer (e.g., carbamazepine, phenytoin, phenobarbital, primidone) and not taking valproic acid

Levetiracetam

DRUG	DOSING	SAFETY/SIDE EFFECTS/MONITORING
Levetiracetam *(Keppra, Keppra XR, Elepsia XR, Spritam)* Tablet, ODT, oral solution, injection	**Initial:** 500 mg BID or 1,000 mg daily (XR) **Maximum:** 3,000 mg/day **CrCl ≤ 80 mL/min:** ↓ dose IV:PO ratio 1:1	**WARNINGS** Psychiatric reactions, including psychotic symptoms, somnolence, fatigue, aggression, anxiety and suicidal behavior; anaphylaxis, angioedema, coordination difficulties, severe skin reactions (SJS/TEN), multiorgan hypersensitivity reactions (DRESS), hematologic abnormalities (mainly anemias), loss of seizure control during pregnancy **SIDE EFFECTS** Somnolence, dizziness, weakness, asthenia **NOTES** No significant drug interactions

Topiramate

DRUG	DOSING	SAFETY/SIDE EFFECTS/MONITORING
Topiramate *(Topamax, Topamax Sprinkle, Eprontia)* Topiramate extended-release *(Qudexy XR, Trokendi XR)* Capsule, extended-release capsule, tablet, oral solution Also used for migraine prophylaxis	**Initial:** Week 1: 25 mg BID (IR) or 50 mg daily (XR) Weeks 2-4: ↑ by 25 mg BID (IR) or 50 mg daily (XR) each week Week 5 and on: ↑ by 100 mg weekly until max dose or therapeutic effect **Maximum:** 400 mg/day **CrCl < 70 mL/min:** ↓ dose by 50%	**CONTRAINDICATIONS** *Trokendi XR* only: alcohol use 6 hours before or after dose, *Qudexy XR* only: patients with metabolic acidosis who are taking metformin **WARNINGS** Hyperchloremic non-anion gap metabolic acidosis, oligohidrosis (reduced perspiration)/hyperthermia (mostly in children), nephrolithiasis (kidney stones), acute myopia and secondary angle-closure glaucoma, hyperammonemia (alone and with valproic acid), visual problems (reversible), fetal harm **SIDE EFFECTS** Somnolence, dizziness, psychomotor slowing, difficulty with memory/concentration/attention, weight loss, anorexia, paresthesia **MONITORING** Electrolytes (especially bicarbonate), renal function, hydration status, eye exam (intraocular pressure) **NOTES** *Topamax Sprinkle*: swallow whole or open and sprinkle on a small amount of soft food (do not chew; swallow immediately)

Topiramate Drug Interactions

- Topiramate is a weak inhibitor of CYP2C19 and inducer of CYP3A4.

- Phenytoin, carbamazepine, valproic acid and lamotrigine can ↓ topiramate levels.

- Topiramate can ↓ effectiveness of oral contraceptives, (especially with doses ≥ 200 mg/day). Non-hormonal contraception is recommended.

- Topiramate can ↓ the INR in patients on warfarin; monitor closely.

Valproate

DRUG	DOSING	SAFETY/SIDE EFFECTS/MONITORING
Valproic acid Capsule, syrup Valproate sodium IV **Divalproex (Depakote, Depakote ER, Depakote Sprinkle)** *Depakote* – delayed-release (DR) tablet *Depakote ER* – extended-release (ER) tablet *Depakote Sprinkle* – capsules can be opened and sprinkled on food Also used for bipolar disorder and migraine prophylaxis	**Initial:** 10-15 mg/kg/day **Maximum:** 60 mg/kg/day **Therapeutic range:** 50-100 mcg/mL (total level) If albumin is low (< 3.5 g/dL), the free (unbound) concentration of valproic acid may be elevated while the total concentration appears normal or low (see the Pharmacokinetics chapter) DR and ER formulations are not bioequivalent; ↑ total daily dose 8-20% when converting from DR to ER tablets	**BOXED WARNINGS** Hepatic failure: usually during first 6 months of therapy, children < 2 years old and patients with mitochondrial disorders are at ↑ risk; fetal harm (neural tube defects and ↓ IQ scores); pancreatitis **CONTRAINDICATIONS** Hepatic disease, urea cycle disorders, prophylaxis of migraine in pregnancy, certain mitochondrial disorders if < 2 years of age **WARNINGS** Hyperammonemia (treat with carnitine in symptomatic adults only), hypothermia, dose-related thrombocytopenia (↑ bleeding risk), multiorgan hypersensitivity reactions (DRESS) **SIDE EFFECTS** Alopecia (supplement with biotin, selenium and zinc), nausea/vomiting, weight changes (gain > loss), headache, anorexia, abdominal pain, dizziness, somnolence, tremor, edema, diplopia, blurred vision **MONITORING** LFTs (baseline and frequently in the first 6 months), CBC with differential (especially platelets), serum valproate levels, serum ammonia **NOTES** Divalproex is a valproic acid derivative The term "valproate" is used to refer to any formulation of valproic acid, valproate sodium or divalproex

Valproate Drug Interactions

- Valproate is an inhibitor of CYP2C9 (weak) and UGT, a substrate of CYP2C19 and 2E1 (minor) and can displace certain drugs from protein-binding sites (e.g., warfarin).

- Valproate can ↑ levels of lamotrigine, phenobarbital, phenytoin, warfarin and zidovudine.

- Salicylates displace valproate from albumin (↑ levels).

- Carbapenem antibiotics can ↓ levels of valproate.

- Estrogen-containing hormonal contraceptives can ↓ valproate levels.

- Use caution with valproate and lamotrigine due to risk of serious rash; use lower starting dose of lamotrigine and titrate slowly.

- Use with topiramate can lead to hyperammonemia with or without encephalopathy.

COMMON NARROW-SPECTRUM ANTISEIZURE MEDICATIONS

Lacosamide

DRUG	DOSING	SAFETY/SIDE EFFECTS/MONITORING
Lacosamide (Vimpat) C-V Tablet, oral solution, injection	**Initial:** 50-100 mg BID **Maximum:** 400 mg/day **CrCl < 30 mL/min:** Maximum dose is 300 mg/day IV:PO ratio 1:1	**WARNINGS** Prolongs PR interval and ↑ risk of arrhythmias; obtain an ECG prior to use and after titrated to steady state in patients with or at risk of cardiac conduction problems; multiorgan hypersensitivity reactions (DRESS), syncope, dizziness, ataxia **SIDE EFFECTS** Dizziness, headache, diplopia, blurred vision, ataxia, tremor, euphoria **MONITORING** ECG (baseline and at steady state) in at-risk patients

Lacosamide Drug Interactions

- Lacosamide is a substrate of CYP2C19 (minor), 2C9 (minor), 3A4 (minor) and an inhibitor of CYP2C19 (weak). Caution with inhibitors of 2C19, 2C9 and 3A4 (can ↑ lacosamide).

- Use caution with medications that prolong the PR interval (e.g., beta-blockers, calcium channel blockers, digoxin) due to the risk of AV block and bradycardia.

Carbamazepine

DRUG	DOSING	SAFETY/SIDE EFFECTS/MONITORING
Carbamazepine **(Tegretol, Tegretol XR,** *Carbatrol, Epitol)* Capsule, tablet, chewable, oral suspension *Equetro* – for bipolar disorder Also used for trigeminal neuralgia	**Initial:** 200 mg BID (or 100 mg QID for suspension) **Maximum:** 1,600 mg/day (some patients can require more) **Therapeutic range:** 4-12 mcg/mL	**BOXED WARNINGS** Serious skin reactions, including SJS/TEN: HLA-B*1502 allele testing is required for patients of Asian descent prior to starting treatment; if positive for this allele, carbamazepine cannot be used (unless benefit clearly outweighs risk); aplastic anemia and agranulocytosis; discontinue if significant myelosuppression occurs **CONTRAINDICATIONS** Myelosuppression, hypersensitivity to TCAs, use of MAO inhibitors within past 14 days, use with nefazodone or non-nucleoside reverse transcriptase inhibitors (NNRTIs) that are substrates of CYP3A4 **WARNINGS** Risk of developing a hypersensitivity reaction ↑ in patients with the variant HLA-A*3101 allele, multiorgan hypersensitivity reactions (DRESS), hyponatremia (SIADH), hypothyroidism, ↑ intraocular pressure, cardiac conduction abnormalities, liver damage, fetal harm **SIDE EFFECTS** Dizziness, drowsiness, ataxia, N/V, pruritus, photosensitivity, blurred vision, rash, ↑ LFTs, alopecia, renal impairment **MONITORING** CBC with differential (including platelets) prior to and during therapy, LFTs, rash, eye exam, thyroid function tests, serum Na, renal function Monitor carbamazepine levels within 3-5 days of initiation and after 4 weeks due to autoinduction **NOTES** Enzyme inducer, autoinducer – ↓ level of other drugs and itself

Carbamazepine Drug Interactions

- Carbamazepine is an autoinducer and will ↓ its own levels.

- Carbamazepine is a strong inducer of CYP3A4 and also induces CYP1A2, 2B6, 2C19, 2C9 and P-glycoprotein (P-gp). It can ↓ the levels of many drugs, including other antiseizure medications, aripiprazole, levothyroxine, warfarin and hormonal contraceptives. Use of an alternative, non-hormonal contraceptive is recommended.

- Carbamazepine is a major CYP3A4 substrate; inhibitors will ↑ carbamazepine levels and inducers will ↓ carbamazepine levels. Do not use with nefazodone or NNRTIs.

- Carbamazepine suspension should not be taken with other liquid medications, as precipitates can form.

Oxcarbazepine

DRUG	DOSING	SAFETY/SIDE EFFECTS/MONITORING
**Oxcarbazepine *(Trileptal,* *Oxtellar XR)* Tablet, oral suspension *(Trileptal)* Extended-release tablet *(Oxtellar XR)*	**Initial:** 300 mg BID *(Trileptal)*; 600 mg daily *(Oxtellar XR)* **Maximum:** 2,400 mg/day **CrCl < 30 mL/min:** Start 300 mg daily Carbamazepine to oxcarbazepine dose conversion: 1.5x carbamazepine dose	**CONTRAINDICATIONS** Hypersensitivity to eslicarbazepine **WARNINGS** ↑ risk for serious skin reactions (SJS/TEN), consider screening patients of Asian descent for HLA-B*1502 prior to initiating therapy, multiorgan hypersensitivity reactions (DRESS) Hyponatremia, hypothyroidism, potential worsening of generalized seizures **SIDE EFFECTS** Somnolence, dizziness, N/V, abdominal pain, diplopia, visual disturbances, ataxia, tremor **MONITORING** Serum Na (especially during the first 3 months of treatment), thyroid function, CBC **NOTES** Structurally similar to carbamazepine *Trileptal* oral suspension: use within 7 weeks once original container is opened XR tablet: take on empty stomach 1 hour before or 2 hours after a meal

Oxcarbazepine Drug Interactions

- Oxcarbazepine is a weak CYP3A4 inducer and CYP2C19 inhibitor but is not an autoinducer. Strong CYP3A4 inducers can ↓ oxcarbazepine levels. Oxcarbazepine can ↑ levels of fosphenytoin, phenytoin and phenobarbital.

- Oxcarbazepine can significantly ↓ hormonal contraceptive levels; non-hormonal contraception is recommended.

Phenytoin/Fosphenytoin

DRUG	DOSING	SAFETY/SIDE EFFECTS/MONITORING
Phenytoin (Dilantin, Dilantin Infatabs, Phenytek) Capsule, chewable, oral suspension, injection (IV only)	**Loading dose:** 15-20 mg/kg (dose can be divided) **Maintenance dose:** Up to 300-600 mg/day **Therapeutic range:** 10-20 mcg/mL (total level) 1-2 mcg/mL (free level) Fraction of unbound (free) drug is higher with renal or hepatic failure or ↓ albumin IV:PO ratio 1:1	**BOXED WARNINGS** Phenytoin IV administration rate should not exceed 50 mg/minute and fosphenytoin IV should not exceed 150 mg PE/minute or 2 mg PE/kg/min (use the slower rate); if given faster, hypotension and cardiac arrhythmias can occur **CONTRAINDICATIONS** Previous hepatotoxicity due to phenytoin **WARNINGS** Extravasation (leading to purple glove syndrome, characterized by edema, pain and bluish discoloration of the skin, which can sometimes lead to tissue necrosis) Avoid phenytoin in patients with a positive HLA-B*1502 test and in patients who have had a severe rash with carbamazepine Multiorgan hypersensitivity reactions (DRESS), fetal harm, bradycardia, ↑ risk of serious skin reactions (SJS/TEN), blood dyscrasias, cardiac arrest (caution in cardiac disease), hepatic and renal impairment, hypothyroidism
Fosphenytoin (Cerebyx) Injection (IV/IM) Prodrug of phenytoin	Fosphenytoin is dosed in phenytoin equivalents (PE): 1 mg PE = 1 mg phenytoin (fosphenytoin 1.5 mg = 1 mg PE)	**SIDE EFFECTS** **Dose-related (toxicity):** Nystagmus, ataxia, diplopia/blurred vision, slurred speech, dizziness, somnolence, lethargy, confusion or delirium **Chronic:** Gingival hyperplasia, hepatotoxicity, hair growth, morbilliform rash (measles-like), rash, peripheral neuropathy, ↑ BG, metallic taste, connective tissue hyperplasia **MONITORING** Serum phenytoin concentration, LFTs, CBC with differential IV: continuous cardiac (ECG, BP, HR) and respiratory function **NOTES** See adjusting phenytoin doses for low albumin later in the chapter

Phenytoin/Fosphenytoin Drug Interactions

- Phenytoin and fosphenytoin are strong inducers of several enzymes, including 2C19, 2C8/9, 3A4, P-gp and UGT1A1; they are substrates of CYP2C19 (major), 2C9 (major) and 3A4 (minor). Phenytoin and fosphenytoin can ↓ the concentration of many drugs, including other ASMs, contraceptives and warfarin.

- Use of an alternative, non-hormonal contraceptive is recommended with chronic phenytoin treatment.

- Both have high protein binding and can displace or be displaced by other highly protein-bound drugs. This can cause an ↑ in free drug levels and lead to toxicity.

PHENYTOIN/FOSPHENYTOIN ADMINISTRATION

IV Phenytoin
- Do not exceed 50 mg/minute (slow infusion)
- Monitor BP, respiratory function and ECG
- Requires a filter
- Dilute in NS, stable for 4 hours, do not refrigerate

NG-tube Phenytoin
- Enteral feedings (e.g., tube feeds) ↓ phenytoin absorption
- Hold feedings 1-2 hours before and after administration

IV Fosphenytoin
- Do not exceed 150 mg PE/minute
- Monitoring same as above
- Lower risk of purple glove syndrome than phenytoin

Phenytoin Monitoring

The metabolism of phenytoin can become saturated; when there are no enzymes available to metabolize the drug, a small increase in the dose can lead to a large increase in the drug concentration. See the Study Tip Gal on adjusting phenytoin doses. It is important to monitor levels and make dose changes carefully.

CASE SCENARIO

A patient has a total phenytoin level of 13 mcg/mL and recent labs as follows: SCr 1.1 mg/dL, albumin 3.1 g/dL. What is the corrected phenytoin level (round to the nearest TENTH)?

Phenytoin correction = 13 / (0.2 x 3.1) + 0.1

Phenytoin correction = 18.1 mcg/mL

ADJUSTING PHENYTOIN DOSES

Phenytoin follows Michaelis-Menten kinetics, also called saturable kinetics.

If the enzymes have become saturated, a small ↑ in dose can cause a large ↑ in drug level.

If albumin is low (< 3.5 g/dL) and CrCl ≥ 10 mL/min, adjust the total level with the formula:

$$\text{Phenytoin correction} = \frac{\text{Total phenytoin measured}}{(0.2 \times \text{albumin}) + 0.1} \quad †$$

Free levels do not require correction. See the Pharmacokinetics chapter for more details.

† Use serum phenytoin in mcg/mL and albumin in g/dL

Phenobarbital

DRUG	DOSING	SAFETY/SIDE EFFECTS/MONITORING
Phenobarbital (*Sezaby*) C-IV Tablet, elixir, injection *Sezaby* – injectable formulation for neonatal seizures in infants (preservative free)	**Initial:** 50-100 mg BID or TID **Therapeutic range:** 20-40 mcg/mL (adults) 15-40 mcg/mL (children)	**CONTRAINDICATIONS** Severe hepatic impairment, dyspnea or airway obstruction, previous addiction to sedative-hypnotics, intraarterial administration **WARNINGS** Caution in substance use disorder (potential for drug dependency), respiratory depression, fetal harm, paradoxical reactions including hyperactive or aggressive behavior (in acute pain and pediatric patients), hypotension when given IV, serious skin reactions (SJS/TEN) **SIDE EFFECTS** Physiological dependence, tolerance, residual sedation (i.e., hangover effect), somnolence, cognitive impairment, dizziness, ataxia, depression, folate deficiency **MONITORING** LFTs, CBC with differential **NOTES** Primidone is a prodrug of phenobarbital

Phenobarbital Drug Interactions

- Phenobarbital (and primidone, which is the prodrug) is a strong inducer of several enzymes, including 3A4 and P-gp. They can ↓ the levels of many drugs metabolized by these enzymes, such as other ASMs.

- Phenobarbital and primidone can significantly ↓ hormonal contraceptive levels. Use of an alternative, non-hormonal contraceptive is recommended.

ASM COUSINS

Some ASMs have "family members" with similar side effects and safety considerations.

- Carbamazepine, oxcarbazepine and eslicarbazepine
  - ❏ Hyponatremia, rash, enzyme induction
- Gabapentin and pregabalin
  - ❏ Weight gain, peripheral edema, mild euphoria
  - ❏ Used primarily for neuropathic pain

- Phenobarbital and primidone (prodrug of phenobarbital)
  - ❏ Sedation, dependence/tolerance/overdose risk, enzyme induction
- Topiramate and zonisamide
  - ❏ Weight loss, metabolic acidosis
  - ❏ Nephrolithiasis and oligohidrosis/hyperthermia (in children)

OTHER ANTISEIZURE MEDICATIONS

DRUG	SAFETY/SIDE EFFECTS/MONITORING
Benzodiazepines, including: Lorazepam (*Ativan*) Clobazam (*Onfi, Sympazan*) Diazepam (*Diastat AcuDial, Valtoco*) Midazolam (*Nayzilam*) Tablet, suspension, oral film, nasal spray, rectal gel C-IV	**BOXED WARNINGS** Use with opioids can result in profound sedation, respiratory depression and death **WARNINGS** Serious skin reactions (SJS/TEN), paradoxical reactions including hyperactive or aggressive behavior, anterograde amnesia **NOTES** Clobazam is used for Lennox-Gastaut syndrome or refractory epilepsy; all others are used to stop an active seizure Causes physiological dependence, tolerance, drooling, pyrexia, nasal/throat irritation (nasal formulations)
Brivaracetam (*Briviact*) Tablet, oral solution, injection C-V	**WARNINGS** Behavioral reactions including psychotic symptoms, irritability, depression, aggressive behavior and anxiety; bronchospasm and angioedema **MONITORING** Somnolence and fatigue, caution driving or operating machinery **NOTES** No added therapeutic benefit when used in combination with levetiracetam
Cannabidiol (*Epidiolex*) Oral solution	**WARNINGS** Somnolence and sedation (risk is ↑ when used with clobazam); hepatotoxicity (monitor LFTs), risk is ↑ when used with valproic acid or clobazam **NOTES** For seizures associated with Lennox-Gastaut syndrome, Dravet syndrome or tuberous sclerosis complex; can ↓ appetite
Cenobamate (*Xcopri*) Tablet C-V	**WARNINGS** Multiorgan hypersensitivity reactions (DRESS), shortening of the QT interval, somnolence, gait disturbance, visual changes (diplopia, blurred vision) **MONITORING** Eye exam, serum K (can become elevated)
Eslicarbazepine (*Aptiom*) Tablet Oxcarbazepine – active metabolite	**NOTES** Same warnings/side effects as oxcarbazepine including ↓ Na (monitor) plus a warning for drug-induced liver injury (monitor LFTs) Inducer of CYP3A4 (moderate)
Ethosuximide (*Zarontin*) Capsule, oral solution Used for absence seizures	**WARNINGS** Serious skin rash (SJS/TEN), blood dyscrasias, multiorgan hypersensitivity reactions (DRESS) **SIDE EFFECTS** N/V, abdominal pain, weight loss, hiccups, dizziness, somnolence **MONITORING** LFTs, CBC with differential, urinalysis, platelets, signs of rash, trough serum concentration
Felbamate (*Felbatol*) Tablet, oral suspension	**BOXED WARNINGS** Aplastic anemia, hepatic failure **MONITORING** LFTs, CBC, serum levels of other ASMs **NOTES** Informed consent needs to be signed by patient and prescriber prior to dispensing
Fenfluramine (*Fintepla*) Oral solution	**BOXED WARNING** Valvular heart disease, pulmonary hypertension (available only through a restricted distribution program/REMS) **WARNINGS** ↓ appetite/weight loss, serotonin syndrome (contraindicated with MAO inhibitors), ↑ BP, angle-closure glaucoma **MONITORING** Echocardiogram required before, during and after treatment, weight, BP

DRUG	SAFETY/SIDE EFFECTS/MONITORING
Gabapentin (Neurontin) Capsule, tablet, oral solution, oral suspension *Gralise* – postherpetic neuralgia (PHN) *Horizant* (gabapentin enacarbil) – PHN and restless legs syndrome	**WARNINGS** Angioedema **SIDE EFFECTS** Dizziness, somnolence, peripheral edema, weight gain, ataxia, diplopia, blurred vision, dry mouth, mild euphoria **MONITORING** Edema/weight gain **NOTES** Often used for neuropathic pain treatment See the Pain chapter for more details
Perampanel *(Fycompa)* Tablet, oral suspension C-III	**BOXED WARNING** Neuropsychiatric events (dose-related) including irritability, aggression, anger and paranoia, mainly in the first 6 weeks **NOTES** Substrate of CYP3A4 (major)
Pregabalin (Lyrica) C-V	**NOTES** Warnings, side effects and monitoring are the same as gabapentin Also used for diabetic or spinal cord injury neuropathic pain, PHN and fibromyalgia See the Pain chapter for more details
Primidone *(Mysoline)*	**NOTES** Prodrug of phenobarbital and phenylethylmalonamide (PEMA) – both are active metabolites See phenobarbital drug table for more details
Rufinamide *(Banzel)* Tablet, oral suspension	**CONTRAINDICATIONS** Patients with familial short QT syndrome due to QT shortening (dose-related) **NOTES** Take with food
Stiripentol *(Diacomit)* Capsule, oral suspension	**WARNINGS** Loss of appetite/weight loss, delirium/hallucinations (rare) **MONITORING** CBC and hepatic function, weight, mood **NOTES** To be taken with clobazam to treat seizures associated with Dravet syndrome
Tiagabine *(Gabitril)* Tablet	**WARNINGS** Worsening of seizures/new-onset seizures when used off-label for other indications, serious skin reactions (SJS/TEN) **NOTES** Take with food
Vigabatrin *(Sabril, Vigadrone)* Tablet, packet for solution	**BOXED WARNING** Causes permanent vision loss ($\geq$ 30% of patients) **MONITORING** Eye exam at baseline, every 3 months during therapy and 3-6 months after discontinuation **NOTES** Only available through a restricted program called the Vigabatrin REMS Program
Zonisamide *(Zonegran, Zonisade)* Capsule, oral suspension	**CONTRAINDICATIONS** Hypersensitivity to sulfonamides **WARNINGS** Same as topiramate except no hyperammonemia warning and there is a risk of serious skin reactions (SJS/TEN); multiorgan hypersensitivity reactions (DRESS) **SIDE EFFECTS** Similar to topiramate, including oligohidrosis/hyperthermia (typically in children) and risk of nephrolithiasis

MONITORING

All ASMs require monitoring of seizure frequency (to ensure efficacy) and mental status (to minimize adverse effects). Some ASMs (e.g., phenytoin, valproic acid, carbamazepine, phenobarbital) also have therapeutic drug level ranges that are monitored to control seizures and keep the toxic effects to a minimum. Drug levels are obtained when treatment is started, at dose adjustments, with suspected toxicity and to monitor adherence periodically.

DRUG INTERACTIONS

ASMs can cause drug interactions through protein binding or enzyme-mediated effects. Some ASMs are highly protein-bound (e.g., phenytoin, valproate, clobazam) and can interact with other protein-bound drugs by displacing them from protein binding sites; this creates more free (unbound) drug and increases the risk of toxicity. Some ASMs may induce or inhibit enzymes responsible for drug metabolism (e.g., CYP, UGT) or transporter proteins (e.g., P-glycoprotein).

Many ASMs are enzyme inducers and lower the concentration of other medications, including other ASMs (see Study Tip Gal).

Valproic acid is an enzyme inhibitor that increases the levels of substrates, such as lamotrigine. Higher lamotrigine levels increase the risk of severe rash; dose adjustments are required when using valproic acid and lamotrigine together to decrease this risk.

SELECT ASMs WITH ENZYME INDUCTION OR INHIBITION

Enzyme Inducers

- Carbamazepine
- Oxcarbazepine
- Phenytoin
- Fosphenytoin
- Phenobarbital
- Primidone

Enzyme Inhibitor

- Valproic acid (↑ lamotrigine)

SPECIAL POPULATIONS

Use in Pregnancy

Several older ASMs (e.g., clonazepam, phenobarbital, primidone, phenytoin, fosphenytoin, carbamazepine, valproic acid) have known teratogenic risk. Valproic acid has the highest risk, causing neural tube defects and impaired cognitive function in the child (decreased IQ). Levetiracetam has the lowest risk and is preferred in pregnancy; lamotrigine also has a low risk and can be considered during pregnancy. The risk profiles of newer ASMs are not well defined; most have some degree of risk in pregnancy.

Congenital malformations occur more commonly in children exposed to ASMs *in utero*. Most are minor, but some are not (e.g., cardiac defects, urogenital defects, neural tube defects). Neural tube defects occur most commonly in children born to mothers taking carbamazepine or valproic acid. Women of childbearing age on ASMs should receive daily folate supplementation.

Women of childbearing age on ASMs should avoid unplanned pregnancy. Pre-pregnancy counseling should be done to ensure that a plan is in place to maintain good seizure control. Many ASMs reduce the efficacy of oral hormonal contraceptives and require the use of non-hormonal contraceptives while on treatment (see the Contraception & Infertility chapter).

ASMs contribute to bone loss. During pregnancy, the mother provides calcium for fetal bone growth. This leads to a need for extra calcium. Adequate calcium and vitamin D supplementation is required for pregnant patients taking an ASM.

Blood levels of ASMs can change throughout pregnancy and postpartum. Monitoring drug levels throughout this time frame is very important. ASM levels decline during pregnancy, with some being more affected than others. Low ASM levels can lead to seizures, which can be harmful to the baby; dose increases may be needed. In the postpartum period, ASM levels increase, and decreased doses are commonly needed. Monitoring ASM levels during the postpartum period is required to minimize side effects and better control seizures.

Use in Children

In addition to cognitive impairment and coordination difficulty, there are drug-specific risks in children taking ASMs. Topiramate and zonisamide can cause reduced sweating (i.e., hypohidrosis) in young children. This means that sun exposure should be limited to minimize the risk of hyperthermia. Lamotrigine-induced rash with risk of fatality occurs more commonly in children.

Administering medications to children can be difficult as many are unable to swallow tablets and capsules. ASMs used in children often come in formulations that are easy to swallow (e.g., lamotrigine ODT or chewable tablets, levetiracetam ODT or oral solutions).

KEY COUNSELING POINTS

See the Drug Formulations and Patient Counseling chapter for counseling language/layman's terminology.

ALL ANTISEIZURE MEDICATIONS

- Can cause:
  - ❏ Suicidal thoughts or behaviors.
  - ❏ Drowsiness.
- Seizures can become worse when the drug is suddenly stopped. The dose must be gradually decreased.
- Many drug interactions, including drugs that worsen drowsiness (e.g., benzodiazepines and opioids) and drugs that lower the seizure threshold.
- Supplement with calcium and vitamin D while taking this medication.

Carbamazepine

- Can cause:
  - ❏ Severe rash.
  - ❏ Rare but serious blood disorders. You will need to have your blood checked while on this medication.
- Avoid in pregnancy (teratogenic).

Lamotrigine

- Can cause:
  - ❏ Severe rash (most likely in the first 2 to 8 weeks of treatment).
- Chewable tablets can be swallowed whole, chewed or mixed in water or diluted juice. If mixed, drink the whole amount right away.

Oxcarbazepine

- Can cause:
  - ❏ Low sodium levels. Contact your healthcare provider if you experience fatigue, headache, nausea or confusion.
  - ❏ Severe rash.
- Take extended-release (*Oxtellar XR*) on an empty stomach at least one hour before or two hours after food.
- Shake oral suspension for 10 seconds before using. It can be mixed in a small glass of water.

Phenytoin

- Can cause:
  - ❏ Severe rash.
  - ❏ Gingival hyperplasia.
  - ❏ Changes in vision (e.g., double vision).
  - ❏ Abnormal eye movements.
- Avoid in pregnancy (teratogenic).

Phenobarbital

- Abuse and dependence can occur.
- Avoid in pregnancy (teratogenic).

Topiramate

- Can cause:
  - ❏ Problems with concentration, attention, memory or speech.
  - ❏ Eye damage.
  - ❏ Decreased sweating and increased body temperature (especially in children).
  - ❏ Weight loss.
- Sprinkle capsules can be swallowed whole or opened and sprinkled on a teaspoon of soft food. Swallow whole; do not chew. Follow with a glass of water.
- Drink plenty of fluids to prevent kidney stones.
- Avoid in pregnancy (teratogenic).

Valproic Acid

- Can cause:
  - ❏ Liver damage.
  - ❏ Weight gain.
- Avoid in pregnancy (teratogenic).
- Take with food to help avoid stomach upset.

Diazepam Rectal Gel

- The green "READY" band should be visible before leaving the pharmacy.

- Administration instructions (detailed administration instructions can be found at https://diastat.com/):

    ❑ Put the person on their side in a safe location (where they can't fall).

    ❑ Get medication syringe and lubricating jelly.

    ❑ Remove syringe cap (and seal pin) by pushing up with thumb.

    ❑ Apply lubricating jelly to syringe tip.

    ❑ Turn the person on their side facing you and bend upper leg forward to expose the rectum.

    ❑ Separate buttocks and gently insert syringe tip into the rectum until the rim is snug against the rectal opening.

    ❑ Slowly count to 3 while gently pushing the plunger until it stops.

    ❑ Count to 3 before removing syringe from rectum.

    ❑ Remove the syringe and count to 3 again while holding buttocks together to prevent leakage.

    ❑ Make note of the time given and observe.

- Call 911 if the seizure continues 15 minutes after giving the medication.

- To dispose of any medication remaining in the syringe, first remove the plunger from syringe, then replace it. Aim the application tip over the sink or toilet. Push the plunger down to remove any remaining medication in the syringe.

Select Guidelines/References

Evidence-Based Guideline: Treatment of Convulsive Status Epilepticus in Children and Adults: Report of the Guideline Committee of the American Epilepsy Society. *Epilepsy Curr.* 2016;16(1):48-61.

Operational Classification of Seizure Types by the International League Against Epilepsy. 2017 Update. *Epilepsia.* 58(4):522-530.

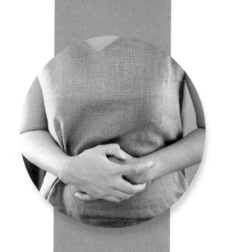
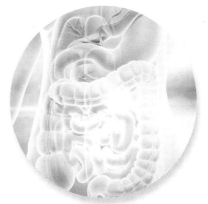
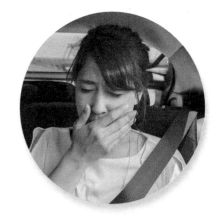

GASTROINTESTINAL CONDITIONS

CONTENTS

CONTENT LEGEND

 = Study Tip Gal
 = Key Drug Guy

CHAPTER 71

GASTROESOPHAGEAL REFLUX DISEASE (GERD) & PEPTIC ULCER DISEASE (PUD)

GASTROESOPHAGEAL REFLUX DISEASE

BACKGROUND

Parietal cells in the epithelial lining of the stomach secrete hydrochloric acid (HCl) through the H^+/K^+-adenosine triphosphatase (ATPase) pump, known as the proton pump. The pump, and secretion of HCl, is stimulated by histamine, acetylcholine and the hormone gastrin, which has the added role of stimulating stomach muscle contractions to aid in digestion. Acidic gastric contents are normally prevented from backflow into the esophagus by a protective ring of muscle fibers called the lower esophageal sphincter (LES). Patients with gastroesophageal reflux disease (GERD) have reduced LES pressure (muscle tone), and gastric contents can backflow into the esophagus.

SCREENING AND DIAGNOSIS

Typical GERD symptoms include heartburn (daytime or nocturnal), hypersalivation and regurgitation of acidic contents into the mouth or throat. Less common symptoms include epigastric pain, nausea, cough, sore throat, hoarseness or chest pain, which can be difficult to distinguish from cardiac pain.

Diagnosis is based on patient-reported symptoms (duration, daytime and/or nocturnal occurrence), frequency (≥ 2 times per week) and risk factors (e.g., family history, diet and eating habits, sleep position); invasive testing is not required when typical symptoms are present.

GERD can decrease quality of life and lead to esophageal erosion, strictures, bleeding and Barrett's esophagus (abnormal cell growth in the esophageal lining which can lead to esophageal cancer). If a patient has alarm symptoms (see next page) or there is concern for a more serious condition, endoscopy can be performed to further investigate the problem. Patients who are refractory to GERD treatment may benefit from 24-hour esophageal pH monitoring.

KEY DRUGS THAT CAN WORSEN GERD SYMPTOMS

Aspirin/NSAIDs	Fish oil products	Steroids
Bisphosphonates	Iron supplements	Tetracyclines
Dabigatran	Nicotine replacement therapy	
Estrogen products		

GERD Treatment Algorithm

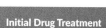

Lifestyle Modifications

- Weight loss (if overweight or recently gained weight)*
- Elevate the head of the bed with foam wedges or blocks
- Avoid eating high fat meals within 2-3 hours of bedtime
- Avoid foods/beverages that trigger reflux (patient-specific): caffeine, chocolate, acidic/spicy foods, carbonated beverages

Initial Drug Treatment

PPI once daily for 8 weeks

- Can increase to twice daily if partial response or if nocturnal symptoms are present

Stop treatment at 8 weeks; if symptoms return, start maintenance therapy

Maintenance Treatment

- 1st line: PPI at the lowest effective dose**
- Alternative: H2RA, if there is no erosive esophagitis and it relieves symptoms
- Not recommended: metoclopramide or sucralfate

*Weight loss has the best evidence for improvement of symptoms
**Can include intermittent or on-demand dosing (see PPI section of text)*

TREATMENT PRINCIPLES

The vast majority of patients self-treat GERD symptoms with OTC products and do not seek medical attention unless this fails; a pharmacist is often the first healthcare encounter. Patients should be referred for further evaluation if they do not respond to lifestyle modifications and/or two weeks of self-treatment with OTC products, or if alarm symptoms are present [e.g., odynophagia (painful swallowing), dysphagia, frequent nausea and vomiting, hematemesis, black or bloody stools, unintentional weight loss].

Treatment should include lifestyle modifications and drugs. Infrequent heartburn (< 2 times/week) can be treated with as needed OTC antacids or histamine-2 receptor antagonists (H2RAs). For frequent (≥ 2 times/week) or severe GERD symptoms, an eight-week course of a proton pump inhibitor (PPI) is the initial treatment of choice and is used to heal any erosive esophagitis. After eight weeks, interrupt treatment and start maintenance therapy if symptoms return. Vonoprazan, an oral potassium-competitive acid blocker, was recently approved for the treatment of erosive esophagitis caused by GERD, though its place in therapy is not yet well defined.

DRUG TREATMENT

Antacids

Antacids work by neutralizing gastric acid (producing salt and water), which increases gastric pH. Since antacids do not require systemic absorption, they provide relief within minutes, but the duration of relief is short (30 – 60 minutes). Antacids can be purchased OTC and are suitable for mild, infrequent symptoms. Patients using antacids containing aspirin (e.g., *Alka-Seltzer)* should be made aware of the serious bleeding risk if used too frequently.

DRUG	DOSING	SAFETY/SIDE EFFECTS/MONITORING
Calcium carbonate (Tums, others) **+ magnesium (Mylanta Supreme,** others) **+ simethicone** (anti-gas) **(Maalox Advanced Maximum Strength,** others) **Magnesium hydroxide (Milk of Magnesia,** others) + aluminum (Mag-Al, others) **+ aluminum + simethicone (Mylanta Maximum Strength,** others) **Sodium bicarbonate/aspirin/ citric acid (Alka-Seltzer,** others)**	Many formulations including suspensions, chewable tablets, capsules Dosing varies by product; many require administration 4-6 times per day	**WARNINGS** Aluminum and magnesium: can accumulate with severe renal dysfunction (not recommended if CrCl < 30 mL/min); risk of bleeding with aspirin-containing products **SIDE EFFECTS** Unpleasant taste Calcium: constipation, bloating, belching Aluminum: constipation, hypophosphatemia Magnesium: loose stools (use with aluminum may counter-balance) **NOTES** Calcium-containing antacids may be preferred in pregnancy (see Drug Use in Pregnancy & Lactation chapter) *Alka-Seltzer* contains > 500 mg Na per tablet which can worsen edema in patients with heart failure or cirrhosis

Histamine-2 Receptor Antagonists

H2RAs reversibly inhibit H2 receptors on gastric parietal cells, which decreases gastric acid secretion. They are used PRN for infrequent or mild heartburn but have a slower onset than antacids. H2RAs can be used as maintenance treatment for GERD, after the initial eight weeks of PPI therapy, if there are no esophageal erosions and the patient can remain symptom-free. Use of an H2RA for maintenance treatment could decrease side effects associated with long-term use of PPIs (see Risks Associated with PPI section). If H2RAs are used for ulcer healing or hypersecretory conditions (e.g., Zollinger-Ellison syndrome), higher doses are needed.

DRUG	DOSING	SAFETY/SIDE EFFECTS/MONITORING
Famotidine **(Pepcid AC, Zantac 360,** others) Rx and OTC: tablet, chewable tablet, suspension Rx: injection + calcium carbonate and magnesium hydroxide (Pepcid Complete) OTC: chewable tablet + ibuprofen (Duexis) Rx: tablet	**OTC** 10-20 mg 1-2 times daily PRN **Rx** 20 mg BID CrCl < 60 mL/min: decrease dose	**WARNINGS** Confusion, usually reversible [risk factors: elderly, severely ill, renal impairment (see Notes)] Vitamin B12 deficiency with prolonged use (≥ 2 years) Famotidine: ECG changes (QT prolongation) with renal dysfunction **SIDE EFFECTS** Headache, agitation/vomiting in children < 1 year Cimetidine (high doses): gynecomastia, impotence **NOTES** Onset of relief: within 60 minutes; duration: 4-10 hours
Cimetidine (Tagamet HB) Rx and OTC: tablet, oral solution	**OTC** 200 mg 1-2 times daily PRN **Rx** 400 mg Q6H	May be used in pregnancy when clinically indicated Decrease dose when CrCl < 50 mL/min (nizatidine) or CrCl < 30 mL/min (cimetidine) Cimetidine can ↑ SCr, without causing renal impairment Avoid cimetidine due to drug interactions and side effects
Nizatidine Rx: capsule	**Rx** 150 mg BID	To relieve symptoms, take PRN; to prevent symptoms, take PRN 30-60 minutes before food or beverages that cause heartburn Tachyphylaxis (tolerance to effects) can occur if used on a scheduled basis

All ranitidine products (previously branded Zantac) were removed from the market in April 2020.

Proton Pump Inhibitors

PPIs irreversibly bind to the gastric H^+/K^+-ATPase pump (the proton pump) in parietal cells. This shuts down the pump and blocks gastric acid secretion. PPIs are the most effective medications for GERD, and an eight-week course of treatment is recommended for relief of symptoms and to heal erosions that may be present. All PPIs have similar efficacy, though an individual patient may respond better to one drug over another. If used long-term as maintenance treatment, the lowest effective dose should be used and the need for treatment should be assessed regularly. Intermittent use (PPI taken for a short time after relapse of GERD symptoms) and on-demand use (PPI taken only when symptoms occur) are additional options.

Recommended Administration of Oral PPIs

DRUG	MEAL	TIMING
Esomeprazole (Nexium)		At least 60 minutes before
Lansoprazole (Prevacid, Prevacid SoluTab)		Time not specified
Omeprazole (Prilosec)	Before breakfast	Time not specified
Omeprazole + sodium bicarbonate (Zegerid)		60 minutes before (can control nocturnal symptoms if given at bedtime)
Dexlansoprazole (Dexilant)		Without regard to meals
Pantoprazole (Protonix)	Formulation-specific	Tablet: without regard to meals Oral suspension: 30 minutes before a meal
Rabeprazole (Aciphex)		Tablet: without regard to meals Capsule sprinkles: 30 minutes before meal

Proton Pump Inhibitor Products

DRUG	DOSING	SAFETY/SIDE EFFECTS/MONITORING
Dexlansoprazole (Dexilant) Rx: capsule	**Rx** 30-60 mg daily	**WARNINGS** C. difficile-associated diarrhea (CDAD), hypomagnesemia, vitamin B12 deficiency with prolonged use (≥ 2 years), osteoporosis-related bone fractures with high doses or long-term (≥ 1 year) use, acute interstitial nephritis (hypersensitivity reaction), cutaneous and systemic lupus erythematosus
Esomeprazole (Nexium, Nexium 24HR, Nexium I.V., others) Rx and OTC: capsule, tablet Rx: injection, packet for oral suspension **+ naproxen (Vimovo)** Rx: tablet	**OTC** 20 mg daily **Rx** 20-40 mg daily	PPIs may diminish the therapeutic effect of clopidogrel, do not use omeprazole and esomeprazole while taking clopidogrel; rabeprazole or pantoprazole have less risk IV Protonix: thrombophlebitis, severe skin reactions (SJS/TEN)
Lansoprazole (Prevacid, Prevacid SoluTab, Prevacid 24HR, others) Rx and OTC: capsule, ODT	**OTC** 15 mg daily **Rx** 15-30 mg daily	**SIDE EFFECTS** Generally well-tolerated, can cause headache, abdominal pain, nausea, diarrhea
Omeprazole (Prilosec, Prilosec OTC) Rx and OTC: capsule, tablet Rx: packet for oral suspension OTC: ODT **+ sodium bicarbonate (Konvomep, Zegerid)** Rx and OTC: capsule, packet for oral suspension **+ aspirin (Yosprala)** Rx: tablet	**OTC** 20 mg daily **Rx** 20-40 mg daily	**NOTES** Onset: 1-3 hours; duration > 24 hrs for most PPIs May be used in pregnancy when clinically indicated Pantoprazole and esomeprazole are the only PPIs available IV Do not crush, cut, or chew tablets or capsules Dexlansoprazole, esomeprazole, lansoprazole, omeprazole and rabeprazole capsules can be opened (not crushed), mixed in applesauce and swallowed immediately (without chewing) Zegerid 20 mg and 40 mg have the same Na bicarbonate content (1,100 mg); do not substitute two 20 mg capsules/packets for one 40 mg capsule/packet because the patient will receive twice the amount of Na; caution in patients on Na-restricted diet (e.g., heart failure, cirrhosis)
Pantoprazole (Protonix) Rx: tablet, injection, packet for oral suspension	**Rx** 40 mg daily	Suspension compounding kits are available that contain pre-measured powdered drug, suspension liquid (with flavoring) and mixing tools
Rabeprazole (Aciphex) Rx: tablet, capsule sprinkle	**Rx** 20 mg daily	

Risks Associated with PPI Therapy

Long-term use of PPIs causes chronic changes in gastric pH. This can promote growth of microorganisms and increase the risk of GI infections, including C. difficile and possibly pneumonia (due to reflux of gastric contents beyond the oral cavity). PPIs also increase the risk of osteoporosis and fractures. The Beers Criteria recommend that PPIs not be used beyond eight weeks in elderly patients unless there is a clear indication (e.g., high risk for GI bleed due to chronic NSAID use, demonstrated need for maintenance treatment).

H2RA AND PPI FORMULATIONS TO KNOW

- H2RAs and PPIs are very common medications. Sometimes suspensions, solutions or ODT formulations are needed (e.g., infants, children, adults unable to swallow tablets/capsules). Non-oral formulations are used when patients are NPO.

	OTC	ODT	ORAL SOLUTION/SUSPENSION	INJECTION
H2RA	Cimetidine Famotidine		Cimetidine Famotidine	Famotidine
PPI	Esomeprazole Lansoprazole Omeprazole	Lansoprazole Omeprazole	**Packets for suspension:** Esomeprazole Omeprazole Pantoprazole	Esomeprazole Pantoprazole

Metoclopramide and Other Medications

Other medications historically used for GERD treatment include the cytoprotective drugs, misoprostol and sucralfate, and the prokinetic drug, metoclopramide. There is currently no role for these medications in the management of GERD and they are not recommended by guidelines. Misoprostol and sucralfate can be used for peptic ulcer disease, which is discussed later in the chapter. Metoclopramide and erythromycin are most commonly used when patients have coexisting gastroparesis.

Metoclopramide is a dopamine antagonist. At higher doses, it blocks serotonin receptors in the chemoreceptor zone of the CNS which helps nausea and vomiting (see the Oncology chapter). Metoclopramide enhances the response to acetylcholine in the upper GI tract, causing increased motility, accelerated gastric emptying (peristaltic speed) and ↑ LES tone.

DRUG	DOSING	SAFETY/SIDE EFFECTS/MONITORING
Metoclopramide (*Reglan*, *Gimoti*) Tablet, ODT, oral solution, injection, nasal solution	10-15 mg QID 30 min before meals and at bedtime Short duration of action (food must be present in the gut) Not recommended for use > 12 weeks CrCl < 60 mL/min: decrease dose 50% (to avoid side effects, including CNS/EPS side effects)	**BOXED WARNING** Can cause tardive dyskinesia (a serious movement disorder, often irreversible); there is increased risk with high doses, long-term treatment (> 12 weeks) and in elderly patients **CONTRAINDICATIONS** GI obstruction, perforation or hemorrhage, history of seizures, pheochromocytoma, use in combination with other drugs likely to increase extrapyramidal symptoms (EPS) **WARNINGS** EPS (including acute dystonia), parkinsonian-like symptoms, rare neuroleptic malignant syndrome (NMS), depression, suicidal ideation Avoid use in patients with Parkinson disease **SIDE EFFECTS** Drowsiness, restlessness, fatigue, hypertension, pro-arrhythmic, diarrhea

DRUG INTERACTIONS

There are many types of interactions between acid-suppressing drugs and other medications. This section highlights the most important interactions for antacids, H2RAs and PPIs, but it is not all-inclusive. As appropriate, refer to other chapters (e.g., HIV, Hepatitis & Liver Disease, Infectious Diseases).

Antacids, H2RAs and PPIs

- Some drugs require an acidic gut for absorption, including enteric-coated or delayed-release products that can dissolve and release drug prematurely if the gastric pH is increased. The Key Drugs Guy to the right shows some important drugs that can have decreased absorption when given concurrently with antacids, H2RAs and PPIs.

  - Due to the short duration of action of antacids, this type of interaction can often be alleviated by separating administration of the interacting drugs (see Antacids section on next page).

  - The following should be avoided completely when taking H2RAs or PPIs: dasatinib, pazopanib and the delayed-release formulation of risedronate (*Atelvia*). Erlotinib, rilpivirine and velpatasvir/sofosbuvir (*Epclusa*) are additional medications that should be avoided in combination with PPIs.

KEY DRUGS WITH DECREASED ABSORPTION

Drugs that require an acidic gut (absorption ↓ by antacids, H2RAs and PPIs)
- Antiretrovirals: rilpivirine (NNRTI), atazanavir (PI)
- Antivirals: ledipasvir, velpatasvir/sofosbuvir
- Azole antifungals: *Sporanox* (itraconazole capsules), ketoconazole, posaconazole oral suspension*
- Cephalosporins (oral): cefpodoxime, cefuroxime
- Iron products
- Risedronate delayed-release
- Tyrosine kinase inhibitors: dasatinib, erlotinib, pazopanib

Oral drugs/drug classes that antacids bind
- Antiretrovirals (INSTIs): bictegravir, dolutegravir, elvitegravir, raltegravir
- Bisphosphonates
- Isoniazid
- Levothyroxine
- Mycophenolate
- Quinolones
- Sotalol
- Steroids (especially budesonide)
- Tetracyclines

NNRTI = non-nucleoside reverse transcriptase inhibitor, PI = protease inhibitor, INSTI = integrase strand transfer inhibitor
*Absorption decreased by H2RAs and PPIs only

Antacids

- Antacids can decrease the absorption of some drugs by binding or adsorbing to them. It is necessary to separate administration of antacids from select drugs (see Key Drugs Guy on previous page). The timing of separation varies; for most products, avoiding antacids 2 – 4 hours before or 2 – 6 hours after is recommended.

H2RAs

- Use caution with CNS depressants (especially in the elderly) due to the risk of additive delirium, dementia and cognitive impairment. Use lower doses in patients with renal impairment.

- Do not use famotidine with highest risk QT-prolonging drugs (see the Arrhythmias chapter).

- Cimetidine is an inhibitor of CYP450 enzymes (e.g., CYP2C19, CYP3A4, CYP1A2). Avoid use with dofetilide and use caution with other drugs, including amiodarone, calcium channel blockers, clopidogrel, phenytoin, SSRIs, theophylline and warfarin.

PPIs

- All PPIs inhibit CYP2C19; most are weak inhibitors but omeprazole and esomeprazole are moderate inhibitors. PPIs can ↑ the levels of citalopram, phenytoin, tacrolimus, voriconazole and warfarin. Do not use PPIs with nelfinavir.

- Omeprazole and esomeprazole can ↓ the effectiveness of clopidogrel (a prodrug) through CYP2C19 inhibition. Do not use these drugs together.

- PPIs can inhibit renal elimination of methotrexate, leading to ↑ serum levels and risk of methotrexate toxicities.

Metoclopramide

- Do not use in patients receiving medications for Parkinson disease (antagonistic effect). Do not use in combination with antipsychotic drugs, droperidol or promethazine due to an increased risk of adverse effects. When used in combination with SSRIs, SNRIs or TCAs, monitor for possible EPS, NMS and serotonin syndrome.

PEPTIC ULCER DISEASE

BACKGROUND

Peptic ulcer disease (PUD) occurs when there is mucosal erosion within the gastrointestinal tract. Unlike gastritis, the ulcers in PUD extend deeper into the mucosa. Most ulcers occur in the duodenum, but a small percentage occur in the stomach. Ulcers can be observed with an upper gastrointestinal endoscopy. The three most common causes of PUD are *Helicobacter pylori (H. pylori)*-positive ulcers, non-steroidal anti-inflammatory drug (NSAID)-

induced ulcers and stress ulcers, which occur in critically ill and mechanically-ventilated patients (see the Acute & Critical Care Medicine chapter). *H. pylori*, a spiral-shaped, pH-sensitive, gram-negative bacterium that lives in the acidic environment of the stomach, is responsible for the majority of peptic ulcers (70 – 95%). Less common causes of PUD are hypersecretory states (e.g., increased gastric acid in Zollinger-Ellison syndrome), viral infections (e.g., cytomegalovirus), radiation therapy and infiltrative diseases (e.g., Crohn's Disease).

Under normal conditions, a physiologic balance exists between gastric acid secretion and the gut's mucosal defense and repair mechanisms, which include mucus and bicarbonate secretion, mucosal blood flow, prostaglandin synthesis, cellular regeneration and epithelial cell renewal. These mechanisms protect the GI mucosa from damage caused by NSAIDs (including aspirin), *H. pylori*, acid, pepsin and other GI irritants.

Symptoms

The primary symptom of PUD is dyspepsia, a gastric pain that can feel like a gnawing or burning sensation in the middle or upper stomach. If the ulcer is duodenal (usually caused by *H. pylori*), pain is typically worse 2 – 3 hours after eating (when the stomach is empty); eating food or taking antacids lessens the pain. With gastric ulcers (primarily from NSAIDs), eating generally worsens the pain. Other symptoms include heartburn, belching, bloating, cramping, nausea and anorexia.

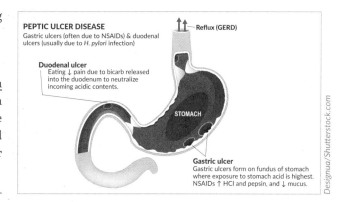

PEPTIC ULCER DISEASE
Gastric ulcers (often due to NSAIDs) & duodenal ulcers (usually due to *H. pylori* infection)

↑↑ — Reflux (GERD)

Duodenal ulcer
Eating ↓ pain due to bicarb released into the duodenum to neutralize incoming acidic contents.

STOMACH

Gastric ulcer
Gastric ulcers form on fundus of stomach where exposure to stomach acid is highest. NSAIDs ↑ HCl and pepsin, and ↓ mucus.

Designua/Shutterstock.com

H. PYLORI DETECTION AND MANAGEMENT

Diagnostic Tests

Common, non-invasive, diagnostic tests for *H. pylori* include the urea breath test (UBT), which detects gas (CO_2) produced by the bacteria, and the fecal antigen test, which detects *H. pylori* in the stool. PPIs, bismuth and antibiotics should be discontinued two weeks prior to these tests to avoid false negative results. The infection should be treated if testing is positive.

Drug Treatment

H. pylori infection, if left untreated, can lead to gastric cancer. There are several combination regimens available to treat *H. pylori* (see the table below). Due to failure rates with triple therapy (often caused by clarithromycin resistance), the American College of Gastroenterology (ACG) guidelines recommend quadruple therapy first-line. The use of triple therapy first-line is only recommended if clarithromycin resistance rates are low (< 15%) and the patient has no previous history of taking a macrolide antibiotic (for any reason).

Do not make drug substitutions in *H. pylori* eradication regimens. H2RAs should not be substituted for a PPI, unless the patient cannot tolerate a PPI. Other antibiotics within a class should not be substituted (for example, do not use ampicillin instead of amoxicillin). If the PPI is continued beyond 14 days, this is to help ulcer healing; it should not be continued indefinitely.

First-Line *H. pylori* Treatment Regimens

DRUG REGIMEN	NOTES
Bismuth Quadruple Therapy: Take for 10-14 Days Use first-line, especially if local resistance rates to clarithromycin are high (≥ 15%), the patient has had a previous macrolide exposure or a penicillin allergy, or triple therapy failed (if used first)	
Bismuth subsalicylate 300 mg QID +	Tinidazole may be substituted for metronidazole
Metronidazole 250-500 mg QID +	If the patient cannot tolerate a PPI, substitute an H2RA (e.g., famotidine 40 mg daily, nizatidine 150 mg BID)
Tetracycline 500 mg QID +	Swallow all capsules in the *Pylera* regimen (3 capsules per dose)
PPI BID	
Or use a (3-in-1) combination product + PPI:	**Alcohol Use** Do not use metronidazole
Pylera (bismuth subcitrate potassium 420 mg + metronidazole 375 mg + tetracycline 375 mg) QID + PPI BID	**Pregnancy/Children** Do not use tetracycline during pregnancy or in children < 8 years of age
	Salicylate Allergy Do not use bismuth subsalicylate
Concomitant Therapy: Take for 10-14 Days Use only if local resistance rates to clarithromycin are low (< 15%) and the patient has had no previous exposure to a macrolide; preferred over clarithromycin triple therapy if previous macrolide exposure	
Amoxicillin 1,000 mg BID +	Tinidazole may be substituted for metronidazole
Clarithromycin 500 mg BID +	
Metronidazole 500 mg BID +	
PPI BID	
Clarithromycin Triple Therapy: Take for 14 Days Use only if local resistance rates to clarithromycin are low (< 15%) and the patient has had no previous exposure to a macrolide	
Amoxicillin 1,000 mg BID +	Penicillin allergy: replace amoxicillin with metronidazole 500 mg TID or use quadruple therapy (see above)
Clarithromycin 500 mg BID +	*Prevpac* contains all medications on one blister card; take the entire contents of one card (divided BID) every day for 14 days
PPI BID (or esomeprazole 40 mg daily)	*Omeclamox-Pak* is a combination package, swallow capsules and tablets whole
Or use a (3-in-1) combination product with PPI:	
Prevpac (amoxicillin + clarithromycin + lansoprazole)	
Omeclamox-Pak (amoxicillin + clarithromycin + omeprazole)	

Other *H. pylori* Treatments

Sequential therapy (PPI + amoxicillin for 5 - 7 days, followed by a PPI, clarithromycin and metronidazole for the remaining 5 - 7 days), hybrid therapy (PPI + amoxicillin for 7 days, followed by a PPI, amoxicillin, clarithromycin and metronidazole for 7 days) and quinolone-based regimens are other options in the guidelines, though with a weaker level of evidence.

Talicia (rifabutin + amoxicillin + omeprazole) is an FDA-approved treatment for *H. pylori*. Vonoprazan (see GERD Treatment Principles earlier in the chapter) is also indicated for *H. pylori* treatment in combination with an appropriate antibiotic regimen and can be used in place of a PPI (though its place in therapy is not yet clear). It is available in combination with amoxicillin (*Voquezna Dual Pak)* and amoxicillin + clarithromycin (*Voquezna Triple Pak)*.

NON-STEROIDAL ANTI-INFLAMMATORY DRUG-INDUCED ULCERS

Background

NSAIDs, including aspirin, can cause gastric mucosal damage by two mechanisms: direct irritation of the gastric epithelium and systemic inhibition of prostaglandin synthesis (by inhibiting COX-1). The chronic use of NSAIDs increases the risk for gastric (GI) ulcers. Patients are at high risk if they have any of the risk factors shown in the box to the right.

RISK FACTORS FOR NSAID-INDUCED ULCERS
Age > 60 years
History of PUD (including *H. pylori*-induced)
High-dose NSAIDs
Using > 1 NSAID (e.g., ibuprofen plus aspirin)
Concomitant use of anticoagulants, steroids, SSRIs or SNRIs

Prevention and Treatment

All NSAIDs elevate blood pressure and decrease renal blood flow; they should be used with caution in any person with cardiovascular or renal disease. When selecting an NSAID, it is important to weigh these risks with the risks for GI ulcers and bleeding. NSAIDs with selective inhibition of COX-2 (e.g., celecoxib) have decreased GI risk but increased cardiovascular (CV) risk compared to non-selective NSAIDs. NSAIDs that approach the selectivity of celecoxib are meloxicam, nabumetone, diclofenac and etodolac.

Patients with high GI risk (or a history of ulcers) who take non-selective NSAIDs can use a PPI to prevent or decrease the risk of ulcers and bleeding, but the long-term risks need to be considered (see Risks of PPI Therapy section). The cytoprotective drug, misoprostol, is an alternative option to a PPI, but diarrhea, cramping and its four times per day dosing contribute to poor patient adherence. Combination products specifically marketed to reduce the risk of NSAID-induced ulcers include naproxen/esomeprazole *(Vimovo)*, ibuprofen/famotidine *(Duexis)* and diclofenac/misoprostol *(Arthrotec)*; these are indicated to relieve symptoms of osteoarthritis and rheumatoid arthritis in patients at risk of GI ulcers. *Yosprala*, a combination of aspirin and omeprazole, is approved for secondary prevention of cardiovascular and cerebrovascular events in patients at risk for aspirin-associated ulcers.

If possible, both non-selective NSAIDs and COX-2 selective drugs should be avoided in patients with both high GI and high CV risk. Naproxen may be the preferred NSAID in patients with low-moderate GI risk and high CV risk. A COX-2 selective drug, with or without a PPI, can be used in patients who do not have CV risk factors.

If an ulcer develops, it should be treated with a PPI for eight weeks, and NSAIDs should be discontinued. If PPIs cannot be used, high-dose H2RAs or sucralfate are other options.

Cytoprotective Drugs

Misoprostol is a prostaglandin E1 analog that replaces the gastro-protective prostaglandins removed by NSAIDs. Sucralfate is a sucrose-sulfate-aluminum complex and can interact with albumin and fibrinogen to form a physical barrier over an open ulcer. This protects the ulcer from further insult by HCl acid, pepsin and bile, and allows it to heal.

DRUG	DOSING	SAFETY/SIDE EFFECTS/MONITORING
Misoprostol *(Cytotec)* + diclofenac 50 mg *(Arthrotec)*	200 mcg PO QID with food; if not tolerated, may ↓ to 100 mcg QID; take with meals and at bedtime	**BOXED WARNING** Misoprostol: an abortifacient, do not use to ↓ NSAID-induced ulcers in females of childbearing potential unless capable of adhering to effective contraceptive measures; warn patients not to give this drug to others *Arthrotec*: NSAIDs ↑ risk of serious GI events (e.g., bleeding and ulceration) and CV disease (e.g., MI and stroke) **SIDE EFFECTS** Diarrhea, abdominal pain **NOTES** Use of psyllium *(Metamucil)* can help decrease diarrhea
Sucralfate *(Carafate)* Tablet, suspension	1 gram PO QID before meals (empty stomach) and at bedtime	**WARNING** Caution in renal impairment; sucralfate is in an aluminum complex and can accumulate **SIDE EFFECTS** Constipation **NOTES** Drink adequate fluids and use laxatives PRN for constipation Difficult to use due to binding interactions (separate antacids by 30 minutes and take other drugs 2 hrs before or 4 hrs after)

KEY COUNSELING POINTS

See the Drug Formulations and Patient Counseling chapter for counseling language/layman's terminology.

ANTACIDS, H2RAs AND PPIs

- Seek urgent or emergency care if you have trouble or pain when swallowing, bloody stools or vomit with blood or material that looks like coffee grounds.
- Drug interactions due to binding and high gastric pH.

Antacids

- Can cause bleeding [antacids with aspirin (e.g., *Alka Seltzer)*].

H2RAs

- Can cause confusion, dizziness or memory loss in the elderly, especially with kidney disease.

PPIs

- Can cause diarrhea.
- Can increase the risk of bone fractures, especially if taking longer than a year. Supplemental calcium and vitamin D may be needed. Calcium citrate is the preferred calcium supplement.

Prevacid SoluTab

- Contains phenylalanine. Do not use if you have phenylketonuria (PKU).

METOCLOPRAMIDE

- Can cause drowsiness.
- Can cause unusual body movements. Contact your healthcare provider immediately if you have symptoms that include shakiness, stiffness or uncontrollable movements of the mouth, tongue, cheeks, jaw, arms or legs.

H. PYLORI TREATMENTS

- Some components can cause:
  - ❏ Allergy/anaphylaxis (antibiotics).
  - ❏ Bleeding/bruising (bismuth subsalicylate).
  - ❏ Diarrhea (antibiotics, PPIs).
  - ❏ Headache (PPIs).
  - ❏ Bad taste in the mouth (metronidazole).
  - ❏ Dark tongue and stool (bismuth subsalicylate).
- If treatment includes metronidazole, avoid alcohol during treatment and for at least three days after stopping, as you may have headaches, flushing, cramps and an upset stomach.

Prevpac

- Each card has your dose (four pills) for the morning and the evening. Take your dose before breakfast and before dinner.

Pylera

- Use *Pylera* with a separate acid-reducing medication.
- Take *Pylera* (three capsules) four times each day with a full glass of water (after breakfast, lunch, dinner and at bedtime). Swallow the capsules whole.

Select Guidelines/References

Katz PO, Dunbar KB, Schnoll-Sussman FH, et al. American Colleg of Gastroenterology (ACG) clinical guideline for the diagnosis and management of gastroesophageal reflux disease. *Am J Gastroenterol.* 2022;177:27-56.

Chey, WD, Leontiadis, G, Howden, CW. American College of Gastroenterology (ACG) clinical guideline: treatment of *Helicobacter pylori* infection. *Am J Gastroenterol.* 2017;112:212-238.

CONTENT LEGEND

 = Study Tip Gal   = Key Drug Guy

iStock.com/Tharakorn

CHAPTER 72
CONSTIPATION & DIARRHEA

CONSTIPATION

BACKGROUND

Constipation is defined as infrequent bowel movements (less than three per week) or difficulty passing stools (e.g., straining, lumpy/hard stools, pushing for more than 10 minutes, stool requiring digital evacuation or the sensation of incomplete evacuation). Constipation can be caused by diet, lifestyle, drugs (see Key Drugs Guy on the next page), pregnancy, GI disorders and other medical conditions (see box below). When constipation persists for several weeks or longer and the cause is unknown, it is termed chronic idiopathic constipation (CIC). Patients with CIC should be screened for alarm symptoms, such as weight loss or gastrointestinal bleeding, prior to starting treatment. If alarm symptoms are present, diagnostic testing should occur. Idiopathic constipation associated with chronic or recurrent abdominal discomfort that is relieved by defecation is termed irritable bowel syndrome with constipation (IBS-C).

MEDICAL CONDITIONS THAT CAN CAUSE CONSTIPATION	
Irritable bowel syndrome (constipation-predominant)	Parkinson disease
	Pregnancy
Anal disorders (fissures, fistulae, rectal prolapse)	Spinal cord tumors
Multiple sclerosis	Diabetes
	Hypothyroidism
Cerebrovascular events	

NON-DRUG TREATMENT

Non-drug treatments are preferred for constipation. These include increasing fluid intake (64 oz daily recommended), limiting caffeine and alcohol intake (to avoid dehydration) and increasing physical activity. Replacing refined foods with whole grain products, bran, fruits, vegetables, beans and other foods high in fiber can help prevent constipation. Drugs that are constipating should be discontinued, if possible. It is important to use the bathroom as soon as the urge to defecate arises. For young children, a scheduled bathroom time may be needed.

DRUG TREATMENT

If constipation does not improve with lifestyle modifications, or if a constipating drug cannot be stopped, one or more drug treatments can be used. Most medications are available OTC and can be tried for the initial treatment of IBS-C, CIC or opioid-induced constipation (OIC). If constipation is not improved after seven days of OTC treatment, a healthcare provider should be consulted for further evaluation and, if appropriate, prescription medication can be considered.

Most drug treatments act to stimulate the muscles of the digestive tract or soften the stool, which results in quicker bowel movements; thus, the most common side effects are diarrhea and abdominal cramping.

- Bulk-forming drugs (e.g., soluble fiber such as psyllium) and dietary fiber are the first-line treatments in most cases and the treatment of choice in pregnancy. They absorb water in the intestine, which adds bulk to the stool. This increases peristalsis and decreases stool transit time.

- Osmotics [e.g., polyethylene glycol (PEG)] contain large ions or molecules that are poorly absorbed. They draw fluid into the bowel lumen through osmosis, which distends the colon and increases peristalsis. For CIC, these can be given in addition to fiber or as monotherapy.

- Stimulants (e.g., senna, bisacodyl) directly stimulate neurons in the colon, causing peristaltic activity. Patients who use chronic opioids, all of which are constipating, often require a stimulant laxative, because opioids reduce peristalsis and prolong stool transit time. A stool softener can be given with a stimulant laxative if the stool is hard. If the stool is not hard, but the patient cannot push it out, a stimulant alone is the usual treatment.

- Stool softeners (e.g., docusate) are emollients that reduce the surface tension of the stool, allowing more water to mix with the stool. This softens the fecal mass and makes defecation easier. These are frequently used by patients taking iron supplements, which make the stool hard and compact.

- Lubricants (e.g., mineral oil) coat the bowel and stool with a waterproof film. This keeps moisture in the stool and makes defecation easier.

DRUGS THAT ARE CONSTIPATING

KEY DRUGS

Antidiarrheals

Anticholinergic drugs
Antihistamines (e.g., diphenhydramine)
Antispasmodics (e.g., baclofen)
Phenothiazines (e.g., prochlorperazine)
TCAs (e.g., amitriptyline)
Incontinence drugs (e.g., oxybutynin)

Cation-containing drugs
Antacids with aluminum or calcium
Iron
Sucralfate

Colesevelam

Opioids

Select antihypertensives
Clonidine
Non-DHP calcium channel blockers
(especially verapamil)

Others:
5-HT3 receptor antagonists (e.g., ondansetron)

Antipsychotics (esp. clozapine)

Milnacipran

Phentermine/ topiramate

Ranolazine

Tramadol, tapentadol

Varenicline

WHICH OTC TO RECOMMEND FOR CONSTIPATION

Most adults
Fiber

Iron-induced or hard stool
Stool softener (e.g., docusate) or bulk-forming drug

Opioid-induced
Stimulant (e.g., senna, bisacodyl) or osmotic (e.g., polyethylene glycol) laxative

Pregnancy
Fiber

Fast relief needed
Adults: bisacodyl or glycerin (more gentle) suppository
Children: glycerin suppository

If no improvement in 7 days, refer patient to a healthcare provider.

COMMON DRUGS USED FOR CONSTIPATION

DRUG	DOSING	SAFETY/SIDE EFFECTS/MONITORING
Bulk-Forming Drugs		
Psyllium (Metamucil, others) Capsule, powder OTC	2.5-30 g/day in divided doses	**CONTRAINDICATIONS** Fecal impaction and GI obstruction (psyllium) **SIDE EFFECTS** Flatulence, abdominal cramping, bloating, bowel obstruction (if strictures present), choking (if powder forms are not taken with enough liquid)
Calcium polycarbophil (FiberCon, others) Caplet, chewable tablet OTC	1,250 mg 1-4 times/day	**NOTES** Onset of action 12-72 hrs
Methylcellulose (Citrucel, others) Caplet, powder OTC	1-6 g/day	Adequate fluids are required; use caution if fluid restricted (e.g., heart failure), if difficulty swallowing (e.g., Parkinson disease) or if at risk for fecal impaction (e.g., intestinal ulcerations, stenosis)
Wheat dextrin (Benefiber) Tablet, chewable tablet, powder OTC	4 g (2 teaspoons) in 4-8 oz of liquid or soft food TID	Calcium is a polyvalent cation; separate calcium polycarbophil from select drugs due to a binding interaction Sugar-free options available Psyllium modestly improves cholesterol and blood glucose levels
Osmotics		
Magnesium hydroxide (Milk of Magnesia, others), magnesium citrate, magnesium sulfate Chewable tablet, suspension OTC	Magnesium hydroxide: 2.4-4.8 g QHS or in divided doses	**CONTRAINDICATIONS** Anuria (sorbitol), low galactose diet (lactulose), GI obstruction (MiraLax) **SIDE EFFECTS** Electrolyte imbalance, abdominal cramping, abdominal distention, flatulence, dehydration, rectal irritation (suppository)
Polyethylene glycol 3350 (MiraLax, GaviLax, GlycoLax, others) Powder OTC	17 g in 4-8 oz of water daily	**NOTES** Onset of action 30 mins to 96 hrs (oral), 5-30 mins (rectal)
Glycerin (Fleet Liquid Glycerin Supp, Pedia-Lax, others) Suppository: adult & pediatric sizes OTC	PR: insert 1 daily	Magnesium-containing products: caution with renal impairment and do not use if severe renal impairment Lactulose: used commonly for hepatic encephalopathy
Lactulose (Constulose, Enulose, Generlac, Kristalose) Crystal packet, solution Rx	PO: 10-20 g daily Oral solution can be diluted and administered rectally	Glycerin suppository used commonly in children who need to defecate quickly
Sodium phosphates (Fleet Enema, others) Enema OTC	PR: insert contents of one 4.5 oz enema as a single dose	
Sorbitol Enema, oral solution OTC	PO: 30-150 mL (70% solution) as a single dose PR (enema): 120 mL (25-30% solution)	

DRUG	DOSING	SAFETY/SIDE EFFECTS/MONITORING
Stimulants		
Senna (*Ex-Lax, Senokot,* others) Tablet, chewable tablet, liquid, syrup OTC **+ docusate (*Senna S, Senokot S, Senna Plus,* others)** Tablet OTC	17.2-50 mg daily-BID	**WARNINGS** Avoid use with stomach pain, N/V or a sudden change in bowel movements that lasts > 2 weeks **SIDE EFFECTS** Abdominal cramping, electrolyte imbalance, rectal irritation (suppository) **NOTES** Onset of action 6-12 hrs (oral), 15-60 mins (rectal)
Bisacodyl Enteric-coated tablet, suppository (*Dulcolax,* others) Enema (*Fleet Bisacodyl,* others) OTC	PO: 5-15 mg daily, do not take within 1 hr of dairy products or antacids PR (enema, suppository): 10 mg daily, cool suppository in the fridge or cold water first if too soft to insert	Take oral products at bedtime to induce a bowel movement the following morning; can give 30 mins after a meal to enhance peristalsis Chronic opioid use often requires a stimulant laxative
Emollients (Stool Softeners)		
Docusate sodium (*Colace,* others), docusate calcium, docusate potassium Capsule, tablet, enema, liquid, syrup OTC **+ senna (*Senna S, Senokot S, Senna Plus,* others)** Tablet OTC	Docusate sodium: PO: 50-360 mg daily or in divided doses PR (enema): 283 g/5 mL daily-TID	**CONTRAINDICATIONS** Abdominal pain, N/V, use with mineral oil, OTC use > 1 week **SIDE EFFECTS** Abdominal cramping, throat irritation (liquid) **NOTES** Onset of action 12-72 hrs (oral), 2-15 mins (rectal) Preferred when straining should be avoided (e.g., postpartum, post-MI, anal fissures, hemorrhoids) Use when stool is hard or dry Do not take docusate and mineral oil together (it increases the absorption of mineral oil)
Lubricants		
Mineral oil Oral liquid, enema OTC	PO: 15-45 mL daily or in divided doses PR (enema): 118 mL as a single dose	**CONTRAINDICATIONS** Age < 6 years, pregnancy, bedridden patients, elderly, use > 1 week, difficulty swallowing **SIDE EFFECTS** Abdominal cramping, nausea, incontinence, rectal discharge **NOTES** Onset of action 6-8 hrs (oral), 2-15 mins (rectal) Oral formulation generally not recommended due to safety concerns (e.g., risk of aspiration and lipid pneumonitis) Take a multivitamin at a different time due to malabsorption of fat-soluble vitamins Do not take docusate and mineral oil together (it increases the absorption of mineral oil)

OTHER DRUGS USED FOR CONSTIPATION

Prescription medications can be used if constipation is not relieved with OTC drugs or lifestyle modifications.

- The chloride channel activator lubiprostone acts on chloride channels in the gut, leading to increased fluid secretion and peristalsis.

- Guanylate cyclase C agonists (e.g., linaclotide) increase chloride and bicarbonate secretion into the lumen of the intestines, increasing the speed of GI transit and reducing abdominal pain.

- Peripherally-acting mu-opioid receptor antagonists (PAMORAs) (e.g., alvimopan) act on mu-opioid receptors in the GI tract, decreasing constipation.

- Serotonin 5-HT4 receptor agonists (e.g., prucalopride) release acetylcholine which causes muscle contractions and increases gastrointestinal motility.

PRESCRIPTION DRUGS BY LABELED INDICATION

	CIC	IBS-C	OIC	SURGERY
Lubiprostone	X	X*	X	
Linaclotide, Plecanatide	X	X		
Alvimopan				X
Methylnaltrexone, Naloxegol, Naldemedine			X	
Prucalopride	X			

*IBS-C in adult women

DRUG	DOSING	SAFETY/SIDE EFFECTS/MONITORING
Chloride Channel Activator		
Lubiprostone (Amitiza) Capsule CIC, OIC, IBS-C in adult women	CIC & OIC: 24 mcg BID IBS-C: 8 mcg BID ↓ dose with moderate-severe liver impairment	**CONTRAINDICATIONS** Mechanical bowel obstruction **SIDE EFFECTS** Nausea, diarrhea, abdominal pain, abdominal distension, headache **NOTES** Take with food and water to decrease nausea Consider alternative treatment with methadone (↓ lubiprostone effects)
Guanylate Cyclase C Agonists		
Linaclotide (Linzess) Capsule CIC, IBS-C	CIC: 145 mcg daily IBS-C: 290 mcg daily Take ≥ 30 mins before breakfast on an empty stomach	**BOXED WARNING** Do not use in pediatric patients; high risk of dehydration that can cause death **CONTRAINDICATIONS** Age < 6 years, mechanical GI obstruction **SIDE EFFECTS** Diarrhea, abdominal pain, flatulence
Plecanatide (Trulance) Tablet CIC, IBS-C	3 mg daily	**NOTES** Swallow Linzess capsules whole; if needed, can open the capsule and mix contents with applesauce or room temp water; swallow mixture immediately Trulance tablets can be crushed
Peripherally-Acting Mu-Opioid Receptor Antagonists (PAMORAs)		
Alvimopan (Entereg) Capsule For hospitalized surgery patients to decrease risk of post-operative ileus	12 mg, 30 min-5 hrs prior to surgery, then 12 mg BID for up to 7 days total (maximum 15 doses)	**BOXED WARNING** Potential risk of MI with long-term use; available only for short-term inpatient use through a REMS program **CONTRAINDICATIONS** Therapeutic doses of opioids for > 7 consecutive days immediately prior to use **SIDE EFFECTS** Dyspepsia
Methylnaltrexone (Relistor) **Naloxegol (Movantik)** Naldemedine (Symproic)		**NOTES** Only used in patients taking opioids who have OIC (see Pain chapter)

DRUG	DOSING	SAFETY/SIDE EFFECTS/MONITORING
Serotonin 5-HT4 Receptor Agonist		
Prucalopride *(Motegrity)* Tablet CIC, used off-label for OIC	CIC: 2 mg daily CrCl < 30 mL/min: 1 mg daily Avoid use in ESRD with HD	**CONTRAINDICATIONS** Gastrointestinal obstruction, bowel perforation, ileus, severe inflammatory conditions of the GI tract (Crohn's disease, ulcerative colitis, toxic megacolon) **WARNINGS** Suicidal ideation **SIDE EFFECTS** Diarrhea, headache, nausea, abdominal pain **MONITORING** Worsening of depression or emergence of suicidal thoughts; rectal bleeding, blood in stool, severe abdominal pain

LAXATIVES USED FOR WHOLE BOWEL IRRIGATION

Several laxatives are specifically designed to prep the bowel before a colonoscopy. Some of these drugs contain the same active ingredients as those used for constipation. For example, PEG is available OTC under the brand name *MiraLax* to treat constipation, but also by prescription under the name *GoLytely* for bowel prep before a colonoscopy. Although usually safe and well-tolerated, laxatives for whole bowel irrigation can cause fluid and electrolyte losses. These can be critical in some patients and with select products (e.g., oral sodium phosphates such as *OsmoPrep)*. Use extra caution in patients with cardiovascular disease, renal insufficiency or if taking loop diuretics (due to additional fluid loss) or NSAIDs.

DRUG	DOSING	SAFETY/SIDE EFFECTS/MONITORING
Polyethylene glycol-electrolyte solution (Colyte, GoLytely, NuLytely, GaviLyte-G, GaviLyte-N, MoviPrep, Plenvu)	Drink 240 mL every 10 mins until 4 liters are consumed *MoviPrep:* the evening before, drink 240 mL every 15 mins until 1 liter is consumed, then drink 480 mL clear liquid; repeat in the morning *Plenvu:* the evening before, drink 480 mL over 30 mins, then drink 480 mL clear liquid over 30 mins; repeat in the morning	**BOXED WARNING** *OsmoPrep:* nephropathy **CONTRAINDICATIONS** Ileus, gastrointestinal obstruction, gastric retention, bowel perforation, toxic colitis, toxic megacolon *OsmoPrep:* acute phosphate nephropathy, gastric bypass or stapling surgery *Clenpiq:* severe renal impairment **WARNINGS** Arrhythmias, electrolyte abnormalities, seizures **SIDE EFFECTS** Abdominal discomfort, bloating, N/V
Sodium phosphates (OsmoPrep)	Take 4 tablets (with 8 oz of clear liquid) every 15 mins (5 doses the evening before and 3 doses 3-5 hrs before the procedure)	**NOTES** Onset of action 1-6 hrs
Sodium sulfate, potassium sulfate and magnesium sulfate (Suprep Bowel Prep Kit)	Evening before: drink 480 mL followed by 960 mL clear liquid over 1 hr; repeat in the morning	Bowel prep regimens typically require doses the evening before colonoscopy and the morning of colonoscopy to completely evacuate the bowel
Sodium picosulfate, magnesium oxide, and citric acid *(Clenpiq)* Combination of a stimulant and osmotic laxative (enables lower fluid intake)	Evening before: drink 160 mL; repeat 5 hrs before the procedure	A clear liquid diet is required the day prior to colonoscopy and can include: water, clear broth (beef or chicken), juices without pulp (apple, white cranberry, white grape, lemonade), soda, coffee or tea (without milk or cream), clear gelatin (without fruit pieces), popsicles (without fruit pieces or cream) Do not consume the following: solid or semi-solid foods, anything with red or blue/purple food coloring (including gelatin and popsicles), milk, cream, tomato, orange or grapefruit juice, alcoholic beverages, cream soups

DIARRHEA

BACKGROUND

Diarrhea is an increase in the number of bowel movements or stools that are more watery and loose than normal. When the intestines push stools through the bowel too rapidly (i.e., before water in the stool can be reabsorbed), diarrhea occurs. Abdominal cramps, nausea, vomiting or fever can be present.

Diarrhea can be idiopathic or caused by diseases, drugs (see Key Drugs Guy below) or consuming contaminated food/water. Most cases of diarrhea are viral, have a quick onset and resolve within a few days without treatment. E. coli is the most common bacterial cause. Infectious diarrhea is discussed in the Travelers and Infectious Diseases II chapters.

Recurrent idiopathic diarrhea associated with chronic or reoccurring abdominal discomfort that is relieved by defecation is termed irritable bowel syndrome with diarrhea (IBS-D).

Diarrhea that occurs after consuming milk or milk products could be due to lactose intolerance. Lactose intolerance can be confirmed through testing or eliminating dairy intake to see if diarrhea resolves.

NON-DRUG TREATMENT

Management of diarrhea includes fluid and electrolyte replacement, especially in moderate-severe cases and in children, older adults or adults with chronic medical conditions. Dehydration from diarrhea in infants is dangerous; care should be overseen by a healthcare provider (see Pediatrics chapter for more information). Replace fluid and electrolytes with oral rehydration solutions (ORS), such as *Pedialyte* or *Enfamil Enfalyte*, which are available over the counter. *Gatorade* or similar products can be used as alternatives.

DRUG TREATMENT FOR DIARRHEA

Most patients with non-infectious diarrhea who require symptomatic relief can use short-term bismuth subsalicylate *(Pepto-Bismol)* or loperamide as needed. Bismuth subsalicylate has both antisecretory and antimicrobial effects when used as an antidiarrheal. Loperamide and diphenoxylate are antimotility drugs that slow intestinal motility, prolonging the time for water absorption. Pain and abdominal discomfort associated with IBS-D can be managed with antispasmodics (e.g., dicyclomine) and antidepressants in select cases.

Eluxadoline *(Viberzi)* is indicated for IBS-D when other treatments have failed. It is a mixed mu-opioid receptor agonist (in contrast to the PAMORAs, which are mu-receptor antagonists). While the PAMORAs compete and displace the binding of opioids to receptors in the periphery to reduce constipation, eluxadoline binds to the opioid receptors as an agonist to treat diarrhea.

SELECT DRUGS THAT CAN CAUSE DIARRHEA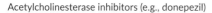

Acetylcholinesterase inhibitors (e.g., donepezil)

Antacids containing magnesium

Antibiotics (especially broad-spectrum drugs), diarrhea may be infectious (e.g., C. difficile)

Antidiabetics (e.g., metformin, GLP-1 agonists)

Antineoplastics (e.g., irinotecan, capecitabine, fluorouracil, methotrexate, TKIs)

Colchicine

Drugs used for constipation (e.g., laxatives)

Misoprostol

Mycophenolate

Prokinetic drugs (e.g., metoclopramide, cisapride)

Protease inhibitors (especially nelfinavir)

Quinidine

Roflumilast

DRUG	DOSING	SAFETY/SIDE EFFECTS/MONITORING
Antidiarrheals		
Bismuth subsalicylate (Pepto-Bismol, others) Suspension (262 mg/15 mL) Chewable tablet (262 mg) OTC	524 mg (30 mL or 2 tablets) every 30-60 mins PRN or 1,050 mg (60 mL or 4 tablets) every 60 mins PRN Max: 4,200 mg/day for up to 2 days	**CONTRAINDICATIONS** Salicylate allergy, taking other salicylates (e.g., aspirin), GI ulcer, bleeding problems, black/bloody stool **WARNINGS** Children and teenagers who are recovering from the flu, chickenpox or other viral infections should not use this drug due to the risk of Reye's syndrome **SIDE EFFECTS** Black tongue/stool (temporary and harmless), salicylate toxicity if used excessively (tinnitus, metabolic acidosis), nausea, abdominal pain **NOTES** Can cause an increased risk of bleeding when used with anticoagulants, antiplatelets (e.g., aspirin) or NSAIDs Use caution in those with renal insufficiency or in combination with other nephrotoxic drugs
Loperamide (Imodium A-D, *Anti-Diarrheal, Diamode*) Capsule, tablet, liquid, suspension OTC 1 tab/cap = 2 mg	4 mg PO after the first loose stool, then 2 mg after each subsequent loose stool Max: 8 mg/day (self-care) or 16 mg/day (under healthcare supervision)	**BOXED WARNING** Torsades de pointes, cardiac arrest and sudden death with doses higher than recommended; do not exceed the recommended dose Do not use in children < 2 years **CONTRAINDICATIONS** Acute dysentery (bloody diarrhea and high fever), pseudomembranous colitis (*C. difficile*), bacterial enterocolitis caused by invasive organisms (toxigenic *E. coli*, *Salmonella*, *Shigella*), abdominal pain without diarrhea, acute ulcerative colitis **SIDE EFFECTS** Constipation, abdominal cramping, nausea, QT prolongation **NOTES** Self-treatment: do not use > 48 hrs Loperamide can be abused, as it causes a mild opioid-like "high" in large quantities To encourage safe use, the FDA requires use of blister packs or other single-dose packaging for tablets and capsules, and the number of doses per package is limited to no more than 48 mg (24 tablets/capsules)
Diphenoxylate/atropine (Lomotil) Liquid, tablet C-V Diphenoxylate inhibits excessive GI motility and propulsion; atropine is used to discourage abuse	Diphenoxylate 5 mg (2 tablets) up to 4 times daily Max: 20 mg/day Improvement is usually seen within 48 hrs; if not seen within 10 days, discontinue	**CONTRAINDICATIONS** Risk of respiratory and CNS depression in children [do not use if < 2 years of age (or < 6 years of age for tablets)], diarrhea caused by enterotoxin-producing bacteria or pseudomembranous colitis (*C. difficile*), obstructive jaundice **SIDE EFFECTS** Mild euphoria due to diphenoxylate, possible anticholinergic effects (see Notes) **NOTES** Liquid formulation is recommended in children < 13 years Anticholinergic effects due to atropine (e.g., constipation, dry mouth, sedation, tachycardia, flushing, urinary retention, blurred vision); these are mild at recommended doses
Antispasmodic		
Dicyclomine (Bentyl) Capsule, injection, solution, tablet	20 mg QID Max: 80 mg/day for < 2 weeks (can increase to 40 mg QID after 1 week, if symptoms respond)	**CONTRAINDICATIONS** Gastrointestinal obstruction, severe ulcerative colitis, reflux esophagitis, acute hemorrhage with cardiovascular instability, obstructive uropathy, narrow-angle glaucoma, myasthenia gravis, breastfeeding women, infants < 6 months of age **WARNINGS** Anticholinergic (caution in patients ≥ 65 years, per Beer's Criteria), caution in mild-moderate ulcerative colitis (can cause toxic megacolon or paralytic ileus) **SIDE EFFECTS** Dizziness, dry mouth, nausea, blurred vision, somnolence, weakness, nervousness

DRUG	DOSING	SAFETY/SIDE EFFECTS/MONITORING
Peripherally-Acting Mixed Mu-Opioid Receptor Agonist		
Eluxadoline *(Viberzi)* Tablet <u>C-IV</u> IBS-D	100 mg PO BID Decrease to 75 mg BID if unable to tolerate 100 mg dose Take with food	**CONTRAINDICATIONS** <u>Patients without a gallbladder</u>, biliary duct obstruction, sphincter of Oddi dysfunction/disease, pancreatic disease (including history of pancreatitis), alcoholism or > 3 alcoholic drinks/day, severe hepatic impairment (Child-Pugh class C), history of severe constipation, gastrointestinal obstruction **WARNINGS** CNS depression **SIDE EFFECTS** Constipation, nausea, abdominal pain **MONITORING** S/sx of pancreatitis or sphincter of Oddi spasm (e.g., abdominal pain that radiates to the back or shoulder, nausea and vomiting), LFTs

OTHER ORAL MEDICATIONS FOR DIARRHEA

Other available treatments shown in the table below have advantages and disadvantages and are used less commonly.

DRUG CLASS	COMMENTS
Antibiotic Rifaximin *(Xifaxan)* IBS without constipation	Costly, and relapse often occurs within several months of treatment.
Serotonin 5-HT3 Receptor Antagonist Alosetron *(Lotronex)* IBS-D	Approved for women only; has a boxed warning regarding risk of ischemic colitis.

KEY COUNSELING POINTS

See the Drug Formulations and Patient Counseling chapter for counseling language/layman's terminology.

ALL CONSTIPATION PRODUCTS

- Can cause diarrhea and/or abdominal cramping.
- If no improvement after one week of OTC treatment, contact a healthcare provider.

Bulk-Forming Drugs

- Drug interactions due to binding.

ALL DIARRHEA PRODUCTS

- Contact a healthcare provider for any of the following: age < 6 months, pregnancy, high fever (> 101°F), severe abdominal pain or blood in the stool.
- Can cause constipation.

Bismuth Subsalicylate

- Do not take for longer than two days without the approval of your healthcare provider.
- Can cause:
  - Bleeding/bruising.
  - Dark tongue and stool; this is normal.

Loperamide

- Do not take for longer than two days without the approval of your healthcare provider.

Diphenoxylate/Atropine

- Can cause anticholinergic effects.

Dicyclomine

- Can cause anticholinergic effects.

Select Guidelines/References

Chang L, Chey WD, Imdad A, et al. American Gastroenterological Association-American College of Gastroenterology Clinical Practice guideline: Pharmacological management of chronic idiopathic constipation. *Gastroenterology.* 2023;164(7):1086-1106.

American College of Gastroenterology (ACG) Clinical Guideline: Management of Irritable Bowel Syndrome. *Gastroenterology.* 2021;116:17-44.

CONTENT LEGEND

= Study Tip Gal

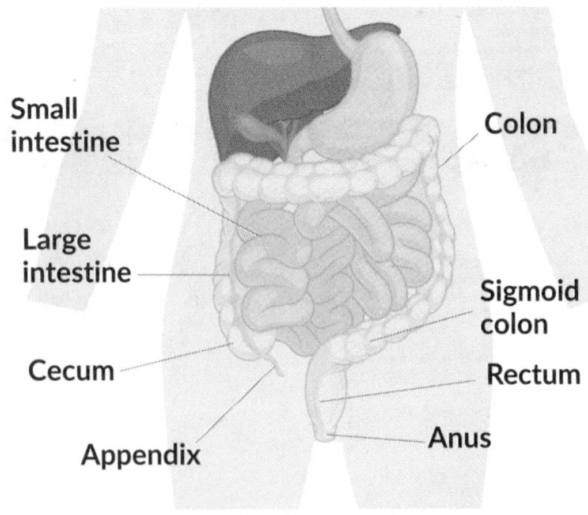

iStock.com/BluezAce

CHAPTER 73

INFLAMMATORY BOWEL DISEASE

BACKGROUND

Inflammatory bowel disease (IBD) is a group of inflammatory conditions of the colon and small intestine. The major types of IBD are ulcerative colitis and Crohn's disease. The classic symptom is bloody diarrhea. Other symptoms include rectal urgency, tenesmus (a feeling of having to pass stools, even if the colon is empty), abdominal pain, fatigue and, in some cases, weight loss, night sweats, nausea, vomiting and constipation. IBD is a chronic, intermittent disease; symptoms can be mild to severe during flares (or exacerbations) and minimal or absent during periods of remission. Flares can occur at any time and can be triggered by infections, use of NSAIDs or certain foods. Food triggers are patient-specific but can include fatty foods and gas-producing foods (e.g., lentils, beans, legumes, cabbage, broccoli, onions). Food triggers can be avoided or food can be prepared in a way that improves tolerability.

IBD can be mistaken for irritable bowel syndrome (IBS), as they have similar symptoms (e.g., abdominal pain, bloating, gas, and either constipation or diarrhea). Unlike IBD, IBS does not cause inflammation and is not as serious of a condition. Drugs used to treat IBS primarily treat constipation or diarrhea; refer to the Constipation & Diarrhea chapter for drug specifics.

ULCERATIVE COLITIS

Ulcerative colitis (UC) is characterized by mucosal inflammation confined to the rectum and colon with superficial ulcerations. When UC is limited to the descending colon and rectum, it is called distal disease and can be treated with topical (rectal) treatment. Inflammation limited to the rectum is called proctitis. The larger the affected area (e.g., extensive UC), the worse the symptoms. When the disease flares, patients can have numerous stools per day, often with pain, which can significantly decrease quality of life. UC is classified as mild, moderate, severe or fulminant. Moderate disease is characterized by > 4 stools per day with minimal signs of toxicity, and patients with severe disease have ≥ 6 bloody stools per day with evidence of toxicity [fever, tachycardia, anemia, or an elevated erythrocyte sedimentation rate (ESR)]. Fulminant disease refers to patients with > 10 stools per day and severe symptoms (e.g., continuous bleeding, abdominal pain, distension and acute, severe toxic symptoms including fever and anorexia). These patients are at risk of progressing to toxic megacolon and bowel perforation.

CROHN'S DISEASE

Crohn's disease (CD) is characterized by deep, transmural (through the bowel wall) inflammation that can affect any part of the GI tract. The ileum and colon are most commonly affected. Damage to the bowel wall can cause strictures (narrowing of the bowel) and fistulas (abnormal connections or openings in the bowel). Symptoms of CD include chronic diarrhea (often nocturnal), abdominal pain and weight loss. Perianal symptoms [e.g., bleeding, fissures (tears)] can be present before bowel symptoms.

CD AND UC COMPARISON

CLINICAL FEATURES	CD	UC
Diarrhea	Bloody or non-bloody	Bloody
Fistulas/ Strictures	Common	Uncommon
Location	Entire GI tract (especially the ileum & colon)	Colon (especially the rectum)
Depth	Transmural	Superficial
Pattern	Non-continuous, "cobblestone" appearance	Continuous

DIAGNOSIS

IBD can be difficult to diagnose because the symptoms mimic other common conditions (e.g., constipation, diarrhea, infections, anorexia/bulimia and peptic ulcer disease). These conditions must be ruled out before a diagnosis is made. Laboratory blood tests (for inflammatory markers, such as CRP) and stool testing (e.g., fecal calprotectin test) can be helpful, but usually a colonoscopy with tissue biopsy is needed to make the diagnosis. A colonoscopy allows the healthcare provider to visualize the entire colon. A sigmoidoscopy might be used for UC, which is similar to a colonoscopy but only evaluates the end part of the intestine, closest to the rectum. Endoscopy (scope through the mouth) might be used if upper GI symptoms are present. Imaging tests (e.g., CT, MRI) can be helpful for diagnosis as well.

LIFESTYLE MEASURES, SUPPORTIVE CARE AND NATURAL PRODUCTS

As previously mentioned, patients with IBD should adapt their diet to avoid foods that are more likely to trigger flares. In general, eating smaller, more frequent meals that are low in fat and dairy products can be helpful. Fiber should be added to the diet, as tolerated. It is usually best to drink plenty of water. Alcohol and caffeinated beverages that can stimulate the GI tract should be avoided, as well as carbonated beverages that can be gas-producing. The patient should watch for avoidable problems; both sorbitol and lactose are excipients that are present in various medications. Sorbitol is often used as a sweetener in some diet foods; it has laxative properties and can cause considerable GI distress in some patients. Lactose will worsen GI symptoms if the patient is lactose-intolerant.

Some patients may use antidiarrheals or antispasmodic drugs [e.g., dicyclomine (Bentyl)] to help manage symptoms of diarrhea; these should be used cautiously, and under the supervision of a healthcare provider, as they need to be avoided in select patients with IBD (e.g., severe disease, acute exacerbations, post-bowel resection). Generally, opioid use should be avoided due to the side effect of constipation and an increased risk of developing toxic megacolon in this population. See the Constipation & Diarrhea and Pain chapters for more information on these products. Vitamin supplements (e.g., B12, folate, vitamin D, calcium, iron, zinc) can help prevent deficiencies related to malabsorption. Nicotine and cigarette smoking have been shown to worsen CD but can be protective in UC. Nicotine patches have been used as an adjunct therapy for UC, but adverse effects (e.g., nausea, dizziness) limit the benefits.

The probiotics Lactobacillus or Bifidobacterium infantis can reduce abdominal pain, bloating, urgency, constipation or diarrhea in some patients. Fish oils with EPA and DHA (omega-3 fatty acids) can help fight inflammation, although the evidence for benefit is minimal. Some natural products that might be useful include peppermint (in oils or teas), chamomile, horehound and wheatgrass.

DRUG TREATMENT

Treatments for IBD are used to induce remission (they treat exacerbations or active disease) and/or maintain remission. Short courses of oral or IV steroids are commonly used to treat acute exacerbations in both UC and CD. Systemic steroids are not recommended for maintenance of remission and will usually be tapered over 8 – 12 weeks once remission is achieved.

In general, treatment options that are used for induction can be continued for maintenance of remission for both UC and CD, with the exception of steroids (due to the risk of long-term side effects). For mild disease, budesonide is used for induction in CD and mesalamine (oral and/or rectal) with or without a steroid is used for induction in UC. A biologic (e.g., anti-tumor necrosis factor (TNF) drug, IL receptor antagonist) with or without an immunomodulator (e.g., a thiopurine) is used for induction in moderate to severe CD and UC.

For maintenance therapy of mild disease, aminosalicylates (active component is 5-aminosalicylic acid, or 5-ASA) are used for UC and oral budesonide is used for up to 3 months in CD (afterwhich it is discontinued or changed to a thiopurine or methotrexate). For maintenance therapy of moderate-severe UC and CD, immunosuppressive medications (e.g., thiopurines, anti-TNF drugs) are recommended (see Study Tip Gal below). Steroids might be needed for severe cases of CD.

Some of the more common drugs used to treat UC and CD are shown in the tables on the following pages. Additional medications [e.g., IV steroids, anti-TNF agents (infliximab, adalimumab, certolizumab), methotrexate, interleukin receptor antagonists (ustekinumab)] are discussed fully in the Systemic Steroids & Autoimmune Conditions chapter.

OVERVIEW OF MEDICATIONS USED FOR TREATMENT OF CD AND UC BASED ON SEVERITY

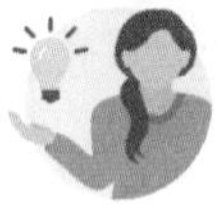

CROHN'S DISEASE

Mild disease of the ileum and/or right colon
- Oral budesonide for ≤ 3 months, then discontinue or change to a thiopurine or methotrexate

Moderate-severe disease
- Preferred treatments include:
  - ❏ Anti-TNF agent with or without methotrexate or a thiopurine
  - ❏ IL receptor antagonist
  - ❏ Integrin receptor antagonist
- Alternative options (not responding to above):
  - ❏ Janus kinase inhibitor
  - ❏ Integrin receptor antagonist

ULCERATIVE COLITIS

Mild disease
- Mesalamine (5-ASA)
  - ❏ Distal disease: rectal preferred
  - ❏ Extensive disease: rectal ± oral

Moderate-severe disease
- Preferred treatments include:
  - ❏ Anti-TNF agent with or without a thiopurine
  - ❏ IL receptor antagonist
  - ❏ Integrin receptor antagonist
- Alternative options (not responding to above):
  - ❏ Janus kinase inhibitor
  - ❏ Oral sphingosine-1-phosphate receptor modulators

STEROIDS

DRUG	DOSING	SAFETY/SIDE EFFECTS/MONITORING
Oral Steroids		
Prednisone Tablet Oral solution (*Prednisone Intensol*) Delayed-release tablet (*Rayos*)	5-60 mg PO daily	**CONTRAINDICATIONS** Systemic fungal infections, live vaccines **SIDE EFFECTS** Short-term: ↑ appetite/weight gain, emotional instability (euphoria, mood swings, irritability), insomnia, fluid retention, indigestion, higher doses can cause an ↑ in BP and blood glucose Long-term: adrenal suppression/Cushing's syndrome, impaired wound healing, ↑ BP, ↑ blood glucose, cataracts, osteoporosis, others; refer to the Systemic Steroids & Autoimmune Conditions chapter **NOTES** **All Steroids**
Budesonide **(Entocort EC, Uceris)** *Entocort EC*: 3 mg extended release capsule (for CD only) *Uceris*: 9 mg extended release tablet (for UC only)	**Induction (CD and UC):** 9 mg PO once daily in the morning for up to 8 weeks **Maintenance (CD only):** 6 mg PO once daily for 3 months, then taper	For management of acute flares; avoid long-term use if possible Can use alternate day therapy (ADT) to ↓ adrenal suppression and other adverse effects If used longer than 2 weeks, must taper to avoid withdrawal symptoms If long-term use is required, assess bone density (optimize calcium and vitamin D intake and consider bisphosphonates if needed) **Budesonide** Undergoes extensive first-pass metabolism; ↓ systemic exposure than other oral steroids Swallow whole – do not crush or chew; can open *Entocort EC* capsules and sprinkle on applesauce
Rectal Steroids		
Hydrocortisone (*Cortenema, Cortifoam*) Enema, rectal foam	**Induction and/or Maintenance** *Cortenema*: 1 enema (100 mg) QHS for 21 days or until remission, then taper *Cortifoam*: 1 applicatorful (90 mg) 1-2 times daily for 2-3 weeks, then every other day thereafter; taper after long-term therapy	**CONTRAINDICATIONS** *Cortifoam*: obstruction, abscess, perforation, peritonitis, fresh intestinal anastomoses, extensive fistulas and sinus tracts *Cortenema*: ileocolostomy in immediate/early post-op period **NOTES** Rectal steroids are indicated for UC only Not proven effective for maintenance of remission; maintenance use is limited to mild-moderate distal UC as an alternative to aminosalicylates
Budesonide rectal foam (*Uceris*)	**Induction** 1 metered dose PR BID x 2 weeks, then 1 metered dose daily x 4 weeks (1 metered dose = 2 mg budesonide)	Budesonide rectal foam: propellant is flammable; avoid fire and smoking during and after use

Budesonide Drug Interactions

- Budesonide is a major substrate of CYP450 3A4. Avoid strong and moderate inhibitors of CYP3A4, including grapefruit juice and grapefruit products.

- Use of steroids with other immunosuppressants can increase the risk of serious adverse events.

- Antacids can cause enteric coated oral budesonide to dissolve prematurely due to ↑ gastric pH. Separate administration of antacids by two hours.

AMINOSALICYLATES

Aminosalicylates are indicated for treatment of UC; the mechanism of action is unknown, but they appear to have a topical anti-inflammatory effect in the gastrointestinal tract. Mesalamine (5-ASA) is the primary aminosalicylate used in the U.S.; it is well tolerated and available in both oral and rectal formulations. The other aminosalicylates (sulfasalazine, balsalazide, olsalazine) are available in oral form only and must be converted to mesalamine to have an effect. Sulfasalazine is used less commonly due to the many side effects associated with the sulfapyridine component.

DRUG	DOSING	SAFETY/SIDE EFFECTS/MONITORING
Mesalamine ER ER capsules **(Pentasa,** Apriso, Delzicol) ER tablets **(Asacol HD***, Lialda) Enema **(Rowasa)** Suppository **(Canasa)**	**Induction** *(oral therapy for 6-8 weeks and/or rectal therapy for 3-6 weeks)* *Asacol HD*: 1.6 g PO TID *Delzicol*: 800 mg PO TID *Lialda*: 2.4-4.8 g PO daily *Pentasa*: 1 g PO QID Suppository: 1 g rectally QHS, retain for at least 1-3 hours Enema: 4 g rectally QHS, retain in the rectum overnight for approximately 8 hours **Maintenance** *Apriso*: 1.5 g PO daily *Delzicol*: 1.6 g PO in 2-4 divided doses *Lialda*: 2.4 g PO daily *Pentasa*: 1 g PO QID Enema: 2 g rectally QHS, or 4 g QHS every 2-3 days	**CONTRAINDICATIONS** Hypersensitivity to salicylates or aminosalicylates **WARNINGS** Acute intolerance syndrome (cramping, acute abdominal pain, bloody diarrhea); caution in patients with renal or hepatic impairment; delayed gastric retention (e.g., due to pyloric stenosis) can delay release of oral products in the colon; hypersensitivity reactions (including myocarditis, pericarditis, nephritis, hematologic abnormalities and other internal organ damage) – more likely with sulfasalazine than mesalamine; ↑ risk of blood dyscrasias in patients > 65 years of age, photosensitivity *Apriso* contains phenylalanine; do not use in patients with phenylketonuria (PKU) *Rowasa* enema contains potassium metabisulfite, may cause an allergic-type reaction **SIDE EFFECTS** Abdominal pain, nausea, headache, flatulence, eructation (belching), nasopharyngitis **MONITORING** Renal function, CBC, hepatic function, s/sx of IBD **NOTES** Mesalamine is better tolerated than other aminosalicylates Rectal mesalamine is more effective than oral mesalamine and rectal steroids for distal disease/proctitis in UC; can use oral and topical formulations together *Asacol* and *Delzicol*: can leave a ghost tablet in the stool Swallow capsules/tablets whole; do not crush, chew or break due to delayed-release coating *Apriso*: do not use with antacids (dissolution is pH-dependent)
Sulfasalazine Tablets *(Azulfidine)* ER tablets *(Azulfidine EN-tabs)*	**Induction** 3-4 g PO divided TID or QID, titrate to 4-6 g PO daily divided QID **Maintenance** 2 g PO daily divided TID or QID	Refer to the Systemic Steroids & Autoimmune Conditions chapter **CONTRAINDICATIONS** Salicylate allergy, sulfa allergy, intestinal or urinary obstruction, porphyria **NOTES** Doses should be taken at ≤ 8 hour intervals Can reduce dose if GI intolerance occurs
Balsalazide *(Colazal)* Capsule	**Induction** *Colazal*: 2.25 g (three 750 mg capsules) PO TID for 8-12 weeks	**CONTRAINDICATION** Salicylate allergy **WARNINGS** Gastric retention (e.g., due to pyloric stenosis) can delay release of drug in the colon; acute intolerance syndrome; caution in patients with renal or hepatic impairment, photosensitivity **SIDE EFFECTS** Headache, abdominal pain, N/V/D **MONITORING** Renal function, LFTs, s/sx of IBD **NOTES** *Colazal* capsule can be opened and sprinkled on applesauce; beads are not coated, so mixture can be chewed if needed; when used this way, it can cause staining of the teeth/tongue
Olsalazine *(Dipentum)* Capsule	**Maintenance** 500 mg PO BID Take with food	**CONTRAINDICATION** Salicylate allergy **SIDE EFFECTS** Diarrhea, abdominal pain **MONITORING** CBC, LFTs, renal function, symptoms of IBD

*Brand discontinued but name still used in practice.

THIOPURINES

The thiopurines, azathioprine and mercaptopurine, are immunosuppressive drugs, sometimes referred to as "immunomodulators." They do not have an FDA indication for IBD but are recommended as an option in guidelines for induction and maintenance of remission, often in combination with other drugs.

DRUG	DOSING	SAFETY/SIDE EFFECTS/MONITORING
Azathioprine (*Azasan, Imuran*) Tablet, injection	1.5-2.5 mg/kg/day IV or PO CrCl < 50 mL/min: adjustment required PO: taking after meals or in divided doses may ↓ GI side effects	**BOXED WARNINGS** Chronic immunosuppression ↑ risk of malignancy in patients with IBD (especially lymphomas); mutagenic potential; risk for hematologic toxicities **WARNINGS** Hematologic toxicities (e.g., leukopenia, thrombocytopenia, anemia); patients with a genetic deficiency of thiopurine methyltransferase (TPMT) are at ↑ risk for myelosuppression GI hypersensitivity reactions (severe N/V/D, rash, fever, ↑ LFTs), serious infections, hepatotoxicity **SIDE EFFECTS** N/V/D, rash, ↑ LFTs **MONITORING** LFTs, CBC (weekly for 1st month), renal function, s/sx of malignancy **NOTES** Consider TPMT genetic testing before starting (see Pharmacogenomics chapter) Azathioprine is metabolized to mercaptopurine; do not use the thiopurines in combination Aminosalicylates inhibit TPMT; caution with use in combination Allopurinol inhibits a pathway for inactivation of azathioprine; azathioprine dose reduction required if used in combination
Mercaptopurine (*Purixan*) Tablet, oral suspension	1-1.5 mg/kg/day CrCl ≤ 50 mL/min: adjustment required	Same as azathioprine above (except no boxed warning) plus: **NOTES** Take on an empty stomach Avoid old terms "6-mercaptopurine" and "6-MP"; they ↑ the risk of overdose due to administration of doses 6-fold higher than normal

METHOTREXATE AND CYCLOSPORINE

Methotrexate is an immunosuppressive drug with anti-inflammatory properties. It does not have an FDA indication for IBD, but it is recommended by guidelines for induction and maintenance of remission in moderate-severe CD in patients who cannot tolerate azathioprine. It is dosed once weekly by IM or SC injection. See the Systemic Steroids & Autoimmune Conditions chapter for information on methotrexate.

Cyclosporine is an immunosuppressive drug reserved for severe acute UC refractory to steroids. It can be given orally or via IV continuous infusion. See the Transplant chapter for more information on cyclosporine.

OTHER ORAL TREATMENT OPTIONS

The following are oral treatment options for moderate to severe IBD, but are considered second-line to biologics.

Janus Kinase Inhibitors

Janus kinase (JAK) enzymes are involved in stimulating immune cell function. Approved JAK inhibitors include upadacitinib (*Rinvoq*) for UC and CD and tofacitinib (*Xeljanz*) for UC.

Sphingosine 1-Phosphate (S1P) Receptor Modulators

S1P receptor modulators block lymphocytes from exiting the lymph nodes, reducing lymphocytes in the intestines. Drugs in this class include ozanimod (*Zeposia*) and etrasimod (*Velsipity*), both approved for UC.

BIOLOGIC TREATMENT OPTIONS

Anti-TNF Monoclonal Antibodies

The anti-TNF agents (e.g., infliximab, adalimumab) are monoclonal antibodies that bind to human TNF-alpha, preventing induction of proinflammatory cytokines (e.g., interleukins). They are used in patients with moderate-severe UC or CD, often in combination with a thiopurine. See the Systemic Steroids & Autoimmune Conditions chapter for more information.

Interleukin Receptor Antagonists

There are several interleukin receptor antagonists used for IBD with varied targets, which are used to treat moderate-severe disease. They include ustekinumab (*Stelara*) and its biosimilar *Wezlana* for UC and CD, risankizumab (*Skyrizi*) for CD and mirikizumab-mrkz (*Omvoh*) for UC.

Integrin Receptor Antagonists

The following are monoclonal antibodies that bind to subunits of integrin molecules, blocking the ability of integrin to interact with adhesion molecules and preventing inflammatory cells from migrating into gastrointestinal tissue. They are indicated for induction and maintenance of remission in patients with moderate to severe IBD.

DRUG	DOSING	SAFETY/SIDE EFFECTS/MONITORING
Natalizumab (Tysabri) Injection Approved for Crohn's disease and multiple sclerosis Biosimilar: *Tyruko*	300 mg IV over 1 hour every 4 weeks Discontinue if no response by 12 weeks	**BOXED WARNING** Progressive multifocal leukoencephalopathy [(PML), an opportunistic viral infection of the brain that leads to death or severe disability]; monitor for mental status changes; risk factors include: anti-JCV antibodies, ↑ treatment duration and prior immunosuppressant use Only available through the REMS TOUCH Prescribing Program **WARNINGS** Herpes encephalitis and meningitis, hepatotoxicity, hypersensitivity (antibody formation), immunosuppression/infections **SIDE EFFECTS** Infusion reactions, headache, fatigue, arthralgia, nausea, rash, depression, gastroenteritis, abdominal/back pain **NOTES** Rarely used for CD due to risk of PML Cannot be used with other immunosuppressants Stable in NS only; do not shake If taking steroids when initiating *Tysabri*, begin tapering when the onset of benefit is observed; stop *Tysabri* if patient cannot taper steroids within 6 months of initiation
Vedolizumab (Entyvio) Injection Approved for Crohn's disease and ulcerative colitis	300 mg IV over 30 min at 0, 2, and 6 weeks, then every 8 weeks Discontinue if no benefit by week 14	**WARNINGS** Infusion reactions, hypersensitivity reactions, infections, liver injury, PML All immunizations must be up to date before starting; avoid live vaccines during treatment **SIDE EFFECTS** Headache, nasopharyngitis, arthralgia, antibody development **MONITORING** LFTs, s/sx of infection, hypersensitivity, neurological symptoms (to monitor for PML), routine TB screening **NOTES** Risk of PML is lower than with natalizumab Refrigerate and store in original packaging to protect from light Swirl during reconstitution, do not shake Cannot be used with other immunosuppressants

KEY COUNSELING POINTS

See the Drug Formulations and Patient Counseling chapter for counseling language/layman's terminology and instructions for suppository and enema administration.

MESALAMINE

- Select ER products can cause a ghost tablet.

Mesalamine Enemas and Suppositories

- Administer in the evening, just before bedtime. Try not to have a bowel movement until morning.

- Can cause staining of surfaces, including clothing and other fabrics.

Select Guidelines/References

American College of Gastroenterology (ACG) Clinical Practice Guidelines on the Medical Management of Moderate to Severe Luminal and Perianal Fistulizing Crohn's Disease. *Am J Gastroenterol* 2021;160:2496–2508.

American Gastroenterological Association (AGA) Clinical Practice Guidelines on the Management of Mild-to-Moderate Ulcerative Colitis. *Gastroenterology* 2019;156:748-764.

American Gastroenterological Association (AGA) Clinical Practice Guidelines on the Management of Moderate-to-Severe Ulcerative Colitis. *Gastroenterology* 2020;158:1450-1461.

DEFINITIONS

Nausea

The uncomfortable, queasy feeling that one may vomit.

Treatment

The chemoreceptor trigger zone (CTZ) in the CNS contains receptors for dopamine (DA), serotonin (5-HT) and acetylcholine (Ach). Each receptor can set off a chemical pathway leading to nausea and vomiting. Blocking the receptors reduces nausea, such as:

- Blocking 5-HT with 5-HT3 receptor antagonists (e.g., ondansetron)

- Blocking DA with phenothiazines (e.g., prochlorperazine)

- Blocking 5-HT and DA with metoclopramide (a prokinetic that moves food through the gut)

Nausea due to chemotherapy is treated with 5-HT3 receptor antagonists and various other medications; see the Oncology chapter.

Vertigo

Dizziness, with the sensation that the environment is moving or spinning. Vertigo is typically due to an inner ear condition that affects balance.

Treatment
- Vestibular (inner-ear) suppressants, including antihistamines (e.g., meclizine, dimenhydrinate) and benzodiazepines

5-HT3 receptor antagonists are not useful for vertigo because they do not affect the inner ear.

Motion Sickness

Dizziness, with a sensation of being off-balance and woozy due to repetitive motions, such as a boat moving over waves or an airplane flying in turbulent weather.

Treatment
- Anticholinergics (e.g., scopolamine) and antihistamines (e.g., meclizine)

iStock.com/NiwatSingsamarn

CONTENT LEGEND

✷ = Study Tip Gal

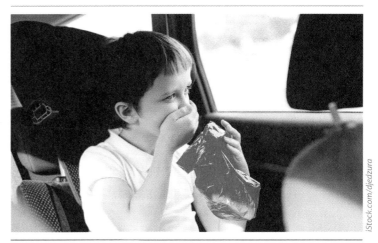

iStock.com/djedzura

CHAPTER 74
MOTION SICKNESS

BACKGROUND

Motion sickness (kinetosis) is a common condition that is also called travel/car sickness, seasickness or airsickness. Symptoms include nausea, dizziness and fatigue. People can get motion sickness on a moving boat, airplane, car or amusement park ride. Symptoms can be triggered in some patients by movies or video games.

NON-DRUG TREATMENT

Some patients find benefit with a wrist band that presses on an acupuncture point located on the inside of the wrist, about the length of 2 fingernails up the arm from the center of the wrist crease. One popular brand is *Sea-Band*.

Ginger, in teas or supplements, is used commonly for nausea. Some people also find it helpful for motion sickness. Peppermint may also be helpful. The best way to stop motion sickness, if possible, is to stop the motion.

DRUG TREATMENT

Antihistamines and anticholinergics are recommended for motion sickness. Scopolamine *(Transderm Scop)*, an anticholinergic, is most commonly prescribed. It is not more effective than generically-available OTC drugs, but is applied topically (behind the ear) and is taken less frequently (lasts three days).

Antihistamines used for motion sickness include diphenhydramine *(Benadryl)*, dimenhydrinate *(Dramamine)* and meclizine *(Dramamine Less Drowsy, Bonine)*. Oral medications must be taken 30 – 60 minutes prior to the needed effect. Dimenhydrinate and meclizine are long-acting piperazine antihistamines and are a little less sedating than other antihistamines. All of the antihistamines have anticholinergic effects similar to scopolamine.

Medications for motion sickness cause drowsiness and impair judgment. Pilots, ship crew members, or anyone operating heavy equipment or driving a car should not take them. Sometimes combinations of products (such as scopolamine to reduce nausea, taken with a stimulant, such as dextroamphetamine, to counteract the drowsiness from the scopolamine) are used, but these combinations have significant risk and should not be routinely recommended.

Traditional antiemetics are discussed in the Oncology chapter. Promethazine is prescription only; for motion sickness, use is generally reserved for patients that do not respond to antihistaminess. It should not be used in children due to the risk of respiratory depression; all promethazine products carry a boxed warning to avoid use in children less than 2 years old and to strongly caution against use in children age 2 and older (see the Pediatric Conditions and Allergic Rhinitis, Cough & Cold chapters). Metoclopramide and the 5-HT3 receptor antagonists (e.g., ondansetron) are generally not effective for motion sickness.

MOTION SICKNESS DRUGS

DRUG	DOSING	SAFETY/SIDE EFFECTS/MONITORING
Scopolamine *(Transderm Scop)*	**Motion Sickness** Apply 1 patch behind the ear at least 4 hrs before the effect is needed. May use a new patch every 3 days PRN. **Preoperative (e.g., cesarean section)** Apply 1 patch the night before surgery or 1 hr prior to surgery. Remove patch 24 hrs after surgery.	**CONTRAINDICATIONS** Hypersensitivity to belladonna alkaloids, closed-angle glaucoma **SIDE EFFECTS** Dry mouth, CNS effects [drowsiness, dizziness, confusion (can be significant in elderly, frail), hallucinations (rare)], stinging of the eyes and pupil dilation (if eyes are touched after handling), risk of ↑ IOP, tachycardia (rare), withdrawal symptoms (e.g., diaphoresis, dizziness, fatigue, headache, nausea) after discontinuation (can last several days) **NOTES** Refer to counseling section (on the following page) Remove the patch before an MRI (contains metal) Avoid alcohol while wearing the patch Primarily for motion sickness, occasionally used inpatient Do not use in children
Dimenhydrinate *(Dramamine)* Tablet, injection	**Motion Sickness** Oral: 50-100 mg Q4-6 hrs **Nausea and Vomiting** IM, IV: 50-100 mg Q4 hrs	**WARNINGS** CNS depression (may impair physical or mental abilities, caution in elderly), worsening of BPH symptoms, ↑ IOP (glaucoma) **SIDE EFFECTS** Dizziness, drowsiness, dry mouth, blurry vision, tachycardia **NOTES** There are various OTC formulations of *Dramamine* with different ingredients. *Dramamine* contains only dimenhydrinate. *Dramamine Less Drowsy* contains only meclizine.
Meclizine *(Dramamine Less Drowsy, Bonine)*	25-50 mg PO 1 hour before travel, can repeat Q24 hrs PRN	**WARNINGS** CNS depression (may impair physical or mental abilities, caution in elderly), worsening of BPH symptoms, ↑ IOP (glaucoma) **SIDE EFFECTS** Drowsiness, dry mouth, dry/blurry vision, tachycardia **NOTES** Commonly used for vertigo; it was previously branded as *Antivert*

KEY COUNSELING POINTS

See the Drug Formulations and Patient Counseling chapter for counseling language/layman's terminology.

SCOPOLAMINE PATCH *(TRANSDERM SCOP)*

- See <u>Study Tip Gal</u> to the right for application instructions.
- Can cause:
  - ❏ Drowsiness.
  - ❏ Dry mouth.
  - ❏ Vision changes, such as blurry vision and widening of the pupils.
- Withdrawal symptoms after discontinuation are more likely with prolonged use (3 days or longer).
- Remove patch before an MRI.

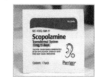

SCOPOLAMINE *(TRANSDERM SCOP)* PATCH

For N/V due to motion sickness or anesthesia/ surgery

- Apply at least 4 hours before needed or the night before surgery
- Press firmly to skin behind ear for 30 seconds
- Try to avoid placing the patch over hair, or when the patch is removed, the hair may be removed, too
- Lasts 3 days; if continued treatment needed, remove the first patch and place a new patch behind the other ear
- Wash hands after applying

Do not drive: high level of drowsiness, dizziness and confusion. These anticholinergic side effects are worse, and not well-tolerated, in elderly patients (avoid use when possible).

Arne Beruldsen/Shutterstock.com

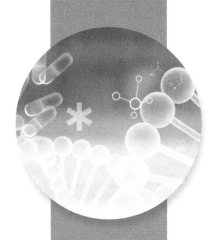
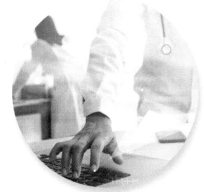
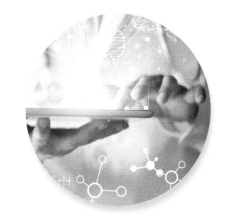

PHARMACY FOUNDATIONS PART 2

CONTENTS

CONTENT LEGEND

☀ = Study
    Tip Gal

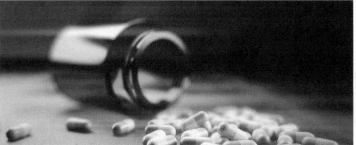

iStock.com/peshkov

CHAPTER 75

MEDICATION SAFETY & QUALITY IMPROVEMENT

BACKGROUND

A report published by the Institute of Medicine (IOM), *To Err is Human* (1999), increased awareness of the prevalence of medical errors. The study found that up to 98,000 Americans die each year in U.S. hospitals due to preventable medical errors, with 7,000 from medication errors alone. These numbers understated the problem because they did not include preventable deaths due to medical treatments outside of hospitals. Since the release of the IOM study, there has been a greater focus on the quality of healthcare provided in the U.S.

HOW TO APPROACH MEDICATION SAFETY

The term "medication safety" is defined as <u>freedom from preventable harm</u> due to <u>medication use</u>. It is an essential component of all areas of pharmacy practice and is therefore encompassed throughout most chapters in this course book (see examples in the table below). This chapter is intended to set the foundation and discuss some of the core elements of medication safety.

TOPIC*	SELECT CHAPTERS
Collaborative practice	Diabetes
	Anticoagulation
	Contraception & Infertility
Transitions of care and continuity of care	Answering Case-Based Exam Questions
	Drug Formulations & Patient Counseling
Disease prevention and stewardship	Immunizations
	Human Immunodeficiency Virus
	Hypertension
Vulnerable populations	Drug Use in Pregnancy & Lactation
	Pediatrics
	Oncology
Pharmacy informatics	Drug References
	Lab Values & Drug Monitoring

*Adapted from Area 6 of the NAPLEX Competency Statements

MEDICATION ERRORS

The National Coordinating Council for Medication Error Reporting and Prevention (NCC MERP) defines a medication error as "any preventable event that may cause or lead to inappropriate medication use or patient harm while the medication is in the control of the healthcare professional, patient or consumer." Medication errors can occur at any step of the medication use process (see diagrams later in this chapter).

Do not confuse medication errors with adverse drug reactions (ADRs). ADRs are usually not preventable, although they may be more likely to occur if the drug is given to a patient at high risk for certain complications. Furthermore, the severity of some ADRs can be reduced with changes in care, such as if additional monitoring was performed (refer to the Lab Values & Drug Monitoring and Drug Allergies & Adverse Drug Reactions chapters for more information).

EXAMPLE OF AN ADR (NOT A MEDICATION ERROR)

A 55-year-old female has a history of herpes zoster. She reports considerable "shingles pain" and received a prescription for pregabalin. She returned to the clinic with complaints of ankle swelling, which required drug discontinuation.

This is not a medication error made by the prescriber of pregabalin or by the pharmacist who dispensed it. Rather, this is a side effect that can occur with the use of this drug.

A close call (also called a near miss) is when an error or situation occurred but was corrected before reaching the patient (e.g., a patient picks up a prescription for levothyroxine, but notices the tablets are a different color from previous prescriptions and alerts the pharmacist before taking the medication).

A sentinel event is a patient safety event that results in death, severe harm (of any duration) or permanent harm (regardless of severity) of a patient. When a sentinel event occurs, it is important to find out what went wrong and implement measures to prevent it from happening again.

Errors can be further divided into errors of omission and commission. Errors of omission occur when something was left out that is needed for safety (e.g., failing to use a pharmacist double-check system for chemotherapy orders). Errors of commission occur when something was done incorrectly (e.g., prescribing bupropion to a patient with a history of seizures).

MEDICATION ADMINISTRATION ERRORS

Many medication errors occur when at least one of the "five rights" was not upheld (see image). These rights reflect aspects of medication administration where potential errors can occur and serve as a quick double-check every time a medication is administered. In this context, "right" means "correct," as in the correct patient, dose, route, etc. These rights represent the goals of medication safety at the most basic level, and must be combined with other system-based error prevention methods to be successful (discussed later in this chapter).

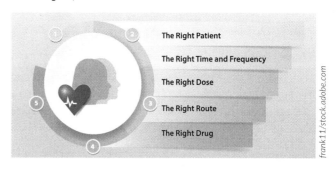

The Right Patient

The Right Time and Frequency

The Right Dose

The Right Route

The Right Drug

CAUSES OF MEDICATION ERRORS

There are many causes of medication errors (see the box below), as human error is inevitable and unpredictable. Errors occur unintentionally because of the way we navigate high-stress and intricate work environments and perform complex tasks. Though humans commit errors, they are usually caused by problems with the system (referred to as "system-based" errors). However, human error must be distinguished from at-risk and reckless behaviors:

- At-risk behaviors: a behavioral choice when an individual has lost the perception of risk, or mistakenly believes the risk to be insignificant or justified. Examples include developing "workarounds" for time-consuming or tedious processes, like failing to scan a medication's barcode prior to patient administration because it has a high rate of scanning failures.

- Reckless behaviors: a conscious disregard of a substantial and unjustifiable risk. Examples include working under the influence of drugs or alcohol and drug diversion.

CAUSES OF COMPROMISED PATIENT SAFETY

- Low patient health literacy
- Insufficient training, lack of experience or unfamiliarity with tasks
- Breakdowns in communication
  - ❏ Hesitancy to speak up or question authority/other professions
  - ❏ Rushed communication
- Competing priorities in the face of stress, fatigue or burnout
  - ❏ Running on "autopilot"
- Fast-paced, high-volume environment with time constraints
  - ❏ Frequent interruptions, lapses in concentration
- Complex technology and processes
  - ❏ Creation of "workarounds" to subvert complexity

ORGANIZATIONS FOCUSED ON PATIENT SAFETY

Organizations that specialize in error prevention can analyze the system-based causes of errors and make recommendations. They also help in setting standards and best practices for patient safety.

THE INSTITUTE FOR SAFE MEDICATION PRACTICES (ISMP)

The ISMP is a nonprofit organization dedicated to the prevention of medication errors across all healthcare settings. Since errors that occur in one organization are likely to occur in another, the ISMP releases Medication Safety Alert newsletters to share information across healthcare organizations, so that process improvements can be implemented proactively to prevent future events. Every pharmacist should routinely read medication error reports such as this one and evaluate the potential for the same error within their own institution.

Part of the ISMP is the national Medication Errors Reporting Program (MERP), which is a confidential, voluntary reporting program. It provides expert analysis of the system causes of medication errors and provides recommendations for prevention.

Medication errors and close calls can be reported on the ISMP website (www.ismp.org). Professionals and consumers should be encouraged to report medication errors using this site even if the error was reported internally. When there are many reports of a particular error, the manufacturer may be required to take measures to increase drug safety (e.g., REMS program, name change, packaging change).

THE JOINT COMMISSION (TJC)

The Joint Commission on Accreditation of Healthcare Organizations (TJC) is an independent, not-for-profit organization that accredits and certifies more than 20,000 healthcare organizations and programs in the U.S., including hospitals, healthcare networks, long-term care facilities, home care organizations, office-based surgery centers and independent laboratories. TJC focuses on the highest quality and safety of care and sets standards that institutions must meet to be accredited. An accredited organization must undergo regular on-site surveys, which are usually unannounced.

National Patient Safety Goals

National Patient Safety Goals (NPSGs) are set annually by TJC for different types of healthcare settings (e.g., ambulatory care, behavioral health, hospital). Each goal includes defined measures that must be met, called "Elements of Performance."

These are often included in institutional protocols. Important NPSGs for pharmacists are described below.

- Use at least two patient identifiers when providing care, treatment and services.
  - ❑ Appropriate patient identifiers include name, medical record number and date of birth.
  - ❑ Inappropriate patient identifiers include zip code, room number and physician name.
- Reduce the likelihood of patient harm associated with the use of anticoagulant therapy.
  - ❑ There are many important elements to this goal, including the requirements to use approved dosing protocols and programmable pumps (e.g., for heparin) and to provide education to patients and families. Protocols should include starting dose ranges, alternate dosing strategies to address drug-drug interactions, communication with the dietary department to address drug-food interactions, general monitoring requirements and monitoring for bleeding and heparin-induced thrombocytopenia (HIT).
- Maintain and communicate accurate patient medication information.
  - ❑ This includes medication reconciliation, providing written information to the patient and conducting discharge counseling. The medication name, dose, frequency, route and indication (at a minimum) should be confirmed. Refer to the section on Medication Reconciliation later in this chapter.

SELECT NATIONAL PATIENT SAFETY GOALS

Identify patients correctly: use at least two patient identifiers when providing care, treatment and services (NPSG 01.01.01).

Improve staff communication: report critical results of tests and diagnostic procedures on a timely basis (NPSG 02.03.01).

Use medications safely:

- Label all medications, medication containers (e.g., syringes) and other solutions on and off the sterile field in perioperative and other procedural settings (NPSG 03.04.01).
- Reduce the likelihood of patient harm associated with the use of anticoagulant therapy (NPSG 03.05.01).
- Maintain and communicate accurate patient medication information (NPSG 03.06.01).

Use clinical alarms safely: improve the safety of clinical alarm systems (NPSG 06.01.01).

Prevent infections: comply with either the Centers for Disease Control (CDC) or World Health Organization (WHO) hand hygiene guidelines (NPSG 07.01.01).

CENTER FOR MEDICAID AND MEDICARE SERVICES (CMS)

CMS (part of the U.S. Department of Health and Human Services) surveys hospitals seeking reimbursement for Medicare and Medicaid patients. In order to bill to Medicare, hospitals must meet standards of patient safety set by CMS. Many of these standards are similar to measures developed by TJC.

OTHER ACCREDITING ORGANIZATIONS

Other organizations that accredit and certify healthcare programs include:

- National Association of Boards of Pharmacy (NABP): accredits many pharmacy settings (e.g., community, compounding)
- Accreditation Association for Ambulatory Health Care (AAAHC)
- Accreditation Commission for Health Care (ACHC)
- Center for Improvement in Healthcare Quality (CIHQ)
- Utilization Review Accreditation Commission (URAC)

Similar to TJC, each organization has specific standards that must be met to obtain accreditation. The approaches to accreditation are different, and institutions can select the accrediting organization that best matches their needs.

COMMON METHODS TO REDUCE MEDICATION ERRORS

IMPLEMENT JUST CULTURE

When medication errors occur, blame is often placed on the individual who committed the error. This type of punitive response causes individuals to be hesitant about reporting errors or mistakes, which prevents identification of potential hazards and allows the danger to other patients to persist. Instead, organizations should implement a culture of safety by doing the following:

- Acknowledge the high-risk nature of healthcare and be determined to achieve safe operations.
- Implement a blame-free environment where individuals are able to report errors and near misses without fear of reprimand or punishment (often referred to as "just culture").
- Encourage collaboration across disciplines and levels of authority to seek patient safety solutions.
- Dedicate resources to track, monitor and address safety concerns.

ANALYZE ERRORS USING A SYSTEMS-BASED APPROACH

A systems-based approach to patient safety seeks to identify situations or factors that are likely to give rise to human error, as well as recommend changes to different aspects of care to avoid or reduce the frequency of future errors. Most errors result from multiple, smaller errors at different steps in the process (often referred to as the "Swiss Cheese" model). In this model, each layer represents a wall of defense and the holes represent the deficiencies of each layer that could allow an error to pass through (see illustration). When the holes align, it allows for a hazard to reach the end of the process (in this case, a medical error to reach the patient).

After the investigation of an error, recommendations include implementing mitigation strategies to prevent the reoccurrence of the error, such as human factors engineering strategies (see the table on the next page). Often, strategies need to be employed at multiple steps in the process, as no single intervention is 100% effective or reliable.

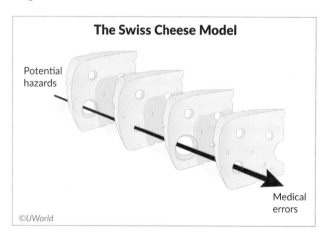

The Swiss Cheese Model

Potential hazards

Medical errors

©UWorld

Human Factors Engineering Strategies

STRATEGY	DESCRIPTION AND EXAMPLES
High Reliability	
Forcing functions	Create hard stops in a design or process to eliminate the risk of incorrect use
	■ Example: require specific fields to be completed during order entry
Computerized automation	Utilize automated processes to remove human effort and variations that cause error
	■ Example: use a computerized order entry system to prevent transcription errors
Human machine redundancy	Create a repetitive step to confirm a correct action in an error-prone process
	■ Example: electronically scan the barcode of medications in addition to visual inspection
Medium Reliability	
Standardization and simplification	Align processes to minimize variation, complexity and learning curve
	■ Example: every pharmacist follows the same approved renal dosing protocol
Environment and physical layout	Design workspaces to facilitate correct action and minimize error and/or distractions
	■ Example: stock medications prone to error separately from each other
Reminders and alerts	Develop processes and prompts to notify clinicians to check actions to reduce errors
	■ Example: alerts for patient allergies and drug-drug interactions
Double checks	Engage a second person to independently review a high-risk process
	■ Example: require two pharmacists to individually review chemotherapy
Low Reliability	
Education and training	Provide regular instruction on medication errors
	■ Example: monthly review of recent medication errors with staff
Policy changes	Develop a policy to address general work flows, error-prone processes and best practices
	■ Example: a policy outlining the multidisciplinary review of medication errors that occur in the facility

MANAGE CARE TRANSITIONS EFFECTIVELY

Care transitions refers to the movement of patients from one setting to another, such as from the intensive care unit to the medical ward or when being discharged from the hospital to home. Every transition poses a risk of an error occurring, especially with medications.

An important aspect of managing care transitions is to perform patient counseling, as poor health literacy increases the risk for medication errors. Patients can play a vital role in preventing medication errors when they have been encouraged to ask questions and seek satisfactory answers about their medications before drugs are dispensed. If a patient questions any part of the medication dispensing process (e.g., the drug's appearance, dose) the pharmacist must be receptive and responsive (not defensive). All patient inquiries should be thoroughly investigated before the medication is dispensed.

Written information that is provided about medications should be at a reading level that is appropriate for the patient. It may be necessary to provide pictures or other means of instruction to patients who do not speak English or are unable to read English. Attempts must be made to communicate to the patient in their language, using on-site staff or dial-in translation services.

Medication Reconciliation

Medication reconciliation ("med rec") should be performed at every care transition and aims to prevent harm from the administration of unnecessary or potentially inappropriate medications (see steps below). This reconciliation is done to avoid medication errors such as omissions, duplications, dosing errors or drug interactions during transitions of care.

The medication reconciliation process comprises of five steps:

- Develop a list of current medications (including OTC) and dietary supplements
- Develop a list of medications to be prescribed
- Compare the medications on the two lists
- Note discrepancies and make decisions to continue, stop or hold medications based on the comparison and clinical status of the patient
- Communicate the new list to the patient, caregivers and other health professionals involved in the patient's care

Medication reconciliation is most effective when complete and accurate information is entered into the patient's medical record. When information (e.g., weight or past medical history) is unavailable in the computer system, errors can result. For this reason, pharmacists are often actively involved in documenting home medication use and performing medication reconciliation. In many hospitals, admission orders for a patient cannot be entered into the electronic system until medication reconciliation is completed.

Discharge medication reconciliation is an opportunity for the prescriber to address any of the patient's home medications that were "on hold" during the hospitalization and which medications used during the hospitalization should be continued when the patient goes home. Medication reconciliation is equally important in ambulatory care, as many patients receive prescriptions from more than one outpatient provider and may go to several pharmacies.

Include Indications and Proper Instructions on Prescriptions

An indication for use written on the prescription (such as lisinopril 10 mg once daily for hypertension) helps pharmacists ensure appropriate prescribing and drug selection.

Using the term "as directed" is not acceptable on prescriptions because the patient often will not know what this means, and the pharmacist cannot verify a proper dosing regimen. Occasionally, this phrase is used on the label along with a separate dosing calendar (e.g., with warfarin). It is preferable to write "use per instructions on the dosing calendar" since the patient may not understand how to take the medication and may not be aware that a separate dosing calendar exists.

EXAMPLE OF THE BENEFIT OF MEDICATION RECONCILIATION

AN is an 82-year-old female. Her only medication for the previous ten years has been atenolol 25 mg daily. She recently developed influenza, began to have trouble breathing and was taken to the hospital. It was discovered that she had pneumonia and heart failure. She was prescribed sacubitril/valsartan, carvedilol, dapagliflozin and furosemide. AN was discharged to transitional care and received the new medications plus her home medication (atenolol). A consultant pharmacist conducted a medication review to reconcile the medications and, after discussion with the physician, the pharmacist wrote an order to discontinue the atenolol.

UTILIZE MEDICATION THERAPY MANAGEMENT

Errors may be discovered during a medication therapy review (MTR) as part of the medication therapy management (MTM) process. MTM involves the preparation of a personal medication record (PMR) and a medication-related action plan (MAP), preferably by a pharmacist-led team. The next steps involve interventions or referrals, documentation and plans for follow-up. Patients targeted for MTM include those with multiple chronic conditions who are taking multiple drugs and are likely to incur annual costs for covered drugs that exceed a predetermined level. Computer databases are used to identify patients with certain high-risk conditions (such as heart failure or uncontrolled diabetes) and assign a pharmacist to review profiles for proper medication use.

These reviews may identify missing therapy (e.g., lack of an ACE inhibitor or ARB in patients with diabetes and albuminuria, missing beta-blocker therapy post-MI) or result in de-prescribing (i.e., stopping unncessary medications). A popular MTM initiative is to improve nonadherence in patients with heart failure due to the high rate of ED visits. MTM is also used to identify cost savings, by promoting switches to generics or more affordable brands (often initiated by the patient's insurance company), or by suggesting patient assistance programs or low-income subsidies for eligible individuals.

IMPLEMENT INTERDISCIPLINARY TEAMS

An interdisciplinary team involves clinicians from different backgrounds (e.g., nurses, pharmacists, physicians, physical therapists, respiratory therapists) that work collaboratively to provide patient care. This team approach allows clinicians to share expertise, resources and skills to improve outcomes. A team may work together under a formal relationship (e.g., a collaborative practice agreement between a physician and pharmacist) or as a less formal team (e.g., an interdisciplinary rounding service at a hospital). Stewardship is an interdisciplinary process that involves reviewing patient medications to optimize safety and efficacy as well as to ensure appropriate use. Stewardship activities often target drug classes with a high risk of adverse outcomes; some common examples include antimicrobials, anticoagulants and opioids.

Collaborative Practice Agreements (CPAs)

CPAs allow pharmacists to perform advanced care activities (e.g., order and monitor therapeutic drug levels, modify medication doses). Incorporating pharmacists in this manner ensures a focus on medication safety and improved patient outcomes. The requirements for CPAs differ based on the legal jurisdiction (i.e., state laws) and specific institution.

DEDICATE PHARMACISTS TO HIGH-RISK AREAS

Making pharmacists more available in certain high-risk areas (e.g., intensive care units, pediatric units, emergency departments) is a common strategy to improve medication safety. This is also known as "decentralization." In many cases, these settings have a high incidence of preventable medication errors. With better visibility and accessibility, pharmacists working directly with providers on these units can assist in many facets of the medication use process and develop solutions to prevent medication errors proactively.

EDUCATE STAFF

Staff education, including "in-services" or electronic competency activities, should be provided whenever new high-alert drugs are being used in the facility, to introduce new guidelines or process changes aimed at preventing medication errors and upon hiring of new employees. Many organizations require annual competency activities to re-train employees on important initiatives.

DEVELOP ORGANIZATIONAL POLICIES FOR HIGH-RISK SCENARIOS AND ERROR-PRONE PRACTICES

Healthcare organizations will often create policies and protocols that include best practices for high-risk scenarios and/or to address error-prone activities. In general, policies are the least effective strategy to reduce errors, because individuals must be aware of them, which is why employees require initial and regular training about existing policies for them to be effective. The following examples are common policies that an organization should maintain for safety.

Medication Error Policy

A medication error policy commits resources and a standard process for responding to medication errors as well as reporting when errors occur. Policies will often also address tracking errors and developing an interdisciplinary team to investigate errors.

Response

Institutions should have a plan in place for responding to medication errors. The plan should address the following:

- Internal notification: who should be notified within the institution and within what time frame?
- External reporting: who should be notified outside of the institution?
- Disclosure: what information should be shared with the patient/family? Who will be present when this occurs?
- Investigation: what is the process for immediate and long-term internal investigation of an error?
- Improvement: what process will ensure that immediate and long-term preventative actions are taken?

Reporting

Medication errors, preventable adverse drug reactions, hazardous conditions and "close calls" or "near misses" (even when they do not reach the patient) should be reported. Medication errors are reported so that changes can be made to the system to prevent similar errors in the future. Without reporting, these events may go unrecognized and will likely happen again because others will not learn from the incident.

The staff member who discovers the error should immediately report it to the appropriate authority (e.g., corporate office, the owner of an independent pharmacy, designated hospital office) using the established reporting structure. Many state boards of pharmacy require quality assurance programs to promote pharmacy processes that prevent medication errors. Error investigations need to take place quickly (within 48 hours of the incident) so that the sequence of events remains clear to those involved. Many states mandate the ethical requirement that errors be reported to the patient and the prescriber as soon as possible.

Most medication error reporting systems within hospitals are electronic. The hospital's Pharmacy and Therapeutics (P&T) committee and Medication Safety Committee (or similar entity) should be informed of the error.

Evaluation and Quality Improvement

Evaluation and quality improvement can be performed prospectively, retrospectively or continuously.

- Prospective

  - A failure mode and effects analysis (FMEA) is a proactive method used to reduce the frequency and consequences of errors. FMEA is used to analyze the design of the system in order to evaluate the potential for failures and to determine what potential effects could occur when the medication delivery system changes in any substantial way or if a potentially dangerous new drug will be added to the formulary.

- Retrospective

  - A root cause analysis (RCA) is a retrospective investigation of an event that has already occurred, which includes reviewing the sequence of events that led to the error. The information obtained in the analysis is used to design changes that will hopefully prevent future errors. The TJC requires that an RCA is performed after a sentinel event.

- Continuous

  - Continuous quality improvement (CQI) is the goal for most healthcare settings. CQI programs improve efficiency, quality and patient satisfaction while reducing costs. Examples include Lean and Six Sigma, which are often used together (and used for other CQI initiatives beyond medication errors). Lean focuses on minimizing waste, while Six Sigma focuses on reducing defects. Six Sigma uses the DMAIC (define, measure, analyze, improve, control) process.

Unsafe Abbreviations

Abbreviations are unsafe and contribute to many medical errors. The minimum list of "Do Not Use" abbreviations per TJC is shown in the table below. ISMP also publishes a list of error-prone abbreviations, symbols and dosage designations which includes those on TJC's list and many others. All institutions accredited by TJC are required to have a list of abbreviations that should not be used in the facility. This list must include all of the abbreviations from the TJC "Do Not Use" list and any additional abbreviations selected by the institution (e.g., those that have resulted in significant errors in the past). The unapproved abbreviation list should be readily accessible in the institution (e.g., wall charts, pocket cards). It is best to try to avoid abbreviations entirely. In addition, electronic prescribing can eliminate errors associated with poor handwriting. See the Study Tip Gal below.

DO NOT USE	POTENTIAL PROBLEM	USE INSTEAD
U, u (unit)	Mistaken for "0" (zero), the number "4" (four) or "cc"	Write "unit"
IU (international unit)	Mistaken for IV (intravenous) or the number 10 (ten)	Write "international unit"
Q.D., QD, q.d., qd (daily)	Mistaken for each other	Write "daily"
Q.O.D., QOD, q.o.d., qod (every other day)	Period after the Q mistaken for "I" and the "O" mistaken for "I"	Write "every other day"
Trailing zero (X.0 mg) Lack of leading zero (.X mg)	Decimal point is missed resulting in a 10-fold dosing error	Write X mg Write 0.X mg
MS MSO$_4$ and MgSO$_4$	Can mean morphine sulfate or magnesium sulfate Confused with one another	Write "morphine sulfate" Write "magnesium sulfate"

DO NOT USE ABBREVIATIONS

Potassium Chloride
10 mEq po Q.D
Humalog 4/2/6u
Lantus 80 units SQHS
Coumadin 10 mg QD

How often should the potassium be given?

Is that 8 or 80 units of *Lantus*?

Coumadin 1 or 10 mg? Once daily or four times per day?

Look-Alike, Sound-Alike Medications

Tall Man Lettering

Look-alike, sound-alike ("LASA") medications are a common cause of medication errors. Poor handwriting and similar product labeling aggravate the problem. Drugs that are easily mixed up should be labeled with tall man letters. For example:

- *CeleXA, CeleBREX*
- predniSONE, prednisoLONE

Tall man lettering mixes upper and lower case letters to draw attention to the dissimilarities in drug names. The letters that are upper case are the ones that are different between the two look-alike, sound-alike drugs. Safety-conscious organizations (e.g., ISMP, FDA, TJC) have promoted the use of tall man letters as one means of reducing confusion between similar drug names. Information from the FDA and ISMP on approved tall man lettering is available at: https://www.ismp.org/recommendations/tall-man-letters-list.

Drug dictionaries (also known as drug libraries) within computer systems and automated dispensing cabinets (ADCs) often have alerts that prompt the provider to confirm that the correct medication is being ordered or withdrawn. For example, a warning may appear on the screen of the ADC that will state: "This is *DILAUDID*. Did you want HYDROmorphone?" to avoid confusion with morphine.

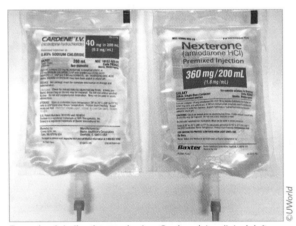

Example of similar drug packaging: Cardene (nicardipine), left; Nexterone (amiodarone), right

Medications With Similar Packaging

Look-alike packaging can contribute to errors. If unavoidable, separate look-alike drugs in the pharmacy and patient care units, or repackage. Never rely on the package appearance (e.g., color, design) to identify the right drug product. Pharmacies frequently have to purchase products from different manufacturers (and these may look vastly different).

High-Alert Medications

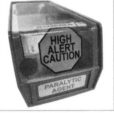

©UWorld

Drugs with a heightened risk of causing significant patient harm if used in error should be designated as high-alert (see Study Tip Gal below). The ISMP "high-alert" list for acute care settings is available online. ISMP's list represents the most common agents that are high risk, but an institution's list may include additional drugs based on experience in that setting.

High-alert medications can be used safely by developing polices, protocols or order sets for use, using premixed products whenever possible, limiting concentrations available in the institution and stocking high-alert products only in the pharmacy. See examples of safe use precautions for insulin and potassium chloride on the following page. Protocols for high-alert drugs increase appropriate prescribing and reduce the chance of errors from inappropriate prescribing.

SELECT HIGH-ALERT MEDICATIONS

- Anesthetics, inhaled or IV (e.g., propofol)
- Antiarrhythmics, IV (e.g., amiodarone)
- Anticoagulants/antithrombotics (e.g., heparin, warfarin)
- Chemotherapeutics (e.g., methotrexate)
- Epidural/intrathecal drugs
- Hypertonic saline (greater than 0.9% NaCl)
- Immunosuppressants (e.g., cyclosporine)
- Inotropics (e.g., digoxin)
- Insulins (e.g., insulin aspart, insulin U-500)
- Magnesium sulfate injection
- Neuromuscular blocking agents (e.g., vecuronium)
- Opioids
- Oral hypoglycemics (e.g., sulfonylureas)
- Parenteral nutrition
- Potassium chloride and phosphates for injection
- Sterile water for injection

Any drug that is high-risk for significant harm if dispensed incorrectly can be placed in a medication bin that provides a visual alert (e.g., a high-alert sticker) to the person accessing the medication. The bin can be labeled with warnings and include materials (placed inside the bin) that should be dispensed with the drug (such as oral syringes or MedGuides).

Examples of Safe-Use Precautions

DRUG	PRECAUTIONS
Insulin	All insulin orders should be reviewed by a pharmacist prior to dispensing
	Standardize all insulin infusions to one concentration
	Develop protocols for insulin infusions, transition from infusion to SC and sliding scale orders; use standard orders for management of hypoglycemia
	Do not use "U" for units; always label with "units" or "units = mL," but never just "mL"
	If U-500 is stocked, specify conditions under which it is to be used, which product will be stocked (vials and U-500 syringes vs. pens) and how doses will be supplied; ideally U-500 should be kept in the central pharmacy
Potassium Chloride	Remove all KCl vials from floor stock; prepare all KCl infusions in the pharmacy
	Use premixed containers
	Use protocols for KCl delivery which include indications for IV administration, maximum rate of infusion, maximum allowable concentration, guidelines for when cardiac monitoring is required, a stipulation that all KCl infusions must be given via a pump, prohibition of multiple simultaneous KCl solutions (e.g., no IV KCl while KCl is being infused in another IV)
	Allow for automatic substitution of oral KCl for IV KCl, when appropriate
	Label all fluids containing potassium with a "Potassium Added" sticker

Drug Recalls

Drugs can be recalled for several reasons, including inaccurate labeling, the presence of undeclared ingredients or contamination, a newly found risk to the patient or if the product is defective (e.g., does not dissolve properly). Since recalls occur regularly, healthcare organizations and pharmacies need to be prepared to remove recalled medications from stock and prevent dispensing of a recalled product to a patient (which usually only affects certain lots or batches). A drug recall policy will outline the process for identifying recalls, removing a drug from distribution and informing prescribers/patients as necessary.

Use of the Metric System

Healthcare organizations will often have a policy that requires measurements to be recorded using the metric system only. For example, prescribers should use metric units to express all weights (g, kg) and volumes (mL, L). Computer systems generally have a drop-down menu for selecting the correct units (e.g., lb vs. kg) and easily converting between units. It is critical to record the correct units since many calculations (CrCl or eGFR) and dosing checks are performed automatically by the EHR system based on the height and/or weight recorded for the patient. It is not uncommon to care for patients weighing 100 kg (or more), but serious errors can occur if this weight was intended to be 100 lb. Another common error with measurements is confusing "teaspoon" or "tablespoon" for milliliters (e.g., giving 3.5 tsp vs. 3.5 mL). Standard use of milliliters is preferred, with education to patients/caregivers.

Multiple-Dose Vials and Products

A policy for the use of multiple-dose vials and products in institutional settings is important because of the risk for cross-contamination (infection) and overdosing. Examples include insulin vials and inhalers. If used, they should be designated for a single patient and labeled appropriately. The remainder should be discarded when the medication is discontinued or the patient is discharged.

Emergency Medications/Crash Carts

Staff must be properly trained to handle emergencies and use crash cart medications. The medications should be in unit-dose packaging (i.e., contains a single dose) and be age-specific, including doses for pediatric patients. If a unit-dose medication is not available, prefilled syringes and premixed drips are best (if possible) because codes are high-stress situations and mistakes are likely. A standardized drug reference sheet should be available during emergencies, including a quick reference with weight-based dosing (e.g., Broselow tape) for trays used in a pediatric unit. Emergency medications should be stored in sealed or locked containers and replaced as soon as possible after use (so that the area is not left without required medications). Drug expiration dates should be monitored. Trained pharmacists should be present at codes when possible.

CODE BLUE

A code blue refers to a patient requiring emergency medical care, typically for cardiac or respiratory arrest. The overhead announcement and/or paging system will provide the patient's location. The code team (often including a pharmacist) will rush to the room and begin immediate resuscitative efforts. During the code, closed-loop communication (i.e., repeating back for verification) is used and careful documentation is completed.

TECHNOLOGY AND AUTOMATED SYSTEMS TO REDUCE ERRORS

The integration of medication-related knowledge with technology and automation is called pharmacy informatics. Some of the more common systems integrated into the medication-use process are described in the sections below. In most institutions, pharmacists are actively involved in creating, monitoring and improving use of these tools.

COMPUTERIZED PROVIDER ORDER ENTRY AND CLINICAL DECISION SUPPORT

Computerized physician/provider order entry (CPOE) is a process that allows direct entry of medical orders by prescribers into the computer system. This has the benefit of reducing errors by minimizing the ambiguity resulting from handwritten orders. A greater benefit is seen when CPOE is combined with clinical decision support (CDS) tools. Clinical guidelines and patient labs can be built into the CPOE system, and alerts can notify a prescriber if the drug is inappropriate, or if labs indicate that the drug could be unsafe (such as a high potassium level and a new order for a potassium-sparing diuretic). For example, one of the ISMP's best practice recommendations is to program the CPOE system to default to a weekly frequency for oral methotrexate orders to prevent accidental selection of daily dosing, and require an oncologic indication to be entered for daily dosing.

CPOE can include standard order sets, clinical decision pathways and protocols (e.g., standardized initial dosing recommendations for heparin based on indication). An example of an on-screen alert from a CDS system is shown below. This alert appears when a prescriber attempts to order a citalopram dose > 40 mg/day. In addition to medication orders, CPOE is used for laboratory orders and procedures.

One aspect of CQI is monitoring, reporting trends and addressing alert overrides. While alerts in the EHR can help reduce errors, an overabundance of alerts can lead to alert fatigue (i.e., desensitization to alerts due to frequency or low-importance alerts, leading to excessive overrides).

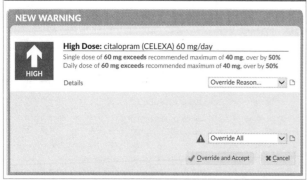

©UWorld

BARCODING

Barcoding may be the most important medication error reduction tool currently available. Regardless of the setting (i.e., outpatient vs. inpatient), the barcode follows the drug through the medication-use process to ensure it is properly stocked (such as in the right space in the pharmacy or in the right pocket in the dispensing cabinet), through compounding (if required) and dispensing/administration to the right patient. It also helps to prevent diversion of drugs that are commonly abused.

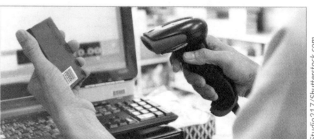

In the hospital, the barcode is used at the bedside to ensure that the correct drug (by scanning the barcode on the drug's packaging) is going to the right patient (by scanning the barcode on the patient's wristband) and to confirm that the dose is being given at the right time (by matching to the order in the system). The nurse is often signed into the electronic medical record (or scans the barcode on their name tag) while barcode scanning, which records who administered the dose.

Barcodes are now on many infusion pumps and can prevent errors involving medications being given IV. This includes identifying drugs that are not meant to be administered via this route, auto-programming that pulls infusion parameters from the EHR (i.e., manual entry not required) and auto-documentation (which records dose/rate changes for others to review/confirm in the EHR).

When a medication is scanned and administered using barcode technology, the administration can automatically populate on the medication administration record (MAR), thus avoiding the time associated with manually charting medication administration.

AUTOMATED DISPENSING CABINETS

Common automated dispensing cabinets (ADCs) include *Pyxis, Omnicell, ScriptPro* and *Accudose*. Many hospitals utilize ADCs to replace the more labor-intensive patient cassettes, which require at least once daily filling and exchange.

Practical Benefits of ADCs

Drug inventory and medication replenishment can be automated when drugs are stocked in or removed from the cabinet. ADCs provide enhanced security of controlled drugs by recording detailed information about transactions (e.g., who gained access to the controlled medications). The drugs are easily available at the unit and do not require individual delivery from the pharmacy. ADCs permit barcoding and provide alerts and usage reports.

Methods to Improve ADC Safety

- TJC requires that the pharmacist review the order before the medication can be removed from the ADC for a patient, except in special circumstances (an override). The override function should be limited to a select list of medications. Overrides for medications used for reversal of adverse events (e.g., naloxone, flumazenil) should be investigated.

- The most common error associated with ADC use is giving the wrong drug or dose to a patient. The patient's MAR should be accessible to practitioners while they are removing medications from the ADC. The use of barcode scanning improves ADC safety.

- Look-alike, sound-alike medications should be stored in different locations within the ADC. Using computerized alerts can help reduce error risk (e.g., require confirmation when selecting drugs with high potential for mix-up).

- Certain medications should not be put into ADCs, including U-500 insulin, warfarin and high-dose narcotics (such as hydromorphone 10 mg/mL and morphine 25 mg/mL).

- Nurses should not be permitted to put medications back into the medication compartment because they might be placed in the wrong area; it is best to have a separate drawer for all "returned" medications.

- If the machine is in a busy, noisy environment, or in one with poor lighting, errors increase.

STERILE COMPOUNDING TECHNOLOGY

Several technologies have been developed to assist with reducing errors during sterile compounding (e.g., automated compounding devices, IV workflow management systems, IV robots). These should interface with the EHR to eliminate transcription errors from manual entry into one system from another. See the Sterile Compounding chapter for more information.

PATIENT CONTROLLED ANALGESIA DEVICES

Opioids are effective medications for moderate to severe post-surgical pain. They may be administered with patient-controlled analgesia (PCA) devices, where the patient can self-administer doses of medication with the push of a button (see image). The dose and dose limits are ordered by the physician. The PCA will not allow the patient to take more medication than ordered. PCAs allow the patient to treat pain quickly (there is no need to call the nurse and wait for the dose to arrive) and allow the administration of small doses, which helps reduce side effects (particularly over-sedation).

PCA drug delivery can mimic the pain pattern more closely and provide good pain control. PCAs can be administered with anesthetics for a synergistic benefit.

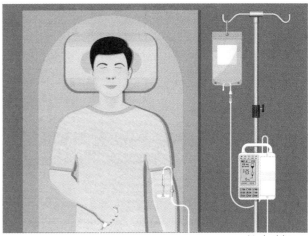

rumruay/stock.adobe.com

PCA Safety Considerations

- The devices can be complex and require setup and programming. This is a significant cause of preventable medication errors. PCAs should be used only by well-coordinated healthcare teams.

- Patients may not be appropriate candidates for PCA treatment. They should be cooperative and should have a cognitive assessment prior to using the PCA to ensure that they can follow instructions.

- Friends and family members should not administer PCA doses. This is a TJC requirement.

- PCAs do not frequently cause respiratory depression, but the risk is present. Advanced age, obesity and concurrent use of CNS depressants (in addition to higher opioid doses) increase the risk.

PCA Safety Steps

- Limit the opioids available outside of ADCs. Use standard order sets (set drug dosages, especially for opioid-naïve patients) so that safe doses of drugs are selected.

- Educate staff about HYDROmorphone and morphine mix-ups.

- Implement PCA protocols that include independent double-checking of the drug, pump setting and dosage. The concentration on the MAR should match the PCA label.

- Use barcoding technology. Some infusion pumps incorporate barcoding technology. Scanning the barcode on the PCA would help ensure the correct concentration is entered during PCA programming. It will also ensure that the right patient is getting the medication.

- Assess the patient's pain, sedation and respiratory rate on a scheduled basis.

SUMMARY OF STEPS AND SAFETY CHECKS IN THE MEDICATION USE PROCESS

The following diagrams show a summary of common steps needed in order to get a medication from the drug supplier to a patient in the inpatient and outpatient settings. Underneath the steps are a list of safety checks and methods to reduce the risk of errors. Errors can occur at any point in the medication use process (e.g., purchasing, storage, prescribing, preparation/ dispensing, administration). Multiple layers of safety checks help to reduce the risk of an error reaching the patient.

INPATIENT MEDICATION USE PROCESS

Drug ordered from supplier

- Limit available drugs to those on formulary (P&T committee)
- Limit the concentrations stocked

Drug arrives in pharmacy and is checked into inventory

- Barcode scanning ensures the correct drug was received and allows for inventory tracking

Drug added to pharmacy stock

- Separate look-alike, sound-alike drugs and use tall man lettering
- Clearly label high-alert medications

Medication order placed for patient

- CPOE and CDS decrease errors – verbal or handwritten orders can be misinterpreted
- Avoid abbreviations

Pharmacist reviews drug order

- The patient-specific dose, frequency, route and risk for drug interactions are assessed for appropriateness
- CDS provides safety double-check

Drug compounding (if needed)

- Use good compounding practices (see Compounding chapters)

Drug delivered to patient care unit

- Several routes for drug delivery
  - Drug prepared and labeled in pharmacy, checked by pharmacist, then delivered to the unit (pneumatic tube systems can be used for some medications)
  - Drug stocked by pharmacy in ADC on unit; nurse removes drug from ADC once the order is approved/verified
- Barcode scanning ensures correct drug/dose was selected for the correct patient

Drug administered to patient

- Five rights checked (typically with barcode scanning): right patient (two identifiers needed), right drug, right route, right dose, right time

ADC = automated dispensing cabinet, CDS = clinical decision support,
CPOE = computerized physician/provider order entry,
P&T = Pharmacy and Therapeutics

OUTPATIENT MEDICATION USE PROCESS

Drug ordered from supplier

Drug arrives in pharmacy and is checked into inventory

- Barcode scanning ensures the correct drug was received and allows for inventory tracking

Drug added to pharmacy stock

- Separate look-alike, sound-alike drugs and use tall man lettering
- High-alert medications should be labeled

Prescription is received

- CPOE and CDS decrease errors – verbal or handwritten orders can be misinterpreted
- Avoid abbreviations

Pharmacy staff processes order

- CDS provides safety double-check

Drug compounding (if needed)

- Use good compounding practices (see Compounding chapters)

Prescription filled

- Barcode scanning used to make sure the correct drug was pulled from pharmacy stock
- Drugs may be stored in an ADS in the pharmacy; drug counted and vial filled using automated technology to reduce errors

Pharmacist reviews drug order

- The patient-specific dose, frequency, route and risk for drug interactions are assessed for appropriateness
- CDS and barcode scanning provide safety double-checks

Drug dispensed to patient

- Proper counseling needed to decrease error risk
- Two identifiers needed for pick up to ensure delivery to correct recipient

ADS = automated dispensing system, CDS = clinical decision support, CPOE = computerized physician/provider order entry

INFECTION CONTROL IN HOSPITALS

More than one million infections are acquired in hospitals annually – about one infection for every thirty patients. Hospital infections cause avoidable illness and death, and add enormous financial costs. Many of these infections are preventable if proper techniques are followed. Many states now require hospitals to report infection rates, and Medicare can refuse reimbursement for hospital-acquired infections that are largely avoidable.

It is important to properly clean surfaces, including bed rails, eating trays and other room surfaces. Healthcare professionals should be careful not to be sources of infection from contaminated clothing (including white coats and ties). Organisms that spread via surface contact include VRE, *C. difficile*, noroviruses and other intestinal tract pathogens.

COMMON TYPES OF HOSPITAL-ACQUIRED (NOSOCOMIAL) INFECTIONS

- Urinary tract infections from indwelling catheters; remove the catheter as soon as possible
- Bloodstream infections from IV lines (central lines have the highest risk) and catheters
- Surgical site infections (see Infectious Diseases II chapter)
- *Clostridioides difficile*, other GI infections
- Pneumonia (mostly due to ventilator use)

UNIVERSAL PRECAUTIONS TO PREVENT TRANSMISSION

Universal precautions is an approach to infection control that treats human blood and bodily fluids as if they are infected with HIV, HBV and other bloodborne pathogens. Contact with bodily fluids should be avoided by wearing gloves, performing good hand hygiene and, in select cases, the use of gowns, masks or patient isolation.

The following sections describe the three categories of transmission-based precautions defined by the CDC.

Contact Precautions

- Intended to prevent transmission of infectious agents which are spread by direct and indirect contact with the patient and the patient's environment.
- Single patient rooms are preferred. If not available, keep ≥ 3 feet spatial separation between beds to prevent inadvertent sharing of items between patients.
- Healthcare personnel caring for these patients should wear a gown and gloves for all interactions that may involve contact with the patient or contaminated areas in the patient's room.
- Contact precautions are recommended for patients colonized or infected with MRSA and VRE and patients with *C. difficile* infection.

Droplet Precautions

- Intended to prevent transmission of pathogens spread through close respiratory contact with respiratory secretions.
- Single patient rooms are preferred. If not available, keeping ≥ 3 feet spatial separation and drawing a curtain between beds is especially important for diseases transmitted via droplets.
- Healthcare personnel should wear a mask (a respirator is not necessary) for close contact with the patient. The mask is donned upon entry to the patient's room.
- Droplet precautions are recommended for patients with active *B. pertussis*, influenza virus, respiratory syncytial virus (RSV), adenovirus, rhinovirus, *N. meningitidis*, and group A streptococcus (for the first 24 hours of antimicrobial therapy).

Airborne Precautions

- Intended to prevent transmission of infectious agents that remain infectious over long distances when suspended in the air.
- The patient should be placed in an airborne infection isolation room (AIIR). An AIIR is a single-patient room that is equipped with special air and ventilation handling systems. The air is exhausted directly to the outside or re-circulated through HEPA filtration before being returned.
- Healthcare personnel should wear a mask or respirator (N95 level or higher), depending on the disease, which is donned prior to room entry.
- Airborne precautions are recommended for patients with active pulmonary tuberculosis, measles or varicella virus (chickenpox).

CATHETER-RELATED BLOODSTREAM INFECTIONS

- The most important and cost-effective strategy to minimize catheter-related bloodstream infections (CRBSI) is use of aseptic technique during catheter insertion, including proper handwashing and utilization of standard protocols/ catheter insertion checklist.

- It is also important to minimize use of intravascular catheters, if possible, through intravenous to oral route conversion protocols and setting appropriate time limits for catheter use. For example, peripheral catheters should be removed/replaced every 2 – 3 days to minimize risk for infection.

- Other strategies shown to reduce the risk of CRBSI include the use of skin antiseptics (2% chlorhexidine), antibiotic impregnated central venous catheters, and antibiotic/ ethanol lock therapy, but use must be weighed against the potential risk for increased rates of resistance.

HAND HYGIENE

Numerous studies show that proper hand hygiene by those working in healthcare settings reduces the spread of nosocomial infection. Alcohol-based hand rubs (gel, rinse or foam) or soap and water are options; depending on the situation, one method may be preferred over the other (see the following discussion). Fingernails should be clipped short, and no jewelry should be worn under gloves (this can harbor bacteria and tear the gloves).

Antimicrobial hand soaps that contain chlorhexidine (Hibiclens, others) may be preferable to reduce infections in healthcare facilities. Triclosan may also be beneficial, but this compound gets into the water supply and has environmental concerns.

When to Perform Hand Hygiene

- Before entering and after leaving patient rooms and between patient contacts if there is more than one patient per room.

- Before donning and after removing gloves (use new gloves with each patient).

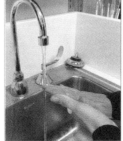

- Before handling invasive devices, including injections.

- After coughing or sneezing.

- Before handling food and oral medications.

©UWorld

- Whenever hands are visibly soiled.

Use Soap and Water (not Alcohol-Based Rubs) in These Situations

- Before eating.

- After using the restroom.

- Anytime there is visible soil (anything noticeable on the hands).

- After caring for a patient with diarrhea or known *C. difficile* or spore-forming organisms; alcohol-based hand rubs have poor activity against spores. Handwashing with soap and water physically removes spores and washes them down the drain.

- Before caring for patients with food allergies.

Soap and Water Technique

- Wet both sides of hands, apply soap, rub together for at least 15 seconds.

- Rinse thoroughly.

- Dry with paper towel and use the towel to turn off the water.

Alcohol-Based Hand Rubs Technique

- Use enough gel (2 – 5 mL or about the size of a quarter).

- Rub hands together until the gel dries (15 – 25 seconds).

- Hands should be completely dry before putting on gloves.

Hand-Hygiene for Sterile Compounding

- Refer to the Compounding chapters.

SAFE INJECTION PRACTICES

Safe injection practices are necessary to prevent the reuse of syringes in multiple patients and contamination of IV bags with used syringes. See the Study Tip Gal on the next page for safe injection practices.

If a needle-stick (percutaneous exposure) occurs with a used needle, contact the proper department at a healthcare facility immediately. If post-exposure prophylaxis (PEP) is required (for HIV and/or hepatitis), acting quickly is important. PEP regimens are more likely to be effective the sooner they are started. In the outpatient setting, instruct the patient to wash the area right away with soap and water and contact their healthcare provider. See the Human Immunodeficiency Virus chapter for details on PEP medication regimens.

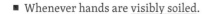

SAFE INJECTION PRACTICES FOR HEALTHCARE FACILITIES

- Never administer an oral solution/suspension intravenously; fatal errors have occurred. Use oral syringes (which are difficult or impossible to attach to a needle for IV injection) and label oral syringes "for oral use only."

- Never reinsert used needles into a multiple-dose vial or solution container. Single-dose vials are preferred over multiple-dose vials, especially when medications will be administered to multiple patients.

- Needles used for withdrawing blood or any other bodily fluid, or used for administering medications or other fluids, should preferably have "engineered sharps protection," which reduces the risk of an exposure incident by a mechanism such as drawing the needle into the syringe barrel after use.

- Never touch the tip or plunger of a syringe to avoid contamination.

- Lancing ("fingerstick") devices should not be used in more than one patient. Ideally, glucometers should not be shared; if sharing a glucometer among multiple patients in an institutional setting, they should be cleaned and disinfected after every use.

- Disposable needles that are contaminated (e.g., with drugs, chemicals or blood products) should never be removed from their original syringes, unless no other option is available. Throw the entire needle/syringe assembly (needle attached to the syringe) into the red plastic sharps container.

- Immediately discard used disposable needles or sharps into a sharps container without recapping.

- Sharps containers should be easily accessible and not allowed to overfill; they should be routinely replaced.

SHARPS DISPOSAL

Patients who use injectable medications should have a disposal container and be instructed to put needles and other sharps in the container immediately after use (see Study Tip Gal). Sharps should be disposed of in an FDA-cleared sharps container, which is puncture resistant, labeled or color-coded appropriately, closeable and leak-proof. They are marked with a line that indicates when the container should be considered full (about ¾ full). Never compress or "push down" on the contents of any sharps container.

If an FDA-cleared container is not available, some community guidelines recommend using a heavy-duty plastic household container as an alternative (e.g., a plastic laundry detergent container). The container must be leak and puncture-resistant with a tight-fitting lid.

The entire needle/syringe assembly is discarded. The only time that recapping a needle is permitted is when the sharps container is not immediately available; in that case, use the one-hand method to recap until the sharps container can be reached:

- Place the cap on a table or counter next to something firm to push the cap against.

- Hold the syringe with the needle attached and slip the needle into the cap without using the other hand.

- Push the capped needle on the firm surface to "seat" the cap onto the needle using only the one hand.

Sharps disposal guidelines and programs vary. The local trash removal service or health department should have the available services, and the pharmacy can provide this information to patients. Services include drop boxes or supervised collection sites (such as in a hospital, pharmacy, police or fire station), household hazardous waste collection sites, mail-back programs and residential special waste pick-up services.

Select Guidelines/References

Institute for Safe Medication Practices. www.ismp.org (accessed 2024 Jan 10).

The Joint Commission. www.jointcommission.org (accessed 2024 Jan 10).

Agency for Healthcare Research and Quality (AHRQ). Patient Safety 101. https://psnet.ahrq.gov/patient-safety-101 (accessed 2024 Jan 10).

MMWR Guideline for Hand Hygiene in Health-Care Settings October 25, 2002, 51(RR16);1-44.

DEFINITIONS

Mild or Severe Reactions to Histamine Release

Urticaria (hives)
A rash with red/pinkish raised patches. The patches have varied shapes and sizes.

Pruritus (itching)
Any rash or reaction that causes itching can be referred to as pruritus.

Erythema
Redness on the skin from superficial (near the surface) capillaries, often due to inflammation with pruritus. When pressed down, the red skin will blanch (whiten) temporarily because the blood flow is blocked. Erythematous refers to an area on the skin, such as a patch, with erythema.

Angioedema
Swelling caused by edema in the deeper dermal, cutaneous and submucosal tissue.

Morbilliform
Macular or maculopapular rash (or both), with 1-10 mm lesions and healthy skin between the lesions.

CONTENT LEGEND

 Study Tip Gal   Key Drug Guy

---

designua/stock.adobe.com

Mast cell · IgE · Antigen · Histamine · Gastric acid secretion · Blood vessels dilate · Itchiness · Contraction of respiratory ways

CHAPTER 76

DRUG ALLERGIES & ADVERSE DRUG REACTIONS

BACKGROUND

Adverse drug reaction (ADR) is a term that encompasses all unintended pharmacologic effects of a drug when it is administered correctly and used at recommended doses. ADRs should not be confused with medication errors, which can include overdose and administration mistakes, and are discussed in the Medication Safety & Quality Improvement chapter. ADRs result in substantial morbidity and mortality, and ADR reports are increasing; over one million reports with serious outcomes (including over 150,000 deaths) are logged with the FDA each year.

Although side effects or adverse effects can occur in anyone, some patients are more susceptible than others. For example, some degree of renal damage can occur with use of an aminoglycoside for longer than seven days. However, in patients with underlying renal impairment, nephrotoxicity is more likely to occur and may happen after a shorter duration of treatment.

ADVERSE DRUG REACTIONS VS. ERRORS

Adverse Drug Reaction (ADR)
Effects from a drug when it is administered correctly. ADRs are typically dose-related; the ADR severity increases with higher doses/reduced clearance.

The new drug you are taking causes "urinary retention" which means it can take longer to pee when you use the restroom.

Medication Error
Something wrong occurred, such as giving a medication dose to the wrong person.

This patient got a 2-fold overdose of insulin??!!

Hi Mrs. Smith, I received a *Celebrex* prescription for you for joint pain. Weren't you hospitalized recently for a stroke?

iStock.com/Irina_Strelnikova

ADVERSE DRUG REACTIONS

ADRs are categorized into two types: predictable (type A) and unpredictable (type B) reactions.

TYPE A REACTIONS

Type A reactions are dose-dependent, related to the known pharmacologic properties of the drug, can occur in any patient and can range from mild to severe. Type A reactions are most common and account for an estimated 85% of ADRs. Examples of type A reactions:

- Orthostatic hypotension with doxazosin (minimized and/ or prevented by dose titration)
- Nephrotoxicity with aminoglycosides
- Tachycardia with albuterol

TYPE B REACTIONS

Type B reactions are not dose-dependent, are unrelated to the pharmacologic actions of the drug and can be influenced by patient-specific factors (e.g., genetics). The majority of type B reactions are caused by exposure to the active ingredient, but excipients (inactive ingredients) can be implicated too. Type B reactions are categorized as immediate (occurring within 60 minutes after exposure) or delayed (occurring days to months after exposure).

Type B reactions include:

- Drug allergies, which are reactions that have a definite immune mechanism (e.g., antibody- or T cell-mediated). The types of drug allergies are described in the top right box on this page. In general, allergies are not hereditary (e.g., if a patient's mother has anaphylaxis to penicillin, it does not mean that the patient cannot receive penicillin).
- Drug hypersensitivity reactions (DHRs), which clinically resemble drug allergy but may or may not be immune-mediated. DHRs do not always result in a contraindication to future administration, such as histamine release when vancomycin is infused too quickly. DHRs can be linked to genetics, such as reactions that occur with specific human leukocyte antigen (HLA) alleles (see the Pharmacogenomics chapter).
- Idiosyncratic reactions, which arise from genetic differences (e.g., select medications are more likely to cause drug-induced hemolytic anemia in patients with G6PD deficiency).

TYPES OF DRUG ALLERGIES

Type I Reactions - Immediate
- IgE-mediated, ranging from minor local reactions to severe systemic reactions
  - ❑ Examples: urticaria, bronchospasm, angioedema, anaphylaxis

Type II Reactions - Delayed
- Antibody-mediated, usually occurring 5-8 days after exposure
  - ❑ Examples: hemolytic anemia, thrombocytopenia

Type III Reactions - Delayed
- Immune-complex reactions, occurring ≥ 1 week after exposure
  - ❑ Example: serum sickness

Type IV Reactions - Delayed
- T cell-mediated, occurring 48 hours to weeks after exposure
  - ❑ Example: Stevens-Johnson syndrome

INTOLERANCES AND IDIOSYNCRATIC REACTIONS

CHARACTERIZING AN ADVERSE DRUG REACTION

When patients report an adverse drug reaction, pharmacists must ask the right questions in order to determine whether an adverse reaction is an intolerance or a drug allergy:

- What reaction occurred (e.g., mild rash, severe rash with blisters, trouble breathing)?
- When did it occur? About how old were you?
- Can you use similar drugs in the class? For example, for a penicillin allergy, ask if cephalexin has ever been used.
- Do you have any food allergies or a latex allergy?

INTOLERANCE OR ALLERGY?

Gather enough information to determine the type of reaction.

Example:
A patient reports getting a stomach ache from varenicline.

Scenarios:
I did not eat anything until dinner because varenicline made me nauseous. (Intolerance)

I got nauseous, felt dizzy and had trouble breathing. (Allergy)

Intolerances are less serious complaints, such as nausea or constipation. Since the drug bothers the patient, it should be avoided, if possible.

Allergies are an immune system response and range from mild (e.g., pruritus) to severe (e.g., anaphylaxis). Allergies can present in different ways, for example:

- Facial swelling, bronchoconstriction and/or drop in BP
- Weakness, fever and severe rash

STOMACH UPSET/NAUSEA

Stomach upset or nausea (in the absence of other hypersensitivity symptoms) is often incorrectly reported as an allergy. It should be listed on the patient profile because the drug bothered the patient and, if possible, should be avoided in the future, but this is not an allergy and should not prevent drugs in the same class from being used. This is more accurately categorized as an intolerance. Electronic medical records allow for documentation of intolerances separate from allergies. An example of an intolerance is the patient who has stomach upset with codeine (but not hydrocodone or other opioids) or erythromycin (but not azithromycin).

EXAMPLE: INTOLERANCE REPORTED INCORRECTLY AS A DRUG ALLERGY

CG received acetaminophen 300 mg/codeine 30 mg for pain relief after a dental extraction. She got very nauseated from the medication. When she was admitted to the hospital several years later for a left hip replacement, she reported that she was "allergic" to codeine. The reaction was not clarified, which led the physician to order fentanyl with a patient-controlled analgesia device for postoperative pain control, instead of hydrocodone. The prescriber used a less desirable option for pain control because of the reported allergy.

PHOTOSENSITIVITY

Photosensitivity can occur when sunlight reacts with a drug in the skin and causes tissue damage that looks like a severe sunburn on sun-exposed areas; this occurs within hours of sun exposure.

When dispensing medications that can cause photosensitivity (see Key Drugs Guy below), it is important to advise the patient and/or their caregivers to limit sun exposure and to use broad-spectrum sunscreen that blocks both UVA and UVB radiation.

DRUGS MOST ASSOCIATED WITH PHOTOSENSITIVITY

KEY DRUGS

Amiodarone

Diuretics (thiazide and loop)

Methotrexate

Oral and topical retinoids

Quinolones

St. John's wort

Sulfa drugs

Tacrolimus

Tetracyclines

Voriconazole

Others:

Antihistamines (1st generation)

Chloroquine

Coal Tar

Fluorouracil

Griseofulvin

NSAIDs

Quinidine

Tigecycline

THROMBOTIC THROMBOCYTOPENIC PURPURA

Thrombotic thrombocytopenic purpura (TTP), sometimes referred to as drug-induced thrombotic microangiopathy (DITMA), is a blood disorder in which clots form throughout the body. The clotting process consumes platelets and leads to bleeding under the skin and the formation of purpura (bruises) and petechiae (dots) on the skin. TTP can be fatal and should be treated immediately with plasma exchange. Common drugs that can cause TTP include oral P2Y12 inhibitors (e.g., clopidogrel) and sulfamethoxazole.

SPOTS AND RASHES

Papules
Raised spots

Macules
Flat spots

Purpura
Red/purple skin spots (lesions) due to bleeding underneath the skin. Purpura includes small and large spots:

Petechiae — Pinpoint in size

Ecchymosis — Large bruised area

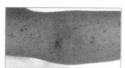

Purpura, with petechiae and ecchymoses (TTP rash)

National Heart, Lung, and Blood Institute; National Institutes of Health; U.S. Department of Health and Human Services.

Hematoma
A collection of blood under the skin due to trauma (injury) to a blood vessel, resulting in blood leaking into the surrounding tissue. Drugs that can cause a hematoma include heparin, low molecular weight heparin (LMWH), other anticoagulants and phytonadione (vitamin K) if given mistakenly as an IM injection.

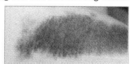

Hematoma
SneSivan/Shutterstock.com

DRUG HYPERSENSITIVITY REACTIONS AND ALLERGIES

This section describes specific drug hypersensitivity and allergic reactions and their treatment, but keep in mind that similar treatment can be used for non-drug allergies, including food allergies (e.g., soy, peanut). All allergies should be noted in the patient medical record, including latex allergies because some drugs require tubing, have latex vial stoppers or require gloves for administration.

Anyone with severe drug or food allergies should wear a medical identification bracelet to alert emergency responders. A reaction without breathing difficulty can sometimes be treated by stopping the offending drug. Antihistamines can be used to counteract the histamine release that causes itching, swelling and rash. Systemic steroids, and sometimes NSAIDs, can be used to decrease swelling. Severe swelling may necessitate a steroid injection. Epinephrine is used to reverse bronchoconstriction if the patient is wheezing or has other signs of breathing trouble.

NON-IMMUNE DRUG HYPERSENSITIVITY REACTIONS

Many drugs can cause reactions that clinically mimic drug allergy, but are not immune-mediated. These can be both immediate and delayed in onset. Examples:

- Opioids can cause a non-IgE-mediated release of histamine from mast cells in the skin, causing itching and hives. This is particularly apparent after inpatient surgery, when opioid-naïve patients receive them or when non-naïve patients receive higher than normal doses. This type of reaction, if not severe, can be reduced or avoided by premedicating with an antihistamine, such as diphenhydramine.

- Vancomycin, when infused too rapidly, can cause a direct release of histamine from cutaneous mast cells, causing flushing, hives and sometimes hypotension. In most cases, this reaction can be avoided by slowing the infusion rate.

HUMAN LEUKOCYTE ANTIGEN-ASSOCIATED HYPERSENSITIVITY REACTIONS

For some drugs, the presence of specific HLA alleles increases the risk of delayed-type hypersensitivity syndromes. Reactions range from severe cutaneous adverse reactions (described below) to drug-specific syndromes. For example, patients positive for HLA-B*5701 are at an increased risk for abacavir hypersensitivity, which is a unique syndrome presenting with fever, malaise, gastrointestinal or respiratory symptoms and rash. See the Pharmacogenomics chapter for details regarding medications with HLA-specific testing recommendations.

SEVERE CUTANEOUS ADVERSE REACTIONS

There are several severe cutaneous adverse reactions (SCARs) that can be caused by drugs, including Stevens-Johnson syndrome (SJS), toxic epidermal necrolysis (TEN) and drug reaction with eosinophilia and systemic symptoms (DRESS). All of these are categorized as delayed drug allergies. They can be life-threatening and require prompt treatment. While many drugs have SCARs listed in their prescribing information, the drugs most commonly associated with these reactions are listed in the Key Drugs Guy to the right.

Stevens-Johnson Syndrome and Toxic Epidermal Necrolysis

SJS and TEN involve epidermal detachment and skin loss that is equivalent to third-degree burns. They generally occur 1 – 3 weeks after drug exposure and can result in severe mucosal erosions, a high body temperature, major fluid loss and organ damage (eyes, liver, kidney, lungs).

SJS and TEN are commonly classified by the percent of skin detachment. The key to treating both is to stop the offending agent as soon as possible, replace fluids and electrolytes, perform wound care and administer pain medications. Systemic steroids are contraindicated with TEN, but may be used for SJS, though the benefit is controversial. Due to the severity of mucosal involvement, antibiotics are often necessary to prevent or treat an infection. A history of SJS/TEN to a medication is a contraindication to receiving it again.

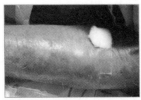
Patient with Stevens-Johnson syndrome
Pawarit Khunkrai/Shutterstock.com

Drug Reaction with Eosinophilia and Systemic Symptoms (DRESS)

DRESS can include a variety of skin eruptions accompanied by systemic symptoms such as fever, hepatic dysfunction, renal dysfunction and lymphadenopathy, but it rarely involves mucosal surfaces. Treatment consists of stopping the offending drug, although symptoms may continue to worsen for a period of time after the drug has been discontinued.

ANAPHYLAXIS

Anaphylaxis is a severe, life-threatening allergic reaction that usually happens within 1 hour of drug exposure, and involves multiple organs (most commonly the skin/mucosal tissue, and the cardiovascular, respiratory and gastrointestinal systems). Anaphylaxis typically occurs after an initial exposure and subsequent immune response, but some drugs can cause anaphylaxis with the first exposure. A patient experiencing anaphylaxis usually has a combination

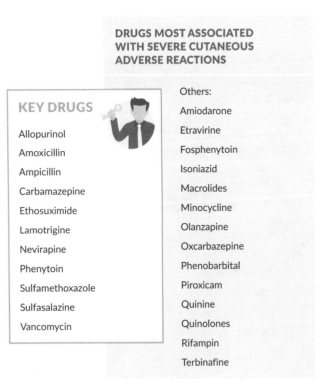

DRUGS MOST ASSOCIATED WITH SEVERE CUTANEOUS ADVERSE REACTIONS

KEY DRUGS

Allopurinol
Amoxicillin
Ampicillin
Carbamazepine
Ethosuximide
Lamotrigine
Nevirapine
Phenytoin
Sulfamethoxazole
Sulfasalazine
Vancomycin

Others:
Amiodarone
Etravirine
Fosphenytoin
Isoniazid
Macrolides
Minocycline
Olanzapine
Oxcarbazepine
Phenobarbital
Piroxicam
Quinine
Quinolones
Rifampin
Terbinafine

of symptoms, including generalized underline(urticaria (hives), swelling of the mouth and throat, difficulty breathing or wheezing sounds, severe gastrointestinal symptoms) (e.g., repetitive vomiting, severe abdominal cramping) and/or hypotension (which can cause dizziness, lightheadedness or loss of consciousness). Because symptoms can develop quickly, treatment must be administered immediately.

Anaphylaxis Treatment

An anaphylactic reaction requires immediate emergency medical care. The patient or family should be instructed to call 911 if anaphylaxis occurs. Treatment includes an epinephrine injection ± diphenhydramine ± steroids ± IV fluids. To avoid

blocking the airway, nothing should be placed under the head or in the mouth. Swollen airways can be quickly fatal.

Patients with a history of anaphylaxis (particularly to foods or insect bites) should carry a single-use epinephrine auto-injector (*EpiPen, EpiPen Jr, Auvi-Q, Symjepi* or a generic equivalent) as they may be at future risk. These are generally available as epinephrine 1 mg/mL (previously labeled as underline(1:1000)) in doses of 0.3 mg (adult dose) or 0.15 mg (pediatric dose). The 0.15 mg dose is for patients 15 – 30 kg (*EpiPen Jr*). *Auvi-Q* is also available in 0.1 mg (for patients weighing 7.5 – 14 kg). The patient's emergency kit should also include emergency contact information and diphenhydramine tablets (25 mg x 2), which should be taken only if there is no tongue/lip swelling.

KEY COUNSELING POINTS FOR EPINEPHRINE AUTO-INJECTORS

- Tell family, caregivers and others where the epinephrine auto-injector is kept and how to use it, as you may not be able to speak in an emergency.

- It is important to keep the thumb, fingers and hand away from the needle end of the device, as accidental injection can cause vasoconstriction and necrosis.

- When injecting an uncooperative child, hold the leg firmly to avoid bending or breaking the needle.

- Skin infections can occur. Report any prolonged redness, swelling, warmth or tenderness at the injection site.

For *Symjepi*:
- Pull off the cap, holding the syringe with the fingers (avoiding the needle).

- Inject in the middle of the outer thigh, hold needle firmly in place for two seconds, then massage area for 10 seconds.

- After injection, slide the safety guard out over the needle.

For *Auvi-Q*:
- Pull off the outer case, then follow the voice instructions to administer. Hold the needle firmly in place on the thigh for five seconds.

EPINEPHRINE AUTO-INJECTOR ADMINISTRATION

EpiPen:
- Remove from the carrying case and pull off the blue safety release.

- Keep thumb, fingers and hand away from the orange (needle) end of the device.

- To inject, jab the orange end into the middle of the outer thigh at a 90 degree angle.

- Hold the needle firmly in place while counting to 3.

- Remove the needle and massage the area for 10 seconds.

- After the injection, the orange tip will extend to cover the needle. If the needle is visible, it should not be reused.

All epinephrine auto-injectors:
- It is normal to see liquid remaining in the device after injecting.

- Call for emergency help because additional care may be needed.

- A second dose (in the opposite leg) may be given, if needed, prior to the arrival of medical help.

- Refrigeration is not required.

- All products can be injected through clothing.

- Check the device periodically to make sure the medication is clear and not expired.

COMMON DRUGS ASSOCIATED WITH ALLERGIC REACTIONS

While any drug can lead to an allergic reaction, some are known to do so more than others. Drugs that commonly cause allergies are discussed below. Often the drug that caused a reaction can be replaced with another drug. Patch testing performed in the outpatient setting by an allergist is a reliable way to determine if a person is truly allergic to a drug.

BETA-LACTAMS

Beta-lactam antibiotics (includes several classes) are the most commonly implicated medications in drug allergies. Reactions range from mild rash to anaphylaxis and severe delayed reactions (e.g., SJS).

Penicillins have many related compounds within the class (e.g., ampicillin, piperacillin). Anyone who is <u>allergic to one</u> is typically presumed to be <u>allergic to others in the class</u>. In such cases, the <u>entire class</u> should be <u>avoided</u>, unless they have been evaluated by a healthcare provider.

Cephalosporins and carbapenems are <u>structurally related</u> to penicillin. A penicillin allergy history carries a small risk of experiencing an allergic reaction to a cephalosporin or carbapenem. While the risk of cross-reactivity is low, <u>on the NAPLEX, beta-lactams should be avoided</u> with a stated allergy to another beta-lactam. A notable <u>exception</u> is in <u>acute otitis media</u> (AOM); the American Academy of Pediatrics recommends a 2nd- or 3rd-generation <u>cephalosporin</u> in patients with a <u>non-severe penicillin allergy</u> (e.g., delayed-onset mild rash), due to the toxicities and decreased efficacy of alternative AOM therapies in children (see the Infectious Diseases II chapter). <u>Aztreonam</u> (a monobactam) is considered <u>safe</u> in patients with an immediate-type <u>penicillin allergy</u>.

Beta-lactams can cause a <u>delayed-onset mild rash</u> (benign exanthem), often described as morbilliform and/or maculopapular in appearance. In the absence of other severe symptoms of anaphylaxis, this mild rash is not a contraindication to recieving the drug again or drugs from similar classes.

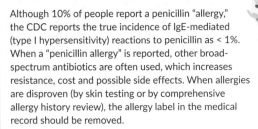

A PENICILLIN ALLERGY, OR NOT?

Although 10% of people report a penicillin "allergy," the CDC reports the true incidence of IgE-mediated (type I hypersensitivity) reactions to penicillin as < 1%. When a "penicillin allergy" is reported, other broad-spectrum antibiotics are often used, which increases resistance, cost and possible side effects. When allergies are disproven (by skin testing or by comprehensive allergy history review), the allergy label in the medical record should be removed.

For immediate-type reactions (e.g., anaphylaxis), a skin test can assess risk:

- Patients with a negative result should be given an oral drug "challenge" dose before the full treatment dose.

- Patients with a positive test should avoid use of the drug.

  - ❏ Remember: penicillin is the only acceptable treatment in pregnant or non-adherent patients with syphilis. If a skin test is positive, temporarily desensitize and administer penicillin.

- Skin testing should not be performed for severe cutaneous adverse reactions (e.g., SJS/TEN).

Many cephalosporins can be safely tolerated in patients with a mild penicillin allergy. In acute otitis media patients with an allergy to penicillin/amoxicillin, give cefdinir, cefpodoxime, ceftriaxone or cefuroxime.

SULFA DRUGS

Sulfa reactions are most commonly reported with <u>sulfamethoxazole</u> (in *Bactrim*). Other drugs that should be <u>avoided</u> in patients with a sulfa allergy include <u>sulfasalazine</u> and <u>sulfadiazine</u>.

The package labeling for "non-arylamine" sulfonamides [<u>thiazide</u> diuretics, <u>loop</u> diuretics (except ethacrynic acid), <u>sulfonylureas, acetazolamide, zonisamide and celecoxib</u>], as well as cidofovir, <u>darunavir</u>, fosamprenavir and tipranavir contain <u>warnings or contraindications</u> for use in patients with a sulfa allergy, but in practice the risk of cross-reactivity with sulfamethoxazole is low. Even so, the patient should be aware to watch for a possible reaction and on the NAPLEX, drugs with a possible risk for causing a reaction should be recognized. <u>Sulfite or sulfate allergies do not cross-react</u> with sulfonamides.

OPIOIDS

Opioid hypersensitivity reactions due to histamine release are common; however, a true opioid allergy is uncommon. Antihistamines can be used to reduce or avoid non-severe reactions thought to be due to histamine release. See the Pain chapter for information on treatment options in patients with opioid allergies.

HEPARIN

See the Anticoagulation chapter for information on heparin-induced thrombocytopenia (HIT).

BIOLOGICS

Biologics (e.g., rituximab) can cause hypersensitivity reactions and other ADRs. Desensitization to some agents is possible in patients who need a biologic and have had a prior reaction. See the next page for more information regarding desensitization procedures.

ASPIRIN AND NSAIDs

Aspirin and NSAIDS can cause many different types of hypersensitivity reactions, the most common being respiratory in nature (e.g., asthma, rhinorrhea) and urticaria/angioedema. Up to 20% of patients with asthma are sensitive to aspirin and other NSAIDs. Aspirin should be avoided in patients with a history of asthma, nasal polyps and prior respiratory reactions to NSAIDs.

RADIOCONTRAST MEDIA

Radiocontrast media (used in some imaging studies) can cause immediate and delayed hypersensitivity reactions, which can be immune- or non-immune-mediated. The type of radiocontrast agent used and patient-specific factors (e.g., asthma history) influences the frequency and severity of these reactions.

PEANUTS AND SOY

It is important for pharmacists to be aware if a patient has a peanut allergy. Parents of children with peanut allergies should have ready access to an epinephrine auto-injector. An oral immunotherapy [peanut allergen powder (Palforzia)] is indicated to mitigate allergic reactions to peanuts, including anaphylaxis. Soy is used in some medications; peanuts and soy are in the same family and can have cross-reactivity. Drugs that are contraindicated with a soy allergy include clevidipine (Cleviprex) and propofol (Diprivan).

EGGS

If a patient has a true allergy to eggs, they cannot use clevidipine (Cleviprex), propofol (Diprivan) or the yellow fever vaccine (eggs are used in vaccine production). For influenza vaccines, ACIP states that even patients who have had severe symptoms when consuming eggs can receive any indicated inactivated vaccine (though Flublok and Flucelvax are egg-free options). If a severe reaction to an influenza vaccine occurs, the patient should not receive further doses of any influenza vaccine. For further discussion, refer to the Immunizations chapter.

SKIN TESTING, DESENSITIZATION AND DELABELING ALLERGIES

PENICILLIN SKIN TESTING

Some patients report a penicillin "allergy" when their reaction was more properly categorized as an intolerance (e.g., nausea, diarrhea). In other cases, patients may have had a true allergic reaction to penicillin in the past, but over time, the antibodies can wane and the patient may be able to safely receive penicillins. Due to concerns of cross-reactivity with cephalosporins and carbapenems, a penicillin allergy can severely limit the selection of antibiotics available to treat infectious diseases, leading to use of broad-spectrum antibiotics that have an increased risk for C. difficile (e.g., quinolones) or other toxicities (e.g., vancomycin). The goal of penicillin skin testing is to identify patients who are at the greatest risk of a type I hypersensitivity reaction if exposed to a systemic penicillin.

The penicillin skin test uses the components of penicillin that most often cause an immune (allergic) response, such as the diagnostic agent Pre-Pen (benzylpenicilloyl polylysine injection), with very dilute solutions of penicillin G. A step-wise skin test is performed, beginning with a skin prick test followed by intradermal testing. This process includes a positive control (histamine) and negative control (saline) for comparison.

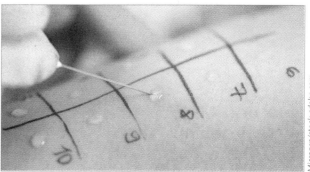

Microgen/stock.adobe.com

A localized reaction around the *Pre-Pen* or penicillin G test site larger than the negative control indicates a high risk of a reaction to systemic penicillin and the patient should not receive it. A patient with a negative skin test (no reaction to the test solution) is then given an oral drug challenge, and if tolerated, the patient can safely receive penicillin. Skin testing is only appropriate for suspected IgE-mediated reactions. Skin testing is contraindicated for severe delayed reactions (e.g., SJS or TEN) and patients should not be challenged.

TEMPORARY INDUCTION OF DRUG TOLERANCE (DESENSITIZATION)

In many cases when a drug allergy is present, an alternative medication can be chosen. When no acceptable alternative is available, induction of drug tolerance (often referred to as desensitization) may be recommended. For example, if a pregnant patient has syphilis and a penicillin allergy, the CDC recommends desensitization and penicillin treatment (see the Infectious Diseases II chapter).

Desensitization is a step-wise process that begins by administering a very small dose of the medication and then incrementally increasing the dose at regular intervals up to a target dose. This modifies the patient's response to the medication and temporarily allows safe treatment. The desensitization procedure must take place in a medical setting where emergency care can be provided if a serious reaction occurs. Treatment with the drug must start immediately following desensitization and must not be interrupted. If doses are missed, the drug-free period allows the immune system to re-sensitize to the drug and serious hypersensitivity reactions (including anaphylaxis) could occur with subsequent doses.

Desensitization does not "cure" the patient of an allergy, and the reaction should not be removed from the patient's medical record. If the drug is required on a separate occasion, the desensitization process must be repeated. Desensitization protocols exist for a number of antimicrobial agents, some biologics and a few other medications (e.g., aspirin). Desensitization should never be attempted if a drug has previously caused SJS or TEN.

DELABELING ALLERGIES

Patients with allergy labels on their profile are often prescribed less effective and more expensive antibiotics, which is linked to worse outcomes and higher healthcare costs. When allergies are found to be disproven (by skin testing, drug challenge or otherwise), the allergy label should be removed from the patient's profile (known as "delabeling"). Furthermore, patients should be counseled so that disproven allergies are not re-added to the profile at a future encounter. This practice should help improve treatment of future infections and reduce costs.

ASSESSING CAUSALITY OF AN ADVERSE DRUG REACTION

When an ADR occurs, the Naranjo Scale (a validated causality assessment scale) can help determine the likelihood that a drug caused the adverse reaction. Based on the questionnaire, a probability score is calculated. A score ≥ 9 = definite ADR; 5 – 8 = probable ADR; 1 – 4 = possible ADR; 0 = doubtful ADR.

QUESTION	YES	NO	DO NOT KNOW
Are there previous conclusive reports on this reaction?	+1	0	0
Did the adverse event appear after the suspected drug was given?	+2	–1	0
Did the adverse reaction improve when the drug was discontinued or a specific antagonist was given?	+1	0	0
Did the adverse reaction appear when the drug was readministered?	+2	–1	0
Are there alternative causes that could (on their own) have caused the reaction?	–1	+2	0
Did the reaction reappear when a placebo was given?	–1	+1	0
Was the drug detected in any body fluid in toxic concentrations?	+1	0	0
Was the reaction more severe when the dose was increased or less severe when the dose was decreased?	+1	0	0
Did the patient have a similar reaction to the same or similar drugs in any previous exposure?	+1	0	0
Was the adverse event confirmed by any objective evidence?	+1	0	0

ADR REPORTING

Side effects, adverse events and allergies to drugs, biologics, medical devices, nutritional products and some cosmetics should be reported to the FDA Adverse Event Reporting System (FAERS, also known as the FDA MedWatch program). Vaccine reactions are reported under a different program called VAERS (see the Immunizations chapter for more information).

When drugs are studied in clinical trials, high-risk patients are typically excluded, though in a real-life setting, high-risk patients may receive the medication. The FDA can require Phase IV trials (post-marketing safety surveillance programs) for approved drugs and biologics, to collect and analyze ADR reports and better understand a drug's safety profile in a real-world setting. Post-marketing reports also help identify side effects that occur less frequently. If a drug causes a reaction in 1 out of every 3,000 people, the problem may not be apparent in a smaller clinical trial. For this reason, community-based ADR reporting is critical.

EXAMPLE: ADR INCIDENCE IN REAL LIFE VS. A CLINICAL TRIAL

When spironolactone was studied in heart failure patients during the RALES trial, patients with renal insufficiency or elevated potassium levels were excluded due to the known risk of additional hyperkalemia from the use of spironolactone. The drug was found to have benefit in advanced heart failure patients and doctors in the community began to use it in their heart failure patients. In this real-life setting, patients with renal insufficiency or elevated potassium were occasionally prescribed spironolactone, and arrhythmias and sudden death due to hyperkalemia were reported.

Reporting is voluntary but has important implications for safe medication use. Healthcare professionals and patients can report adverse events to the drug manufacturer, who is required by law to send the report to the FDA. The MedWatch form used for reporting can be found online. Reports can also be made by calling the FDA directly.

If the FDA receives enough reports that a drug is linked to a particular problem, the manufacturer can be required to update the labeling (e.g., package insert). In especially risky cases, a drug safety alert is issued to prescribers, usually before the labeling is changed.

EXAMPLE: ADR REPORTS LEAD TO FDA REQUIREMENT FOR SAFETY LABELING CHANGES

Oseltamivir (Tamiflu) was initially marketed without any warning of unusual behavior in children. The FDA received enough reports that they issued a warning to prescribers in 2006. In 2008, after many more reports, the FDA required the manufacturer to update the prescribing information to include a precaution about hallucinations, confusion and other strange behavior in children.

FDA TOOLS TO REDUCE ADVERSE DRUG REACTIONS

BOXED WARNINGS

A boxed warning indicates a risk of death or permanent disability from a drug (e.g., increased risk of venous thromboembolism and death from stroke with raloxifene).

The risk of fatality can be due to prescribing or dispensing errors. For example, conventional amphotericin B deoxycholate has a boxed warning not to exceed 1.5 mg/kg. Fatalities have been caused by using the lipid amphotericin dosing (typically 3 – 6 mg/kg) for conventional amphotericin, resulting in a more than two-fold overdose.

CONTRAINDICATIONS, WARNINGS AND PRECAUTIONS

Contraindications indicate that the drug cannot be used in that patient. The risk will outweigh any possible benefit (e.g., a history of venous thromboembolism is a contraindication to the use of raloxifene). If there are no known contraindications for a drug, the section of the package insert will state "None."

> Mrs. Jones, you cannot get *Evista* because you had a DVT in the past.

Warnings and precautions include serious reactions that can result in death, hospitalization, medical intervention, disability or teratogenicity (e.g., raloxifene has a warning for venous thromboembolism). Warnings and precautions may or may not change a prescribing decision.

> Mrs. Smith, you could get a DVT from *Evista* if you are immobile most of the day.

ADVERSE REACTIONS

Adverse reactions refer to undesirable, uncomfortable or dangerous effects from a drug (e.g., arthralgia from raloxifene). The risk-benefit assessment is patient-specific (e.g., arthralgia from raloxifene will be more of a concern in a patient with chronically sore joints versus a patient with no sore joints).

> Mrs. Ngo, you are starting *Evista*. You might get hot flashes and achy joints.

RISK EVALUATION AND MITIGATION STRATEGIES

Risk Evaluation and Mitigation Strategies (REMS) are required by the FDA for some drugs. They are developed by the manufacturer and approved by the FDA to ensure the benefits of a drug outweigh the risks. REMS programs can include a medication guide or patient package insert, communication plan, elements to assure safe use or an implementation system.

For example, the REMS for a drug could require prescribers or pharmacies to have a special certification to prescribe or dispense the drug, enroll patients in a registry so that ADRs can be tracked, or evaluate lab tests before dispensing. Examples include the clozapine REMS, the isotretinoin iPLEDGE program and the REMS to reduce misuse of long-acting opioids.

MEDICATION GUIDES

Medication Guides (or MedGuides) are FDA-approved patient handouts that detail a drug's important adverse events in non-technical language; they are considered part of the drug's labeling. If a medication has a MedGuide, it must be dispensed with the original prescription and with each refill. It is not necessary to dispense a drug's MedGuide for hospitalized patients because the patient is being monitored, though the MedGuide should be available to the patient or family upon request.

MedGuides are required for many individual drugs and, in some cases, entire classes of medications (e.g., anticonvulsants, antidepressants, long-acting opioids, NSAIDs, ADHD stimulants).

Select Guidelines/References

Food and Drug Administration MedWatch program http://www.fda.gov/Safety/MedWatch/ (accessed 2023 Dec 11)

Drug Allergy: A 2022 Practice Parameter Update. *J Allergy Clin Immunol.* 2022 Dec;150(6):1333-1393.

Steady State

With Loading Dose

No Loading Dose
(Maintenance Dose Only)

Time

(y-axis: Concentration)

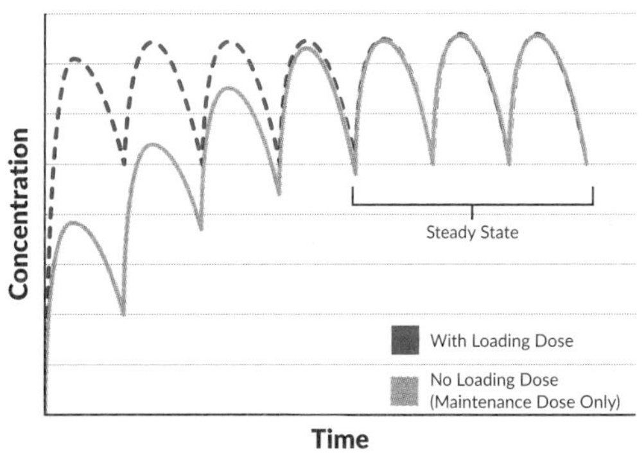

CHAPTER 77

PHARMACOKINETICS

BACKGROUND

Pharmacokinetics is what the human body does to a drug during the processes of drug absorption, distribution, metabolism and excretion (often abbreviated ADME). Mathematical relationships are used to describe these processes, which clinicians use to assess drug levels and optimize drug therapy. Pharmacodynamics, what the drug does to the human body, refers to the relationship between the drug concentration at the site of action, and both therapeutic and adverse effects.

ABSORPTION

When a drug is given intravascularly (e.g., intravenously or intra-arterially), absorption is not required because the drug enters directly into the bloodstream (systemic circulation). If a drug is administered extravascularly, drug absorption occurs as the drug moves from the site of administration to the bloodstream (see the Study Tip Gal on the next page). Some examples of drug formulations with extravascular administration include oral, sublingual, buccal, intramuscular, subcutaneous, transdermal, inhaled, topical, ocular, intraocular, intrathecal and rectal products.

When a drug is given orally, it passes from the stomach to the intestine. Most oral drug absorption occurs in the small intestine because of the large surface area and permeable membrane. After gut absorption, the drug enters the portal vein and travels to the liver. Some drugs are extensively metabolized in the liver before reaching the systemic circulation; this is called first-pass metabolism (discussed later). Some drugs are transported through the bile back to the gut where they can be reabsorbed. This is called enterohepatic recycling (see the Drug Interactions chapter).

Absorption of oral drugs occurs via two primary processes: passive diffusion across the gut wall or active transport. Passive diffusion is movement of drugs from an area of high concentration (e.g., the gut lumen) to an area of lower concentration (e.g., the blood). Energy is not required for passive diffusion. Active transport occurs when drugs are moved across the gut wall via transporter proteins that are normally used to absorb nutrients from food.

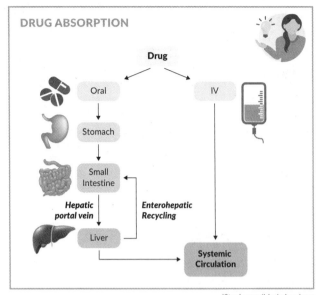

DRUG ABSORPTION

iStock.com/MariaAverburg
Mechanic Design, winnievinzence/Shutterstock.com

LOCAL VS. SYSTEMIC EFFECTS

Drugs administered extravascularly can be divided into two categories: drugs intended for local effects and drugs intended for systemic effects. Drugs intended for local effects are often applied topically where the drug effect is needed. Examples of this include eye drops for glaucoma (e.g., latanoprost), dermal preparations for psoriasis (e.g., coal tar preparations) and nasal sprays for allergies (e.g., fluticasone nasal spray). Topical administration of a drug can produce therapeutic effects while minimizing systemic toxicity due to lower systemic exposure.

Drugs intended for systemic effects are formulated to facilitate some percentage of drug absorption from the site of administration into the circulatory system. Examples include oral tablets for seasonal allergies (e.g., loratadine), suppositories for fever (e.g., acetaminophen), sublingual tablets for angina (e.g., nitroglycerin SL) and transdermal patches for pain (e.g., fentanyl patch).

DISINTEGRATION, DISSOLUTION AND DRUG SOLUBILITY

When a solid oral dosage form is ingested, it breaks into smaller pieces in the gastrointestinal (GI) tract, which is called disintegration. The smaller pieces then dissolve, and the active ingredient is released from the dosage form (typically a compressed tablet or a capsule). This is called dissolution. The rate of dissolution is described by the Noyes-Whitney equation. The rate of disintegration and dissolution depend on the inactive ingredients used to make the dosage form. Some drugs are made using polymers that help slow down the release of the drug in a controlled way. This can provide less variability in drug concentrations and reduce the dosing frequency.

Sublingual (SL) and orally-disintegrating tablet (ODT) formulations generally have fast absorption. In general, the rate of absorption by dosage form will follow this order (fastest to slowest): IV, SL, ODT, immediate-release tablet, extended-release tablet.

Most immediate-release formulations dissolve and get absorbed rapidly, but some can be destroyed in the gut (primarily by hydrolysis, or lysis with water) making them less available for absorption. Drug formulations have been developed with protective coatings to limit drug degradation in the stomach (acidic) and permit dissolution in the intestine (basic). Drugs with this type of enteric-coated formulation include *Dulcolax* and budesonide.

If a drug has poor absorption, one of the methods used to increase the dissolution rate is to reduce particle diameter, which increases surface area. Drugs with very small particle diameters are referred to as micronized, which usually means the diameter was measured in micrometers but sometimes refers to even smaller particle sizes measured in nanometers. Progesterone and fenofibrate are examples of drugs with poor oral absorption that have been developed in micronized formulations.

Following disintegration, the released drug can dissolve in GI fluids. The rate and extent to which the drug dissolves depends on the drug's solubility. Poorly soluble drugs are generally lipophilic, or lipid-loving. Freely soluble drugs are generally hydrophilic, or water-loving. As a drug moves through the GI tract, only dissolved drug is absorbed into the bloodstream. Poorly soluble drugs generally have poor systemic absorption, and highly soluble drugs often have good systemic absorption.

BIOAVAILABILITY

The extent of drug absorption into the systemic circulation is called bioavailability. Bioavailability is reported as a percentage (from 0 to 100%) and reflects the percentage of drug absorbed from extravascular (e.g., oral) compared to intravascular administration (e.g., IV). Bioavailability is affected by solubility, dissolution, route of administration and other factors.

A drug with good absorption has high bioavailability (> 70%), while a drug with poor absorption has low bioavailability (< 10%). For example, levofloxacin and linezolid have high bioavailability; nearly 100% of the oral dose is absorbed, and the oral and IV doses are the same. In many hospitals, these drugs are automatically converted from IV to the same oral dose using a therapeutic interchange or IV to PO protocol. Bisphosphonates, like ibandronate, have low oral bioavailability, so the oral dose (150 mg PO monthly) is much higher than the IV dose (3 mg IV every 3 months) to produce a similar therapeutic effect.

Bioavailability can be calculated using the area under the plasma concentration time curve, or AUC. The AUC represents the total systemic exposure to the drug following administration.

Absolute bioavailability, represented by F, is calculated using the following equation:

$$F\,(\%) \;=\; 100 \;\times\; \frac{AUC_{extravascular}}{AUC_{intravenous}} \;\times\; \frac{Dose_{intravenous}}{Dose_{extravascular}}$$

---

1. **A pharmacokinetic study of an investigational drug was conducted in healthy volunteers. Following an IV bolus dose of 15 mg, the AUC was determined to be 4.2 mg x hr/L. Subjects were later given an oral dose of 50 mg and the AUC was determined to be 8 mg x hr/L. Calculate the absolute bioavailability of the investigational drug. Round to the nearest whole number.**

$$F\,(\%) \;=\; 100 \;\times\; \frac{\dfrac{8\ mg \times hr}{L}}{\dfrac{4.2\ mg \times hr}{L}} \;\times\; \frac{15\ mg}{50\ mg} \;=\; 57\%$$

Different dosage forms of the same drug (e.g., tablet vs. solution) may have different bioavailabilities. The formula below can be used to calculate an equivalent dose of a drug when the dosage form is changed:

$$\frac{\text{Dose of New}}{\text{Dosage Form}} \;=\; \frac{\text{Amount Absorbed from Current Dosage Form}}{\text{F of New Dosage Form}}$$

DISTRIBUTION

Distribution is the process by which drug molecules move from the systemic circulation to various tissues and organs. Distribution can occur with intravascular and extravascular routes of administration and depends on the physical and chemical properties of the drug molecule and interactions with membranes and tissues throughout the body. Factors that impact distribution include drug lipophilicity, molecular weight, solubility, ionization status and the extent of protein binding. Factors that favor passage across membranes and greater drug distribution to the tissues include high lipophilicity, low molecular weight, unionized status and low protein binding.

Human plasma contains many proteins, and albumin is the primary protein responsible for drug binding. Only the unbound (free) form of a drug can interact with receptors, exert therapeutic or toxic effects and be cleared from the body. If a drug is highly protein-bound (> 90%) and serum albumin is low (< 3.5 g/dL), then a higher percentage of the drug will be in the unbound form and the patient may experience therapeutic or even adverse effects at what appears to be a normal or subtherapeutic level.

Many drug assays cannot differentiate between bound and unbound (active) drug. When assessing levels of highly protein bound compounds (e.g., phenytoin, calcium) in a patient with low serum albumin, an adjustment (correction) of the total level is required. The correction formulas allow us to determine what the concentration would be if albumin was normal. With hypoalbuminemia, the corrected level of a highly protein bound drug will be higher than the total level reported by the lab. This is discussed further in the Calculations III and Seizures/Epilepsy chapters.

The issue described above can be overcome by obtaining a "free" phenytoin level or ionized calcium level. Free phenytoin and ionized calcium only measure the unbound portion, so no adjustment is required for hypoalbuminemia.

CALCIUM AND PHENYTOIN CORRECTION FORMULAS

$$Ca_{corrected} \text{ (mg/dL)} = calcium_{reported \text{ (serum)}} + [(4.0 - albumin) \times (0.8)] \dagger$$

$$\text{Phenytoin corrected (mcg/mL)} = \frac{\text{Total phenytoin measured}}{(0.2 \times albumin) + 0.1} \ddagger$$

† *Use serum calcium in mg/dL and albumin in g/dL (standard units in the U.S.) in the corrected calcium formula.*
‡ *Use serum phenytoin in mcg/mL and albumin in g/dL (standard units in the U.S.) in the corrected phenytoin formula.*

2. **A pharmacist receives a call from a provider asking for assistance with two patients in the clinic. Both patients have a seizure disorder and are taking phenytoin. Patient A is seizure free, but is experiencing symptoms of toxicity. Patient B has a higher phenytoin level and is doing fine. Both patients have normal renal function. Which of the following statements is/are true of this scenario? (Select ALL that apply.)**

LAB	REFERENCE RANGE	PATIENT A	PATIENT B
Phenytoin level (total)	10-20 mcg/mL	14.3	17.8
Albumin	3.5-5 g/dL	2.1	4.2

    A. Patient B's corrected phenytoin level will be lower than the total level reported.

    B. Patient A's corrected phenytoin level will be lower than the total level reported.

    C. Patient A's corrected phenytoin level will be higher than the total level reported.

    D. Patient A has a greater percentage of bound phenytoin.

    E. Patient A has a greater percentage of unbound phenytoin.

The correct answers are (C) and (E). The corrected phenytoin level for Patient A (using the formula provided) is 27.5 mcg/mL. Increased unbound phenytoin is contributing to the patient's side effects.

VOLUME OF DISTRIBUTION

The volume of distribution (V or Vd) reflects how large of an area in the patient's body the drug has distributed into and is based on the properties of the drug (discussed previously). The volume of distribution relates the amount of drug in the body to the concentration of the drug measured in plasma (or serum). The equation for volume of distribution is:

> **SUBSCRIPTS IN FORMULAS**
>
> Vd can be written as V_d and ke can be written as k_e. Subscripts are not used in this chapter for simplicity.

$$Vd = \frac{\text{Amount of drug in body}}{\text{Concentration of drug in plasma}}$$

The Vd is determined from the amount of drug in the body immediately after an IV dose is given.

3. **A 500 mg dose of gentamicin is administered to a patient, and a blood sample is drawn. The concentration of gentamicin is measured as 25 mcg/mL (which is the same as 25 mg/L). What is the volume of distribution of gentamicin in this patient?**

$$Vd = \frac{500 \text{ mg}}{25 \text{ mg/L}} = 20 \text{ L}$$

Vd is a theoretical value, which is why it is sometimes called the "apparent" volume of distribution. Vd is not an exact physical volume that is measured, but is a helpful parameter used to make inferences regarding how widely a drug distributes throughout the body.

METABOLISM

Metabolism is the process by which a drug is converted from its original chemical structure into other forms to facilitate elimination from the body. The original chemical form is called the parent drug and the additional forms are called metabolites. Metabolism can occur throughout the body. The gut and liver are primary sites for drug metabolism due to high levels of metabolic enzymes in these tissues.

Blood from the gut travels to the liver before it reaches the rest of the body. First-pass metabolism is the metabolism of a drug before it reaches the systemic circulation, which can dramatically reduce the bioavailability of an oral formulation. First-pass metabolism of lidocaine is so extensive that the drug cannot be given orally – it must be given IV. Some drugs with extensive first-pass metabolism can be given orally, but in much higher doses than IV doses (e.g., propranolol). Many non-oral, extravascular methods of administration (e.g., transdermal, buccal, sublingual) bypass first-pass metabolism entirely. Rectal administration partially avoids first-pass metabolism.

Drug metabolism involves Phase I reactions (oxidation, reduction and hydrolysis), followed by Phase II reactions (e.g., conjugation). Phase I reactions provide a reactive functional group on the compound that permits the drug to be attacked by Phase II enzymes. For example, breaking carbon bonds or adding a hydroxyl group to a drug makes the drug more hydrophilic – this means more of the drug stays in the blood; the blood then passes through the kidneys, and the drug is renally excreted. Glucuronidation and other Phase II reactions create compounds that are more readily excreted in the urine and bile. Cytochrome P450 (CYP450) enzymes, located mainly in the liver and intestines, metabolize the majority of drugs. Refer to the Basic Science Concepts chapter for further discussion of hydrolysis and oxidation as they relate to drug degradation.

EXCRETION

Excretion is the process of irreversible removal of drugs from the body. Excretion can occur through the kidneys (urine), liver (bile), gut (feces), lungs (exhaled air) and skin (sweat). The primary route of excretion for most drugs is the kidneys (renal excretion). Renal excretion can be increased by adjusting the acidity of the urine. For a weak base, increase excretion by acidifying the urine. For a weak acid, increase excretion by alkalinizing the urine.

P-glycoprotein (P-gp) efflux pumps in the gut play a role in the absorption and excretion of many drugs (see the Drug Interactions chapter). Renal excretion is discussed in the Renal Disease and Calculations IV chapters.

CLEARANCE AND AREA UNDER THE CURVE

Clearance (Cl) describes the rate of drug removal in a certain volume of plasma over a certain amount of time. Since the liver and kidneys clear most of the drug (and these organs do not usually speed up or slow down), most drug elimination occurs at a steady rate (called the rate of elimination). This is true of drugs that follow first-order kinetics (discussed later in the chapter). Clearance is the efficiency of drug removal from the body and is described by the following equation:

$$Cl = \frac{Rate\ of\ Elimination\ (Re)}{Drug\ Concentration}$$

4. A dose of gentamicin is given to a patient, and urine is collected from the patient for 4 hours after drug administration. It is determined that 300 mg of gentamicin was eliminated during that time period, and the measured plasma concentration at the midpoint of the collection was 12.5 mg/L. Calculate the patient's gentamicin clearance.

$$Cl = \frac{300 \text{ mg of gentamicin} / 4 \text{ hours}}{12.5 \text{ mg/L}} = 6 \text{ L/hr}$$

or

$$Cl = \frac{300 \text{ mg of gentamicin}}{4 \text{ hours}} \times \frac{L}{12.5 \text{ mg}} = 6 \text{ L/hr}$$

The rate of elimination (Re) has units of mass per time (e.g., mg/hr), and drug concentration has units of amount per volume (e.g., mg/L); units of mass (mg) cancel out and clearance has units of volume per time (e.g., L/hr). Because the rate of elimination is difficult to assess clinically, another method is used to calculate the clearance of a drug from the body:

$$F \times Dose = Cl \times AUC$$

The AUC is the most reliable measurement of a drug's bioavailability because it directly represents the amount of the drug that has reached the systemic circulation. The clearance for extravascular administration is calculated with this formula:

$$Cl = \frac{F \times Dose}{AUC}$$

Following IV administration, bioavailability (F) = 1, which can be inserted into the previous equation to determine clearance for a drug given intravenously:

$$Cl = \frac{Dose}{AUC}$$

5. A patient is currently receiving 400 mg of gentamicin IV once daily and, based on measured serum concentrations, the AUC is determined to be 80 mg x hr/L. Calculate the patient's gentamicin clearance.

$$Cl = \frac{400 \text{ mg}}{80 \frac{\text{mg} \times \text{hr}}{L}} = 5 \text{ L/hr}$$

ZERO VS. FIRST-ORDER PHARMACOKINETICS

Most drugs follow first-order elimination or "first-order kinetics," where a constant percentage of drug is removed per unit of time. For example, a 325 mg dose of acetaminophen is eliminated at the same rate as a 650 mg dose. With zero-order elimination, a constant amount of drug (mg) is removed per unit of time, no matter how much drug is in the body. The following table provides an example of zero-order and first-order elimination of a 2 gram dose of a drug.

Hour	ZERO-ORDER			FIRST-ORDER		
	Amount of Drug (mg)	Percent Removed in Previous Hour	Amount (mg) Removed in Previous Hour	Amount of Drug (mg)	Percent Removed in Previous Hour	Amount (mg) Removed in Previous Hour
0	2,000			2,000		
1	1,700	15	300	1,600	20	400
2	1,400	17.65	300	1,280	20	320
3	1,100	21.43	300	1,024	20	256

MICHAELIS-MENTEN KINETICS

Phenytoin, theophylline and voriconazole exhibit Michaelis-Menten kinetics (also called saturable, mixed order or non-linear kinetics). The maximum rate of metabolism is defined as the Vmax (see figure on the right). The concentration at which the rate of metabolism is half maximal is defined as the Michaelis-Menten constant (Km). At very low concentrations (much less than the Km), the rate of metabolism mimics a first-order process.

At most concentrations approaching and exceeding the Km, the rate of metabolism becomes mixed. At even higher concentrations relative to the Km, the rate of metabolism approaches zero-order (e.g., Vmax). Throughout this process, an increase in dose leads to a disproportionate increase in drug concentration at steady state. The rate of phenytoin metabolism approaches the maximum at accepted therapeutic concentrations. Because of this, phenytoin dose adjustments should be made in small increments (30 – 50 mg) when the serum concentration is > 7 mcg/mL. See the Study Tip Gal.

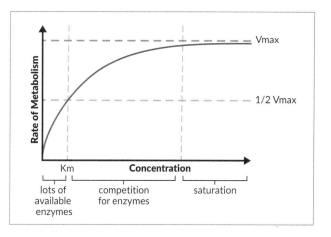

DOSE ADJUSTMENTS FOR MICHAELIS-MENTEN KINETICS

Most drugs follow first-order (linear) kinetics.

- At steady state, doubling the dose approximately doubles the serum concentration.

Some drugs (phenytoin, theophylline and voriconazole) follow Michaelis-Menten (also called non-linear, saturable or mixed-order) kinetics.

- Doubling the dose of these drugs can more than double the serum concentration.

  ❏ Using a proportion to calculate a new dose is not appropriate.

  ❏ Dosing adjustments must be made cautiously to avoid toxicity.

6. **A patient has been using phenytoin 100 mg three times daily. A phenytoin level was drawn and found to be 8.8 mcg/mL (reference range 10 - 20 mcg/mL). The dose was doubled to 200 mg three times daily. The patient started to slur her words, felt fatigued and returned to the clinic. The level was repeated and found to be 23.7 mcg/mL. Which of the following statements is accurate regarding the most likely reason for the change in phenytoin level?**

   A. Phenytoin half-life is reduced at higher doses.

   B. Phenytoin volume of distribution increases at higher doses.

   C. The patient's serum albumin level likely increased.

   D. Phenytoin bioavailability can decrease at higher doses.

   E. Phenytoin metabolism can become saturated at higher doses.

   The correct answer is (E). The most likely explanation for the increase in phenytoin level is that when the dose was doubled, the metabolism became partially or completely saturated, and the steady-state level increased dramatically.

ELIMINATION RATE CONSTANT

The <u>elimination rate constant (ke)</u> is the fraction of the drug that is eliminated (cleared) per unit of time. It is calculated from the Vd and the clearance:

$$ke = \frac{Cl}{Vd}$$

7. **A drug has the following pharmacokinetic parameters: Vd = 50 liters and Cl = 5,000 mL/hour. Calculate the elimination rate constant of the drug.**

$$ke = \frac{5\ L/hr}{50\ L} = 0.1\ hr^{-1}$$

   Be certain that the values are converted to units that properly cancel out in the equation. The ke is 0.1 hr^{-1} (meaning that <u>10% of the drug remaining is cleared per hour</u>).

Predicting Drug Concentrations

The ke can be used to predict the concentration of a drug at any time (t) after the dose using the calculations below. The second formula is derived from the first.

$$C_2 = C_1 \times e^{-kt}$$

$$ke = \frac{\ln(C_1/C_2)}{t}$$

Where C1 = the first or higher drug concentration (sometimes the peak concentration), C2 = the second (or lower) drug concentration (at time = t) and e = the base of the natural log.

8. **A patient received a dose of gentamicin. A short time after the end of the infusion, it is known that the drug level was 10 mg/L, and the patient's ke = 0.22 hr^{-1}. Calculate the predicted concentration after 8 hours.**

$$C_2 = 10\ mg/L \times e^{-0.22 \times 8}$$

$$C_2 = 10\ mg/L \times 0.172 = 1.72\ mg/L$$

9. A patient being treated with vancomycin had a supratherapeutic trough level of 28 mcg/mL. If ke = 0.15 hr^{-1}, predict how long it will take for the trough to decrease to the goal therapeutic trough (15 mcg/mL). Round to the nearest hour.

$$0.15 \text{ hr}^{-1} = \frac{\ln(28/15)}{t} = 4.16 \text{ hr, or 4 hours}$$

HALF-LIFE (t½) AND STEADY STATE

The time required for a drug concentration (and drug amount) to <u>decrease by 50%</u> is called the elimination <u>half-life</u> ($t_{1/2}$). For example, it takes 5 hours for theophylline concentrations to fall from 16 to 8 mg/L. The half-life of theophylline is 5 hours. It takes 5 more hours for the drug concentration to fall from 8 mg/L to 4 mg/L. Half-life is independent of the drug concentration for drugs exhibiting first-order kinetics.

Half-life is more clinically meaningful than ke. The half-life of a drug can be calculated from the ke:

$$t_{1/2} = \frac{0.693}{ke}$$

The half-life of a drug can be used to calculate the time required for drug washout (complete elimination) or the time required to achieve steady-state (refer to the table below). When a fixed dose is administered at regular intervals, the drug accumulates until it reaches steady state where the rate of <u>drug intake equals</u> the rate of <u>drug elimination</u>. The time required to reach steady state depends on the elimination half-life of the drug. It takes <u>~5 half-lives to reach steady state</u>, assuming the drug follows first-order kinetics (described previously) in a one-compartment distribution model (the drug is rapidly and evenly distributed throughout the body) and no loading dose has been given. Similarly, <u>5 half-lives are required to eliminate more than 95% of the drug</u> if no additional doses are given. The most clinically useful information is obtained from drug levels collected at <u>steady state</u>.

# OF HALF-LIVES	ELIMINATION (NO ADDITIONAL DOSES GIVEN) % OF DRUG REMAINING IN THE BODY	ACCUMULATION (MULTIPLE DOSES GIVEN) % OF STEADY-STATE ACHIEVED
1	50	50
2	25	75
3	12.5	87.5
4	6.25	93.8
5	3.13	96.9

10. Tetracycline has a clearance of 7.014 L/hr and a Vd of 105 L. Calculate the half-life of tetracycline (round to the nearest tenth) and the time required for elimination of greater than 95% of the drug from the body.

$$ke = \frac{Cl}{Vd} = \frac{7.014 \text{ L/hr}}{105 \text{ L}} = 0.0668 \text{ hr}^{-1}$$

$$t_{1/2} = \frac{0.693}{ke} = \frac{0.693}{0.0668 \text{ hr}^{-1}} = 10.4 \text{ hours}$$

The time required is 10.4 hours × 5 half-lives = 52 hours

11. **The serum concentration of Drug A over time is plotted in the figure below. What is the half-life of Drug A?**

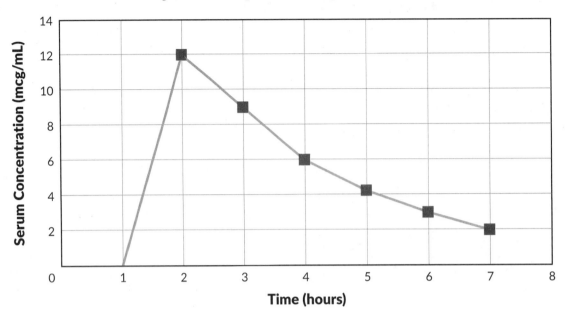

The drug concentrations can be presented in a figure (as shown) or in a list. <u>Identify two times</u> (in hours) where the <u>drug concentration has decreased by half</u> to find the half-life:

- At 2 hours the concentration is 12 mcg/mL and at 4 hours the concentration is 6 mcg/mL.
- It takes 2 hours for the concentration to decrease by 50%, so the half-life is 2 hours.

The equations under "Predicting Drug Concentrations" can also be used to calculate half-life and drug levels on a concentration curve like this. Plotting out the levels and time can be useful for solving many types of pharmacokinetic problems.

---

12. **A patient was receiving Drug B for 1 week. The drug was held on June 1st due to an elevated serum concentration. Based on the serum concentrations obtained after the drug was held (shown below), what is the half-life of Drug B?**

TIME	CONCENTRATION OF DRUG B
1400	12 mcg/mL
1500	8.5 mcg/mL
1600	6 mcg/mL
1700	4.3 mcg/mL
1900	2.1 mcg/mL

The drug concentration fell by 50% (from 12 mcg/mL to 6 mcg/mL) in 2 hours, so the half-life of Drug B is 2 hours. This is a different way of presenting the same information from the previous problem.

---

13. **A patient receives 200 mg of a drug with a half-life of 5 hours. How much of the drug remains after 10 hours?**

- 10 hours = 2 half-lives
- 50 mg of the drug remains after 10 hours

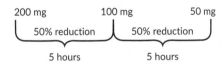

LOADING DOSE

Administration of a loading dose can be necessary to rapidly achieve therapeutic concentrations of a drug. When the half-life of a drug is long relative to the frequency of administration, several doses must be administered before steady state is achieved.

14. **A patient will be started on daily oral digoxin for management of atrial fibrillation. The following pharmacokinetic parameters for oral digoxin are known: F = 0.6, Vd = 500 L and Cl = 120 L/day. When would steady state be reached? Round to the nearest day.**

$$ke \ = \ \frac{Cl}{Vd} \ = \ \frac{120 \ L/day}{500 \ L} \ = \ 0.24 \ days^{-1} \qquad t_{1/2} \ = \ \frac{0.693}{ke} \ = \ \frac{0.693}{0.24 \ days^{-1}} \ = \ \sim2.89 \ days$$

$$Steady \ State \ = \ 5 \ half\text{-}lives \times 2.89 \ days \ = \ \sim14 \ days$$

It is beneficial to administer a loading dose to achieve the targeted levels more quickly in this case. The loading dose can be determined with the following equation:

$$Loading \ Dose \ = \ \frac{Desired \ Concentration \times Vd}{F}$$

15. **Using the pharmacokinetic parameters provided in the previous question, what oral loading dose of digoxin is appropriate to rapidly achieve a peak concentration of 1.5 mcg/L?**

$$Loading \ Dose \ = \ \frac{Desired \ Concentration \times Vd}{F} \ = \ \frac{1.5 \ mcg/L \times 500 \ L}{0.6} \ = \ 1,250 \ mcg \ or \ 1.25 \ mg$$

THERAPEUTIC DRUG MONITORING

Some medications are monitored with drug levels to reach dosing goals and avoid toxicity (see the Lab Values & Drug Monitoring chapter). If drug levels are too <u>high, toxicity</u> can occur. If drug levels are too <u>low</u>, the patient's condition might <u>not</u> be <u>treated</u> adequately. To prevent either toxicity or inadequate treatment, an adjustment of the dosing regimen is needed.

The <u>peak</u> level is the highest concentration in the blood the drug will reach. With intravenous drugs, peaks are typically drawn 30 minutes after the end of the infusion to allow for drug distribution to occur (e.g., aminoglycosides). The <u>trough</u> level is the lowest concentration reached by the drug before the next dose is given; it is drawn <u>immediately before</u> (or <u>within 30 minutes</u> before) the <u>dose</u> is due. When adjusting a dosing regimen, changing the dose generally affects the peak, and changing the interval/frequency generally affects the trough.

Therapeutic drug monitoring optimizes drug therapy by enhancing efficacy (e.g., overcoming resistance) and reducing toxicity associated with overdosing or drug accumulation. Antibiotic dosing strategies are dictated by certain pharmacodynamic parameters [e.g., peak to minimum inhibitory concentration (MIC) ratio, AUC to MIC ratio or time above the MIC]. This is discussed in the Infectious Diseases I chapter.

16. A patient is receiving tobramycin 120 mg IV every 8 hours at 0600, 1400 and 2200. The drug is being infused over 30 minutes. A tobramycin level drawn at 1500 was 9.8 mcg/mL. A trough level scheduled for 2200 was inadvertently drawn at 1830 and was 5.6 mcg/mL. What would the expected level (extrapolated trough) be at 2200? Round to the nearest tenth.

$$k_e = \frac{\ln(9.8 / 5.6)}{3.5} = 0.1599 \ hr^{-1}$$

$$C_2 = 5.6 \ mcg/mL \times e^{-0.1599 \times 3.5}$$

$$C_2 = 5.6 \ mcg/mL \times 0.5714 = 3.2 \ mcg/mL$$

CALCULATING TIME (t)

Determining the correct value to use for time (t) can be challenging. Try creating your own concentration-time curve and plotting the values you are given.

Either measured level (9.8 mcg/mL or 5.6 mcg/mL) can be used in the second step of the problem. If 9.8 mcg/mL was used, time (t) would be 7 hours. In this case, the regimen should be adjusted due to an elevated trough (goal < 2 mcg/mL) by increasing the dosing interval.

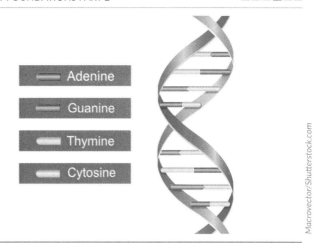

Macrovector/Shutterstock.com

- Adenine
- Guanine
- Thymine
- Cytosine

CHAPTER 78

PHARMACOGENOMICS

BACKGROUND

Pharmacogenomics is the science of examining inherited variations in genes that determine a patient's response to a drug. It is estimated that genetic factors are responsible for 20 – 40% of the differences in drug metabolism and response between patients. The goal of pharmacogenomics is to identify these factors and design treatments with improved efficacy and reduced adverse reactions.

Pharmacogenomics is called "personalized medicine" because drugs can be avoided entirely or used preferentially, based on a person's genotype. The genotype is an individual's unique genetic instructions (the coding in the DNA), which can determine response and tolerability of drugs.

Pharmacogenomics is Becoming Mainstream

Medication prescribing has historically been hit-or-miss (e.g., it has not always been possible to predict a patient's response to or tolerability of medications). Today, pharmacogenomic testing is more accessible, and assessing the presence or lack of genes that

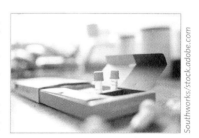

Southworks/stock.adobe.com

influence efficacy (response) and the likelihood of adverse events can guide prescribing.

Many tests are conducted on DNA extracted from a sample of saliva. Health insurance plans cover the cost of some pharmacogenetic tests if prescribed by a healthcare provider.

CONTENT LEGEND

 = Study Tip Gal    = Key Drug Guy

DOMINANT AND RECESSIVE TRAITS

Dominant and recessive genotypes describe the inheritance patterns of certain traits. They can be used to determine how likely it is for a certain phenotype (an observable trait) to pass from parent to offspring.

Each parent contributes one copy (an allele) of each gene to the offspring. The differences in each allele cause variations in protein production (expression), which determines the phenotype (e.g., brown or blonde hair). The phenotype will also be influenced by the offspring's environment.

A dominant allele produces a dominant phenotype in individuals who have one copy of the allele from one parent. For a recessive allele to produce a recessive phenotype, the individual must have two copies, one from each parent (see figure).

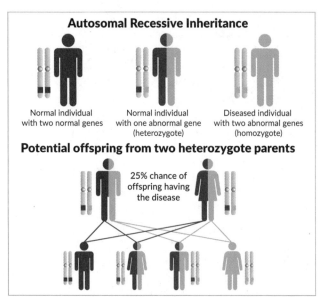

Ali/stock.adobe.com

DEFINITIONS

TERM	DEFINITION
Deoxyribonucleic acid (DNA)	The genetic information inherited from both parents that is present in two long chains of nucleotides, joined together by hydrogen bonds and twisted into a double helix. DNA is the main component of chromosomes.
Nucleotide	A subunit of the nucleic acids DNA and RNA (ribonucleic acid). Each nucleotide contains a nitrogen base, a five-carbon sugar (deoxyribose in DNA, and ribose in RNA) and a phosphate group. In DNA, the bases consist of two purines (adenine and guanine) and two pyrimidines (thymine and cytosine). In RNA, uracil is present instead of thymine.
Chromosome	A tightly packed structure within the cell nucleus, consisting of DNA and proteins. Chromosomes contain genes. Human cells contain 23 pairs of chromosomes.
Gene	A specific sequence of nucleotides that code (i.e., provide instructions) for a single protein. A gene is similar to a recipe, or a set of instructions, on how to make a protein. Since proteins make up the entire life form, genes are referred to as the "blueprint" of life.
Allele	The specific form of a gene. Alleles are either wild-type or variants. Wild-type is usually the most commonly occurring allele.
Genotype	The set of unique genes that determine a specific trait in an individual. Two identical alleles make up a homozygous genotype (e.g., CYP450 2C19*1/*1) and two different alleles make up a heterozygous genotype (e.g., CYP2C19*1/*3).
Phenotype	An observable trait (outward expression) of the genotype, even if it is not outwardly visible. Examples include physical traits (e.g., eye color), genetic diseases (e.g., sickle cell disease, cystic fibrosis) and changes in metabolism (e.g., poor metabolizer of a drug).
Haplotype	A group of genes or DNA variations inherited from a single parent that exist on the same chromosome and are likely to be inherited together.
Polymorphism	An inherited variation in the DNA sequence (such as a single nucleotide polymorphism).

SINGLE NUCLEOTIDE POLYMORPHISM

A single nucleotide polymorphism (SNP; pronounced "snip") occurs when there is a change in a single base pair in a genetic sequence (e.g., C replaced by G). SNPs are the most common genetic alteration in DNA. A SNP can be harmless, or it can lead to a disease or altered response to a drug. For example, in cystic fibrosis, a SNP results in defective coding for a protein involved in sweat and mucus production. SNPs are responsible for the majority of individual variability in response to a drug.

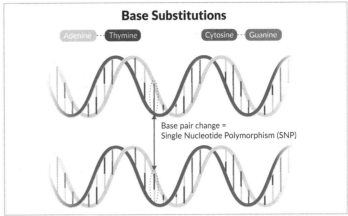

Base Substitutions

Base pair change =
Single Nucleotide Polymorphism (SNP)

Julee Ashmead/stock.adobe.com

CYTOCHROME P450 ENZYMES

CYP ENZYMES ARE POLYMORPHIC

The CYP450 enzymes are polymorphic, which means there are different forms of the same enzyme (due to a SNP in the DNA that codes for the enzyme). A SNP can cause the enzyme activity or production in an individual to increase or decrease, which will increase or decrease the rate of drug metabolism and, consequently, the serum level of the substrate drug. The major types of CYP enzyme variations impacting activity (i.e., rate of metabolism) are classified into 5 groups (see table below): ultrarapid metabolizer (UM), rapid metabolizer (RM), normal metabolizer (NM), intermediate metabolizer (IM) and poor metabolizer (PM).

- PMs have significantly reduced or no enzyme activity of a particular enzyme.
  - ❏ For example, a person who is a CYP2D6 PM has reduced or no metabolism of a drug metabolized by CYP2D6.
  - ❏ In this case, drug levels increase (or in the case of a prodrug, less will be metabolized to the active form).
  - ❏ This might mean a patient should avoid drugs metabolized by that enzyme or use a modified dose to prevent adverse effects.
- IMs have lower enzyme activity that falls between NMs and PMs.
- NMs have fully functional enzyme activity, which typically results in an expected drug response.
- UMs and RMs have a higher enzyme activity compared to NMs.
  - ❏ This leads to faster metabolism of a drug through that enzyme, causing drug levels to decrease.
  - ❏ Patients could quickly metabolize a prodrug to its active form and/or eliminate an active drug faster than expected.

PHENOTYPE	ENZYME ACTIVITY	EXAMPLE CYP2C19
Poor metabolizer	Very low or none	CYP2C19*2/*2
Intermediate metabolizer	Low	CYP2C19*1/*2
Normal metabolizer	Normal	CYP2C19*1/*1
Rapid Metabolizer	High	CYP2C19*1/*17
Ultrarapid metabolizer	Very high	CYP2C19*17/*17

CYP Enzymes Vary by Ethnicity and Among Individuals

Gene variants are most often inherited, and the variant enzyme expression can be measured among ethnic groups. Using CYP2D6 as an example, PMs are more commonly found in Europeans, while a significantly higher frequency of UMs are found in Pacific Islanders.

PHARMACOGENOMIC TESTING AND PHARMACIST ACTION

DRUG	TEST	SIGNIFICANCE/POPULATION	RESULT/ACTION
Human leukocyte antigen (HLA) testing: the major histocompatibility complex, class I, B (HLA-B) is an important gene in the immune system.			
Abacavir *(Ziagen)* and abacavir-containing combination drugs (e.g., **Triumeq, Epzicom**)	HLA-B*5701	Patients who are HLA-B*5701 positive are at ↑ risk for a hypersensitivity reaction. Test all patients prior to starting. Serious and fatal hypersensitivity reactions have occurred.	If positive, do not use.
Allopurinol *(Zyloprim, Aloprim)*	HLA-B*5801	Patients testing positive for HLA-B*5801 have an increased risk of Stevens-Johnson syndrome (SJS). Discontinue at the first sign of an allergic reaction, including skin rash. Consider testing high-risk individuals (African, Asian and Native Hawaiian/Pacific Islander ancestry).	If positive, do not use.
Carbamazepine *(Tegretol,* others) **Oxcarbazepine** *(Trileptal)* **Phenytoin** *(Dilantin,* others) **Fosphenytoin** *(Cerebyx)*	HLA-B*1502	The HLA-B*1502 allele (more common in Asian populations) ↑ the risk of serious skin reactions including SJS and toxic epidermal necrolysis (TEN). Test all Asian patients before starting carbamazepine; testing is suggested for oxcarbazepine and is optional for phenytoin and fosphenytoin.	If positive, do not use (unless benefit clearly outweighs risk).
Select drugs impacted by CYP450 polymorphisms: polymorphisms of various CYP450 enzymes may be responsible for much of the variability in medication response. These polymorphisms could affect any population, but are not yet routinely tested.			
Citalopram *(Celexa)*	CYP2C19	Citalopram is metabolized by CYP2C19 to inactive metabolites. The CYP2C19*1 allele is fully functional, whereas the *2 and *3 alleles indicate reduced metabolism. Patients with CYP2C19*2 or *3 alleles are poor metabolizers and are at risk of QT prolongation.	If the patient is known to have the CYP2C19*2 or *3 alleles, citalopram should be limited to 20 mg/day.
Clopidogrel *(Plavix)*	CYP2C19	Clopidogrel is a prodrug. It must be converted to an active metabolite by CYP2C19. The CYP2C19*2 and *3 alleles indicate reduced metabolism (less active metabolite formed). Patients with CYP2C19*2 or *3 alleles are poor metabolizers and have ↑ cardiovascular events.	If the patient is known to have the CYP2C19*2 or *3 alleles, consider alternative treatment.
Codeine	CYP2D6	Codeine (a prodrug) is metabolized to morphine via CYP2D6. Ultrarapid metabolizers are at ↑ risk of opioid overdose due to extensive conversion to morphine. Over-production of morphine can cause ↑ CNS effects, including respiratory depression. Infant deaths have occurred when nursing mothers who were ultrarapid metabolizers took codeine for pain. Excessive morphine was passed to the infant through breast milk.	If a known CYP2D6 ultrarapid metabolizer, do not use (toxicity risk). If a known CYP2D6 poor metabolizer, do not use (lack of efficacy).
Warfarin	CYP2C9*2 and *3, VKORC1	Increased bleeding risk due to reduced function of alleles and haplotypes (CYP2C9*2 and *3) and VKORC1 G > A variant.	If these allele variations are known to be present, start with a lower dose.

DRUG	TEST	SIGNIFICANCE/POPULATION	RESULT/ACTION
Other pharmacogenomic tests			
Trastuzumab (Herceptin) and other HER2 inhibitors (see Oncology chapter)	HER2 gene expression	These drugs require overexpression of HER2 for efficacy. HER2 negative status and those with weakly positive (1+) tumors do not respond well to treatment.	If tumor is HER2 negative, drugs are not effective.
Cetuximab (Erbitux) and other EGFR inhibitors (see Oncology chapter)	KRAS mutation	Only patients who are KRAS mutation-negative (i.e., are wild-type) should receive these medications. They are not effective in patients with colorectal cancer who are positive for the KRAS mutation (~40% of patients).	If positive for a KRAS mutation, do not use.
Azathioprine (Azasan, Imuran)	Thiopurine methyltransferase (TPMT)	Low/absent TPMT activity ↑ the risk of severe, life threatening myelosuppression (↓ WBCs, ↓ RBCs, ↓ platelets); patients with intermediate TPMT activity are also at ↑ risk for myelosuppression, but with lower severity.	If TPMT activity is low/absent, start at a very low dose or use an alternative treatment.
Capecitabine (Xeloda) **Fluorouracil**	DPD deficiency	Dihydropyrimidine dehydrogenase (DPD) deficiency ↑ risk of severe toxicity (diarrhea, neutropenia, neurotoxicity).	If DPD deficient, do not use.

Refer to the Key Drugs Guy below for drugs with required or strongly recommended pharmacogenomic testing per the package labeling.

DOES A POSITIVE OR NEGATIVE TEST REQUIRE ACTION?

Avoid the drug when these pharmacogenomic tests are POSITIVE

- HLA-B: a positive test indicates ↑ risk of hypersensitivity
- KRAS mutation: a positive test (often called "KRAS mutant") predicts a poor response

Avoid the drug when this pharmacogenomic test is NEGATIVE

- HER2 expression: a negative result indicates a poor response

SELECT DRUGS WITH PHARMACOGENOMIC IMPLICATIONS

KEY DRUGS

Testing required or strongly recommended:
Abacavir and any combination products containing abacavir

Azathioprine

Carbamazepine

Cetuximab and other EGFR inhibitors

Trastuzumab and other HER2 inhibitors

May consider testing, though not routine:
Allopurinol

Capecitabine and fluorouracil

Clopidogrel

Codeine

Phenytoin and fosphenytoin

Warfarin

Select Guidelines/References
Clinical Pharmacogenetics Implementation Consortium (CPIC) Guidelines. https://cpicpgx.org/guidelines.

CHAPTER CONTENT

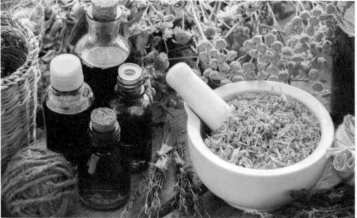

iStock.com/ChamilleWhite

CHAPTER 79

DIETARY SUPPLEMENTS, NATURAL & COMPLEMENTARY MEDICINE

BACKGROUND

Complementary medicine refers to health practices (e.g., dietary supplements, acupuncture) that are used with conventional medicine (e.g., healthcare provider visits, prescription medications). In the last decade, yoga and meditation had the largest increases in use. Complementary medicine is used commonly in the United States.

The term alternative medicine is used when conventional medicine is not used.

NATURAL MEDICINE

'Natural medicine' is a general umbrella term that includes herbals (plant products), vitamins, minerals and many substances that are not plant-derived but exist in nature, such as glucosamine from shellfish. The FDA uses the term "dietary supplements," which will be used here.

Dietary supplements are regulated by the Dietary Supplement Health and Education Act (DSHEA) of 1994. DSHEA requires the manufacturer to ensure that their products are safe before they are marketed. In contrast, drugs must be proven safe and effective before they can be sold. Once the supplement is marketed, the FDA must show it is "unsafe" before it can restrict use or remove it from the marketplace. The company selling or distributing the supplement must forward adverse event reports to the FDA. Adverse events from supplements can be reported to the FDA's Safety Reporting Portal, which sorts safety issues to the correct FDA site. The National Institutes of Health (NIH) has a Dietary Supplements Label Database that provides health information about dietary supplements for consumers and health professionals. Information on natural medicines can also be found in general drug references and the *Natural Medicines Database*.

DIFFERENCES BETWEEN DIETARY SUPPLEMENTS AND DRUGS

Supplement safety is the manufacturer's responsibility, which should be proven prior to release. After release, the FDA can remove a supplement if it is found to be unsafe.

- In contrast, drugs must be proven safe and effective to the FDA prior to release.

Supplements cannot claim to treat, cure or mitigate (lessen) a condition (e.g., "melatonin treats insomnia" is not appropriate).

- In contrast, drug claims are based on FDA approval (e.g., "zolpidem treats insomnia" is appropriate).

SUPPLEMENTS
- The Supplement Facts label is similar to the label required on food products. It includes the ingredients, quantities, serving size, servings/container, calories, calories from fat, total fat and saturated fat, cholesterol, sodium, carbohydrate, dietary fiber, sugars, protein, vitamin A, vitamin C, calcium and iron, when present in measurable amounts.

OTC DRUGS
- The OTC Drug Facts label includes ingredients, purpose, uses, warnings, instructions, excipients and allergic reaction alerts/warnings. OTC drugs can include a package insert similar to prescription drugs; this depends on the product's approval process.

PRESCRIPTION DRUGS
- The package insert contains much more detailed information; see the Drug References chapter.

Manufacturers cannot make claims that the product treats or cures a condition. Health claims are limited to the nutrient content, the relationship to health and the impact on normal body structure or function, such as "calcium builds strong bones," and "fiber maintains bowel regularity." Products that make claims on the structure or function of the body (e.g., antioxidants maintain cell integrity) must state in a "disclaimer" that the FDA has not evaluated the claim. The United States Pharmacopeia (USP) establishes standards for dietary supplements. Pharmacists can help consumers choose a reputable product with the USP Verified Mark on the product label.

Supplements can pose safety risks in certain patients. Four areas of particular concern are situations where supplements interact with prescription drugs, increase bleeding risk or cause hepatotoxicity or cardiotoxicity. Risks with natural products are usually dose-dependent; higher doses have a higher risk.

DIETARY SUPPLEMENT LABELING

The claims on supplement labels are limited (see Study Tip Gal above) because the supplements have not had rigorous trials to determine safety and efficacy. The Supplement Facts label includes the recommended daily intake (RDI) and the amount of each ingredient in the product.

INTERACTIONS WITH PRESCRIPTION DRUGS

St. John's Wort

St. John's wort (SJW) has several important drug interactions to be aware of.

- SJW induces the CYP450 3A4, 2C19, 2C9 and 1A2 enzymes and p-glycoprotein (P-gp), which decreases the level of other drugs (with possible treatment failures).
  - ❏ Avoid use of SJW with other medications, especially oral contraceptives, transplant drugs and warfarin.
- SJW is serotonergic and is often implicated in serotonin syndrome.
  - ❏ Do not use with MAO inhibitors, including linezolid.
  - ❏ Concurrent use with other serotonergic drugs can be dangerous, especially at higher doses, including SSRIs and SNRIs.
- SJW causes photosensitivity and requires counseling on sun protection and avoidance.
  - ❏ Photosensitivity risk increases when taken with other photosensitizing drugs, including diuretics, retinoids, quinolones, sulfamethoxazole, tetracyclines and transplant drugs (e.g., tacrolimus); see Drug Allergies & Adverse Drug Reactions chapter.
- SJW may lower the seizure threshold. Caution is required when taking SJW with other drugs known to lower the seizure threshold (e.g., bupropion, quinolones, tramadol, penicillin, carbapenems) as well as in patients with a history of seizures; see Seizures/Epilepsy chapter.

SUPPLEMENTS THAT INCREASE BLEEDING RISK

Several natural medicines have the potential to increase bleeding risk.

- The "5 Gs": garlic, ginger, ginkgo, ginseng and glucosamine
- Fish oils (at higher doses)
- Vitamin E
- Dong quai
- Willow bark (a salicylate); do not use with anticoagulants.

Other supplements should not be given concurrently with warfarin; see Anticoagulation chapter.

SUPPLEMENTS WITH RISK OF LIVER TOXICITY

Natural products can be hepatotoxic.

- Black cohosh (used for menopausal symptoms)
- Kava (used for stress/anxiety)
- Chaparral, comfrey
- Green tea "extracts" may be a health concern; see below

SUPPLEMENTS WITH RISK OF CARDIAC TOXICITY

Cardiotoxic supplements will have a higher risk in patients with cardiac conditions, but can cause toxicity in anyone.

- Ephedra was removed from the market due to reports of cardiac toxicity. Bitter orange (Citrus aurantium or synephrine) replaced ephedra in many products.
  - ❑ Ephedra and bitter orange/synephrine are stimulants with dose-dependent cardiac toxicity. They increase blood pressure and heart rate. There are reports of myocardial infarction, stroke and arrhythmias.
- DMAA (dimethylamylamine) is an amphetamine derivative used in body-building or performance-enhancement products, including powdered supplement mixtures.
  - ❑ DMAA causes cardiotoxicity, including increasing blood pressure and heart rate.
- Licorice contains glycyrrhizin; artificially flavored licorice products do not contain this compound.
  - ❑ Glycyrrhizin, taken in excess, can lower potassium and increase blood pressure.
- Yohimbe is used to increase libido and for erectile dysfunction.
  - ❑ Yohimbine, the alkaloid derived from yohimbe, raises blood pressure, increases heart rate and has a risk of seizures.

Caffeine and Health Risks

Caffeine taken in usual doses is not harmful; in excessive doses, caffeine can raise blood pressure and increase heart rate.

- Caffeine is present in supplements for weight loss, energy and body-building. Many have high caffeine content.
- Caffeine is present in black tea, green tea, cocoa (including chocolate), yerba mate, guarana and kombucha (fermented tea).
- Green tea "extract" (with various unknown contents) has been linked to liver damage in body-building products.

Caffeine and Health Benefits

Caffeine is not all bad; it is the most popular drug in the world, with several benefits.

- Caffeine increases alertness, helps with weight management and can be useful in treating headaches.
- Green tea, in reasonable amounts, helps lower LDL and triglycerides. The table on the following page includes other supplements with beneficial cardiovascular effects.

MEDICAL FOODS

Medical foods are not medications, nor are they supplements. They are compounds used to meet a nutritional need, which should be used under medical supervision, yet not all require a prescription. Medical foods are not covered by most insurance plans.

FDA Requirements for Medical Foods

The FDA requires medical foods to be:

- Taken enterally (i.e., by mouth or with an enteral feeding tube).
- Taken under the supervision of a healthcare professional.
- Intended to treat a condition with a known nutritional requirement.

Medical Food Use is Increasing

Commonly used medical foods include L-methylfolate, an active form of folate (Deplin) used for depression, B6 and B12 (Metanx) used for neuropathic pain and phosphatidylserine conjugated to different forms of enriched omega-3 fatty acids used for mild cognitive impairment.

Generally Recognized As Safe

Some of the supplements in the following table (e.g., chamomile, cinnamon, synephrine) are used in food products. The FDA labels food additives as Generally Recognized As Safe (GRAS) when the additive is considered safe when used as intended. When used in doses that are higher than the intended dose, the safety profile will change and could include toxicity. All ingredients in a medical food must be GRAS.

COMMONLY USED SUPPLEMENTS

CONDITION	TREATMENT
Anxiety	Valerian
	Passionflower
	Kava
	St. John's wort
	Chamomile
	5-Hydroxytryptophan (5-HTP)
Cold Sores (Aphthous Ulcers/Canker Sores)	L-lysine
Colds and Flu	Echinacea
	Zinc
	Vitamin C (ascorbic acid)
	Eucalyptus oil, used for nasal congestion, allergies
	Probiotics (e.g., *Bifidobacterium animalis*, *Lactobacillus acidophilus*)
Dementia/ Memory	Ginkgo
	Vitamin E (alpha-tocopherol)
	Vitamin D
	Acetyl-L-carnitine
	Vinpocetine, used for memory, neuroprotection, weight loss
Depression	St. John's wort
	SAMe (S-adenosyl-L-methionine), used for depression, osteoarthritis
	5-HTP
	Valerian
Diabetes	Alpha lipoic acid, used for diabetic neuropathy, memory, neuroprotection
	Chromium
	Cassia cinnamon
	Magnesium
	American ginseng
	Panax ginseng

CONDITION	TREATMENT
Dyslipidemia	Red yeast rice (contains a natural form of lovastatin)
	Omega-3 fatty acids, "fish oils"
	Garlic (controversial benefit; small ↓ TC and LDL)
	Plant sterol (beta-sitosterol)
	Fiber (barley, psyllium, oat bran)
	Artichoke extract
Dyspepsia	Calcium
	Magnesium
	Peppermint
	Chamomile
Energy/Weight Loss	Bitter orange (synephrine component)
	Caffeine
	Guarana, green tea powder (contain caffeine)
	Garcinia cambogia
Erectile Dysfunction	Ginseng
	L-arginine
	Yohimbe
Heart Failure, Heart Health (general)	Coenzyme Q10 (ubiquinone), used as adjunctive treatment with HF medications
	Hawthorn
	Omega-3 fatty acids, "fish oils"
Hypertension	Omega-3 fatty acids, "fish oils"
	Garlic (controversial benefit; small ↓ in systolic BP)
	Fiber (barley, psyllium, oat bran)
	Potassium
Gastrointestinal Health	Fiber (barley, psyllium, oat bran), used for diarrhea, constipation
	Chamomile
	Probiotics (*Lactobacillus, Saccharomyces boulardii, Bifidobacterium infantis* strains)
	Ginger, used for nausea
	Peppermint
	Horehound, used for GI health, constipation
	Wheatgrass, used for GI health, detoxification
Inflammation	Omega-3 fatty acids, "fish oils"
	Flax seeds/oil (converted to DHA and EPA)
	Turmeric

CONDITION	TREATMENT
Insomnia/Sleep	Melatonin, used for sleep (taken QHS) and to help prevent/treat jet lag (0.5 to 2 mg taken pre-flight and higher doses, such as 5 mg, post-flight)
	Valerian
	Chamomile
	Lemon balm
	Passionflower
	5-HTP and L-tryptophan
Liver Disease	Milk thistle
Menopause	Black cohosh
	Dong quai
	Evening primrose oil [provides essential fatty acids (gamma-lineloic acid, or GLA)]
	Soy, red clover, Panax ginseng [contain mild phyto-(plant) estrogens]
Migraine, Prophylaxis	Feverfew
	Butterbur
	Magnesium
	Riboflavin (vitamin B2)
	Coenzyme Q10
	Guarana (for caffeine) or other caffeine sources
Motion Sickness	Ginger
	Peppermint

CONDITION	TREATMENT
Osteoarthritis	Glucosamine (best evidence with sulfate salts)
	Chondroitin
	SAMe (S-adenosyl-L-methionine), used for depression, osteoarthritis
	Turmeric, used to ↓ inflammation/pain
Osteoporosis	Calcium
	Vitamin D
	Soy
	Ipriflavone
Prostate Health	Saw palmetto
	Lycopene
	Pygeum
	Pumpkin seed (contains beta-sitosterol)
Skin Conditions	Tea tree oil, for acne, dandruff, fungal infections
	Aloe vera, for lichen planus, psoriasis, HSV, burns
	Topical vitamin D, for psoriasis, seborrheic keratosis (vitamin A & D ointment for diaper rash)
	Biotin, for hair loss, ↑ nail/hair thickness
UTI	Cranberry
	Yogurt
	Probiotics (*Bifidobacteria*, *Lactobacillus* strains)

SAFETY ISSUES WITH COMMON SUPPLEMENTS

TREATMENT	NOTES, SAFETY ISSUES
5-HTP	Serotonergic, ↑ risk with other serotonergic drugs
Artichoke extract	Allergic reactions (uncommon); due to possible allergenic cross-reactivity, patients with allergies to asters, echinacea, chamomile, chrysanthemums and ragweed should avoid artichoke extract
Beta-carotene	↑ risk of lung cancer (in smokers or asbestos exposure), ↑ cardiovascular mortality
Bitter melon	↓ blood glucose (BG); caution with hypoglycemic drugs
Bitter orange (synephrine component)	Stimulant; dose-related ↑ BP, ↑ HR, arrhythmia risk
Black cohosh	May be hepatotoxic Do not use with medications for heart failure: ACE inhibitors, ARBs, beta-blockers, amiodarone
Caffeine (including guarana and green tea powder)	Dose-related (with high doses) dizziness, agitation, irritability, ↑ BP, ↑ HR
Chamomile	Allergic reactions (uncommon); due to possible allergenic cross-reactivity, patients with allergies to asters, echinacea, chrysanthemums and ragweed should avoid chamomile
Chondroitin	Bleeding risk at higher doses, ↑ INR with warfarin

TREATMENT	NOTES, SAFETY ISSUES
Dong quai	Increased bleeding risk (e.g., with concurrent use of anticoagulants, antiplatelets, salicylates)
Echinacea	Controversial safety with autoimmune disorders; due to allergenic cross-reactivity, patients with allergies to artichoke, asters, chamomile, chrysanthemums, and ragweed should avoid echinacea
Feverfew	Mouth ulceration (inflammation of the oral cavity/tongue), increased bleeding risk (e.g., with concurrent use of anticoagulants, antiplatelets, salicylates)
Fiber (barley, psyllium, oat bran)	GI effects (e.g., bloating, cramping, flatulence)
Garlic	
Ginger	Known as the "5 Gs"
Ginkgo	↑ bleeding risk; risk is further increased with concurrent use of other drugs known to increase bleeding risk (e.g., SSRIs, SNRIs, anticoagulants, antiplatelets, salicylates)
Ginseng	Discontinue in advance of surgery
Glucosamine	
Hawthorn	Positive inotrope; avoid concurrent use with digoxin (additive effect), ↓ BP; caution for additive effect with BP-lowering drugs
Kava	Avoid due to hepatotoxicity
L-arginine	L-arginine converts into nitric oxide, ↓ BP and ↑ dizziness, caution for additive effect with BP-lowering drugs; avoid concurrent use with nitrates
Melatonin	When used chronically for sleep, endogenous melatonin can be decreased, resulting in dependency for sleep
Omega-3 fatty acids, "fish oils"	↑ bleeding risk with high doses, can ↑ LDL
Passionflower	QT prolongation; avoid with QT risk/other QT-prolonging drugs
Potassium	Potassium levels should be measured in a lab, and dosed accordingly (not with OTC supplements)
Probiotics	Separate use from oral antibiotics, safety concern with use of live bacteria in immunocompromised states
Red yeast rice	CYP450 inhibitors (e.g., amiodarone) will ↑ red yeast rice level; red yeast rice ↓ coenzyme Q10, which may ↑ myopathy risk; do not use with statins
SAMe (S-adenosylmethionine)	Serotonergic, ↑ risk with other serotonergic drugs ↑ bleeding risk, do not use in bipolar disorder due to ↑ risk manic behavior
Soy, red clover, Panax ginseng	Contain mild phyto-(plant) estrogens; soy might increase breast cancer risk in postmenopausal women who are not producing estradiol
St. John's wort	Many drug interactions, mainly due to enzyme induction (results in ↓ levels of other drugs, except ↑ levels of prodrugs); serotonergic, photosensitivity
Valerian	Sedation, CNS depressant; risk with concurrent CNS depressants
Vinpocetine	Vinpocetine is semi-synthetic and derived from a plant product; FDA issued a warning for fetal harm
Vitamin C (ascorbic acid)	Nephrolithiasis with high doses, false-negative stool occult blood 48 to 72 hours after ascorbic acid ingestion
Vitamin E (alpha-tocopherol)	Do not exceed 400 IU daily; bleeding risk
Yohimbe	↑ BP, ↑ HR, seizure risk
Zinc	Nasal products can cause loss of smell

VITAMIN SUPPLEMENTATION

People who consume a balanced diet typically do not require supplementation with vitamins. Many people have poor diets that are low in nutritional value and may require a vitamin supplement to prevent nutrient deficiencies. Vitamin supplementation may also be needed in select age groups (e.g., folate in women of childbearing age) or conditions (e.g., thiamine in alcohol use disorder).

VITAMINS	NAMES
Vitamin A	Retinol
Vitamin B1	Thiamine
Vitamin B2	Riboflavin
Vitamin B3	Niacin
Vitamin B6	Pyridoxine
Vitamin B9	Folic Acid
Vitamin B12	Cobalamin
Vitamin C	Ascorbic Acid
Vitamin D2	Ergocalciferol
Vitamin D3	Cholecalciferol
Vitamin E	Alpha-tocopherol

Pharmacists are part of the solution to problems associated with vitamin deficiencies, and it is important to know their common names (see table above). Some drugs may deplete nutrients, require a supplement to work properly or require a supplement to reduce toxicity (see table on the following page).

CALCIUM & VITAMIN D

Calcium and vitamin D intake remains insufficient for the majority of adults and children. Low levels of vitamin D impairs calcium absorption. Patients who do not receive enough vitamin D from the sun or diet can benefit from supplementation with both calcium and vitamin D. Calcium and vitamin D supplementation is an essential topic for pharmacists since they often recommend OTC products. Product type and selection are discussed in the Osteoporosis, Menopause & Testosterone Use chapter.

The American Academy of Pediatrics (AAP) makes the following recommendations for infants and children:

- Exclusively breastfed infants or babies drinking less than 1 liter of baby formula need 400 IU of vitamin D daily. *Poly-Vi-Sol* products (discussed later) or generics are acceptable.

- Older children who do not drink at least 4 cups of vitamin D fortified milk per day also need vitamin D supplementation.

For all prescription medications for low bone density (osteopenia or osteoporosis), adequate calcium and vitamin D supplementation should be recommended if dietary intake is inadequate.

FOLIC ACID (FOLATE)

Folate intake among women of childbearing age can be insufficient. Folate deficiency causes birth defects of the brain and spinal cord (neural tube defects). With the FDA update for RDI labeling, folic acid will have units listed on labels in dietary folate equivalents (DFE) instead of in micrograms:

- Folic acid 600 mcg DFE ≅ 360 mcg of folic acid daily.

All women of childbearing age should obtain 400 mcg DFE/day of folic acid. During pregnancy, folate requirements increase to 600 mcg DFE/day. Folate should be taken at least one month before pregnancy and continued for the first 2 – 3 months of pregnancy. Once pregnant, the patient will likely take a prescription prenatal vitamin which is continued throughout the pregnancy since it also contains calcium (not enough, about 200 mg) and some iron. Folate is in many healthy foods, including fortified cereals (some of which are not healthy), dried beans, leafy green vegetables and orange juice. Multivitamins usually contain an amount in the recommended range. Prescription prenatal vitamins usually contain 1,000 mcg, or 1 mg, of folate. The birth control pills *Beyaz*, *Safyral* and *Tydemy* contain folate (as levomefolate). However, it is less expensive to use a different birth control pill with a separate supplement.

VITAMIN E

It is unusual to have a vitamin E deficiency since it is present in many foods. Vitamin E in foods is considered healthy, but excess intake of supplements is considered a health risk; patients should not exceed 400 IU daily. Vitamin E supplementation is not recommended for prevention of cardiovascular disease or cancer due to a lack of benefit in either condition.

THIAMINE

Thiamine (vitamin B1) deficiency is common in alcohol use disorder and malabsorptive states such as Crohn's disease, following bariatric surgery, advanced HIV and several other conditions. Thiamine deficiency can cause Wernicke's encephalopathy. Symptoms of Wernicke's include mental confusion, ataxia, tremor and vision changes. As the symptoms of Wernicke's fade, Korsakoff syndrome tends to develop (also called Korsakoff psychosis), which is permanent neurologic (mental) damage.

IRON

AAP Iron Recommendations

AGE	PREVENTION
0 – 4 months	Supplemental iron is not required.
4 – 6 months	Formulas contain adequate iron; supplementation is not required. Breastfed babies need 1 mg/kg/day from 4-6 months old and until consuming iron-rich foods. At about 6 months, most breastfed babies get about half their calories from other foods, which may be adequate.
6 – 12 months	Need 11 mg/day of iron. Food sources are preferred; supplement as-needed.
1 – 3 years	Need 7 mg/day of iron. Food sources are preferred; supplement as-needed.

Pre-Term Infants

- Preterm (< 37 weeks) breastfed infants should receive 2 mg/kg/day of elemental iron supplementation from age 1 – 12 months. Most preterm formula-fed infants receive enough iron from formula, but some still require supplementation.

Adolescent Girls

- Adolescent girls are at risk of anemia once menstruation begins. During this time, females should consume a diet high in iron-rich foods such as beans, eggs, fortified cereals and meats. Some will need an oral iron supplement.

Iron-Only Supplements (generics available)

Check the label on iron drops because the amount of iron provided by the dropper ranges from 10 – 15 mg.

- *Fer-In-Sol* Iron Supplement Drops
- *Feosol* tablets and caplets

Vitamin Supplements with Iron

- *Poly-Vi-Sol* Vitamin Drops with Iron: use if both vitamin D and iron are needed
- Others: *Flintstones* Children's Chewable Multivitamin plus Iron, store brands

DRUGS THAT CAUSE NUTRIENT DEPLETION

DRUG	DEPLETED NUTRIENT	CHAPTER
Amphotericin B	Magnesium, potassium	Infectious Diseases III
Antiseizure medications* (including carbamazepine, lamotrigine, oxcarbazepine, phenobarbital/primidone, phenytoin, topiramate, valproic acid/divalproex, zonisamide)	Calcium	Seizures/Epilepsy, Bipolar Disorder, others
Isoniazid	Vitamin B6	Infectious Diseases II (for neuropathy prevention)
Loop Diuretics	Potassium	Hypertension, Chronic Heart Failure
Metformin	Vitamin B12	Diabetes
Methotrexate	Folate	Systemic Steroids & Autoimmune Conditions, Oncology
Orlistat	Beta-carotene, fat-soluble vitamins	Weight Loss
Proton Pump Inhibitors	Magnesium, vitamin B12 (> 2 years of treatment)	GERD & PUD

*A supplement is needed for most patients using these drugs. Calcium should be given with vitamin D, if needed.

CONDITIONS WITH RECOMMENDED SUPPLEMENTS

CONDITION	RECOMMENDED SUPPLEMENT	CHAPTER
Alcohol Use Disorder	Vitamin B1, folate	Hepatitis & Liver Disease
Bariatric Surgery	Various; patient-specific	Weight Loss
Crohn's Disease (possibly ulcerative colitis)	Patient-specific, depends on levels; can require iron, zinc, folate, calcium, vitamin D, B vitamins	Inflammatory Bowel Disease
Chronic Kidney Disease	Vitamin D	Renal Disease, Bipolar Disorder (for lithium side effect)

CONDITION	RECOMMENDED SUPPLEMENT	CHAPTER
Goiter	Iodine (iodized salt)	Thyroid Disorders
Macrocytic Anemia	Vitamin B12 and/or folate	Anemia
Microcytic Anemia	Ferrous sulfate	Anemia
Pregnancy	Folate, calcium, vitamin D, pyridoxine (for nausea)	Pregnancy
Osteopenia/Osteoporosis	Calcium, vitamin D	Osteoporosis, Pregnancy

CANNABIDIOL (CBD)

Cannabidiol (CBD) is one cannabinoid found in the cannabis plant (marijuana is a type of cannabis plant). CBD does not cause the "high" that can come from marijuana use, and it does not appear to cause physical or psychological dependence. Tetrahydrocannabinol (THC) is generally extracted from marijuana; ingestion of THC may result in a "high." CBD is used in a variety of health issues (some with proof of efficacy and some without), including childhood epilepsy (Dravet syndrome and Lennox-Gastaut syndrome), anxiety, insomnia and chronic pain. While generally well-tolerated, it can cause nausea, diarrhea, fatigue and irritability.

The legality of CBD is evolving and can be confusing. Currently, it is illegal to market CBD as a food or dietary supplement because it is available as a prescription drug (*Epidiolex* used in certain childhood seizures). This means nonprescription CBD products are not FDA-approved. CBD can be extracted from the hemp plant, and federal law removed hemp from the definition of marijuana. Hemp-derived CBD products are still considered illegal in some states, while some states have legalized marijuana (and CBD) with various restrictions.

HOMEOPATHIC PRODUCTS

Homeopathy is based on "the law of similars" or the concept that "like is cured by like." This is when very small amounts of an active substance are given to stimulate the body to react against similar symptoms produced by that same substance when given at a higher dose. For example, homeopathic medicine made from the coffee bean relieves sleeplessness with agitation and racing thoughts. Although there is some evidence supporting the clinical use of homeopathic medicines, more research is needed before it can be considered a conventional medicine option.

Most homeopathic medicines are made from diluted amounts of the active substance, reported in X or C dilution scales. An X represents a 1:10 dilution, and C represents a 1:100 dilution of solute:solvent. The number in front of the X or C is the number of dilutions. A low dilution (e.g., 6C) could be seen to treat more localized symptoms such as a sore throat. A high dilution (e.g., 30C) could be seen in the treatment of more systemic symptoms (e.g., fever) or psychologic or behavioral symptoms (e.g., insomnia). The more dilute a substance is, the more "potent" it is considered.

The official compendium for homeopathic medicines is the Homeopathic Pharmacopoeia of the United States (HPUS), which is recognized by the FDA and equivalent to the United States Pharmacopoeia (USP). The HPUS publishes standards for homeopathic substances, including the identity, origin and quality assurance methods. The HPUS also determines what dilution of each medicine can be sold over the counter or with a prescription.

Since homeopathic medicines do not require FDA approval, manufacturers could distribute products with false claims, poor quality, measurable concentrations of drugs, nutrients or dietary supplements. In 2010, *Hyland's Teething Tablets* were recalled due to cases of belladonna toxicity. The amount of belladonna could be measured and was unsafe. In 2022, the FDA issued guidance on how to approach and prioritize regulatory actions for homeopathic products. It listed a risk-based and enforceable approach focusing on homeopathic products with the greatest risk to patients (e.g., products/ingredients with reported safety concerns, those with claims to treat or prevent serious medical conditions, and products with significant quality issues).

Select Guidelines/References

United States Pharmacopoeia. Choosing for Quality: Dietary Supplements. https://www.usp.org/sites/default/files/usp/document/about/convention-membership/usp-ds-qual-pharmacists-fact-sheet.pdf (accessed 2023 Nov 29).

National Center for Complementary and Integrative Health (NCCIH). National Health Interview Survey 2017. https://nccih.nih.gov/research/statistics/NHIS/2017 (accessed 2023 Nov 29).

Baker RD, Greer FR. Diagnosis and prevention of iron deficiency and iron-deficiency anemia in infants and young children (0-3 years of age). *Pediatrics*. 2010;126(5):1040-50.

U.S. Food and Drug Administration (FDA). Homeopathic Drug Products Guidance for FDA Staff and Industry. https://www.fda.gov/media/163755/download?utm_medium=email&utm_source=govdelivery (accessed 2023 Nov 29).

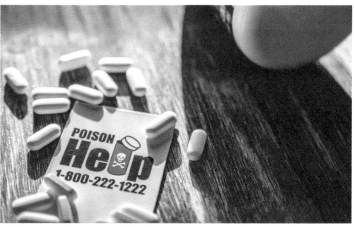

Lost_in_the_Midwest/Shutterstock.com

CHAPTER 80
TOXICOLOGY & ANTIDOTES

EMERGENCY PREPAREDNESS

Pharmacy staff are involved in the response to a disaster (e.g., natural disasters, industrial accidents, biological and chemical threats). They collaborate with federal, regional/state and local agencies to develop emergency response plans, including for drug distribution and stockpiling.

Pharmacy staff involved in emergency preparation should be well-informed about likely threats in their locality and should be familiar with emergency protocols for their institution or workplace, including those for evacuation, disaster preparedness, mass dispensing and poisoning emergencies. Legal issues regarding dispensing a drug during an emergency are discussed in the UWorld RxPrep MPJE and CPJE courses.

Communication concerning emergency planning and response requires a network of hospital pharmacy department directors and community pharmacies that can meet increased needs. Pharmacists should be familiar with the recommendations of the American Society of Health-System Pharmacists (ASHP).

The CDC pages on Emergency Preparedness and Response include recommendations for exposure to biological agents, information on current disease outbreaks and treatment for chemical and radiation exposure. One of the antidotes (KI, potassium iodide) for exposure to radioactive iodine is reviewed in the Thyroid Disorders chapter.

CONTENT LEGEND

 = Study Tip Gal

TOXICOLOGY

Toxicology is the study of the adverse effects of chemical exposures, including drugs used at unsafe doses. Children are the most common victims of accidental poisoning in the U.S. The top categories of exposures in children include cosmetics/personal care products, analgesics and cleaning substances. Accidental poisoning is common among the elderly, primarily due to mental or physical impairment, the use of multiple drugs and reduced elimination of drugs from the body.

Poisoning can be due to illicit drug use, or the use of FDA-approved drugs (e.g., opioids) taken alone or in combination with other drugs. Poisoning can be intentional, such as with attempted suicide or a drug-facilitated sexual assault. General drug information resources (e.g., Micromedex, Lexicomp) often contain toxicology information.

PREVENTION OF ACCIDENTAL OVERDOSE

To reduce accidental poisoning in children, child-resistant (C-R) packaging, also known as special packaging (e.g., push-and-turn or squeeze-and-turn caps), is helpful. This packaging is required for most prescription drugs unless

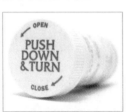

Jorge Salcedo/Shutterstock.com

waived by the patient or the provider (in accordance with state and federal law). Some drugs are excluded from this requirement, such as nitroglycerin sublingual tablets.

Non-prescription (OTC) drugs that require C-R containers include diphenhydramine, iron, acetaminophen, salicylates, NSAIDs and drugs that have been switched from prescription to OTC status. Non-drug compounds that are dangerous if swallowed require C-R packaging, such as turpentine. A list of drugs that must have C-R packaging is provided in the UWorld RxPrep MPJE Course, since this is a federal legal requirement per the Poison Prevention Packaging Act (PPPA).

INITIAL OVERDOSE MANAGEMENT

If poisoning is suspected, anyone can contact Poison Control by phone (1-800-222-1222) to receive guidance and recommendations. Basic first aid for poisonings should be initiated immediately after the exposure.

- For topical exposure, remove contaminated clothing and wash skin with soap and water for at least 15 minutes to remove the poison from the skin.

- For ocular exposure, remove contact lenses and rinse eyes with a gentle stream of water for at least 15 minutes.

- For oral ingestion, remove any remaining substances from the mouth. If there are symptoms of burning or irritation, drink a small amount of water or milk immediately.

- For inhaled exposure, move to fresh air immediately. Stay away from toxic fumes and/or gases.

- For ingestion of button batteries, give two teaspoons of honey every 10 minutes while seeking immediate medical care. Ingestion can be fatal within hours, and honey or sucralfate can slow damage to the esophagus and airway.

Ipecac syrup, used previously to induce emesis for certain exposures, is no longer recommended or commercially available.

If a patient is unconscious, having difficulty breathing, appears agitated or is having a seizure, call 911. While waiting for emergency help to arrive, initiate basic life support (BLS). The first step of "CAB" (circulation, airway, breathing) is to evaluate if the patient has a pulse. If pulseless, immediately start cardiopulmonary resuscitation (CPR) with chest compressions. Give two breaths for every 30 chest compressions. At a minimum, hands-only CPR is encouraged. Once medical personnel arrive, supportive care (e.g., blood pressure support, airway management) will be initiated.

HOSPITAL OVERDOSE MANAGEMENT

Correct identification of the ingested substance (or substances) is helpful to optimize treatment and support the patient. Pharmacists can assist with the identification by interviewing family members or calling the patient's pharmacy. For some substances, specific antidotes or dialysis may be used. Antidotes for common overdoses are discussed later in the chapter. In many cases of overdose, more than one drug is involved and more than one antidote may be required.

If the specific cause of the overdose remains unknown, patients are treated with supportive care and symptomatic treatment (see Study Tip Gal later in the chapter). Some overdoses have specific symptoms that can help healthcare providers identify the exposure or ingestion (see Additional Antidotes table later in the chapter).

Several dangerous compounds do not cause immediate symptoms after exposure. The clinician should consider the formulation, quantity and timing of ingestion of these substances. For example, in an acetaminophen overdose, the patient can remain asymptomatic or have non-specific symptoms (such as nausea, abdominal pain, fatigue) until end organ toxicity (liver failure) becomes apparent.

DECONTAMINATION WITH ACTIVATED CHARCOAL

Activated charcoal is used in the emergency room treatment of certain <u>orally ingested drugs</u> or chemicals and is an early step in some overdose protocols. Although it is available <u>OTC</u> (e.g., for gas/bloating, odor control, toothbrushing), at-home administration for an overdose is <u>not recommended</u>.

Activated charcoal is most effective when used <u>within one hour</u> of ingestion to decrease the absorption of as much of the drug as possible while it is still in the gut. The <u>charcoal adsorbs</u> the <u>drug</u>, which prevents GI absorption and systemic toxicity. The <u>dose</u> of activated charcoal is <u>1 g/kg</u>. Typically, only one dose of activated charcoal is administered. Multiple doses should only be considered if a patient has ingested a life-threatening amount of carbamazepine, dapsone, phenobarbital, quinine or theophylline.

<u>Prior</u> to using activated charcoal, the <u>airway</u> should be <u>protected</u> (with intubation, if needed) to <u>prevent aspiration</u>. Aspiration or inhalation of activated charcoal can cause lung irritation, leading to respiratory failure, infection or death. Some ingested compounds, such as <u>hydrocarbons</u> (petroleum products including gasoline and paint thinner) can <u>increase</u> the <u>risk of aspiration</u>. Care must be taken to protect the airway from these ingestions.

Activated charcoal is <u>contraindicated</u> in these situations:

- When the <u>airway</u> is <u>unprotected</u>, including when the patient:
  - ❏ Is unconscious
  - ❏ Cannot clear their throat
  - ❏ Cannot hold their head upright
- With intestinal obstruction
- When the gastrointestinal tract is not intact or when there is decreased peristalsis

Other potential complications of activated charcoal administration include transient constipation, bowel obstruction and regurgitation.

ANTIDOTES FOR COMMON POISONS

Antidotes reduce the harmful effects of the poison or overdosed drug. Many are used off-label. According to 2020 data from the American Association of Poison Control Centers (AAPCC), the most commonly ingested substances by adults are analgesics, sedative hypnotics, antipsychotics and antidepressants. Analgesics include both prescription (e.g., opioids) and non-prescription (e.g., acetaminophen) medications. The antidotes for acetaminophen and opioid overdoses are reviewed individually since these are frequent overdoses.

ACETAMINOPHEN

Acetaminophen is the most common cause of drug-induced liver injury (DILI). Excessive ingestion can lead to <u>hepatotoxicity</u>; limiting acetaminophen from all sources to <u>< 4,000 mg</u> per day can reduce this risk.

Hepatotoxicity is a dose-dependent adverse effect caused by the increased metabolism of acetaminophen by <u>CYP450 2E1</u> to N-acetyl-p-benzoquinone imine (<u>NAPQI</u>) (see figure on next page). NAPQI can bind to liver cell proteins and cause liver injury, and ultimately, <u>liver failure</u>. Acetaminophen overdose presents in four phases:

- Phase 1 (<u>1 – 24 hours</u>): commonly <u>asymptomatic</u> or non-specific symptoms, such as <u>nausea</u> and <u>vomiting</u>.
- Phase 2 (<u>24 – 72 hours</u>): hepatotoxicity evident on labs (e.g., <u>elevated INR, AST/ALT</u>); any symptoms from phase 1 usually subside.
- Phase 3 (<u>72 – 96 hours</u>): <u>fulminant hepatic failure</u> (e.g., <u>jaundice, coagulopathy, renal failure</u> and/or <u>death</u>).
- Phase 4 (<u>> 96 hours</u>): the patient <u>recovers</u> or receives a <u>liver transplant</u>.

In order to prevent hepatotoxicity, acetaminophen overdose must be identified early and the <u>antidote, N-acetylcysteine (NAC), given quickly</u> (preferably within 8 hours). The <u>acetaminophen level</u> (drawn 4 – 24 hours after ingestion) is used as the basis for treatment.

The level is plotted on the <u>Rumack–Matthew nomogram</u> to determine the risk of hepatotoxicity. If there is possible or probable hepatotoxicity, NAC should be started (see <u>Study Tip Gal</u> below). NAC is available in both <u>oral and IV</u> formulations, but the IV form is used more often due to intolerance (e.g., foul odor, vomiting) to the oral form.

N-ACETYLCYSTEINE (NAC) TREATMENT

- N-acetylcysteine (*Acetadote*) mechanism: free radical scavenger and precursor to glutathione (GSH). Ultimately increases GSH, which converts NAPQI to non-toxic metabolites.
- Treatment: use the Rumack-Matthew nomogram to determine the need for NAC (IV or oral).
  - ❏ Oral NAC (using injectable or inhalation solution): high dose given once, then lower dose for 17 doses. Repeat the dose if emesis occurs within 1 hour of administration.
  - ❏ IV NAC: three infusions over a total of 21 hours.

Acetaminophen Metabolism and Use of N-acetylcysteine (NAC)

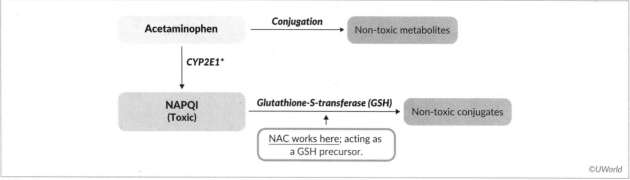

*CYP pathway only activated with excessive acetaminophen levels
NAPQI: N-acetyl-p-benzoquinone imine*

OPIOIDS

Opioid overdose and related deaths have become an epidemic in the U.S. Acute opioid overdose can lead to life-threatening respiratory depression and sedation. The effects of opioids can be reversed if the appropriate antidote, naloxone or nalmefene, is administered quickly. There are minimal to no adverse effects associated with giving naloxone to a patient who did not ingest any opioids. Various opioid reversal products are covered in the Pain chapter.

ADDITIONAL ANTIDOTES

DRUG OVERDOSE/POISON	SYMPTOMS/TREATMENT
Anticholinergics: atropine, diphenhydramine, dimenhydrinate, scopolamine, *Atropa belladonna* (deadly nightshade), jimson weed	Symptoms: "red as a beet" (flushing), "dry as bone" (dry skin and mucous membranes), "blind as a bat" (mydriasis with double or blurry vision), "mad as a hatter" (altered mental status), "hot as a hare" (fever)
	Primarily supportive care, rarely physostigmine is given; physostigmine inhibits the enzyme acetylcholinesterase, which breaks down acetylcholine (ACh); this ↑ ACh and ↓ anticholinergic toxicity
Anticoagulants: warfarin, direct thrombin inhibitors, factor Xa inhibitors, heparin, low molecular weight heparins	Symptoms: bleeding
	Treatment is agent specific: see the Anticoagulation chapter for more details
	Andexanet alfa (*Andexxa*): apixaban, rivaroxaban
	Idarucizumab (*Praxbind*): dabigatran
	Phytonadione (vitamin K): warfarin
	Protamine: heparin, low molecular weight heparin
	Prothrombin complex concentrate (e.g., *Kcentra*): warfarin
Antipsychotics	Symptoms: seizures
	Primarily supportive care, benztropine can be given for dystonia, benzodiazepines can be given for seizures and bicarbonate can be given if there is QRS-interval widening
Benzodiazepines	Flumazenil: can cause seizures when used in patients taking benzodiazepines chronically; sometimes used for non-benzodiazepine hypnotic overdose (e.g., zolpidem), but not routinely recommended
Beta-blockers	Supportive care (e.g., fluids, vasopressors), glucagon (if unresponsive to supportive treatment)
	High-dose insulin with dextrose may be used in patients refractory to glucagon
	Lipid emulsion to enhance elimination of some lipophilic drugs
Calcium channel blockers	Same as beta-blockers plus:
	IV calcium (chloride or gluconate): avoid fast infusion, monitor ECG, do not infuse calcium in same line as phosphate-containing solutions
Cyanide: smoke inhalation, nitroprusside in high doses/long durations/renal impairment	Hydroxocobalamin (*Cyanokit*)
	Sodium thiosulfate + sodium nitrite (*Nithiodote*)
Digoxin, oleander, foxglove	Digoxin immune Fab (*DigiFab*)
	Each *DigiFab* 40 mg vial binds ~0.5 mg digoxin; when the amount ingested or digoxin level is unknown, the max adult dose is 20 vials
	Interferes with digoxin levels drawn after it has been given

DRUG OVERDOSE/POISON	SYMPTOMS/TREATMENT
Ethanol (alcoholic drinks)	Can cause an ↑ anion gap If chronic alcohol use suspected, administer thiamine (vitamin B1) to prevent Wernicke's encephalopathy (neurological damage)
5-fluorouracil (5-FU), capecitabine	Uridine triacetate (Vistogard)
Heavy metals: arsenic, copper, gold, lead, mercury, thallium	Dimercaprol: arsenic, gold, mercury Dimercaprol +/- EDTA +/- succimer (Chemet, DMSA): lead Ferric hexacyanoferrate ["Prussian blue" (Radiogardase)]: thallium Penicillamine: copper
Hydrocarbons: petroleum products, gasoline, kerosene, mineral oil, paint thinners	Do not induce vomiting; keep patient NPO due to aspiration risk
Insulin, hypoglycemics (e.g., sulfonylureas)	Dextrose injection or infusion, oral glucose (do not administer if the patient is unconscious) Glucagon (when IV dextrose cannot be administered) Sulfonylurea-induced hypoglycemia: octreotide (Sandostatin)
Isoniazid	Symptoms: seizures, altered mental status IV pyridoxine (vitamin B6) and benzodiazepines Oral pyridoxine 10–50 mg is used daily with isoniazid to prevent neuropathy
Iron and aluminum	Deferoxamine (Desferal): iron and aluminum Deferiprone (Ferriprox) or deferasirox (Exjade, Jadenu): iron overload from blood transfusions
Local anesthetics (bupivacaine, mepivacaine, ropivacaine) and other lipophilic drugs	IV lipid emulsion 20%
Methotrexate	IV sodium bicarbonate (to alkalinize the urine) Leucovorin (a reduced form of folic acid) or levoleucovorin (Fusilev, Khapzory): "rescue" therapy after high-dose cancer treatment Glucarpidase (Voraxaze): rapidly lowers methotrexate levels in patients with acute kidney injury and delayed methotrexate clearance
Methemoglobinemia from topical benzocaine (in OraGel or teething products), dapsone, nitrates or sulfonamides	Methylene blue (ProvayBlue) Methylene blue is contraindicated in patients with G6PD deficiency; avoid administration with SSRIs and SNRIs (risk for serotonin syndrome)
Mushrooms (amatoxin-containing)	Treat severe muscarinic symptoms (bradycardia) with atropine
Neostigmine, pyridostigmine	Pralidoxime (Protopam): counteracts the muscle weakness and/or respiratory depression secondary to overdose of acetylcholinesterase inhibitors used to treat myasthenia gravis Atropine or glycopyrrolate can be given to prevent bradycardia from neostigmine
Nicotine, including e-cigarettes	Early symptoms: abdominal pain, nausea, diaphoresis, tachycardia, tremors Later symptoms: bradycardia, dyspnea, lethargy, coma, seizures Supportive care (e.g., atropine for symptomatic bradycardia, benzodiazepines for seizures)
Organophosphates (OPs), including insecticides (e.g., malathion) and nerve gases (e.g., sarin)	Symptoms: OPs block acetylcholinesterase, which ↑ ACh levels and causes cholinergic "SLUDD" symptoms (salivation, lacrimation, urination, diarrhea/defecation, see Study Tip Gal on next page) Atropine: anticholinergic which blocks the effects of ACh to reduce the cholinergic SLUDD symptoms Pralidoxime (Protopam): treats muscle weakness and relieves paralysis of respiratory muscles by reactivating acetylcholinesterase Atropine and pralidoxime (DuoDote)
Paralytics (e.g., rocuronium bromide, vecuronium bromide, pancuronium bromide)	To reverse the effects of neuromuscular blockade in adults undergoing surgery: Neostigmine methylsulfate (Bloxiverz): rocuronium, vecuronium and pancuronium Sugammadex (Bridion): rocuronium and vecuronium
Salicylates	Sodium bicarbonate: alkalinizes the urine, which ↓ drug reabsorption and ↑ the excretion of salicylates

DRUG OVERDOSE/POISON	SYMPTOMS/TREATMENT
Stimulants: amphetamines, including ADHD and weight loss drugs, cocaine, ephedrine, caffeine, theophylline, MDMA (ecstasy)	Benzodiazepines for agitation or seizures
Toxic alcohols: ethylene glycol (antifreeze), diethylene glycol, methanol	Can cause an ↑ anion gap Fomepizole is preferred; ethanol (if fomepizole is unavailable)
Tricyclic antidepressants (TCAs)	Overdose can quickly cause fatal arrhythmias Sodium bicarbonate: to ↓ a widened QRS complex Benzodiazepines for agitation or seizures Vasopressors for hypotension
Valproic acid or topiramate-induced hyperammonemia	Levocarnitine (*Carnitor*)

ORGANOPHOSPHATE OVERDOSE

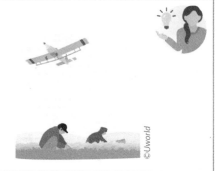

SLUDD SYMPTOMS	TREATMENT	CAUSES
Salivation **L**acrimation **U**rination **D**iarrhea **D**efecation	Atropine: blocks the effects of acetylcholine Pralidoxime (*Protopam*): reactivates acetylcholinesterase Atropine and pralidoxime (*DuoDote*)	Organophosphates include pesticides. People working on farms are at risk.

©UWorld

SYMPTOMATIC TREATMENT OF OVERDOSE/POISONING

In overdose situations, it is not always known what substance was taken or if it was more than one substance. Symptoms and labs (sometimes referred to as toxidromes) guide the treatment until more information is known.

Possible Actions

- Support circulation, airway and breathing as impairments can be life-threatening.

  ❏ Use fluids and vasopressors for hypotension, atropine for bradycardia and mechanical ventilation for a compromised airway.

  ❏ Shallow breathing with somnolence and pinpoint pupils could be an opioid overdose. Administer naloxone.

- Treat seizures, severe agitation or tachycardia with benzodiazepines.

- Treat hypoglycemia with oral carbohydrates (if patient is alert), IV dextrose or SC glucagon.

- If an ECG demonstrates QT prolongation or QRS widening, administer sodium bicarbonate.

- Check an acetaminophen level and use the Rumack-Matthew nomogram to determine if NAC should be given.

ANTIDOTES FOR COMMON BITES AND STINGS

TOXIN	ANTIDOTE	COMMENTS
Mammal bites	Rabies vaccine (*RabAvert, Imovax Rabies*) + human rabies immune globulin (*HyperRAB S/D, Imogam Rabies-HT*)	Clean wound with soap and water. Tetanus vaccine is required if it has been at least 10 years since the last booster vaccine. High-risk mammal bites or exposure (no previous rabies vaccination): give vaccine and human rabies immune globulin (HRIG). Vaccine given IM in the deltoid (adults) or thigh (children, infants) on days 0, 3, 7, 14 and immune globulin 20 units/kg is given on day 0, infiltrated around wound site and a location separate from vaccine site. HRIG is not useful after day 7 of vaccine or in previously immunized individuals. See the Immunizations chapter for more details.
Black Widow spider bites	Antivenin for *Latrodectus mactans*	The primary treatment is supportive care (opioids for pain management and benzodiazepines for muscle spasms). Antivenin may be administered for severe symptoms unresponsive to supportive care.
Scorpion stings	Antivenin immune Fab *Centruroides* (*Anascorp*)	Scorpions with venom potent enough to cause clinically severe symptoms are found mainly in the southwest.
Snake bites (copperhead, cottonmouth and rattlesnake)	Crotalidae polyvalent immune Fab (*CroFab*) Crotalidae Immune F(ab')$_2$ (*Anavip*)	Do not use ice; do not cut/suck out venom; transport patient to healthcare facility.

Select Guidelines/References

American Heart Association. Update for cardiopulmonary resuscitation and emergency cardiovascular care. *Circulation.* 2020;142:S337-S357.

Lexicomp Toxicology Database. http://online.lexi.com/lco/action/home/tox.

CDC, Emergency Preparedness. http://emergency.cdc.gov.

Poison Control Center. http://poison.org.

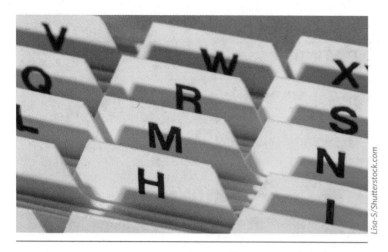

INDEX

Image Credits

Some images have been modified from their original state. All images are being used for illustrative purposes only. Any person depicted in the content is a model.

Front cover:

Gorodenkoff/stock.adobe.com

natagolubnycha/stock.adobe.com

pikselstock/stock.adobe.com

Images used in the design of the book:

iStock.com/Ae11615

iStock.com/ArnaPhoto

iStock.com/Chaliya

iStock.com/bearsky23

iStock.com/blueringmedia

iStock.com/Christoph Burgstedt

iStock.com/Dr_Microbe

iStock.com/francescoch

iStock.com/_human

iStock.com/image_jungle

iStock.com/ipopba

iStock.com/jacklooser

iStock.com/Kateryna Kon

iStock.com/metamorworks

iStock.com/Mohammed Haneefa Nizamudeen

iStock.com/Olivier Le Moal

iStock.com/scyther5

iStock.com/stockdevil

iStock.com/Sudowoodo

iStock.com/SbytovaMN

iStock.com/t:yodiyim

iStock.com/Tharakorn

iStock.com/VolodymyrV

Ann in the uk/Shutterstock.com

Buravleva stock/Shutterstock.com

Crevis/Shutterstock.com

David Fossler/Shutterstock.com

Explode/Shutterstock.com

hernan ceballos/Shutterstock.com

Mark Mondaini/Shutterstock.com

metamorworks/Shutterstock.com

Motortion Films/Shutterstock.com

Palsur/Shutterstock.com

PopTika/Shutterstock.com

Prostock-studio/Shutterstock.com

Roman Zaiets/Shutterstock.com

sciencepics/Shutterstock.com

thodonal88/Shutterstock.com

Tyler Olson/Shutterstock.com

Zern Liew/Shutterstock.com

7activestudio/stock.adobe.com

Chinnapong/stock.adobe.com

freshidea/stock.adobe.com

lufeethebear/stock.adobe.com

MarekPhotoDesign.com/stock.adobe.com

melita/stock.adobe.com

pathdoc/stock.adobe.com

peterschreiber.media/stock.adobe.com

SciePro/stock.adobe.com

Sondem/stock.adobe.com

sudok1/stock.adobe.com

topvectors/stock.adobe.com

REQUIRED FORMULAS

Calculations

Liquid (Volume) Conversions p. 105
1 tsp (t) = 5 mL, 1 tbsp (T) = 15 mL
1 fl oz = 30 mL
1 cup = 8 oz, 240 mL
1 pint = 16 oz, 480 mL
1 quart = 2 pints, 960 mL
1 gallon = 4 quarts, 3,840 mL

Solid (Weight) Conversions p. 105
1 kg = 2.2 pounds (lbs)
1 oz = 28.4 grams (g)
1 lb = 454 g, 16 oz
1 grain = 65 mg
mEq to mmol is 1:1 for monovalent ions, 1:0.5 for divalent ions

Height Conversions p. 105
1 inch (in) = 2.54 centimeters (cm)
1 meter (m) = 100 cm

Percentage Strength p. 117

$$\% \text{ w/v} = \frac{X\ g}{100\ mL} \qquad \% \text{ v/v} = \frac{X\ mL}{100\ mL} \qquad \% \text{ w/w} = \frac{X\ g}{100\ g}$$

Ratio Strength p. 121
Percentage strength = 100 / Ratio strength
Ratio strength = 100 / Percentage strength

Parts Per Million (PPM) p. 123
PPM → Percentage strength   Move the decimal left 4 places
Percentage strength → PPM   Move the decimal right 4 places

Specific Gravity (SG) p. 124

$$SG = \frac{\text{weight of substance (g)}}{\text{weight of equal volume of water (g)}} \quad or \quad SG = \frac{g}{mL}$$

Dilution & Concentration (Changing Strength or Quantity) p. 125
Q1 x C1 = Q2 x C2   Q1 = old quantity   Q2 = new quantity
C1 = old concentration   C2 = new concentration

Alligation p. 126

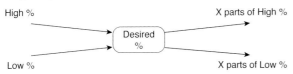

High % → Desired % → X parts of High %
Low % → Desired % → X parts of Low %

Use proportions to calculate amount of high % and/or low % required

Osmolarity p. 129

$$mOsmol/L = \frac{\text{Wt of substance (g/L)}}{\text{MW (g/mole)}} \times (\text{\# of particles}) \times 1,000$$

Isotonicity (E Value) p. 132

$$E = \frac{(58.5)(i)}{(\text{MW of drug})(1.8)}$$

Moles and Millimoles p. 133

$$mols = \frac{g}{MW} \quad or \quad mmols = \frac{mg}{MW}$$

Milliequivalents p. 135

$$mEq = \frac{mg \times valence}{MW} \quad or \quad mEq = mmols \times valence$$

Enteral Nutrition Calories p. 141
Carbs, Protein = 4 kcal/gram   Fat = 9 kcal/gram

Parenteral Nutrition Calories p. 141
Dextrose monohydrate = 3.4 kcal/gram   ILE 10% = 1.1 kcal/mL
Amino acid solutions = 4 kcal/gram   ILE 20% = 2 kcal/mL
                                        ILE 30% = 3 kcal/mL

Determining Fluid Needs p. 139
When weight > 20 kg: 1,500 mL + (20 mL)(weight in kg − 20)
Can estimate using 30-40 mL/kg/day

Total Energy Expenditure p. 140
TEE = BEE x activity factor x stress factor

Grams of Nitrogen From Protein p. 142

$$\text{Nitrogen (g)} = \frac{\text{protein intake (g)}}{6.25}$$

Corrected Calcium for Albumin < 3.5 (not needed with ionized Ca) p. 149
$Ca_{corrected}$ (mg/dL) = $calcium_{reported(serum)}$ + [(4.0 − albumin) x (0.8)]

Body Mass Index (BMI) p. 158

$$BMI\ (kg/m^2) = \frac{\text{weight (kg)}}{[\text{height (m)}]^2} \quad or \quad \frac{\text{weight (lbs)}}{[\text{height (inches)}]^2} \times 703$$

Ideal Body Weight (IBW) p. 159
IBW (males) = 50 kg + (2.3 kg)(number of inches over 5 feet)
IBW (females) = 45.5 kg + (2.3 kg)(number of inches over 5 feet)

Adjusted Body Weight (AdjBW$_{0.4}$) p. 159
$AdjBW_{0.4}$ = IBW + 0.4(TBW − IBW)

Which Weight to Use for Drug Dosing (mg/kg) p. 160
All drugs (if underweight)   Total Body Weight (TBW)
Most drugs (if normal weight or obese)   TBW
Exceptions
Acyclovir, Aminophylline, Levothyroxine,   IBW
Theophylline (normal weight, obese)
Aminoglycosides (obese) $AdjBW_{0.4}$

Flow Rates/Drop Factor (drops/min) p. 161 & p. 164

$$\frac{\text{\# drops}}{mL} \times \frac{mL}{hr} \times \frac{hr}{60\ min} = \frac{\text{\# drops}}{min}$$

Dehydration p. 166
BUN:SCr > 20:1

Cockcroft-Gault Equation p. 167

$$\begin{array}{l}CrCl \\ (mL/min)\end{array} = \frac{140 - (\text{age of patient})}{72 \times SCr} \times \text{weight (kg) (x 0.85 if female)}$$

Arterial Blood Gas (ABG) p. 169
ABG: pH/pCO_2/pO_2/HCO_3/O_2 Sat
1. pH < 7.35 → acidosis, pH > 7.45 → alkalosis
2. Respiratory: pCO_2 < 35 → alkalosis, pCO_2 > 45 → acidosis
   Metabolic: HCO_3 > 26 → alkalosis, HCO_3 < 22 → acidosis
3. Which abnormal value (pCO_2 or HCO_3) matches the pH from Step #1?
   Ex: ↓ pH + ↑ pCO_2 → respiratory acidosis
   Ex: ↓ pH + ↓ HCO_3 → metabolic acidosis

Anion Gap p. 170
Anion gap (AG) = Na − Cl − HCO_3

pH Calculations p. 171
Weak acid   Weak base

$$pH = pK_a + \log\left[\frac{salt}{acid}\right] \qquad pH = pK_a + \log\left[\frac{base}{salt}\right]$$

Percent Ionization p. 174
Weak acid   Weak base

$$\% \text{ ionization} = \frac{100}{1+10^{(pKa-pH)}} \qquad \% \text{ ionization} = \frac{100}{1+10^{(pH-pKa)}}$$

Absolute Neutrophil Count (ANC) p. 176
ANC (cells/mm^3) = WBC x [(% segs + % bands)/100]

Answering Case-Based Exam Questions
Temperature Conversions (Fahrenheit ↔ Celsius) p. 97
°C = (°F − 32)/1.8   °F = (°C x 1.8) + 32

Common Skin Conditions
Time to Burn (TTB) p. 532
TTB (with sunscreen in min) = SPF x TTB (without sunscreen)

Biostatistics

Mean, Median and Mode p. 192
Mean - average value
Median - value in the middle of an ordered list
Mode - value that occurs most frequently

Risk, Relative Risk (RR) p. 197, Relative Risk Reduction (RRR), Absolute Risk Reduction (ARR) p. 198

$$Risk = \frac{\text{Number of subjects in group with an unfavorable event}}{\text{Total number of subjects in group}}$$

$$RR = \frac{\text{Risk in treatment group}}{\text{Risk in control group}}$$

$$RRR = \frac{(\% \text{ risk in control group} - \% \text{ risk in treatment group})}{\% \text{ risk in the control group}}$$

ARR = (% risk in control group) − (% risk in treatment group)

Number Needed to Treat or Harm (NNT, NNH) p. 199-200

$$\text{NNT or NNH} = \frac{1}{\text{ARR*}}$$

*expressed as decimal

Odds Ratio (OR) p. 200

Exposure	Outcome Present	Outcome Absent
Present	A	B
Absent	C	D

$$OR = \frac{AD}{BC}$$

Hazard Ratio (HR) p. 201

$$HR = \frac{\text{Hazard rate in the treatment group}}{\text{Hazard rate in the control group}}$$

Incremental Cost-Effectiveness Ratio p. 211

$$\text{Incremental cost ratio} = \frac{(C_2 - C_1)}{(E_2 - E_1)}$$

C = costs, E = effects

Tobacco Cessation

Pack-Year Smoking History p. 569

Pack-year smoking history = Cigarette packs / day x years smoked

Diabetes

Initiating Basal-Bolus Insulin in Type 1 Diabetes p. 589
1. Calculate total daily dose (TDD) of 0.5 units/kg/day using TBW.
2. Divide into 1/2 basal & 1/2 rapid-acting.
3. Split rapid-acting among meals.

Insulin-to-Carbohydrate Ratio: Rule of 450 for Regular Insulin p. 591

$$\frac{450}{\text{total daily dose of insulin (TDD)}} = \text{grams of carbohydrate covered by 1 unit of regular insulin}$$

Insulin-to-Carbohydrate Ratio: Rule of 500 for Rapid-Acting Insulin p. 591

$$\frac{500}{\text{total daily dose of insulin (TDD)}} = \text{grams of carbohydrate covered by 1 unit of rapid-acting insulin}$$

Correction Factor: 1,500 Rule for Regular Insulin p. 591

$$\frac{1,500}{\text{total daily dose of insulin (TDD)}} = \text{correction factor for 1 unit of regular insulin}$$

Correction Factor: 1,800 Rule for Rapid-Acting Insulin p. 591

$$\frac{1,800}{\text{total daily dose of insulin (TDD)}} = \text{correction factor for 1 unit of rapid-acting insulin}$$

Correction Dose p. 591

$$\frac{(\text{blood glucose now}) - (\text{target blood glucose})}{\text{correction factor}} = \text{correction dose}$$

Dyslipidemia

Friedewald Equation p. 395

$$LDL = TC - HDL - \frac{TG^*}{5}$$

*do not use if TG > 400

Nonsterile Compounding

Minimum Weighable Quantity (MWQ) p. 216

$$MWQ = \frac{\text{Sensitivity requirement}}{\text{Acceptable error rate (usually 0.05)}}$$

Oncology

Body Surface Area (Mosteller) p. 763
(review use of Du Bois and Du Bois)

$$BSA\ (m^2) = \sqrt{\frac{Ht\ (cm)\ x\ Wt\ (kg)}{3,600}}$$

Pharmacokinetics

Bioavailability (F) p. 919

$$F\ (\%) = 100 \times \frac{AUC_{extravascular}}{AUC_{intravenous}} \times \frac{Dose_{intravenous}}{Dose_{extravascular}}$$

Volume of Distribution (Vd) p. 920

$$Vd = \frac{\text{Amount of drug in body}}{\text{Concentration of drug in plasma}}$$

Clearance p. 922 & p. 924

$$Cl = \frac{F \times dose}{AUC} \quad \text{or} \quad Cl = ke \times Vd$$

Elimination Rate Constant (ke) p. 924

$$ke = \frac{Cl}{Vd}$$

Predicting Drug Concentrations p. 924

$$C_2 = C_1 \times e^{-kt} \qquad ke = \frac{\ln (C_1/C_2)}{t}$$

Half-Life (t½) p. 925

$$t_{1/2} = \frac{0.693}{ke}$$

Loading Dose (LD) p. 927

$$LD = \frac{\text{Desired concentration} \times Vd}{F}$$

Acute & Critical Care Medicine

Mean Arterial Pressure (MAP) p. 685

MAP = [(2 x diastolic pressure) + systolic pressure] / 3

Seizures/Epilepsy

Phenytoin (Total) Correction for Albumin < 3.5 p. 853

$$Phenytoin_{corrected}\ (mcg/mL) = \frac{\text{Total phenytoin measured}}{(0.2 \times albumin) + 0.1}$$

DRUG-DOSE CONVERSIONS

KCl Solution (Oral) to Tablets p. 136 (see problem #61)
KCl 10% = 20 mEq/15 mL

Calcium Salts p. 175
Calcium carbonate = 40% elemental calcium
Calcium citrate = 21% elemental calcium

Aminophylline ↔ Theophylline p. 175
Aminophylline to **T**heophylline: **M**ultiply by 0.8 (remember: **ATM**)
Theophylline to Aminophylline: Divide by 0.8

Statins p. 398
Pitavastatin	2 mg	Lovastatin	40 mg
Rosuvastatin	5 mg	Pravastatin	40 mg
Atorvastatin	10 mg	Fluvastatin	80 mg
Simvastatin	20 mg		

Metoprolol p. 417
IV:PO = 1:2.5

Loop Diuretics p. 443
Ethacrynic acid	50 mg	Bumetanide	1 mg
Furosemide	40 mg	Furosemide	IV:PO = 1:2
Torsemide	20 mg	Other Loops	IV:PO = 1:1

Insulin p. 592
Usually, 1:1 conversion
Exceptions:
NPH dosed BID → glargine dosed daily, use 80% of NPH dose
Toujeo → other forms of glargine or detemir, use 80% of *Toujeo* dose

Levothyroxine p. 601
IV:PO = 0.75:1

Steroids p. 608
Cortisone	25 mg	Methylprednisolone	4 mg
Hydrocortisone	20 mg	Triamcinolone	4 mg
Prednisone	5 mg	Dexamethasone	0.75 mg
Prednisolone	5 mg	Betamethasone	0.6 mg

Opioids (methodology) p. 732

Lithium p. 813
5 mL lithium citrate syrup = 300 mg lithium carbonate = 8 mEq Li+ ion